MANUAL OF NUTRITIONAL THERAPEUTICS

Sixth Edition

Editors

David H. Alpers, MD
William B. Kountz Professor of Geriatrics in Medicine
Assistant Director, Center for Human Nutrition
Washington University School of Medicine
St. Louis, Missouri

Beth E. Taylor, DCN, RDN, LD, CNSC, FCCM
Nutrition Support Specialist, Surgical Intensive Care Unit
Barnes-Jewish Hospital
St. Louis, Missouri

Dennis M. Bier, MD
Professor of Pediatrics
Baylor College of Medicine
Director USDA/ARS Children's Nutrition Research Center
Houston, Texas

Samuel Klein, MD
William H. Danforth Professor of Medicine and Nutritional Science
Director, Center for Human Nutrition and Atkins Center of
Excellence in Obesity Medicine
Washington University School of Medicine
St. Louis, Missouri

Wolters Kluwer

Philadelphia • Baltimore • New York • London
Buenos Aires • Hong Kong • Sydney • Tokyo

Executive Editor: Rebecca Gaertner
Senior Product Development Editor: Kristina Oberle
Senior Production Project Manager: Alicia Jackson
Design Coordinator: Teresa Mallon
Marketing Manager: Stephanie Kindlick
Senior Manufacturing Coordinator: Beth Welsh
Prepress Vendor: S4Carlisle Publishing Services

Sixth Edition

Copyright © 2015 Wolters Kluwer

© 2008, 2002, 1995, 1988 by Lippincott Williams & Wilkins; 1983 by Little Brown and Company

All rights reserved. This book is protected by copyright. No part of this book may be reproduced or transmitted in any form or by any means, including as photocopies or scanned-in or other electronic copies, or utilized by any information storage and retrieval system without written permission from the copyright owner, except for brief quotations embodied in critical articles and reviews. Materials appearing in this book prepared by individuals as part of their official duties as U.S. government employees are not covered by the above-mentioned copyright. To request permission, please contact Wolters Kluwer at Two Commerce Square, 2001 Market Street, Philadelphia, PA 19103, via email at permissions@lww.com, or via our website at lww.com (products and services).

9 8 7 6 5 4 3 2 1

Printed in China

Library of Congress Cataloging-in-Publication Data
Alpers, David H., author.
  Manual of nutritional therapeutics / David H. Alpers, Beth E. Taylor, Dennis M. Bier, Samuel Klein. — Sixth edition.
    p. ; cm.
  Preceded by: Manual of nutritional therapeutics / David H. Alpers ... [et al.]. 5th ed. c2008.
  Includes bibliographical references and index.
  ISBN 978-1-4511-9187-5 (alk. paper) — ISBN 1-4511-9187-1 (alk. paper)
  I. Taylor, Beth E., author. II. Bier, Dennis M., author. III. Klein, Samuel, 1953- , author. IV. Title.
  [DNLM: 1. Nutrition Therapy. WB 400]
  RM217.2
  615.8'54—dc23

2014036982

This work is provided "as is," and the publisher disclaims any and all warranties, express or implied, including any warranties as to accuracy, comprehensiveness, or currency of the content of this work.

This work is no substitute for individual patient assessment based upon healthcare professionals' examination of each patient and consideration of, among other things, age, weight, gender, current or prior medical conditions, medication history, laboratory data, and other factors unique to the patient. The publisher does not provide medical advice or guidance, and this work is merely a reference tool. Healthcare professionals, and not the publisher, are solely responsible for the use of this work, including all medical judgments and for any resulting diagnosis and treatments.

Given continuous, rapid advances in medical science and health information, independent professional verification of medical diagnoses, indications, appropriate pharmaceutical selections and dosages, and treatment options should be made and healthcare professionals should consult a variety of sources. When prescribing medication, healthcare professionals are advised to consult the product information sheet (the manufacturer's package insert) accompanying each drug to verify, among other things, conditions of use, warnings, and side effects and identify any changes in dosage schedule or contraindications, particularly if the medication to be administered is new, infrequently used or has a narrow therapeutic range. To the maximum extent permitted under applicable law, no responsibility is assumed by the publisher for any injury and/or damage to persons or property, as a matter of products liability, negligence law or otherwise, or from any reference to or use by any person of this work.

LWW.com

To our fathers, who taught us both respect for knowledge
and concern for the individual.

Preface

MANUAL OF NUTRITIONAL THERAPEUTICS, SIXTH EDITION

The information on nutritional topics that is useful for health-care workers continues to increase at a steady pace. This manual was conceived as a source of information for physicians, nurses, dietitians, and other health professionals in various disciplines, and for students at all levels. The continued use of this manual has supported the need for such an information source, filtered by the authors to focus on the information we find useful for the practice of medicine and surgery. We assume that the health-care worker has knowledge of the underlying diseases that might benefit from nutritional intervention. Thus, this edition of the *Manual of Nutritional Therapeutics*, which was developed in collaboration with the Center for Human Nutrition at Washington University School of Medicine in St. Louis, similar to its predecessors, is not intended to be a textbook of nutrition. It should be used to obtain the information that is needed in managing the nutritional needs of adults, adolescents, and older children. We have tried to be practical and to provide explanations for the recommendations provided. In many cases, new systematic reviews of an increasing number of randomized, controlled clinical trials have provided a much more solid evidence base for these recommendations.

The chapters on individual nutrient components (5–7) and chapter 12 on diets have retained their form subdivided by sections that deal with many different individual nutrients and/or diets. The original outline form has been modified for many of the other chapters to better fit the more narrative needs of those chapters. Several chapters are completely new. Chapter 8 (Dietary Supplements) contains revised material that was formerly in chapters on individual nutrients and on diet, to which have been added sections on many other supplements. Chapter 14 (Obesity) is completely rewritten. Dr. William F. Stenson, a valued contributor to the first five editions, has not been able to continue in this role, because of other commitments. We are very grateful to him for his many contributions over the years. We have added a new author, Samuel Klein, an internationally renowned expert in obesity and metabolic diseases, and the director of the National Institutes of Health Nutrition & Obesity Research Center at Washington University in St. Louis.

The information is as current as possible given the lag time involved in publishing a book. But nutrient preparations can change rapidly, or are replaced by other products; so the reader should always check the local availability of any given preparation. URLs for many websites containing nutritional information are included, not only for convenience and to update information not included in the manual but also to provide sources of information that the authors use and trust.

The authors are gratified by the reception the book has enjoyed, and hope that its readers, old and new, will derive as much benefit from it as we, the authors, have received in revising it. We are grateful to our colleagues at Wolters Kluwer (especially Kristina Oberle) for editorial support and advice. Especially, we thank our spouses and families for their support in allowing us the time needed to create the sixth edition of this book.

David H. Alpers, MD
Beth E. Taylor, DCN, RDN, LD, CNSC, FCCM
Dennis M. Bier, MD
Samuel Klein, MD

Contents

Preface   iv

Section I General Concepts in Nutrition   1

1 Recommendations for Healthy Young Adults   1

2 Recommendations for Healthy Elderly Adults   13

3 Pregnancy and Lactation   34

4 Approach to Nutrient Deficiency   51

Section II Individual Nutrient Components   81

5 Protein and Calories: Requirements, Intake, and Assessment   81

6 Vitamins   123

7 Minerals   245

8 Dietary Supplements   361

Section III Therapeutic Nutrition   399

9 Nutritional Support Decision Making   399

10 Enteral Nutritional Therapy   411

11 Parenteral Nutritional Therapy   453

12 Use of Diets and Dietary Components in Clinical Practice 483

Section IV Nutritional Management of Specific Diseases 571

13 Dietary Management of Diabetes, Renal Disease, and Hyperlipidemia 571

14 Obesity 631

15 Nutritional Considerations in Chronic Diseases 657

Appendix A: Facts and Formulas Commonly Used in Nutritional Therapeutics 683
Appendix B: Food Labeling 686
INDEX 693

SECTION I
General Concepts in Nutrition

1 Recommendations for Healthy Young Adults

INTRODUCTION

Despite the extensive availability of diverse, often conflicting, information on nutrition, diet, and health on the Internet or sold in bookstores, virtually all expert scientific panels reporting guidelines for good nutritional practice have devised remarkably consistent dietary recommendations for healthy adults. Further, despite impressions generated by almost daily media reports of new dietary fads, the principles of healthy eating have not fundamentally changed over at least the last 50 years, and many of these principles were promoted more than a century ago. The most widely disseminated general recommendations for healthy adults are included in several reports. The first, which represents the combined recommendations of the US Department of Agriculture and the US Department of Health and Human Services, is called *Dietary Guidelines for Americans, 2010* (1). In 2015, the current guidelines will be updated, although it is unlikely that these will contain any additions that will change the fundamental principles that have been the foundation of the *Dietary Guidelines for Americans*, since they were first issued in 1980. The current guidelines, the 2015 updates when they are issued, and copies of every prior version of the *Dietary Guidelines for Americans* can be found at *http://health.gov/dietaryguidelines/dga2010/dietaryguidelines2010.pdf*. Additional authoritative dietary guidelines for health maintenance and disease prevention include the *2013 American Heart Association/American College of Cardiology Guideline on Lifestyle Management to Reduce Cardiovascular Risk* (2) and the *American Cancer Society Guidelines on Nutrition and Physical Activity for Cancer Prevention* (3).

CONSOLIDATED RECOMMENDATIONS

Despite somewhat different approaches to the issues, various assessments of the data, and distinct formats for translating the findings to dietary recommendations (Tables 1-1, 1-2, and 1-3), the authoritative bodies (1–3) nevertheless come to common guiding principles and an overall similarity of the resulting recommendations. Moreover, all guidelines emphasize consuming adequate amounts of the known essential nutrients as *whole foods* in healthful dietary patterns accompanied by lifestyle practices found to promote health and reduce the risks of developing chronic diseases. Taken together, these authoritative sets of dietary guidelines can be consolidated as follows:

Do Not Become Obese

Obesity is the most significant form of malnutrition in the United States today. Data obtained over the last 40 years in the National Health and Nutrition Examination Surveys (NHANES), consecutive, representative samples of individuals across the United States, have documented disturbing trends in body weight. From 1976 to 1980, 15% of adults aged 20 to 74 years were obese and 47.1% were either overweight or obese. In 2011 to 2012, obese adults constituted

TABLE 1-1 Dietary Guidelines for Americans, 2010[a]

Balancing Calories to Manage Weight
- Prevent and/or reduce overweight and obesity through improved eating and physical activity behaviors.
- Control total calorie intake to manage body weight. For people who are overweight or obese, this will mean consuming fewer calories from foods and beverages.
- Increase physical activity and reduce time spent in sedentary behaviors.
- Maintain appropriate calorie balance during each stage of life—childhood, adolescence, adulthood, pregnancy and breastfeeding, and older age.

Foods and Food Components to Reduce
- Reduce daily sodium intake to less than 2,300 milligrams (mg), and further reduce intake to 1,500 mg among persons who are 51 and older and those of any age who are African American or have hypertension, diabetes, or chronic kidney disease. The 1,500-mg recommendation applies to about half of the US population, including children and the majority of adults.
- Consume less than 10% of calories from saturated fatty acids by replacing them with monounsaturated and polyunsaturated fatty acids.
- Consume less than 300 mg/day of dietary cholesterol.
- Keep *trans*-fatty acid consumption as low as possible by limiting foods that contain synthetic sources of *trans*-fats, such as partially hydrogenated oils, and by limiting other solid fats.
- Reduce the intake of calories from solid fats and added sugars.
- Limit the consumption of foods that contain refined grains, especially refined grain foods that contain solid fats, added sugars, and sodium.
- If alcohol is consumed, it should be consumed in moderation—up to one drink per day for women and two drinks per day for men—and only by adults of legal drinking age.

Foods and Nutrients to Increase
Individuals should meet the following recommendations as part of a healthy eating pattern while staying within their calorie needs.
- Increase vegetable and fruit intake.
- Eat a variety of vegetables, especially dark green and red and orange vegetables and beans and peas.
- Consume at least half of all grains as whole grains. Increase whole grain intake by replacing refined grains with whole grains.
- Increase intake of fat-free or low-fat milk and milk products, such as milk, yogurt, cheese, or fortified soy beverages.
- Choose a variety of protein foods, which include seafood, lean meat and poultry, eggs, beans and peas, soy products, and unsalted nuts and seeds.
- Increase the amount and variety of seafood consumed by choosing seafood in place of some meat and poultry.
- Replace protein foods that are higher in solid fats with choices that are lower in solid fats and calories and/or are sources of oils.
- Use oils to replace solid fats where possible.
- Choose foods that provide more potassium, dietary fiber, calcium, and vitamin D, which are nutrients of concern in American diets. These foods include vegetables, fruits, whole grains, and milk and milk products.

Recommendations for Specific Population Groups
Women Capable of Becoming Pregnant
- Choose foods that supply heme iron, which is more readily absorbed by the body, additional iron sources, and enhancers of iron absorption such as vitamin C–rich foods.
- Consume 400 mcg/day of synthetic folic acid (from fortified foods and/or supplements) in addition to food forms of folate from a varied diet.

TABLE 1-1   Dietary Guidelines for Americans, 2010 *(Continued)*

Women Who are Pregnant or Breastfeeding
- Consume 8–12 ounces of seafood per week from a variety of seafood types.
- Owing to their high methyl mercury content, limit white (albacore) tuna to 6 ounces per week, and do not eat the following four types of fish: tilefish, shark, swordfish, and king mackerel.
- If pregnant, take an iron supplement, as recommended by an obstetrician or other healthcare provider.

Individuals Age 50 Years and Older
- Consume foods fortified with vitamin B_{12}, such as fortified cereals, or dietary supplements.

Building Healthy Eating Patterns
- Select an eating pattern that meets nutrient needs over time at an appropriate calorie level.
- Account for all foods and beverages consumed, and assess how they fit within a total healthy eating pattern.
- Follow food safety recommendations when preparing and eating foods to reduce the risk of foodborne illnesses.

[a]http://health.gov/dietaryguidelines/dga2010/dietaryguidelines2010.pdf

TABLE 1-2   American Heart Association Dietary Guidelines[a]

- Balance the number of calories you eat and physical activity to maintain a healthy body weight (this means not eating more calories than you need).
- Make your diet rich in fruits and vegetables. A typical adult should try for 9–10 servings (4.5 cups) of fruits and vegetables every day.
- Choose whole grains and high-fiber foods (three 1-oz servings per day). A diet rich in fiber can help manage your weight because fiber keeps you feeling fuller longer, so you eat less.
- Eat fish, especially oily fish like salmon or albacore tuna, twice a week to get omega-3 fatty acids.
- Limit saturated and *trans*-fat and cholesterol by choosing lean meats, selecting fat-free (skim), 1% and low-fat dairy products, and avoiding hydrogenated fats (margarine, shortening, cooking oils and the foods made from them).
  - A person needing 2,000 calories each day should consume less than 16 g saturated fat, less than 2 g *trans*-fat and between 50 and 70 g of total fat, and limit cholesterol to no more than 300 mg each day.
- Limit the amount of added sugars you consume to no more than half of your daily discretionary calorie allowance. For most American women, this is no more than 100 calories per day and no more than 150 calories per day for men (or approximately 6 tsp/day for women and 9 tsp/day for men).
  - Limit sugar-sweetened beverages to no more than 450 calories (36 oz) per week.
- Choose and prepare foods with little or no salt (sodium) to maintain a healthy blood pressure. Keep sodium intake to 1,500 mg/day or less.
  - Limit processed meat (such as sandwich meat, sausage, and hot dogs) to fewer than two servings per week.
- Try to eat four servings per week of nuts, seeds, or legumes (beans).
- If you choose to consume alcohol, do so in moderation. This means an average of one to two drinks per day for men and one drink per day for women.
- If you eat out, pay attention to portion size and the number of calories in your meal.

[a]http://www.heart.org/HEARTORG/GettingHealthy/NutritionCenter/HealthyCooking/Healthy-Diet-Guidelines_UCM_430092_Article.jsp
Reprinted with permission Article copyright © 2014 American Heart Association. For more articles and simple, quick and affordable recipes, visit heart.org/simplecooking.

TABLE 1-3 Summary of The American Cancer Society Guidelines on Nutrition and Physical Activity[a]

ACS Recommendations for Individual Choices

Achieve and Maintain a Healthy Weight Throughout Life.
- Be as lean as possible throughout life without being underweight.
- Avoid excess weight gain at all ages. For those who are overweight or obese, losing even a small amount of weight has health benefits and is a good place to start.
- Get regular physical activity and limit intake of high-calorie foods and drinks as keys to help maintain a healthy weight.

Be Physically Active.
- Adults: Get at least 150 minutes of moderate-intensity or 75 minutes of vigorous-intensity activity each week (or a combination of these), preferably spread throughout the week.
- Children and teens: Get at least 1 hour of moderate- or vigorous-intensity activity each day, with vigorous activity on at least 3 days each week.
- Limit sedentary behavior such as sitting, lying down, watching TV, and other forms of screen-based entertainment.
- Doing some physical activity above usual activities, no matter what one's level of activity, can have many health benefits.

Eat a Healthy Diet, With an Emphasis on Plant Foods.
- Choose foods and drinks in amounts that help you get to and maintain a healthy weight.
- Limit how much processed meat and red meat you eat.
- Eat at least 2½ cups of vegetables and fruits each day.
- Choose whole grains instead of refined grain products.

If You Drink Alcohol, Limit Your Intake.
- Drink no more than one drink per day for women or two per day for men.

ACS Recommendations for Community Action

Public, private, and community organizations should work together at national, state, and local levels to apply policy and environmental changes that:
- Increase access to affordable, healthy foods in communities, places of work, and schools, and decrease access to and marketing of foods and drinks of low nutritional value, particularly to youth.
- Provide safe, enjoyable, and accessible environments for physical activity in schools and workplaces, and for transportation and recreation in communities.

[a] http://www.cancer.org/acs/groups/cid/documents/webcontent/002577-pdf.pdf

34.9% of the population and 68.5% of adults were either overweight or obese (4). In 1995, no state had an obesity prevalence rate of greater than 20% whereas in 2012, no state had a prevalence rate of less than 20% and obesity prevalence in 13 states topped 30% (5).

Obesity is associated with a wide variety of increased health risks, as discussed more fully in Chapter 14. These include an increased risk of morbidity and mortality from coronary heart disease, hypertension, type II diabetes mellitus, arthritis, gallstones, and certain forms of cancer. Recent analysis of pooled data from 97 prospective cohort studies that included 1.8 million subjects found that each increment of five BMI units was associated with a 27% increased risk of coronary heart disease and an 18% increment in stroke (6). Forty-six percent of the increased coronary heart disease risk and 76% of the elevated stroke risk appeared to reflect the associated confounders of elevated blood pressure, elevated cholesterol, and increased blood glucose that accompany elevations in BMI. In overweight and obese individuals, 50% and 44%, respectively, of the excess risk of coronary heart disease was a reflection of these three mediators, and their contributions to the increased risk of stroke was even greater, 98% and 69%, respectively (6).

All guidelines advocate maintaining a healthy weight by balancing calorie intake with regular physical activity. The first step in devising a dietary plan is to set one's energy intake at a level to maintain a BMI within the normal adult range of 18.5 to 25. Remember, however, that all initial estimates of dietary energy intake for an individual person are just that, crude estimates, and must be refined upward or downward on the basis of the person's body weight response to the initial approximation. An individual's estimated energy requirement (EER) in kilocalories per day can be estimated from his or her age, body weight in kilograms, and height in meters according to the following equations (7,8):

Men:
$$EER = 662 - (9.53 \times age) + PA \times [(15.91 \times wt) + (539.6 \times ht)]$$

Women:
$$EER = 354 - (6.91 \times age) + PA \times [(9.36 \times wt) + (726 \times ht)]$$

PA is the subject's physical activity quotient. The value of PA assigned to the activities of usual daily living is 1.0. PA increases to 1.11 to 1.12 (for women and men, respectively) for the activities of daily life *plus* an additional 30 to 60 minutes of moderate activity daily; to 1.25 to 1.27 for at least an *additional* 60 minutes of moderate daily activity; and to 1.45 to 48 for the activities of daily life plus an *additional* 180 minutes of moderate activity or at least an *additional* 60 minutes of moderate daily activity plus an *additional* 60 minutes of vigorous activity (9,10). Since most people do not have very active lifestyles, when initially estimating an individual's energy expenditure, it is best to estimate the PA quotient on the low side.

Be Physically Active on a Daily Basis

Avoid a sedentary lifestyle. Regular physical activity burns calories. Additionally, it improves cardiovascular fitness and reduces the risk for heart disease, hypertension, colon cancer, and type 2 diabetes, while maintaining muscle strength and endurance, maintaining bone health and reducing osteoporosis, and promoting psychological well-being, including reducing symptoms of depression (1–3,11). As for the *Dietary Guidelines for Americans*, the Nation's most authoritative recommendations on physical activity are included in a similarly detailed report *2008 Physical Activity Guidelines for Americans* (11), freely available at www.health.gov/paguidelines. It is critical for everyone to avoid inactivity and spending most of their time in sedentary activities. To achieve measurable health benefits, adults should do at least 150 minutes of moderate-intensity or 75 minutes of vigorous-intensity aerobic physical activity per week (11). Additional health benefits can be achieved by doubling the above durations and/or by adding moderate to high-intensity resistance exercise to the program on two or more days weekly (11). Calories expended in hourly bouts of common physical activities are shown in Table 1-4. It is imperative to remember that these physical activity recommendations are made in the context of persons who do not exceed their recommended calorie intakes and maintain adequate hydration. It is also important to remember that, to ensure safety, an older individual should consult his/her physician before beginning moderate or intensive physical activity programs.

Enjoy a Wide Variety of Foods

No single food can supply all the known essential nutrients in sufficient amounts. For this reason, it is imperative to consume a wide variety of foods, both within and among the different food groups. The USDA defines the basic food groups as grains; vegetables; fruits; milk, yogurt and cheese; and meat, poultry, fish, dry beans, eggs, and nuts. The Dietary Approaches to Stop Hypertension (DASH) diet plan is available at http://www.nhlbi.nih.gov/health/resources/heart/hbp-dash-index.htm. Promoted by the National Heart, Lung, and Blood Institute because of its demonstrated effectiveness in lowering high blood pressure and improving blood lipids, the DASH diet emphasizes fruits, vegetables, and low- or nonfat dairy products, but includes whole grains, fish, poultry, beans, seeds, and nuts (12). Since each food group contributes one or more of the essential nutrients necessary to constitute a nutritionally adequate diet, it is necessary to include all food groups in one's regular diet. Furthermore, variety enhances the enjoyment of eating. Nonetheless, in our society, where an abundance of affordable food is readily available, persons who expend relatively low amounts of energy on a daily basis are at increased risk for becoming obese. To maintain a healthy weight, particular attention must also be paid to portion

TABLE 1-4 Calories Expended for Each Hour of Common Physical Activities

Moderate Physical Activity	Calories/H
Hiking	370
Light gardening/yard work	330
Dancing	330
Golf (walking and carrying clubs)	330
Bicycling (<10 mph)	290
Walking (3.5 mph)	280
Weight lifting (general light workout)	220
Stretching	180
Vigorous Physical Activity	
Running/Jogging (5 mph)	590
Bicycling (>10 mph)	590
Swimming (slow freestyle laps)	510
Aerobics	480
Walking (4.5 mph)	460
Heavy yard work (chopping wood)	440
Weight lifting (vigorous effort)	440
Basketball (vigorous)	440

Approximate energy expended, calculated for a person who weighs 70 kg. The values will be higher for those who weigh more and lower for individuals who weigh less.

size and to the energy and nutrient densities of the foods consumed. Energy-dense foods are those that supply calories, but relatively few essential nutrients. Nutrient-dense foods are those that provide a substantial amount of essential nutrients like vitamins and minerals, but contain relatively fewer calories than energy-dense foods. In today's environment, foods that are low in energy but relatively nutrient-dense (e.g., fruits and vegetables) are preferable to energy-dense foods that are relatively nutrient-poor (e.g., fats, oils, and alcohol), both for helping to maintain energy balance and for providing what are known to be health-promoting nutrients.

Consume a Variety of Fruits, Vegetables, and Grain Products Daily

In the context of the statements immediately above, dietary patterns characterized by the consumption of large amounts of fruits, vegetables, and whole grains have been associated with decreased risks of cardiovascular disease, stroke, hypertension, and certain cancers (1–3). In addition, because they are rich in nutrients (Table 1-5) but low in caloric density, these foods help one to maintain a healthful weight. Moreover, since they are also high in fiber, they may promote satiety, enhance bowel function, and modestly lower blood cholesterol levels.

For a reference 2,000 calorie diet, approximately 2.5 cups of fruits and 2.5 cups of vegetables are recommended daily (1). Obviously, the recommended amounts increase or decrease proportionately, depending on a person's actual calorie intake. Further, because different types of vegetables supply different nutrients (Table 1-5), recommendations tend to distribute vegetable intake categories approximately as dark green vegetables (1.5 cups weekly), legumes (1.5 cups weekly), red and orange vegetables (5.5 cups weekly), starchy vegetables (5 cups weekly), and other vegetables (4 cups weekly). One should also drink three cups fat-free, low-fat, or equivalent milk products on a daily basis. Additionally, 6 ounces of grains should be consumed daily, with more than 3 ounces as whole grain products (1). It is important to remember that whole grain products are only those *that are specifically labeled as whole grain* wheat, oats, corn, rye and barley, oatmeal, popcorn, brown rice, wild rice, buckwheat, bulgur, millet, quinoa, and sorghum. Whole grains are excellent sources of dietary fiber, and Dietary Reference Intakes for total fiber have been set at 14 grams per 1,000 kcal per day. Less than about 6 ounces of fish, lean meats, or poultry should be consumed daily, with fish eaten at least twice weekly. Four to

TABLE 1-5 Selected Nutrients in Fruits and Vegetables

Sources of Vitamin A (carotenoids)
- Bright orange vegetables like carrots, sweet potatoes, and pumpkin
- Tomatoes and tomato products, red sweet pepper
- Leafy greens such as spinach, collards, turnip greens, kale, beet and mustard greens, green-leaf lettuce, and romaine
- Orange fruits like mango, cantaloupe, apricots, and red or pink grapefruit

Sources of Vitamin C
- Citrus fruits and juices, kiwi fruit, strawberries, guava, papaya, and cantaloupe
- Broccoli, peppers, tomatoes, cabbage (especially Chinese cabbage), brussels sprouts, and potatoes
- Leafy greens such as romaine, turnip greens, and spinach

Sources of Folate
- Cooked dry beans and peas
- Oranges and orange juice
- Deep green leaves like spinach and mustard greens

Sources of Potassium
- Baked white or sweet potatoes, cooked greens (such as spinach), winter (orange) squash
- Bananas, plantains, many dried fruits, oranges and orange juice, cantaloupe, and honeydew melons
- Cooked dry beans
- Soybeans (green and mature)
- Tomato products (sauce, paste, puree)
- Beet greens

---

five servings of nuts and/or seeds should be consumed weekly (serving size varies according to the product).

When possible, fresh fruits and vegetables should be included in the diet, although frozen and canned fruits and vegetables remain excellent sources of essential nutrients that should be used when fresh products are not readily or cheaply available. When vegetables are cooked, a minimal amount of water should be used and the vegetables cooked only until tender to limit the loss of vitamins and nutrients. Legumes are good sources of vegetable protein in addition to fiber. Because most fruits, vegetables, and grains are also low in fat, they are good alternatives to high-fat foods.

Choose a Diet Low in Saturated Fats

More than 40 years of extensive epidemiologic research have shown that heart disease is increased in populations and persons who consume diets high in saturated fats, *trans*-fats and, to a lesser extent, cholesterol (1,2). For this reason, it is prudent to limit one's combined intake of dietary saturated fats to less than 10% of total energy intake (1), aiming for 5% to 6% as an ultimate goal (2). The intake of *trans*-fatty acids should be as low as possible. Although there is insufficient evidence that reducing dietary cholesterol will convincingly lower LDL cholesterol (2), some guidelines (1) continue to recommend limiting dietary intake to less than 300 mg per day to "maintain normal blood cholesterol levels" (1) and less than 200 mg per day to "further help individuals at high risk of cardiovascular disease" (1). In the past, these recommendations were part of a general recommendation to reduce the total dietary fat intake. More recently, however, dietary guidelines have recognized that diets rich in mono- and polyunsaturated fats are beneficial in reducing the risks of adverse cardiovascular events, particularly when the mono- or polyunsaturated fats replace dietary saturated fats (2). What has also become clear is that the macronutrient that replaces dietary saturated fats when intake of the latter is reduced is not a simple matter as far as long-term health risks are concerned (2,13). (For further discussion, see Chapter 12.) Thus, current dietary recommendations focus on the overall healthful pattern of the *whole diet* with fat intake recommendations allowed to range widely from 20% to 35% of energy intake as long as the fats consumed are weighted to those associated with long-term health maintenance and reduction of disease risk. Nonetheless, it is important to recognize that, for some individuals, reducing dietary fat intake may aid in preventing excessive consumption of dietary energy and thus help maintain body weight. The evidence that low-fat diets reduce the risk of developing various cancers is no longer compelling (14).

Beef, pork, liver and other organ meats, processed meats and cold cuts, whole milk, nondairy creamers, cheese, ice cream, eggs, butter, margarine, mayonnaise, lard, shortening, salad and cooking oils, deep-fried foods of all types, pastries, doughnuts, cookies, pie crusts, and cakes are the major sources of fat and saturated fat in the American diet. The *Dietary Guidelines for Americans* notes that saturated fats are largely solid fats, so the recommendation is made to limit the consumption of foods containing solid fats. Further, various prepared foods often contain significant amounts of "hidden" fat. An informed consumer *always* reads the label. A good rule of thumb for reducing total and saturated fat intake is to limit one's daily intake of lean meat, fish, and poultry to two to three servings (cooked weight of no more than about 5 to 6 oz).

Exercise Moderation in Salt and Sugar Consumption

Across a wide range of intakes in populations, there is an association between increasing dietary sodium and increasing blood pressure. Further, a large number of randomized clinical trials and meta-analyses support the fact that lower sodium intakes lead to lower blood pressures, especially in individuals with elevated blood pressures (9,10,15–17). The most compelling evidence that lowering dietary salt intake is an important factor in maintaining a normal blood pressure and reducing blood pressure in hypertensive individuals is the DASH sodium trial (18). Based on these data, the Dietary Guidelines for Americans recommends limiting sodium intake to less than 2,300 mg per day (approximately 1 tsp of table salt) and even further to 1,500 mg per day in individuals older than 51 years of age or in people of any age who are African American, or who have hypertension, diabetes, or chronic renal disease (1). Achieving this goal, however, can be very difficult because the principal sources of salt are processed and prepared foods, over which the consumer has little control other than nonconsumption. Moreover, recent evidence has questioned this lower limit in groups at risk for complications of very low sodium intakes. Thus, recent data have indicated that both excessively low and excessively high sodium intakes are associated with increased mortality (9,15,17,19). These data have stirred an intensive discussion of the rationale for guidelines that severely limit dietary sodium intake, but guidelines that support modest reduction in dietary sodium remain defensible. On average, Americans consume about 3.5 g of sodium daily, not far below the average global population consumption of about 4.0 g of sodium per day, but significantly less than some Asian populations that consume 5 to 6 g of sodium daily (20). Thus, dietary sodium intake reductions aimed at approaching the 2,300 mg per day level are surely reasonable in the context of American dietary lifestyles, but are not necessarily readily achievable goals given the habitual nature of individual eating patterns and preferences.

The debate about dietary sugar intake is particularly vocal, although the data indicating that dietary sugars are harmful to health are far less compelling than those for salt. The most convincing medical consequence of excessive sugar intake is the development of dental caries (21), but even here sugar intake is only one of many contributing factors, and the evidence supporting a benefit of severe restriction of sugars intake "was judged to be of very low quality." There is no evidence that sugars per se cause many of the problems commonly attributed to them, such as hyperactivity, obesity, and diabetes. Although the evidence supports a temporal association of increased dietary sugars consumption and increased body weight (22) and despite variously postulated mechanisms for the role of sugars in obesity-associated comorbidities (22), formal systematic data assessments do not support a unique role of sugars, per se, on the causal pathway. Thus, in isocaloric feeding studies or when total energy intake is accounted for, sugars have no unique effect on body weight (23–26). Similarly, when the relationships of sugars intake to blood pressure, blood lipids, and hepatic lipids were examined, either no or very minor effects were found (27–30). One study assessed the effects of added sugars intake on cardiovascular diseases mortality in American adults using data from the NHANES study (31). While this study demonstrated an association between sugars intake and increased cardiovascular disease risk, there was no change in all-cause mortality across the entire range of added sugars intake, a finding that raises questions about the net public health benefit of reducing added sugars intakes. This is especially the case when nearly all of those consuming sugars below about 15% of total energy intake would have to restrict their sugars intake but only very few people would achieve a beneficial reduction in cardiovascular risk (31).

Additionally, no evidence indicates that "added sugars" produce effects different from those of intrinsic sugars, and no controlled intervention studies have demonstrated long-term beneficial effects of low-sugar diets at any level. Because dietary sugars are often consumed in foods that have a lower density of other nutrients, the principal reasons for recommending moderate sugar consumption are to prevent the over consumption of unnecessary calories, to allow for consumption of more healthful, nutrient-dense foods by reducing the contribution of sugars to satiety, thus limiting "dilution" of the intake of other essential nutrients in the diet. Nonetheless, these arguments also apply to selective overconsumption of the other macronutrients, especially fat, and are not unique to sugars alone.

Drink Alcoholic Beverages in Moderation, If at All, and Do Not Smoke

The evidence for the detrimental effects of smoking on health is overwhelming. Although data now suggest that one and two alcoholic drinks daily for women and men, respectively, may reduce the risk of cardiovascular disease, far more ample evidence indicates that excessive consumption of alcohol has significant detrimental effects on health, including increased risks for hypertension, stroke, liver disease, accidents, violent behavior, suicide, and cancers of pharynx, mouth, esophagus, liver, colorectum, and breast (1,3). For these reasons, one should consider whether any consumption of alcoholic beverages is prudent. Further, because the risks of alcohol consumption during embryogenesis and fetal development are well established, pregnant women and women of childbearing age who may become pregnant should not consume alcohol.

Moderate Your Protein Intake

The Estimated Average Requirement for protein in adults of both sexes is 0.66 g/kg/day, with a corresponding Recommended Dietary Allowance (RDA) of 0.8 g/kg/day (7,8). The RDA for protein represents about 10% of dietary energy intake for young adults. There is no evidence to indicate that intakes above the RDA have any benefit, although modest increments, representing about 12% to 15% of total energy intake or 1.0 to 1.2 g/kg/day, are more likely to be consistent with current lifestyle and dietary habits in the United States. These increments should be from plant protein sources rather than from animal proteins. Sources of animal protein are not only more expensive as a rule, but are also generally high in fat calories, saturated fat, and cholesterol. Additionally, prolonged high intakes of animal protein are suspected to contribute to renal failure, reduced bone density, and cancers of the breast and colon, although the evidence is not compelling. However, elimination of all animal sources of protein is not necessarily desirable because these foods are the only source of vitamin B_{12}, the best source of readily absorbable iron, and a good source of zinc.

Maintain an Adequate Intake of Calcium

Adequate cellular function, skeletal growth, and proper bone and dental mineralization require the essential nutrient calcium. All but about 1% of total body calcium is found within bones and teeth. Accelerated rates of calcium deposition occur at or near the onset of puberty and continue during the adolescent growth spurt. The net gain of bone calcium during early adolescence is a critical determinant in the prevention of osteoporosis much later in life. After menarche, net bone calcium deposition rates fall, and by the age of about 20, bone calcium accretion is essentially complete. Thus, consumption of adequate dietary calcium intake is especially important for teenagers, particularly girls. An adequate intake (AI) of calcium is 1,300 mg daily for adolescent boys and girls 9 to 18 years of age (8). Similarly, maintaining optimal bone mineralization during young adult life is equally important. For adult men and women between the ages of 19 and 50, the calcium AI is 1,000 g per day (8). Pregnancy or lactation does not alter the values for adolescent or adult women (8) (see Chapter 3).

The principal dietary sources of calcium are milk and milk products, and selected food sources ranked by their calcium contents can be found in the appendix of the *Dietary Guidelines for Americans* (1) and many other sources available on the Internet. To maintain the dietary objective of reduced saturated fat intake, the best approach to achieving adequate calcium intake is consumption of low-fat or nonfat milk and milk products in addition to fruit juices and soy products with added calcium. Although calcium is also found in various dark green leafy vegetables, the oxalic acid in some of these vegetables (e.g., spinach) makes the calcium less bioavailable. Ensuring adequate calcium and vitamin D intakes is critical for preventing osteoporotic fractures, and food sources of dietary calcium are preferred. There is only marginal evidence that consuming calcium (or calcium plus vitamin D) at intake levels above the recommended AI has additional protective effects against such fractures (32,33). Long-term clinical trials using calcium supplements are bedeviled by low rates of compliance, and there is some indication of potential harm (33). There is surely no reason to exceed the 2.5 g per day tolerable upper intake level (UL) of calcium (8).

Do Not Take Unnecessary Dietary Supplements in Excessive Amounts

Except for selected persons in special circumstances, nutritional needs can be met with ordinary foods. Approximately half of adults in the United States take a vitamin or mineral supplement with some regularity. A single daily multivitamin and mineral supplement containing 100% of the RDA is not known to be harmful, but neither is it known to be beneficial for the vast majority of persons already meeting their nutritional needs by consuming a regular diet. By and large, persons who take supplements are those who are more likely to consume an adequate diet. Little evidence is available to indicate that such persons will reap a sizable health "dividend" from this form of nutrition "insurance." At the present time, there is no convincing evidence that the consumption of "pharmacologic" amounts of vitamins, minerals, antioxidants, and other food constituents of unknown or dubious function has any direct, long-term effect of preventing chronic disease in persons who consume a balanced diet containing essential nutrients at the RDA level (34–36). In fact, the evidence is just the opposite, and consuming large amounts of some supplements has been shown to increase mortality in randomized trials (36).

IMPLEMENTATION GUIDANCE

For many years, the USDA used its well-recognized Food Guide Pyramid to provide practical guidance on how individuals might implement the nutritional recommendations in the Dietary Guidelines for Americans. In 2011, following release of the current guidelines, the USDA released a revised tool called MyPlate. This implementation tool is readily available at www.choosemyplate.gov and includes various applications such as a nutrient database, a food tracker, a physical activity tracker, BMI calculator, energy expenditure calculator, weight management aids, and various recipes.

Similarly, the American Heart Association diet plan can be found at http://www.heart.org/HEARTORG/GettingHealthy/NutritionCenter/HealthyEating/The-American-Heart-Associations-Diet-and-Lifestyle-Recommendations_UCM_305855_Article.jsp a site that includes both diet and lifestyle advice and various helpful tools. The corresponding guidelines site hosted by the American Cancer Society is located at http://www.cancer.org/healthy/eathealthygetactive/acsguidelinesonnutritionphysicalactivityforcancerprevention/nupa-guidelines-toc.

It is important to realize that alternative approaches to dietary guidance exist as well. Based on extensive data from many large epidemiologic studies conducted worldwide that relate dietary intake patterns to health outcomes, the Harvard School of Public Health has devised an alternative guidance system designed to promote a healthy lifestyle that is located at the following URL: http://www.hsph.harvard.edu/nutritionsource/pyramid-full-story/. This approach is called "The Healthy Eating Plate." In addition to a figure "scampering across the bottom" of the placement to emphasize the need to keep active, the Harvard School of Public Health plan emphasizes the following rules for filling one's plate in a healthy fashion:

1. Fill half your plate with vegetables and fruit.
2. Save a quarter of your plate for whole grains—not just any grains.
3. Pick a healthy source of protein to fill a quarter of your plate.
4. Enjoy healthy fats.
5. Drink water, coffee, or tea.

Overall, the bulk of this message is the same as that of other expert groups discussed earlier, but emphasizes more forcefully the position of the Harvard School of Public Health that other recommendations are not as aggressive as they should be in promoting whole grains, are not as aggressive in restricting red meat and processed meats, and are more supportive of recommending excessive dairy intake than is warranted.

SUGGESTIONS FOR IMPLEMENTATION

The following are various practical suggestions for achieving the dietary guidelines outlined earlier.

1. **Cook at home as frequently as possible.** At home, you can best control the composition of your diet. Restaurant food, particularly "fast food," tends to be high in saturated fat, cholesterol, and salt. If you eat out, ask the chef to prepare food the way you want it. After all, that is his or her job, and you are paying the bill.

2. **Start shopping in the supermarket produce department.** Continue around the perimeter of the store, where fresh foods, unprocessed foods, fish, poultry, and dairy products are generally located. Avoid processed foods, and be careful not to consume too many foods that can contribute more calories to your diet than nutrients.

3. **Always read the label. Repeat: always read the label.** With the present vast array of food technologies and the plethora of foods prepared accordingly and obtainable in today's supermarket, it is impossible to know the actual composition of a processed food without reading the label—specifically the label on the back or side of the package. By statute, virtually all processed foods must carry two label panels: the nutrition facts panel and the ingredients panel. The information in the nutrition facts panel provides a good guide to the calories in a product, in addition to the content of fat, saturated and *trans*-fat, protein, carbohydrate and total sugars, sodium, calcium, iron, and vitamins A and C. Reading the label will help you identify hidden sources of dietary fat. The ingredients label must list all the product's ingredients, in order of weight. Thus, a product that lists water as its first ingredient has more water in the product than it does for the next ingredients listed. Likewise, a product that is called raspberry juice but shows its apple juice as the first entry on the ingredients label is primarily apple juice.

4. **Understand the difference between grams of fat and percentage of calories from fat.** The dietary guidelines discussed earlier include moderating total fat intake between 20% and 35% of total calorie intake. While 8 oz of plain yogurt made from whole milk contains 8 g of fat and 150 calories, nearly 50% of the calories in the yogurt come from fat because 8 g of fat provides 72 calories.

5. **Steam, broil, bake, or microwave foods** to avoid increasing the fat content. Use nonstick cookware and very little oil when sautéing. Stir-frying is an additional acceptable alternative because proper stir-frying techniques require intense heat but almost no fat. However, stir fried foods obtained in many Asian restaurants are often not low in fat because excessive oil is used in the frying process.

6. Slowly **wean yourself from adding salt** while cooking or eating. Proper seasoning with herbs and spices helps reduce the need for salt. The taste for salt is largely acquired, and once you adapt to the taste of unsalted food, you will find salted food "too salty." Adopt a diet high in fresh fruits and vegetables. This will not only reduce your salt intake, it will increase your intake of potassium, an additional beneficial factor in lowering blood pressure.

7. **Maintain calcium intake** by consuming low-fat or nonfat dairy products. Although dairy products are the best source of dietary calcium, full-fat dairy products are also the second-largest source of saturated fats after meats, the leading source. However, a very large array of reduced-fat or nonfat dairy products of all descriptions is now available in supermarkets, in addition to a variety of calcium-fortified juices and other products. These facilitate attaining the adult AI for calcium without jeopardizing the goals for fat reduction.

8. **Avoid fads and "magic bullets."** Excellent nutritional health can be achieved by following the sensible dietary guidelines discussed previously. No fad diet has ever been shown to provide better nutrition, and many have been shown to provide less than adequate nutrition. Similarly, no individual plant, animal, biochemical, or chemical "magic bullet" has ever been shown to achieve effects beyond those provided by a nutritionally adequate diet alone.

REFERENCES

1. U.S. Department of Agriculture and U.S. Department of Health and Human Services. *Dietary Guidelines for Americans 2010.* U.S. Government Printing Office, December 2010.
2. Eckel RH, Jakicic M, Ard JD, et al. 2013 AHA/ACC guideline on lifestyle management to reduce cardiovascular risk: a report of the American College of Cardiology/American Heart Association Task Force on Practice Guidelines. *Circulation.* 2014;129:(25 Suppl 2):S1–S45.
3. Kushi LH, Doyle C, McCullough M, et al. American Cancer Society Guidelines on Nutrition and Physical Activity for cancer prevention: reducing the risk of cancer with healthy food choices and physical activity. *CA Cancer J Clin.* 2012;62:30–67.
4. Ogden CL, Carroll MD, Kit BK, et al. Prevalence of childhood and adult obesity in the United States, 2011–2012. *JAMA.* 2014;311(8):806–814.
5. Department of Health and Human Services. National Center for Health Statistics. *U.S. Obesity Trends 1985–2005.* http://www.cdc.gov/obesity/data/adult.html
6. Global Burden of Metabolic Risk Factors for Chronic Diseases Collaboration (BMI Mediated Effects), Lu Y, Hajifathalian K, et al. Metabolic mediators of the effects of body-mass index, overweight, and obesity on coronary heart disease and stroke: a pooled analysis of 97 prospective cohorts with 1.8 million participants. *Lancet.* 2014;383(9921):970–983.
7. Food and Nutrition Board, Institute of Medicine, National Academy of Sciences. *Dietary Reference Intakes for Energy, Carbohydrate, Fiber, Fat, Fatty Acids, Cholesterol, Protein, and Amino Acids.* Washington, DC: National Academy Press, 2005.
8. Institute of Medicine, National Academy of Sciences. *Dietary Reference Intakes: The Essential Guide to Nutrient Requirements.* Washington, DC: National Academy Press, 2006.
9. Kyu S. Dietary salt intake and hypertension. *Electrolyte Blood Press.* 2014;12:7–18.
10. He FJ, Li J, MacGregor GA. Effect of longer term modest salt reduction on blood pressure: cochrane systematic review and meta-analysis of randomised trials. *BMJ.* 2013;346:f1325.
11. U.S. Department of Health and Human Services. *2008 Physical Activity Guidelines for Americans.* www.health.gov/paguidelines
12. Lin P-H, Aickin M, Champagne C, et al. Perspectives in practice. Food group sources of nutrients in the dietary patterns of the DASH-sodium trial. *J Am Diet Assoc.* 2003;103:488–496.
13. Bier DM. Saturated fats and cardiovascular disease: interpretations not as simple as they once were. *Crit Rev Food Sci Nutr.* In press.
14. Schwab U, Lauritzen L, Tholstrup T, et al. Effect of the amount and type of dietary fat on cardiometabolic risk factors and risk of developing type 2 diabetes, cardiovascular diseases, and cancer: a systematic review. *Food Nutr Res.* 2014;58:2545.
15. Kotchen TA, Cowley AW Jr, Frohlich ED. Salt in health and disease—a delicate balance. *N Engl J Med.* 2013;368:1229–1237.
16. Koliaki C, Katsilambros N. Dietary sodium, potassium, and alcohol: key players in the pathophysiology, prevention, and treatment of human hypertension. *Nutr Rev.* 2013;71:402–411.
17. Aaron KJ, Sanders PW. Role of dietary salt and potassium intake in cardiovascular health and disease: a review of the evidence. *Mayo Clin Proc.* 2013;88:987–995.
18. Sacks FM, Svetkey LP, Vollmer WM, et al, for the DASH-Sodium Collaborative Research Group. Effects on blood pressure of reduced dietary sodium and the dietary approaches to stop hypertension (DASH) diet: DASH-Sodium Collaborative Research Group. *N Engl J Med.* 2001;344:3–10.
19. Graudal N, Jürgens G, Baslund B, et al. Compared with usual sodium intake, low- and excessive-sodium diets are associated with increased mortality: a meta-analysis. *Am J Hypertens.* 2014;27(9):1129–1137.
20. Powles J, Fahimi S, Micha R, et al, on behalf of the Global Burden of Diseases Nutrition and Chronic Diseases Expert Group (NutriCoDE). Global, regional and national sodium intakes in 1990 and 2010: a systematic analysis of 24 h urinary sodium excretion and dietary surveys worldwide. *BMJ Open.* 2013;3:e003733.
21. Moynihan PJ, Kelly SAM. Effect on caries of restricting sugars intake: systematic review to inform WHO guidelines. *J Dent Res.* 2014;93:8–11.
22. Bray GA, Popkin BM. Dietary sugar and body weight: have we reached a crisis in the epidemic of obesity and diabetes? Health be damned! Pour on the sugar. *Diabetes Care.* 2014;37:950–956.
23. Te Morenga L, Mallard S, Mann J. Dietary sugars and body weight: systematic review and meta-analyses of randomised controlled trials and cohort studies. *BMJ.* 2012;345:e7492.
24. Malik VS, Pan A, Willett WC, et al. Sugar-sweetened beverages and weight gain in children and adults: a systematic review and meta-analysis. *Am J Clin Nutr.* 2013;98:1084–1102.

25. Sievenpiper JL, de Souza RJ, Mirrahimi A, et al. Effect of fructose on body weight in controlled feeding trials—a systematic review and meta-analysis. *Ann Intern Med*. 2012;156:291–304.
26. Kahn R, Sievenpiper JL. Dietary sugar and body weight: have we reached a crisis in the epidemic of obesity and diabetes? We have, but the pox on sugar is overwrought and overworked. *Diabetes Care*. 2014;37:957–962.
27. Te Morenga L, Howatson AJ, Jones RM, et al. Dietary sugars and cardiometabolic risk: systematic review and meta-analyses of randomized controlled trials of the effects on blood pressure and lipids. *Am J Clin Nutr*. 2014;100:65–79.
28. Ha V, Sievenpiper JL, de Souza RJ, et al. Effect of fructose on blood pressure – a systematic review and meta-analysis of controlled feeding trials. *Hypertension*. 2012;59:787–795.
29. Wang DD, Sievenpiper JL, de Souza RJ, et al. Effect of fructose on postprandial triglycerides: a systematic review and meta-analysis of controlled feeding trials. *Atherosclerosis*. 2014;232:125–133.
30. Chiu S, Sievenpiper JL, de Souza RJ, et al. Effect of fructose on markers of non-alcoholic fatty liver disease (NAFLD): a systematic review and meta-analysis of controlled feeding trials. *Eur J Clin Nutr*. 2014;68:416–423.
31. Yang Q, Zhang Z, Gregg EW, et al. Added sugar intake and cardiovascular diseases mortality among US adults. *JAMA Intern Med*. 2014;174:516–524.
32. Tang BMP, Eslick GD, Nowson C, et al. Use of calcium or calcium combination in combination with Vitamin D supplementation to prevent fractures and bone loss in people aged 50 years and older: a meta-analysis. *Lancet*. 2007;370:657–666.
33. Bauer DC. Calcium supplements and fracture prevention. *N Engl J Med*. 2013;369:1537–1543.
34. Macpherson H, Pipingas A, Pase MP. Multivitamin-multimineral supplementation and mortality: a meta-analysis of randomized controlled trials. *Am J Clin Nutr*. 2013;97:437–444.
35. Fortmann SP, Burda BU, Senger CA, et al. Vitamin and mineral supplements in the primary prevention of cardiovascular disease and cancer: an updated systematic evidence review for the U.S. Preventive Services Task Force. *Ann Intern Med*. 2013;159:824–834.
36. Guallar E, Stranges S, Mulrow C, et al. Enough is enough: stop wasting money on vitamin and mineral supplements. *Ann Intern Med*. 2013;159:850–851.

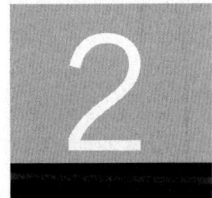

Recommendations for Healthy Elderly Adults

INTRODUCTION
Definitions

Aging is a continuous function, and one does not suddenly pass from young to elderly at any specific. Furthermore, chronologic age alone is not a particularly precise indicator of biologic or functional age because of differences in genotypes, individual characteristics, such as physical ability and mental health, and environmental circumstances, all of which vary widely among people as they age. No uniform legal criteria exist. At age 60, a person can participate in the benefits of the Older Americans Act, but the same person does not receive Medicare or full Social Security benefits until age 65. The US Census Bureau recognizes the demographic heterogeneity of the elderly by classifying them into three groups: ages 65 through 74, 75 through 84, and 85 or older.

Society has its own arbitrary definition. Age 60 defines an old age pensioner in the United Kingdom. Many banks, theaters, shops, and service organizations in the United States offer discounts or special services to senior citizens, but the eligibility criteria for the designation "senior citizen" vary widely. At age 50, a person can join the largest information, advocacy, and service group for older adults in the United States, the AARP (formerly the American Association of Retired Persons).

Population Trends

In the year 2010, the most recent US census reported that the median age of the US population reached 37.2 years, the highest in the nation's history. At the time, 13% of the population were 65 years of age or older and 1.8% of the population were 85 years of age or older (1). Given that the US population is now approximately 308 million people, more than 40 million Americans are aged 65 or older and 5.5 million are 85 years of age or older (1). In fact, nearly 2 million people are over the age of 90 and more than 53,000 centenarians live in the United States (2). By the year 2050, demographers project that 80 million people in the United States will be 65 years of age or older (3).

Even more importantly, the elderly population is getting older. Persons who are 85 years of age or older, the "oldest old," represent the most rapidly growing group of elderly people. Twenty years ago, the 1 million "oldest old" in the United States constituted 1% of the entire population and 10% of the elderly. Today, the "oldest old" accounts for nearly 2% of the population and their number is expected to grow to 19 million in 2050. If the projections prove correct, the "oldest old" will then account for 24% of the elderly population and 5% of the entire US population (3). Similar trends occur in aging populations worldwide, although the aging population is growing proportionately even faster in the developing world compared with the growth rate observed in developed countries due to a decline in birth rates as well as improvement of life span.

Life Expectancy

During the 20th century, the average life expectancy of an American has increased dramatically. In 1900, average life expectancy was 47 years and only 0.03% of people survived to the age of 100. In 2010, life expectancy was 78.7 years and a person aged 65 today can expect to live an additional 19.1 years (4). During the first half of the 20th century, the principal contributor to the gain in life span reflected the improved survival of infants and children because of immunization, treatment of infectious diseases, and public health sanitary measures, including safe food and water supplies. In 1900, only 87.6% of infants survived the first year, while today, this figure is well above 99%. In the latter half of the 20th century, the principal gains in survivorship occurred mostly in the elderly population. Today's average 65-year-old lives 2 to 3 years longer than a person who reached the age of 65 in 1990.

Nonetheless, there remain significant disparities in life expectancy. On average, women live 4 to 5 years longer than men (2,4) and life expectancy remains significantly different among Black, White, and Hispanic individuals of either gender (4). On average, White and Hispanic women live to ages 81 to 83, but Black women have a life expectancy that is slightly below 78 years. The life expectancy of Hispanic and Caucasian men is between 76.4 and 78.5 years, but Black men live only to 71.5 years on average. The reasons for these disparities are discussed elsewhere (5). The remarkable change in the age distribution of populations in developed and developing countries is shown in Figure 2-1 (6).

Dietary Intakes

The National Health and Nutrition Examination Surveys (NHANES) have collected successive, cross-sectional data on the health and nutritional status of representative adults from across the nation for four decades. Since 1999, the data are collected on an annual basis, but full data reporting tends to lag by several years. In persons over the age of 60, dietary energy intake declines with increasing age and the median energy intakes for both men and women are below the estimated energy requirements (EERs) for sedentary adults (7). On average, elderly subjects consume about 33% of their dietary energy as fat, with about 10% coming from saturated fats (7,8). Median cholesterol intake is less than 200 mg per day (7,8). About 16% of dietary energy comes from the intake of protein (7), a percentage equivalent to approximately 60 to 70 g of dietary protein. An estimated 12% of elderly men and 20% of elderly women consume inadequate amounts of protein (9).

Average calcium intake, however, is only about 60% to 70% of the adequate intake (AI) level (9), and the important medical issues relating to adequate calcium intake are discussed further below. Vitamin E intake is only about 60% of the estimated average requirement (EAR) level (7,10,11), and more than 90% of elderly adults are estimated to have inadequate vitamin E

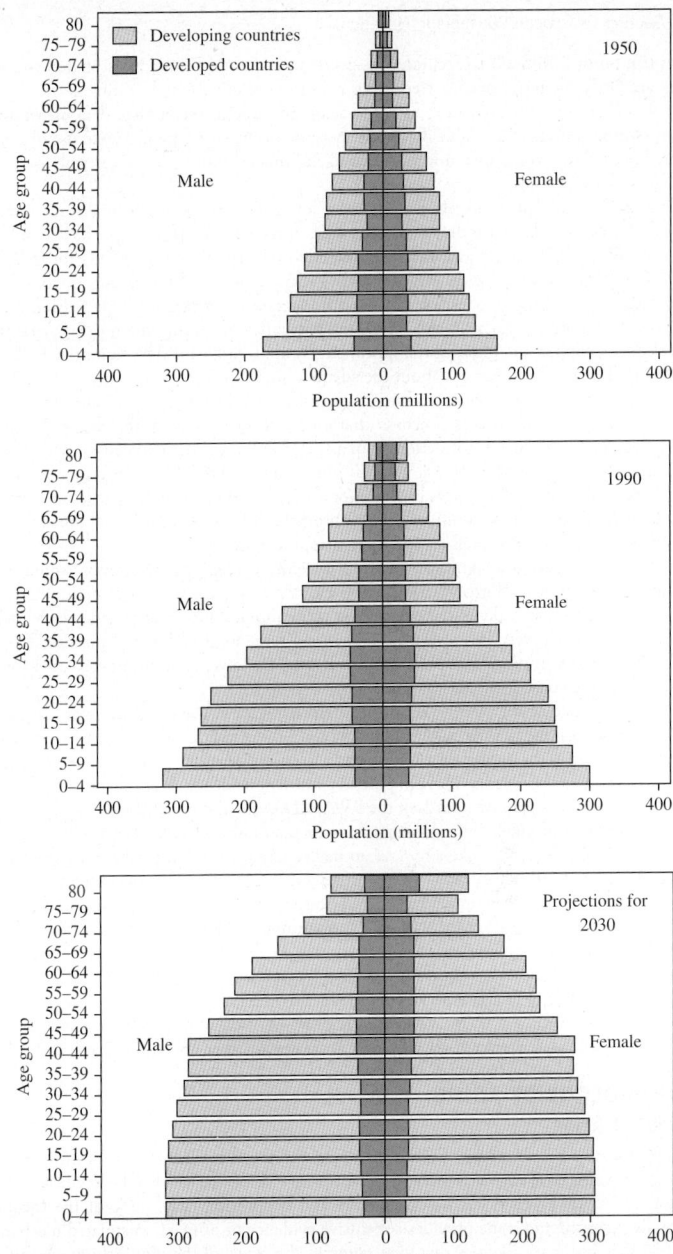

Figure 2-1 Population age distribution for developing and developed countries, by age group and sex—worldwide, 1950, 1990, and 2030. (From Centers for Disease Control and Prevention. Trends in aging—United States and worldwide. *MMWR Morb Mortal Wkly Rep*. 2003;52:101–104, 106. Data from United Nations, 1999, and US Bureau of the Census, 2000.)

intakes (9), but it is difficult to accurately assess dietary vitamin E intake. Estimated vitamin E intakes are likely the result of underreporting because of the inability to estimate the amounts and types of fats and oils used in food preparation and due to incomplete data on vitamin E content of food sources in available databases. Because of the currently increased use of polyunsaturated oils, which contain vitamin E, the intake of this vitamin is almost certainly more than sufficient in most persons.

Vitamin D levels are routinely found to be low in elderly adults who do not consume vitamin D–fortified dairy products. The average intake of potassium in elderly individuals is only about 50% to 60% of the recommended dietary allowance (RDA) for potassium (7,9,10,11). This is a particularly important deficit because AIs of potassium, in conjunction with avoidance of excessive sodium intakes, are important for control of hypertension and the prevention of strokes. Median intakes of thiamin, riboflavin, niacin, vitamin B_{12}, vitamin A, iron, selenium, copper, and phosphorus appear largely appropriate for their respective EAR levels (7,9,10,11). There is disagreement about the adequacy of intakes of pyridoxine, vitamin A, folic acid, magnesium, and zinc. Some assessments estimate largely adequate consumption of these nutrients (7,10,11), while others conclude that a significant fraction of the elderly population have inadequate intakes (9). Information from assorted other studies on dietary intakes of folate and vitamin B_{12} supports the fact that a significant minority of elderly adults does not consume these vitamins in adequate amounts or does not absorb them adequately. The latter is particularly relevant in the case of vitamin B_{12}, since absorption of the vitamin is well documented to be impaired in elderly individuals secondary to atrophic gastritis.

All surveys show that a significant fraction of elderly adults consume more sodium than recommended by almost all expert committees. However, recently the risk/benefit ratio of very low sodium intakes, especially in the elderly, has come into question and is under active debate. New data suggest that very low sodium intakes yield little additional blood pressure–lowering benefit compared with more modest intakes, but that the lower sodium intakes are associated with more adverse consequences (12–18).

Nonetheless, one of the considerations in interpreting the adequacy of nutrient intake levels based on the RDAs is the fact that adults should be consuming less than the RDAs because these are set at the upper end of the normal distribution curve to ensure adequacy in nearly all persons. A convenient, conventional population index of potential nutrient inadequacies is the fraction of the population consuming less than two-thirds of the RDA. RDAs are not intended to be used to estimate inadequacy of nutrient intakes in individuals. However, an individual who is generally consuming more than the RDA is very unlikely to have an inadequate intake of a specific nutrient. The best estimate for assessing the adequacy of nutrient intakes in an individual is to compare the average observed nutrient intakes of an individual with the respective EARs for those nutrients, when EAR values for the nutrient(s) are known. Nonetheless, the amount of a nutrient necessarily adequate for an individual elderly adult is not known accurately or precisely without specific biochemical testing. As a practical, general clinical guideline, however, elderly persons are more likely to be nutritionally deficient as they advance in age, especially those older than 85, if they are poor, if they suffer from significant chronic medical problems (particularly gastrointestinal or neurological disorders), if they are taking multiple prescription drugs, or if they are hospitalized or institutionalized.

PATHOBIOLOGY OF AGING
Theories of Aging

Although theories are abundant, we do not know the specific cause(s) of the common forms of aging. A variety of currently debated theories are discussed in detail elsewhere (19–29) (Table 2-1). Although each has its proponents and supporting data, none of the theories is universally accepted and none provides conclusive evidence of primacy. Postulated mechanisms include (a) evolutionary theories that view aging as the result of the diminishing advantage of natural selection that is the consequence of survival beyond the age of reproductive fitness, (b) genetic and epigenetic theories that postulate that aging results from effects at the gene level that cause molecular damage to DNA, alter gene expression, and reduce the accuracy and fidelity of translation and related effects, (c) cellular theories that relate the generation of aging to the consequences of repeated damage to cellular components and metabolic processes, oxidative

TABLE 2-1 Theories of Aging

Biological Level/Theory	Description
Evolutionary	
Mutation accumulation	Mutations that affect health at older ages are not selected against.
Disposal soma	Somatic cells are maintained only to ensure continued reproductive success; after reproduction, soma becomes disposable.
Antagonistic pleiotropy	Genes beneficial at younger age become deleterious at older ages.
Molecular	
Gene regulation	Aging is caused by changes in the expression of genes regulating both development and aging.
Codon restriction	Fidelity/accuracy of mRNA translation is impaired due to inability to decode codons in mRNA.
Error catastrophe	Decline in fidelity of gene expression with aging results in increased fraction of abnormal proteins.
Somatic mutation	Molecular damage accumulates, primarily to DNA/genetic material.
Dysdifferentiation	Gradual accumulation of random molecular damage impairs regulation of gene expression.
Cellular	
Cellular senescence—telomere theory	Phenotypes of aging are caused by an increase in frequency of senescent cells. Senescence may result from telomere loss (replicative senescence) or cell stress (cellular senescence).
Free radical	Oxidative metabolism produces highly reactive free radicals that subsequently damage lipids, protein, and DNA.
Wear and tear	Accumulation of normal injury.
Apoptosis	Programmed cell death from genetic events or genome crisis.
System	
Neuroendocrine	Alterations in neuroendocrine control of homeostasis results in aging-related physiological changes.
Immunologic	Decline of immune function with aging results in decreased incidence of infectious diseases but increased incidence of autoimmunity.
Rate of living	Assumes a fixed amount of metabolic potential for every living organism (live fast, die young).

From Weinert BT, Timiras PS. Physiology of aging. *J Appl Physiol*. 2003;95:1706–1716.

damage to the proteins or the mitochondrial electron transfer system or to mitochondrial DNA, the intracellular accumulation of altered proteins resulting from oxidative damage, glycosylation, or other posttranslational modifications, or to accelerated apoptosis and cell senescence, and (d) system theories that consider aging to be the consequence of slow, but inexorable failure of fine regulatory control within major biological systems such as the neuroendocrine or immunological systems. One of the most consistent and compelling observations, valid across a wide range of species from *Caenorhabditis elegans* to primates, is that animals whose energy intakes are modestly restricted live longer than those consuming a full complement of calories. There are suggestive data that these observations may apply to man as well, but we do not know with any confidence that calorie restriction will extend human life span (30), a hypothesis being tested by the NIH CALORIE (http://calerie.dcri.duke.edu/) that is currently underway. Perhaps the most exciting insight into a common mechanism responsible for the aging process came with the discovery of the underlying molecular defect in the Hutchinson–Gilford progeria syndrome, a disease of accelerated aging that has many similarities with common aging (31–33). Progeria, and a variety of related syndromes, have been shown to be the result of mutations in the *LMNA* gene responsible for encoding the inner nuclear membrane proteins, lamin A and lamin C, so the resulting diseases are now often referred to as laminopathies (31–33). Although individuals with progeria do not have deterioration of the nervous system, they do manifest a wide range of the clinical signs of common aging, and progerin, the abnormal lamin found in people with progeria, has now also been identified in aging subjects. Moreover, the lamin defect provides a link that supports DNA–dependent theories of aging and provides potential therapeutic targets for the treatment of progeria that may have relevance to the slowing of common aging (33).

PATHOPHYSIOLOGIC CONSEQUENCES OF AGING

Body Composition

Lean body mass declines approximately 6% per decade after age 30. To a significant extent, this decrement is a consequence of diminished physical activity rather than of the aging process itself. Muscle, a principal component of lean mass, is altered both structurally and functionally as one ages (34), largely on the basis of reduced mitochondrial energy production through ATP. These changes result in frailty and disability. One additional consequence of the decline in lean body mass is a corresponding increase in fat mass. Many elderly persons are overweight or frankly obese. Others who fit within normal weight-for-height ranges are relatively obese—that is, for the same BMI as young adults, elderly adults have a disproportionate increase in adipose tissue. Nonetheless, data across a wide variety of studies support the observation that a BMI in the overweight range is not associated with increased mortality in elderly individuals and BMIs in the obese range are associated with only a modest increase in mortality compared with the risk found at younger ages (35–36).

Protein and Energy Metabolism

Rates of whole body protein turnover (synthesis and breakdown) decline slightly with age. When corrected for the age-related changes in lean body mass, however, protein turnover rates are relatively constant throughout adult life. No consistent body of evidence indicates that protein needs are altered by aging. Even though the rates of protein synthesis and breakdown are slowed, body net nitrogen balance is achieved at the same levels of dietary protein intake in aging persons. For these reasons, the dietary reference intake (DRI) values for protein are not altered in elderly adults and there appears little reason to do so for active elderly individuals who are less than, perhaps, age 75 or so. However, some expert groups argue that the RDA for protein in elderly individuals should be increased based on their assessment of the reported potential benefits of supplemental amino acid and protein intakes on a variety of aging physical processes and comorbidities (37–40).

Energy is expended principally by the metabolically active lean tissues. Because lean body mass declines with age, energy expenditure declines correspondingly. Thus, to maintain energy balance, an elderly person must consume fewer calories. This is the most uniform and consistent nutritional consequence of aging. DRI equations for estimating the energy requirements of elderly individuals are provided below.

Organ System Function

During aging, a generalized decline in organ function involves the gastrointestinal system, but not primarily its absorptive or nutrient assimilation properties. Aging is associated with diminished smell and taste, particularly the loss of sweet and salty tastes. A reduction in salivary flow, loss of teeth, and disturbances of swallowing and esophageal dysfunction may be noted. Many persons experience various forms of discomfort associated with eating, including heartburn, gas, and constipation. Approximately 10% to 30% of persons over age 60 have atrophic gastritis, and its prevalence reaches about 40% over age 80. Although originally thought to be a consequence of aging, atrophic gastritis is principally the consequence of infection with *Helicobacter pylori*. Reductions in gastric acid, pepsin, and intrinsic factor lead to slower emptying of mixed meals and diminished absorption of iron, folate, and vitamin B_{12}. Bacterial overgrowth in the proximal small bowel is sometimes an accompanying feature. Pancreatic secretion is usually normal, but some people have a reduced hepatic function that is secondary to reduced blood flow, not to altered hepatocyte function. Nonetheless, except for the vitamins and iron mentioned above, absorption of macronutrients, vitamins, and minerals is generally normal. Aging is also associated with declining cardiac, pulmonary, and renal function and with diminished secretion of growth hormone, which some believe contributes to the decline in lean body and muscle mass (sarcopenia) that accompanies aging, although growth hormone replacement does not convincingly rectify the problem. Furthermore, a decrease in cell-mediated immunity is manifested by decreased numbers of circulating T cells and defective cell-mediated immune responses, which may contribute to the morbidity associated with aging. Humoral immunity is generally less severely affected, but the incidence of autoimmune disorders is increased. Atherosclerosis, arthritis, osteoporosis, diabetes, assorted cancers, and diminished sight and hearing are all commonly present. To varying degrees, these conditions can limit mobility and access to food, affect mood, and diminish appetite.

NUTRITIONAL ISSUES IN ELDERLY PERSONS
Food Access and Selection

1. **Economics.** A reduced income generally accompanies aging. This reduction often entails alterations in dietary habits, including the elimination of relatively high-priced items such as meat. In the United States, the prevalence of food insecurity is approximately 15% and food insecurity is a significant issue in maintenance of nutritional health in elderly adults whose incomes are limited (41–42). This problem is compounded when elderly individuals have to deal with the cost of medications. Nearly 20% of adults with chronic illnesses in the National Health Interview Survey reported food insecurity, and nearly one-quarter were unable to buy all of the medications they required (43).
2. **Mobility.** Because of physical infirmities, various illnesses, and, especially, loss of a means of transportation, the mobility of elderly adults is often limited. Along with the economic constraints discussed immediately above, such physical limitation can directly or indirectly restrict access to food purchase. It is particularly important for a medical caregiver to know whether elderly individuals under their care have the ability to travel to places where they can purchase food. Access to food and food affordability are critical determinants of dietary intake (44).
3. **Psychosocial and neurologic problems**, such as depression and mental deterioration, may lead to loss of the desire to shop, a diminished appetite, forgetfulness about meals, or frank inability to eat. Bereavement and living alone are additional critical determinants of dietary intake in the elderly. A medical caregiver must carefully assess an elderly patient's mental state and evaluate the practical consequences of functional inadequacies.

Bone Health: Calcium, Phosphorus, Vitamin D, and Vitamin K

Osteopenia secondary to osteoporosis and osteomalacia is a significant problem in the elderly, particularly elderly women (45–47). The resultant increased incidence of fractures is responsible for a very high level of physical and psychosocial disabilities in addition to substantial financial costs. Obligatory calcium losses increase, but calcium intake and absorption decline with age. Reduced absorption may be a consequence of decreased vitamin D function, in turn caused by the combined effects of reduced dietary intake, decreased exposure to sunlight and capacity of the aged skin to synthesize vitamin D, reduced intestinal absorption of the vitamin, and reduced hepatic and renal ability to hydroxylate vitamin D to its active form. As discussed earlier, the average calcium intake in women over age 51 is only about 50% to 60% of the AI level (7,9,10). The calcium intake of men over age 51 is somewhat better, but still well below the AI level. Based on the most recent assessment of the reference intakes for calcium, the RDA for calcium has been set at 1,200 mg per day for women over 51 years of age, 1,000 mg daily for men between 51 and 70 years of age, and 1,200 mg per day for men over the age of 70 (48) because of increasing evidence that increasing calcium intake in the elderly is a factor in maintaining bone density when accompanied by an AI of vitamin D (47–50), including meta-analyses of randomized controlled trials (48). Correspondingly, the RDA for vitamin D has been set at 15 μg cholecalciferol daily (600 IU vitamin D) for adults aged 51 through 70 years and 20 μg per day (800 IU vitamin D) for adults older than age 70 (48), although dissenting experts believe that these intake levels are not sufficient to ensure optimal vitamin D status in aged individuals. Several of these experts, however, were members of the committee issuing the Endocrine Society Clinic Practice Guidelines on Vitamin D (51) in which the recommended intakes of vitamin D for individuals above the age of 51 were identical to the values above from the Institute of Medicine (48).

Nonetheless, while one recent analysis of pooled studies of vitamin D dose and fracture prevention concluded that vitamin D supplementation greater than or equal to 800 IU per day "was somewhat favorable in the prevention of hip fracture and any nonvertebral fracture in persons 65 years of age of older" (52), alternative expert committee assessments were unable to support an effect of vitamin D supplementation on fracture prevention (53,54). Similar assessments of the potential beneficial effects of vitamin D on cancer risk, cardiovascular risk and all-cause mortality have produced provocative, often conflicting data, but have been unable overall to demonstrate convincing evidence of benefit (48, 54–60), at least to the degree necessary to satisfy ongoing debate about the potential benefits (or lack thereof) of higher intakes of vitamin D.

Phosphorus intake is generally higher than calcium intake, and most diets provide ample phosphorus. Data from various NHANES show that elderly generally meet the current estimated average intake levels of phosphorus of 580 mg per day or the RDA of 700 mg per day (49,61).

Other than its function in blood coagulation, vitamin K also functions as a cofactor for the vitamin K–dependent carboxylase that catalyses the posttranslational formation of γ-carboxylated bone proteins such as osteocalcin (62). The AI levels for vitamin K have been set at 120 μg per day for men and at 90 μg per day for women (61,63). Although initial observational studies suggested that vitamin K supplementation may help prevent osteoporotic fractures, recent assessments based on the findings of a limited number of small randomized trials can find no support for this hypothesis (64,65). Only large-scale clinical trials will be able to settle this issue with any degree of confidence.

Antioxidants

The theory that highly reactive free radicals, generated during normal oxidative metabolic processes, contribute to the tissue deterioration of aging is a highly popular one. The free radicals damage tissue through membrane lipid peroxidation, oxidation of proteins and carbohydrates, and abnormal DNA cross-linking. Considerable experimental evidence indicates that these events occur at the cellular level during normal metabolism. Therefore, to prevent or ameliorate the consequences of aging, many people consume increased quantities of antioxidants: vitamins E and C, β-carotene, selenium (a cofactor for glutathione peroxidase), and cofactors of the superoxide dismutase system, including copper, zinc, and manganese. However, repeated randomized, controlled trials have failed to confirm benefit of antioxidant supplements (or vitamin supplements in general) in preventing atherosclerosis and most cancers, or in improving bone-mineral density, cognitive function, or mood, and various expert panels have concluded that there is no convincing evidence to support recommendations for antioxidant or other vitamin supplementation in humans (66–94). In fact, there are now data supporting the fact that β-carotene, vitamin A, and vitamin E supplement users have increased, rather than decreased, risk of mortality (85,94–96). Nonetheless, there are some data that high intakes of antioxidants either as dietary constituents or as supplements may not prevent the onset of age-related macular degeneration (97) but may help delay its progression (98), although the largest randomized controlled trial in this area (AREDS) was unable to show that antioxidant supplements prevented visual acuity loss or cataract development in this condition, except in a subset of approximately 25% of the subjects (99). Unfortunately, there is no prospective way to identify those who will benefit. A long-term follow-up of the trial subjects after the trial ended revealed a reduction in the development of moderate vision loss (100), although the "relentless loss of vision" in individuals with this disease continued (101). However, precisely because age-related macular degeneration is a relentless condition leading to blindness, and since it is not possible to identify those who will benefit from treatment beforehand, it is now common clinical practice to prescribe the AREDS "cocktail" to essentially all individuals with this disease with the hope of preventing visual deterioration in a quarter of the patients. Proprietary products are available based on the original AREDS formulation and/or on modifications to the formulation made later. The principal components are 500 mg of vitamin C, 400 IU of vitamin E, 25 or 80 mg of zinc oxide, 2 mg of copper as cupric oxide, and either 15 mg β-carotene or 10 mg lutein plus 2 mg of zeaxanthin.

What is particularly important in evaluation of the role of various vitamins with respect to their roles in the consequences of aging is that observational trials often show inverse associations among nutrient status and clinical state. However, these associations cannot prove cause and effect. Moreover, observational associations do not address the critical issue of "the chicken or the egg." That is, individuals with the early stages of illness, cognitive decline, etc., may have subtle covariate consequences that impair access to foods or reduce desire or ability to consume adequate healthy diets. In other words, the slow relentless progression of aging and of its associated medical problems may contribute to nutrient inadequacy and not the other way round.

The levels of vitamin C in plasma and leukocyte levels decline with age, apparently as a function of intake, as absorption, metabolism, and excretion do not change consistently with age. Data on saturation of the vitamin C body pool (http://calerie.dcri.duke.edu/) have led to the recommendation of an EAR for vitamin C of 60 mg per day in women and 75 mg per day in men. Corresponding RDA are 75 mg per day in women and 90 mg per day in men (61,75).

As discussed, vitamin E intakes are repeatedly reported as low in dietary surveys. Vitamin E deficiency is not a clinical problem in the United States. The dietary survey results are the combined effect of inadequate accounting for all the vitamin E present in foods and some debate over whether the DRI recommendations for vitamin E are too high (102). The EAR for vitamin E in the elderly is 12 mg per day of α-tocopherol, and the RDA is set at 15 mg per day of α-tocopherol (61,75).

Selenium is an essential cofactor for the antioxidant enzyme glutathione peroxidase and dietary selenium requirements are based the intake levels that maximize plasma glutathione peroxidase levels (75). No evidence has been found that selenium requirements or biochemical markers of selenium status are affected by age (75). Selenium intake varies enormously among populations according to the selenium content of the soils. Although various surveys have reported low selenium intakes in elderly adults, NHANES III, which evaluated more than 6,000 persons over the age of 51, showed a mean selenium intake of 134 µg in men between the ages of 51 and 70, and 112 µg in men over the age of 70. Corresponding values for women were 94 µg and 83 µg. The fifth percentile intake levels in all groups were at or above the current RDA of 55 µg per day for men and women over the age of 50 years (75). There is also no reason to suspect selenium deficiency on the basis of dietary intake information, food composition data, or available metabolic indices. Selenium deficiency is a problem only in areas of the world where food is grown in soil with extremely low selenium content and in patients undergoing long-term parenteral nutrition with selenium-deficient solutions. As discussed above, there is no compelling reason to consume excess dietary selenium to improve cardiovascular function or prevent cancer. Because selenium is stored in the body, excessive consumption can result in toxicity, and an upper intake level (UL) of 400 µg has been established (75). Additionally, although selenium supplements have been advocated for the prevention of prostate cancer, there is no evidence that such supplementation prevents prostate cancer (84) and by far the largest randomized trial that tested the selenium and vitamin E supplements for the prevention of prostate cancer not only found that selenium, vitamin E, or both in combination were ineffective in preventing prostate cancer, it uncovered the fact that vitamin E supplementation increased the risk of developing prostate cancer (85).

Fiber

Dietary fibers are the nondigestible, nonabsorbable carbohydrates and lignin present in food plants, principally fruits, vegetables, legumes, and grains. Increasing the intake of dietary fiber is an important adjunct in the treatment of constipation in the elderly, although abdominal discomfort, flatulence, and potentially decreased absorption of iron and zinc may be the unwanted side effects of excess consumption. The mechanism by which dietary fiber improves gastrointestinal mobility is unknown, but presumably related to its bulking effects. A high intake of dietary fiber is also associated with a modest reduction in serum LDL cholesterol and may reduce circulating triglyceride concentrations and attenuate the blood glucose response to meals. Epidemiological studies have demonstrated that high fiber intakes are associated with a reduced risk of diabetes, coronary heart disease, and colon cancer, but data on the protective effects of dietary fiber intakes on the risks of developing breast, endometrial, ovarian and prostate cancers are not compelling (103). The protective effect of fiber intake on development of cancers of the gastrointestinal tract has been supported by recent meta-analyses (104–106). However, because fiber is an essential component of fruits, vegetables, and whole grains, the cancer-protective effects associated with fiber intake are difficult to attribute solely to fiber.

Nonetheless, improving the intake of foods high in dietary fiber is a healthful nutritional option for elderly adults because these foods contain important vitamins and minerals. The AI level of 14 g/1,000 kcal/day for dietary fiber in adults was set primarily on the intake level in epidemiological studies that were associated with a protective effect against coronary heart disease (103).

Folic Acid, Vitamin B_{12}, and Pyridoxine

Vitamin B_{12} levels are often low in elderly adults, although aging, per se, does not alter vitamin B_{12} absorption. However, B_{12} malabsorption is more frequent in elderly adults because of an increased prevalence of pernicious anemia and atrophic gastritis. The absorption of vitamin B_{12} is altered in atrophic gastritis not because of any abnormal intrinsic factor, but because dissociation of the vitamin from food proteins is limited by inadequate acid digestion. Additionally, because of bacterial overgrowth in the proximal small intestine secondary to atrophic gastritis, some vitamin B_{12} that reaches the small bowel is metabolized by bacteria rather than absorbed. Vitamin B_{12} is found only in animal products, and some elderly adults have low levels of B_{12} because of their decreased consumption of meat, fish, poultry and dairy products. Often, this is for economic reasons, although the prevalence of B_{12} deficiency is not increased in the low-income elderly. Elderly vegetarians are particularly at risk for vitamin B_{12} deficiency (107). The subject of vitamin B_{12} deficiency has recently been reviewed at length (108), and is covered in detail in Chapter 6.

The current RDA for vitamin B_{12} is 2.4 mg per day for elderly men and women (61,109), and nearly all elderly Americans consumed this level in NHANES III. However, because atrophic gastritis is present in about 10% to 30% of elderly adults (110), the vitamin B_{12} present in food may not be absorbed adequately in many elderly people. Thus, elderly individuals are advised to meet their vitamin B_{12} requirements by consumption of food products fortified with vitamin B_{12} or by taking a dietary supplement containing vitamin B_{12} (109–110). This is one of the very few circumstances in human nutrition in which supplements are recommended in preference to foods to satisfy nutrient requirements. Nonetheless, even though vitamin B_{12} inadequacy is known to impair cognition and other neurological functions, and to increase the circulating level of homocysteine, a known risk factor for cardiovascular disease and osteoporotic fractures, various randomized trial conducted over the last decade provide no support for the fact that lowering homocysteine levels with supplemental B_{12}, folic acid, pyridoxine, or multivitamin combinations that include these vitamins can improve cardiovascular risks, prevent fractures, or slow the progression of cognitive decline as cited in the related discussion earlier in this chapter (76,77,79, 80,82,83,86,87,90) and affirmed by a variety of additional trials (111–115).

Folate is widely distributed in foods, although the amounts and bioavailability of folate in various foods are the subject of some debate because of analytical issues. However, synthetic folic acid, the form found in supplements and fortified food products, is nearly twice as bioavailable (>85%) as naturally occurring food folate (~50%). National dietary survey data show that average folate intakes in elderly individuals are within the range of the EAR, but red blood cell folate levels, the best clinical index of folate status, show diminished folate status in a small fraction of elderly adults. The prevalence of low folate nutriture is higher in persons with low incomes, whose intake of foods high in folate is reduced. Although folate absorption is limited by the atrophic gastritis often found in elderly adults, a compensatory increase in folate production occurs in bacterial overgrowth in the proximal small bowel. Folate is required to convert homocysteine to methionine, and folate intakes below 400 μg per day are associated with elevated homocysteine levels, an independent risk factor for coronary artery and cerebrovascular disease as discussed above. Even though more recent trials fail to show a clinical benefit of reducing homocysteine levels alone, nearly a decade ago the RDAs for folate were revised upward to 400 μg of dietary folate equivalents in elderly men and women (60,96). Dietary folate equivalents take into account the fact that synthetic folic acid is more bioavailable than dietary food folates, particularly when taken without food. Thus, one dietary folate equivalent equals 1 μg of food folate, 0.6 μg of folic acid from fortified foods or from a folic acid supplement taken with food, or 0.5 μg of a folic acid supplement taken on an empty stomach (61,109). Because grain products are now fortified with folic acid and because many elderly adults consume other folic acid fortified products as well as take dietary supplements containing folic acid, there is concern that some elderly adults who take supplements are at greater risk for exceeding the tolerable UL of folate (1 mg per day) than they are at risk for folate inadequacy. This is particularly important, since many individuals are consuming dietary folate supplements to reduce plasma homocysteine levels, but a recent meta-analysis of randomized control trials could not show benefit on folic acids supplementation on the risk of cardiovascular disease or cognitive decline as discussed earlier.

Pyridoxine (vitamin B_6) intakes appear to vary widely, although incomplete vitamin B_6 food composition data limit our ability to quantify them with any precision. Although the data are very limited, vitamin B_6 needs appear to increase with age (109) and estimated average intakes for individuals over the age of 50 are 1.4 mg per day for men and 1.3 mg per day for women. The corresponding RDAs are 1.7 mg per day for men and 1.5 mg per day for women (61,109). Although various earlier nutrition surveys and biochemical assessments of vitamin B_6 status suggest that vitamin B_6 intake may be inadequate in a significant fraction of elderly men and women, the most recent national survey data show that median pyridoxine intakes in men exceed and median pyridoxine intake in women approximate the EAR and clinical evidence of vitamin B_6 deficiency is rare.

Thiamin, Riboflavin, and Niacin

Thiamin status, measured by the erythrocyte transketolase assay, has been highly variable and reported to be low in small to significant fractions of elderly adults. In NHANES III, only about 10% of elderly Americans consumed less than the RDA of thiamin. The most significant clinical cause of thiamin deficiency in aging adults is alcohol consumption coupled with decreased dietary intake. The current EAR for thiamin is 0.9 mg per day in women and 1.0 mg per day in men, with corresponding RDAs of 1.1 and 1.2 mg per day (61,109).

Riboflavin absorption and metabolism are unaffected by aging, and riboflavin status appears to be normal in most aging adults. In NHANES III, only about 10% of American men and women consumed less than the RDA for riboflavin set at 1.1 mg per day and 1.3 mg per day, respectively (61,109). The corresponding EAR for riboflavin is 0.9 mg per day in women and 1.0 mg per day in men (61,109). Milk and other dairy products (except butter) are the best and most convenient dietary sources of riboflavin for elderly adults.

Niacin requirements do not change with age. In NHANES III, only about 10% of elderly Americans consumed less than the RDA of niacin, which has been set at 14 mg per day for elderly women and 16 mg per day for elderly men (61,109). Corresponding EARs are 11 mg per day and 12 mg per day (61,109).

Vitamin A

Vitamin A requirement does not increase with age, and there is evidence that elderly individuals retain vitamin A in liver, and fat stores longer than in younger people. Vitamin A intakes also appear to increase with age. Thus, vitamin A status appears adequate in the majority of elderly men and women, although about one-third of Americans older than 70 questioned in NHANES III reported that they consume less than two-thirds of the current RDA for vitamin A. This apparent contradiction is explained by the fact that the RDA may be excessive for elderly adults, since vitamin A absorption appears to be increased and plasma clearance of vitamin A decreased in elderly persons. The EARs for vitamin A are 500 µg retinol activity equivalents (RAEs) daily for women and 625 µg RAE per day for men, with corresponding RDAs of 700 µg RAE and 900 µg RAE daily for women and men (61,63).

Except in special circumstances, vitamin A supplementation is to be avoided because it has known, serious toxicity. Further, although initial data from observational studies raised the hypothesis that excess vitamin A intake might increase the risk of osteoporotic fractures, a more recent interventional study in more than 2,000 individuals consuming high-dose retinol supplements for up to 16 years was unable to confirm this hypothesis (116).

Magnesium, Iron, Zinc, Iodine, and Other Minerals

Magnesium intake in about 50% of elderly adults is generally below two-thirds of the current RDA levels (49). Because magnesium occurs in many foods and in drinking water (albeit at highly variable concentrations), and because clinical magnesium deficiency is rare, the EAR (265 mg per day for women, 350 mg per day for men), and the RDA (320 mg per day for women; 420 mg per day for men) may be set at a very generous levels, particularly in light of the fact that the RDAs were based on the results of magnesium balance studies in a limited number of elderly men and the results of a single study in young adult women extrapolated to elderly women (49). Subsequent to determination of the RDA, additional pooled data from 27 controlled balance studies provided experimental support for the lowering of the DRI values for magnesium (117). In elderly persons, however, one must be aware that digoxin, diuretics, and impaired renal tubular function may enhance magnesium loss. Laxatives also can augment intestinal magnesium loss, but magnesium-containing laxatives and antacids are common sources of excessive magnesium intake in the elderly. Recently, there has been renewed interest in the clinical consequences of low magnesium status since a number of observational studies have shown an inverse association between magnesium status and cardiovascular disease risk (118–121). However, as we learned earlier, hypotheses generated from observational associations do not always define events on the causal pathway. For this reason, one must interpret cautiously the clinical significance of the reported association between low magnesium status and increased cardiovascular risk. Only a large-scale, randomized clinical trial will allow determination of whether magnesium contributes directly to cardiovascular risk.

Iron absorption does not diminish with age, and iron status understandably improves in women following the cessation of menses. Most anemia in the elderly is the result of iron deficiency, chronic inflammation or chronic renal disease in approximately equal amounts (122) but anemia due to a deficient dietary intake of iron is not the most prevalent cause of iron-deficiency anemia. Goodnough and Schrier (122) provide a detailed discussion of the systematic diagnostic workup and management of anemia in the elderly. When iron deficiency occurs in the elderly, one must first eliminate possible causes of chronic occult blood loss and the reduction of nonheme iron absorption associated with atrophic gastritis, which account for most cases of iron deficiency, before searching for other reasons related to inadequate dietary iron intake. NHANES show that iron intake averages about 13 to 14 mg per day in elderly men and about 9 to 10 mg per day in elderly women. The EAR for iron is 5 mg per day in postmenopausal women and 6 mg per day in men (61,63). The corresponding RDA values are 8 mg per day in both elderly men and women (61,63).

Zinc absorption declines with age, but endogenous zinc losses also decline, so zinc balance is preserved. Various dietary intake surveys show that many elderly adults generally consume less than two-thirds the current RDA levels for zinc, set at 11 mg per day for men and 8 mg per day for women (61,63). Nonetheless, normal plasma zinc levels are generally maintained, and only a very small percentage of elderly adults have plasma zinc levels in a deficient range. Little clinical evidence of zinc deficiency has been found in elderly adults, although some have questioned whether a lowered zinc status may contribute to the altered immune competence of the elderly, since zinc is important to maintaining immune function. Given this consideration, it appears prudent to aim for the current zinc RDA intake levels, although there is little cause for concern is zinc intakes are above the EAR levels of 6.8 mg per day for women and 9.4 mg per day for men (61,63).

Iodine has only a single essential function, which is thyroid hormonogenesis. Iodine levels in the United States have declined slightly during the last decade. However, since the introduction of iodized salt in 1924, the use of iodate dough oxidizers in bread making, and recent patterns of increased seafood consumption, there has been little evidence of clinical iodine deficiency. The EARs for iodine in elderly individuals are not different from those in young adults, 95 μd for both men and women (46,47). The current RDA for iodine is set at 150 μg per day for both sexes (61,63). One gram of iodized salt provides 76 μg of iodine.

The DRI values for other micronutrient minerals are the same in young and elderly adults. The RDA for copper is 900 μg per day and for molybdenum is 45 μg per day. (61,63). The AI level set for manganese is 2.3 mg per day in men and 1.8 mg per day in women (61,63).

Table 2-2 provides a summary of the RDAs for individuals above the age of 51 years.

Drugs

Elderly adults use almost 25% of the over-the-counter drugs sold in the United States, and the vast majority of elderly adults take at least one prescription drug daily. Many elderly adults take multiple medications daily. Some common drugs known to affect nutritional status are listed in Table 3-2. Conversely, nutrients affect drug absorption, as shown in Table 3-3. Thus, both

TABLE 2-2 Recommended Nutrient Intakes for Persons 51 Years of Age and Older

	Recommended Dietary Allowances	
	Men	Women
Energy (kcal)	2,300	1,900
Protein (g)	63	50
Vitamin A (µg RAE)[a]		700
Vitamin C (mg)	90	75
Vitamin E (mg)[c]	15	15
Vitamin K (µg)	120	90
Thiamin (mg)	1.2	1.1
Riboflavin (mg)	1.3	1.1
Niacin (mg)[d]	16	14
Vitamin B_6 (mg)	1.7	1.5
Folate (µg)	400	400
Vitamin B_{12} (µg)[e]	2.4	2.4
Iron (mg)	10	10
Zinc (mg)	15	12
Phosphorus (mg)	700	700
Magnesium (mg)	420	320
Selenium (µg)	55	55
Iodine (µg)	150	150
Calcium (mg) 51–70 yrs	1,000	1,200
Calcium (mg) >70 yrs	1,200	1,200
Vitamin D (ug)[b]	15	15
Vitamin D (µg)[b]	20	20

[a] Retinol activity equivalents: 1 RAE = 1 µg all-*trans* retinol or 6 µg β-carotene = 24 µg α-carotene and β-cryptoxanthin.
[b] As cholecalciferol: 1 µg cholecalciferol = 40 IU of vitamin D. Above the age of 70 years, the daily recommended intake for vitamin D increases to 15 µg/d.
[c] As α-tocopherol, including *RRR*-α-tocopherol, the natural food form, and the 2*R*-stereoisomeric forms that occur in fortified foods and supplements, but not the 2*S*-stereoisomers that are also found in fortified foods and supplements.
[d] As niacin equivalents: 1 NE = 1 mg niacin or 60 mg dietary tryptophan.
[e] Because elderly individuals may malabsorb food-bound vitamin B_{12}, it is advisable for the elderly to meet the requirement by consuming foods fortified with vitamin B_{12} or with a supplement containing vitamin B_{12}.
Data from References 48 and 61.

physicians and the elderly adults under their care are responsible for assessing potential nutrient–drug interactions. The physician must be alert to potentially detrimental nutritional effects of the prescribed therapeutic regimen. Likewise, the patient must pay close attention to the package insert and physician's instructions regarding the timing of drug ingestion relative to the consumption of food and drink. Tables 2-3 and 2-4, respectively, provide examples of the effects of vitamins and minerals on drug actions and of the effects of drugs on food intake.

PRACTICAL NUTRITIONAL ADVICE FOR ELDERLY ADULTS

The principal biologic factor underlying the altered nutrient needs of the elderly adult is the decline in energy expenditure secondary to a reduction of lean body mass. Because of this decline, less macronutrient intake is needed to satisfy energy needs; concomitantly, the intake of various vitamin and mineral constituents of the diet is diminished. Additional physical infirmities, dentures, neuropsychological disorders, social conditions, and economic constraints may aggravate further the inability to consume diets adequate in quantity or quality. In this context, then, elderly individuals should consume foods that are nutrient-dense, that is those that have a high ratio of nutrients to energy.

TABLE 2-3 Effects of Drugs on Nutrients

Drug	Effect
Anti-Infective Agents	
Amikacin, gentamicin, sisomicin, tobramycin	Hypokalemia, hypomagnesemia, and hypocalcemia; increased urinary potassium and magnesium loss
Aminosalicylic acid	Decreased vitamin B_{12} and fat absorption
Amphotericin B	Increased urinary excretion of potassium and decreased serum potassium and magnesium levels
Capreomycin	Hypokalemia, hypomagnesemia, and hypocalcemia
Cycloserine	Decreased serum folate
Isoniazid	Pyridoxine deficiency
Neomycin	Decreased absorption of carotene, iron, vitamin B_{12}, and cholesterol
Rifampin	Decreased serum 25-hydroxycholecalciferol level
Sulfasalazine	Folate deficiency
Tetracycline	Decreased absorption of Ca, Mg, Fe, Zn
Anticoagulants	
Warfarin	Decreased vitamin K–dependent coagulation factors
Cardiovascular Drugs	
Colestipol	Decreased absorption of fat-soluble vitamins and folic acid
Hydralazine	Pyridoxine deficiency
Sodium nitroprusside	Decreased total serum vitamin B_{12}
Thiazides, ethacrynic acid	Increased urinary loss of Na, K, Mg, Zn, P
Triamterene, spironolactone	Increased urinary loss of K, Ca, Mg, Zn
CNS Drugs	
Alcohol	Increased urinary loss of Mg, Zn, Ca
Aspirin	Decreased serum folate
Monoamine Oxidase Inhibitors	
Isocarboxazid	Decreased leukocyte and platelet ascorbic acid levels
Pargyline	Increased iron loss
Phenelzine	Increased sensitivity to tyramine-containing foods; possible development of hypertensive crisis
Tranylcypromine	Pyridoxine deficiency
Phenobarbital	Decreased serum vitamin K_1
Phenytoin	Decreased serum folate, calcium, 25-hydroxycholecalciferol levels
Electrolyte Drugs	
Potassium chloride, slow release	Decreased vitamin B_{12} absorption
Gastrointestinal Drugs	
Aluminum hydroxide	Decreased absorption of iron, phosphate, vitamin B_{12}
Cholestyramine	Decreased absorption of vitamins A, D, E, K, and B_{12} and folate along with decreased absorption of inorganic phosphate and fat
H_2-receptor antagonists, proton pump inhibitors	Decreased absorption of protein-bound vitamin B_{12}
Laxatives	Increased fecal loss of Na, K, Ca, Mg
Mineral oil	Decreased absorption of vitamins A, D, E, and K
Hormones	
Glucocorticoids	Increased urinary loss of K, Ca; increased Na absorption
Oral contraceptives	Decreased serum folate, pyridoxine deficiency, riboflavin deficiency
Other Agents	
Colchicine	Decreased absorption of vitamin B_{12}, sodium, potassium, fat, nitrogen
Penicillamine	Pyridoxine deficiency

From Weinsier RL, Morgan SL. *Fundamentals of Clinical Nutrition*. St. Louis: Mosby, 1993:186, with permission.

TABLE 2-4   Effects of Nutrients on Drugs

Food can change the absorption characteristics of certain drugs. The mechanisms for the effect include physicochemical interactions with food in the intestinal lumen, changes in gastric emptying, competition between drug and food components for absorption, and altered first-pass hepatic kinetics. These effects can decrease the efficacy of the drug or increase the absorption of the drug, so a greater response to the drug or a side effect results. There can be large differences from one formulation to another, and no drug class effects can be assumed. The reader should check carefully with the literature and the manufacturer's information concerning individual formulations, especially when the therapeutic window is narrow. Listed below are some of the drugs commonly used that can be affected by food and instructions on how to minimize the effects of food on the drug.

Decreased Absorption (Avoid taking these drugs with food. Take at least 1 hour before or 2 hours after a meal.)

Ampicillin	Erythromycin stearate	Levodopa/carbidopa	Quinidine
Atenolol	Ferrous salts	Lisinopril	Sotalol
Calcium carbonate	Folic acid	Methotrexate	Sulfamethoxazole
Captopril	Furosemide	Omeprazole	Tetracycline
Cephalexin	Iron	Penicillin G	Trimethoprim
Cloxacillin	Isoniazid	Penicillin V	Zinc sulfate
Digitalis	Isosorbide	Phenytoin	
Disopyramide	Lansoprazole	Propantheline	

Increased Absorption (Food will alter the amount of the drug absorbed; therefore, the drug should be taken at the same time(s) each day relative to meals.)

Buspirone	Gemfibrozil	Methoxsalen	Propranolol
Carbamazepine	Griseofulvin	Metoprolol	Spironolactone
Chlorothizide	Labetalol	Nifedipine	Sulfadiazine
Diazepam	Lithium	Nitrofurantoin	Trazodone
Dicumarol	Lovastatin	Phenytoin	

Delayed Absorption (Food will delay the absorption of these drugs but not the overall amount absorbed. These drugs should be taken at least 1 hour before or 2 hours after a meal.)

Acetaminophen	Hydrochlorothiazide	Pentobarbital	Suprofen
Aspirin	Hydrocortisone	Pentoxifylline	Tocainide
Cimetidine	Indomethacin	Sulfisoxazole	
Doxycycline	Ketoprofen		

Data from Weinsier RL, Morgan SL. *Fundamentals of Clinical Nutrition*. St. Louis: Mosby, 1993:188, and Utermohlen V. In: Shils ME, Olson JA, Shike M, et al, eds, *Modern Nutrition in Health and Disease*, 9th ed. Baltimore: Williams & Wilkins, 1998:1621.

Although it is clear that significant biologic, physical, and psychosocial differences exist between very old (> 85 years of age) and moderately old (between 70 and 85 years of age) persons, there are no generally agreed upon specific dietary standards for the very old, who often have special needs because of physical disabilities or mental infirmity. However, if elderly adults remain physically and mentally capable of following the dietary guidelines outlined for young adults earlier in this manual, with the relatively minor adjustments discussed below it is unlikely that they will become malnourished. Finally, regular physical exercise and a balanced diet do more to promote and preserve health in elderly adults than all other health supplements, "nutritional" or otherwise. The desire and ability of elderly adults to prepare and consume a wide variety of foods are often enhanced by simple companionship during grocery shopping and meals.

Resting energy expenditure declines as a function of age and lean body mass after age 50. Regular exercise, particularly resistance exercise, can help preserve strength and lean mass. Reduced physical activity further contributes to the loss of lean mass and decline in energy expenditure seen in the elderly. Based on available energy expenditure data, the DRI committee developed equations for daily EER. These are as follows:

Men:

$$EER = 662 - (9.53 \times age\,[y]) + PA \times [(15.91 \times wt[kg]) + (539.6 \times ht\,[m])]$$

Women:

$$EER = 354 - (6.91 \times age\,[y]) + PA \times [(9.36 \times wt[kg]) + (726 \times ht\,[m])]$$

TABLE 2-5 Selected Sources of Reliable Information for Elderly Adults

Administration for Community Living
1 Massachusetts Ave. NW
Washington, DC 20201
Tel. 202-619-0724
www.acl.gov

Alzheimer's Association
225 North Michigan Ave.
Floor 17
Chicago, IL 60601-7633
Tel. 800-272-3900
www.alz.org

AARP
601 E St., NW
Washington, DC 20049
Tel. 888-687-2277
www.aarp.org

American Cancer Society
250 Williams Street, NW
Atlanta, GA 30303
Tel. 800-227-2345
www.cancer.org

American Diabetes Association
1701 North Beauregard St.
Alexandria, VA 22311
Tel. 800-342-2383
www.diabetes.org

American Federation for Aging Research
55 West 39th St., 16th Floor
New York, NY 10018
Tel. 888-582-2327
www.afar.org

American Geriatrics Society
40 Fulton Street
18th Floor
New York, NY 10038
Tel. 212-308-1414
www.americangeriatrics.org

American Heart Association
National Center
7272 Greenville Ave.
Dallas, TX 75231
Tel. 800-242-8721
www.americanheart.org

American Society for Nutrition
9650 Rockville Pike
Bethesda, MD 20814
Tel. 301-634-7050
www.nutrition.org

Department of Agriculture
1400 Independence Ave., SW
Washington, DC 20250
202-720-2791
www.usda.gov

Division of Geriatrics & Clinical Gerontology
National Institute on Aging
31 Center Drive, MSC 2292
Bethesda, MD 20892
Tel. 301-496-6761
www.nia.nih.gov/research/dgcg

National Council on Aging
1901 L. Street, NW
4th Floor
Washington, DC 20036
Tel. 202-479-1200
www.ncoa.org

National Institute on Aging
National Institutes of Health
31 Center Drive, MSC 2292
Bethesda, MD 20892
Tel. 800-222-2225
www.nih.gov/nia

Jean Mayer USDA Human Nutrition
Research Center on Aging at Tufts University
711 Washington St.
Boston, MA 02111
Tel. 617-556-3000
hnrca.tufts.edu

where PA is the subject's physical activity quotient. The values for PA range from 1.0 for the activities of usual daily living to 1.11 to 1.12 for women and men, respectively, for the activities of daily life plus an additional 30 to 60 minutes of moderate activity daily; to 1.25 to 1.27 for at least an additional 60 minutes of moderate daily activity; to 1.45 to 1.48 for the activities of daily life plus an additional 180 minutes of moderate activity or at least an additional 60 minutes of moderate daily activity plus an additional 60 minutes of vigorous activity (61,103). Needless to say, unless there is otherwise clear evidence for a very active lifestyle, it is most prudent to initially estimate the PA quotient in elderly subjects as 1.00 or 1.11 to 1.12. These equations were tested in individuals above the age of 70 and proved to be accurate, although the DRI equations tended to underestimate energy expended in physical activity (123).

However, as with all calorie intake recommendations at any age, the value initially estimated for an individual person must be tailored to the value that maintains body weight within a desirable range. Above the age of 80, and for persons who are physically inactive, either as a result of advanced age or physical incapacity, dietary energy intakes must be reduced correspondingly.

Although there is no systematic evidence that dietary protein needs are increased in elderly adults, dietary protein intake is closely linked to dietary energy intake. Therefore, elderly adults with low energy intakes are also at risk for inadequate protein intakes and medical caregivers should be alert to this possibility.

While there is no consensus that dietary nutrient intakes need to be drastically altered in otherwise healthy elderly adults, based on the risks discussed above, nutritionists commonly recommend that elderly adults consider taking a multivitamin/mineral supplement that contains vitamin B_{12} (12 to 25 µg), vitamin D (400 IU), and up to 100% of the RDAs for the other essential nutrients. Because over-the-counter multivitamin/mineral preparations do not generally contain sufficient calcium to meet the requirements for calcium or enough vitamin D to provide this vitamin at the intake levels recommended by some, nutritionists also often recommend an additional supplement containing 400 to 800 mg of calcium and 200 to 400 U of vitamin D.

RESOURCES

Because of the ever-growing elderly population, a wide variety of public and private societal resources have become available. A selected small number of these are listed in Table 2-5.

REFERENCES

1. U.S. Department of Commerce, US Census Bureau. American Fact Finder. http://factfinder2.census.gov/faces/nav/jsf/pages/community_facts.xhtml
2. Meyer J. Centenarians: 2010. 2010 Census Special Reports. US Department of Commerce, Economics and Statistics Administration, US Census Bureau. December 2012.
3. US Census Bureau Statistical Brief. Sixty-Five Plus in the United States. https://www.census.gov/population/socdemo/statbriefs/agebrief.html
4. Hoyert DL, Xu J. Deaths: preliminary data for 2011. *NVSS*. 2012;61(6).
5. Harper S, MacLehose RF, Kaufman JS. Trends in the black-white life expectancy gap among US states, 1990–2009. *Health Aff*. 2014;33(8):1375–1382.
6. Centers for Disease Control and Prevention. Public health and aging: trends in aging—United States and worldwide. *Morb Mortal Wkly Rep (MMWR)*. 2003;52:101–106.
7. Centers for Disease Control and Prevention. Dietary intake of ten key nutrients for public health, United States: 1999–2000. *Adv Data*. 2003;348:1–6.
8. Ervin RB, Wright JD, Wang CY, et al; Centers for Disease Control and Prevention. Dietary intake of fats and fatty acids for the United States population: 1999–2000. *Adv Data*. 2004;348:1–6.
9. Murphy SP, Yaktine AL, Suitor CW, et al, eds; Committee to Review Child and Adult Care Food Program Meal Requirements, Food and Nutrition Board, Institute of Medicine. *Child and Adult Care Food Program—Aligning Dietary Guidance for All*. Washington, DC: The National Academies Press, 2011.
10. Ervin RB, Wang CY, Wright JD, et al; Centers for Disease Control and Prevention. Dietary intake of selected minerals for the United States population: 1999–2000. *Adv Data*. 2004;341:1–5.
11. Ervin RB, Wright JD, Wang CY, et al; Centers for Disease Control and Prevention. Dietary intake of selected vitamins for the United States population: 1999–2000. *Adv Data*. 2004;339:1–4.
12. Graudal NA, et al. Effects of low sodium diet vs. high-sodium diet on blood pressure, renin, aldosterone, catecholamines, cholesterol, and triglyceride (Cochrane Review). *Am J Hypertens*. 2012;25:1–15.

13. Institute of Medicine. *Sodium Intake in Populations: Assessment of Evidence*. Washington, DC: National Academies Press, 2013. http://www.iom.edu/Reports/2013/Sodium-Intake-in-Populations-Assessment-of-Evidence.aspx
14. Strom BL, Anderson CA, Ix JH. Sodium reduction in populations: insights from the institute of medicine committee. *JAMA*. 2013;310:31–32.
15. Mente A, O'Donnell MJ, Rangarajan S, et al. Association of urinary sodium and potassium excretion with blood pressure. *N Engl J Med*. 2014;371:601–611.
16. O'Donnell MJ, Mente A, Rangarajan S, et al. Urinary sodium and potassium excretion, mortality, and cardiovascular events. *N Engl J Med*. 2014;371:612–623.
17. Mozaffarian D, Fahimi S, Singh GM, et al. Global sodium consumption and death from cardiovascular causes. *N Engl J Med*. 2014;371:624–634.
18. Oparil S. Low sodium intake—cardiovascular health benefit or risk. *N Engl J Med*. 2014;371:677–679.
19. Cefalu CA. Theories and mechanisms of aging. *Clin Geriatr Med*. 2011;27:491–506.
20. Park DC, Yeo SG. Aging. *Korean J Audiol*. 2013;17:39–44.
21. Xi H, Li C, Ren F, et al. Telomere, aging and age-related diseases. *Aging Clin Exp Res*. 2013;25:139–146.
22. Falandry C, Bonnefoy M, Freyer G, et al. Biology of cancer and aging: a complex association with cellular senescence [Epub ahead of print]. *J Clin Oncol*. 2014;32.
23. Ljubuncic P, Reznick AZ. The evolutionary theories of aging revisited—a mini-review. *Gerontology*. 2009;55:205–216.
24. Greaves LC, Turnbull DM. Mitochondrial DNA mutations and ageing. *Biochim Biophys Acta*. 2009;1790:1015–1020.
25. Brewer GJ. Epigenetic oxidative redox shift (EORS) theory of aging unifies the free radical and insulin signaling theories. *Exp Gerontol*. 2010;45:173–179.
26. Pizza V, Agresta A, D'Acunto CW, et al. Neuroinflammation and ageing: current theories and an overview of the data. *Rev Recent Clin Trials*. 2011;6:189–203.
27. Boyd-Kirkup JD, Green CD, Wu G, et al. Epigenomics and the regulation of aging. *Epigenomics*. 2013;5:205–227.
28. Liochev SI. Reflections on the theories of aging, of oxidative stress and of science in general. Is it time to abandon the free radical (oxidative stress) theory of aging? [Epub ahead of print]. *Antioxid Redox Signal*. 2014.
29. Weinert BT, Timiras PS. Physiology of aging. *J Appl Physiol*. 2003;95:1706–1716.
30. Heilbronn LK, Ravussin E. Calorie restriction and aging: review of the literature and implications for studies in humans. *Am J Clin Nutr*. 2003;78:361–369.
31. Worman HJ, Bonne G. "Laminopathies": a wide spectrum of human diseases. *Exp Cell Res*. 2007;313:2121–2133.
32. Ghosh S, Zhou Z. Genetics of aging, progeria and lamin disorders. *Curr Opin Genet Dev*. 2014;26:41–46.
33. Gordon LB, Rothman FG, López-Otin C, et al. Progeria: a paradigm for translational medicine. *Cell*. 2014;156:400–407.
34. Nair KS. Aging muscle. *Am J Clin Nutr*. 2005;81:953–963.
35. Winter JE, MacInnis RJ, Wattanapenpaiboon N, et al. BMI and all-cause mortality in older adults: a meta-analysis. *Am J Clin Nutr*. 2014;99:875–890.
36. Sorkin JD. BMI, age, and mortality: the slaying of a beautiful hypothesis by an ugly fact. *Am J Clin Nutr*. 2014;99:759–760.
37. Volpi E, Campbell WW, Dwyer JT, et al. Is the optimal level of protein intake for older adults greater than the recommended dietary allowance? *J Gerontol A Biol Sci Med Sci*. 2013;68:677–681.
38. Bauer J, Biolo G, Cederholm T, et al. Evidence-based recommendations for optimal dietary protein intake in older people: a position paper from the PROT-AGE Study Group. *J Am Med Dir Assoc*. 2013;14:542–559.
39. Wolfe RR. Perspective: optimal protein intake in the elderly. *J Am Med Dir Assoc*. 2013;14:65–66.
40. Ferrando AA, Paddon-Jones D, Hays NP, et al. EAA supplementation to increase nitrogen intake improves muscle function during bed rest in the elderly. *Clin Nutr*. 2010;29:18–23.
41. Wellman NS, Weddle DO, Kranz S, et al. Elder insecurities: poverty, hunger, and malnutrition. *J Am Diet Assoc*. 1997;97:S120–S122.
42. Rose D. Economic determinants and dietary consequences of food insecurity in the United States. *J Nutr*. 1999;129:517S–520S.
43. Berkowitz SA, Seligman HK, Choudhry NK. Treat or eat: food insecurity, cost-related medication underuse, and unmet needs. *Am J Med*. 2014;127:303–310.

44. Minaker LM, Raine KD, Wild TC, et al. Objective food environments and health outcomes. *Am J Prev Med.* 2013;45:289–296.
45. Siris ES, Brenneman SK, Barrett-Connor E, et al. The effect of age and bone mineral density on the absolute, excess, and relative risk of fracture in postmenopausal women aged 50–99: results from the National Osteoporosis Risk Assessment (NORA). *Osteoporos Int.* 2006;17:565–574.
46. Khosla S, Melton LJ. Osteopenia. *N Engl J Med.* 2007;356:2293–2300.
47. Heaney RP. Bone health. *Am J Clin Nutr.* 2007;85:300S–303S.
48. Ross CA, Taylor CL, Yaktine AL, et al, eds. Committee to Review Dietary Reference Intakes for Vitamin D and Calcium, Food and Nutrition Board, Institute of Medicine. *Dietary Reference Intakes for Calcium and Vitamin D.* Washington, DC: The National Academies Press, 2011.
49. Food and Nutrition Board, Institute of Medicine, National Academy of Sciences. *Dietary Reference Intakes for Calcium, Phosphorus, Magnesium, Vitamin D, and Fluoride.* Washington, DC: National Academies Press, 1997.
50. NIH Consensus Development Panel on Osteoporosis Prevention, Diagnosis, and Therapy. Osteoporosis Prevention, Diagnosis, and Therapy. *JAMA.* 2001;285:785–795.
51. Holick MF, Binkley NC, Bischoff-Ferrari HA, et al. Evaluation, treatment, and prevention of vitamin D deficiency: an endocrine society clinical practice guideline. *J Clin Endocrinol Metab.* 2011;96:1911–1930.
52. Bischoff-Ferrari HA, Willett WC, Orav EJ, et al. A pooled analysis of vitamin D dose requirements for fracture prevention. *N Engl J Med.* 2012;367:40–49.
53. Moyer VA; on behalf of the US Preventive Services Task Force. Vitamin D and calcium supplementation to prevent fractures in adults: US Preventive Services Task Force Recommendation Statement. *Ann Intern Med.* 2013;158:691–696.
54. Theodoratou E, Tzoulaki I, Zgaga L, et al. Vitamin D and multiple health outcomes: umbrella review of systematic reviews and meta-analyses of observational studies and randomised trials. *BMJ.* 2014;348:g2035.
55. Schöttker B, Jorde R, Peasey A, et al. Vitamin D and mortality: meta-analysis of individual participant data from a large consortium of cohort studies from Europe and the United States. *BMJ.* 2014;348:g3656.
56. Chowdhury R, Kunutsor S, Vitezova A, et al. Vitamin D and risk of cause specific death: systematic review and meta-analysis of observational cohort and randomised intervention studies. *BMJ.* 2014;348:g1903.
57. Bjelakovic G, Gluud LL, Nikolova D, et al. Vitamin D supplementation for prevention of mortality in adults. *Cochrane Database Syst Rev.* 2014;10:CD007470.
58. Kim Y, Je Y. Vitamin D intake, blood 25(OH)D levels, and breast cancer risk or mortality: a meta-analysis. *Br J Cancer.* 2014;110:2772–2784.
59. Yin L, Ordóñez-Mena JM, Chen T, et al. Circulating 25-hydroxyvitamin D serum concentration and total cancer incidence and mortality: a systematic review and meta-analysis. *Prev Med.* 2013;57:763–64.
60. Liu SL, Zhao YP, Dai MH, et al. Vitamin D status and the risk of pancreatic cancer: a meta-analysis. *Chin Med J (Engl).* 2013;126:3356–3359.
61. Institute of Medicine, National Academy of Sciences. *Dietary Reference Intakes: The Essential Guide to Nutrient Requirements.* Washington, DC: National Academy Press, 2006.
62. Berkner KL. The vitamin K-dependent carboxylase. *Annu Rev Nutr.* 2005;25:127–149.
63. Food and Nutrition Board, Institute of Medicine, National Academy of Sciences. *Dietary Reference Intakes for Energy for Vitamin A, Vitamin K, Arsenic, Boron, Chromium, Copper, Iodine, Iron, Manganese, Molybdenum, Nickel, Silicon, Vanadium and Zinc.* Washington, DC: National Academy Press, 2011.
64. Gundberg CM, Lian JB, Booth SL. Vitamin K-dependent carboxylation of osteocalcin: friend or foe? *Adv Nutr.* 2012;3:149–157.
65. Hamidi MS, Gajic-Veljanoski O, Cheung AM. Vitamin K and bone health. *J Clin Densitom.* 2013;16:409–413.
66. Verhagen H, Buijsse B, Jansen E, et al. The state of antioxidant affairs. *Nutr Today.* 2006;41:244–250.
67. Bleys J, Miller ER, Pastor-Barriuso R, et al. Vitamin-mineral supplementation and the progression of atherosclerosis: a meta-analysis of randomized controlled trials. *Am J Clin Nutr.* 2006;84:880–887.
68. Wright ME, Virtamo J, Hartman AM, et al. Effects of α-tocopherol and β-carotene supplementation on upper aerodigestive tract cancers in a large, randomized controlled trial. *Cancer.* 2007;109:891–898.
69. Bjelakovic G, Nagorni A, Nikolova D, et al. Meta-analysis: antioxidant supplements for primary and secondary prevention of colorectal adenoma. *Aliment Pharmacol Ther.* 2006;24:281–291.

70. Reid ME, Duffield-Lillico AJ, Sunga A, et al. Selenium supplementation and colorectal adenomas: an analysis of the nutritional prevention of cancer trial. *Int J Cancer*. 2006;118:1777–1781.
71. Taylor PR, Greenwald P. Nutritional interventions in cancer prevention. *J Clin Oncol*. 2005;23:333–345.
72. Reid IR, Bolland MJ, Grey A. Effects of vitamin D supplements on bone mineral density: a systematic review and meta-analysis. *Lancet*. 2014;383:146–155.
73. Kang JH, Cook N, Manson J, et al. A randomized trial of vitamin E supplementation and cognitive function in women. *Arch Intern Med*. 2006;166:2462–2468.
74. Rayman M, Thompson A, Warren-Perry M, et al. Impact of selenium on mood and quality of life: a randomized, controlled trial. *Biol Psychiatry*. 2006;59:147–154.
75. Food and Nutrition Board, Institute of Medicine, National Academy of Sciences. *Dietary Reference Intakes for Vitamin C, Vitamin E, Selenium, and Carotenoids*. Washington, DC: National Academy Press, 2000.
76. Fortmann SP, Burda BU, Senger CA, et al. Vitamin and mineral supplements in the primary prevention of cardiovascular disease and cancer: an updated systematic evidence review for the US preventive services task force. *Ann Intern Med*. 2013;159:824–834.
77. Grodstein F, O'Brien J, Kang JH, et al. Long-term multivitamin supplementation and cognitive function in men: a randomized trial. *Ann Intern Med*. 2013;159:806–814.
78. Pais R, Dumitraşcu DL. Do antioxidants prevent colorectal cancer? A meta-analysis. *Rom J Intern Med*. 2013;51:152–163.
79. Vollset SE, Clarke R, Lewington S, et al. Effects of folic acid supplementation on overall and site-specific cancer incidence during the randomised trials: meta-analyses of data on 50,000 individuals. *Lancet*. 2013;381:1029–1036.
80. Lamas GA, Boineau R, Goertz C, et al. Oral high-dose multivitamins and minerals after myocardial infarction: a randomized trial. *Ann Intern Med*. 2013;159:797–805.
81. Qin X, Cui Y, Shen L, et al. Folic acid supplementation and cancer risk: a meta-analysis of randomized controlled trials. *Int J Cancer*. 2013;133:1033–1041.
82. Hankey GJ, Ford AH, Yi Q, et al. Effect of B vitamins and lowering homocysteine on cognitive impairment in patients with previous stroke or transient ischemic attack: a prespecified secondary analysis of a randomized, placebo-controlled trial and meta-analysis. *Stroke*. 2013;44:2232–2239.
83. Zhang C, Chi FL, Xie TH, et al. Effect of B-vitamin supplementation on stroke: a meta-analysis of randomized controlled trials. *PLoS One*. 2013;8:E81577.
84. Kristal AR, Arnold KB, Neuhouser ML, et al. Diet, supplement use, and prostate cancer risk: results from the prostate cancer prevention trial. *Am J Epidemiol*. 2010;172:566–577.
85. Klein EA, Thompson IM Jr, Tangen CM, et al. Vitamin E and the risk of prostate cancer: the Selenium and Vitamin E Cancer Prevention Trial (SELECT). *JAMA*. 2011;306:1549–1556.
86. Marti-Carvajal AJ, Solà I, Lathyris D, et al. Homocysteine-lowering interventions for preventing cardiovascular events. *Cochrane Database Syst Rev*. 2013;1:CD006612.
87. Myung SK, Ju W, Cho B, et al. Efficacy of vitamin and antioxidant supplements in prevention of cardiovascular disease: systematic review and meta-analysis of randomised controlled trials. *BMJ*. 2013;346:f10.
88. Ye Y, Li J, Yuan Z. Effect of antioxidant vitamin supplementation on cardiovascular outcomes: a meta-analysis of randomized controlled trials. *PLoS One*. 2013;8:e56803.
89. Jeon Y, Myung S, Lee EH, et al. Effects of beta-carotene supplements on cancer prevention: meta-analysis of randomized controlled trials. *Nutr Cancer*. 2011;63:1196–1207.
90. Ford AH, Almeida OP. Effect of homocysteine lowering treatment on cognitive function: a systematic review and meta-analysis of randomized controlled trials. *J Alzheimers Dis*. 2012;29:133–149.
91. MacPherson H, Pipingas A, Pase MP. Multivitamin-multimineral supplementation and mortality: a meta-analysis of randomized controlled trials. *Am J Clin Nutr*. 2013;97:437–444.
92. Bjelakovic G, Nikolova D, Gluud LL, et al. Antioxidant supplements for prevention of mortality in healthy participants and patients with various diseases. *Cochrane Database Syst Rev*. 2012;3:CD007176.
93. Park S-Y, Murphy SP, Wilkens LR, et al. Multivitamin use and the risk of mortality and cancer incidence—the multiethnic cohort study. *Am J Epidemiol*. 2011;173:906–914.
94. Guallar E, Stranges S, Mulrow C, et al. Enough is enough. *Ann Intern Med*. 2014;160:809–810.
95. Bjelakovic G, Nikolova D, Gluud C. Meta-regression analyses, meta-analyses, and trial sequential analyses of the effects of supplementation with beta-carotene, vitamin A, and vitamin E singly or in different combinations on all-cause mortality: do we have evidence for lack of harm? *PLoS One*. 2013;8:e74558.
96. Bjelakovic G, Nikolova D, Gluud LL, et al. Mortality in randomized trials of antioxidant supplements for primary and secondary prevention: systematic review and meta-analysis. *JAMA*. 2007;297:842–857.

97. Evans JR, Lawrenson JG. Antioxidant vitamin and mineral supplements for preventing age-related macular degeneration. *Cochrane Database Syst Rev.* 2012;6:CD000253.
98. Evans JR, Lawrenson JG. Antioxidant vitamin and mineral supplements for slowing the progression of age-related macular degeneration. *Cochrane Database Syst Rev.* 2012;11:CD000254.
99. Age-Related Eye Disease Study Research Group. A randomized, placebo-controlled, clinical trial of high-dose supplementation with vitamins C and E and beta carotene for age-related cataract and vision Loss: AREDS report no. 9. *Arch Ophthalmol.* 2001;119:1439–1452. Erratum in *Arch Ophthalmol.* 2008;126:1251.
100. Chew EY, Clemons TE, Agrón E, et al. Long-term effects of vitamins C and E, β-carotene, and zinc on age-related macular degeneration: AREDS report no. 35. *Ophthalmology.* 2013;120:1604–1611.
101. Chew EY, Clemons TE, Agrón E, et al. Ten-year follow-up of age-related macular degeneration in the age-related eye disease study: AREDS report no. 36. *JAMA Ophthalmol.* 2014;132:272–277.
102. Horwitt MK. Critique of the requirement for vitamin E. *Am J Clin Nutr.* 2001;73:1003–1005.
103. Food and Nutrition Board, National Institute of Medicine, National Academy of Sciences. *Dietary Reference Intakes for Energy, Carbohydrate, Fiber, Fat, Fatty Acids, Cholesterol, Protein, and Amino Acids.* Washington, DC: National Academy Press, 2005.
104. Ben Q, Sun Y, Chai R, et al. Dietary fiber intake reduces risk for colorectal adenoma: a meta-analysis. *Gastroenterology.* 2014;146:689–699.
105. Zhang Z, Xu G, Ma M, et al. Dietary fiber intake reduces risk for gastric cancer: a meta-analysis. *Gastroenterology.* 2013;145:113–120.
106. Coleman HG, Murray LJ, Hicks B, et al. Dietary fiber and the risk of precancerous lesions and cancer of the esophagus: a systematic review and meta-analysis. *Nutr Rev.* 2013;71:474–482.
107. Pawlak R, Parrott SJ, Raj S, et al. How prevalent is vitamin B(12) deficiency among vegetarians? *Nutr Rev.* 2013;71:110–117.
108. Stabler SP. Vitamin B_{12} deficiency. *N Engl J Med.* 2013;368:149–160.
109. Institute of Medicine, National Academy of Sciences. Folate. *Dietary Reference Intakes for Thiamine, Riboflavin, Niacin, Vitamin B_6, Folate Vitamin B_{12}, Pantothenic Acid, Biotin and Choline.* Washington, DC: National Academy Press, 2006.
110. Bailey LB. Folate and vitamin B_{12} recommended intakes and status in the United States. *Nutr Rev.* 2004;62:S14–S20.
111. Green TJ, McMahon JA, Skeaff CM, et al. Lowering homocysteine with B vitamins has no effect on biomarkers of bone turnover in older persons: a 2-y randomized controlled trial. *Am J Clin Nutr.* 2007;85:460–464.
112. McMahon JA, Green TJ, Skeaff CM, et al. A controlled trial of homocysteine lowering and cognitive performance. *N Engl J Med.* 2006;354:2764–2772.
113. Kang JH, Irizarry MC, Grodstein F. Prospective study of plasma folate, vitamin B_{12}, and cognitive function and decline. *Epidemiology.* 2006;17:650–657.
114. Bazzano LA, Reynolds K, Holder KN, et al. Effect of folic acid supplementation on risk of cardiovascular diseases: a meta-analysis of randomized controlled trials. *JAMA.* 2006;296:2720–2726.
115. Durga J, van Boxtel MPJ, Schouten EG, et al. Effect of 3-year folic acid supplementation on cognitive function in older adults in the FACIT trial: a randomised, double blind, controlled trial. *Lancet.* 2007;369:208–216.
116. Ambrosini GL, Bremner AP, Reid A, et al. No dose-dependent increase in fracture risk after long-term exposure to high doses of retinol or beta-carotene. *Osteoporos Int.* 2013;24:1285–1293.
117. Hunt CD, Johnson LK. Magnesium requirements: new estimations for men and women by cross-sectional statistical analyses of metabolic magnesium balance data. *Am J Clin Nutr.* 2006;84:843–852.
118. Guasch-Ferré M, Bulló M, Estruch R, et al. Dietary magnesium intake is inversely associated with mortality in adults at high cardiovascular disease risk. *J Nutr.* 2014;144:55–60.
119. Peters KE, Chubb SA, Davis WA, et al. The relationship between hypomagnesemia, metformin therapy and cardiovascular disease complicating type 2 diabetes: the Fremantle Diabetes Study. *PLoS One.* 2013;8:e74355.
120. Sakaguchi Y, Fujii N, Shoji T, et al. Hypomagnesemia is a significant predictor of cardiovascular and non-cardiovascular mortality in patients undergoing hemodialysis. *Kidney Int.* 2014;85:174–181.
121. Deng X, Song Y, Manson JE, et al. Magnesium, vitamin D status and mortality: results from US National Health and Nutrition Examination Survey (NHANES) 2001 to 2006 and NHANES III. *BMC Med.* 2013;11:187.
122. Goodnough LT, Schrier SL. Evaluation and management of anemia in the elderly. *Am J Hematol.* 2014;89:88–96.
123. Blanc S, Schoeller DA, Bauer D, et al. Energy requirements in the eighth decade of life. *Am J Clin Nutr.* 2004;79:303–310.

Pregnancy and Lactation

NUTRITION DURING PREGNANCY

Studies in humans and animals indicate that nutrition during pregnancy influences not only the normal development of the fetus and immediate health of the newborn infant, but there are now also compelling data that maternal nutrition prior to becoming pregnant and during pregnancy influence the subsequent morbidity and mortality of the offspring when they are grown adults (1–10). We have long appreciated that low maternal weight before pregnancy, inadequate weight gain during pregnancy, and inadequate intakes of protein and calories by the expectant mother are all associated with the delivery of low-birth-weight infants. Similarly, we have known for some time that low birth weight, in turn, is associated with increased perinatal mortality, impaired neurologic development, and a retarded postnatal growth pattern. More recently, however, compelling evidence has continued to accrue that infants born small, as a consequence of nutritional or other negative influences on fetal growth, are at increased risk for the development of hypertension, coronary artery disease, diabetes, and possibly other conditions during adult life (1–10). Current recommendations for nutrition in women of childbearing age stress the importance of nutritional adequacy and optimal body weight prior to becoming pregnant and emphasize the importance of a proper pattern of weight gain and an adequate intake of calories, protein, vitamins, and minerals during pregnancy to allow for optimal fetal development, the preservation of maternal health, the immediate postnatal health of the infant and the infant's subsequent health as an adult. These recommendations also stress evaluation of the mother, either before conception or early in pregnancy, for the presence of nutritional risk factors that might jeopardize the outcome of the pregnancy.

Energy and Protein Requirements

Resting metabolic rate increases about 5% during the first trimester of pregnancy. As the fetus grows and requires increased energy for its own metabolic demands and because its size and the size of the placenta impose increased energy demands on the mother, resting metabolic rate increases by about 10% during the second trimester and 25% during the third trimester, with the fetus accounting for about half of the increased energy expenditure during the last trimester (11,12). Nonetheless, because the mother's activity declines on the order of 2% to 6% from her prepregnancy levels, a pregnant woman's total daily energy expenditure increases minimally during the first trimester of pregnancy, only 1% to 3% on average, rises modestly by about 5% to 6% during the second trimester. It is only during the third trimester, when maternal energy costs of weight bearing and physical activity increase to a great extent, does maternal energy expenditure rise significantly, averaging about 10% to 20% above that of the mother's prepregnancy total daily energy expenditure (11,12). It is also important to recognize that changes in energy expenditure increase significantly under circumstances of excessive gestational weight gain. Thus, inappropriately increased maternal energy intake leads to augmented deposition of calories as in maternal fat stores, and increases the risk of poor maternal and fetal outcomes (11–13).

Over the entire duration of pregnancy, maternal basal metabolic rate increases by an average of about 106 to 180 kcal per day (11). However, as discussed above, the energy demands of late pregnancy are much higher than those of early pregnancy. Thus, based on total daily energy expenditure data, and accounting for changes in maternal physical activity, dietary energy deposited in fetal tissue accretion and dietary energy deposited in maternal organs supporting the fetus and in maternal fat stores, there is no recommended increase in the mother's estimated energy requirement (EER) during the first trimester of pregnancy, an increase in EER of about 350 kcal per day during the second trimester and of approximately 450 kcal per day during the last trimester (11,14). Hytten has calculated that the total energy cost of pregnancy is a remarkable 85,000 calories (15) (Table 3-1).

The estimated average requirement (EAR) for dietary protein in adult, nonpregnant women is 0.66 g/kg/day, with a recommended dietary allowance (RDA) of 0.80 g/kg/day (14). Over the entire course of pregnancy, the protein RDA increases by about 10 to 15 g per day but no change in maternal EAR or RDA for dietary protein is necessary during the first trimester (14). During the second and third trimesters, protein intake allowances increase modestly to an EAR of 0.88 g/kg/day (an increase of ~20 g of protein daily) and an RDA of 1.1 g/kg/day (an increase of about 25 g per day). The calculated additional intakes of dietary protein are those required to support the deposition of protein in new maternal and fetal tissues (16) (Table 3-2) and account for the efficiency of converting consumed dietary protein to the tissue protein deposited. Based on the limited data available (14), these values average about 20 g of protein per day over the last two trimesters of pregnancy, being somewhat less in the second trimester and somewhat more during the third (14). This level of increased protein intake is achieved easily on the standard middle-class Western diet. However, women from lower socioeconomic groups or women who,

TABLE 3-1 Energy Cost of Pregnancy

	Gestational Weeks				Cumulative Total (kcal)
	0–10	10–20	20–30	30–40	
	Energy Equivalence (kcal/d)				
Protein	3.6	10.3	26.7	34.2	5,186
Fat	55.6	235.6	207.6	31.3	36,329
Oxygen consumption	44.8	99.0	148.2	227.2	35,717
Total net energy	104.0	344.9	382.5	292.7	77,234
Metabolizable energy (+10%)	114	379	421	322	84,957

Data from Hytten FE. Weight gain in pregnancy. In: Hytten FE, Chamberlain G, eds. *Clinical Physiology in Obstetrics.* Oxford: Blackwell Scientific Publications, 1991:173–203.

TABLE 3-2 Tissue and Nutrient Deposition During Pregnancy

	Week of Gestation			
	10	20	30	40
Products of conception				
Fetus (g)	5	300	1,500	3,400
Placenta (g)	20	170	430	650
Amniotic fluid (g)	30	250	750	800
Maternal tissue gain				
Uterus (g)	140	320	600	970
Mammary gland (g)	45	480	360	405
Plasma volume (mL)	50	800	1,200	1,500
Nutrient accretion in mother + fetus				
Fat deposition (g)	328	2,064	3,594	3,825
Protein deposition (g)	36	165	498	925
Iron accretion (g)				565
Calcium accretion (g)				30
Zinc accretion (mg)				100

Data from King JC. Physiology of pregnancy and nutrient metabolism. *Am J Clin Nutr.* 2000;71:1218S–1225S.

by preference, consume a diet low (or absent) in animal protein and/or dairy products may require dietary counseling to meet this level of increased protein intake and assure an adequate intake of high-quality proteins.

Maternal Weight Gain

Severe restriction of weight gain during pregnancy (total weight gain of 16 to 18 lb) was recommended widely until several decades ago in an attempt to prevent preeclampsia and eclampsia. Maternal obesity and insulin resistance strongly predispose a pregnant woman to preeclampsia (17–19); however, the pathogenesis of this disorder remains an enigma (20,21), and the precise role of maternal body weight or body composition in the pathophysiology of preeclampsia is unclear. Nonetheless, maternal pregravid obesity and excessive maternal weight gain during pregnancy convey significant risks to both mother and fetus (11). Given the dramatic secular trend in the rise of obesity prevalence worldwide, the issue of optimal weight gain during pregnancy has become increasingly important.

Likewise, restricted weight gain may affect pregnancy adversely, resulting in an infant with a low or very low birth weight and the consequences of low birth weight may be more encompassing than previously thought, as discussed earlier (1,4,5,10). Limited weight gain during pregnancy, especially when the mother's weight is low before pregnancy, increases the risk for fetal growth retardation. The risk for mortality is markedly increased in infants with a low birth weight, especially in those with a very low birth weight. Similarly, in low-birth-weight infants who survive, many studies over the last several decades had documented an inverse relationship between birth weight and degree of neonatal morbidity and between birth weight and adverse neurologic outcomes.

Because of the observed increased prevalence of maternal obesity during the last two decades and increasing recognition of the adverse consequences of low birth weight in adult life, the Institute of Medicine (IOM) has issued two detailed reports on appropriate weight gain during pregnancy (13,22). These reports differed in several important ways from prior recommendations by recognizing that healthy, normal infants are delivered to mothers whose gestational weight gains vary by as much as 30 lb and that weight accretion during pregnancy is affected by the mother's prepregnancy BMI. Thus, mothers with a low BMI before pregnancy can gain more weight during pregnancy than mothers whose BMI is high before pregnancy. Based on this information, the IOM committees have recommended a set of target ranges of total weight gain and rates of weight gain according to the mother's prepregnancy BMI (13,22) (Table 3-3). Although limited, there is accumulating evidence that the weight gain guidelines proposed by the IOM committees achieve the goals of better outcomes for the infant and the mother. Jain et al. (23) compared pregnancy outcome risks against the IOM maternal weight gain guidelines in a sample of 7,661 women, of whom 18% were obese and 13% were overweight. The data showed that pregnancy outcomes of women who gained 25 to 34 lb during pregnancy were indistinguishable from those of women who gained 16 to 24 lb, thus supporting the recommendations

TABLE 3-3 Recommended Weight Gain in Pregnancy

Prepregnancy Body Mass Index Category	Mothers of Singletons		Mothers of Twins (Provisional)
	Total Weight Gain (lb)	Rate of Weight Gain in the Second and Third Trimesters (lb/wk)	Total Weight Gain at Term (lb)
Under weight (<18.5 kg/m^2)	28–40	1.0 (1.0–1.3)	No guideline available
Normal-weight (18.5–24.9 kg/m^2)	25–35	1.0 (0.8–1.0)	37–54
Overweight (25.0–29.9 kg/m^2)	15–25	0.6 (0.5–0.7)	31–50
Obese (≥ 30.0 kg/m^2)	11–20	0.5 (0.4–0.6)	25–42

From Rasmussen KM, Catalano PM, Yaktine AL. New guidelines for weight gain during pregnancy: what obstetrician/gynecologists should know. *Curr Opin Obstet Gynecol*. 2009;21:521–525.

published by the IOM, while women whose weight gain during pregnancy exceeded 35 lb had dramatically increased rates of macrosomia and cesarean delivery (23). Further, however, when weight gain during pregnancy was controlled for, women who were overweight and obese had significantly higher rates of fetal macrosomia and cesarean section (23). Likewise, in a recent meta-analysis Quinlivan et al. (24) demonstrated that "antenatal dietary interventions in obese pregnancy women can reduce maternal weight gain in pregnancy," and, importantly, another meta-analysis by Nehring et al. (25) confirmed that gestational weight gain consistent with the IOM recommendations "is associated with long-term effects on postprandial weight retention". In other words, mothers who limited their weight gain in pregnancy weighed significantly less after pregnancy than women who did not, even as long as 15 years postpartum (25). Importantly, a meta-analysis by Tie et al. (26) demonstrated that the risk of childhood obesity is significantly greater in women with excessive gestational weight gain and when their analysis was restricted to high-quality studies using IOM guidelines, the relationship was even stronger. Looked at from an "inverse" perspective, the latter data suggest that limiting pregnancy weight gain to the ranges proposed by the IOM will have significant, subsequent effects on the development of childhood obesity.

REQUIREMENTS FOR SPECIFIC NUTRIENTS DURING PREGNANCY

Requirements for individual nutrients in pregnancy have been reviewed by others (11,27,28). The basis for the majority of specific nutrient intake recommendations are the values determined by the various IOM expert committees on *dietary reference intakes* (29).

Iron

Iron requirements are dramatically increased during pregnancy. Hematologic changes during pregnancy profoundly affect iron homeostasis. The maternal red cell volume increases 20% to 30%, so the delivery of an extra 450 to 500 mg of iron to the maternal marrow is required for erythropoiesis (30). This is in addition to the basal losses of iron, averaging about 250 mg, and the 315 to 360 mg of iron transferred to the fetus and placenta (11,28). Thus the additional iron required during pregnancy is on the order of 1,100 mg. Of this increment, approximately 150 to 250 mg of blood iron is trapped in the placenta or lost during delivery, but the mother recovers about 250 to 300 mg when her blood volume diminishes after delivery (31). Thus, the total net iron "debt" during pregnancy is about 750 or 850 mg (1,100 minus 250 to 350). Of this amount, almost all of the extra iron is required during the second and third trimesters of gestation, amounting to approximately 20 mg per day (31). Based on these considerations, the EAR for iron during pregnancy is 22 mg per day and the RDA for iron during pregnancy is 27 mg per day (31). These amounts are on the order of 14 mg per day and 9 mg per day greater than the respective EAR and RDA for nonpregnant women (31).

Only about 10% of dietary iron is absorbed before pregnancy or during the first trimester. Efficiency of absorption increases to about 20% in iron deficiency and may increase up to 15% to 20% during the third trimester. The typical American diet provides only about 1 to 2 mg of absorbed iron each day. Thus, even a diet carefully selected for foods rich in iron may not satisfy the increased iron requirements of the last half of pregnancy and an attempt to provide the total iron RDA with dietary iron is likely to result in excessive calorie intake. For this reason, most women will require an iron supplement to meet the RDA (28,29,32). Importantly, a Cochrane systematic review by Peña-Rosas et al. (33) has provided the evidence that oral iron supplementation benefits both the mother and the infant. The standard recommendation of the Centers for Disease Control and Prevention is a daily supplement of 30 mg of elemental iron (generally in the form of simple iron salts such as ferrous gluconate, ferrous sulfate, or ferrous fumarate) beginning at the first prenatal visit (34) in pregnant women whose hemoglobin and iron stores are normal prior to pregnancy. The WHO recommends a supplementation of 60 mg in settings where iron deficiency is a prevalent problem and 120 mg if the pregnant woman has anemia (32). Thus, pregnant women with confirmed anemia should be carefully evaluated medically for the cause of the anemia and, if due to iron deficiency, should be treated with 60 to 120 mg of supplemental elemental iron daily until the hemoglobin concentration becomes normal, at which time the supplementation can be reduced to 30 mg per day. Commonly used prenatal vitamin and mineral supplements contain 45 to 60 mg of elemental iron per tablet; a 320-mg ferrous sulfate tablet contains 64 mg of elemental iron.

It is important to recognize that oral iron supplements can cause *gastrointestinal side effects,* including heartburn, nausea, constipation or diarrhea, abdominal cramps, and change in stool color. The unpleasant gastrointestinal side effects of iron can be minimized by taking iron supplements after a meal rather than on an empty stomach. Unfortunately, iron ingested with or after a meal is not absorbed as well as iron taken during fasting. Since nausea is a problem for many women early in pregnancy, since this problem may be exacerbated by iron supplements, and since iron requirements do not increase significantly until the second trimester of pregnancy, it is reasonable to defer iron supplementation until the second trimester in women who have nausea that is worsened by iron supplements. The constipation that is commonly associated with oral iron supplementation and can be treated with conventional laxatives and stool softeners, but patients taking iron supplements should be warned that their stools may turn black.

Pregnant women with small children should be warned to keep iron supplements out of reach, a recommendation that must be emphasized by physicians and other health caregivers. Ingestion of maternal prenatal iron supplements is a common cause of significant *iron intoxication in children,* no trivial issue, since iron intoxication is a relatively common cause of fatal poisoning in childhood. Antacids impair the absorption of iron, and the two should not be taken together. This is of some importance because gastroesophageal reflux with heartburn develops frequently in late pregnancy.

Pica, the craving for unnatural foods, particularly dirt and clay, develops occasionally in pregnant women and is often associated with iron-deficiency anemia. However, most individuals with iron deficiency do not exhibit pica and although various explanations have been offered for the occurrence of pica none are either fully satisfactory or proven by experiment. From a clinical-practice perspective, however, pregnant women with iron-deficiency anemia should be asked about pica, and those with pica should be tested for iron-deficiency anemia.

Folic Acid

The role of folic acid in human reproduction has been extensively reviewed (35). Folic acid is the most commonly deficient vitamin during pregnancy. Folate is required for the synthesis of the thymidylate moiety and, thus, for DNA synthesis. Folate, then, is required in increasing amounts during gestation to satisfy the needs of cell division in order to accommodate new growth of maternal and fetal tissues. A principal reason for the markedly increased folate requirement in pregnancy is increased maternal erythropoiesis, since maternal erythrocyte volume increases 20% to 30% during the last two trimesters.

The primary maternal manifestation of severe folate deficiency is megaloblastic anemia. Severe folate deficiency is not commonly seen as a complication of pregnancy in the United States. If, however, depletion of folate stores estimated from red blood cell folate concentrations or from elevation of plasma homocysteine levels are employed to uncover folate insufficiency, then the incidence of inadequate folate status during pregnancy is much higher (35).

Folic acid antagonists, such as aminopterin and methotrexate, have long been recognized as human teratogens. Additionally, commonly prescribed drugs such as phenobarbital, phenytoin, primidone, carbamazepine, trimethoprim, and triamterene, that either inhibit dihydrofolate reductase or interfere with folic acid metabolism by other mechanisms, more than double the relative risk for fetal cardiovascular defects, urinary tract defects, or oral clefts when taken during the second or third month after the mother's last menstrual period, but appear to have no deleterious effects on fetal development when taken in the second or third trimesters (36). The use of folic acid supplements during pregnancy diminished the effects of dihydrofolate reductase inhibitors, but not the teratogenic effects of antiepileptic drugs (36).

As discussed extensively elsewhere (35,37–38), various studies have reported higher incidences of spontaneous abortion, stillbirth, abruptio placentae, preeclampsia, premature rupture of the membranes, preterm delivery, orofacial clefts, Down syndrome, congenital heart defects, impaired fetal growth, and limb defects in association with diminished maternal red cell folate levels. However, each of these consequences remains unproven either because the data are conflicting among studies or because, among other potential confounders, it is difficult in such surveys to isolate the specific effects of low folate status from other manifestations of poor nutrition and low socioeconomic status.

Neural Tube Defects

On the other hand, convincing data from many sources have proven the adverse effects of low-maternal-folate status during the periconceptional period and within the first month of pregnancy on closure of the neural tube with the devastating consequence of an increased incidence of neural tube defects (NTDs; anencephaly and spina bifida) among the offspring (35). Further, and most importantly, overwhelming evidence is now available to indicate that the incidence of NTDs in the offspring of women who take folic acid supplements of at least 400 mg per day before and during the first 4 weeks of pregnancy is approximately 25% to 50% that of women who do not (35,39–40). Nonetheless, despite more than two decades of intensive research on the mechanism(s) for folate's beneficial effects, the precise reason(s) for this effect remain(s) elusive (41) and women who have some polymorphisms in the 5,10-methylenetetrahydrofolate reductase (MTHFR) gene have an increased risk of bearing a child with a NTD, while those carrying other polymorphisms do not (42–44).

The effect of supplemental folic acid is lost after the first month of gestation because embryonic neural tube closure is complete by then. Only about 5% of NTDs are recurrences. Approximately half the women of childbearing age who become pregnant do not plan to do so. In addition, by the time most women realize that they are pregnant, they are at least halfway through the first 4 weeks of gestation. For these reasons, in September of 1992, the Centers for Disease Control and Prevention issued the recommendation that *all women of childbearing age* take supplemental folic acid (45). Further, to help ensure adequate levels of folate in women of childbearing age, cereal grain products in the United States are now fortified with 140 µg of folic acid per 100 g of grain (46), a value calculated to provide individuals with approximately 100 µg of additional folic acid intake daily. This practice has successfully reduced the incidence of NTDs in the countries where the practices were adopted and data have been reported (40,47). As a consequence of the US fortification policy, population blood folate levels have increased without leading to an increase in the prevalence of low vitamin B_{12} status as feared by some (47–49) while achieving the initial fortification goal, a significant reduction in the incidence of NTDs.

Folate Requirements

For adult women of childbearing age who are not pregnant, definition of the folate requirement is based largely on controlled metabolic studies although epidemiological data were used as supportive information. Based on this information, the EAR is defined as 320 µg dietary folate equivalents (DFEs) daily, and the RDA is set at 400 µg DFE per day (50–53). Based on similar controlled metabolic study data, approximately 200 µg of *additional* folate is required daily to maintain folate status in pregnant women (50,52), so the RDA for folate in pregnant women is set at 600 µg of folate equivalents per day (11,28,50–53) (Table 3-4). It is important to realize that this recommendation is made on the basis of different studies from those that led to the Centers for Disease Control and Prevention recommendation of folic acid supplementation to prevent NTDs (45) (see below). The latter recommendation was based both on the minimum tested dose of folic acid supplementation that was effective in preventing NTDs in controlled clinical studies and on the relevant public health consideration that the neural tube is substantially formed before most women know that they are pregnant and seek professional advice.

A "healthful" diet in individuals who do not take dietary supplements contains approximately 700 µg of food folates, of which about half is bioavailable. Thus, while this diet approaches the EAR for folate in women of childbearing age, a slightly substandard diet that is more typical of the current American diet would be deficient in folate. Despite the population increase in serum and red cell folate values following mandatory fortification of grain products in the United States and significant decline in the prevalence of individuals consuming folate at below RDA levels, a small percentage of American women still do not meet the dietary reference intake values for folate. Thus, in women of childbearing age, increased attention should be paid to improving dietary sources of this vitamin. Good dietary sources of folate include dark green leafy vegetables, green and lima beans, orange juice, fortified cereals, yeast, mushrooms,

TABLE 3-4 RDAs for Nonpregnant, Pregnant, and Lactating Women

	Nonpregnant Women	Pregnant Women	Lactating Women
Vitamin A (µg)	800	800	800
Vitamin D (µg)	5	15	15
Vitamin E (mg)	15	15	19
Vitamin C (mg)	75	85	120
Thiamin (mg)	1.1	1.2	1.4
Riboflavin (mg)	1.1	1.4	1.6
Vitamin B_6 (mg)	1.3	1.9	2.0
Niacin (mg NE)	14	18	17
Folate (µg DFE)	400	600	500
Vitamin B_{12} (µg)	2.4	2.6	2.8
Calcium (mg), ≥19 yo	1,000	1,000	1,000
Calcium (mg), 14–18 yo	1,300	1,300	1,300
Phosphorus (mg)	700	700	700
Magnesium (mg)	320	350	310
Iron (mg)	15	30	15
Iodine (µg)	150	175	200
Selenium (µg)	55	60	70

yo, year old.
Data from Institute of Medicine, National Academy of Sciences. *Dietary Reference Intakes: The Essential Guide to Nutrient Requirements*. Washington, DC: National Academy Press, 2006; Food and Nutrition Board, Institute of Medicine, National Academy of Sciences. *Dietary Reference Intakes for Calcium and Vitamin D*. Washington, DC: National Academy Press, 2011.

liver, and kidneys. Root vegetables, eggs, and most dairy products are poor sources of folate. Remember too that dietary folate is markedly influenced by food storage and methods of food preparation. Folate is destroyed by boiling and by various other food-processing methods, including canning.

Normal body stores of folate are in the range of 12 to 18 mg. A pregnant woman consuming a folate-deficient diet could deplete her normal folate stores in a few weeks to a few months, depending on the level of her prior stores and the degree of dietary deficiency. Women consuming a diet chronically deficient in folate (including alcoholics and many from lower socioeconomic groups) have small folate stores that would be depleted even more rapidly. Furthermore, the effects of oral contraceptives on folate metabolism are not completely defined and there are some data indicating that red cell levels of folate are diminished in long-time users of oral contraceptives, drug that have variously been described to interfere with folate absorption and accelerate folate degradation in the liver. Whatever the mechanism, it appears that folate stores may be reduced in women who have used oral contraceptives, and that folate deficiency is more likely to develop in these women during pregnancy.

Folate Supplementation

As discussed earlier, because of accumulating data showing that folic acid supplementation in the periconceptional period profoundly decreased the incidence of NTDs, the US Public Health Service through the Centers for Disease Control and Prevention issued the following recommendation in September 1992: "All women of childbearing age in the United States who are capable of becoming pregnant should consume 0.4 mg of folic acid per day for the purposes of reducing their risk of having a pregnancy affected with spina bifida and other NTDs. Because the effects of high intakes are not well-known but include complicating the diagnosis of B_{12} deficiency, care should be taken to keep total folate consumption under 1 mg per day, except under the supervision of a physician. Women who have a prior NTD-affected pregnancy are at high risk of having a subsequent affected pregnancy. When these women are planning to become pregnant, they should consult their physician for advice" (45).

It is important to realize that the current RDA of 400 μg of DFEs equivalents for nonpregnant women does not strictly conform to the Centers for Disease Control recommendation, since, in clinical studies of the prevention of NTDs, folic acid was taken as a *supplement* to the usual diet containing food folates. Therefore, the Centers for Disease Control and Prevention recommendation, as written, recommends supplementation in the form of folic acid. An important consequence is that the recommended intake of folic acid/folates as DFEs in women capable of becoming pregnant exceeds the RDA. **Thus, the IOM recommends that "women capable of becoming pregnant consume 400 μg of folate daily from supplements, fortified foods, or both, *in addition* to consuming food folate from a varied diet. At this time, the evidence for a protective effect from folate supplements is much stronger than that for food folate"** (50). It is further assumed that "women will continue consuming 400 μg from supplements or fortified foods until their pregnancy is confirmed and they enter prenatal care, which ordinarily occurs after the end of the periconceptional period—the critical time for formation of the neural tube" (29). *Finally, it is important to counsel women who have previously delivered a child with a NTD that considerably higher doses of folic acid (generally in the range of 4 to 5 mg per day) taken as supplements are required to prevent a recurrence of an NTD in subsequent pregnancies.*

Calcium, Phosphorus, Zinc, and Vitamin D

The added calcium requirement of pregnancy is about 25 to 30 g—the amount of calcium in the fetus at term (11,28). Almost all the fetal calcium is added during the last trimester, when the fetus takes up an average of 300 mg per day. In the first half of pregnancy, fetal calcium accretion is only about 50 mg per day.

Unlike maternal iron stores, which are relatively small, maternal calcium stores are large. Almost all the maternal stores are in the skeleton, some of which can be mobilized easily if needed (11,28). The 30-g calcium requirement of a single pregnancy represents only about 2.5% of the total maternal stores. Further increased maternal absorption of dietary calcium easily fulfills the small additional need, and no evidence has been found that maternal bone-mineral density changes during pregnancy in relation to calcium intake. Therefore, the EAR for calcium during pregnancy remains unchanged from the corresponding recommendations for nonpregnant women, 800 mg per day for women above the age of 19 and 1,100 mg per day for adolescent girls aged 18 or less (54) (Table 3-4) with corresponding RDAs of 1,000 mg per day and 1,300 mg per day, respectively (54, Table 3-4). For similar reasons, the ERA and RDA for phosphorus remain unchanged by pregnancy at 580 and 700 mg per day, respectively, in women over the age of 19 and 1,055 mg per day and 1,250 mg per day, respectively, in adolescent girls aged 18 or below (29,54,55).

Adequate dietary calcium intake is easily achieved by women who consume dairy products (1 qt of milk contains 1,000 mg of calcium) and dietary calcium sources from regular or fortified food products are plentiful. Even women who avoid dairy products because of lactose intolerance can achieve an adequate dietary calcium intake. Those who are relatively lactose-deficient may substitute hard cheese for milk. For example, 2 oz of Swiss cheese has twice as much calcium as 8 oz of milk but only one-eleventh as much lactose. Further, a much wider array of calcium fortified food products, such as orange juice, are now widely available. Rare cases of osteomalacia have been reported in multiparous women in underdeveloped countries, who have very low levels of dietary calcium. This has not been a problem in the United States. The calcium intakes recommended for pregnancy are sometimes not achieved with dietary sources alone in some groups having special or selective food preferences and in some African American, Hispanic, and Native American populations. These groups should be encouraged to increase their intake of calcium from acceptable food sources or, less preferably, be given a calcium supplement.

When calcium supplementation is needed, calcium carbonate, citrate, gluconate, or lactate can be given to provide significant extra calcium intake daily and make up the difference between the recommended adequate intake of calcium and the amount of calcium consumed as food in the diet. For example, a 500-mg tablet of calcium carbonate contains 200 mg of elemental calcium. Although there are some data that calcium carbonate may be less bioavailable than calcium salts having an organic anion such as citrate, gluconate, or lactate, calcium bioavailability from calcium carbonate was identical to its bioavailability from calcium citrate in carefully controlled studies. Given its low price, a cost/benefit analysis clearly favors the use of calcium carbonate. The IOM has set the tolerable upper intake limit (UL) for calcium during pregnancy at 2,500 mg per day, a value no different from that advised for nonpregnant women (54,55). When supplements are necessary to treat deficiency, the degree of replacement can be followed by measuring the 24-hour urinary excretion of calcium, although this is rarely done in ordinary clinical circumstances.

As is the case with calcium, the additional zinc required to satisfy the needs of pregnancy, amounting to perhaps 100 mg, is only a small fraction of maternal body zinc stores (11,28,55) and primarily occurs in the last trimester pregnancy, with about half of the extra zinc deposited in the fetus (55). Thus, it is likely that pregnant women can continue to satisfy their zinc requirements from dietary sources, if they are consuming an adequate zinc intake at the RDA level (8 mg per day) prior to becoming pregnant. Nonetheless, to account for the additional daily zinc requirement of about 2.5 mg per day during the last trimester of pregnancy, the IOM has set the RDA for zinc intake in pregnancy at 11 mg per day for adult women and 13 mg per day for adolescent girls.

Vitamin D regulates calcium and phosphorus metabolism after conversion of the parent compound, cholecalciferol, to its active hormonal form, 1,25-dihydroxycholecalciferol. It increases calcium and phosphorus absorption from the small intestine and potentiates bone resorption induced by parathyroid hormone. Maternal vitamin D is transported across the placenta to the fetus. In the United States, despite extensive discussion and debate of what level of vitamin D intake constitutes "marginal intake," frank vitamin D deficiency is rare and routine vitamin D supplementation during pregnancy is not currently recommended. The EAR for vitamin D in pregnant women is 10 μg of cholecalciferol (400 IU of vitamin D) and the RDA for vitamin D is 15 μg of cholecalciferol (600 IU of vitamin D) (54). The EAR and RDA are the same as the intakes recommended for nonpregnant women (54).

However, it is important to recognize several important issues about vitamin D nutrition. First, vitamin D does not occur naturally in almost all foods eaten by humans, except for that in certain oily fish and their livers, cod liver oil, and a small amount in egg yolks. Vitamin D obtained from dietary food sources is almost exclusively due to fortification. In the United States, for example, milk is fortified with 400 IU vitamin D per quart, and margarine, some cereals, yoghurts, and orange juice are also fortified. Second, relatively short exposures of skin to sunlight allow the synthesis of all the vitamin D required by man, although more exposure is required in dark skinned individuals and in those living in northern latitudes. Unfortunately, increasingly restrictive outdoor environmental practices, the wearing of protective clothing and the widespread use of sunscreen lotions has reduced the amount of vitamin D that individuals now obtain via skin synthesis. Third, a wide variety of studies measuring blood levels of 25-hydroxycholecalciferol (25-OHD), an index of vitamin D status, have found levels that some consider low to marginal and have led some to propose that a significant fraction of the population is marginally deficient in vitamin D. Because vitamin D is necessary for a ubiquitous range of molecular and cellular functions, the resulting thesis is that marginal vitamin D status is responsible for a wide range of detrimental health consequences on various organs and increases the risk of a variety of chronic diseases, including cancers. These data have led some to question the adequacy of the IOM's current adequate intake recommendations for vitamin D for the population and for women who are pregnant and lactating (56–60). Nonetheless, the most recent IOM assessment of vitamin D dietary reference intakes was unable to find convincing evidence to support any of the health and disease claims that might have led to a significant increase in the recommended intakes for vitamin D (54). The controversial issues surrounding vitamin D requirements are discussed in considerably more detail in Chapter 6.

Evidence suggests that maternal vitamin D deficiency can result in fetal vitamin D deficiency, manifested by neonatal hypocalcemia (61). Vitamin D deficiency is usually the result of a very low dietary intake combined with minimal exposure to sunlight. Daily supplementation with 5 to 10 μg of vitamin D should be considered for complete vegetarians and for persons who avoid sunlight or vitamin D–fortified milk, but these should only be taken on the advice of the individual's physician. Excessive maternal intake of vitamin D may result in severe infantile hypercalcemia. The precise amount of ingested vitamin D and the duration of exposure to this dose that is necessary to induce hypervitaminosis D is not known with any degree of certainty.

For this reason, the tolerable UL for vitamin D intake during pregnancy has been cautiously set at 50 µg (2,000 IU) (54).

Requirements for Selected Other Nutrients

The EAR for magnesium in nonpregnant adult women is about 255 to 265 mg per day with a corresponding RDA for magnesium set in the range of 310 to 320 mg per day (55). The data available to set a dietary reference intake for magnesium in pregnancy are very limited. The EAR for magnesium is calculated to increase by an additional 35 mg per day based on estimates of magnesium accretion in maternal and fetal lean body mass, corrected for bioavailability. Thus, the magnesium EAR in pregnancy is calculated as 290 to 300 mg per day and the pregnancy RDA for magnesium is increased to 50 to 360 mg per day for pregnant women, although no direct experimental data are available to support the increased need (55).

The adult woman's RDA for vitamin C is 75 mg per day (62). During pregnancy, this value is increased to 85 mg per day on the basis of declining maternal plasma vitamin C levels and the necessary transfer of vitamin C to the fetus (62). However, no direct experimental data support the need for additional vitamin C during pregnancy. Because vitamin C is actively transported from the maternal to the fetal circulation, because there are no proven benefits of vitamin C intake above the RDA intake levels, and because of uncertainty of potential harm to the fetus of pharmacological exposures to vitamin C, a tolerable UL for vitamin C intake in pregnancy has been set at 1,800 to 2,000 mg (62).

With very limited experimental data, and from calculations based largely on changes in maternal metabolism during pregnancy and estimates of fetal nutrient accretion, the RDAs for thiamin, riboflavin, niacin, vitamin A, vitamin B_6, vitamin B_{12}, and selenium have been modestly increased for pregnant women, as have the RDAs for copper, iodine, and molybdenum and the adequate intake recommendations for chromium and manganese (29) (Table 3-4). The RDA for vitamin E and biotin remain unchanged by pregnancy (29).

Assessment of Nutritional Status During Pregnancy

A pregnant woman should be assessed for nutritional risk factors that would jeopardize the outcome of her pregnancy. A history of previous pregnancies should be obtained, with attention to complications, duration of pregnancy, birth weight and length, and development of the child after delivery. A history of eclampsia, abortion, low-birth-weight infant, hyperemesis, or anemia during past pregnancies has implications for the outcome of the present pregnancy. A nutritional assessment also should include the patient's weight, a brief diet history (including alcohol intake and smoking), and a history of the use of medications that might affect nutrient absorption (e.g., folic acid antagonists, anticonvulsants, thyroid medications, vitamins).

NUTRITIONAL RISK FACTORS AT THE ONSET OF PREGNANCY
Adolescence

An adolescent who becomes pregnant within 3 years of menarche is at special risk for a poor outcome of pregnancy. The nutritional demands of pregnancy are added to the needs of a mother who may still be still growing. The demands for calories, protein, and calcium are all increased and the corresponding RDA during pregnancy is higher than those for adult women. Further, adolescents are more likely than adults to have inadequate diets, and so special attention must be paid to the diet of pregnant adolescents. Pregnant adolescents are also more likely to come from low socioeconomic groups, among which poor nutrition is common.

Three or More Pregnancies within 2 Years

Multiple pregnancies at close intervals deplete stored nutrients, including iron and folate. Iron deficiency is an especially significant problem in this group.

Poor Reproductive Performance

A past history of low-birth-weight infants, abortions, or perinatal loss may reflect nutritional deficiency. The factor most highly correlated with the delivery of a low-birth-weight infant is the past history of a low-birth-weight infant.

Economic Deprivation

The diets of patients with low incomes are more likely to be deficient in iron, folate, protein, and B vitamins.

Food Restriction and Fadism

Women who are on unusual diets, diets designed to significantly achieve a healthy body weight or diets that are deficient in specific nutrients are at risk for adverse outcomes during pregnancy.

Women who are underweight at the beginning of pregnancy (BMI <18.5) are at risk for having low-birth-weight babies. Underweight mothers also may be at increased risk for toxemia. If a woman who is underweight before pregnancy does not gain enough weight during pregnancy, the risks are increased further. Obviously, the optimal time for dealing with the underweight woman is before pregnancy. An underweight woman who is considering pregnancy should be encouraged to gain weight first. When an underweight woman does become pregnant, she should be encouraged to gain more weight than is recommended for the woman who enters pregnancy at a normal weight. Protein–calorie supplements may be necessary to correct previous nutritional deficits and provide for the needs of pregnancy. Very low calorie, restrictive diets during the periconceptional period may limit the ability to become pregnant and may diminish the success of in vitro fertilization efforts in mothers undergoing such procedures. Further, mothers on aggressive weight loss programs during pregnancy, especially severely carbohydrate-restricted diets that result in ketosis, are at risk for a poor outcome. The reasons to avoid severe calorie restriction during pregnancy are compelling. When caloric intake is severely restricted, inadequate intakes of calcium, iron, folate, B vitamins, and protein result. If ingested protein is to be used in the synthesis of maternal and fetal proteins, total energy intake must also be adequate. If caloric intake is inadequate, ingested proteins are catabolized for energy needs. Furthermore, severe restriction of total caloric intake, especially when carbohydrate intake is also restricted, results in ketosis. Studies of diabetic women indicate that ketosis is poorly tolerated by the fetus. Ketosis may be associated with a reduction in uterine blood flow. Ketone bodies are concentrated in the amniotic fluid and taken up by the fetus. The mental development of the offspring of mothers who have had ketonuria during pregnancy, as a consequence of either diabetes or starvation, may be compromised. Whether this is a direct effect of fetal ketosis or the effect of an associated metabolic problem is not clear.

Strict vegans may be deficient in vitamin B_{12} and riboflavin in addition to iron. These problems are readily preventable by careful dietary choices as discussed in more detail on Chapter 6.

The ingestion of vitamins in excessive quantities (megavitamin therapy) may have harmful effects on the fetus. "Rebound" scurvy has been reported in the infants of mothers who have taken massive doses of vitamin C (>5 g per day). The fetus becomes metabolically dependent on high levels of vitamin C that are provided by the mother in utero but not by the infant's diet after birth. Studies in rats have shown unequivocally that high doses of vitamin A are teratogenic, 13-*cis*-retinoic acid has been demonstrated to be teratogenic in humans (63), and several epidemiological studies support possible teratogenicity due to high intakes of preformed vitamin A (31). Pregnant women are advised not to take more than 800 μg of retinol equivalents per day.

Smoking, Drug Addiction, and Alcoholism

Maternal smoking during pregnancy "accounts for 20% to 30% of low birth weight, up to 14% of preterm births and approximately 10% of all infant deaths in the United States," (64) and a meta-analysis has shown that even environmental exposure to tobacco smoke during pregnancy reduces average birth weight (65). In addition, smoking may increase a woman's chance of having placenta previa and placental abruption (64) and there is some evidence that infants born to smoking mothers are at increased risk for sudden infant death syndrome (66–68). The Centers for Disease Control and Prevention estimates that smoking during pregnancy is the single most preventable cause of illness and death among mothers and infants. (68). The full contraindications to smoking are both more comprehensive and independent of those occurring in of pregnancy, but pregnancy surely adds one more immediately, compelling reason for adult women who smoke to stop doing so.

Heavy maternal drinking is associated with prenatal growth retardation. Heavy alcohol consumption is associated with a diet deficient in B vitamins, folate, and protein. Maternal alcoholism is associated with fetal toxicity in addition to nutritional deficiencies. Animal studies show that alcohol is a teratogen. Fetal abnormalities associated with heavy maternal alcohol ingestion in humans (fetal alcohol syndrome) include microcephaly, cleft palate, and micrognathia. Moderate to high alcohol intakes during pregnancy have significant detrimental effects on the neuropsychological outcomes of the child born from these pregnancies (69), and milder fetal exposures to alcohol have suggestive detrimental consequences (69). The effects of limited or occasional alcohol intake are undefined and it is not known whether a minimum alcohol intake exists below which risk is not increased. For this reason, essentially all authoritative, expert organizations advise against drinking during pregnancy.

Chronic Systemic Disease

Pregnant diabetic women must be diligent to avoid both hypoglycemia and hyperglycemia with ketosis. Diabetes in pregnancy is associated with resistance to insulin and an increased insulin requirement. On the other hand, fetal glucose utilization may cause maternal fasting hypoglycemia. Diseases associated with malabsorption may cause problems during pregnancy. Primary diseases of the small intestine, such as Crohn disease, may result in malabsorption of many nutrients or malabsorption of selected nutrients, such as vitamin B_{12} or iron. Chronic pancreatic disease is associated with malabsorption of fats and, to a lesser extent, fat-soluble vitamins. Usually, malabsorption can be managed either by treating the underlying disease or by appropriate nutritional supplementation.

NUTRITIONAL RISK FACTORS THAT DEVELOP DURING PREGNANCY
Anemia

Beginning at 3 months' gestation, the maternal blood volume increases markedly. The increase in blood volume precedes the increase in red cell mass, which begins at 6 months, and the increase in blood volume is proportionally greater than the increase in red cell mass. This dilutional anemia is characterized by decreased "normal" values for hemoglobin and hematocrit. The decrease begins at 3 to 5 months of gestation. Hemoglobin and hematocrit continue to fall until 5 to 8 months. They begin to rise at term and are normal by 6 weeks after delivery. In many pregnant women, a nutritional anemia develops along with the normal dilutional anemia. In the vast majority of cases, nutritional anemia is a consequence of inadequate iron intake. The hemoglobin levels of up to 40% of women who are not given supplemental iron drop below 11 g per dL. With iron supplementation, a hemoglobin level this low is uncommon. Nutritional megaloblastic anemia secondary to folate deficiency also occurs, but much less often.

Inadequate Weight Gain

The normal pattern of weight gain is a total of about 6 lb during the first trimester, followed by a relatively steady gain of almost a pound per week during the second and third trimesters. Inadequate weight gain (<2 lb per month during the second and third trimesters) is associated with low birth weight, intrauterine growth retardation, and fetal jeopardy. Failure of fetal growth frequently correlates with inadequate weight gain. Negative discrepancy in gestational age versus uterine size or in biparietal diameter of the fetal head as measured by sonography is signs of intrauterine growth retardation. Women with inadequate weight gain or actual weight loss should be evaluated. A careful diet history should be taken to determine if protein and calorie intake are adequate, and supplements should be given if needed.

Excessive Weight Gain

Rapid weight accumulation (>1.5 to 2 lb per week) is usually a sign of fluid retention. Fluid retention is associated with toxemia, although it does not cause toxemia. Not everyone who retains fluid becomes toxemic, and fluid retention in the absence of hypertension or proteinuria is not an indication for salt restriction or diuretic therapy. Women who retain fluid should be observed for other signs of toxemia. Edema in the lower extremities is commonly seen in the later stages of pregnancy; it is caused by the accumulation of interstitial fluid secondary to obstruction of the pelvic veins. The edema can be treated by elevating the legs and wearing support hose. Excessive weight gain during pregnancy may be caused by fat deposition rather than fluid retention. The consequences of excessive weight gain in pregnancy have been discussed earlier, and these should be assessed and managed according to accepted obstetrical practices.

GASTROINTESTINAL PROBLEMS IN PREGNANCY

Nausea and Vomiting

Nausea and vomiting are common in early pregnancy. Eating foods high in carbohydrate, such as crackers, bread, or dry cereal, before rising in the morning may help. Drinking liquids between meals should be encouraged. Fatty foods and caffeine should be avoided.

Constipation

Constipation is common in pregnancy and is caused by pressure of the enlarging uterus, hormonal changes, and iron supplements. Constipation can be treated with increased exercise, increased fluid intake, and either increased dietary fiber or the use of a supplemental psyllium or polycarbophil preparations.

Heartburn

Reflux esophagitis is common in pregnancy secondary to increased abdominal pressure caused by the enlarging uterus. Hormonal changes may loosen the lower esophageal sphincter. The initial approach is very similar to that used in nonpregnant patients with reflux esophagitis.

- Elevate the head of the bed four inches with bed blocks.
- Avoid eating within the two to three hours before retiring.
- Avoid alcohol, especially before retiring.
- Eat frequent small meals.
- Take antacids as needed. Be alert to their effects on iron absorption.

Nutrition During Lactation

Human milk is the optimal food for human infants (70–72). It contains a plethora of unique dietary components and host resistance factors that cannot be provided by conventional commercial formulas (70–72). Every authoritative source recommends that infants be exclusively breast-fed for the first 4 to 6 months of life and, preferably, continued for the first year of life in combination with appropriate complementary foods. Virtually all women in the United States are capable of breast-feeding their infants adequately. In 1993, a National Academy of Sciences expert panel extensively reviewed the nutritional needs during lactation (73).

Maternal nutritional status is not related to milk volume in the United States and other industrialized countries. Average milk volumes of 750 to 800 mL per day are comparable among thin, normal-weight, and obese women despite large differences in dietary intakes. Regular exercise also does not appear to affect milk volume. Milk volume is primarily regulated by infant demand and the nutritional quality of human milk is not usually affected adversely by modest deficiencies in maternal nutrition, even in those mothers who lose weight during lactation, although there is no consistent effect of breast-feeding on maternal body weight (71). Milk from frankly malnourished women may provide an infant with adequate calories, proteins, vitamins, and minerals, although not necessarily in the amounts provided by adequately nourished mothers. The levels of many nutrients in milk are maintained at the expense of maternal stores and maternal dietary intake does not dramatically alter the macronutrient contents of milk, although the type and amount of specific fatty acids (omega-3 fatty acids, for example) are strongly influenced by the nature of the maternal diet. Milk calcium, phosphorus, sodium, potassium, and magnesium contents are not altered by the maternal diet, although the levels of iodine and selenium in milk tend to parallel maternal intake. The concentrations of vitamins in human milk depend on the mother's stores and her current intake. However, within usual dietary intake levels, these differences are not generally practically important for the infant. The levels of pyridoxine and vitamins A, D, and B_{12} in milk are the most likely to decline as a result of sustained maternal malnutrition. Conversely, increasing maternal nutrient intakes above the RDA level usually does not result in correspondingly high nutrient levels in milk, with the exception of iodine, selenium, vitamin D, and pyridoxine. Thus, excessive maternal calorie intake is not only of no benefit to the infant, but consequent development of obesity can be an adverse effect in the mother. Further, there is substantial evidence that obesity itself impairs lactation performance (74).

NUTRIENT REQUIREMENTS DURING LACTATION

Nutritional requirements in lactation are largely set on the amount of calories and nutrients removed from maternal stores due to their net loss in human milk (produced in the amount of about 750 ml per day) plus the metabolic costs to the mother of producing the milk. In the first 4 to 5 months of life, the average, exclusively breast-fed infant gains about the same weight as the average fetus accrues during 9 months of term gestation. It is easy to appreciate, then, that the requirements for most nutrients consumed by a lactating mother exceed those for the pregnant woman. Thus, on average during the first 6 months postpartum, the total dietary energy requirements of a lactating woman are increased by about 500 kcal per day (71), but a lactating woman mobilizes about 170 kcal per day as energy stored in her body fat stores during pregnancy (71). Thus, the net EER of lactating women averages an additional 330 kcal per day above their non-pregnant, nonlactating energy requirement (i.e., +500 to 170 kcal).

Similarly, during lactation the RDAs for many nutrients, including vitamin A, vitamin E, thiamin, riboflavin, zinc, iodine, and selenium, are increased above those necessary during pregnancy (Table 3-4), as is the RDA for protein, which is set at 1.3 g/kg/day, largely on the basis of the amount of nitrogen lost in milk (14).

The lactating woman mobilizes calcium and phosphorus from her skeleton to supply milk with these minerals. There is no evidence that increasing dietary calcium or phosphorus intakes prevent this process (54). For this reason, the RDA for dietary calcium and phosphorus during lactation are identical to those of both pregnant and nonpregnant, nonlactating women (54) (Table 3-4). Likewise, iron requirements of the lactating mother are not significantly increased compared with the nonlactating woman (Table 3-4) because the amount of iron secreted into milk is less than that normally lost during menstruation. It is common obstetric practice, however, to prescribe an iron supplement.

During lactation, the RDA for folate is based principally on the extra amount of folate necessary to supply milk folate (50). Thus, the lactation daily RDA for folate (500 μg DFE) remains above that of the nonlactating woman (400 μg DFE), but is less than that of the pregnant woman (600 μg DFE) because the folate demands for new tissue synthesis are significantly greater during pregnancy (50,71) (Table 3-4). Likewise, the RDA for vitamin C and the other water-soluble B vitamins are increased somewhat to account for the maternal vitamins lost into her milk (71) (Table 3-4).

SPECIAL CONSIDERATIONS

Lactating women should be educated to obtain adequate nutrition from a well-balanced diet rather than through the use of nutritional supplements. Further, almost all women can breast-feed their infants successfully. Thus, a mother who is having problems with lactation should seek the professional help of individuals who have extensive experience helping women with these problems. Lactation counseling is widely and freely available throughout the nation, both from public (state and local government) and private sources. Trained lactation consultants will have the initials CLC (certified lactation consultant) or IBCLC (international board–certified lactation consultant) after their name. A directory of CLCs can be found at the website of the International Lactation Consultant Association (http://www.ilca.org), and extensive help with breast-feeding issues can be obtained from La Leche League International (http://www.llli.org).

Women with specialized dietary habits, such as strict vegans, should receive competent nutritional advice from trained professionals to ensure the adequate nutritional health of themselves and their infants during lactation. There is absolutely no reason to discourage breast-feeding in women with unique dietary patterns. Rather, appropriate educational advice should be provided to ensure she consumes adequate amounts of essential nutrients from acceptable foods. If necessary, dietary supplements can provide limiting nutrients.

As is the case for any human being, substance abuse and the use of illicit drugs should be actively discouraged in pregnant and lactating women as well. Perhaps it is more appropriate to say especially discouraged or absolutely contraindicated for the health and normal development of the fetus and infant. Addicted persons should be actively encouraged to enter appropriate treatment programs. Lactating women should not smoke. Besides the known long-term health risks, smoking reduces milk volume. Modest consumption of coffee and alcohol, less than one to two cups and one to two drinks daily, respectively, is not known to affect lactation or the health of the infant adversely.

Women with HIV/AIDS in developed, high-income countries like the United States should not breast-feed their infants when safe alternatives are available. Approximately 50% of HIV infections are transmitted to the infant at the end of pregnancy, and approximately 50% are transmitted after birth in breast-fed populations (75). In 2005, an estimated 280,000 to 360,000 infants were infected through breast-feeding (76). The rate of HIV transmission from mother to infant ranges from about 3 to 9 transmissions per 100 child years of breast-feeding, resulting in a cumulative probability of HIV transmission to infants breast-fed for 18 months on the order of 9% (77,78), with a rate that may be as high as 25% if breast-feeding is prolonged to 2 years of age (77,78). **In high-income countries where the risk of HIV transmission by breast-feeding is greater than the risk of alternative formula feeding, women infected with HIV should not breast-feed their infants and receive appropriate antiretroviral therapy. On the other hand, in less-well-developed, low-income countries where the formula-feeding risks due to unclean water and poor sanitation are greater than the risks of HIV transmission via breast-feeding, HIV–infected mothers should continue to breast-feed their infants, according to WHO guidelines, and receive appropriate antiretroviral therapy when available.**

A discussion of the breast-feeding issues and policies in high- and low-income countries can be found at http://www.avert.org/hiv-and-breastfeeding.htm.

REFERENCES

1. Gluckman PD, Hanson MA, Cooper C, et al. Effect of in utero and early-life conditions on adult health and disease. *N Engl J Med*. 2008;359:1.
2. Waterland RA, Michels KB. Epigenetic epidemiology of the developmental origins hypothesis. *Ann Rev Nutr*. 2007;27:363–388.
3. Duncan EJ, Gluckman PD, Dearden PK. Epigenetics, plasticity, and evolution: how do we link epigenetic change to phenotype? *J Exp Zool*. 2014;322B:208–220.
4. Alexander BT, Dasinger JH, Intapad S. Effect of low birth weight on women's health. *Clin Ther*. 2014 (in press).
5. Kelishadi R, Poursafa P. A review the genetic, environmental, and lifestyle aspects of the early-life origins of cardiovascular disease. *Curr Probl Pediatr Adolesc Health Care*. 2014;44:54–72.
6. Low FM, Gluckman PD, Hanson MA. Developmental plasticity and epigenetic mechanisms underpinning metabolic and cardiovascular diseases. *Epigenomics*. 2011;3:279–294.
7. Sellayah D, Cagampang FR, Cox RD. On the evolutionary origins of obesity: a new hypothesis. *Endocrinology*. 2014;155(5):1573–1588.
8. Dennison EM, Harvey NC, Cooper C. Programming of osteoporosis and impact on osteoporosis risk. *Clin Obstet Gynecol*. 2013;56:549–555.
9. Barouki R, Gluckman PD, Grandjean P, et al. Developmental origins of non-communicable disease: implications for research and public health. *Environ Health*. 2012;11:42.
10. Ojha S, Robinson L, Symonds ME, et al. Suboptimal maternal nutrition affects offspring health in adult life. *Early Hum Dev*. 2013;89:909–913.
11. American Academy of Pediatrics Committee on Nutrition. Butte NF. Nutrition During Pregnancy. In: Kleinman RE, ed. *Pediatric Nutrition Handbook*. 6th ed. Elk Grove Village, IL: American Academy of Pediatrics, 2009:249–273.
12. Butte NF, Wong WW, Treuth MS, et al. Energy requirements during pregnancy based on total energy expenditure and energy deposition. *Am J Clin Nutr*. 2004;79:1078–1087.
13. Food and Nutrition Board, Institute of Medicine, National Academy of Sciences. *Nutrition During Pregnancy*. Washington, DC: National Academy Press; 1990.
14. Food and Nutrition Board, Institute of Medicine, National Academy of Sciences. *Dietary Reference Intakes for Energy, Carbohydrate, Fiber, Fat, Fatty acids, Cholesterol, Protein, and Amino Acids*. Washington, DC: National Academy Press; 2005.
15. Hytten FE. Weight gain in pregnancy. In: Hytten FE, Chamberlain G, eds. *Clinical Physiology in Obstetrics*. Oxford, UK: Blackwell Scientific Publications; 1991:173–203.

16. King JC. Physiology of pregnancy and nutrient metabolism. *Am J Clin Nutr.* 2000;71:1218S–1225S.
17. O'Brien TE, Ray JG, Chan WS. Maternal body mass index and the risk of preeclampsia: a systematic overview. *Epidemiology.* 2003;14:368–374.
18. Duckitt K, Harrington D. Risk factors for pre-eclampsia at antenatal booking: systematic review of controlled studies. *Br Med J.* 2005;330(7491):549–550.
19. Wang Z, Wang P, Liu H, et al. Maternal adiposity as an independent risk factor for pre-eclampsia: a meta-analysis of prospective cohort studies. *Obes Rev.* 2013;14:508–521.
20. Masoura S, Kalogiannidis A, Gitas G, et al. Biomarkers in pre-eclampsia: a novel approach to early detection of the disease. *J Obstet Gynecol.* 2012;32:609–16.
21. Roberts JM, Bell MJ. If we know so much about preeclampsia, why haven't we cured the disease? *J Reprod Immunol.* 2013;99:1–9.
22. Rasmussen KM, Yaktine AL, eds; Committee to Reexamine IOM Pregnancy Weight Guidelines; Institute of Medicine; National Research Council. *Weight Gain During Pregnancy: Reexamining the Guidelines.* Washington, DC: National Academies Press, 2009. http://www.nap.edu/catalog.php?record_id=12584
23. Jain NJ, Denk CE, Kruse LK, et al. Maternal obesity: can pregnancy weight gain modify risk of selected adverse pregnancy outcomes? *Am J Perinatology.* 2007;24:291–298.
24. Quinlivan JA, Julania S, Lam L. Antenatal dietary interventions in obese pregnant women to restrict gestational weight gain to institute of medicine recommendations: a meta-analysis. *Obstet Gynecol.* 2011;118:1395–1401.
25. Nehring I, Schmoll S, Beyerlein A, et al. Gestational weight gain and long-term postpartum weight retention: a meta-analysis. *Am J Clin Nutr.* 2011;94:1225–1231.
26. Tie H-T, Xia Y-Y, Zeng Y-S, et al. Risk of childhood overweight or obesity associated with excessive weight gain during pregnancy: a meta-analysis. *Arch Gynecol Obstet.* 2014;289:247–257.
27. Turner RE. Nutrition during pregnancy. In: Shils ME, Shike M, Ross AC, et al, eds. *Modern Nutrition in Health and Disease.* 10th ed. Philadelphia, PA: Lippincott, Williams & Wilkins, 2006;771–782.
28. Allen LH. Maternal nutrient metabolism and requirements in pregnancy and lactation. In: Erdman JW, MacDonald IA, Zeisel SH, eds. *Present Knowledge in Nutrition.* 10th ed. Washington, DC: International Life Sciences Institute, 2012:608–623.
29. Institute of Medicine, National Academy of Sciences. *Dietary Reference Intakes: The Essential Guide to Nutrient Requirements.* Washington, DC: National Academy Press, 2006.
30. Food and Agriculture Organization of the United Nations/World Health Organization. *Requirements of Vitamin A, Iron, Folate and Vitamin B_{12}.* FAO Food and Nutrition Series No. 23. Rome: Food and Agriculture Organization of the United Nations, 1988:33–50.
31. Food and Nutrition Board, Institute of Medicine, National Academy of Sciences. *Dietary Reference Intakes for Energy for Vitamin A, Vitamin K, Arsenic, Boron, Chromium, Copper, Iodine, Iron, Manganese, Molybdenum, Nickel, Silicon, Vanadium and Zinc.* Washington, DC: National Academy Press, 2001.
32. WHO. *Guideline: Daily Iron and Folic Acid Supplementation in Pregnant Women.* Geneva: World Health Organization, 2012.
33. Peña-Rosas JP, De-Regil LM, Dowswell T, et al. Daily oral iron supplementation during pregnancy. *Cochrane Database Syst Rev.* 2012;12:CD004736.
34. Center for Disease and Prevention. CDC Recommendations to prevent and control iron deficiency in the United States. *MMWR Recomm Rep.* 1998;47:1–29.
35. Tamura T, Picciano M. Folate and human reproduction. *Am J Clin Nutr.* 2006;83:993–1016.
36. Hernández-Díaz S, Werler MM, Walker AM, et al. Folic acid antagonist during pregnancy and the risk of birth defects. *N Engl J Med.* 2000;343:1608–1614.
37. Kalter H. Folic acid and human malformations: a summary and evaluation. *Reprod Toxicol.* 2000;14:463–476.
38. Bailey LB, Berry RJ. Folic acid supplementation and the occurrence of congenital heart defects, orofacial clefts, multiple births, and miscarriage. *Am J Clin Nutr.* 2005;81:1213S–1217S.
39. De-Regil LM, Fernández-Gaxiola AC, Dowswell T, et al. Effects and safety of periconceptional folate supplementation for preventing birth defects. *Cochrane Database Syst Rev.* 2010;10:CD007950.
40. Castillo-Lancellotti C, Tur JA, Uauy R. Impact of folic acid fortification of flour on neural tube defects: a systematic review [Erratum in *Public Health Nutr.* 2013;16(8):1527]. *Public Health Nutr.* 2013;16(5):901–911.
41. Wallingford JB, Niswander LA, Shaw GM, et al. The continuing challenge of understanding, preventing, and treating neural tube defects. *Science.* 2013;339:1222002.
42. Wang XW, Luo YL, Wang W, et al. Association between MTHFR A 1298C polymorphism and neural tube defect susceptibility: a metaanalysis. *Am J Obstet Gynecol.* 2012;206(3):251.e1–251.e7.

43. Zhang T, Lou J, Zhong R, et al. Genetic variants in the folate pathway and the risk of neural tube defects: a meta-analysis of the published literature. *PLoS One*. 2013;8(4):e59570.
44. Yadav U, Kumar P, Yadav SK, et al. Polymorphisms in folate metabolism genes as maternal risk factor for neural tube defects: an updated meta-analysis [Epub ahead of print]. *Metab Brain Dis*. 2014.
45. Center for Disease and Prevention. Recommendations for the use of folic acid to reduce the number of cases of spina bifida and other neural tube defects. *MMWR Recomm Rep*. 1991;41:1.
46. Federal Register. *Food Standards: Amendment of the Standards of Identity for Enriched Grain Products to Require Addition of Folic Acid*. Final rule. (Codified at 21 CFR parts 136, 137, and 139). Washington, DC: Food and Drug Administration, 1996;61:8781.
47. Crider KS, Bailey LB, Berry RJ. Folic acid food fortification—its history, effect, concerns, and future directions. *Nutrients*. 2011;3:370–384.
48. Pfeiffer CM, Hughes JP, Lacher DA, et al. Estimation of trends in serum and RBC folate in the U.S. population from pre- to postfortification using assay-adjusted data from the NHANES 1988-2010. *J Nutr*. 2012;142(5):886–893.
49. Qi YP, Do AN, Hamner HC, et al. The prevalence of low serum vitamin B-12 status in the absence of anemia or macrocytosis did not increase among older U.S. adults after mandatory folic acid fortification. *J Nutr*. 2014;144(2):170–176.
50. Institute of Medicine, National Academy of Sciences. Folate. In: *Dietary Reference Intakes for Thiamin, Riboflavin, Niacin, Vitamin B_6, Folate Vitamin B_{12}, Pantothenic Acid, Biotin and Choline*. Washington, DC: National Academy Press, 2006.
51. Suitor CW, Bailey LB. Dietary folate equivalents: interpretation and application. *J Am Diet Assoc*. 2000;100:88–94.
52. Bailey LB. New standard for dietary folate intake in pregnant women. *Am J Clin Nutr*. 2000;71:1304S–1307S.
53. Bailey LB. Folate and vitamin B_{12} recommended intakes and status in the United States. *Nutr Rev*. 2004:62:S14–S20.
54. Food and Nutrition Board, Institute of Medicine, National Academy of Sciences. *Dietary Reference Intakes for Calcium and Vitamin D*. Washington, DC: National Academy Press; 2011.
55. Food and Nutrition Board, Institute of Medicine, National Academy of Sciences. *Dietary Reference Intakes for Calcium, Phosphorus, Magnesium, Vitamin D and Fluoride*. Washington, DC: National Academy Press; 1997.
56. Hollis BW. Circulating 25-hydroxyvitamin D levels indicative of vitamin D sufficiency: implications for establishing a new effective dietary intake recommendations for vitamin D. *J Nutr*. 2005;135:317–322.
57. Holick MF. High prevalence of vitamin D inadequacy and implications for health. *Mayo Clinic Proc*. 2006;81:353–373.
58. Brouwer-Brolsma EM, Bischoff-Ferrari HA, Bouillon R, et al. Vitamin D: do we get enough? a discussion between vitamin D experts in order to make a step towards the harmonisation of dietary reference intakes for vitamin D across Europe. *Osteoporosis Int*. 2013;24(5):1567–1577.
59. Pramyothin P, Holick MF. Vitamin D supplementation: guidelines and evidence for subclinical deficiency. *Curr Opin Gastroenterol*. 2012;28(2):139–150.
60. Hollis BW, Wagner CL. Assessment of dietary vitamin D requirements during pregnancy and lactation. *Am J Clin Nutr*. 2004;79:717–726.
61. Kovacs CS. Vitamin D in pregnancy and lactations: maternal, fetal, and neonatal outcomes from human and animal studies. *Am J Clin Nutr*. 2008;88(Suppl):520S–528S.
62. Food and Nutrition Board, Institute of Medicine, National Academy of Sciences. *Dietary Reference Intakes for Vitamin C, Vitamin E, Selenium, and Carotenoids*. Washington, DC: National Academy Press, 2000.
63. Lammer EJ, Chen DT, Hoar RM, et al. Retinoic acid embryopathy. *N Engl J Med*. 1985; 313:837–841.
64. Brown HL, Graves CR. Smoking and marijuana use in pregnancy. *Clin Obstet Gynecol*. 2013;56(1):107–113.
65. Leonardi-Bee J, Smyth A, Britton J, et al. Environmental tobacco smoke and fetal health: systematic review and meta-analysis. *Arch Dis Child Fetal Neonatal Ed*. 2008;93:F351–F361.
66. Mitchell EA, Milerad J. Smoking and the sudden infant death syndrome. *Rev Environ Health*. 2006;21(2):81–103.
67. Zhang K, Wang X. Maternal smoking and increased risk of sudden infant death syndrome: a meta-analysis. *Leg Med (Tokyo)*. 2013;15(3):115–121.

68. Centers for Disease Control and Prevention. *Maternal and Infant Health: Smoking During Pregnancy.* http://www.cdc.gov/reproductivehealth/MaternalInfantHealth/related/SmokingPregnancy.htm
69. Flak AL, Su S, Bertrand J, et al. The association of mild, oderate, and binge prenatal alcohol exposure and child neuropsychological outcomes: a meta-analysis. *Alcohol Clin Exp Res.* 2014;38(1):214–226.
70. American Academy of Pediatrics Committee on Nutrition. Breastfeeding. In: Kleinman RE, Greer FR, eds. *Pediatric Nutrition.* 7th ed. Elk Grove Village: American Academy of Pediatrics, 2013: 41–60.
71. Butte NF. Maternal nutrition during lactation. In: Kaplan SL, Stapleton FB, eds. *UpToDate Pediatrics.* Wolters Kluwer, 2014.
72. O'Connor DL, Picciano MF. Lactation. In: Ross AC, Caballero B, Cousins RJ, et al, eds. *Modern Nutrition in Health and Disease.* 11th ed. Philadelphia, PA: Wolters Kluwer/LippincottWilliams & Wilkins; 2014:698–711.
73. Committee on Nutritional Status During Pregnancy and Lactation, Food and Nutrition Board, Institute of Medicine, National Academy of Sciences. *Nutrition During Lactation.* Washington, DC: National Academy Press, 1993.
74. Rasmussen KM. Association of maternal obesity before conception with poor lactation performance. *Ann Rev Nutr.* 2007;27:103–121.
75. Kourtis AP, Lee FK, Abrams EJ, et al. Mother-to-child transmission of HIV-1: timing and implications for prevention. *Lancet Infect Dis.* 2006;6:726–732.
76. Coovadia HM, Rollins NC, Bland RM, et al. Mother-to-child transmission of HIV-1 infection during exclusive breastfeeding in the first 6 months of life: an intervention cohort study. *Lancet.* 2007;369:1107–1116.
77. The Breastfeeding and HIV International Transmission Study Group. Late postnatal transmission of HIV-1 in breast-fed children: an individual data meta-analysis. *J Infect Dis.* 2004;189:2154–2166.
78. De Cock KM, Fowler MG, Mercier E, et al. Prevention of mother-to-child HIV transmission in resource-poor countries. *JAMA.* 2000;283:1175–1182.

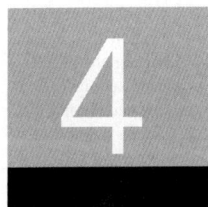

Approach to Nutrient Deficiency

The medical use of nutrients to rectify states of deficiency depends on an appropriate knowledge base. This chapter outlines some general areas that involve both macronutrients (energy, protein, lipids) and micronutrients (vitamins, minerals). The subjects covered include (a) definitions of the nutrient requirement, (b) the concept of dietary goals and guidelines, along with food composition and preparation, (c) the role of food supplements, additive, and fortification, (d) the assessment and identification of general and individual nutrient deficiency, (e) the concept of subclinical nutrient deficiency, (f) the concept of diet therapy, (g) the relationship of food and individual nutrients with drug absorption (and vice versa), and (h) the interpretation and use of nutritional data in translating to clinical practice. Subsequent chapters expand on many of these topics in more detail, and the reader is referred to these chapters when appropriate. This discussion is not meant to include all possible variants on these themes but rather highlights some common examples.

DEFINITIONS OF NUTRIENT SUFFICIENCY
Recommended Dietary Allowance

The recommended dietary allowance (RDA) for many years was the most widely publicized of the definitions of nutrient sufficiency in the United States. It was based on available scientific knowledge and deliberation by experts, and was approved by the Food and Nutrition Board of the National Academy of Sciences Committee on Dietary Allowances. The RDA outlined the levels of intake of essential nutrients judged to be adequate to meet the known nutritional needs of practically all healthy persons. The RDA is currently defined as the average daily dietary nutrient level sufficient to meet the requirement of nearly all (97% to 98%) healthy individuals in a particular gender and life stage group, and so exceeded the requirements of most persons. It is important to remember that the RDA cannot be relied on for a precise estimate of the needs of patients with medical illness, particularly if malabsorption is present. The RDA was revised most recently in 1989. Values quite similar to the RDA have been developed for the basal requirements of the inhabitants of many other countries (1,2).

Nonetheless, these guidelines have been deemed insufficient for many reasons. New understanding has been acquired of nutrient requirements and of the role of food components in reducing the risk for chronic diseases (e.g., cancer, heart disease, and osteoporosis) and preventing classic deficiency syndromes. RDAs were previously developed with only the latter goal in mind. Moreover, RDAs were formerly based on the assumption that all nutrients are derived from natural foods; currently, however, dietary tablets, fortified foods, and food supplements are important sources of some nutrients. Thus, the governments of the United States and Canada together have formulated the dietary reference intake (DRI; see Appendix B).

Dietary Reference Intake

DRI is now a collective term that includes the estimated average requirement (EAR), RDA, adequate intake (AI), and tolerable upper intake level (UL). The DRI has replaced the RDA. It is the undertaking of the Standing Committee on the Scientific Evaluation of Dietary Reference Intakes of the Food and Nutrition Board, Institute of Medicine, National Academy of Sciences (www.nas.edu), in collaboration with Health Canada. It has been developed for 12 life stages, and many volumes have appeared thus far, six covering the nutrients themselves: calcium, vitamin D, magnesium, and phosphorus (3); the B vitamins niacin, biotin, and choline (4); antioxidant micronutrients, including vitamins C and E, selenium, and carotenoids (5); vitamins A and K, iron, zinc, and trace minerals (6); water, potassium, chloride, and sulfate (7); and energy, carbohydrate, fiber, fat, fatty acids, cholesterol, protein, and amino acids (8). Other volumes published by the National Academy Press (http://www.nap.edu) cover guiding principles of nutrition labeling and fortification, applications in dietary planning, applications in dietary assessment, proposed definition of dietary fiber, proposed definition and plan for review of dietary antioxidants and related compounds, risk assessment method for establishing ULs for nutrients, research methods to assess dietary intake in child day care, a volume on DRI for calcium and vitamin D only, the development of DRIs, and a volume on the human microbiome, diet, and health. The Tufts Evidence-based Practice Center at the request of the United States and Canadian sponsors of the DRIs performed a systematic review of the DRI process (9). The Center identified several key issues, that is, the selection of critical health outcomes, documentation of the limitations of relying on existing systematic reviews, the translation of results from studies not designed to address issues relevant to establishing DRIs, and the need to develop quality assessment tools to aid in decision making for DRIs.

The EAR is the daily intake value estimated to meet the requirements of 50% of persons in a normal life stage and gender group. It is used to set the RDA and plan recommendations for intake in various groups. The RDA is the intake level sufficient to meet the daily requirements of most people in a specific life stage and gender group and is set at two standard deviations above the EAR. This estimate also includes a coefficient of variation of 10% if the data do not permit the calculation of standard deviations. If not enough data are available to calculate an EAR, AI is used. AI is based on approximations of average nutrient intake by an age- or gender-defined subgroup. The tolerable UL is the maximum amount of a daily nutrient intake that is unlikely to pose a health threat for persons within an age and gender subgroup. This term was deemed important because so many nutrients are now ingested from supplements at levels far exceeding those possible in the diet. Compromises within the DRI recommendation must be made, both because these values are often not precisely known and because the new recommendation may be used to prevent onset of disease (e.g., fracture risk) rather than clinical deficiency (rickets). Table 4-1 outlines some of the suggested population-based reference intakes that have been recommended to prevent cancer and heart disease, and those levels recommended by the World Health Organization (WHO) and the Commission of

TABLE 4-1 Population Reference Intakes/Guidelines of Dietary Constituents for Prevention of Chronic Diseases in Adults, Aged 20–50

	WCRF[a]	WHO[b]	AHA[c]	PRI/goal[d]
Constituent Macronutrients				
CHO (% kcal)	55–75	55–75	55–60	45–55
Starch (%)	50–70	50–70	55–60	—
Sugar, nonmilk (%)	<10	<10	Low	10
Insoluble fiber (g/day)	20–35	16–24	20–25	39
Fats (% kcal)	15–30	15–30	≤30	20–30
Polyunsaturated	2–10	3–7	≤10	2.5
Monounsaturated	3–10	—	≤15	—
Saturated	0–10	<10	<7	10
Cholesterol (mg/day)	100–130	<300	<300	—
Protein (% kcal)	9–12	10–15	—	—
Vegetable	6–12	—	—	—
Animal	0–3	—	—	—
Alcohol (% kcal)	<2	—	<2 oz	—
Micronutrients				
Carotenoids (mg/day)	9–18	—	—	—
Vitamin C (mg/day)	175–400	30	—	40–45
Folate (µg/day)	250–450	200	—	200
Vitamin D (µg/day)	0 (sun)–10	2.5	—	20
Vitamin E (mg/day)	4–7	—	—	<4
Calcium (mg/day)	500–750	400–500	—	700
Selenium (µg/day)	75–125	30–40	—	55
Iodine (µg/day)	125–150	120–150	—	130
Iron (mg/day)	15–25	16	—	8–20
Potassium (g/day)	1.6–3.2	—	—	3.1
Sodium (g/day)	<4	<4	1.5 g	0.58–3.5
Zinc (mg/day)	11–13	7.1–9.5	—	7.1–14

[a]WCRF (World Cancer Research Fund/American Institute for Cancer Research). *Food, Nutrition, and the Prevention of Cancer: A Global Perspective.* Washington, DC: WCRF/AICR, 1997. Provides estimates of probable range of dietary constituents consumed as a result of following recommendations of the report.
[b]Diet, Nutrition, and the prevention of Chronic Disease. WHO (World Health Organization), 1990. http://whqlibdoc.who.int/trs/WHO_TRS_797_(part1).pdf?ua=1
[c]Lichtenstein AH, Appel LJ, Brands M, et al; American Heart Association Nutrition Committee. Diet and lifestyle recommendations revision 2006. *Circulation.* 2006;114:82–96. 2012 guidelines summarized in http://www.heart.org/HEARTORG/GettingHealthy/NutritionCenter/HealthyDietGoals/Healthy-Diet-Goals_UCM_310436_SubHomePage.jsp.
[d]PRI/goal, population reference intake ranges (female–male) for young European adults (aged 19 to 50), Commission of the European Community. *Report of the Scientific Commission for Food (31st Series): Nutrient and Energy Intakes.* Luxembourg: Office for Official Publications of the European Communities, 1993, or ultimate European goals (James WPT. *Healthy Nutrition.* European series 24. Copenhagen, Denmark: WHO Regional Office for Europe, 1988). Brouwer-Brolsma EM, Bischoff-Ferrari HA, Bouillon R, et al. Vitamin D, do we get enough? *Osteoporos Int.* 2013;24:1567–1577; Doets EL, Cavelaars AE, Dhonukshe-Rutten RA, et al. Explaining the variability in recommended intakes of folate, vitamin B12, iron and zinc for adults and elderly people. *Public Health Nutr.* 2012;15:906–915.

the European Community for young, healthy adults. It takes many years to develop new guidelines, and the American Heart Association is the only one with relatively recent published modifications.

Daily Reference Values

The RDAs were standards set by the U.S. Food and Drug Administration (FDA) in 1973 for purposes of food labeling. *Daily value* and *percent daily value* are the current reference terms on the nutrition label. The term *daily value* encompasses two sets of reference values: daily reference values (DRVs) and the old reference daily intakes (RDIs), now called *DRIs*. DRVs are provided for total and saturated fat, cholesterol, total carbohydrates, dietary fiber, sodium, potassium, and protein. They are based on current nutritional recommendations for adults and children aged 4 or older. RDIs are the same as the current US RDAs for 19 vitamins and minerals. The terms DRV and RDI do not appear on the nutrition label. What do appear are daily values, reflecting DRVs and RDIs for a 2,000-cal reference diet (Table 4-2). (see http://iom.edu/Activities/

TABLE 4-2 Daily Values for Adults and Children Aged 4 or Older

Food Component	Daily Value[a]	Percentage of Total Caloric Intake
Total fat	65 g[b]	30
Saturated fat	20 g[b]	10
Cholesterol	300 mg	—
Sodium	2,400 mg	—
Potassium	3,500 mg	—
Chloride	3,400 mg	—
Total carbohydrate	300 g[b]	60
Dietary fiber	25 g[c]	—
Protein	50 g[b]	10
Vitamin A	5,000 IU	—
Vitamin C	60 mg	—
Calcium	1 g	—
Iron	18 mg	—
Vitamin D	400 IU	—
Vitamin E	30 IU	—
Vitamin K	80 µg	—
Thiamine	1.5 mg	—
Riboflavin	1.7 mg	—
Niacin	20 mg	—
Vitamin B_6	2.0 mg	—
Folate	0.4 mg	—
Vitamin B_{12}	6.0 µg	—
Biotin	0.3 mg	—
Pantothenic acid	10 mg	—
Phosphorus	1 g	—
Chromium	120 µg	—
Iodine	150 µg	—
Magnesium	400 mg	—
Manganese	2 mg	—
Selenium	70 µg	—
Zinc	15 mg	—
Copper	2.0 mg	—
Molybdenum	75 µg	—
Chloride	3.4 g	—

[a]Based on daily reference values and reference daily intakes.
[b]Daily value based on a 2,000-cal reference diet.
[c]Daily value based on 12.5 g/1,000 cal.
From http://www.fda.gov/Food/GuidanceComplianceRegulatoryInformation/GuidanceDocuments/FoodLabelingNutrition/FoodLabelingGuide/ucom064928.htm.

Nutrition/SummaryDRIs/~/media/Files/Activity%20Files/Nutrition/DRIs/5_Summary%20
TTable%20Tables%201-4.pdf for summary DRI Tables.)

Reference Weights
Reference weights and heights are used when the average values provided by age and life stage categories are not appropriate and more specific information is needed. Because overweight and obesity are so prevalent, the older reference values based on the Third National Health and Nutrition Examination Survey (NHANES III) in the United States have been updated (8). Table 4-3 shows the old and newer body mass index (BMI) calculated from available reference data for children and young adults.

Estimated Adequate Intake for Healthy Persons
For some nutrients (Na, Cl, K), the daily requirements appear to be much lower than the content in an average US diet. Thus, the concept of RDA is replaced by that of an AI (Table 4-4). For other nutrients also, the information is insufficient for EAR to be calculated and actual recommendations to be made. These nutrients include vitamin K, biotin, calcium, chromium, fluoride, and manganese. AI is also used to estimate the needs of children for most nutrients (see Appendix B for details). Many vitamins and minerals have been reported to cause toxicity when taken in excess (Table 4-5). This concern is the major reason for the newer concept of UL recommendations

TABLE 4-3 Reference BMI for Children and Adults in the United States

Male (y)	Median BMI (kg/m²)	Female (y)	Median BMI (kg/m²)
4–8	15.3	4–8	15.3
9–13	17.2	9–13	17.4
14–18	20.5	14–18	20.4
19–30[a]	22.5	19–30	21.5

[a]Because no evidence indicates that weights should change with aging, provided that activity is maintained, the reference weights of this group are applicable to all adults.
Data are taken from male and female median BMI from the Centers for Disease Control and Prevention/National Center for Health Statistics growth charts, adapted from *Dietary Reference Intakes: Guiding Principles for Nutrition Labeling and Fortification.* Washington, DC: National Academies Press, 2003:75.

TABLE 4-4 Estimated AI for Healthy Persons for Sodium, Chloride, and Potassium

Age	Weight (kg)	Weight (lb)	Sodium (g/day)	Chloride (g/day)	Potassium (g/day)
Up to 6 mo	4.5	10	0.12	0.18	0.4
7–12 mo	8.9	20	0.37	0.57	0.7
1–3 y			1.0	1.5	3.0
4–8 y			1.2	1.9	3.8
9–13 y			1.5400	2.3	4.5
14–18 y			1.5	2.3	4.7
19–50 y	70	154	1.5	2.3	4.7
51–70 y			1.3	2.0	4.7
>70 y			1.3	1.8	4.7

Data from the Standing Committee on the Scientific Evaluation of Dietary Reference Intakes, Food and Nutrition Board, Institute of Medicine. *Dietary Reference Intakes for Water, Potassium, Sodium, Chloride, and Sulfate.* Washington, DC: National Academies Press, 2005; Standing Committee on the Scientific Evaluation of Dietary Reference Intakes, Food and Nutrition Board, Institute of Medicine. *Dietary Reference Intakes for Energy, Carbohydrate, Fiber, Fat, Fatty acids, Cholesterol, Protein, and Amino Acids.* Washington, DC: National Academies Press, 2005.

TABLE 4-5 Vitamin and Mineral Toxicity

Nutrient	Symptoms of Toxicity	Minimal Intake
Vitamin B_1	Headache, irritability, insomnia	Probably >50 mg/day
	Fast heart rate, weakness, occasional severe allergic reaction (anaphylaxis)	
Vitamin B_2	Yellow-orange color of urine	Safe up to 10 mg/day
Vitamin B_6	Peripheral sensory neuropathy (numbness)	2–6 g/day
Niacin	Flushing, burning of hands and face	>1 g/day
	Nausea, vomiting, diarrhea, abnormal heart rhythm, exacerbation of gout, rash, itching, glucose intolerance, abnormal liver blood chemistries	>3 g/day
Folate	Convulsions if on phenytoin (Dilantin)	>40 mg
	In pregnancy can compete with Zn and Fe for absorption, rare allergy (rash, itching, fever, wheezing)	
Vitamin B_{12}	None	
Vitamin C	False-positive sugar in urine, false low sugar in blood, false-negative test for blood in stool, diarrhea	2–6 g/day
	Dental erosions, increased oxalate, kidney stones, interference with anticoagulation from warfarin (Coumadin)	4–9 g/day
Biotin	None	
Pantothenic acid	Diarrhea	10–20 mg/day
Vitamin A	Nausea, vomiting, skin desquamation	50,000–100,000 IU/day
	Fatigue, hair loss, bone pain, anorexia, irritability	Chronic ingestion
	Vomiting, bulging fontanelles, growth failure, optic atrophy, sixth nerve palsy	>4,000 IU/kg/day
	Newborn microcephaly, dilated ventricles	15,000 IU/day if taken between 14 and 40 days of gestation
Vitamin D	Increased calcium in blood and urine, nausea, anorexia, itching, increased urine, thirst, abdominal pain, constipation, bone pain, kidney stones, weight loss, pancreatitis, hypertension, abnormal heart rhythm	>1,000 IU/day in nongrowing adults, depends on Ca intake
Vitamin E	Any symptoms, occasional weakness, fatigue, hypertension, nausea, increased effect of warfarin (Coumadin)	800–900 IU/day
Vitamin K	Jaundice in newborn	>10 mg/day to infant or pregnant mother
Na	Edema	If retaining sodium (heart, liver disease)
	Confusion	If very excessive intake
K	Weakness, confusion, abnormal heart rhythm	If renal function low and 50–100 mEq/day in supplements, drugs
Ca	Nausea, vomiting, weakness, constipation, dry mouth, increased urine, abnormal heart rhythm, kidney stones	Especially if vitamin D >400 IU/day and supplement >1–2 g/day
Mg	Nausea, vomiting, hypertension, drowsiness	If renal function low and Mg given IV
P	Symptoms not related to low calcium	Only in renal failure

TABLE 4-5 Vitamin and Mineral Toxicity *(continued)*

Nutrient	Symptoms of Toxicity	Minimal Intake
Fe	Nausea, vomiting, diarrhea, abdominal pain	>20 mg/kg/day
Zn	Copper deficiency (anemia), decreased immune function, nausea, vomiting, rash, dehydration, gastric ulceration	>450 mg/day
Cu	Nausea, vomiting, diarrhea, cramps	>15 mg/day
I	Decreased thyroid function	>2,000 µg/day
F	Spine and muscle pain, weakness	20–80 mg/day
Mn	None	Up to 10 mg/day
Cr	None recognized	
Se	Hair and nail loss, skin lesions, tooth decay	>5 mg/day
	Nausea, vomiting, fatigue, hair loss, diarrhea, irritability	>20 mg/day

Compiled from Standing Committee on the Scientific Evaluation of Dietary Reference Intakes, Food and Nutrition Board, Institute of Medicine. *Dietary Reference Intakes for Calcium, Phosphorus, Magnesium, Vitamin D, and Fluoride.* Washington, DC: National Academies Press, 1997; Standing Committee on the Scientific Evaluation of Dietary Reference Intakes, Food and Nutrition Board, Institute of Medicine. *Dietary Reference Intakes for Thiamin, Riboflavin, Niacin, Vitamin B_6, Folate, Vitamin B_{12}, Pantothenic Acid, Biotin, and Choline.* Washington, DC: National Academies Press, 2000; Standing Committee on the Scientific Evaluation of Dietary Reference Intakes, Food and Nutrition Board, Institute of Medicine. *Dietary Reference Intakes for Vitamin E, Vitamin C, Selenium, and Carotenoids.* Washington, DC: National Academies Press, 2000; Standing Committee on the Scientific Evaluation of Dietary Reference Intakes, Food and Nutrition Board, Institute of Medicine. *Dietary Reference Intakes for Vitamin A, Vitamin K, Arsenic, Boron, Chromium, Copper, Iodine, Iron, Manganese, Molybdenum, Nickel, Silicon, Vanadium, and Zinc.* Washington, DC: National Academies Press, 2001.

(see Appendix B). Most cases of nutrient toxicity are associated with supplementation, not food intake. Estimated toxic levels range from as low as 5 times (selenium) to 25–50 times (folate, vitamins C and E) the recommended dietary intake. The best-documented toxicities from nutrients involve vitamins A, B_3 (niacin), B_6, and D, iron, and selenium. Besides direct toxicity, significant problems can arise when high doses of some nutrients interact with other nutrients. For example, high doses of calcium can interfere with iron absorption, high doses of zinc can impair copper absorption, and high doses of vitamin E can impair vitamin K action.

DIETARY GUIDELINES AND FOOD COMPOSITION
Guidelines

Based in part on the nutritional assessments listed above, guidelines have been developed for average normal persons and to prevent chronic diseases (Tables 4-1 and 4-6; see also Chapter 1). These guidelines generally advise that a normal weight be achieved and maintained. In addition, total fat intake should be limited to about 30% of calories, cholesterol intake decreased, intake of complex carbohydrates and fiber increased, excess intake of salt avoided, and alcohol ingested only in moderation.

The *U.S. Dietary Guidelines for Americans (DGAs)*, 2005 (10) emerged from a scientific analysis conducted by the Dietary Guidelines Advisory Committee (DGAC) appointed by the U.S. Department of Health and Human Services and the U.S. Department of Agriculture (USDA) (www.health.govdietary guidelines/dga2005/report/). The recommendations in the Dietary Guidelines are for Americans over age 2, and are written to be flexible enough to include food preferences for different racial, ethnic, and vegetarian groups. The key recommendations have been limited to those that reflect generally agreed-upon scientific evidence. Thus, they are not quite as specific as earlier versions of the Dietary Guidelines.

The DGAs are revised every 5 years. The 2010 revision is a response to focus group sessions and food marketing strategies, and as a result is based on two concepts: (a) to maintain caloric balance over time that achieves and sustains healthy weight and (b) to focus on decreasing consumption of nutrient-dense foods and beverages (11). The key recommendations are listed in

Chapter 12 (Table 12-6), along with the translation of these recommendations to MyPlate, the online successor to MyPyramid, that allow individuals to develop their own dietary program.

Food Composition

Practical application of the dietary guidelines is based on knowledge of food composition. Many guides are available, some of which are listed in Table 4-6. These sources differ in the type of information offered. All cover most vitamins and minerals and macronutrients (water, proteins, lipids, and carbohydrate, including total or crude fiber). McCance and Widdowson (Table 4-6) also cover total dietary fiber, oligosaccharides, selenium, manganese, iodine, nonstarch polysaccharides, and fatty acids for every food. All these sources list the nutrient contents of foods by different food groups (fats and oils, meats, nuts, legumes). Each source can be valuable depending on the clinical need.

The USDA produces a regularly updated Home & Garden bulletin of the *Nutritive Value of Foods*. More details can be found in the USDA *National Database for Standard Reference-release 18*, available on the internet at www.ars.usda.gov/services/. Table 4-7 lists some general sources of information on nutrition available on the internet. A Food Composition Resource List for Professionals has been updated to 2009 by the USDA Food and Nutrition Information Center, www.nal.usda.gov/fnic/pubs/bibs/gen/foodcomp.pdf. This contains links to general databases, special interest databases, international food composition resources, books and other publications, conference proceedings, journals and newsletters, selected journals, and nutrient content of foods. Additional lists of food tables, food composition organizations, and journals are offered by the Arbor Nutrition Guide, http://arborcom.com/frame/food_comp.htm.

Food Processing

The data included in the *Nutritive Value of Foods* document the differences in the composition of raw and processed foods, but the enormous variety of changes that occur during processing

TABLE 4-6 Selected Food Composition Guides

Authors	Title	Year, edition	Publisher
Pennington JAT, Spungen JS	Bowes & Church, Food Values of Portions Commonly Used	2009, 19th	Lippincott Williams & Wilkins
McCance and Widdowson	The Composition of Foods	7th available late 2013	Institute of Food Research (IFR)
Souci SW, Fachmann W, Kraut H	Food Composition and Nutrition Tables	2008, 7th	CRC Press
USDA, Human Nutrition Information Service	Nutritive Value of Foods (Home & Garden Bull No.72) (HG-72 in pdf)	October 2002	U.S. Government Printing Office www.ars.usda.gov
USDA	USDA National Nutrient Database for Standard Reference	2011, release 25	www.ars.usda.gov/services/doc.htm?docid=8964
American Dietetic Association	Manual of Clinical Dietetics	2000, 6th	American Dietetic
Nelson J, Moxness KE, Gastineau CF, Jenson MD	Mayo Clinic Diet Manual	1994, 7th	Mosby-Year Book
Duyff RL	ADA Complete Food and Nutrition Guide	2012, 3rd	American Dietetic Association
31 European Countries	Food Composition Databases	Various	EuroFIR www.eurofir.nte/Food_information/Food_composition.databases

TABLE 4-7 Nutrition-Related Internet Sites

Organization	Internet Address
American Council on Science and Health (consumer education consortium)	www.acsh.org/nutrition/index.html
American Dietetic Association	www.eatright.org
American Heart Association	www.americanheart.org
American Society for Nutrition	www.asnutrition.org
American Society for Parenteral and Enteral Nutrition	www.clinnutr.org
Council for Responsible Nutrition (trade organization for supplement industry)	www.crnusa.org
Department of Agriculture/Agriculture Research Service	www.ars.usda.gov
Dietary Guidelines for Americans, 2005	www.health.gov/dietaryguidelines/dga2005/
Food and Drug Administration	www.fda.gov
Food and Nutrition Information Center	www.nal.usda.gov/fnic
FNIC Food Supplements	www.nal.usda.gov/fnic/IBIDS
FDA, Center for Food Safety and Applied Nutrition	www.cfsan.fda.gov
FDA, *Report Adverse Effects of Supplements*	www.fda.gov/medwatch/
Healthcare professionals	report/hcp.htm
Consumers	report/consumer/consumer.htm
International Food Information Council	foodinside.org
National Center for Complementary and Alternative Medicine	nccam.nih.gov
National Health Information Center	nhic-nt.health.org
NIH Office of Dietary Supplements	ods.od.nih.gov
National Products Alert Database, University of Illinois	pcog8.pmmp.uic.edu/mcp/nap1.html
Office of Dietary Supplements	dietary-supplements.info.nih.gov
Office of Disease Prevention & Health Promotion	odphp.osophs.dhhs.gov
USDA, Dietary Guidelines Advisory Commission	www.usda.gov/dgac
United States Pharmacopeia	www.usp.org
World Health Organization/Food & Agriculture Organization	www.fao.org

cannot be covered. Foods are affected by the type of processing (freezing, canning, concentration), the length of the processing procedure, during which nutrients can be lost or inactivated, and the effects of storage. The factors most likely to render nutrients unstable in food are heating, oxidation, and pH (Table 4-8).

Most processed foods are usually less stable than dry foods because of a lesser degree of oxidation and the possibility of microbial contamination. Fresh produce must be kept moist to prevent wilting and loss of nutrients through cell damage. In modern practice, the characteristics of a controlled environment maintained to retard ripening (as for apples, pears, tomatoes) can play a major role in nutrient stability. The percentage of nutrients lost can be significant, and also varies for enriched versus unenriched foods. Examples are given in Table 4-9 from the tables of the USDA. The USDA periodically updates its Table of Nutrient Retention Factors, calculated by the True Retention Method (%TR), requiring data on the content of nutrient of raw and cooked food. The most recent table, release 6 (2007), includes data on 16 minerals and vitamins, including lycopene and choline (12).

Other specific examples of the effects of food processing are provided in Chapters 6 and 7 in the sections on individual vitamins and minerals. For the most part, water-soluble vitamins and minerals are lost when foods are boiled and are better preserved when foods are broiled, sautéed, or steamed.

TABLE 4-8 Factors Rendering Nutrients Unstable (U) in Foods or Having Little Effect (S)

Nutrients	Heat	Oxygen or Air	Light	pH Acid	pH Neutral	pH Alkaline	Moisture[a]
vitamins							
Vitamin A or carotenes	U	U	U	U	S	S	U
Ascorbate (C)	U	U	U	S	U	U	U
Biotin	U	S	S	S	S	S	—
Choline	S	U	S	S	S	S	—
Cobalamin (B_{12})	S	U	U	S	S	S	—
Vitamin D	U	U	U	S	S	U	U
Folic acid	U	U	U	U	U	S	—
Inositol	U	S	S	S	S	S	—
Vitamin K	S	S	U	U	S	U	—
Niacin	S	S	S	S	S	S	—
Pantothenate	U	S	S	S	S	U	—
Pyridoxine (B_6)	U	S	U	S	S	S	—
Riboflavin	U	S	U	S	S	U	U
Thiamine	U	U	S	S	U	U	U
Tocopherols (E)	U	U	U	S	S	S	U
Amino acids							
Isoleucine	S	S	S	S	S	S	—
Leucine	S	S	S	S	S	S	—
Lysine	U	S	S	S	S	S	—
Methionine	S	S	S	S	S	S	—
Phenylalanine	S	S	S	S	S	S	—
Threonine	U	S	S	U	S	U	—
Tryptophan	S	S	U	U	S	S	—
Valine	S	S	S	S	S	S	—
Fatty acids polyunsaturated	S[b]	U	U	S	S	U	—

[a]Moist processed foods are always less stable than dry because of greater risk of oxidation, effects of heat, and possibilities for microbial growth. In fresh produce, however, adequate moisture to prevent wilting is important in nutrient stability.

[b]If not excessive, such as when dripped on hot coals. Data from Harris RS, Karmas E. *Nutritional Evaluation of Food Processing*. 2nd ed. Westport, CT: AVI, 1975.

The %TR is the most reliable method of nutrient analysis in food, but it is costly and time consuming. Therefore, calculation methods have been developed (13). The method used by EuroFIR combines data on raw food components with weight changes during food preparation to calculate the content per 100 g of cooked food for each nutrient, and then applies a retention factor to adjust for nutrient content changes. These assessments of nutrient content will become more important with time, as processed foods are making an increased contribution to American diets (14), and their nutrient content is becoming the basis for nutrient profiling of foods.

Food Supplements, Fortifiers, and Additives

The need for considering nutrient supplementation derives from the observations from national intake studies that intakes of several vitamins (especially vitamin D) are below recommendations in a significant proportion of the population in Western countries, for example, the United States, Germany, United Kingdom, and the Netherlands (15). The data for supplying some nutrients, such as folic acid, to the entire population support the value of this approach in

TABLE 4-9 Retention of Nutrients in Cooked Vegetables[a]

	Ascorbic Acid (%)	Thiamine (%)	Riboflavin (%)	Niacin (%)	Vitamin B₆ (%)	Folacin (%)	Vitamin A (%)
Potatoes							
Prepared from raw							
Baked in skin	80	85	95	95	95	90	—
Boiled in skin	75	80	95	95	95	90	—
Boiled without skin	75	80	95	95	95	75	—
Fried	80	80	95	95	95	75	—
Hashed-brown[b]	25	40	85	80	—	65	—
Mashed	75	80	95	95	95	75	—
Scalloped and au gratin	80	80	95	95	95	75	—
Prepared from frozen							
French fried, heated	50	75	95	95	95	75	—
Baked, stuffed, heated	80	85	95	95	95	80	—
Hashed-brown	80	80	95	95	95	80	—
Other vegetables[c]							
Prepared from raw, drained							
Greens, dark and leafy	60	85	95	90	90	65	95
Roots, bulbs, other vegetables of high starch and/or sugar content[d]	70	85	95	95	95	70	90
Other[e,f]	80	85	95	90	90	70	90
Prepared from frozen, drained							
Greens, dark and leafy[c]	60	90	95	90	90	55	95
Roots, bulbs, other vegetables of high starch and/or sugar content[d]	70	90	95	95	95	70	90
Other[e,f]	80	90	95	90	90	70	90

[a] Percent true retention = nutrient content per gram of cooked food × grams of food after cooking/nutrient content per gram of raw food × grams of food before cooking × 100.
[b] Potatoes were pared, boiled, and held overnight before hash-browning.
[c] Cooked in small or moderate amount of water until tender.
[d] Vegetables such as beets, carrots, green peas, lima beans, onions, parsnips, rutabagas, salsify, turnips, summer and winter squash, and other immature seeds of the legume group.
[e] Vegetables such as asparagus, bean sprouts, broccoli, brussels sprouts, cabbage, cauliflower, eggplant, kohlrabi, okra, and sweet peppers.
[f] Because of limited data, values are based on nutrient retention data from other cooked plant products.
From *Composition of Foods—Raw, Processed, Prepared, 1990 Supplement*. Agriculture Handbook No. 8. Washington, DC: U.S. Department of Agriculture, Human Nutrition Information Service, 1990.

prevention of neural tube disorders (see Chapter 6). However, the wisdom of providing many other nutrients to the general population continues to be questioned, as randomized controlled trials (RCTs) have not consistently shown benefit in preventing chronic disease (16). A particular nutrient can be added to the diet of a population in several ways. These include (a) providing supplements containing the nutrient, (b) fortifying food samples with the nutrient, and (c) increasing the intake of foods rich in the nutrient. The benefit of supplements is that only appropriate groups are targeted. The consumption of table foods is more natural and conducive to a good diet, but if the nutrient is needed in doses close to or exceeding the upper limit of the DRI (e.g., folic acid to prevent neural tube defects), diet alone may be inadequate. The advantage of fortification is that the nutrient reaches many more people. Although supplements, fortifiers, and additives are defined separately, it is sometimes difficult to distinguish between them, as all are added to foods (Table 4-10). In fact, the USDA brochure on food additives (17) categorizes food additives as outlined in Table 4-10 and defines them broadly as "any substance the intended use of which results or may reasonably be expected to result—directly or indirectly—in

TABLE 4-10 Common Food Additives

Additive Function	Additive Type	Additive Form	Foods Likely Used
Maintain nutrition	B vitamins	Thiamine, riboflavin, niacin, pyridoxine, folate, B_{12}	Cereals, pasta, flour, breads, corn meals, rice
	Fat-soluble vitamins	Vitamins A, D	Milk, milk products
	Minerals	FeEDTA, Zn oxide Ca citrate, carbonate iodide	Cereals, breads Juices, flour, cereal, salt, premature infant formulas
Enhance flavor	Sweeteners	Aspartame, saccharine, acesulfame-K, sucralose, fructose, sugar alcohols, honey, cane juice, molasses, yeast extract	Beverages, yogurt, desirability gelatin desserts, candies, chewing gum
	Fat substitute	Egg white/milk protein blend (Simplesse) Sucrose-triglyceride (Olestra)	Frozen desserts Potato/corn chips
	Glutamates	MSG	Soups
	Stimulants	Caffeine	Soft drinks
Maintain palatability	Preservatives	Ascorbate, BHA, BHT, benzoates, Na nitrite, Na sulfite, propionic acid	Bread, cheese, meat, frozen/dried fruit, margarine, chips
Control pH	Acids/bases	$NaHCO_3$, citric acid, phosphoric acid, tartrazine	Soft drinks, cakes, chocolates, butter
Improve consistency	Bulk agents	Lecithin, mono- and diglycerides, pectin, carrageenan, guar gum, alginates	Baked goods, salad dressing, ice cream, processed cheese
Preservatives	Antimicrobials, antioxidants	Ascorbate, citric acid, sodium benzoate/nitrate, Ca/K sorbate, EDTA	Fruit sauces/jellies, cured meats, baked goods, cereals
Moisture adjusters	Leavening and anticaking agents	Baking soda, calcium carbonate, calcium silicate, silicon dioxide	Breads, baked goods, salt, baking powder

EDTA, ethylenediamine-tetraacetic acid; MSG, monosodium glutamate; BHA, butylated hydroxyanisole; BHT, butylated hydroxytoluene. More details are available in http://www.fda.gov/food/foodingredientspackaging/ucm094211.htm and in Chapter 12 (caffeine, fat substitutes).

its becoming a component or otherwise affecting the characteristics of any food." By this definition, a nutrient fortifier is considered an additive. However, each category is regulated differently and should be considered separately.

Food/Nutrient Supplements

The FDA first regulated supplements as foods "for special dietary use" (1938), and vitamins, minerals, and other dietary substances were included. In 1994, the Dietary Supplement Health and Education Act (DSHEA) became law and provided for some regulation of supplements, while prohibiting their regulation as drugs or food additives. A dietary supplement was defined as a product intended to supplement the diet that contains a vitamin, mineral, herb, amino acid, a substance meant to increase the total dietary intake, or any metabolites, constituents, or combinations of the above. Like conventional foods, they are not subject to premarket approval by the FDA and are exempt from food additive regulations. In other words, clinical studies are not required to demonstrate their efficacy, safety, or possible interactions. Safety issues are handled by public warnings or recalls. Because the law separated supplements from additives, ingredients on the market before 1994 were considered safe. Supplements introduced after 1994 must be accompanied by evidence that the ingredient is "reasonably expected to be safe." Hundreds of supplements have not been approved (18). The situation in Europe is not quite so clear. The European Union Supplements Directive of 2002 required that supplements be safe and pure (19). This directive has been challenged in court, but has been supported to date by the European Court. Individual micronutrient supplements are discussed in Chapters 6 and 7, and other types of nutrient supplements in Chapter 8.

Nutrient Fortification

The addition of nutrients during processing to improve the nutritional qualities of foods is initiated legislatively and regulated by the FDA. The most common nutrients in the United States that are regulated as additives are thiamine, niacin, riboflavin, iron (all in fortified flour since the 1950s), and folate (in cereal grain products and ready-to-eat cereals since 1998) (Table 4-11).

TABLE 4-11	FDA-Recommended Fortification Levels Based on a Caloric Standard	
Nutrient	US RDA	Level of Nutrients Per 100 kcal
Vitamin A, IU	5,000	250
Vitamin C, mg	60	3
Thiamine, mg	1.5	0.075
Riboflavin, mg	1.7	0.085
Niacin, mg	20	1.0
Calcium, g	1	0.05
Iron, mg	18	0.9
Vitamin D, IU	400	20[a]
Vitamin E, IU	30	1.5
Vitamin B_6, mg	2.0	0.1
Folic acid, mg	0.4	0.02
Vitamin B_{12}, µg	6	0.3
Phosphorus, g	1	0.05
Iodine, µg	150	7.5[a]
Magnesium, mg	400	20
Zinc, mg	15	0.75
Copper, mg	2.0	0.1
Biotin, mg	0.03	0.015
Pantothenic acid, mg	10	0.5

[a]Optional.
IU, international unit.
Data from Miller SA, Stephenson MF. Food fortification. *Bibl Nutr Dieta*. 1987;40:82.

The increased intake of these nutrients, documented in the 1997 report *Nutrient Content of the U.S. Food Supply* (USDA Center for Nutrition Policy and Promotion), is a consequence of the fortification of grains. The increased intake of vitamins A and C and carotene is the result of the consumption of larger amounts of fruits and vegetables. These changes reflect a shift from animal fat to vegetable oils and other plant products. Increased intake of calcium and phosphorus is largely a consequence of greater cheese consumption.

Food fortification also prevents the deficiency of nutrients whose major dietary contribution is from only selected foods (e.g., iron or vitamin D), exemplified by the principles used in iron fortification (USDA, *Food Technology,* April 1989). A need for the nutrient must be demonstrated in a defined population (e.g., vitamin D in milk for infants and the elderly), use of the product must not lead to toxicity, the vehicle to which nutrients are added must be appropriate (e.g., addition of iron to cereal to prevent deficiency in children), and use of the product must not be confusing to consumers. Although the amount of added nutrient can vary widely when analyzed, and there is a risk of overconsumption of some nutrients in certain subgroups, there is yet not much evidence to substantiate this risk (20). Analysis of nutrient intake in the NHANES IV survey will determine whether the wide availability of nutrients in supplements has led to overconsumption.

Food Additives

Additives are becoming nearly ubiquitous in processed foods. Although some of these substances have no nutrient value per se, they carry the potential for toxicity and thus can affect the acceptance or availability of a prepared food to which they have been added. The original Food and Agriculture Organization (FAO)/WHO definition of an additive (1955) was "nonnutritive substances added intentionally to food, generally in small quantities, to improve its appearance, flavor, texture, or storage properties." Now the definition of the Codex Alimentarius (sponsored by WHO) includes "any substance not normally consumed as a food by itself and not normally used as a typical ingredient of the food, whether or not it has nutritive value, the intentional addition of which to food for a technological purpose in the manufacturing, processing, preparation, treatment, packing, packaging, transport, or holding of such food results . . . in it or its by-products becoming a component of . . . such foods."

The use of additives is governed by the Food and Drug Act of 1906, which prevented the manufacture of adulterated foods; by the Food, Drug, and Cosmetic Act of 1938, which allowed the government to remove adulterated foods from the market but did not regulate food additives; and by the Food Additives Amendment to the Federal Food, Drug, and Cosmetic Act of 1958. This amendment required that a new preservative or new use or amount of preservative be approved by the FDA before use, and that the compound be safe for humans. The preservative may not be used to make a product appear other (e.g., fresher) than it is. This is the rationale for not allowing sulfites to be added to meats. The additive must also be of food grade. Nearly 3,000 additives are used in food processing. Most recently, the Food Additives Amendment (Delaney clause) has provided that "no additive shall be deemed to be safe if it is found to produce cancer in man or animal." Direct food additives are those added to a food for a specific purpose, such as texture, and these are identified in the label. Indirect food additives are those compounds that become part of the food in trace amounts during packaging, storage, or handling. Such substances must be proved to be safe before their use is permitted by the FDA (21).

Additives are used (a) to improve nutritional value (vitamin D in milk, vitamin A in margarine, iodine in table salt, B vitamins and iron in refined breads and cereals); (b) to make food more appealing (colors, flavor enhancers, and sweeteners, most often sugar, salt, and corn syrup or their substitutes); (c) to maintain palatability and freshness (sodium nitrates to protect cured foods, vitamin C to prevent uncooked fruit from browning); (d) to control pH (in baking mixes, soft drinks); and (e) to improve consistency or aid in processing (carrageenan to give consistency to peanut butter, leavening agents to make baked goods rise) (Table 4-10).

Two major categories are exempt from testing and approval. About 700 additives are "generally recognized as safe" (GRAS) because past experience indicates that they have no known harmful effects. "Prior sanctioned substances," approved for use in food before 1958, also are exempt. New evidence can reopen testing on an additive, however. For example, butylated hydroxyanisole (BHA) and sulfites have been reviewed and approval continued (Food and Drug Administration, June 1998).

Similar regulations have been applied by the Joint Expert Committee for Food Additives of the FAO/WHO. Additives are classified for safety by acceptable daily intake (ADI) from 0 mg per kg to some upper limit (World Health Organization, 1987). The ADI is calculated by dividing the highest dose with no observable adverse effect in animals by a safety factor, usually 100. This improved approach to safety factor determination has been validated in a number of cases, including BHA, saccharine, and the coloring agent erythrosine (22).

ASSESSMENT OF NUTRITIONAL STATUS

A person's nutritional status can be altered by any illness that affects nutrient intake, absorption, or utilization, or increases loss of micronutrients or turnover rates of macronutrients. Evaluation of nutritional status should be a part of any general medical examination or evaluation for a medical disorder. The assessment comprises recording anthropomorphic data (see also Chapter 5), clinical observation (including history and physical examination), laboratory tests, and evaluation of the diet. Many of the details of these components are covered in subsequent chapters, but the general outline is considered here. The purpose of the nutritional evaluation is to determine whether malnutrition is present or to obtain data that will help to estimate risk for clinical outcome that might not be related to malnutrition per se.

The Concept of Malnutrition

It is difficult to separate malnutrition that is correctable by the addition of nutrients from altered status of body stores that results from the underlying disease. In many cases, these two conditions overlap. When the nutritional deficiency is limited to specific micronutrients, these can be individually examined by appropriate tests. Deficiencies are more common in the elderly patient who often presents with insufficient dietary intake, poor appetite, muscle wasting, and weight loss. Common deficiencies in such patients include vitamins A, B_{12}, D, and E, calcium, and zinc. When the deficiency is global, however, it may be more difficult to distinguish from the effects of the underlying disease and enhanced catabolic rate, as exemplified by the differences noted between starvation and cachexia (discussed further in Chapter 15).

Anthropomorphic Measurements

The most useful of these measurements include body weight and height, available as BMI, calculated online or as part of the electronic medical record. Midarm circumference and triceps skin folds as measures of protein and fat stores, respectively, are sometimes used, more for research studies. These measurements are important in estimating the general nutritional status by a comparison with "normal" clinical guidelines (see Chapter 5), and height is also important in assessing energy needs and determining BMI. Percentage of weight loss in the last month ("normal" is <5%) or in the last 6 months (<10%) are often helpful parameters.

Nutritional History and Evaluation of Diet

The history should be focused on identifying possible causes of altered nutrient intake or absorption and of increased losses or requirements (Table 4-12).

Special attention should be paid to changes in body weight (see Chapters 5 and 15), alcohol intake, causes of nutrient loss (bleeding, diarrhea), intercurrent illness, and medication that might affect intake or nutrient losses. Key questions should become a routine part of the history, including the following: (a) Has the patient's weight changed recently? By how much and how rapidly? (b) Has the patient's appetite changed? (c) Is the appetite change caused by altered taste or smell, problems with chewing or swallowing, poorly fitting dentures, or depression? (d) Who prepares meals for the patient, and has that changed recently? (e) Who shops and pays for food? (f) Are symptoms of gastrointestinal disease present? (g) Does the patient consume alcohol, medications, or dietary supplements or herbal remedies? (h) Is the patient on a restricted diet of any sort?

Decreased or altered taste (dysgeusia) is a common symptom that often is overlooked or incompletely assessed. Many common causes of taste perception are not related to nutrient status, for example, as menopause, depression, or poor dental hygiene. Deficiencies of vitamins A and

TABLE 4-12 Nutritional History Screen

Mechanism of Deficiency	If History of	Suspect Deficiency of
Inadequate intake	• All foods, ask about alcoholism, weight loss, poverty, dental disease, AIDS, taste changes	Calories, protein, thiamine, niacin, folate, pyridoxine, riboflavin
	• Fruit, vegetables, grains	Vitamin C, thiamine, niacin, folate, dietary fiber
	• Meat, dairy products, eggs	Protein, vitamin B_{12}
	• Food idiosyncrasies, allergy	Lactose
Inadequate absorption	• Drugs (especially antacids, anticonvulsants, cholestyramine, laxatives, neomycin, alcohol)	Selected vitamins and minerals
	• Malabsorption (diarrhea, weight loss, steatorrhea)	Vitamins A, D, and K, calories, protein, iron, calcium, magnesium, zinc
	• AIDS	Vitamin B_{12}
	• Surgery e.g.	
	Gastrectomy	Vitamin B_{12}, iron
	Resection of small intestine	Vitamin B_{12}, bile salts (if >100 cm of distal ileum), all others (if jejunal)
Increased losses	• Alcohol abuse	Magnesium, zinc, phosphorus
	• Blood loss	Iron
	• Diabetes, poorly controlled	Calories
	• Diarrhea	Protein, zinc, electrolytes
	• Draining abscesses, wounds	Protein
	• Peritoneal dialysis or hemodialysis	Protein, water-soluble vitamins, zinc
	• Drugs (especially diuretics, laxatives)	Potassium, magnesium
Increased requirements	• Fever	Calories
	• Hyperthyroidism	Calories
	• Increased physiologic demands (infancy, adolescence, pregnancy, lactation)	Various nutrients
	• Surgery, trauma, burns, infection	Calories, protein

B_{12} and perhaps zinc may also alter taste. Medications are among the most common causes of decreased or altered taste, especially chloride salts, which are secreted by salivary glands and drugs with anticholinergic effects, which produce xerostomia (see list of drugs in Table 4-13) (23).

Obtaining a clinically valid dietary history is time consuming and requires the skills of a trained dietitian. Nonetheless, the practicing physician should be able to recruit from the patient a general pattern of the diet, focusing on changes in the intake of disease-associated food parameters, such as calories, protein, fat, carbohydrate, free sugar, sodium, and alcohol. By using the Power Plate depiction, one can roughly assess the intake of food groups considered to be healthy by the Physicians Committee for Responsible Medicine (PCRM), that is, fruits, grains, legumes, and vegetables (http://pcrm.org/health/powerplate). Alternatively, the FDA program of MyPlate provides a similar guidance (www.choosemyplate.gov/food-groups/). Recall of diet is generally poor; so the purpose of a preliminary dietary evaluation is to discover major changes in intake and weight.

Clinical Features and Physical Examination

Tissues that proliferate rapidly (skin, oral and gastrointestinal mucosa, hair, bone marrow) are most likely to manifest signs of nutrient deficiency. Some are accessible to the physical examination; some (gastrointestinal mucosa) are manifested by history (diarrhea); and others (bone

TABLE 4-13 Common Drug-Induced Oral Manifestations

Candidiasis
Antibiotics
Antineoplastics
Corticosteroids
Immunosuppressives
Steroid inhalers

Contact Hypersensitivity
Iodine, mouthwashes, cosmetics, antiseptic lozenges, chewing gum, food additives
Menthol, toothpastes (esp. those containing cinnamaldehyde, formalin, and herbal components), dental materials (amalgam, steel wires, acrylic components)
Thymol
Topical analgesics
Topical antibiotics

Erythema Multiforme
Anticonvulsants
Antimalarials
Barbiturates
Busulfan
Chlorpropamide, estrogens/progestins, ginseng, gold compounds, iodine mouthwashes
Isoniazid
Meprobamate
Minoxidil
Penicillins
Phenolphthalein
Phenylbutazone, phenytoin
Propylthiouracil, rifampicin
Salicylates
Sulfonamides
Tetracyclines, tolbutamide, verapamil

Fixed Drug Eruptions
Barbiturates, gold, indomethacin, lidocaine, penicillamine, salicylates
Chlordiazepoxide
Sulfonamides
Tetracyclines

Gingival Hyperplasia
Cotrimoxazole, cyclosporine, erythromycin, ketoconazole, lamotrigine, lithium
Nifedipine, phenobarbital
Phenytoin sodium, sertraline, sodium valproate, topiramate, vigabatrin

Hairy/black Tongue
Antibiotics, antidepressants
Corticosteroids, griseofulvin, lansoprazole
Sodium peroxide, tobacco, tetracyclines

Intraoral Bleeding, Petechiae, Purpura
Antiarrhythmics
Phenylbutazone
Potassium chloride
Sulfonamides
Thiocyanate
Thiouracil
Warfarin sodium

Ulcerations, Mucositis, Stomatitis, Glossitis
ACE inhibitors, antiarrhythmics, antibiotics
Antineoplastics, antidepressants, atorvastatin

(continued)

TABLE 4-13 Common Drug-Induced Oral Manifestations *(continued)*

Aspirin
D-Penicillamine, gabapentin, ganciclovir
Gold salts, interferons
Lamotrigine
Lithium
Meprobamate
Mercurial diuretics
Methotrexate
Methyldopa
NSAIDs
Phenylbutazone
Potassium chloride
Propranolol, propylthiouracil, protease inhibitors, proton pump inhibitors
Spironolactone
Thiazide diuretics
Tolbutamide, zidovudine

Xerostomia
Anorexiants
Antiarrhythmics
Antibiotics (broad-spectrum)
Anticholinergics
Anticoagulants
Anticonvulsants
Antidepressants
Antidiarrheals
Antihistamines, anti-HIV protease inhibitors
Antihypertensives
Antinauseants
Antineoplastics
Antiparkinsonism agents
Antispasmodics
Aspirin
Benzodiazepines
Bronchodilators
CNS stimulants
Decongestants
Diuretics
Ganglion-blocking agents, omeprazole, tramadol

Salivary Gland Enlargement or Pain
Antipsychotics, clonidine, H2-receptor antagonists
Iodides
Isoproterenol
Methyldopa
Hypnotics
Lithium
Monoamine oxidase inhibitors
Muscle relaxants
Narcotics, nitrofurantoin
NSAIDs
Sympathomimetics
Tranquilizers, warfarin

ACE, angiotensin converting enzyme; NSAID, nonsteroidal anti-inflammatory drug; CNS, central nervous system.

Sources: Chernoff R. *Geriatric Nutrition.* Gaithersburg, MD: Aspen Publishers, 1991; Abdollahi M, Radfar M, A review of drug-induced oral reactions. *J Contemp Dent Pract.* 2003;4:10.

marrow failure) present indirectly. The examination can be approached in one of four ways: assessment of the general physical findings to identify the nutrient deficiency, a search for relevant specific signs of nutrient deficiency suspected from the history (24), or oral examination (a neglected area of the physical examination), or the use of screening tools that incorporate elements of history, physical examination, and laboratory tests (24).

Dehydration
Deficiencies of Na, Cl, and H_2O lead to dehydration (see also discussion of sodium in Chapter 7). In adult patients, the manifestations of dehydration (including sunken eyeballs, mucosal xerosis, low blood pressure, and mental confusion) are less striking and specific than in children and infants. One or none may be present in any individual case.

Nutrient Deficiency
An important part of the physical examination is the search for signs of nutrient deficiency. Table 4-14 lists the most common signs and the nutrient deficiencies frequently associated with them. Table 4-15 lists physical examination findings according to the individual nutrient that is lacking (25).

Oral Mucosa
Because the oral mucosa regenerates rapidly, it can be a sensitive indicator of nutrient deficiency. Table 4-16 lists the oral manifestations commonly associated with individual nutrient deficiencies. Oral manifestations are not specific for nutrient deficiency, and the same conditions can be caused in particular by medication (see Table 4-13).

Clinical Assessment of Overall Nutritional Status Using Screening Instrument
Because determination of overall nutritional status must include components that are not specific for malnutrition or the underlying disease status, a number of screening assessments have been developed to estimate disease risk and outcome, with the thought that these assessments are in some way related to underlying nutritional status. The 2011 A.S.P.E.N. guidelines "recommend" 12 different instruments that utilize anthropomorphic measurements (e.g., weight loss, BMI) and plasma proteins (mostly albumin) to assess initial "nutritional" status (26) (Table 4-17). In addition, two more detailed nutrition assessment tools are suggested, as discussed in Chapter 5: the Mini Nutritional Assessment, MNA (Table 5-21), and the Subjective Global Assessment, SGA (Figure 5-1). However, the evidence for recommending such screening for hospitalized patients is weak, although there is somewhat better evidence for recommending nutrition support for patients identified to be at risk by these tools (26). Some authors have suggested using tools designed for risk assessment in critically ill patients (e.g., Acute Physiology and Chronic Health Evaluation [APACHE II] and Simplified Acute Physiologic Score [SAPS]) in addition to more traditional nutritional measurements, but find these additions no more helpful than the SGA (27).

Laboratory Tests
When the history and physical examination findings suggest a deficiency, it is often appropriate to assess the status of individual nutrients by specific tests. One must be careful to use the proper test, depending on whether one is assessing total body stores or recent intake (Tables 4-18 and 4-19). Each of these tests is discussed in detail in Chapters 6 and 7.

Many of the tests listed in Tables 4-18 and 4-19 measure static vitamin and mineral content. Only few tests measure actual function and allow a direct assessment of nutrient status. Measurements to estimate the nutritional status of protein and fat are discussed in Chapter 5.

DIET THERAPY
Diets are used for many purposes, only some of them therapeutic. Some diets are recommended to prevent the onset of chronic diseases, such as atherosclerosis or obesity (see Chapters 13 and 14). The data regarding the efficacy of such diets are incomplete. Other diets are used to manage medical illnesses, such as diabetes, hyperlipidemia, and renal disease (see Chapter 13). Still others are used for one specific aspect of overall management, such as the addition of calcium-containing foods for osteopenia (see Chapter 7). A few diets are used to eliminate or treat specific disorders, such as low-fat, low-lactose, low-sodium, or gluten-free diets (see Chapter 12).

TABLE 4-14 Signs and Symptoms of Nutritional Deficiency in Adult Patients

Sign or Symptom	Possible Nutrient Deficiency
General	
Wasted, skinny (especially temporal muscles)	Protein–calorie
Abdomen	
Distension	Protein–calorie
Hepatomegaly	Protein–calorie
Extremities	
Edema	Protein, thiamine
Decubitus ulcers, poor wound healing	Protein, vitamin C, zinc
Bone tenderness	Vitamin D
Bone ache, joint pain	Vitamin C
Muscle wasting and weakness	Protein, calorie, vitamin D
Muscle tenderness, muscle pain	Thiamine
Skin	
Pallor	Folate, iron, vitamin B_{12}
Follicular hyperkeratosis	Vitamins A and C
Perifollicular petechiae (especially after raised venous pressure)	Vitamin C
Flaking dermatitis, scaling	Protein, calories, niacin, riboflavin, zinc, vitamin A
Bruising, purpura	Vitamins C and K and essential fatty acids
Pigmentation changes, desquamation of semiexposed areas	Niacin, protein–calorie
Scrotal dermatosis	Riboflavin
Cellophane appearance	Protein (also corticosteroid use, aging)
Hair	
Sparse and thin	Protein, zinc, biotin
Easy to pull out	Protein
Corkscrew hairs, coiled hair	Vitamins C and A
Nails	
Spooning	Iron
Transverse lines	Protein
Eyes	
History of night blindness (especially impaired visual recovery after glare)	Vitamin A
Photophobia, blurring, conjunctival inflammation	Riboflavin, vitamin A
Mouth	
Glossitis (slick red tongue)	Riboflavin, niacin, folic acid, vitamin B_{12} protein
Gums—bleeding, receding, spongy, ulcers, hypertrophic	Vitamins C, A, and K; folic acid, niacin
Cheilosis (dry, cracking, ulcerated lips)	Riboflavin, pyridoxine, niacin
Angular stomatitis	Riboflavin, pyridoxine, niacin
Hypogeusia	Zinc, vitamins A and B_{12}
Tongue fissuring	Niacin
Burning, sore mouth and tongue	Vitamins B_{12}, B_6, and C, niacin, folic acid, iron
Leukoplakia	Vitamins A, B_{12}, and B complex; folic acid, niacin

TABLE 4-14 Signs and Symptoms of Nutritional Deficiency in Adult Patients *(continued)*

Sign or Symptom	Possible Nutrient Deficiency
Neck	
Goiter	Iodine
Parotid enlargement	Protein (also alcohol excess, starch chewing)
Sign or symptom	Possible nutrient deficiency
Neurologic	
Tetany	Calcium, magnesium
Peripheral neuropathy (paresthesias)	Thiamine, pyridoxine
Loss of reflexes, wrist drop, foot drop (loss of vibratory and position sense)	Vitamins B_{12} and E
Dementia, disorientation	Niacin, vitamin B_{12}
Confabulation	Thiamine
Ophthalmoplegia	Thiamine, vitamin E
Depression	Biotin, folic acid, vitamin B_{12}

TABLE 4-15 Clinical Manifestations of Nutrient Deficiency States in Adults

Nutrient	Major Causes of Deficiency	Clinical Deficiency Symptoms
Thiamine	Inadequate intake, alcoholism	*Neurologic*—mental confusion, irritability, sensory loss and paresthesias (peripheral neuropathy), weakness, anorexia *Eyes*—ophthalmoplegia *Cardiac*—tachycardia, cardiomegaly, congestive heart failure *Other*—constipation, sudden death, muscle tenderness and pain
Riboflavin	Inadequate intake	*Skin*—nasolabial seborrhea, fissuring and redness around eyes and mouth, magenta tongue, genital dermatosis *Eyes*—corneal vascularization
Pyridoxine	Inadequate intake, old age, alcoholism	*Skin*—nasolabial seborrhea, glossitis, cheilosis *Neurologic*—paresthesias, peripheral neuropathy *Other*—anemia
Niacin	Inadequate intake, alcoholism, carcinoid syndrome	*Skin*—nasolabial seborrhea, fissuring eyelid corners, angular fissures around mouth, papillary atrophy, pellagrous dermatitis (sun-exposed areas), burning mouth or tongue *Neurologic*—mental confusion *Other*—diarrhea
Folic acid	Inadequate intake, alcoholism, malabsorption, pregnancy, hemolysis, drugs (anticonvulsants, sulfasalazine, methotrexate)	*Skin*—pallor *Oral*—glossitis, hyperpigmentation of tongue *Neurologic*—depression *Other*—diarrhea, anemia

(continued)

TABLE 4-15 Clinical Manifestations of Nutrient Deficiency States in Adults *(continued)*

Nutrient	Major Causes of Deficiency	Clinical Deficiency Symptoms
Cobalamin (B_{12})	Malabsorption, pernicious anemia, vegetarian diets	*Skin*—hyperpigmentation, pallor *Oral*—glossitis *Neurologic*—ataxia, optic neuritis, paresthesias, peripheral neuropathy, mental disorders *Other*—anemia, anorexia, diarrhea
Vitamin C	Alcoholism, inadequate intake	*Skin*—petechiae, purpura, swollen bleeding gums, delayed wound healing, flaking dermatosis *Other*—bone pain, depression, anorexia
Biotin	Total parenteral nutrition	*Skin*—pluckable sparse hair, pallor, seborrheic dermatitis *Neurologic*—depression *Other*—anemia, fatigue
Vitamin A	Fat malabsorption, alcoholism	*Eyes*—Bitot's spots, conjunctival and corneal xerosis (dryness), keratomalacia, poor dark adaptation *Skin*—follicular hyperkeratosis, xerosis *Hair*—coiled, keratinized
Vitamin D	Fat malabsorption, lack of sunlight, breast-fed newborn	*Bone*—bowlegs, beading of ribs, bone pain, epiphyseal deformities, vertebral fractures, muscle pain
Vitamin E	Premature infants, fat malabsorption, cystic fibrosis, chronic biliary obstruction	*Neurologic*—peripheral neuropathy, ophthalmoplegia
Vitamin K	Fat malabsorption, excessive warfarin dose	*Skin*—subcutaneous hemorrhage, ecchymoses
Zinc	Diarrhea, diuretics, chronic renal disease	Psoriatic dermatitis in hands and feet
Protein energy malnutrition	Malabsorption, chronic disease, anorexia nervosa, renal dialysis patients	Dry wrinkled skin, circumoral pallor, peripheral edema, angular stomatitis

Some diets are advertised commercially as providing nutritional remedies (usually unproven) for serious illness (most commonly cancer) and preventing cancer or obesity. One must keep in mind the strong placebo effect of all treatments, including diets. The greatest caution must be exercised in regard to unproven nutritional remedies for cancer because of the highly charged emotional situation in which these treatments are undertaken. The claims made for these diets can best be countered by promoting the diet recommended for cancer prevention (1) (see Chapter 15), which is very similar to that recommended for all healthy adults (see Chapter 1). In both these diets, the primary goal is achieving and maintaining a normal weight.

Following a U.S. Court of Appeals decision (*Pearson v Shalala*), the FDA revoked the regulations codifying its policy not to allow health claims for four substances and their relationship to disease to appear on food labels. These claims are for dietary fiber and cancer, antioxidant vitamins and cancer, ω-3 fatty acids and coronary artery disease, and 0.8-mg folate supplements to reduce neural tube defects versus lower amounts of folate in conventional food. However, reversal of the FDA policy is not the equivalent of eliminating the need for claims by the FDA regarding substance–disease relationships. Such claims must now be individually assessed.

TABLE 4-16   Nutritional Deficiencies and Related Oral Manifestations

Nutrient Deficiency	Oral Manifestations
Vitamin A	Candidiasis *Gingivae*—hypertrophy, inflammation *Oral mucosa*—keratosis, leukoplakia Periodontal disease
Vitamin B complex	*Lips*—angular cheilosis *Oral mucosa*—leukoplakia Periodontal disease *Tongue*—papillary hypertrophy, magenta color, fissuring, glossitis
Vitamin B_2 (riboflavin)	Filiform papillae—atrophic Fungiform papillae—enlarged *Lips*—shiny, red, angular cheilosis *Tongue*—magenta color, soreness
Vitamin B_3 (niacin)	*Lips*—angular cheilosis *Oral mucosa*—intense irritation/inflammation, red, painful, denuded, ulcerated, mucositis/stomatitis *Tongue*—glossitis; tip/borders—red, swollen, beefy; dorsum—smooth, dry Ulcerative gingivitis
Vitamin B_6 (pyridoxine)	*Oral mucosa*—burning/sore mouth *Lips*—angular cheilosis *Tongue*—glossitis, glossodynia
Vitamin B_{12} (cobalamin)	*Lips*—angular cheilosis Burning/sore mouth *Oral mucosa*—ulcerations (aphthous type), mucositis/stomatitis *Tongue*—beefy red, glossy, smooth, glossitis, glossodynia, loss of papillae
Vitamin C (megavitamin C withdrawal)	Burning/sore mouth Candidiasis *Gingivae*—friability, raggedness, swelling, redness Hemorrhagic tendency—petechiae, subperiosteal Periodontal disease *Teeth*—marked mobility, spontaneous exfoliation
Vitamin D	Periodontal disease
Vitamin K	*Gingivae*—bleeding
Folic acid	*Oral mucosa*—mucositis/stomatitis, ulcerations (aphthous type) Burning/sore mouth Candidiasis Filiform/fungiform papillae—atrophic *Gingivae*—inflammation *Lips*—angular cheilosis *Tongue*—glossitis; tip/borders—red swollen; dorsum—slick, bald, pale, or fiery red
Iron	Dental caries—increased susceptibility Filiform papillae—atrophic *Lips*—angular cheilosis, pallor *Oral mucosa*—pallor, sore mouth, ulcerations (aphthous type) Oral paresthesias, burning *Tongue*—atrophic, pale; glossitis Xerostomia
Protein	*Oral mucosa*—fragility, burning sensation *Lips*—angular cheilosis Periodontal disease

Data from Chernoff R. *Geriatric Nutrition*. Gaithersburg, MD: Aspen Publishers, 1991.

TABLE 4-17 Selected Nutrition Screening Tools

Instrument	Anthropomorphy	Illness Severity	Reference
Birmingham Nutrition Risk Score	Weight loss, BMI, appetite, ability to eat	Stress factor	Reilly HM. *Clin Nutr.* 1995
Malnutrition Screening Tool	Appetite, weight loss unintentional		Ferguson M. *Nutrition.* 1999
Malnutrition Universal Screening Tool	BMI, weight change	Presence of acute disease	Elia M. *Br Assoc Ent Parent Nutr.* 2003
Maastricht Index	% ideal body weight	Albumin, prealb, lymphocyte count	Kuzu MA. *World J Surg.* 2006
Nutrition Risk Classification	Weight loss, % ideal body weight, dietary intake	GI function	Kovacevich DS. *Nutr Clin Pract.* 1997
Nutritional Risk Index	Present/usual weight	Albumin	VA TPN Cooperative Group. 1991
Nutritional Risk Screening 2002	Weight loss, BMI, food intake	Diagnosis	Kondrup J. *Clin Nutr.* 2003
Prognostic Inflammatory & Nutritional Index		Albumin, prealb, Creactive protein, α_1-acid glycoprotein	Igenbleek Y. *Int J Vitam Nutr Res.* 1985
Prognostic Nutritional Index	Triceps skin fold	Albumin, transferrin skin sensitivity	Buzby GP. *Am J Surg.* 1980
Simple Screening Tool	BMI & weight loss	Albumin	Laporte M. *J Nutr Health Aging.* 2001
Short Nutrition Assessment Questionnaire	Recent weight loss, appetite, use of oral supplement		Kruizenga HM. *AJCN.* 2005

Modified from Mueller C, Compher C, Ellen DM; American Society for Parenteral and Enteral Nutrition (A.S.P.E.N.) Board of Directors. A.S.P.E.N. clinical guidelines: nutrition screening, assessment, and intervention in adults. *JPEN J Parenter Enteral Nutr.* 2011;35:16–24.

NUTRIENT–DRUG INTERACTIONS
Effects of Foods on Absorption of Drugs

There are multiple ways in which food or its components can interact with a coadministered drug, namely during absorption or during drug distribution, metabolism, or elimination. Most interactions occur during absorption and/or metabolism of the drug. Absorption can be decreased, delayed, increased, or accelerated by foods that alter absorption (28). The mechanism of such food effects may be related to the content and timing of meals, to changes in intraluminal pH, rate of gastric emptying, site and route of absorption (portal vein vs. lymphatic), or competition for epithelial transporters. The most important variable is the drug itself (and its formulation). Although highly lipid-soluble drugs are more often associated with a food effect, there is no common scientific basis to predict a food effect. Formulation may improve solubility and release of water-insoluble drugs, as with nanoparticles or controlled-release technology (29). Herbals have been implicated in altering drug metabolism by cytochrome P450 inhibition or induction, but the data for these interactions is rather incomplete. Weak effects have been found for *Ginkgo biloba*, milk thistle/sylmarin, goldenseal/berberine, and *Echinacea* (30).

Disease or surgical removal of a significant portion of the intestine might alter drug absorption. However, the effects are variable and not easily predictable (31). This is true even for gastric bypass bariatric surgery, in which drugs that undergo presystemic and hepatic clearance by CYP3A4 may show increased bioavailability, but drugs that depend on transport mediators (e.g., ampicillin) in

TABLE 4-18 Clinical Laboratory Tests for Detection of Vitamin Deficiency

Vitamin	Test	Fluid	Reference Range (units)[a] Marginal	Deficient	Usefulness
B_1	Transketolase ratio	RBC	1.16–1.24	>1.25	+ when severe
	Thiamine	Serum		<12.7 (nmol/L)	Direct measure
	Thiamine	Urine		<27 (μg/g creat.)	
B_2	GSH reductase ratio	Serum	1.20–1.40	>1.40	Body stores
	Riboflavin	Urine	27–79	<27 (μg/g creat.)	Recent intake
B_6	AST activity ratio	RBC	1.70–1.85	>1.85	Body stores
	Pyridoxal-5-PO_4	Plasma	20–30	<20 (nmol/L)	Stores, sensitive
	4-Pyridoxic acid	Urine		<3.0 (μmol/day)	Recent intake
	Total vitamin B_6	Urine		<0.5 (μmol/day)	Recent intake
Niacin	N-methylnicotinamide	Urine	0.5–2.5	<0.5 (mg/g creat.)	Recent intake
	2-Pyridone	Urine	2.0–3.9	<2.0 (mg/g creat.)	Recent intake
Folate	Folic acid	Plasma	3.0–5.9	<3.0 (ng/mL)	Stores + intake
	Folic acid	RBC	140–159	<140 (ng/mL)	Body stores
Folate or B_{12}	Homocysteine	Plasma	12–15	>15 (μmol/L)	Function
	Cobalamin	Serum	150–200	<150 (pg/mL)	Body stores
	Methylmalonic acid	Serum		>376 (nmol/L)	Function
	Holotranscobalamin II	Serum	40–60	>60 (pg/mL)	Stores, sensitive
C	Ascorbic acid	Serum	11–23	<11 (μmol/L)	Recent intake
	Ascorbic acid	WBC	10–20	<10 (μg/108 cells)	Stores
A	Retinol	Plasma	10–19	<10 (μg/dL)	Stores + intake
	Retinol-binding protein	Plasma		<50 (mg/L)	Function
D	25-OH vitamin D	Serum	12–25	<12 (nmol/L)	Body stores
	1,25-$(OH)_2$ vitamin D	Serum	48–65	<48 (pmol/L)	Function
E	α-Tocopherol	Serum	5.0–7.0	<5 (μg/mL)	Body stores
	α-Tocopherol/total lipid	Serum	0.8–1.0	<0.8	Stores preferred
	H_2O_2 hemolysis	RBC	10–20	>20 (%)	Function
K	Prothrombin time	Plasma	1.5–2.0	>2.0 (sec. over function control)	Function
	Phylloquinone			<0.35 (nmol/L)	Recent intake

[a]Check local laboratory for variations from ranges.
GSH, glutathione; AST, aspartate amino transferase.

the upper intestine show decreased exposure (32). However, these effects have been studied in small numbers of patients, and the clinical significance of the pharmacokinetic changes is not clear.

Effects of Drugs on Micronutrient Metabolism

The clinical importance of many such effects is often not apparent because the drugs are used for only a limited time. Information on these multiple interactions is available from the NIH Clinical Center and the Drug–Nutrient Interaction Task Force (www.cc.nih.gov/patient_education/drug_nutrient/), and from books (33).

Effects of Vitamins and Minerals on Drug Action

Although large doses of micronutrients are usually required to produce a clinical effect, the mechanism by which some sources of vitamins (e.g., grapefruit juice) affect drug metabolism

TABLE 4-19 Clinical Laboratory Detection of Micronutrient Mineral Deficiency

Nutrient	Test	Method	Reference Range (units)[a]	Usefulness
Iron	Iron (serum)	Colorimetric	50–200 (mg/dL)	Poor measure of body stores
	Total iron binding (serum)	Colorimetric	245–400 (mg/dL)	
	Iron-binding capacity (TIBC)	Calculation	15–50 (%)	Insensitive for iron status
	Transferrin (serum)	Immunoturbidimetric	200–400 (mg/dL)	Preferred over TIBC if available
	Ferritin (serum)	Immunoturbidimetric	18–300 (ng/mL)	Measures body stores: high specificity when low, poor sensitivity
Zn	Zinc (plasma)	Flame atomic absorption	20–130 (mg/dL)	Poor specificity for body stores
	Zinc tolerance test (plasma Zn)	Flame atomic absorption	>Twofold increase over baseline at 2 h	For malabsorption
Cu	Copper (serum)	Flame atomic absorption	55–175 (mg/dL)	Insensitive for body stores
	Ceruloplasmin (plasma)	Immunoturbidimetric	10–60 (mg/dL)	Independent of body stores
Selenium	Selenium (serum)	Fluorometry	100–340 (ng/mL)	Insensitive for body stores
	Glutathione peroxidase (plasma)	Spectrophotometric	455–800 (U/L)	More sensitive for body stores

[a]Check local laboratory for variation from ranges.

(decreasing the area under the curve following absorption) differs from the effect of the micronutrient itself (Table 4-20). Further details on the effect of fruit juices and beverages on drug absorption can be found in Chapter 12.

Drug-Induced Alterations of Food Intake

Many drugs (including alcohol) decrease appetite, especially in persons with chronic illness. Some drugs, especially tricyclic antidepressants, increase appetite in depressed and also nondepressed persons. Amitriptyline is the most active of this group and causes weight gain, perhaps in part through hyperphagia. Drugs are the most common cause of dysgeusia. Most chloride salts (or other halides) are secreted in saliva and may affect taste. Drugs with anticholinergic effects cause dry mouth and may affect appetite. Table 4-21 lists some drugs that commonly affect food intake.

INTERPRETATION OF DATA IN NUTRITIONAL STUDIES

Proper interpretation of available data is essential for knowing what information to use in practice. In this book, we have tried to include mostly trustworthy data that have stood the test of time, but to identify less reliable data when those were all that were available. These data come in many instances from epidemiological studies, utilizing large databases, but also come from double-blind randomized controlled trials (DBRCT) or from systematic reviews of such trials. These studies are subject, however, to overinterpretation, due either to lack of attention to distinguishing causation from association, from preconceived biases, and from inadequate study design.

TABLE 4-20 Dietary Supplements That Affect Drug Action

Supplement	Drug	Effect
Vitamins		
Vitamin A	Alcohol	Hypervitaminosis A may enhance hepatotoxicity of alcohol.
	Isotretinoin	Additive toxic effects may result from combination therapy with vitamin A or other supplements containing vitamin A.
	Tetracycline	Combination therapy may enhance drug-induced intracranial hypertension (severe headache).
Vitamin D	Digoxin	Vitamin D-induced hypercalcemia may potentiate the effects of the drug and result in cardiac arrhythmias.
Vitamin E	Warfarin	May enhance anticoagulant response to warfarin.
	Aspirin	↑ Antithrombotic effect
Vitamin K	Warfarin	Vitamin K in liquid food supplements may inhibit the hypoprothrombotic effect of drug.
Ascorbic acid	Fluphenazine	Large doses may interfere with drug absorption and result in a return of manic behavior.
	Warfarin	Megadoses may decrease prothrombin time.
Folacin	Methotrexate	Folacin or its derivatives in vitamin preparations may alter responses to drug.
	Phenytoin	May decrease anticonvulsant action of drug.
Pyridoxine	Levodopa	Reverses antiparkinsonism effect of drug.
	Phenytoin	Large doses may reduce phenytoin levels.
	Hydralazine, isoniazid, penicillamine	May correct drug-induced peripheral neuropathy.
Minerals		
Calcium, iron	Tetracycline	Concurrent use may decrease drug absorption.
Magnesium, zinc, iron	Penicillamine	Concurrent use may decrease drug effectiveness.

Data from Pemberton CM. *Mayo Clinic Diet Manual*. 6th ed. Toronto, ON: Decker, 1988.

The inference for causation was outlined by Hill's criteria (Table 4-22) (34). These include the realization that a strong association is more likely causal than a weak one, that any causal factor should precede the effect, that a scientific justification should exist between cause and effect, and that the hypothetical cause should be supported by RCTs. These key issues are often overlooked, as in the proposed associations between food ingredients and cancer risk. Those risks are weak even in single studies and disappear in meta-analyses (35). Biases do exist in the nutrient-cancer (and other) literature. And biased research interpretation is common, with a variety of intentional, motivational, and even simple cognitive determinants (36).

Observational studies often make assertions about effects on the basis of $p < 0.05$. The assumption underlying such a conclusion is that there is only a 5% probability that the observed effect might be seen by chance, when there is no true effect. In observational studies, much more than in RCTs, residual systematic error is usually not corrected in the analysis; so that biases and confounding factors may render the traditional p value interpretation untenable. An analysis of 4,970 articles reported observational health care data, in which the standard error was back calculated (by including estimates of negative control populations to derive an empirical null population), and the p value recomputed under various assumptions of bias (37). The not-so-surprising result was that at least half of the significant findings were rendered nonsignificant.

Bias can occur even in placebo-controlled trials, a trend that can be overcome in part by high-quality methods (38). But the magnitude of bias is in general small in RCTs, and is constrained by a large body of information. One way to increase transparency and to limit bias is to have transparent registries of raw data; another is to conduct clinical trials to prove hypotheses.

TABLE 4-21 Examples of Drug-Induced Alteration of Food Intake

Hypophagic Drugs	Hyperphagic Drugs	Drugs Producing Hypogeusia/Dysgeusia
Alcohol	Amitriptyline hydrochloride	Amphetamines, acarbose, acetaminophen, ACE inhibitors, acetazolamide, acyclovir, antibiotics, antidepressants, β-blockers, benzodiazepines, carbimazole, chlorhexidine, chlorpromazine, cisplatin, clofibrate, D-penicillamine, dicyclomine, encainide, ethionamide, etidronate, 5-fluorouracil, ganciclovir, granisetron, gold salts, griseofulvin, isotretinoin, lansoprazole, levodopa, lithium carbonate, methimazole, methocarbamol, methylthiouracil, oxyfedrine, penicillin, pentamidine, phytonadione, propylthiouracil, quinidine, ranitidine, ritonavir, selegiline, statins, tamoxifen, topiramate, triptans, ursodiol, vitamins (high-dose)
Amphetamines	Anabolic steroids	
Cisplatin	Benzodiazepines	
Cocaine	Buclizine hydrochloride	
Diethylpropion hydrochloride	Chlortetracycline	
Fenfluramine hydrochloride	Cyproheptadine hydrochloride	
Hydroxyurea	Glucocorticoids	
Methotrexate	Phenothiazines	
Metformin	Reserpine	
Phenmetrazine hydrochloride	Sulfonylureas	
SSRIs	other tricyclic and heterocyclic (SNRI) antidepressants	

SSRI, selective serotonin reuptake inhibitor.
Source (in part): Abdollahi M, Radfar M. A review of drug-induced oral reactions. *J Contemp Dent Pract.* 2003;4:1.

Even with this support, however, randomized trials can have design flaws that prevent testing the hypothesis. This can take the form of a lack of considering nutrient levels in inclusion criteria for studies testing the effect of a nutrient (39). Or it can involve the lack of a valid reference instrument for estimating dietary measurement errors in protein (and other nutrient) intake (40).

Equally important to obtaining reliable answers to questions is to ask an appropriate question involving the proper patient population (41). This factor is often lacking in the way secondary questions are asked of large epidemiological databases. Lack of a good question with an appropriate population is a consistent issue in studies of ICU patients (42). There is no doubt

TABLE 4-22 Hill's Criteria for Causal Inference

Criterion	Rationale
Strength of association	Strong association more likely to be causal than weak one.
Consistency	Association should be consistent across study designs.
Specificity	Assumption that one cause is responsible for one effect, but redundancy exists in many biological systems.
Biologic gradient	A causal effect should show a dose-response relationship.
Plausibility	Is there a scientific justification for the cause and effect?
Coherence	The central relationship fits with what else is known.
Experimental evidence	i.e., Randomized controlled trials
Analogy	A soft criterion

Adapted from Bruemmer B, Harris J, Gleason P, et al. Publishing nutrition research: a review of epidemiologic methods. *J Am Diet Assoc.* 2009;109:1728.

that the ICU population is difficult to study, and many confounding factors limit the ability to do high-quality studies, but then the reader needs to be cautious in interpreting such studies.

What is readily apparent, however, is that historical, nutritional epidemiological observations have generated seminal hypotheses. These hypotheses, when tested, have proven invaluable to nutritional health globally. Additionally, what is equally apparent is that various other hypotheses generated from such observational studies have not survived following critical intervention testing. This is, in fact, as it should be, and confirms that epidemiological associations may lead to hypotheses about cause and effect relationships, but that these need to be tested in order to confirm their validity. While testing these hypotheses in nutrition is, admittedly, a difficult task, not testing them leaves the question of their validity open. New epidemiological tools, such as Mendelian Randomization, independent markers of dietary foods and nutrient intakes, validated surrogate markers of long-term consequences, etc., are likely to further contribute to the importance of nutritional epidemiology. It is good to keep the Hill criteria in mind as one reads the literature. These were designed for epidemiological studies, but are relevant to all clinical studies.

REFERENCES

1. World Cancer Research Fund/American Institute for Cancer Research. *Food, Nutrition, and the Prevention of Cancer: A Global Perspective*. Washington, DC: WCRF/AICR, 1997.
2. World Health Organization. *Trace Elements in Human Nutrition and Health*. Prepared in collaboration with the Food and Agriculture Organization of the United Nations and the International Atomic Energy Agency. Geneva: WHO, 1996.
3. Standing Committee on the Scientific Evaluation of Dietary Reference Intakes, Food and Nutrition Board, Institute of Medicine. *Dietary Reference Intakes for Calcium, Phosphorus, Magnesium, Vitamin D, and Fluoride*. Washington, DC: National Academies Press, 1997.
4. Standing Committee on the Scientific Evaluation of Dietary Reference Intakes, Food and Nutrition Board, Institute of Medicine. *Dietary Reference Intakes for Thiamin, Riboflavin, Niacin, Vitamin B6, Folate, Vitamin B12, Pantothenic Acid, Biotin, and Choline*. Washington, DC: National Academies Press, 2000.
5. Standing Committee on the Scientific Evaluation of Dietary Reference Intakes, Food and Nutrition Board, Institute of Medicine. *Dietary Reference Intakes for Vitamin E, Vitamin C, Selenium, and Carotenoids*. Washington, DC: National Academies Press, 2000.
6. Standing Committee on the Scientific Evaluation of Dietary Reference Intakes, Food and Nutrition Board, Institute of Medicine. *Dietary Reference Intakes for Vitamin A, Vitamin K, Arsenic, Boron, Chromium, Copper, Iodine, Iron, Manganese, Molybdenum, Nickel, Silicon, Vanadium, and Zinc*. Washington, DC: National Academies Press, 2001.
7. Standing Committee on the Scientific Evaluation of Dietary Reference Intakes, Food and Nutrition Board, Institute of Medicine. *Dietary Reference Intakes for Water, Potassium, Sodium, Chloride, and Sulfate*. Washington, DC: National Academies Press, 2005.
8. Standing Committee on the Scientific Evaluation of Dietary Reference Intakes, Food and Nutrition Board, Institute of Medicine. *Dietary Reference Intakes for Energy, Carbohydrate, Fiber, Fat, Fatty Acids, Cholesterol, Protein, and Amino Acids*. Washington, DC: National Academies Press, 2005.
9. Chung M, Balk EM, Ip S, et al. Systematic review to support the development of nutrient reference intake values: challenges and solutions. *Am J Clin Nutr*. 2010;92:273–276.
10. Dietary Guidelines for Americans, 2005. http://www.health.gov/dietaryguidelines/dga2005.
11. Dietary Guidelines for Americans, 2010. http://www.health.gov/dietaryguidelines/dga2010/DietaryGuidelines2010.pdf.
12. USDA, Nutrient Data Laboratory. USDA Table of Nutrient Retention Factors, Release 6. http://www.ars.usda.gov/nutrientdata.
13. Eurofir.org. How Do Recipes and Composite Foods Come to Their Nutritional Values? http://www.eurofir.net/compiler_network/guidelines/recipe_calculation.
14. Eicher-Miller HA, Fulgoni VL III, Keast DR. Contributions of processed foods to dietary intake in the US from 2003–08: a report of the Food and Nutrition Science solutions join task force of the Academy of Nutrition and Dietetics, American Society for Nutrition, Institute of Food Technologists, and International Food Information Council. *J Nutr*. 2012;142:2065S.
15. Troesch B, Hoeft B, McBurney M, et al. Dietary surveys indicate vitamin intakes below recommendation are common in representative Western countries. *Br J Nutr*. 2012;108:602–608.
16. McCormick DB. Vitamin/mineral supplements: of questionable benefit for the general population. *Nutr Rev*. 2010;68:207–213.

17. U.S. Department of Agriculture, Food and Drug Administration. *Food Additives*. Washington, DC: U.S. Government Printing Office, 1992.
18. Fletcher RJ, Bell IP, Lambert JP. Public health aspects of food fortification: a question of balance. *Proc Nutr Soc*. 2004;63:605.
19. European Commission. Food Safety-Labeling & Nutrition-Health & Nutrition Claims. http://ec.europa.edu/food/food/labellingnutrition/claims/index_en.htm.
20. Sarubin A. *The Health Professional's Guide to Popular Dietary Supplements*. 2nd ed. Chicago, IL: The American Dietetic Association, 2003.
21. FDA. Food Ingredients & Packaging. http://www.fda.gov/food/foodingredientspackaging/ucm094211.htm.
22. Pascal G. Safety assessment of food additives and flavoring substances. In: van der Heijden K, Younes M, Fishbein L, et al, eds. *International Food Safety Handbook*. New York, NY: Marcel Dekker, 1999:239.
23. Femiano F, Lanza A, Buonaiuto C, et al. Oral manifestations of adverse drug reactions: guidelines. *J Eur Acad Dermatol Venereol*. 2008;22:681–691.
24. WHO Monograph No. 53. Clinical assessment of nutritional status. *Am J Public Health*. 1973;63(11 suppl):18–27.
25. Jen M, Yan AC. Syndromes associated with nutritional deficiency and excess. *Clin Dermatol*. 2010;28:669–685.
26. Mueller C, Compher C, Ellen DM; American Society for Parenteral and Enteral Nutrition (A.S.P.E.N.) Board of Directors. A.S.P.E.N. clinical guidelines: nutrition screening, assessment, and intervention in adults. *JPEN J Parenter Enteral Nutr*. 2011;35:16–24.
27. Sungurtckin H, Sungertckin U, Oner O, et al. Nutrition assessment in critically ill patients. *Nutr Clin Pract*. 2008;23:635–641.
28. Singh BN. Effects of food on clinical pharmacokinetics. *Clin Pharmacokinet*. 1999;37:213.
29. Parott N, Lukacova V, Fraczkiewicz G, et al. Predicting pharmacokinetics of drugs using physiologically based modeling—applications to food effects. *AAPS J*. 2009;11:45.
30. Haermann R, von Richter O. Clinical evidence of herbal drugs as perpetrators of pharmacokinetic drug interactions. *Planta Med*. 2012;78:1458.
31. Tandra S, Chalasani N, Jones DR, et al. Pharmacokinetic and pharmacodynamic alterations in the Roux-en-Y gastric bypass recipients. *Ann Surg*. 2013;258:262.
32. Chan LN. Drug therapy-related issues in patients who received bariatric surgery (part I and II). *Pract Gastroenterol*. 2010;34:26 (July) and 24 (August).
33. Boulleta JI, Armenti VT. *Handbook of Drug-Nutrient Interactions*. Towata, NJ: Humana Press, 2004.
34. Bruemmer B, Harris J, Gleason P, et al. Publishing nutrition research: a review of epidemiologic methods. *J Am Diet Assoc*. 2009;109:1728.
35. Schoenfeld JD, Ioannides JP. Is everything we eat associated with cancer? A systematic cookbook review. *Am J Clin Nutr*. 2013;97:127.
36. MacCoun RJ. Biases in the interpretation and use of research results. *Annu Rev Psychol*. 1998;49:259.
37. Schuemie MJ, Ryan PB, DuMouchel W, et al. Interpreting observational studies: why empiricial calibration is needed to correct p-values. *Stat Med*. 2014;33:209.
38. Shang A, Huwiler-Munterer K, Nartey L, et al. Are the clinical effects of homeopathy placebo effects? Comparative study of placebo-controlled trials of homeopathy and allopathy. *Lancet*. 2005;366:726.
39. Morris MC, Tangney CC. A potential design flaw of randomized trials of vitamin supplements. *JAMA*. 2011;305:1348.
40. Kipnis V, Midthune D, Freedman L, et al. Bias in dietary-report instruments and its implications for nutritional epidemiology. *Public Health Nutr*. 2002;5:915.
41. Moher D, Tricco AC. Issues related to the conduct of systematic reviews: a focus on the nutrition field. *Am J Clin Nutr*. 2008;88:1191.
42. Preiser JC, Chiolero R, Wernerman J. Nutritional papers in ICU patients: what lies between the lines? *Intensive Care M*ed. 2003;29:156.

SECTION II
Individual Nutrient Components

Protein and Calories: Requirements, Intake, and Assessment

ESTIMATION OF NORMAL DAILY REQUIREMENTS

The physician is often faced with patients who are losing or gaining weight, are undergoing surgery, or have a disease that increases or decreases their usual energy needs. To ensure the proper caloric intake, a reasonable estimate of energy needs must be made. Most of these estimates rely on the carefully measured and standardized determination of the basal metabolic rate (BMR) and of energy utilization during exercise. The general principles behind the estimation of energy requirements have been reviewed in detail (1,2).

Energy Equation

It is impossible to predict daily energy use precisely because of the complex factors involved. The methods used to determine energy needs experimentally are flawed, including diet recall and metabolic rates. Current recommendations do not allow for diversity in body composition, dietary intake, or level of activity. Nonetheless, if the principles involved in deriving the recommendations are understood, one can use the various methods to estimate energy needs. Energy requirements in humans are defined by the following formula:

$$\text{TEE} = \text{BMR} (60\% - 75\%) - \text{EEA} (15\% - 30\%) + \text{TEF} (\sim 10\%)$$

where TEE, total energy expenditure; BMR, basal metabolic rate, or BEE, basal energy expenditure; EEA, energy expenditure of activity; TEF, thermal effect of food.

BMR is a measure of the amount of energy expended to maintain a living state while at rest and asleep approximately 12 hours after a meal; synonyms for this measurement are *basal energy requirement* (BER), *basal energy expenditure* (BEE), *resting metabolic rate* (RMR), and *resting energy expenditure* (REE), though REE is not usually measured under resting but awake basal conditions. In practice, BMR and REE differ by less than 10%. The BMR or RMR is proportional to the fat-free mass (FFM) but is influenced by age, sex, body composition, and genetics. It decreases about 2% to 3% per decade and is greater in men than in women of equal weight. In the current dietary reference intake (DRI) volume covering energy (2), the BEE and TEE are assessed from a doubly labeled water (DLW) database, because this provided more reliable data than the older methods that relied either on factorial approaches or on food intake data. By following the decay in labeled body water ($^{3}\text{H}_2{}^{18}\text{O}$) for 1 to 2 weeks, one can calculate the rate of carbon dioxide production and estimate total daily energy needs in free-living individuals.

EEA, or thermal effect of activity (TEA), is a measure of the energy expended by the body to support a variety of physical activities. This is the most variable item in the energy equation, ranging from about 100 kcal per day in sedentary persons to about 3,000 kcal per day in moderately active persons. The EEA decreases with age and loss of FFM and is greater in men than in women of equal weight. In the derivation of DRI energy estimates (2), the EEA is replaced

TABLE 5-1 PAL Categories and Walking Equivalence

PAL Category	PAL Range	PAL	Light (44 kg)	Medium (70 kg)	Heavy (120 kg)
			(Mean Walking Equivalence [miles/day at 3–4 mph])		
Sedentary	1.0–1.39	1.25	~0	~0	~0
Low active	1.4–1.59	1.5	2.9	2.2	1.5
Active	1.6–1.89	1.75	9.9	7.3	5.3
Very active	1.9–2.49	2.2	22.5	16.7	12.3

Sources: Adapted from Standing Committee on the Scientific Evaluation of Dietary Reference Intakes, Food and Nutrition Board, Institute of Medicine. *Dietary Reference Intakes for Energy, Carbohydrate, Fiber, Fat, Fatty Acids, Cholesterol, Protein and Amino Acids.* Washington, DC: The National Academies Press, 2005:161.

by a physical activity level (PAL). The PAL is defined as the ratio of TEE to BEE. Thus, the impact of PAL on TEE depends on body size and age, as these are factors that affect the BEE. The data for PAL have been derived from the DLW database for BEE and from the multiples of an individual's resting oxygen uptake (metabolic equivalents [METs]) for a variety of activities (see Section III, Energy Requirements). A range of PALs has allowed individuals to be classified as sedentary, low active, active, or very active (Table 5-1). Because walking is the most significant activity in the lives of most people, this is taken as the reference activity.

The PAL can be envisioned by equating the various PAL levels with an estimated walking distance for individuals of various builds, assuming that all of their activity would be performed by walking.

TEF is an estimate of the number of calories produced during the ingestion and metabolism of food, also called the *specific dynamic action of food* (SDA). The obligatory components of the TEF represent the energy needed for absorption and transport of nutrients plus synthesis and storage. Ingesting protein increases energy expenditure by 12% of consumed calories, carbohydrate by 6%, and fat by 2%. A mixed diet causes an increase in energy expenditure by 6% of consumed calories, but 10% is the usual figure used for simplicity. The lower the TEE, the greater the relative importance of the caloriogenic effect in determining total energy requirements. The caloriogenic effect of food occurs even after food is administered intravenously. The TEF decreases with age and insulin resistance. In hypermetabolic or infected, febrile patients, the SDA is lower than normal because heat production is already increased. Thus, the figure used to calculate additional energy requirements for these patients should be 5% rather than 10%. The estimated energy requirement (EER) derived in the DRI (2) comprises a number based on BEE obtained from the DLW database, plus the PAL coefficient, with age, height, and weight factored in.

DRI equations for estimating EER include TEE, PAL, and a factor for energy deposition for ages up to 18, but only TEE and PAL for older ages. Energy is reported in kilocalories (kcal) for DRIs, but the World Health Organization (WHO) has adopted kilojoules, the mechanical equivalent of heat, as their unit of energy: $4.184 \text{ kJ} = 1 \text{ kcal}$, or $1 \text{ kJ} = 0.239 \text{ kcal}$.

For ages 0 to 36 months:

0–3 months	$(89 \times \text{weight [kg]}) - 100) + 175 \text{ kcal}$
4–6 months	$(89 \times \text{weight [kg]}) - 100) + 56 \text{ kcal}$
7–12 months	$(89 \times \text{weight [kg]}) - 100) + 22 \text{ kcal}$
13–36 months	$(89 \times \text{weight [kg]}) - 100) + 20 \text{ kcal}$

For ages 3 to 8 years:

Boys $135.3 - [30.8 \times \text{age (y)}] + \text{PA} \times [10.0 \times \text{weight (kg)} + 903 \times \text{height (m)}] + 20 \text{ kcal}$
Girls $135.3 - [30.8 \times \text{age (y)}] + \text{PA} \times [10.0 \times \text{weight (kg)} + 934 \times \text{height (m)}] + 20 \text{ kcal}$

PA is based on PAL status and = 1.0 for sedentary, 1.13 (M) or 1.16 (F) for low active, 1.31 (F) or 1.26 (M) for active, and 1.56 (F) or 1.42 (M) for very active.

For ages 9 to 18:

Boys 88.5 − [61.99 × age (y)] + PA × [26.7 × weight (kg) + 903 × height (m)] + 25 kcal
Girls 135.3 − [30.8 × age (y)] + PA × [10.0 × weight (kg) + 934 × height (m)] + 25 kcal

PA is based on PAL status as noted for ages 3 to 8.

For ages 19 and older:

Men 662 − [9.53 × age (y)] + PA × [15.91 × weight (kg) + 539.6 × height (m)]
Women 354 − [6.91 × age (y)] + PA × [9.36 × weight (kg) + 726 × height (m)]

PA is based on PAL status (Table 5-1) and = 1.0 for sedentary, 1.11 (M) or 1.12 (F) for low active, 1.25 (M) or 1.27 (F) for active, and 1.48 (M) or 1.45 (F) for very active. An online spreadsheet is available to calculate EER based on PAL (http://www.cdc.gov/pcd/issues/2006/OCT/06_0034.htm).

Choice of Method

Although the DRI estimates of EER are considered the most accurate that can be made using current technology, more easily derived numbers are used for clinical purposes. The physician can be confused by the large number of empirically derived methods for estimating the three components of the daily energy requirement. More than 190 methods have been reported to predict energy expenditures (3). The following sections outline a number of the available methods. It is important to use a single method of calculation for each of the three components and to understand the limitations of that method. It is not necessary to learn multiple methods for calculating the BMR or any of the other components because the methods all provide only an estimate and not a precise calculation.

ASSESSMENT OF BASAL METABOLIC RATE

Measurement of BMR by Using Indirect Calorimetry

The metabolic pathways that consume oxygen produce carbon dioxide and heat. Indirect calorimetry involves measuring oxygen uptake ($\dot{V}O_2$) and carbon dioxide output ($\dot{V}CO_2$) at the mouth. Most clinical equipment utilizes the open-circuit method, in which a set of one-way valves directs expired air into a collecting bag. At the end of a timed period, both the volume and composition of expired air are measured and the rates of oxygen consumption and carbon dioxide production are calculated by the difference between the concentrations in the inspired air and the gas collected. The REE is determined from these data by using the respiratory quotient, ($\dot{V}CO_2$)/($\dot{V}O_2$) This method requires the use of a metabolic cart and trained personnel but is generally quite accurate. Breath-by-breath systems now allow measurement of the REE even in ventilator patients receiving high levels (>80%) of inspired oxygen (4). If only oxygen consumption data are available, the REE can be estimated by multiplying the oxygen consumption in milliliters per minute by a factor of 7.

The Fick equation can be used to calculate energy expenditure in patients who have a pulmonary artery catheter in place (5). The calculation is based on ($\dot{V}O_2$) alone, with the use of the known caloric value of oxygen (4.86 kcal per L for an estimated respiratory quotient of 0.85). Oxygen consumption is calculated from the Fick equation with measurements of cardiac output (CO), hemoglobin level (Hb), and arterial (SaO_2) and mixed venous ($S\dot{V}CO_2$) oxygen saturations.

$$REE \text{ (kcal/day)} = CO \times Hb \times (SaO_2 - S\dot{V}O_2) \times 95.18$$

This method appears to be as accurate as indirect calorimetry and uses data available in most intensive care units. In mechanically ventilated nonsurgical patients without sepsis, the Harris–Benedict estimate was comparable (6). In patients with sepsis, an additional requirement of about 20% is appropriate.

Although the equipment for measuring BMR is not complicated, the actual measurement is time-consuming, and considerable variability is involved unless the conditions maintained during measurement are carefully standardized. It has become accepted practice that estimates of BMR are derived from carefully collated data from normal subjects obtained under controlled conditions. Additional energy requirements attributed to the TEF, growth (in children), and illness are estimated independently and added to the calories required for the BMR.

In mechanically ventilated patients, reliable measurements of energy expenditure can be made by using indirect calorimetry if trained personnel are available who are able to use the equipment properly and to interpret the results (7). System leaks must be avoided, FIO_2 must be greater than 80% and stable, and multiple samples of 15 to 30 minutes should be taken to extrapolate a mean REE over a 24-hour day (4). Confounding factors that lead to instability of VO_2 include multiple trauma, burns, multisystem organ failure, sepsis, ARDS, oversedation, or large or multiple open wounds. Although underfeeding is often associated with a RQ less than 0.85, it is important to realize that RQ does not always reflect substrate use, especially in the face of underlying pulmonary disease, acid/base abnormalities, or pharmacologic agents. All these confounders limit the use of indirect calorimetry, even when accurate assessment of REE is most needed, for example, for critically ill patients

Methods for Calculating BMR

The BMR can be estimated in a variety of ways by using calculations based on (a) body size (height and weight), (b) weight alone, (c) body size and age, (d) weight and sex, and (e) weight, height, age, and sex. Not surprisingly, the BMR values based on different individual parameters are not identical for each method in the same person. In regard to clinical usefulness, all these methods are satisfactory. The first group of methods presented requires the use of tables to estimate the BMR. Shorter methods not requiring tables are reasonably accurate for estimating the BMR over the entire range of existing body sizes and are currently in widespread use.

The cells of the body require oxygen for their integrity; the greater the number of cells, the greater the oxygen consumption. Adipose cells are relatively inert from a metabolic point of view; they constitute about 20% of the body mass but account for only 2% to 4% of the BMR. Thus, in overweight persons, whose adipose cells are increased in number and size, the correlation between weight alone and oxygen consumption is not linear, and oxygen consumption per pound of extra weight is not equivalent to that per pound of lean body weight. Instead of the old, portable BMR apparatus, DLW ($^3H_2^{18}O$) is used. Body surface area is a more reasonable determinant of lean body mass (LBM)—that is, metabolically active tissues. Muscle makes up 35% to 40% of body weight but contributes only 20% to the BMR. The brain, heart, kidneys, and liver require high levels of energy but change less with body size than does muscle mass. The increase in BMR per kilogram of body weight or per square meter of surface area depends primarily on the relative proportions of skeletal muscle and adipose tissue and their metabolic activity (different for various states of conditioning). Thus, oxygen consumption increases at the same rate in any person for every unit of increase in body surface area (BSA). As body weight increases over normal, when adipose tissue is the major component of body tissue added, the rate of increase in oxygen consumption declines. It is more accurate to have an estimation of BMR that accounts for these changes rather than one based on weight alone.

BMR Estimate Based on Body Surface Area

This estimate is made according to the following steps:

a. Determine BSA. This is most easily accomplished using an online site, such as MedCalc (http://medcalc.com/body.htm. The BSA can be calculated at this site by one of five methods (Mosteller, DuBois & DuBois, Haycock, Gehan & George, and Boyd); all give similar results. The BMR is expressed in square meters (m^2).

b. Identify the metabolic rate for any individual from predicted averages for age and sex (Table 5-2). These rates are given as kilocalories per square meter per day ($kcal/m^2/day$), an energy equivalent derived from the rate of oxygen consumption. The BMR is highest per square meter in the first few years of life and then steadily declines, although a slight increase occurs at puberty.

c. The BMR (kcal per day) equals the metabolic rate ($kcal/m^2/day$) given in (Table 5-2) times surface area (m^2). Basal metabolism may not be constant throughout the day, and the final calculated estimate does not account for such variations. Nonetheless, it provides a clinically useful guide.

TABLE 5-2 Standard BMRs Based on BSA for Age and Sex

Metabolic Rate (kcal/m²/day)

Age (y)	Men	Women
1	1,272	1,272
2	1,258	1,258
3	1,231	1,229
4	1,207	1,195
5	1,183	1,162
6	1,160	1,128
7	1,135	1,090
8	1,111	1,051
9	1,085	1,027
10	1,056	1,020
11	1,032	1,008
12	1,020	991
13	1,015	967
14	1,010	941
15	1,003	910
16	994	886
17	979	871
18	960	862
19	941	852
20	926	847
25	900	845
30	883	842
35	876	840
40	871	838
45	869	828
50	859	814
55	850	799
60	838	785
65	826	773
70	811	761
75 and over	797	751

Sources: Data from Fleish A. Le métabolisme basal standard et sa determination au moyen du "Metabocalculator" [in German]. *Helv Med Acta.* 1951;18:23.

Method Based on Sex, Height, Age, and Weight (Harris–Benedict Equation)

An estimate based on indirect calorimetry was devised by J. A. Harris and F. G. Benedict (8). This method has gained wide acceptance because it requires no tables and is reasonably accurate in comparison with measurements of oxygen consumption (REE prediction is accurate to ±14%). However, malnutrition is associated with an increase in resting oxygen consumption, apparently only when it is expressed per predicted body mass (9). In malnutrition, a greater preservation of visceral than of skeletal components leads to an increase in REE (BMR) per body cell mass. The underestimation of BMR by the Harris–Benedict equation in malnourished patients is about 20%, but no constant factor can be applied to all patients. This inaccuracy would be true for all methods of estimating BMR but has been examined most carefully for the Harris–Benedict equation. A similar overestimation occurs in obese patients (10).

For normally nourished persons, the BMR can be calculated from the following formulas:

$$\text{BMR women} = 665 + (9.6 \times W) + (1.8 \times H) - (4.7 \times A)$$

$$\text{BMR men} = 66 + (13.8 \times W) + (5 \times H) - (6.8 \times A)$$

where *W* is actual or usual weight (kg); *H*, height (cm); and *A*, age (years).

The Harris–Benedict data have been reevaluated, and data for a wider age range, but still for normally nourished people, have been added (9).

For overweight persons, an adjusted body weight can be used, based on usual body weight (10):

$$\text{Adjusted body weight} = \left[(\text{actual weight} - \text{ideal weight}) \times 0.25\right] + \text{ideal body weight}$$

Alternatively, ideal body weight may be estimated by using the Hamwi formula (11): For males, 106 lb for the first 60 in of height plus 6 lb for each additional inch; for females, 100 lb for the first 60 in of height plus 5 lb for each additional inch. Add 10% for a large frame size; subtract 10% for a small frame size.

To determine frame size, wrist measurements are used. Small and large frames fall outside the ranges for a medium frame. A medium frame for males taller than 165 cm (65 in) is defined as a wrist circumference of 16.5 to 19 cm. Comparable figures for wrist circumference for females are 14 to 14.5 cm for a height of less than 157 cm (62 in), 15 to 16 cm for a height of 157 to 165 cm, and 16 to 16.5 cm for a height above 165 cm.

More simply, ideal body weight can also be calculated after input of body weight and height on various websites (e.g., http://www.medcalc.com/body.htm).

World Health Organization/Food and Agriculture Organization Equations

These equations for REE (BMR) are simpler than those of Harris and Benedict and are based on more comprehensive data. The sample used includes persons who are thin (body mass index [BMI] > 25). People of the same weight but different heights have similar BMRs, but among adults of the same height but different weights, those with lighter weights have higher BMRs per kilogram because of the difference in body composition. For this reason, the simpler formula based only on body weight, age, and sex is reasonable. The equations to be used are as follows:

Age (y)	Male	Female
0–3	$(60.9 \times W^a) - 54$	$(61.0 \times W) - 51$
3–10	$(22.7 \times W) - 495$	$(22.5 \times W) + 499$
10–18	$(17.5 \times W) + 651$	$(12.2 \times W) + 746$
18–30	$(15.3 \times W) + 679$	$(14.7 \times W) + 996$
30–60	$(11.6 \times W) + 879$	$(8.7 \times W) + 829$
>60	$(13.5 \times W) + 987$	$(10.5 \times W) + 596$

[a] Weight in kilograms.

With such formulas, one can derive daily REE values for persons of different weights (Table 5-3). The values differ from the 1973 WHO standards mostly for females, in whom an overestimation of weight above 40 kg reached nearly 18% by the end of the scale. For both sexes, the earlier standards underestimated values between 15 and 20 kg. The overestimation of BMR for healthy women over 40 kg was confirmed in a careful study of 44 women aged 18 to 65 years (12). This study found that other currently available tables and regression equations (including Harris–Benedict) overestimate the BMR of healthy women by 7% to 14%. The authors offered the following equations:

For persons who are not athletes:

$$\text{BMR} = 795 + 7.18 \times W\,(\text{kg})$$

For athletes:

$$\text{BMR} = 50.4 + 21.1 \times W\,(\text{kg})$$

TABLE 5-3   BMRs According to Weight and Sex

	Metabolic Rate (kcal/24 h)	
Body Weight (kg)	Males	Females
3.0	120	144
4.0	191	191
5.0	239	239
6.0	287	311
7.0	357	383
8.0	431	431
9.0	478	502
10.0	550	550
11.0	622	622
12.0	670	670
13.0	718	718
14.0	765	765
15.0	813	813
16.0	861	837
17.0	885	861
18.0	909	885
19.0	933	909
20.0	957	933
22.0	1,005	957
24.0	1,058	981
26.0	1,100	1,005
28.0	1,124	1,055
30.0	1,172	1,076
32.0	1,196	1,100
34.0	1,244	1,124
36.0	1,268	1,148
38.0	1,316	1,172
40.0	1,340	1,172
42.0	1,363	1,196
44.0	1,387	1,220
46.0	1,435	1,220
48.0	1,459	1,244
50.0	1,483	1,268
52.0	1,507	1,268
54.0	1,531	1,292
56.0	1,579	1,316
58.0	1,603	1,316
60.0	1,627	1,340
62.0	1,650	1,363
64.0	1,674	1,387
66.0	1,698	1,411
68.0	1,722	1,435
70.0	1,746	1,459
72.0	1,746	1,459
74.0	1,770	1,483
76.0	1,794	1,507
78.0	1,818	1,507
80.0	1,842	1,532
82.0	1,866	1,555
84.0	1,890	1,579

Sources: MJ/24 h has been converted to kcal/24 h as follows: 1,000 kcal = 4.18 MJ (Kleiber M. Joules VS. Calories in nutrition. *J Nutr.* 1972;102:307). These figures are not applicable to the elderly. See text for a formula to use for persons older than 60 years.
Data from James WPT. Basal metabolic rate: comments on the new equations. *Hum Nutr Clin Nutr.* 1985;39C(suppl 1):5.

The WHO/ Food and Agriculture Organization equations offer realistic and comprehensive estimates. One should remember, however, that the predicted BMR in nonathletes may overestimate or underestimate the measured values by 20% to 30% for any individual.

Method Based on Body Size and Age

The BMR declines with age by almost 2% per decade in adults 20 to 75 years of age (13). The metabolic rate data compiled by Fleish (Table 5-2) can be converted to Wilmore's equation, which allows the rate to be calculated without consulting the table (14). If one assumes a metabolic rate of 55 kcal/m²/hour at birth, then the following equations apply:

From birth to age 19 years:

$$BMR (kcal/m^2/h) = 55 - age (y)$$

For age 20 years or more:

$$BMR (kcal/m^2/h) = 37 - [(age - 20) + 10]$$

Estimated BEE for Most Hospitalized Patients

The goal for caloric intake for most patients is between 25 and 35 kcal/kg/day, or 125% to 175% of the BEE (BMR). The range of TEE for healthy nonelderly US adults, by comparison, is 167 ± 14% of the BEE (2). To avoid excess provision of glucose, fat, or amino acids, reasonable goals for nonprotein kilocalories per day are as follows: glucose, ≤5 g/kg/day; lipid, ≤1 g/kg/day; and amino acids, 0.75 to 1.5 g/kg/day from a mixed protein diet, depending on the status of protein stores and the need to replace protein losses.

A simple method for estimating total daily energy requirements in hospitalized patients is based on the BMI (kg per m²) (Table 5-4). Increments in energy requirements are inversely proportional to the BMI. The lower range in each category should be considered in patients who are insulin resistant or critically ill, unless they are depleted of body fat, to decrease the risk for hyperglycemia and infection associated with overfeeding.

The total energy requirement in illness in hospitalized patients on total *parenteral nutrition* (TPN) rarely exceeds by much the basal rate of the same patient in health. This is because both starvation and catabolic states (cachexia) lead to a relative conservation of body tissues. Starvation produces a fall in nearly all metabolic processes, whereas cachexia increases catabolism. But the net effect on TEE is minimal or even negative.

Because the energy of activity is quite low in immobilized patients, the total energy requirement in severe illness usually does not exceed the estimated BMR by more than 25% (15). Therefore, although the total energy requirement in patients with illness has been estimated by adding to the REE additional energy requirements for activity, stress, and fever, it is probably most accurate to base the REE on Harris–Benedict equation or WHO equations using actual body weight. Equations have been developed for use in estimating the REE of hospitalized patients

TABLE 5-4 Estimate of Energy Requirements for Patients Based on BMI[a]

	Energy Requirements (kcal/kg/day)	
BMI (kg/m²)	Critically Ill Patients (RMR)	Other Patients (RMR + TEF + TEA)
<15	35–40	35–40 + 20%
15–19	30–35	30–35 + 20%
20–29	20–25	20–25 + 20%
≥30	15–20[b]	15–20

[a]Use Harris–Benedict or WHO equations to estimate requirement for patients whose estimate by this method is <1,200 kcal/day.
[b]Do not exceed 2,000 kcal/day.
BMI, body mass index; RMR, resting metabolic rate; TEF, thermal effect of food; TEA, thermal effect of activity.

TABLE 5-5 Estimation of REE in Hospitalized Patients

For Ventilator-Dependent Patients:

REE(s) = 1784 − 11(A) + 5(W) + 244(S) + 239(T) + 804(B)

For Spontaneously Breathing Patients:

REE(s) = 629 − 11(A) + 25(W) − 609(O)

REE, resting energy expenditure (kcal/d); A, age (y); W, body weight (kg); S, sex (male = 1, female = 0); T, diagnosis of trauma (present = 1, absent = 0); B, diagnosis of burn (present = 1, absent = 0); O, obesity (present = 1, absent = 0).
Sources: From Malone AM. Methods of assessing energy expenditure in the intensive care unit. *Nutr Clin Pract.* 2002;17:21.

when indirect calorimetry is not available and when more precision is desired than is provided by the Harris–Benedict equation (10,16). These equations were developed for both ventilator-dependent and spontaneously breathing patients by correlating indirect calorimetry results and other variables by means of multivariate regression analysis (Table 5-5). Increases above those determined for REE can be estimated, even for medically ill patients. For severely catabolic or malnourished hospitalized patients or for those with high fever or sepsis, an increase of 20% to 25% can be added. Overestimation should be avoided, however, because increased feeding with high-glucose infusions can cause hyperglycemia, hypokalemia, edema, and fatty liver.

THE ENERGY EXPENDITURE OF ACTIVITY/PHYSICAL ACTIVITY LEVEL

The EEA can vary from 1.1 to 10.3 kcal/kg/hour. In fact, a correct calculation of energy requirement over 24 hours would include sleep time (about 90% of BMR) and the metabolic rate per hour of different types of work. In some types of work (e.g., gardening), certain muscle groups become fatigued without a large number of calories being used. Usually, any exercise in which the body leaves the ground (e.g., running) uses a large number of calories. However, one should not overestimate the contribution of sports to overall daily energy use because sports activities generally last for a short time and are followed by a much longer period of inactivity. Table 5-6 provides a more detailed analysis of activity-related energy expenditures. A number of methods are used to estimate or calculate the EEA.

Calculation Based on Level of Activity

A calculation, albeit imprecise, can be used if the typical activity pattern is known. An average daily activity factor can be calculated from the estimated level of activity, weighted for the time spent in each activity. Average estimates for different levels of activity are given in Table 5-7 as METs measured by the rate of oxygen consumption relative to basal conditions. The ΔPAL is calculated from the BEE using the reference body weights and heights for adults (Table 5-8). The difficulty with assigning a level of activity to individuals without a daily diary is due to the large variability in the duration and intensity of physical activity. The determination of the level of PAL (sedentary, low active, active, very active) is determined by the type of activity and how sustained it is. A truly valid estimate would consider activity patterns over days or weeks. An easy approach to calculating EER has been presented, linked to the concept of PAL (17). This article can be accessed online (http://www.cdc.gov/pcd/issues/2006/oct/06_0034.htm). At the end of the article, there is a link to an Excel spreadsheet that will calculate the BEE for men and women after input of age, weight (kg), and height (m). A list of activities is presented, and by altering the duration of each, the template will then calculate the PAL and deliver the TEE for the individual. This template can be used for both healthy subjects and those with illness.

While TEE decreases in the elderly as a function of decreased body mass and PAL, the presence of disease may increase energy expenditure. An accurate estimation of the BMR, or REE, of patients in intensive care units is important because both overfeeding and underfeeding may produce adverse effects. The calculation made from equations can be inaccurate in critically ill patients (18). Moreover, the effects of stress and infection are difficult to estimate. Therefore,

TABLE 5-6 Calories Used for 10 Minutes of Activity

Activity	\multicolumn{5}{c}{Body Weight (lb)}				
	125	150	175	200	250
Sedentary					
Sleeping	10	12	14	16	20
Sitting	10–15	12–18	14–21	16–24	18–30
Standing	12	14	16	19	24
Dressing or washing	26	32	37	42	53
Light office work	25	30	34	39	50
Standing (light activity)	20	24	28	32	40
Typing 40 words per minute	25	30	34	39	50
Locomotion					
Walking, downstairs	56	67	78	88	111
Walking, upstairs	146	175	202	229	288
Walking, 2 mph	29	35	40	46	58
Walking, 4 mph	52	62	72	81	102
Running, 5.5 mph	90	108	125	142	178
Running, 7 mph	118	141	164	187	232
Cycling, 5.5 mph	42	50	58	67	83
Cycling, 13 mph	89	107	124	142	178
Light Work					
Domestic work	34	41	47	53	68
Weeding garden	49	59	68	78	98
Shoveling snow	65	78	89	100	130
Lawn mowing, power	34	41	47	53	67
Assembly work in factory	20	24	28	34	40
Auto repair	35	46	48	54	69
House painting	29	35	40	46	58
Heavy Work					
Chopping wood	60	73	84	96	121
Pick and shovel	56	67	78	88	110
Dragging logs, lifting heavy materials	158	189	220	252	315
Recreation					
Baseball (except pitching)	39	47	54	62	78
Basketball	58	70	82	93	117
Dancing (moderate)	35	42	48	55	69
Football	69	83	96	110	137
Golfing	33	40	48	55	68
Racketball, squash	75	90	104	117	144
Skiing, downhill	80	96	112	128	160
Skiing, cross-country	98	117	138	158	194
Swimming, crawl (20 yd/min)	40	48	56	63	80
Tennis	56	67	80	92	115
Volleyball	43	52	65	75	94

Sources: Data from Brownell KD. *The Partnership Diet Program.* New York, NY: Rawson-Wade, 1980.

other methods have been used to provide more accurate assessments. It is not yet certain whether this degree of accuracy is required for patients in intensive care units because the WHO and Harris–Benedict equations are useful in determining the REE in many cases. In addition, determinations must be made when the patient's clinical condition is stable. It is unlikely that the risk of providing too much (or too little) energy to critically ill patients will justify the expense of calorimetric measurements. The risks of nutrient provision more often involve fluid and

TABLE 5-7 Impact of Various Activities on PAL Estimations

Activity	METs	ΔPAL/h	Activity	METs	ΔPAL/h
Mild → moderate			**Vigorous**		
Lying quietly	1.0	0	Chopping wood	4.9	0.22
Riding in a vehicle	1.0	0	Tennis (doubles)	5.0	0.23
Light activity, sitting	1.5	0.03	Dancing (fast)	5.5	0.26
Playing piano	2.3	0.07	Skating, ice	5.5	0.26
Walking (2 mph)	2.5	0.09	Cycling, moderate	5.7	0.27
Watering plants	2.5	0.09	Dancing, aerobic	6.0	0.29
Golf (with cart)	2.5	0.09	Skating, roller	6.5	0.31
Dancing, ballroom	2.9	0.11	Skiing, water/snow	6.8	0.33
Volleyball, casual	2.9	0.11	Climbing hills	6.9	0.34
Walking the dog	3.0	0.11	Swimming	7.0	0.34
Loading/unloading car	3.0	0.11	Climbing w/load	7.4	0.37
Taking out trash	3.0	0.11	Walking (5 mph)	8.0	0.4
Mopping/vacuuming	3.5	0.14	Jogging (10 mph)	10.2	0.53
Lifting, raking lawn	4.0	0.17	Playing squash	12.1	0.63
Calisthenics, no weight	4.0	0.17			
Golf, no cart	4.4	0.19			
Swimming, slow	4.5	0.20			
Walking, 4 mph	4.5	0.20			

METs = multiples of resting oxygen uptake, based on 3.5 mL of O_2/min/kg body weight in adults.
PAL levels are as follows: Sedentary 1.0 to 1.4, Low active 1.4 to 1.6, Active 1.6 to 1.9, Very active 1.9 to 2.5.
Sources: Data from Standing Committee on the Scientific Evaluation of Dietary Reference Intakes, Food and Nutrition Board, Institute of Medicine. *Dietary Reference Intakes for Energy, Carbohydrate, Fiber, Fat, Fatty Acids, Cholesterol, Protein and Amino Acids.* Washington, DC: The National Academies Press, 2005:885–886.

TABLE 5-8 New Median Heights and Weights for Children and Adults in the United States

Gender	Age	Reference Height (cm [in])	Reference Weight (kg [lb])	BMI (kg/m^2)
M, F	2–6 mo	62 (24)	6 (13)	—
	7–12 mo	71 (28)	9 (20)	—
	1–3 y	86 (34)	12 (27)	
	4–8 y	115 (45)	20 (44)	
Male	9–13 y	144 (57)	36 (79)	
	14–18 y	174 (68)	61 (134)	20.5
	19–30 y	177 (70)	70 (154)	22.5
Female	9–13 y	144 (57)	37 (81)	
	14–18 y	163 (64)	54 (119)	20.4
	19–30 y	163 (64)	57 (126)	21.5

Sources: Data from Standing Committee on the Scientific Evaluation of Dietary Reference Intakes, Food and Nutrition Board, Institute of Medicine. *Dietary Reference Intakes for Energy, Carbohydrate, Fiber, Fat, Fatty Acids, Cholesterol, Protein and Amino Acids.* Washington, DC: The National Academies Press, 2005:35.

electrolytes when given in excess. If calorimetry is available, it should be used only for selected patients who are very malnourished or who might tolerate the energy provision poorly, such as those in cardiac or respiratory failure.

SPECIAL ENERGY REQUIREMENTS

There are additional energy requirements in illness. Heat production increases with inflammation and infection. Infection increases basal metabolism. The final caloric expenditure depends on the increase in oxygen consumption caused by fever or new cell production and the decrease in oxygen consumption caused by diminished calorie intake and immobility. An estimate for increasing the REE for fever is the following: (°F $-$ 98.6) $\times$ 0.07 for Fahrenheit, and (°C $-$ 37.0) $\times$ 0.13 for centigrade.

Fasting or very low calorie intake decreases the BMR by approximately 25% by day 20. Although the calculations for BEE probably underestimate the REE for malnourished patients, the total REE falls significantly as weight falls. REE, when adjusted for differences in body weight (20 kcal per kg) and FFM (28 kcal per kg of FFM/day), is similar in healthy and ill elderly people (19). Over the age of 60, however, the effect of sex disappears. The major organs contributing to REE are liver, brain, heart, kidneys, and skeletal muscle, with the latter contribution due to the large mass of muscle. The similarity of REE across age groups is consistent with the fact that age-adjusted energy expenditure attributed to various organs (adjusted for organ size) is similar across the spectrum of adult ages (20).

Many conditions associated with weight loss have been thought to be associated with increased energy needs. However, daily energy expenditure is lower than expected in elderly patients with cachexia (21). This result is consistent with inadequate intake as the cause of weight loss because in the long term, the balance between daily energy expenditure and food intake must determine body composition.

Malabsorption is a special case of an increased energy requirement, in which a loss of nutrients results from incomplete absorption of food. The most accurate way to assess caloric loss would be calorimetry of the feces. However, one can determine daily fat excretion more practically with a 72-hour fecal fat study. Fat accounts for about 40% of caloric intake. If one assumes that protein and carbohydrate are similarly malabsorbed, one then can estimate total calorie malabsorption by multiplying caloric loss from fat by 2.5. Carbohydrate probably is more efficiently absorbed than fat in diseases producing a short-bowel syndrome but not necessarily in diffuse mucosal disease. In practice, no distinction needs to be made between the proportion of macronutrients as caloric sources in the diet and as caloric losses in the feces.

$$\text{Fat excretion (g/day)} \times 9 \text{ kcal/g} = \text{fecal kcal loss from fat malabsorption}$$

$$\text{Fecal kilocalorie loss from fat} \times 2.5 = \text{total kcal lost from diet}$$

The energy requirement for a full-term pregnancy is estimated at 80,000 kcal. The WHO recommends an increased intake for pregnant women of 150 kcal per day over normal during the first trimester and 350 kcal per day over normal during the rest of the pregnancy. This estimate does not take into account any variation in physical activity or weight gain unrelated to gestation. Because the activity of pregnant women in Western societies is usually decreased, an increase of 300 kcal per day is recommended for the second and third trimesters.

The production of 1 dL of human breast milk requires 67 to 77 kcal. Because the efficiency of converting nutrients to milk energy is 80% to 90%, the total energy requirement is 80 to 95 kcal per dL of milk. If 8.5 dL per day is the average rate of milk production for 3 months, the energy needed will be 750 kcal per day. However, extra fat stores are deposited during pregnancy, and it is estimated that these can provide the mother with 200 to 300 kcal per day for 3 months. Thus, the recommended additional caloric requirement for nursing mothers is 500 kcal per day.

ESTIMATION OF CALORIC INTAKE

The estimation of a patient's total daily intake of calories requires a careful dietary history. It is most helpful to use a reference in which the caloric contents of foods are listed according to common package limits or portion sizes (i.e., per ounce or per cup). Sources of such data are readily available to be downloaded from the U.S. Department of Agriculture website for the National Nutrient Database for Standard References (www.ars.usda.gov/Services/docs.htm?docid=8964) (22). Table 5-9 lists the caloric content of some important common foods. Numerous calorie

TABLE 5-9 Caloric Content of Common Foods

Food	Portion Size	Kilocalories
Apple	1 (3/4 lb)	80
Baby foods		
Vegetables, fruits	4 3/4 oz	113–207
Meat	3 1/2-oz jar	99–136
Bacon, cooked	Yield from 1/4 lb	215
Beans, green, cooked	1 cup	35
Beef		
Sirloin steak, cooked	Yield from 1/2 lb	596
Ground beef, lean, cooked	Yield from 1/2 lb	497
Beverages		
Cola	12-oz can	144
Ginger ale, sweet mixers	12-oz can	113
40% Bran flakes	1 cup	106
Bread		
White	1 slice, regular	63–74
Whole wheat	1 slice, regular	56–61
Rye	1 slice, regular	61
Butter or margarine	1 tbs	322
Cake		
Chocolate, no icing	1 piece, 3 × 3 × 2 in	322
White, with chocolate icing	1 piece, 3 × 3 × 2 in	453
Candy		
Chocolate	1 oz	135–144
Chocolate with nuts	1 oz	159
Carrot	1	30
Cheese		
Cheddar	1 slice	96
American	1 oz	113
Cottage (regular)	1 oz	30
Swiss	1 slice	130
Chicken		
Broiled	Yield from 1 lb	273
Fried	Yield from 1 lb	565
	Breast, half	160
	Thigh	122
Cookies		
Brownies	1	97
Chocolate chip	1	52
Sugar	1	46
Corn, cooked	1 ear	70
Crackers		
Saltines	1 cracker	12
Graham	1 cracker	62
Doughnuts		
Raised	1	176
Cake	1	164

(continued)

TABLE 5-9   Caloric Content of Common Foods *(continued)*

Food	Portion Size	Kilocalories
Eggs		
Extra large, fried	1	112
Cooking oil	1 tbs	111–120
Grapefruit	1	80–132
Ice cream		
Regular	1 cup	257
Frozen custard	1 cup	334
Rich (16% fat)	1 cup	329
Jam	1 tbs	54
Milk		
Whole	1 cup	159
Skim	1 cup	88
Low fat	1 cup	145
Noodles, egg	Yield from 4 oz	440
Orange		
Navel	1	45–87
Juice	1 cup	112–122
Pastry, Danish	One 4-in-diameter pastry	274
Peanuts, out of shell	1 oz	166
Peanut butter	1 tbs	94
Peas, canned	1 cup	142
Pies		
Fresh, banana	One 31/2-in piece (1/8 pie)	253
Fresh, pecan		431
Frozen	One 31/2-in piece (1/8 pie)	187–282
Pizza		
Homemade, cheese	1/8 12-in pie	153
Frozen, cheese	1/8 12-in pie	139
Ham, roasted or baked	1/2 lb	848
Pork chops, lean	Yield from 1/2 lb	442
Potatoes		
Boiled with skin	1	173
Boiled without skin	1	122
French fried	Ten 4-in strips	214
Chips	10 chips	114
Rice, white, cooked	1/4 cup	56
Salad dressing, Italian	1 tbs	83
Salmon		
Fresh, broiled	1/2 lb	364
Canned	1/2 lb	320–477
Sausage		
Bologna	1 slice	67–86
Hot dogs, cooked	1	134–170
Pork, cooked	1 link	62
Salami	1 slice	66–88
Spaghetti, cooked, from 21/2 oz dry	1/4 lb	168
Sugar, granulated	1 tsp	15
	1 cup	770
Tuna, canned	7 oz	570

TABLE 5-10 Caloric Content of Food Groups

Nutrient	kcal/g	kJ/g
Carbohydrates		
Monosaccharide	3.75	16
Disaccharide	3.94	16
Starch and glycogen	4.13	17
Total carbohydrate	4	17
Protein	4	17
Long-chain triglyceride	9	37
Medium-chain triglyceride	8.3	34
Alcohol (specific gravity 0.79)	7	29
Intralipid 10% (specific gravity 0.91)	1.1 kcal/mL	4

counters are available online, with estimates related to serving sizes. WebMD offers a calorie counter and calculator for over 37,000 foods and drinks (http://www.webmd.com/diet/health-tool-food-calorie-counter). Similar sites are available for other countries, such as the United Kingdom (http://www.weightlossresources.co.uk/calories/calorie-counter.htm).

Sometimes, the type of food is known to be homogeneous, and the caloric content can be estimated from the volume ingested (Table 5-10).

The caloric content of alcoholic beverages can be calculated as follows: The specific gravity of alcohol is 0.79 (rounded off to 0.8). Thus,

$$\text{Grams of alcohol} = (\text{proof of alcoholic beverage} \div 2) \times 0.8 \times \text{dL of beverage}$$

$$\text{kcal of beverage from alcohol} = \text{grams of alcohol} \times 7 \text{ kcal/g}$$

For example, three 2-oz drinks of 86-proof bourbon yields greater than 400 kcal

$$(86 \div 2) \times 0.8 \times 1.8 = 62 \text{ g} \times 7 \text{ kcal/g} = 434 \text{ kcal}$$

or to approximate the content with more rapidly,

$$\text{kcal from alcohol} = 0.8 \times \text{proof} \times \text{no. of ounces}$$

Using the example above, three drinks (2 oz each) of 86-proof bourbon = $0.8 \times 86 \times 6 = 413$ kcal.

The alcohol content of a unit of common beverages varies from 10 to 13 g (Table 5-11).

To calculate the caloric content of cooking oil:

$$\text{kcal} = \text{mL} \times \text{specific gravity of cooking oil } (0.91) \times 9 \text{ kcal/g}$$

TABLE 5-11 Alcohol and Caloric Content of Standard Drinks

Beverage	Unit	Alcohol Content (g)	kcal/U
Distilled liquor	One jigger		
80 proof		10	70
90 proof		11	80
100 proof		13	90
3.6%–4.0% beer	One 12-oz can	12.6–13.5	140–150
12.5%–14.5% wine	3 1/2-oz glass	10.0–11.6	70–80

for example, 2 tbs of olive oil = 30 × 0.9 × 9 = 243 kcal. To calculate the caloric content of dextrose infusions:

kcal = nutrient % × [volume infused (mL) ÷ 100] × 3.4 kcal/g of hydrated dextrose

for example, 3 L of 5% dextrose in water contains 5 × (3,000 ÷ 100) × 3.4 = 510 kcal.

Methods for Assessing Dietary Intake

Even if one allows for the accurate translation of food units into calories, it is difficult to obtain a reliable dietary history with the methods available. The Committee on Food Consumption Patterns, Food and Nutrition Board, of the National Research Council has compiled many data on the methods for assessing food consumption and its relationship to nutritional status (23).

The 24-hour recall is the simplest method available in that it relies on the patient's ability to remember how much food was eaten in a 24-hour period. The 24-hour dietary recall requires a trained interviewer but has been used with success in the National Health and Nutrition Examination Surveys (NHANESs). It takes a minimum amount of time to complete and can provide reproducible data. Although it is notoriously inaccurate in terms of the actual amount of food the patient has ingested (e.g., the intake of alcohol may be neglected), it is often the only technique available for assessing intake. The inaccuracy is compounded by not knowing the nutrient content of the ingested foods, and by the underreporting of intake in women in comparison with men.

The food history is also based on the patient's ability to recall, but the intake of food is averaged over a period of time. For example, the contents of a patient's average breakfast, lunch, or dinner, or all three, are calculated. The food history method is easy to use but suffers from the same inaccuracy of memory as 24-hour recall.

The patient can keep a written record of the amounts and types of food ingested. This method is accurate if the record is scrupulously maintained, but such thoroughness is rare. Also, people tend to alter their eating behavior during the test period to simplify the record. However, the energy content of foods eaten can be determined accurately, with only moderate overestimates, in a 5-day food record.

The calorie count is useful for the hospitalized patient because it requires the assistance of a dietitian, who understands the need for the calorie count. To ensure the accuracy of the count, no food is ingested by the patient other than what is reported to the dietitian. The tray passer usually estimates the portion of "missing food" when the tray is collected. Daily variations in food preparation and serving portions in the central kitchen can produce some inaccuracies. This method is the best of those available for estimating caloric intake, although it contains many inaccuracies. It combines some direct observation of the food actually ingested with a reasonable degree of control over its preparation. The major disadvantage is that it assesses intake of hospital food rather than home-prepared meals.

The weighed diet is very accurate, but it must be carried out on a metabolic ward where the portions of foods are weighed and most of the food is prepared on the floor. In this way, differences in the processing of foods are minimized, and the actual caloric content of foods is best estimated.

ENERGY BALANCE

Energy balance (kcal per day) equals kilocalories obtained minus kilocalories expended (BEE + EEA). *Calories obtained* refers to an estimate of dietary intake or to a calculation of calories fed enterally or parenterally (it can also refer to a combination of estimation and calculation). *Energy expended* includes that expended in basal metabolism and through physical activity or disease. When the intake of food exceeds the expenditure of energy, weight is gained. When the expenditure of energy exceeds the intake of food, weight is lost. When the energy balance is zero, weight is stable.

Although both water and carbohydrate stores are lost in the first few days of fasting, the loss of cell water is proportionally greater than the loss of glycogen. The mean composition of tissue lost during the first 11 weeks of semistarvation in otherwise healthy subjects is 40% fat, 12% protein, and 48% water. From weeks 12 to 23, the composition of tissue lost is 54% fat, 9% protein, and 37% water. The BMR per square meter falls an average of 31%, and the PAL drops by 55%. Thus, the rate of weight loss diminishes with time because expenditure decreases as intake remains constant.

The mean composition of tissue initially lost from obese subjects is 78% fat and 22% fat-free mass. It appears that obese patients use more adipose tissue as fuel during calorie restriction than do persons of normal weight.

Weight loss during starvation is not the same as during a low-calorie diet and may approach 50% fat and 50% FFM. Thus, during total starvation, the decrease in muscle mass and in BMR is larger than during a low-calorie diet.

To calculate an estimated weight loss on a controlled diet, an allowance must be made for the decreased BMR. To allow for the slowing of weight loss over time, new estimates have been approached by various models. A one-dimensional differential equation model has been developed based on the relationship between FFM and fat mass (FM) derived from a large sample from the Centers for Disease Control (24). The model allows for lack of constancy of weight loss during dieting and accounts for total energy expended in activities of daily living, including those that occur "at rest," such as change of posture or fidgeting. Another method uses frequent measurements of body weight over extended periods (>28 days) to estimate precisely changes in energy intake in free-living individuals (25).

A new "rule of thumb" has been proposed for the average overweight person trying to estimate a weight loss plan: every permanent 10 kcal decrease in energy intake/day will lead to a loss of 1 lb when the body weight reaches a new steady state (e.g., 24 kcal/day per kg of weight change) (26,27). Using this more realistic estimate, it would take approximately 1 year to achieve 50% of the proposed weight loss and approximately 3 years to achieve 95% of the loss. The dynamic energy balance equations needed to estimate time to weight loss require complex calculations, but are available at several sites online. The body weight simulator endorsed by the NIDDK utilizes the method of Hall et al. (25), and requires input of baseline weight, PAL, baseline caloric intake, and the goal weight loss over a set time period (http://bwsimulator.niddk.nih.gov). Calculations can also be made for maintaining a stable weight, or for adding exercise, thereby decreasing the necessary caloric deficit. Another website sponsored by the Pennington Biomedical Research Center uses an approach related to the balance between FFM and FM, derived from body composition values from the NHANES (https://www.pbrc.edu/research-and-faculty/calculators/weight-loss-predictor/). This model has been applied and validated as a method to assess energy intake during weight loss (26). The approach to utilize data-driven calculations to estimate long-term weight loss has been endorsed by a consensus of the American Society for Nutrition and the International Life Sciences Institute, North American branch (27).

Recommended Daily Energy Intake

Energy intake must be balanced according to the needs of age, sex, body size, and physical activity if a desirable body weight is to be maintained.

Despite attempts to estimate energy requirements for groups of adults, a wide range is seen within persons of the same body size and age that reflects differences in activity and individual metabolism. Moreover, it is not possible to establish desirable weights with certainty. For these reasons, the Committee on DRIs of the Food and Nutrition Board has derived a table of mean estimated energy intakes that are related not only to the EER and the level of PAL, but also allows for a decline in these estimates with each year above 18 (Table 5-12). The data included are only for persons of average weight and height (as defined in Table 5-8) who are classified as "active" in the PAL scale.

The energy requirement needed for weight maintenance has been determined by the double-labeled water method, as part of the CALERIE 2 study (28). Subjects under-reported energy intake significantly by approximately 15%, making it more difficult to assess need for maintenance. Using data from 1 month of weight stability, the study derived a regression equation relating total daily energy expenditure (TDEE) to weight as follows:

TDEE (kcal/d) = 1279 + 18.3 (weight, kg) + 2.3 (age, y) − 338 (sex; 1 = female, 0 = male)

Although still only an approximation, perhaps this equation, and its companion using body composition data, will be helpful is estimating free-living requirements of nonobese adults.

TABLE 5-12 Dietary Reference Intake Values for Energy by Active Healthy Americans[a]

Life Stage Group	EER (kcal/d)[b]	
	Male	Female
0–6 mo	570	520 (3 mo)
7–12 mo	743	676 (9 mo)
1–2 y	1,046	992 (24 mo)
3–8 y	1,742	1,642 (6 y)
9–13 y	2,279	2,071 (11 y)
14–18 y	3,152	2,368 (16 y)
>18 y	3,067	2,403 (19 y)
>19 y	Subtract 10 kcal/day/year	Subtract 7 kcal/day/year
Pregnancy 19–50 y	1st/2nd/3rd trimester	2,403/2743/2855 (19 y)
Lactation 19–50 y	1st 6 mo/2nd 6 mo	2,733/2,803 (19 y)

[a]Applies to moderately active (active PAL group) residents of the United States and Canada.
[b]The intake is appropriate for individuals of the reference weight, height, and age who qualify for a PAL designation of "active."
Sources: Data from Standing Committee on the Scientific Evaluation of Dietary Reference Intakes, Food and Nutrition Board, Institute of Medicine. *Dietary Reference Intakes for Energy, Carbohydrate, Fiber, Fat, Fatty Acids, Cholesterol, Protein and Amino Acids.* Washington, DC: The National Academies Press, 2005:5.

ESTIMATION OF PROTEIN REQUIREMENTS

Normally, nitrogen derived from amino acids, the catabolic product of proteins, is excreted in the urine and feces and lost from the skin. Unlike the energy that is retained and stored in triglyceride and glycogen, proteins and amino acids are not stored in the body. Therefore, protein or nitrogen requirements are often estimated by calculating nitrogen losses on a daily rather than a weekly basis. When excess protein is ingested, the amino acids not needed for new protein synthesis are transaminated so that the nonnitrogenous portion of the molecule can be used as a calorie source, as, for example, in pyruvate derived from alanine. The nitrogen that is not needed is converted to urea and excreted in the urine.

Urinary losses of nitrogen urea account for more than 80% of urinary nitrogen. Creatinine, porphyrins, and other nitrogen-containing compounds account for the remaining nitrogen.

$$\text{Urinary nitrogen loss} = [\text{urea N}_{\text{urine}} \text{ (mg/dL)} \times \text{daily urine volume (dL)}] \div 0.8$$

Urinary nitrogen excretion is related to the BMR. The larger the muscle mass in the body, the greater the number of calories needed to maintain it. Also, the rate of transamination is greater as amino acids and carbohydrates are interconverted to fulfill energy needs in the muscle. Between 1 and 1.3 mg of urinary nitrogen is excreted for each kilocalorie required for basal metabolism. Nitrogen excretion also increases during exercise and heavy work.

Fecal and skin losses account for a relatively constant proportion of nitrogen loss from the body in normal conditions, but these may vary widely in disease states. Thus, measurement of urinary nitrogen loss alone may not provide a reliable prediction of the daily nitrogen requirement when it is most needed. Fecal losses are a consequence of the inefficient digestion and absorption of protein (93% efficiency). In addition, the intestinal tract secretes proteins into the lumen from saliva, gastric juice, bile, pancreatic enzymes, and enterocyte sloughing. These sources contribute, respectively, about 3, 5, 1, 8, and 50 g of protein daily to the total protein secreted into the intestinal lumen.

Total nitrogen (N) losses include those from urine, feces, and skin. Fecal nitrogen averages 1 to 2 g per day in the absence of diarrhea. Skin losses average 0.3 g per day. The total fecal and skin losses can be estimated at about 2 g per day.

$$\text{Total N loss (g/day)} = N_{\text{urine}} + N_{\text{stool}} + N_{\text{skin}} \approx N_{\text{urine}} + 2$$

When fecal losses are measured, an estimated nitrogen loss of 1 g per day is used to cover losses in skin and other compartments.

Normal daily protein requirement is based on estimates of N loss and need (weight and extra requirements for growth and pregnancy). Obligatory losses of nitrogen are not altered by differences in age or sex, and urinary losses of nitrogen are proportional to body size and weight. The total losses from all sources are approximately 2 mg of nitrogen per basal kilocalorie. The best estimate of EAR of nitrogen in healthy adults is 105 mg N/kg/day, or 0.66 g/kg/day (29). This is the lowest amount of intake that achieved zero N balance, and was not apparently affected by climate, age, sex, or source of dietary protein. Women have a lower N requirement than men per kilogram of body weight, but they have a higher percentage of FM (28%) compared with men (15%). There is no difference in protein requirements by gender when corrected for LBM (2). The RDA estimated by the DRI Committee was based on the meta-analysis by Rand et al. (29). The amount of protein needed for zero balance in older adults was similar to that for younger adults (2). Minimal nitrogen loss per day has been estimated for adults. In a series of 11 studies reviewed by the WHO, daily obligatory nitrogen losses averaged 53 mg per kg (range: 46 to 69 mg per kg). On the basis of short- and long-term balance studies, the WHO proposed a mean requirement of 0.6 g/kg/day for reference protein (highly digestible, high-quality protein such as eggs, meat, milk, or fish) (30). If a value of 25% above the average is used to meet the needs of 97% of the population, 0.6 × 1.25, or 0.75 g/kg/day, was the RDA in 1989 for young male and female adults, and matches well with the current recommendation of 0.8 mg/kg/day (2) (Table 5-13).

Safe levels of protein intake for adult men and women have been suggested by the WHO, based on the recommendation of 0.8 g/kg/day of protein with a digestibility-corrected amino acid score of 1.0 (high-quality protein). These levels for teenage males and females are 56 and 46 g per day, respectively, and for adult men and women are roughly 56 and 46 g per day (30). Short-term nitrogen balance studies have supported these estimates and that the requirement for total dietary protein is similar in young and older healthy adults (31). The corresponding figures for DRIs for ranges of protein intake that are acceptable are 5 to 20 g per day for children 1 to 3 years of age, 10 to 30 g per day for children 4 to 18 years of age, and 10 to 35 g per day for adults (32). The report may be accessed on www.nap.edu.

Protein requirements are highest during infancy and adolescence. However, total body protein is lowest in infancy, and obligatory losses are greatest, so that protein deficiency is most

TABLE 5-13 Dietary Reference Intake Values for Protein by Life Stage Group

	EAR[a] (g/kg/day)		RDA[b] (g/kg/day)	
Life Stage Group	Males	Females	Males	Females
0–6 mo		1.52[c]		
7–12 mo	1.0	1.0	1.2	1.2
1–3 y	0.87	0.87	1.05	1.05
4–8 y	0.76	0.76	0.95	0.95
9–13 y	0.76	0.76	0.95	0.95
14–18 y	0.73	0.71	0.85	0.85
>18 y	0.66	0.66	0.80	0.80
Pregnancy		0.88		1.1
Lactation		1.05		1.3

[a]EAR = estimated average requirement, the intake that meets the needs of half of the group.
[b]RDA = recommended dietary allowance, intake that meets the needs of nearly all the group.
[c]AI = adequate intake, the amount that sustains a defined health status, such as growth.
Sources: Data from Standing Committee on the Scientific Evaluation of Dietary Reference Intakes, Food and Nutrition Board, Institute of Medicine. *Dietary Reference Intakes for Energy, Carbohydrate, Fiber, Fat, Fatty Acids, Cholesterol, Protein and Amino Acids.* Washington, DC: The National Academies Press, 2005:12–13.

common in infancy. A modified factorial procedure has been developed to calculate the protein needs of infants and children. Starting with a protein requirement of 1.1 g/kg/day for maintenance, an increment was added for growth and increased by 50% to allow for variability. Efficiency of utilization was assumed to be 70%, and a final calculated growth increment was added to the maintenance figure to recommend daily allowances for average US dietary protein (Table 5-13). Another estimate is needed to convert the figures derived for reference proteins. The true digestibility of a mixed US diet is estimated at greater than 90%, varying from 95% for milk, meat, eggs, peanut butter, and refined wheat, to 88% for polished rice, to 86% for oatmeal, whole wheat, corn, and soy flour, to 78% for beans (30).

However, although the need for protein is greater in the first 2 years of life, there is also an increase in protein, as percentage of total energy, from approximately 5% in the breastfed infant to approximately 15% when complementary foods are added. Cow's milk has a high protein content, and stimulates insulin-induced growth factor-1 (IGF-1) secretion. The difference in growth rate between breast- and formula-fed infants may be due in part to the percentage protein intake. This increase may prove to be a risk factor for obesity occurring in later life (33). It is possible that avoiding a very high protein intake by limiting the amount of cow's milk and/or formula may be recommended in future, but there are insufficient data at present to take that position.

About 925 g of protein is synthesized during a pregnancy by the mother for fetal and placental tissues. Protein needs increase as the pregnancy progresses. The amount of protein required for new deposition is 12.6 g per day, assuming that no additional protein is needed for the first trimester. Thus, the increased amount based on average body weight is 12.6 g per day ÷ 57 (reference adult female) = +0.22 g of protein/kg/day. When added to the EAR of a nonpregnant woman, one reaches an EAR of 0.88 g of protein/kg/day or an RDA of 1.1 g/kg/day. Based on the coefficient of variation of 12% seen in lactating women, an additional 0.2 g of protein/kg/day is recommended for lactating women.

CALORIE REQUIREMENT FOR PROTEIN ONLY WHEN ENERGY IS LIMITED

Nitrogen ingested as amino acids without other sources of energy is not efficiently incorporated into protein because the energy consumed in heat loss during metabolism (thermal effect) is especially high for protein. Moreover, the incorporation of amino acids into peptides requires three high-energy phosphate bonds, so that 10 kcal is used for each molecule derived from the hydrolysis of ATP. Any excess of dietary energy over basic needs improves the efficiency of dietary nitrogen utilization. To achieve a positive nitrogen balance when protein intake is barely adequate, a positive energy balance of approximately 2 kcal/kg/day is required (34). In other words, when energy intake is limited, protein balance is negative, even when protein intake seems adequate but is not excessive. The exact amount of extra calories required to produce a positive nitrogen balance depends on a large number of factors, including body energy stores, body protein mass, and the ratio of energy to protein sources in the food. To ensure positive nitrogen balance in the depleted patient, it is advisable to provide an amount of calories near the EER. Excessive calories may not lead to improvement in meaningful LBM.

This situation of inadequate protein occurs in low-energy diets. With a 1,400 kcal per day diet, 15% of calories as protein correspond to 52 g per day of protein. This level is barely adequate for healthy adult males. Thus, when energy is limited, protein needs are proportional to body weight (and tissue mass) and not to energy intake (35). In addition, because protein is not stored, optimal protein intake should be spread evenly over individual meals (35). And because chronic diseases occur in aging populations that might lead to increased protein catabolism or decreased synthetic rate, such adults should ingest more than the protein amount suggested for healthy populations (Table 5-13).

A safe ratio (protein energy to total energy) that avoids protein–calorie malnutrition in children seems to be 1:20 (36)—that is, for every kilocalorie provided by protein, 19 kcal of nonprotein energy is needed to prevent protein–calorie malnutrition in children. Each gram of protein produces 4 kcal of energy, so 4 × 19 or 76 kcal of nonprotein energy is needed per gram of protein during the period of intense growth in children. When protein is present in excess of needs,

TABLE 5-14 Energy Intake Required to Maintain Positive Nitrogen Balance

Type of Patient	Energy (kcal/kg/day)	Nitrogen (mg/kg/day)	kcal/g Nitrogen	kcal/g Protein
TPN postoperative	46.0	250	184	29
TPN septic	43.3	240	180	29
Ambulatory RDA	38.5	128	308	49

TPN, total parenteral nutrition; RDA, recommended daily allowance.
Sources: Data for postoperative patients from Hentley TF, Lee HA. Investigations into optimumnitrogen and caloric requirements and competitive nutritive value of three intravenous amino acid solutions in the post-operative period. *Nutr Metab.* 1975;19:201. Data for patients with septic disorders from Long CL, Crosby F, Geiger JW, et al. Parenteral nutrition in the septic patient: nitrogen balance, limiting plasma amino acids, and calorie to nitrogenratios. *Am J Clin Nutr.* 1976;29:380. Data for ambulatory patients from National Research Council. *Recommended Daily Allowances.* 10th ed. Washington, DC: National Academies Press, 1989, with permission.

even when nonprotein calories are limited, some of the protein is converted to energy that can be metabolized, and the 1:20 ratio is not required. Nitrogen balance studies have demonstrated that increased protein intake, regardless of the energy intake, promoted more nitrogen retention (37). Nitrogen balance was achieved by an intake of 1.2 to 1.5 g protein per day. However, if the protein is being administered as a parenteral amino acid mixture, allowance should be made for the fact that such mixtures deliver 17% of less protein energy than assumed (when hydration is accounted for), so as much as 1.8 g/kg/day of the mixture may be needed (38).

Relative requirements also have been estimated for energy and nitrogen in adult patients maintained in nutritional balance (Table 5-14). These estimates are, not surprisingly, somewhat lower than the estimates for children. Estimates of energy–protein requirements for normal, ambulatory 70-kg persons call for approximately 50 kcal from nonprotein sources per gram of protein, or about 300 kcal per g of nitrogen. This high ratio cannot usually be achieved with parenteral feeding because caloric intake is limited by the volume that must be infused. Therefore, acceptable figures for parenteral nutrition are about 25 to 30 kcal from nonprotein sources per gram of protein, or 150 to 180 kcal per g of nitrogen. These figures, however, should not be used as substitutes for independent estimates of energy and protein requirements. Especially in sick patients, energy and protein requirements may be dissociated to some extent. The protein–calorie ratios are important only insofar as they serve as a reminder of the need of calories along with protein replacement.

ESTIMATION OF PROTEIN REQUIREMENTS IN ILLNESS

Obligatory loss of protein from the body (25 to 40 g per day) represents a small fraction of total protein synthesized by the body, which has been estimated to be from 285 to 340 g per day. Thus, the synthesis of protein can be decreased much more severely than is suggested by daily losses alone. Moreover, normal protein losses from the skin and gastrointestinal tract are only a fraction of what can be lost potentially. The average normal gastrointestinal protein loss is 1.7 g of nitrogen times 6.25, or 10.6 g of protein, some of which is recovered in the colon. The value of 6.25 is usually used for conversion of total nitrogen values to grams of protein because this is the factor for the high-quality protein found in meat, fish, and eggs, and also in corn and beans. A lower factor (5.2 to 5.8) is used for other vegetable proteins and higher values (~6.4) for dairy proteins.

Conditions Characterized by Excessive Protein Loss

Urinary Loss

Loss of protein occurs in nephrosis, chronic renal disease, and states of hypermetabolism with tissue breakdown. The losses from tissue breakdown are accounted for in the usual estimate of urinary nitrogen loss. Estimating urinary urea nitrogen as the sole factor in urinary protein loss is the most logical determination for hypermetabolic conditions, in which body proteins are degraded to urea. Protein loss can be estimated by multiplying urinary nonprotein nitrogen loss times 6.25. When protein per se is lost into the urine (e.g., in nephrosis or chronic renal disease), the protein itself is often measured.

Loss through Other Body Fluids
Nasogastric losses or losses through fistulae can be measured and added to the daily protein loss to allow a better estimate of total protein losses, especially if drainage volumes are large.

Loss through Gastrointestinal Tract, Skin, or Lungs
Nitrogen can be lost from organs with a large surface area of epithelial cells. These organs include the intestine, skin, and lungs. A limited number of observations have been made in illnesses involving these organs. Because the losses vary widely, no formula can be devised to estimate them. Intestinal losses are greatest in disorders associated with either decreased digestion or absorption of protein or increased loss of protein into the lumen. Because the small intestine has the largest surface area and the highest normal rate of protein loss of all the enteric organs (about 50 g of protein per day), diseases of the small intestine have the potential to cause the highest rate of protein loss from the body. These *protein-losing enteropathies* may or may not be accompanied by symptoms.

Estimation of Protein Requirements According to Severity of Illness
Nitrogen losses usually cannot be measured in clinical situations. For a hospitalized, adequately nourished adult receiving high-quality protein intravenously, the basal requirements can be estimated to be about 0.4 to 0.6 g per kg. For an ambulatory patient consuming a standard diet of mixed-quality protein, the basal requirements should be estimated at 0.75 g per kg. The estimates in Table 5-15 are used to calculate protein requirements when excessive loss cannot be measured. In patients with critical illness with prolonged protein catabolism (e.g., sepsis, burn injury, trauma, and multiple organ failure), evidence is limited, but strongly suggests that 2.0 to 2.5 g per kg of body weight should be provided for such patients (39).

ASSESSMENT OF BODY COMPOSITION
Anthropomorphic Assessment by BMI
Assessments are made to describe the nutritional status of populations and individuals. Normal values are descriptive of healthy subject groups and may not relate well to the individual patient undergoing evaluation. No single measure in routine use today can accurately reflect the protein–calorie status. Thus, many different anthropometric laboratory tests may be combined to formulate an overall impression. The advantages, disadvantages, and utility of the tests are described, but their routine use in nutritional therapeutics is not necessarily endorsed. Longitudinal measures can be sensitive indicators of malnutrition before static body compartment measurements become abnormal. In the adult, maintenance of the usual body weight is generally expected. Therefore, weight loss with time is a helpful and simple longitudinal measurement in nutritional assessment. In the child, weight gain with growth is expected, and failure to maintain

Table 5-15 Estimate of Recommended Daily Protein Intake

Clinical Condition	Protein Requirements (g/kg IBW/day)
Normal	0.75
Metabolic "stress/illness/injury"	
Mild/moderate	1.0–1.25
Moderate/severe	1.25–1.5
Severe with extra losses (e.g., skin, urine)	>1.5
Renal failure, acute (undialyzed)	0.8–1.0
Hemodialysis	1.2–1.4
Peritoneal dialysis	1.3–1.5
Hepatic encephalopathy	0.4–0.6

IBW, ideal body weight.

an expected growth rate similarly can be a simple indication of protein and calorie malnutrition. In addition to weight, increases in length and head circumference can be monitored in children because bone is growing.

Height should be measured without shoes in adults with the patient erect. Historical data are often erroneous by 1 to 2 in.

Weight is a simple measure of nutritional status. It can be compared with ideal weights or with usual weights corrected for height, derived from representative values of the adult US population sampled in NHANES surveys.

$$\% \text{ Reference body weight} = \left(\text{actual weight} \div \text{reference body weight}\right) \times 100$$

To calculate weight change:

$$\% \text{ Body weight change} = \left[\left(\text{usual weight} - \text{actual weight}\right) \div \text{usual weight}\right] \times 100$$

A loss of 5% of body weight or less is not usually clinically important unless it occurs within a short time. Clearly, the rate of weight loss also must be considered in judging its significance. Weight changes cannot be an assessment of nutritive status in the face of increased extracellular fluid (edema, ascites, and congestive failure) or during diuretic therapy. Despite these cautions, body weight is probably the best comprehensive estimate of protein–calorie status.

The definition of healthy weight has traditionally been set at the range of weights associated with the lowest mortality. However, many problems have arisen with this approach (40). A problem with standard weight guidelines is that a person can gain considerable weight (even 15 to 20 kg) and still remain within the recommended range. Initially, the concept was that weight gain with age is acceptable. However, some data have suggested that smaller gains in weight (e.g., 5 to 10 kg) during adult life are associated with an increased risk for chronic disease, including cancer, diabetes, hypertension, coronary artery disease, and cholelithiasis (40). Thus, it has been recommended that adults monitor their body weight, best corrected for height as in the BMI, as advocated by both the WHO and the International Obesity Task Force (see also Table 5-16). However, although it still seems likely that overweight and obesity are risk factors for chronic disease, an increased risk of mortality (as opposed to morbidity) is associated only with grade 2 and 3 obesity (BMI $\geq$ 35) (41). In older populations even within the range of "normal" BMI (20 to 22), increased mortality was found compared to a BMI of 22 to 24 (42). Thus, any modifiable causes of weight loss in the elderly should be pursued for medical causation.

The BMI is obtained by dividing weight (kg) by the square of the height (m^2)

$$\text{BMI} = W \div H^2$$

This measure best predicts the percentage of body fat in groups of subjects, but not in individual persons. Because the height is squared, that contributing factor is minimized. Overweight is now defined as a value greater than 25 (43). This figure is based on excess body weight of 15% or more, according to Metropolitan Life Insurance tables of 1983, which offer ideal weights somewhat lower than those found in the NHANES data for the average US population (44). For children, different height–weight data must be used. The BMI may not be representative of some subsets of the population (e.g., elderly, medically ill), and it does not take into account frame size or distribution of fat. The National Institutes of Health Technology Assessment Conference Panel on Methods for Voluntary Weight Loss and Control endorsed use of the BMI to define overweight (45). Its use has been less well documented for identifying conditions associated with weight loss. Simple formulas for calculating the BMI from pounds and inches have been developed:

$$\text{BMI} = [W(\text{lb}) \div H(\text{in})] \div 0.0014192 \text{ (reference 46)}$$
$$\text{BMI} = W(\text{lb}) \div H^2 (\text{in}) \times 703 \text{ (reference 47)}$$

Tables 5-16 and 14-1 provide a quick conversion of height and weight into BMI for most patients. The advantage of the BMI over linear height and weight is that it provides rapid, if oversimplified, estimate of disease risk (Table 5-17). Calculation of BMI is offered in many online sites, for example, http://www.medcalc.com/body.html.

TABLE 5-16 BMI for Overweight Patients

	Overweight							Obesity			
BMI	25	26	27	28	29	30	31	32	33	34	35	40
Height (in)						Weight (lb)						
58	119	124	129	134	138	143	149	153	158	163	167	191
59	124	128	133	138	143	148	154	158	164	169	173	198
60	128	133	138	143	148	153	159	164	169	175	179	204
61	132	137	143	148	153	158	165	169	175	180	185	211
62	136	142	147	153	158	164	170	175	181	186	191	218
63	141	146	152	158	163	169	175	181	187	192	197	225
64	145	151	157	163	169	174	181	187	193	199	204	232
65	150	156	162	168	174	180	187	193	199	205	210	240
66	155	161	167	173	179	186	192	199	205	211	216	247
67	159	166	172	178	185	191	198	205	211	218	223	255
68	164	171	177	184	190	197	204	211	218	224	230	262
69	169	176	182	189	196	203	210	217	224	231	236	270
70	174	181	188	195	202	207	216	223	230	237	243	278
71	179	186	193	200	208	215	222	230	237	244	250	286
72	184	191	199	206	213	221	228	236	244	251	258	294
73	189	197	204	212	219	227	236	243	251	258	265	302
74	194	202	210	218	225	223	241	250	258	265	272	311
75	200	208	216	224	232	240	248	256	264	272	279	319
Height (cm)						Weight (kg)						
147.3	54.0	56.4	58.6	60.9	62.7	65.0	67.7	69.5	71.8	74.1	75.9	86.8
150	56.4	58.2	60.5	62.7	65.0	67.3	70.0	71.8	74.5	76.8	78.6	90
152.4	58.2	60.5	62.7	65.0	67.3	69.5	72.3	74.5	76.8	79.5	81.4	92.7
155	60.0	62.3	65.0	67.3	69.5	71.8	75.0	76.8	79.5	81.8	84.1	95.9
157.5	61.8	64.5	66.8	69.5	71.8	74.5	77.3	79.5	82.3	84.5	86.8	99.1
160	64.1	66.4	69.1	71.8	74.1	76.8	79.5	82.3	85.0	87.3	89.5	102.3
162.5	65.9	68.6	71.4	74.1	76.8	79.1	82.3	85.0	87.7	90.5	92.7	105.5
165	68.2	70.9	73.6	76.4	79.1	81.8	85.0	87.7	90.5	93.2	95.5	109.1
167.6	70.5	73.2	75.9	78.6	81.4	84.5	87.3	90.5	93.2	95.9	98.2	112.3
170.2	72.3	75.6	78.2	80.9	84.0	86.8	90.0	93.2	95.9	99.1	101.4	115.9
172.7	74.5	77.7	80.4	83.6	86.3	89.5	92.7	95.9	99.1	101.8	104.5	119.1
175.3	76.8	80.0	82.7	85.9	89.0	92.3	95.5	98.6	101.8	105.0	107.3	122.7
177.8	79.0	82.3	85.4	88.6	91.8	94.1	98.2	101.4	104.5	107.7	111.0	126.4
180.3	81.4	84.5	87.7	90.9	94.5	97.7	101.4	104.5	107.7	111.0	113.6	130
182.9	83.6	86.8	90.5	93.6	96.8	100.5	103.6	107.3	111.0	114.1	117.3	133.6
185.4	85.9	88.2	92.7	96.4	99.5	103.2	107.3	110.5	114.0	117.3	120.5	137.3
188	88.2	91.8	95.5	99.1	102.3	106.0	109.5	113.6	117.3	120.5	123.6	141.4
190.5	90.9	94.5	98.2	101.8	105.5	109.0	112.7	116.4	120.0	123.6	126.8	145

Body shape (abdominal or hip circumference) has been considered to provide better data than do BMI regarding risk of complications of overweight or obesity. However, using a 3-D body scan in the UK National Sizing survey, BMI was significantly associated with chest and waist in men and with hips and bust in women (48). For any given BMI, waist measurements varied widely, and the differences between sexes disappeared with age. 3-D BMI may be useful for assessing body shape and thus risk of disease.

Fat Stores

Adipose tissue comprises about 25% of body weight, theoretically providing more than 150,000 kcal in the average adult. Although reduction of the fat reserves in comparison with

TABLE 5-17 BMI as a Measure of Associated Disease and Mortality Risk

Weight Category	BMI (kg/m^2)	Disease Risk	Mortality Risk
Extremely underweight	<14.0	Extremely high	Increased
Underweight	14.1–18.4	Increased in smokers, chronic illness	
Normal	18.5–22.99	Normal	Normal or ↑d in elderly
	22–24.99	Normal	
Overweight	25–27.49	Increased	Normal
	27.5–29.99	Increased	
Obesity			
Class I	30.0–34.9	High	Normal
Class II	35.0–39.9	Very high	Increased
Class III	≥40.0	Extremely high	Increased

Sources: Data from National Institute of Diabetes and Digestive and Kidney Diseases. Clinical guidelines on the identification, evaluation, and treatment of overweight and obesity in adults—the evidence report. *Obes Res.* 1998;6:S53; WHO, BMI classification http://apps.who.int/bmi/index.jsp?introPage=intro_3.html; Flegal KM, Kit BK, Orpana H, Graubard BI. Association of all-cause mortality with overweight and obesity using standard body mass index categories: a systematic review and meta-analysis. *JAMA.* 2013;309:71.

those of the normal population is not in itself detrimental, it does suggest inadequate calorie intake for a prolonged period of time and a concomitant protein compartment deficiency. Thus, normal fat reserves in comparison with population standards do not ensure that the protein compartment status is normal. Fat stores can be inferred from the body weight and estimated from subcutaneous fat measurements.

The triceps skin fold thickness (TSF) can be measured in a fold of skin taken over the triceps muscle, using Holtain skin calipers. The measurement is taken at a standardized position at the midpoint of the back of the upper arm with the subject standing upright, arms hanging down, and requires some experience for accuracy and reproducibility. Early studies suggested a positive correlation between TSF and deep body fat, but comparisons with computed tomography have not confirmed a strong correlation. However, for children and adolescents in whom limb fat reflects much more of total body fat, TSF provides a reasonable estimate of body fat. The WHO provides online TSF percentiles for children and adolescents, http://www.who.int/childgrowth/standards/tsf_for_age/en/index.html. Data are also available from the 1971 to 1974 NHANES database for subjects aged 1 to 74 (49).

Older techniques such as subcutaneous fat (skinfold) measurement and mid-arm muscle circumference do not allow for differences in distribution of fat or muscle in parts of the body other than the upper arm. There are now available noninvasive techniques that can measure FFM and FM. Although these methods are to some extent driven by clinical investigation, they are much more informative than the older methods, and should be preferred for evaluation of overall body composition.

Dual-energy X-ray absorptiometry (DEXA) is a reliable technique for measuring body composition. It can be used for both healthy subjects and for patients. Scanning time is now reasonably short (~5 minutes), and the results for a given machine are fairly reproducible. The technique is based on the concept that photon attenuation in vivo is related to body composition, and that the three body components of fat, fat-free, or lean tissue and bone mineral can be distinguished from each other. The software containing the algorithms to produce the resulting information is different for each of the three major manufacturers of scanners, and is proprietary. Although the method assumes that soft tissue is well hydrated to accurately assess the fat and lean tissue masses, in practice fluid shifts seem to have only minor effects on the results. The QDR-4500 and Delphi from Hologic and Prodigy from GE-Lunar are examples of DEXA scanners.

The estimates from these machines are different and were dependent on sex. At higher body fat levels (>25%), the differences were small but became larger, underestimating the FM, in lean individuals with less than 10% body fat. Truncal fat can be measured and correlates with total body fat. These machines are acceptable and sensitive for following longitudinal changes in body composition, and have been used to determine factors associated with clinical outcomes (50).

Bioelectrical impedance analysis (BIA) of body composition is less expensive than DEXA but not as reliable. The method does not measure body composition directly, but the electrical properties recorded are calibrated against other methods to produce equations predicting components of body composition (51). A four-surface electrode is the most common method for BIA used currently. With this apparatus, total body water, extracellular water, FFM, and percentage FM can be predicted from the impedance measurements. The method is valid in healthy young adults who are euvolemic. It is best used to determine estimates within groups, but because the results are derived from comparative equations, clinical applicability to individuals is limited. The best clinical use of BIA may be in following up individuals longitudinally over time. There is yet no single agreed-upon technology for multiple-frequency recordings, and there is still an abundance of instruments and equations in use for clinical research.

Protein "Stores"

The *somatic protein compartment* largely represents muscle mass. Measurements of body weight also reflect the muscle mass because it constitutes approximately 30% of the total body weight. Protein–calorie malnutrition causes a decrease in the muscle mass as well as in body fat stores, both of which are reflected by a decrease in body weight. Comparison of body weight with values from a reference population can suggest somatic protein depletion, but single measurements can underestimate depletion in large patients and overestimate depletion in patients of small build. Recent weight change or weight as a percentage of usual body weight often better suggests protein depletion, even though these parameters do not measure the compartment directly.

Mid-Upper Arm Circumference

The mid-upper arm circumference (MUAC) is useful as a simple measure to assess severe malnutrition in the adult (and child). The measurement in normal adults is 54 U+ 11 and 30 + 7 in normal healthy adult males and females, respectively, http://www.merckmanuals.com/professional/nutritional_disorders/undernutrition/overview_of_undernutrition.html. Severe malnutrition is recognized when these values decrease by 50%. To obtain more accurate assessment of muscle mass, separate from fat, derived measures have been developed, http://en.wikipedia.org/wiki/Anthropometry_of_the_upper_arm. These calculations are based on the assumption that the arm is cylindrical in shape and assumes the geometry of a cylinder. However, the measurements are reasonably accurate for groups of people, excluding those who are obese (overestimate) and elderly (great variability). The MUAC has been shown to be a simple way to classify critically ill patients, and the percentile may prove to be useful in predicting outcomes (52).

Lean Body Mass

LBM is calculated by subtracting body fat weight from total body weight, using a variety of formulas. Those of Mosteller, DuBois & DuBois, Haycock, Gehan & George, and Boyd are used in calculating LBM at http://www.medcalc.com/body/html, and those of Hume are provided at http://en.wikipedia.org/wiki/Lean_body_mass. LBM may be useful in certain circumstances, such as prescribing medications, but is only an estimate based on observations in normal healthy subjects within 2 SD of the mean for the observation used (e.g., height, weight, surface area).

Creatinine–Height Index

Endogenous creatinine production and excretion indirectly reflect the total body muscle mass. Creatinine is a dehydrated end-product of creatine, a complex molecule involved in supplying ATP to muscle cells; it is concentrated in the muscle mass. About 2% of the creatine phosphate in muscle is converted daily into creatinine in an irreversible reaction. Good correlation has been found between LBM measured by radioisotope labeling and by 24-hour creatinine excretion. For purposes of clinical assessment, a patient's creatinine excretion is compared with the expected excretion of a person of similar height and ideal weight. Actual population standards

TABLE 5-18 Ideal 24-Hour Urinary Creatinine Excretion by Adults of Various Heights (for Use in Calculation of the Creatinine–Height Index)

Height		Ideal Creatinine Excretion (mg)	
In	cm	Adult Women	Adult Men
58	147.3	830	—
59	149.9	851	—
60	152.4	875	—
61	154.9	900	—
62	157.5	925	1,288
63	160.0	949	1,325
64	162.6	977	1,359
65	165.1	1,006	1,386
66	167.6	1,044	1,426
67	170.2	1,076	1,467
68	172.7	1,109	1,513
69	175.3	1,141	1,555
70	177.8	1,174	1,596
71	180.3	1,206	1,642
72	182.9	1,240	1,691
73	185.4	—	1,739
74	188.0	—	1,785
75	190.5	—	1,831
76	193.0	—	1,891

Sources: Data from Blackburn GL, Bistrian BR, Maini BS, et al. Nutritional and metabolic assessment of the hospitalized patient. *JPEN J Parenter Enteral Nutr.* 1977;1:11.

for this measurement do not exist. Calculated ideal values are derived from the average 24-hour creatinine excretions of healthy children and adults while on a creatinine- and creatine-free diet; adult values are given in Table 5-18. The creatinine height index (CHI) compares the actual 24-hour creatinine excretion of a patient with the expected value for a person of the same height:

CHI = (actual 24-h creatinine excretion ÷ ideal 24-h creatinine excretion) × 100

The CHI indicates mild or no protein depletion when it is above 80%; moderate protein depletion is indicated at a CHI of 60% to 80%; and severe depletion is indicated by a CHI below 60%. The test is potentially useful when edema or obesity makes the measurement of body weight or BMI unreliable as an estimate of malnutrition. Like other measurements that rely on comparison with reference population standards, the CHI relies on ideal body weight standards for adults and calculated reference standards for children. Estimates of muscle mass may be inaccurate in patients who do not fall into the midrange of ideal body weight for height. The test is not valid in patients whose urine output is impaired or who have undergone amputation. It requires 24-hour urine collection and a constant protein intake. Conditions that alter creatinine excretion include kidney failure, liver failure, sepsis, and trauma. Aging and consumption of a creatinine-free diet also reduce creatinine excretion. Creatinine excretion is increased by vigorous exercise, a diet rich in red meat, corticosteroid and testosterone therapy, and administration of certain antibiotics (some aminoglycosides and cephalosporins). Because so many factors decrease creatinine excretion, the CHI often overestimates muscle mass depletion. For this reason, it is used less frequently than might be expected from its simplicity. However, serum creatinine has been advocated as a reliable measure of muscle mass in chronic renal disease under steady state, if allowance is made for dietary meat intake and the degree of renal dysfunction (53).

3-Methylhistidine Excretion

3-Methylhistidine is a biochemical degradation product of myofibrillar muscle protein metabolism, particularly of actin and myosin. It would be a marker for meat intake, therefore, except that it is also a degradation product of endogenous protein. This amino acid is not recycled into protein, has a long plasma half-life, and is excreted in the urine. However, 3-methylhistidine is not a breakdown product of sarcoplasmic protein, which constitutes about 35% of muscle protein. Like creatinine excretion, 3-methylhistidine excretion is decreased by old age, a decreased protein intake, trauma, or infection, and like the CHI, it overestimates muscle mass depletion.

Functional Body Composition to Supplement BMI

Characterization of individual body components can add to the risk assessment provided by BMI. This is particularly true in assessing the obesity phenotype, by measuring FFM, FM, and liver fat (54). Other subjects with similar BMIs can have different degrees of liver fat and insulin resistance (55). Those obese subjects who were metabolically normal may not carry increased risk of chronic metabolic disease. Likewise, patients with cancer who have muscle depletion have a poor prognosis, regardless of body weight, similar to patients with cachexia by conventional BMI criteria (56). Just as BMI classification has developed subgroups based on mortality risk, it is likely that more "functional" subgroups for chronic disease risks and/or mortality will be described based on body composition data.

Biochemical Assessment of Protein Status (Plasma Proteins)

Serum levels of circulating proteins can be decreased and reflect protein depletion even when other measurements of the protein compartment appear to be normal. Proteins synthesized by the liver have been used as markers for assessing protein status. Presumably, decreased levels of these proteins reflect a decrease in both amino acid precursors and hepatic (and other visceral) mass. Serum levels of some of these protein markers are listed in Table 5-19. The assumption that decreased levels of these proteins are specific for malnutrition is obviously wrong. Levels of liver-dependent circulating proteins reflect not only on adequacy of nutrition but also the synthetic capacity of the liver (not simply in relation to nutrition but also in relation to hepatic disease), rate of metabolic utilization, status of hydration, and excretion. Therefore, no measurable circulating protein is or likely will be specific for assessing visceral protein nutritional status.

Albumin

Albumin is a single-chain polypeptide with 575 amino acid residues. The liver is the exclusive site of albumin synthesis, and the normal adult synthesizes 120 to 200 mg/kg/day (about 12 g per day for the average adult) as part of a total exchangeable pool of 3.5 to 5.0 g per kg of body weight. Only 40% of the pool is located intravascularly. Equilibrium is slow between intravascular and extravascular albumin, about 5% per hour, so the entire mass of plasma albumin is exchanged daily with the extracellular component. Redistribution of the extravascular pool into the circulating compartment can help maintain normal levels despite protein deprivation.

Albumin represents about half the total exported protein synthesized by the liver. Many factors are involved in regulating albumin synthesis and secretion, and amino acid supply is only one. In short-term exogenous amino acid deprivation, albumin synthesis decreases, serum levels fall, and

TABLE 5-19 Serum Proteins Used for Nutritional Assessment

Protein	Half-Life (days)	Reference Range Conventional Units	SI units
Albumin	18–20	3.3–6.1 g/dL	500–860 µmol/L
Transferrin	8–9	0.26–0.43 g/dL	28.6–47.3 µmol/L
Prealbumin	2–3	0.2–0.4 g/L	3.64–7.27 µmol/L
RBP	0.5	30–60 mg/L	1.43–2.86 µmol/L
Fibronectin, soluble	0.16–1	1.66–1.98 g/L	3.77–4.50 µmol/L

SI, Système International.

hepatic albumin degradation decreases such that a new steady state is reached. The total exchangeable albumin pool may decrease to one-third its normal level before a decreased serum albumin concentration is evident. Restoration of amino acid precursors in such cases allows for greater than normal synthesis rates and normalization of serum albumin levels. Long-term protein deprivation results in less rapidly reversible decreases in the translational machinery of the hepatocytes. Providing amino acids only slowly normalizes the albumin-synthesizing capabilities of hepatocytes.

In health, the serum half-life of albumin is 20 days. This long half-life makes albumin a poor marker for rapid changes in metabolic states. Changes in synthesis and degradation rates in addition to body compartment shifts influence the serum level.

Because the serum albumin level correlates with morbidity and mortality in hospitalized patients, the concept has developed that such patients need nutritional support. Arbitrary levels of serum albumin have been suggested as indicators of protein malnutrition. A serum albumin level of 2.8 to 3.4 g per dL is used to diagnose a mild degree of protein malnutrition; moderate depletion is suggested by a serum albumin level of 2.1 to 2.7 g per dL, and severe depletion by a level below 2.1 g per dL.

Albumin levels correlate with disease severity but not necessarily with nutritional status (57). Use of the serum albumin level as an indicator of the protein nutritional state assumes a steady state, which is seldom the case during acute or subacute illness. The long half-life of albumin in serum makes this protein a poor marker of acute changes in nutritional status. Interpretation varies depending on length of protein deprivation. The rapid loss of plasma proteins (e.g., postoperatively, from burns, from the gastrointestinal tract) reduces serum albumin levels but does not necessarily indicate a reduction in protein mass. Therefore, although the serum albumin level does reflect the size of the intravascular albumin pool, it is simplistic to assume that this measurement, especially during acute illness, always reflects the protein mass. Also, a shift away from the intravascular pool of as much as 16% of the total exchangeable pool can occur with a change in body position from sitting to reclining; this further influences longitudinal measurements. Inflammatory disorders can decrease albumin synthesis and degradation or increase capillary leak. Increased nutrition (e.g., TPN) often does not alter albumin levels (58). Thus, even when protein malnutrition is a component of an illness, restoration of a low serum albumin level to normal with protein or amino acid therapy can be slow, and generally lags considerably behind clinical impressions of successful nutritional therapy.

Reduced serum levels are seen in many conditions, including malnutrition, liver disease, ascites, idiopathic edema, nephrosis, protein-losing enteropathies, thermal burns, severe eczema, hypothyroidism, zinc deficiency, malignant diseases, congestive heart failure, acute stress, and age over 70 years. Albumin is not correlated with LBM, skeletal muscle mass, or body cell mass indices, and thus is not suitable as a marker for protein composition in elderly patients (59).

Transferrin

Transferrin is a globulin (molecular weight of approximately 90,000) that binds and transports iron in the plasma. The liver is the principal but not the only site of transferrin synthesis; hepatic synthesis is probably modulated by ferritin within the hepatocytes. Serum levels are similar for men and women and decline only slightly in later life.

The synthetic rate appears to be the predominant factor in determining serum levels, although in acute illness, enhanced degradation can result in depressed levels. The body pool is only about 5 g, and the serum half-life of the protein is 8 to 10 days. Direct measurement of the protein is not always performed routinely, whereas serum total iron-binding capacity (TIBC) is often obtained when anemia is being investigated. Transferrin concentration can be estimated from the TIBC, but the relationship appears to be less constant at lower concentrations of transferrin, and the constants may vary from institution to institution. The attachment of iron to proteins other than transferrin when the latter is more than half-saturated further contributes to the inaccuracy of this estimate, and the readily measured transferrin is preferred.

Arbitrary levels of serum transferrin have been suggested as indicators of protein depletion. Serum transferrin levels of 150 to 200 mg per dL are associated with a mild degree of protein malnutrition; levels of 100 to 150 mg per dL are associated with moderate depletion, and a level below 100 mg per dL is associated with severe depletion.

Like serum albumin levels, serum transferrin levels depend on alterations in synthesis and degradation, both of which are affected by factors other than nutritional status. In particular, the degradation rate increases in acute illness, and synthesis increases in iron deficiency. *Decreased levels* are also seen in pernicious anemia, anemia of chronic disease, liver disease, starvation, burns, iron overload, nephrotic syndrome, and protein-losing enteropathies, and during steroid (glucocorticoid and androgen) therapy. *Increased levels* are observed during hypoxia, pregnancy, and treatment with estrogens or oral contraceptives.

Other Circulating Proteins

Two proteins that are also synthesized by the liver and secreted into the circulation are *retinol-binding protein* (RBP) and *thyroxine-binding prealbumin* (TBPA). Virtually all RBP is bound to TBPA in a 1:1 ratio. Because of their shorter half-lives (10 to 12 hours for RBP, 2 to 3 days for TBPA), and because of the particular amino acid content of TBPA, these two proteins rapidly reflect changes in hepatic protein synthesis. Any value less than the normal range for these proteins may indicate protein depletion.

Unfortunately, levels of both these proteins promptly drop with acute metabolic stress and the accompanying demand for protein synthesis. RBP and TBPA are both metabolized by the kidney, and levels increase in kidney failure. Because of the problems inherent in trying to use the measured level of serum protein to estimate the size and integrity of the organ where it is synthesized, it is unlikely that an ideal circulating protein to assess protein status will be found.

IMMUNOCOMPETENCE IN NUTRITIONAL ASSESSMENT

Abnormalities of the Immune System

Many aspects of the immune system are frequently abnormal in patients with generalized malnutrition, or with malnutrition associated with specific types of disease, such as autoimmune diseases, cancer, eating disorders, etc. Decreased numbers of circulating T cells, decreased numbers of total circulating lymphocytes, and an impaired delayed cutaneous hypersensitivity (DCH) response to skin test antigens in patients with protein depletion or protein–calorie malnutrition indicate concomitant impairment of cell-mediated immunity.

Depressed levels of various complement components (including C3), reduced amounts of secretory immunoglobulin A in external body secretions, and various abnormalities of the nonspecific cellular mechanisms of host resistance have been observed in malnourished laboratory animals and patients and have been reversed with nutritional repletion. Local nonspecific defenses (e.g., epithelial integrity, mucous production, and cilial mobility) are also adversely affected by malnutrition. These adverse effects together make the malnourished patient a likely candidate for infection.

The precise nutritional deficiency that results in an immune-compromised state in the individual malnourished patient is generally unknown. Although the above mentioned abnormalities are most frequently associated with protein malnutrition, most protein- and calorie-deficient patients have multiple nutritional deficiencies, not pure protein depletion. Almost any nutritional deficiency, if sufficiently severe, will adversely affect some aspect of the immune system. Therefore, the discovery of immunologic dysfunction does not necessarily imply protein malnutrition. However, if other indicators of macronutrient malnutrition are also present, then correction of protein nutritional status may normalize immune function.

Tests of Immune System

The most valid measure of an immune-compromised state in any group of patients may be the rate of infection, provided that all other confounding factors related to such risk are equal. When the immune status is compromised, as in cancer therapy or flares of autoimmune disease, the occurrence of infection may reflect overall immune competence (60). Unusual infections or infections in unusual locations provide more clues regarding immune competence. Primary immune responses tend to be affected much more than secondary responses. Thus, immune system competence can be monitored by the response to initial immunization (against influenza or pneumococcus). If T-cell suppression is anticipated, one can test serum for DNA/RNA for EB virus or cytomegalovirus (60).

TABLE 5-20 Methods Used to Assess Nutrient-Immune Interactions

Tissue Tested	Function	Method	Relevance to Nutrient Status
Mononuclear cells	Disease status	Cell count	Nonspecific
	Proliferation	Cultured blood Culture cells	T-lymphocyte response
	Activation	Isolated cells	T- or B-cell response
	Subtypes	Flow cytometry	T- or B-cell subtypes
	NK cell	Cr release	Subtype of T cell
Cytokine	Serum content	ELISA, RIA	Ability to secrete
	IC content	ELISA, RIA	Ability to synthesize
Delayed-type hypersensitivity	Cell-mediated	Skin test	Reflect in vivo immunity
Serum carnitine	Regulate immune cell function	Enzymatic assay	<30 µmol/L suggest deficiency
Serum amino acids	Glutamine and arginine affect immune cell function	Chromatography	Essential aa/nonessential aa ratio ↓ d in severe protein deficiency

NK, natural killer; ELISA, enzyme-linked immunosorbent assay; RIA, radioimmunoassay; IC, intracellular; Cr, chromium.

Many laboratory tests are available to assess immune function, but none are very sensitive or specific (Table 5-20). Two tests of the immune system have been employed most frequently as nonspecific clinical indicators of malnutrition in nutritional assessment: total circulating lymphocyte count and DCH to skin test antigens.

Total Lymphocyte Count

Circulating lymphocytes are mostly T cells. The thymus-dependent immune responses are very sensitive to malnutrition, and involution of tissues that generate T cells occurs early in the course of protein or protein–calorie malnutrition. Reduction in circulating T cells precedes and eventually leads to lymphopenia. The circulating *total lymphocyte count* (TLC) can be calculated from the peripheral *white blood count* (WBC) and the differential:

$$\text{TLC} = \text{WBC (cells/mm}^3\text{)} \times (\% \text{ of lymphocytes} \div 100)$$

Depression of circulating lymphocyte numbers below normal (200 cells per mm^3) is not specific for any particular nutritional deficiency. As a general indicator of malnutrition, the TLC tends to correlate best with other measures of protein status. A TLC of 1,200 to 2,000 per mm^3 correlates with mild malnutrition; a count of 800 to 1,200 is associated with moderate depletion, and a count below 800 is associated with severe depletion.

Infections and immunosuppressant drugs alter the number of circulating lymphocytes. The reason for lymphopenia in chronic or severe disease is generally not specific or identified. The TLC per se does not indicate the adequacy of immune function. Its use is complicated in cases of infection, metabolic stress, malignancy, or treatment with corticosteroids or immunosuppressive drugs. In such cases, the TLC may correlate with disease severity but not with nutritional status.

Delayed Cutaneous Hypersensitivity Reactions

The erythematous, indurated skin response to recall antigens is the standard for studying the cell-mediated immune response in vivo. The DCH reaction results from the following three sequential processes: (a) processing of antigen by macrophages results in the generation of both effector and memory T cells (the afferent limb); (b) recognition of antigen on rechallenge results in blast transformation, cellular proliferation, and generation of lymphokine-producing effector cells (efferent limb); and (c) local erythema and induration of the skin result from release of lymphokines and chemotactic factors at the antigen site.

A primary DCH response to new antigens requires that both afferent and efferent limbs be intact. Generally, the DCH response is tested by using antigens that the patient has previously encountered. Thus, presumably only the efferent aspects of the system are tested. Such antigens often include microbial antigens, such as purified protein derivative (PPD), *Candida albicans, Trichophyton,* and coccidioidin.

Unfortunately, the response to DCH is relatively insensitive and quantification is poor. Failure to react to recall antigens (anergy) has been well described in patients with protein depletion or protein–calorie malnutrition. Unfortunately, many other factors also influence the complex reaction sequence of the normal DCH response. When reactivity to a battery of skin test antigens is examined in relation to circulating liver-dependent proteins and to the TLC, the percentage of patients with anergy increases as protein levels and lymphocyte counts decrease, but anergy cannot be predicted accurately on the basis of any one variable.

The prevalence of nonreactivity to three recall antigens is about 50% in patients with serum albumin levels below 3.0 g per dL but is also reported up to 30% of the time when the serum albumin level is above 3.0 g per dL.

Normal response is represented by an induration greater than 5 mm after 24 to 72 hours to at least one of five skin test recall antigens (e.g., coccidioidin, PPD, *C. albicans, Trichophyton,* SKSD).

Anergy is variably defined but usually implies a failure to respond to any of five skin test antigens (<5 mm of induration). Reactivity is interpreted as a normal DCH response; anergy, or failure of the DCH response, may be the result of protein–calorie malnutrition and reversible with nutritional repletion.

Recall response depends on prior exposure to the antigen. Because 60% or fewer of subjects respond to many of the antigens used, anergy cannot be assumed on the basis of no response to only one or two antigens. In addition, antigens vary in potency in different lots. A rapid response may occur in subjects tested serially with the same antigen (especially if at the same skin site). The reaction may fade by 48 hours, giving a false-negative test result. Sites should be examined at 24 and 48 hours. The primary illness (e.g., lymphoma, sarcoidosis, cancer, liver or kidney failure, immunosuppressive disease) and medications (e.g., immunosuppressive drugs, chemotherapeutic agents, corticosteroids, warfarin, cimetidine, and aspirin) may influence the results. Edema interferes with the local response. Evidence of immune dysfunction on the basis of an impaired DCH response simply cannot be considered to indicate malnutrition.

CLINICAL APPLICATIONS OF NUTRITIONAL STATUS ASSESSMENT
Selection of Malnourished Patients for Intensive Nutritional Therapy

The patients at most risk for malnutrition are those who are critically ill (increased catabolism), or elderly (decreased intake), or those with long-term chronic diseases. A comprehensive assessment of protein and fat nutritional status may detect global malnutrition. However, none of the available tests is specific for malnutrition, and results can be abnormal in chronic or acute illness alone. Nutrition provision may be part of the reason for abnormal test results, but it is usually not possible to identify this factor among many others. No "gold standard" exists for determining nutritional status because no clinical definition of malnutrition is uniformly accepted. Most of the tests discussed below are judged according to their ability to predict clinical outcome. However, this does not necessarily imply that a poor outcome can be reversed by nutrient provision or nutrition support. Deficiencies of individual nutrients are discussed in Chapters 6 and 7.

Height, Weight, and Body Mass Index

The BMI can help to identify patients at increased risk for medical complications (Table 5-16). Therapy should be provided early for those patients who are extremely underweight (BMI <14 kg per m^2). The upper cutoff of 25 for increased risk for disease is well supported by data, but the much smaller population of underweight persons (BMI < 19.0) who do not smoke or who have not lost weight from illness has never been studied. It is possible that such "underweight" persons with stable weight are not at increased risk for illness (30). Of course, a low BMI resulting from unexplained weight loss should signal a search for underlying causes.

The BMI accounts for approximately two-third of the interindividual variability in body adiposity, in part because it does not account for sex, race, age, and differences in fitness. These confounders may explain (in part) the increased mortality associated with BMI greater than 35, but not for BMI between 25 and 30, the lowest range assigned to the classification of obesity (41). However, although similar findings of lower mortality for grade I obesity have been reported using other indicators of obesity, BMI has been challenged as an inadequate measure of obesity, with FM, waist circumference, and waist-to-hip ratio offered as alternatives (61). Similar caveats are probably apt for using BMI as the sole determinant of malnutrition. Because the definition of clinically significant malnutrition based on the individual measurements described in this chapter is yet to be determined, a comprehensive evaluation incorporating many parameters often is of little practical clinical value. Weight change remains the most significant parameter and the one best correlated with nutritional status, but it also may reflect chronic illness in its late stages, when nutritional replacement may not be effective.

Abnormalities in growth and weight maintenance are the most important clinical indicators of protein–calorie malnutrition in the ambulatory patient population. They are the most frequently used indicators because they are simple and inexpensive. For this reason, growth and weight are routinely monitored by physicians treating children and adults, respectively. Weight loss as a predictor of outcome may be more significant when it is combined with other physiologic measurements in critically ill patients (62).

Screening Tests for Malnutrition (see also Chapter 9)

The need for more comprehensive evaluation of protein and fat nutritional status in hospitalized patients is debatable. An "eyeball" assessment of nutritional status with the use of routine clinical information from the history and physical examination provides an accurate estimation in more than 70% of patients (Table 5-17 and reference 63). "Subjective" assessments can predict complications in hospitalized patients (64,65), but the findings correlate better with the severity of the underlying disease than with specific nutritional deficiencies of calories or protein.

While admitting that it is not possible to readily distinguish between starvation and disease-associated cachexia at the bedside, tools have been developed to assess malnutrition in the clinic and to use these to follow the course of the illness. One such test, the *Mini Nutritional Assessment* (MNA) has been designed for use in the elderly population, and has been translated into many languages and validated in many countries around the world. It is composed of simple measurements and questions and can be completed in 10 to 15 minutes (Table 5-21) (66). It utilizes the BMI and mid-arm circumference measurements described previously in this chapter, and can be used along with the Subjective Global Assessment (SGA) for predicting mortality and hospital costs.

TABLE 5-21 Mini Nutritional Assessment

Category	Criteria for Points	Points
Anthropometric Assessment		
1. BMI (kg/m^2)	<19 = 0, 19 to <21 = 1, 21 to <23 = 2, ≥23 = 3	
2. MAC (cm)	<21 = 0, 21 to ≤22 = 0.5, >22 = 1.0	
3. CC (cm)	<31 = 0 points, >31 = 1 point	
4. Weight loss during last 3 months	>3 kg (6.6 lb) = 0, does not know = 1, 1–3 kg = 2, no weight loss = 3	
General Assessment		
5. Lives independently (not in nursing home or hospital)	No = 0 points, yes = 1 point	
6. Takes >3 prescription drugs/day	Yes = 0 points, no = 1 point	

(continued)

TABLE 5-21 Mini Nutritional Assessment *(continued)*

Category	Criteria for Points	Points
7. Has suffered psychological stress or acute disease in past 3 months	Yes = 0 points, no = 2 points	
8. Mobility chair/bed but doesn't go out = 1, goes out = 2	Bed/chair bound = 0, able to get out of	
9. Neuropsychological problems	Severe dementia = 0, mild dementia = 1 no psychological problems = 2	
10. Pressure sores or skin ulcers	Yes = 0, no = 1	
Dietary Assessment		
11. How many full meals are eaten/day	1 meal = 0, 2 meals = 1, 3 meals = 3	
12. Selected consumption markers for protein intake	At least 1 serving of dairy products/day Y or N? ≥2 servings of legumes or eggs/week Y or N? meat, fish, or poultry every day Y or N? 0 or 1 Y = 0 points, 2 Y = 0.5, 3 Y = 1.0	
13. Consumes two or more servings of fruits or vegetables/day	No = 0, yes = 1	
14. Has food intake declined in past 3 months due to loss of appetite, or digestive, chewing, or swallowing difficulties?	Severe loss of appetite = 0, moderate loss of appetite = 1, no loss of appetite = 2	
15. How much fluid is consumed/day	<3 cups = 0, 3–5 cups = 0.5, >5 cups = 1.0	
16. Mode of feeding	unable to eat without assistance = 0, self-fed with some difficulty = 1, self-fed easily = 2	
Self-Assessment		
17. Do they view themselves as having malnutrition problems?	Major malnutrition = 0, does not know or moderate malnutrition = 1, no problem = 2	
18. In comparison with other, how do they consider their health status	Not as good = 0, does not know = 0.5, people of the same age, as good = 1, better = 2	
	Maximum 30 points	**Total**
Malnutrition Indicator Score	>24 points = well nourished	
	17–23.5 points = at risk of malnutrition	
	<17 points = malnourished	

MAC, mid-arm circumference; CC, calf circumference.
Sources: Adapted from Vellas B, Guigos Y, Garry PJ, et al. The mini nutritional assessment (MNA) and its use in grading the nutritional state of elderly patients. *Nutrition.* 1999;15:116.

The SGA determines whether the nutrient status has been altered by decreased food intake or poor digestion/malabsorption, notes the effects on organ function and body composition, and evaluates the course of the patient's disease (67). The findings of the history and physical examination are then weighted to rank patients as well, moderately, or severely malnourished and predict the risk for medical complications (Figure 5-1). The SGA is not completely subjective because

A. History
  1. Weight change
     overall loss in past 6 months: _____kg
     change in past week: increase _____kg
             no change _____
             decrease _____kg
  2. Dietary intake change compared to normal
     no change _____
     change _____: duration of change _____weeks
     type of change: hypocaloric solid diet _____ full liquid diet _____
             hypocaloric liquids _____ starvation _____
  3. Gastrointestinal symptoms, persisting > 2 weeks
     none____ anorexia _____ nausea _____ vomiting _____ diarrhea ____
  4. Functional capacity
     no dysfunction _____
     dysfunction _____: duration _____weeks
     type of dysfunction: working suboptimally _____ ambulatory _____
             bedridden _____
  5. Disease and its relation to nutritional requirements
     primary diagnosis (specify) _____
     metabolic demand (stress): none _____ low _____ moderate _____
             high _____
B. Physical exam (for each trait specify: 0 = normal, 1+ = mild, 2+ = moderate,
     3+ = severe)
   loss of subcutaneous fat (triceps, chest) _____
   muscle wasting (quadriceps, deltoids, temporals) _____
   ankle/sacral edema _____ ascites _____
   tongue or skin lesions suggesting nutrient deficiency _____
C. SGA rating (select one)
   _____A = well nourished (minimal/no restriction of food intake/absorption,
     minimal change in function, weight stable or increasing)
   _____B = moderately malnourished (food restriction, some functional changes,
     little/no change in body mass)
   _____C = severely malnourished (definitely decreased intake, function, and
     body mass)

Figure 5-1. Subjective global assessment of nutritional status. (From Detsky AS, McLaughlin JR, Baker JP. What is subjective global assessment of nutritional status? *JPEN J Parenter Enteral Nutr.* 1987;11:8, with permission.)

percentage of weight loss and serum albumin levels are taken into account. But hypoalbuminemia is a predictor of general risk, and is not specific for malnutrition (57). Although the SGA is highly sensitive (~100%) (68), it is much less specific (~66%), and misclassifies about 15% of patients (69). The SGA does classify patients better than anthropomorphic measurements (70). In general, the SGA performs well as a screening tool for assessing outcome risks (50), and it correlates well with other screening instruments (69). A patient-generated version of the SGA (PG-SGA) has been developed (71). Other screening tools currently in use include the Malnutrition Universal Screening Tool (MUST) (www.bapen.org.uk/the-must.htm) (72), the DETERMINE check list (www.aafp.org/x17367.xml) (73), and the Nutritional Risk Screening (NRS-2002) (www.health.vic.gov.au/hacc/publications/nutrisk-rm.htm) (74). The *European Society for Parenteral and Enteral Nutrition* (ESPEN) has developed guidelines for nutrition screening suggesting the use of BMI as the initial observation, followed by MUST for adults, the NRS-2002 for hospitalized patients, and the MNA for the elderly (75). A self-screening version of MUST has been developed for hospitalized patients (76), and MUST has been found most valid in estimating malnutrition in the elderly (77). However, the American Society for Parenteral and Enteral Nutrition (ASPEN) does not endorse any screening system, feeling that none of them is sufficiently validated. ASPEN prefers to use the SGA, because this tool has been the most validated in a large number of clinical situations (78). More tools will surely be developed, as none of the available instruments is specific for malnutrition, but all serve as prognostic indicators of severity of illness.

Table 5-22 summarizes the available tests for protein and fat status discussed in this chapter.

Specific Indications for Nutritional Support

A consensus conference involving the National Institutes of Health, ASPEN, and American Society of Clinical Nutrition reviewed the data on nutritional support in gastrointestinal diseases, wasting diseases (especially cancer and AIDS), critical illnesses, and in the perioperative period (79). The conclusions are summarized in Tables 5-23 and 5-24. Although this report reviewed data available in 1997, the overall conclusions are still valid. It is important to note that these conclusions identify issues for further study but are not recommendations or practice guidelines. In the use of nutritional support therapy, the integration of data from clinical trials, clinical experience in the illnesses being treated, and clinical expertise in nutrition and nutritional therapy will continue to be essential.

Overfeeding and Refeeding Syndromes

Although nutritional support is valuable in selected critically ill patients, it is not without risks. Metabolic complications resulting from overfeeding such patients can be serious (80). The

TABLE 5-22 Assessment for the Evaluation of Protein and Energy Nutritional Status

Measurement	Compartment Best Reflected by Measurement	Normal Values	Values Suggesting Malnutrition or Severe Disease
Weight (adults)	Fat/protein mass		
% loss in last month		<5%	>5%
% loss in last 6 months		<10%	>10%
Weight (children)	Fat/protein mass		
% drop on weight chart		<20th percentile	>20th percentile
DEXA	FFM/FM	Relative values depend on specific machine used	Decrease in FFM and FM with time suggests malnutrition
Creatinine/height index (%)	Protein mass	>90% (Table 5-18)	Mild = 80%–90% Severe = <60%
Serum albumin (g/dL)	Protein mass	3.5–4.5	Mild = 2.8–3.5 Moderate = 2.1–2.8 Severe = <2.1
Serum transferrin (mg/dL)	Protein mass	220–350	Mild = 150–20 Moderate = 100–150 Severe = <100
TLC per cubic millimeter	Nonspecific	>2,000	Mild = 1,200–2,00 Moderate = 800–1,200 Severe = <800
DCH to skin test antigens	Nonspecific	Reactive to >1/5 antigens	Anergy

TABLE 5-23		Use of Nutrition Support in Gastrointestinal Diseases	
Condition	Assumptions Driving Studies	Either EN or TPN	TPN alone
IBD	Bowel rest/EN helpful	Steroids > EN[b] therapy[a] EN possibly helpful[b] Mono/oligo/polymeric same outcome[a] Compliance limits use of EN formulations[a] EN/TPN promotes growth in children[b]	Not as primary[a]
Pancreatitis	Support helpful if oral intake limited Jejunal feeding >gastric/duodenal	No effect in mild, moderate disease[a] When course is prolonged, timing, route, and formulation unknown[c] EN can be safely given in mild/moderate disease[a]	IV lipid safe if TG 400 mg/dL[a]
Liver disease	Malnutrition can be identified in these patients	EN/TPN improves some parameters in ESLD[a] EN/TPN effect inconclusive in alcoholic ESLD[a]	
	BCAAs improve outcome	BCAA-enriched formulas improve protein intake in intolerant patients[a]	BCAA-rich aid recovery in hepatic encephalitis vs. glutamic acid,[a] untested vs. other amino acids

EN, enteral nutrition; TPN, total parenteral nutrition; IBD, inflammatory bowel disease; BCAA, branched-chain amino acid; ESLD, end-stage liver disease; TG, triglycerides.
[a]Supported by prospective randomized controlled trials of meta-analyses of prospective randomized controlled trial.
[b]Supported by well-designed nonrandomized prospective controlled trials, or by well-designed retrospective or case cohort studies.
[c]Supported by published experience, case reports, or expert opinion.
Sources: Modified from Klein S, Kinney J, Jeejeebhoy K, et al. Nutrition support in clinical practice: review of published data and recommendations for future research directions. *JPEN J Parenter Enteral Nutr.* 1997;21:133.

clinical characteristics of the syndromes associated with overfeeding are listed in Table 5-25. Most of these are commonly recognized and are detected during the routine follow up of patients on enteral or parenteral therapy (see Chapters 10 and 11). Prospective, randomized studies in critically ill patients have in general confirmed the recommendations to avoid overfeeding (and underfeeding) patients (81). Underfeeding can lead to immune depression, muscle depletion, and increased rate of infection and other complications. Overfeeding can lead to hyperglycemia, increased oxidative stress, hepatic steatosis, increased CO_2 production and respiratory failure, and increased rate of infection.

The refeeding syndrome is potentially very serious, can develop rapidly, and, because of its relative rarity, may not be recognized early (82). The clinical characteristics of this syndrome are listed in Table 5-26. Cardiovascular and electrolyte abnormalities need to be carefully documented before critically ill patients are referred. Patients at high risk of developing the refeeding syndrome include those with anorexia nervosa, chronic alcoholism, patients with cancer or who are postoperative, elderly, with uncontrolled diabetes, or with chronic malnutrition or cachexia. Feeding should be restarted slowly, and it should be ascertained that all nutrients, especially

TABLE 5-24 Use of Nutrition Support in Catabolic Conditions

Condition	Assumptions Driving Studies	Either EN or TPN	TPN alone
Cancer/AIDS	Reversing weight loss improves	Routine use doesn't ↓ morbidity/morality w/ chemo-rad Rx[a] May maintain hydration/nutrition, ↑ survival in pts who can't eat/drink[b] Restoring body composition/tissue mass probably good[c] Restores cell mass in AIDS pts w/ ↓ d food, no infection[b]	Infections ↑ w/chemo Rx[a] No ↓ morbidity/mortality in pts w/BMT[a,d] Routine use doesn't ↓ mortality or QOL[b]
Critical illness	Hypermetabolic patients should improve w/support Critical depletion of lean tissue occurs after 14 days	No good studies to support assumption[c] EN ↓ s complications in trauma pts (or ↑ d with TPN?)[b,e] Support should be started in 7–10 days in pts without oral feeding[c] No data available on special additives (e.g., Gln, Arg)	
Perioperative	"Malnourished" pts (weight loss, ↓ plasma protein, SGA) need nutrients for good outcome	EN after hip fracture ↓ s morbidity[a] Post-op patients who can't eat need calories within 5–10 days[c]	7–10 days of pre-op Rx ↓ s complications by 10%[a]. Routine post-op TPN with no pre-op Rx ↑ s complications 10%[a,d]

EN, enteral nutrition; TPN, total parenteral nutrition; QOL, quality of life; BMT, bone marrow transplantation; SGA, subjective global assessment.

[a]Supported by prospective randomized controlled trials or meta-analyses of prospective randomized controlled trials.

[b]Supported by well-designed nonrandomized prospective controlled trials, or by well-designed retrospective or case cohort studies.

[c]Supported by published experience, case reports, or expert opinion.

[d]Supported by meta-analysis in Kortez RL, Lipman TO, Klein S; American Gastroenterological Association. AGA technical review on parenteral nutrition. *Gastroenterology*. 2001;121:970.

[e]Supported by Heyland DK, Dhaliwal R, Dower JW, et al; Canadian Critical Care Clinical Practice Guidelines, Committee. Canadian clinical practice guidelines for nutrition support in mechanically ventilated, critically ill adult patients. *JPEN J Parenter Enteral Nutr*. 2003;27:355.

Sources: Modified from Klein S, Kinney J, Jeejeebhoy K, et al. Nutrition support in clinical practice: review of published data and recommendations for future research directions. *JPEN J Parenter Enteral Nutr*. 1997;21:133.

TABLE 5-25 Clinical Characteristics of Overfeeding Syndromes

Syndrome	Patients at Risk	Management
Azotemia	Age >65, protein intake >2 g/kg, BUN/Cr >15	Provide adequate energy, hydration, protein intake
Fat overload (respiratory distress, bleeding, jaundice)	Lipid intake >3 g/day, onset days to months	Hold lipids for TG >300 mg/dL, monitor PT, PTT, bilirubin
Hepatic steatosis	High CHO, very low fat during parenteral nutrition	Adjust energy and CHO intake, include fat daily
Hypercapnia	Poor ventilatory status	Decrease energy intake, esp. dextrose, add lipid, monitor pCO_2, pH
Hyperglycemia	On steroids, dextrose provision >4 mg/kg/min	Monitor hydration, blood glucose, replace dextrose with lipid
Hyperglycemic, hyperosmolar, nonketotic	High CHO load + diuresis	Monitor CVP, restore intravascular volume, add insulin and K
Hypertonic dehydration	High protein tube feed + fluid loss + old age	↓ Na and protein intake, use isotonic feeding and rehydration
Hypertriglyceridemia	Lipid intake >2 g/day, infection	Maintain TG <300 mg/dL, avoid overfeeding
Metabolic acidosis	Formulas with low kcal/g N ratio (<90:1), elderly	Monitor hydration, renal function, pH, ↓ protein intake
Refeeding	Weight <70% of ideal, rapid replacement	Monitor cardiac status, P, Mg, K, ↓ energy load, hydrate

BUN, blood urea nitrogen; Cr, creatinine; TG, triglyceride; PT, prothrombin time; PTT, partial thromboplastin time; CHO, carbohydrate; CVP, central venous pressure.
Sources: Modified from Klein CJ, Stanek GS, Wiles CE. Overfeeding macronutrients to critically ill adults: metabolic complications. *J Am Diet Assoc.* 1998;98:795.

TABLE 5-26 Clinical Characteristics of The Refeeding Syndrome

Nutrient/Organ System	Clinical Findings
Energy balance	Weight <70% of ideal weight
Cardiovascular system	↓ Cardiac mass, stroke volume, end-diastolic volume, heart rate, blood pressure ↑ Congestive failure, arrhythmias, QT interval
Kidney	↑ Sodium and water retention
Phosphorus	↓ Plasma P, leading to muscle weakness, seizures, acute respiratory failure, tachycardia, death
Potassium/magnesium	↓ Plasma K, Mg because each g of N used to form leads to retention of 3 mEq of K and 0.5 mEq of mg
Gastrointestinal tract	Diarrhea with oral feeding secondary to reduced epithelial mass

nitrogen, phosphorus, potassium, magnesium, and sodium, are adequately provided. The daily intake should be about 20 kcal per kg and should contain about 150 g of carbohydrate and 1.2 to 1.5 g of protein per kilogram. Sodium should be restricted to about 1.5 g per day, but phosphorus, potassium, and magnesium should be liberally provided while weight, electrolytes, and cardiac function are monitored carefully (83).

REFERENCES

1. Pellett PL. Protein requirements in humans. *Am J Clin Nutr*. 1990;51:723.
2. Standing Committee on the Scientific Evaluation of Dietary Reference Intakes, Food and Nutrition Board, Institute of Medicine. *Dietary Reference Intakes for Energy, Carbohydrate, Fiber, Fat, Fatty Acids, Cholesterol, Protein and Amino Acids*. Washington, DC: The National Academies Press, 2005.
3. Foster GD, Knox LS, Dempsey DT, et al. Caloric requirements in total parenteral nutrition. *J Am Coll Nutr*. 1987;6:231.
4. Makk LJ, McClave SA, Creech PW, et al. Clinical application of the metabolic cart to the delivery of total parenteral nutrition. *Crit Care Med*. 1990;18:1320.
5. Liggett SB, St John RE, Lefrak SS. Determination of resting energy expenditure utilizing the thermodilution pulmonary artery catheter. *Chest*. 1987;91:562.
6. Liggett SB, Renfro AD. Energy expenditures of mechanically ventilated nonsurgical patients. *Chest*. 1990;98:682.
7. Branson R, Rodriguez J, Tajchman S, Hooley JA is the final author. Indirect calorimetry in the ventilated patient. 2013. http://clinicalview.gehealthcare.com/download.php?obj_id=231&browser.pdf.
8. Harris JA, Benedict FG. *A Biometric Study of Basal Metabolism*. Publication No. 279. Washington, DC: Carnegie Institution, 1919.
9. Roza AM, Shizgal HM. The Harris–Benedict equation reevaluated: resting energy requirements and the body cell mass. *Am J Clin Nutr*. 1984;40:168.
10. Ireton-Jones C. Adjusted body weight, con: why adjust body weight in energy-expenditure calculations? *Nutr Clin Pract*. 2004;20:474.
11. Hamwi GJ. Therapy: changing dietary concepts. In: Danowski TS, ed. *Diabetes Mellitus: Diagnosis and Treatment*. New York, NY: American Diabetes Association, 1964.
12. Owen OE, Kayle E, Owen RS, et al. A reappraisal of caloric requirements in healthy women. *Am J Clin Nutr*. 1986;44:1.
13. Keys A, Taylor HL, Grande F. Basal metabolism and age of adult men. *Metabolism*. 1973;22:579.
14. Wilmore DW. *The Metabolic Management of the Critically Ill*. New York, NY: Plenum Press, 1977.
15. Baker JP, Detsky AS, Stewart S, et al. Randomized trial of total parenteral nutrition in critically ill patients: metabolic effects of varying glucose–lipid ratios as the energy source. *Gastroenterology*. 1984;87:53.
16. Ireton-Jones CS, Turner WW Jr, Liepa BU, et al. Equations for the estimation of energy expenditures in patients with burns with special reference to ventilatory status. *J Burn Care Rehabil*. 1992;13:330.
17. Gerrior S, Juan WY, Basiotis P. An easy approach to calculating estimated energy requirements. *Prev Chronic Dis* 2006;3:A129.
18. Mann S, Westenskow DR, Houtchens BA. Measured and predicted caloric expenditure in the acutely ill. *Crit Care Med*. 1985;13:173.
19. Gaillard C, Alix E, Salle A, et al. Energy requirements in frail elderly people: a review of the literature. *Clin Nutr*. 2007;26:16.
20. Wang ZM, Ying A, Boxy-Westphal A, et al. Specific metabolic rates of major organs and tissues across childhood: evaluation by mechanistic model of resting energy expenditure. *Am J Clin Nutr*. 2010;92:1369.
21. Toth MJ, Poehlman ET. Energetic adaptation to chronic disease in the elderly. *Nutr Rev*. 2000;58:61.
22. US Department of Agriculture, Agriculture Research Service. *USDA National Nutrient Database for Standard Reference, Release* 25. 2012. Nutrient Data Laboratory Home Page. http://www.ars.usda.gov/ba/bhnrc/ndl.
23. Standing Committee on the Scientific Evaluation of Dietary Reference Intake, Food and Nutrition Board, Institute of Medicine. *Dietary Reference Intakes: Applications in Dietary Assessment*. Washington, DC: The National Academies Press, 2000.
24. Thomas DM, Martin CK, Heymsfield S, et al. A simple model predicting individual weight change in humans. *J Biol Dyn*. 2011;5:579.
25. Hall KD, Sacks G, Chandramahan D, et al. Quantification of the effect of energy imbalance on bodyweight. *Lancet*. 2011;378:826.

26. Thomas DM, Schoeller DA, Redman LA, et al. A computational model to determine energy intake during weight loss. *Am J Clin Nutr*. 2010;92:1326.
27. Hall KD, Heymsfield SB, Kemnitz JW, et al. Energy balance and its components: implications for weight regulation. *Am J Clin Nutr*. 2012;95:989.
28. Redman LM, Kraus WE, Bhapkar M, et al. Energy requirements in nonobese men and women: results from CALERIE. *Am J Clin Nutr*. 2014;99:71.
29. Rand WM, Pellett PL, Young VR. Meta-analysis of nitrogen balance studies for estimating protein requirements in healthy adults. *Am J Clin Nutr*. 2003;77:109.
30. Joint WHO/FAO/UNU Expert Consultation. Protein and amino acid requirements in human nutrition. *World Health Organ Tech Rep Ser*. 2007;(935):1–265.
31. Campbell WW, Johnson CA, McCable GP, et al. Dietary protein requirements of younger and older adults. *Am J Clin Nutr*. 2008;88:1322.
32. Standing Committee on the Scientific Evaluation of Dietary Reference Intake, Food and Nutrition Board, Institute of Medicine. *Dietary Reference Intakes for Energy, Carbohydrate, Fat, Fatty Acids, Cholesterol, Protein, and Amino Acids*. Washington, DC: The National Academies Press, 2005.
33. Michaelsen KF, Larnkjaer A, Molgaard C. Early diet, insulin-like growth factor-1, growth, and later obesity. *World Rev Nutr Diet*. 2013;106:113.
34. Scrimshaw NS. Shattuck Lecture—strengths and weaknesses of the committee approach: an analysis of past and present recommended dietary allowances for protein in health and disease. *N Engl J Med*. 1976;294:198.
35. Layman DK. Dietary guidelines should reflect new understandings about adult protein needs. *Nutr Metab*. 2009;6:12.
36. Waterlow JC, Payne PR. The protein gap. *Nature*. 1975;258:113.
37. Jeejeebhoy K. Parenteral nutrition in the intensive care unit. *Nutr Rev*. 2012;70:623.
38. Hoffer U. How much protein do parenteral amino acid mixtures provide? *Am J Clin Nutr*. 2011;94:1196.
39. Hoffer LJ, Bistrian BR. Appropriate protein provision in critical illness: a systematic and narrative review. *Am J Clin Nutr*. 2012;96:591.
40. Willett WC, Dietz WH, Colditz GA. Guidelines for healthy weight. *N Engl J Med*. 1999;341:427.
41. Flegal KM, Kit BK, Orpana H, et al. Association of all-cause mortality with overweight and obesity using standard body mass index categories: a systematic review and meta-analysis. *JAMA*. 2013;309:71.
42. Winter JE, MacInnis RJ, Wattanapenpaiboon N, et al. Body mass index and all-cause mortality in older adults: a meta-analysis. *Am J Clin Nutr*. 2014;99:875.
43. Schwartz LM, Woloshin S. Changing disease definitions: implications for disease prevalence. Analysis of the Third National Health and Nutrition Examination Survey, 1988–1994. *Eff Clin Pract*. 1999;2:76.
44. Metropolitan Life Insurance Company. Metropolitan Life Insurance Company Tables: Metropolitan Heights and Weights 1999. www.bcbst.com/MPManual/HW.htm.
45. NIH Technology Assessment Conference Panel. Methods for voluntary weight loss and control. *Ann Intern Med*. 1992;116:942.
46. Frankel HM. Determination of body mass index. *JAMA*. 1986;255:1292.
47. Matz R. Calculating body mass index. *Ann Intern Med*. 1993;118:232.
48. Wells JC, Treleaven P, Cole TJ. BMI compared with 3-dimenstional body shape: the UK National Sizing Survey. *Am J Clin Nutr*. 2007;85:419.
49. Frisancho AR. New norms of upper limb fat and muscle area for assessment of nutritional status. *Am J Clin Nutr*. 1981;34:2540.
50. Kyle UG, Genton L, Pichard C. Hospital length of stay and nutritional status. *Curr Opin Clin Nutr Metab Care*. 2005;8:397.
51. Buchholz AC, Bartok C, Schoeller DA. The validity of bioelectrical impedance models in clinical populations. *Nutr Clin Pract*. 2004;19:433.
52. Ravasco P, Camilo ME, Gouveia-Oliveira A, et al. A critical approach to nutritional assessment in critically ill patients. *Clin Nutr*. 2002;21:71.
53. Patel SS, Molnar MZ, Tayek JA, et al. Serum creatinine as a marker of muscle mass in chronic renal disease: results of a cross-sectional study and review of the literature. *J Cachexia Sarcopenia Muscle*. 2013;4:19.
54. Muller MJ, Lagerpusch M, Enderle J, et al. Beyond the body mass index: tracking body composition in the pathogenesis of obesity and the metabolic syndrome. *Obes Rev*. 2012;13(suppl 2):6.
55. Muller MJ, Westphal AB, Heller M. "Functional" body composition: differentiating between benign and non-benign obesity. *Biol Rep*. 2009;1:75.

56. Martin L, Birdsell L, MacDonald N, et al. Cancer cachexia in the age of obesity: skeletal muscle depletion is a powerful prognostic indicator, independent of body mass index. *J Clin Oncol.* 2013;31:1539.
57. Klein S. The myth of serum albumin as a measure of nutritional status. *Gastroenterology.* 1990;99:1845.
58. Gray GE, Megried MM. Can total parenteral nutrition reverse hypoalbuminemia in oncology patients? *Nutrition.* 1990;6:225.
59. Bouillanne O, May P, Liabaud B, et al. Evidence that albumin is not a suitable marker of body composition-related nutritional status in elderly patients. *Nutrition.* 2011;27:165.
60. Looney RJ, Diamond B, Holers YM, et al. Guidelines for assessing immunocomptency in clinical trials for autoimmune diseases. *Clin Immunol.* 2007;123:235.
61. Vina J, Borras C, Gomez-Cabrera MC. Overweight, obesity, and all-cause mortality [letter]. *JAMA.* 2013;309:1679.
62. Windsor JA, Hill GL. Weight loss with physiologic impairment: a basic indicator of surgical risk. *Ann Surg.* 1988;207:290.
63. Windsor JA, Hill GL. Nutritional assessment: a pending renaissance. *Nutrition.* 2991;7:377.
64. Baker JP, Detsky AS, Wesson DE, et al. Nutritional assessment: a comparison of clinical judgment and objective measurements. *N Engl J Med.* 2982;306:969.
65. Detsky AS. Predicting nutrition-associated complications for patients undergoing gastrointestinal surgery. *JPEN J Parenter Enteral Nutr.* 1987;11:440.
66. Hudgens J, Langkamp-Henken B. The mini nutritional assessment as an assessment tool in elders in long-term care. *Nutr Clin Pract.* 2004;19:463.
67. Detsky AS, McLaughlin JR, Baker JP. What is subjective global assessment of nutritional status? *JPEN J Parenter Enteral Nutr.* 1987;11:8.
68. Mourao F, Amado D, Ravasco P, et al. Nutritional risk and status assessment in surgical patients: a challenge amidst plenty. *Nutr Hosp.* 2004;19:83.
69. Pablo AM, Izaga MA, Alday LA. Assessment of nutritional status on hospital admission: a reevaluation. *J Am Diet Assoc.* 1992;93:27.
70. Planas M, Audivert S, Perez-Portabella C, et al. Nutritional status among adult patients admitted to a university-affiliated hospital in Spain at the time of genoma. *Clin Nutr.* 2004;23:1016.
71. Bauer J, Capra S, Ferguson M. Use of the scored patient-generated subjective global assessment (PG-SGA) as a nutrition assessment tool in patients with cancer. *Eur J Clin Nutr.* 2002;56:779.
72. Malnutrition Advisory Group (MAG). *MAG-Guidelines for Detection and Management of Malnutrition.* Redditch, UK: British Association for Parenteral and Enteral Nutrition, 2000. www.bapen.org.uk/the-must.htm.
73. de Groot LC, Beck AM, Schroll M, et al. Evaluating the DETERMINE Your Nutritional Health Checklist and the Mini Nutritional Assessment as tools to identify nutritional problems in elderly Europeans. *Eur J Clin Nutr.* 1998;52:877. www.aafp.org/PreBuilt/NSI_DETERMINE.pdf.
74. Kondrup J, Ramussen HH, Hamberg O, et al. Nutritional risk screening (NRS 2002): a new method based on an analysis of controlled clinical trials. *Clin Nutr.* 2003;22:321.
75. Kondrup J, Allison SP, Elia M, et al. ESPEN guidelines for nutrition screening 2002. *Clin Nutr.* 2003;22:415.
76. Cawood AL, Elia M, Sharp SKE, et al. Malnutrition self-screening by using MUST in hospital outpatients: validity, reliability, and ease of use. *Am J Clin Nutr.* 2012;96:1000.
77. Poulia KA, Yannakoulia M, Karageorgou D, et al. Evaluation of the efficacy of six nutritional screening tools to predict malnutrition in the elderly. *Clin Nutr.* 2012;31:378.
78. ASPEN Board of Directors. *Clinical Guidelines for the Use of Parenteral and Enteral Nutrition in Adult and Pediatric Patients.* Silver Spring, MD: ASPEN Publications, 2002.
79. Klein S, Kinney J, Jeejeebhoy K, et al. Nutrition support in clinical practice: review of published data and recommendations for future research directions. *JPEN J Parenter Enteral Nutr.* 1997;21:133.
80. Klein CJ, Stanek GS, Wiles CE. Overfeeding macronutrients to critically ill adults: metabolic complications. *J Am Diet Assoc.* 1998;98:795.
81. Singer P, Pichard C. Reconciling divergent results of the latest parenteral nutrition studies in the ICU. *Curr Opin Clin Nutr Metab Care.* 2013;16:187.
82. Mehanna HM, Moledina J, Travis J. Refeeding syndrome: what it is, and how to prevent and treat it. *BMJ.* 2008;336:1495.
83. Boateng AA, Sriram K, Meguid MM, et al. Refeeding syndrome: treatment considerations based on collective analysis of literature case reports. *Nutrition.* 2010;26:156.

6 Vitamins

EVALUATION OF VITAMIN INTAKE AND DEFICIENCY

The intake of vitamins (and other nutrients) is calculated in three ways: (a) the amount an individual needs to avoid deficiency (daily requirement), (b) the average daily amount entire population groups should consume in a period of time to prevent deficiency (recommended dietary allowance [RDA] or adequate intake [AI]), and (c) the amount that can be safely ingested when the vitamin is taken to prevent chronic disease (tolerable upper intake level [UL]). Statistically, the RDA is set two standard deviations above the mean requirement, so that it is sufficient for 97% of normal persons. RDAs therefore exceed the needs of many persons and furthermore are established only for healthy persons (1). The RDA takes into account the dietary form of the nutrient, the efficiency of absorption, and other factors, in addition to the estimated daily requirement for the assimilated nutrient. Daily allowances may thus vary, depending on whether the vitamin is to be administered parenterally (see Chapter 11) or by mouth. Discussions of controversial recommended dietary intakes of many vitamins and minerals are included in the publications of the Standing Committee on the Scientific Evaluation of Dietary Reference Intakes, Food and Nutrition Board, Institute of Medicine (2–4). RDAs and dietary reference intakes (DRIs) are not designed to provide guidelines for therapy. They should be used only as estimates for normal intake and perhaps as a starting point for therapy in cases of deficiency.

Does Vitamin Supplementation Offer Benefit to Healthy People Living in Developed Countries?

The major benefit of individual vitamin supplements in healthy populations is to ensure AI of folic acid in young women and of vitamins D and B_{12} in the elderly. Evidence does not support the use of supplements for vitamins A, C, or E on a routine basis (5). Although vitamin E supplements have been associated with increased mortality, the use of multivitamin–multimineral supplements does not appear to carry such a risk (6).

However, the data for using multivitamin preparations (usually including B and "antioxidant" vitamins) is thought to be less certain. This uncertainty may be related to the fact that nutrient intervention trials can never "control" the use of nutrients in either the control or the experimental arm. Moreover, any randomized controlled trial (RCT) is limited in time, and thus cannot identify changes over long periods. However, the 2010 Dietary Guidelines for Americans do not support a recommendation for the use of multivitamin supplements in the prevention of chronic disease, a conclusion supported by many large studies (7). This conclusion has been supported by two large systematic reviews of studies examining the effect of multivitamin and mineral preparations on mortality from cardiovascular disease and cancer (8,9). These studies included 3 RCTs and 24 and 12 cohort studies, respectively. Most relative risks were near or slightly below the null value, but no clear pattern of benefit was found. When the data from the 3 RCTs were pooled, no effect on all-cause mortality was found (8). This pattern has been confirmed by a fourth RCT studying cardiovascular events after myocardial infarction in men (10). However, a few studies have been used to suggest that small benefits might accrue to the use of such supplements. In a large randomized controlled study of male physicians (PHS-II), and in the Supplementation in Vitamins and Minerals Antioxidants Study (SU.VI.MAX), daily supplements showed a very modest reduction in the risk of total cancers in men, but not of any specific cancer (reviewed in Refs. 8 and 9). A post hoc analysis in French subjects in the SU.VI.MAX study showed that subjects with low vitamin C levels at baseline who were nonsmokers showed improved verbal memory with supplements (11).

Many previous studies had shown no correlation between antioxidant vitamin supplements and specific cognitive function, and this conclusion is supported by a RCT as part of the PHS-II (12). One way to interpret such studies is that there is need to identify subgroups of the population whose vitamin status may be insufficient. However, it is probably time to accept the conclusion that multivitamin and mineral supplementation to the general population does not result in prevention of chronic diseases, in particular, cardiovascular disease, cancer, and dementia.

Requirements for Vitamin Nutrition in Selected Groups

It is clear that vitamin deficiencies are overlooked in many patients. Either food intake may become restricted (e.g., vitamin B_{12}), or endogenous production may decrease (e.g., vitamin D production from skin). These factors may occur in physically active people, the elderly, and persons at increased risk for chronic diseases. Although there are markers for body stores of most vitamins, they are not sensitive or specific enough in most cases to identify a subclinical deficiency state, that is, one in which subsequent clinical deficiency will occur that can be prevented by vitamin supplementation (13). Even in the best studied examples of vitamins B_{12} and D, such a diagnosis is still problematic.

Physically Active People

Only about one-third of people in the United States engage in regular physical exercise—mostly walking, swimming, bicycling, running, and step aerobics. A deficiency of certain vitamins adversely affects physical performance (e.g., by causing anemia, muscle weakness, fatigue, or peripheral neuropathy). These include all the B vitamins. Exercise can increase the need for some nutrients, as in the gastrointestinal blood loss seen during prolonged exercise (14). In addition, some vitamins are considered to be important in reducing the risk for cardiovascular disease. These include vitamin E and the vitamins that lower serum homocysteine (Hcy) levels (vitamins B_6, folate, and B_{12}). The role of each of these vitamins is discussed later in the chapter. In physically active people without deficiency, there is no effect of supplemented vitamins and minerals if they are ingesting a balanced diet (15).

Elderly People

The DRIs include separate recommendations for persons over the age of 70 (16) (see Chapter 3). In the Survey in Europe on Nutrition and the Elderly, a Concerned Action (SENECA) Study, evidence of low vitamin intake/deficiency based on serum levels was found in 47% of European elderly persons for vitamin D, 23% for vitamin B_6, 2.7% for vitamin B_{12}, and 1% for vitamin E (17). Neurocognitive function can be decreased in deficiency states of vitamins B_6 and B_{12} and folate (18), the same vitamins that help to regulate Hcy levels. The intake of these vitamins is often inadequate in the elderly. Because on average the elderly ingest only about 50% of the RDA for any vitamin, special care must be taken to ensure that the full RDA (or DRI) is taken. Supplementation with these three B vitamins in patients with mild cognitive impairment has been shown to delay the progression of brain atrophy, an effect that was correlated with plasma Hcy levels (19). However, use of the same three B vitamins has not been effective in preventing stroke, although Hcy levels were altered (20). Even when an effect is noted, it is often not clear which vitamin might be the active compound, and this might depend on the presence of subclinical deficiency. For example, although folate, B_6, and B_{12} may be protective of depressive symptoms in older adults, the data do not support an association with folate, but with B_{12} in diet and supplements, and with B_6 in supplements alone (21). These findings are consistent with subclinical deficiency of these vitamins in the elderly.

Persons at Risk for Chronic Diseases

The data are not yet sufficient to suggest that regular use of these vitamins prevents cancer or nuclear cataracts or cardiovascular disease (22,23). If vitamins and minerals are effective in these settings, guidelines from professional societies and the US government recommend obtaining the micronutrients from food (24). Small amounts of regular and enriched foods improve vitamin concentrations in frail, elderly patients, so deficiency is not a problem of malabsorption (25). However, other disorders such as chronic inflammatory bowel disease (IBD) (26) and gastric bypass surgery for obesity (27) create abnormal intestinal physiology that can lead to altered absorption of vitamins both from the diet and from enterohepatic circulation.

Most healthy people in the United States do not need vitamin supplements. However, supplements should be given to certain groups of patients at high risk for vitamin deficiency. Details are provided in the sections on the individual vitamins.

Infancy.

1. Vitamin K once (0.5 to 1.0 mg intramuscular or 1 to 2 mg orally) to prevent hemorrhagic disease of the newborn.
2. Vitamin E (500 mg per kg daily) to premature infants weighing less than 1.5 kg to prevent hemolytic anemia.
3. Vitamin D (400 IU per day) to breast-fed infants if not exposed to sunlight.
4. Cobalamin (vitamin B_{12}) to breast-fed infants of strict vegetarian mothers.

Pregnancy. Folic acid requirements are increased. A dosage of 400 μg per day is recommended for all pregnant women to decrease the incidence of neural tube defects.

Low-Calorie Intake/Diets. If less than 1,200 kcal is ingested per day, a multivitamin preparation may be used. This is especially true for alcoholics, elderly persons who are poor or homebound, and patients with anorexia nervosa or severe depression.

Gastrointestinal Disorders. Patients with fat malabsorption may require vitamins A and D or, rarely, E. Following ileal resection, vitamin B_{12} is needed (100 μg per month). Folic acid (1 mg per day) is often required, and all water-soluble vitamins must be administered to patients with short-bowel syndrome. The micronutrients often needed in patients with IBD include folate, vitamin D, calcium, magnesium, iron, and zinc, and vitamin B_{12} in Crohn disease (http://www.nih.gov/health/digest/digest.htm#pubs). A proprietary medication has been formulated for IBD patients. Forvia contains vitamin D 800 IU, vitamin E 150 IU, vitamin K 80 μg, vitamin B_{12} 1 mg, other water-soluble vitamins, zinc 22.5 mg, and iron 30 mg (http://www.forvia.com).

Osteodystrophies. Patients in whom activation of vitamin D is defective may require vitamin D, calcifediol (hepatic disease), or calcitriol (renal disease). In otherwise normal subjects, data are accumulating that suggest the need for a larger daily dose of vitamin D to prevent osteoporosis and fractures. A dose of 800 IU per day (twice the DRI) prevents approximately 30% of hip and nonvertebral fractures in adults older than 65 years, corresponding with 25-hydroxyvitamin D (25(OH)D) concentrations more than 74 nmol per L (28).

Human Immunodeficiency Virus (HIV) Disease. Supplemental vitamins A, B-complex, C, and E, and carotene were provided to pregnant women with HIV disease in a double-blind-controlled study and led to a reduced death rate (25% vs. 31%), as well as decreased progression to stage 3 disease or greater, improved CD4+ counts, and lower viral load (29). Vitamin A alone reduced mortality and improved growth in a single hospital sample of HIV-infected children, and reduced diarrhea-associated mortality in another trial in infants (30). However, there was no evidence that micronutrient supplementation reduced morbidity and mortality in HIV-infected adults.

Vitamin Therapy in Conditions Other than Deficiency. Vitamins are administered in many conditions in which deficiencies are not demonstrated, or where the DRI is felt to be inadequate to counter true deficiency (e.g., vitamin D). In most instances, either no effect of the vitamin has been documented, or the data are insufficient to warrant a strong recommendation for their use. Table 6-1 lists some of the clinical areas in which vitamin supplementation has been suggested, along with references that review the accumulated data. Discussions of some of these uses not related to deficiency are included in the sections on the individual vitamins, especially vitamins A and E. Accepted uses of vitamins in states other than deficiency are the administration of pyridoxine to treat pyridoxine-dependent inborn errors of metabolism, and the administration of vitamin A derivatives to treat skin diseases and acute promyelocytic anemia, and niacin for hyperlipidemia.

TABLE 6-1 Proposed Uses of Vitamins at Higher Than Recommended Doses and/or in Nondeficiency States

Vitamin	Condition	Reference
Riboflavin	Migraine	Modi S, Lowder DM. *Am Fam Physician.* 2006;73:72.
Niacin	Hyperlipidemia	Berra K. *J Am Acad Nurse Pract.* 2004;16:526.
Vitamin B_6	Carpal tunnel syndrome	Aufiero E, et al. *Nutr Rev.* 2004;62:96.
	Premenstrual syndrome	Fugh-Berman A, Kronenberg F. *Reprod Toxicol.* 2003;17:137.
	Immune response	Huang YC, et al. *Nutrition.* 2005;21:779.
	Cognition	Malouf R, et al. *Cochrane Database Syst Rev.* 2003;(4):CD004393.
Folate	Depression	Taylor MJ, et al. *Cochrane Database Syst Rev.* 2004;(4):CD003390.
	Prevention of colon cancer	Strohle A, et al. *Int J Oncol.* 2005;26:1449.
Vitamin B_{12}	Cognition	Malouf R, et al. *Cochrane Database Syst Rev.* 2003;(3):CD004326.
Coenzyme Q	Mitochondrial dysfunction	Littarru GP, Tiano L. *Curr Opin Clin Nutr Metab Care.* 2005;8:641.
Vitamin C	Common cold	Douglas RM, et al. *Cochrane Database Syst Rev.* 2004;(3):CD000980.
	Asthma	Ram FSF, et al. *Cochrane Database Syst Rev.* 2004;(3):CD000993.
	Chronic diseases	Jacob RA, Soutoudeh G. *Nutr Clin Care.* 2002;5:66.
Vitamin A	Cancer/leukemia	Njar VC, et al. *Bioorg Med Chem.* 2006;14:4323.
	Measles	Huiming Y, et al. *Cochrane Database Syst Rev.* 2005;(4):CD001479.
Vitamin E	Cardiovascular disease	Pham DQ, Plakogiannis R. *Ann Pharmacother.* 2005;39:1870.
	Premenstrual syndrome	Soares KVS, McGrath JJ. *Cochrane Database Syst Rev.* 2004;(3);CD000209.
	Cataracts	Tabet N, et al. *Cochrane Database Syst Rev.* 2004;(3):CD002854.
	Tardive dyskinesia	
	Alzheimer disease	
Antioxidants (Vitamins C, E, and/or β-carotene)	Cancer prevention Atherosclerosis	See Chapter 15; Aviram M, et al. *Handb Exp Pharmacol.* 2005;170:263.
Vitamin D	Cardiovascular disease	Holick MF. *Mayo Clin Proc.* 2006;81:353.
	Cancer prevention	Garland CF, et al. *Am J Public Health.* 2006;96:252.
Vitamin K	Childhood bone health	Cashman KD. *Nutr Rev.* 2006;81:353.

Bioavailability of Vitamins

Bioavailability of vitamins differs in various foods. *Bioavailability* refers to the fraction of total dietary vitamin that is absorbed and functions in an organism. The assessment of bioavailability involves assays of tissue content and biologic activity. The accuracy of dietary requirements depends on information about food content and its bioavailability. Nutrient content listed under each vitamin is usually well established. Where data exist concerning bioavailability, they are given.

Vitamin Deficiency

A variety of factors other than dietary intake are related to vitamin deficiency. These are listed in Table 6-2. Dietary deficiency is uncommon in the case of the vitamins that are produced endogenously. Enterohepatic circulation of a vitamin is associated with an increased rate of loss during malabsorption because some portion of the body stores must be reabsorbed each day, along with what is derived from the diet. An enterohepatic circulation of vitamins other than those listed in Table 6-2 is possible, but such data are not available at this time. Hepatic stores of vitamin A and cobalamin are decreased most frequently in cirrhosis. All vitamins may be needed in larger amounts during pregnancy and growth, but folic acid is especially important because body stores are small.

Onset of Clinical Vitamin Deficiency

The onset of clinical vitamin deficiency varies, depending on the rate of loss and the size of available body stores. In general, the body stores of water-soluble vitamins are smaller, whereas fat-soluble vitamins are stored in adipose tissue or liver, so that the body stores are larger. Thus, clinical deficiency of fat-soluble vitamins is usually delayed and may take 2 years or more to develop.

Clinical Manifestations of Deficiency of a Given Water-soluble Vitamin

The clinical manifestations of deficiency of a given water-soluble vitamin are relatively late consequences (Table 6-3). Blood levels fall early in the course of deficiency and are thus useful in detecting changes in body stores of the vitamin. This event is followed by altered cell function and finally clinical symptoms. This sequence is not often seen in deficiencies of the fat-soluble vitamins. Vitamin D must be converted to active forms. Thus, even though body stores of the parent vitamin may be normal, activation to the hydroxylated forms may be inadequate. Vitamins A and D are carried in plasma by specific binding proteins, and alterations in the levels of these binding proteins can lead to an erroneous estimate of body stores. The intracellular content of a vitamin sometimes correlates better with body stores than do plasma levels. Thus, the vitamin content of white or red cells is sometimes used to assess body stores.

Therapeutic Supplementation

In many instances, only one or two vitamin deficiencies exist at one time in a patient. However, when generalized malabsorption occurs, extra vitamins are needed each day to prevent deficiencies. This is often best accomplished with one of the multivitamin and mineral preparations. When feeding is only or largely parenteral, multivitamin supplements must be given. (Doses and administration of parenteral therapy are discussed in Chapter 11.)

A major problem in interpreting studies that provide supplemental vitamins for nondeficiency conditions is that these studies have not been accompanied by pharmacokinetic measurements to assess the true exposure of the populations to the vitamins provided, or by pharmacodynamics measurements to ensure that abnormal physiology has been corrected. The kinetics of vitamins A, C, D, and E are complex. Following either oral or parenteral administration, the vitamin enters the blood, from where it is distributed to peripheral compartments, equilibrating rapidly with plasma, red blood cells (RBCs), liver, and kidney, and more slowly with adipose tissue, muscle, and skin. There is no good biomarker for the effect of vitamin D

TABLE 6-2 Pathophysiology of Vitamin Deficiency

Physiologic factor	Vitamins Affected	Comments
Dietary intake	All except K, B_6, biotin	K, B_6, and biotin probably produced by enteric bacteria
Endogenous synthesis	D (skin), K, B_6, biotin	
Enterohepatic circulation	A, polar metabolites of vitamin D, folic acid, cobalamin	
Decreased storage capacity	Cobalamin, A	Stored in liver
Increased utilization	Folic acid	Used in increased amounts during pregnancy, hemolysis
Increased loss from body	All	During malabsorption

TABLE 6-3   Summary of Vitamin Functions and Deficiency States

Vitamin	Functions	Results of Deficiency	Major Food Sources
Thiamine B_1	Transketolase coenzyme, muscle tone, appetite	Moderate: fatigue, apathy, nausea, irritability, numbness Severe: beriberi with CHF, polyneuritis, edema	Enriched grains, most animal and vegetable products
Riboflavin/B_2	Part of FAD, FMN that accept/donate [H+] equivalents	Angular stomatitis, cheilosis, glossitis, seborrheic dermatitis	Organ meats, enriched cereals/flours, cheese, eggs, lean meat
Niacin	Part of NAD, NADP that accept/donate [H+] equivalents	Dermatitis (light-exposed), diarrhea, swollen tongue, delirium, depression	Meat, nuts, dairy products, eggs
Vitamin B_6	Coenzyme in transamination, decarboxylation, trans-sulfuration	Seborrheic dermatitis, red tongue, irritability, weakness, convulsions, neuritis	Grains, seeds, organ meats, lean meats
Pantothenic acid	Part of CoA/acyl carrier protein	Anorexia, nausea, fatigue, numbness, insomnia	Organ meats, cereals/flours, nuts, eggs
Biotin	Coenzyme in decarboxylation, deamination	Scaly dermatitis, anorexia, glossitis, muscle pains	Organ meats, eggs, soy flour
Folate	Formation of purines, pyrimidines, heme, tyrosine, glutamate	Megaloblastic anemia, glossitis, diarrhea	Organ meats, green vegetables, legumes, eggs, fish, nuts, whole-wheat products, enriched flour/cereals
Vitamin B_{12}	Transfer of single carbon units, synthesis of CH_3-	Sore tongue, weakness, neuropathy, mental changes, pernicious anemia	Organ meats, muscle meats, eggs, dairy products, fish
Vitamin C	Collagen formation, iron absorption, metabolism of folate	Weight loss, fatigue, sore gums/joints, petechiae, bone fractures	Citrus fruits, other fruits, green peppers, leafy vegetables
Vitamin A	Visual adaptation, body/bone growth, gene expression	Night blindness, xerosis, xerophthalmia, follicular dermatitis, abnormal teeth	Organ meats, eggs, dairy (fortified) Carotene: yellow vegetables, fruits
Vitamin D	Calcium/phosphorus absorption, bone mineralization	Rickets, osteomalacia, tetany	Vitamin D-fortified foods (cereals, dairy), fish oils
Vitamin E	Antioxidant against free radicals	Hemolysis, ophthalmoplegia, peripheral neuropathy	Vegetable oils, nuts, seeds, eggs, meats; widely distributed (dairy, meat, eggs, fruit, vegetables)
Vitamin K	Synthesis of clotting factors, glutamate	Delayed blood clotting, hemorrhagic disease of the newborn	

CH_3-, methyl groups; CHF, congestive heart failure; FAD, flavin adenine dinucleotide; FMN, flavin mononucleotide; NAD, nicotinamide adenine dinucleotide; NADP, nicotinamide adenine dinucleotide phosphate.

in nonosseous tissues. Thus, the negative data for these antioxidant vitamins on prevention of cardiovascular disease and cancer cannot be evaluated (31).

Assessment of Vitamin Status

Guidelines are given for the interpretation of test results (see Table 1-19 in Chapter 1). However, the precise values vary among laboratories. The reader should ascertain the exact normal values of the laboratory providing the information.

WATER-SOLUBLE VITAMINS

The B-complex vitamins are often considered together because deficiency frequently produces overlapping symptoms. All of these vitamins form coenzymes in metabolic processes. Some characteristics of the vitamins are listed in Table 6-3.

Thiamine (Vitamin B_1)

Requirements

Relation to Energy Intake

Thiamine pyrophosphate is important in key reactions in energy metabolism (e.g., the decarboxylation of pyruvic acid). Therefore, the requirement for thiamine is usually related to energy intake and more specifically to carbohydrate ingestion. The Food and Nutrition Board recommends 0.5 mg per 1,000 kcal for adults, and the same ratio for infants and children, although fewer data are available for them. Allowances are based on the effects of varying dietary thiamine and the relationship of thiamine intake to signs of clinical deficiency and to urinary excretion of thiamine and serum erythrocyte transketolase activity. The requirements are listed in Table 6-4. A minimum of 1.0 mg per day is recommended for all adults, even those consuming fewer than 2,000 kcal daily.

Higher Requirement in Pregnant and Lactating Women

This pattern is repeated for all the vitamins for which data are available. The lactating mother secretes about 0.1 to 0.2 mg per day in milk, which is available for the suckling child.

Food Sources

Thiamine is produced by many plants and microorganisms, including those in the intestinal lumen (in relatively small amounts), but not usually by animals. Thiamine is abundant in all foods except oils, fats, and refined sugars, and is added to many commercial breads and cereals. Rather small quantities of food provide the needed daily requirement. Thiamine is easily removed during the processing of grains or destroyed (10% to 30%) during heating. Because thiamine is water-soluble, much of the content of the vitamin (up to 80%) is extracted in cooking liquid. The method of food preparation must be considered when lists of food content are consulted. Table 6-5 lists the thiamine content of various foods.

Assessment

Intake or Absorption

Thiamine in the urine is assayed either chemically by the thiochrome method or microbiologically with *Lactobacillus viridescens* (32). When thiamine intake equals the requirement of 0.3 to 0.35 mg per 1,000 kcal, the urinary excretion is 40 to 290 mg per day. When intake is less than 0.2 mg per 1,000 kcal, the urinary excretion falls below 25 mg per day. To correct for variations in the collection of urine and allow random samples to be utilized, excretion is usually reported as micrograms of thiamine per gram of creatinine. When expressed in this way, urinary thiamine is quite sensitive in the detection of low intake. However, this measurement does not assess body stores of the vitamin. Table 6-6 provides some guidelines for interpreting the results of this test.

Body Stores

Assessment is either by the direct measurement of thiamine in blood or serum or more commonly by determining the activity ratio of transketolase with and without added thiamine. The direct method is preferred, if available, as it is more specific and sensitive.

TABLE 6-4 Thiamine Dietary Reference Intakes[a]

Life Stage Group	Thiamine (mg/day)
Infants	
0–6 months	0.2[b]
7–12 months	0.3[b]
Children	
1–3 years	0.5
4–8 years	0.6
Males	
9–13 years	0.9
14–18 years	1.2
19–30 years	1.2
31–50 years	1.2
51–70 years	1.2
>70 years	1.2
Females	
9–13 years	0.9
14–18 years	1.0
19–30 years	1.1
31–50 years	1.1
51–70 years	1.1
>70 years	1.1
Pregnancy	
≤18 years	1.4
19–30 years	1.4
31–50 years	1.4
Lactation	
≤18–50 years	1.4

[a]Estimate based on recommended dietary allowances (RDA).
[b]Recommendation given as adequate intake (AI).
Data from Standing Committee on the Scientific Evaluation of Dietary Reference Intakes, Food and Nutrition Board, Institute of Medicine. *Dietary Reference Intakes for Thiamine, Riboflavin, Niacin, Vitamin B6, Folate, Vitamin B12, Pantothenic Acid, Biotin, and Choline*. Washington, DC: National Academies Press, 1998.

High-pressure liquid chromatography (HPLC) with fluorescent detection is most often used (32). Enzymatic degradation of derivatives produces free B1, which is converted to a fluorescent form and separated by HPLC. Mean values in normal adults are 11 to 19 nmol per L in serum, 101 to 191 nmol per L in whole blood, and 132 to 284 nmol per L in erythrocytes. Levels of phosphorylated thiamine in whole blood of infants and adults range from a mean of 120 to 177 nmol per L. Erythrocyte thiamine diphosphate levels correlate well with erythrocyte transketolase measurements (Table 6-6).

Erythrocyte transketolase is a thiamine-requiring enzyme that catalyzes the following reactions in the pentose phosphate pathway:

xylulose-5-PO_4 + ribose-5-PO_4 → sedoheptulose-7-PO_4 + glyceraldehyde-3-PO_4
xylulose-5-PO_4 + erythrose-4-PO_4 → fructose-6-PO_4 + glyceraldehyde-3-PO_4

When thiamine intake is stable for a period of time, the activity of this enzyme correlates with urinary excretion of thiamine. However, a single determination of urinary excretion detects intake only at one time, whereas transketolase activity (and erythrocyte thiamine diphosphate concentration) assesses cumulative intake and therefore body stores.

The assay is performed on hemolyzed whole blood with ribose-5-phosphate as substrate in the absence and presence of added thiamine. Values obtained without added thiamine reflect the

TABLE 6-5 Approximate Thiamine Content of Selected Foods

Food	Portion	Thiamine (mg)	Percentage of RDI (1.5 mg)
Grain Products			
White bread[a]	Slice	0.131	5–12
Whole-wheat bread	Slice	0.1	5–12
Shredded wheat[b]	Biscuit	0.06	
Spaghetti, enriched, cooked	1 cup	0.286	10–24
Rice, white, enriched, cooked	1 cup	0.334	15–30
Meats			
Beef, rib roast, cooked	3 oz	0.056	1–5
Pork, center loin chops, cooked	4 oz	0.52	>40
Chicken, roasted			
Breast	4 oz	0.065	1–5
Dark meat, thigh	4 oz	0.042	1–5
Sausage, pork, cooked	2-oz patty	0.2	10–24
Ham, roasted	3 oz	0.551	>40
Vegetables			
Peas, cooked from fresh	1/2 cup	0.207	10–24
Peanuts or almonds			
Roasted	1 cup	0.364	10–24
Dried	1 cup	0.969	>40
Potato, baked	2 1/3 in	0.164	10–24
Tomato, raw	2 2/3 in	0.073	5–12
Milk and eggs			
Whole milk	1 cup	0.093	5–12
Eggs, large	One	0.05	1–5
Beverages			
Beer	12 oz	0.021	1–5

RDI, recommended dietary intake.
[a]Thiamine is added to all-purpose flour.
[b]Ready-to-eat cereals may be fortified with thiamine; check the label.
Derived in part from Hands ES. *Food Finder.* 2nd ed. Salem, OR: ESHA Research, 1990.

amount of coenzyme present in tissues. The stimulated value gives a measure of the apoenzyme present that lacks coenzyme. Guidelines for interpretation of the test results are as follows (32):

Body Stores of Thiamine	Thiamine Stimulation	Activity Coefficient
Normal	0%–15%	1.0–1.2
Marginal	16%–24%	1.2–1.25
Low	>25%	>1.25

Physiology
Absorption
Thiamine is absorbed by active and passive mechanisms. Specific transporters are expressed in many tissues, including the small intestine, and, to a lesser extent, the colon (33). Two transporters have been identified (THTR-1 and THTR-2), the products of the *SLC19A2* and *SLC19A3* genes, respectively. Both transporters are important in intestinal absorption, and the presence of colonic transporters suggests that production of thiamine by colonic bacteria may be of more

TABLE 6-6 Guidelines for the Interpretation of Thiamine Status

Age of Subjects (Years)	RBC Thiamine Pyrophosphate (nmol/L)	Thiamine Urinary Excretion (μg/g creatinine)	
		Deficient Intake (<0.3 mg/1,000 kcal)	Very Low Intake
1–3	—	<175	<120
4–6	—	<120	<85
7–9	—	<180	<70
10–12	—	<180	<60
13–15	—	<150	<50
15+	>150 (normal) 120–150 (marginal) <120 (deficient)	<65	<27

RBC, red blood cell.
Data from Sauberlich HE. *Laboratory Tests for the Assessment of Nutritional Status.* 2nd ed. Boca Raton, FL: CRC Press, 1999.

importance than previously considered. Defects in the gene for THTR-1 are responsible for thiamine-responsive megaloblastic anemia (TRMA), which presents with normal plasma thiamine levels (33). This may be related to compensatory induction of THTR-2, as has been shown in knockout mice. Induction of thiamine transporters also occurs with dietary thiamine and during development. Thiamine-responsive Wernicke's type encephalopathy is another genetic disorder that is associated with seizures, ataxia, and ophthalmoplegia. It is caused by mutations in the THTR-2 (33). Negative regulation can be shown in rodents with alcohol ingestion and in Caco-2 cells with enteropathogenic E. coli (EPEC), providing another mechanism for thiamine deficiency in those clinical situations. The capacity for absorption of thiamine is approximately 5 mg per day, and approximately 25 to 30 mg is stored in the body.

Function

Thiamine pyrophosphate is a coenzyme in the oxidative decarboxylation of α-ketoacids to aldehydes, and is closely linked with magnesium. Lipoic acid, nicotinamide adenine dinucleotide (NAD), and coenzyme A (CoA) are also requirements for the reaction in animals. The reaction yields acetyl CoA and succinyl CoA. Thiamine also catalyzes transketolase activity in the pentose phosphate cycle. This function results in the production of pentose phosphates used for nucleotide synthesis and supplies NAD phosphate (NADP) for synthetic pathways (i.e., fatty acid synthesis). In thiamine deficiency, blood pyruvate levels rise. Because the vitamin plays such an important role in carbohydrate metabolism, the requirement is increased when carbohydrate intake is increased.

Metabolism

Thiamine is synthesized by plants, is abundant in all foods, and is added to many commercial baked products and cereals. Although intestinal bacteria may make some thiamine, mammals are dependent on dietary intake. The vitamin is rapidly absorbed from the upper small intestine by transporters of the SLC19 folate and thiamine family, specifically the A2 and A3 types, located both apically and basolaterally in polarized cells such as enterocytes (34). At low concentrations absorption is sodium-dependent, but at higher concentrations passive diffusion is the major mechanism. Absorption efficiency is greater than 80%, although efficiency decreases at higher doses. Thiamine phosphorylation probably occurs in the intestinal mucosa. Thiamine accumulates in all body tissues, and no storage site is preferred. About 1 mg is degraded in the tissues daily. At low intake (≤1 mg), much of the vitamin is excreted in the urine as pyrimidine metabolites; at high intake, unmetabolized thiamine is excreted.

Deficiency

Mechanisms

Deficiency may develop from a decrease in intake, an increase in tissue utilization (e.g., pregnancy), or a combination of the two factors. Diets are rarely totally lacking thiamine, so the time needed to develop clinically significant thiamine deficiency varies. The clinical settings most commonly associated with thiamine deficiency include chronic alcoholism, malabsorption syndromes, nausea and vomiting of pregnancy, and anorexia nervosa. The total amount of thiamine in the human body is about 30 mg, with half of this in muscle, largely as thiamine pyrophosphate. With requirements in excess of 1 mg per day, deficiency can develop rapidly within a period of weeks or a few months.

Antithiamine Factors

Antithiamine factors in foods can alter thiamine activity and be a cause of vitamin deficiency. The thermolabile factor found in the viscera of freshwater fish and shellfish and the thermostable factor in tea leaves and other plants have both been reported to cause deficiency when coupled with low-thiamine intake. The thermostable factor is felt to include polyhydroxyphenolic compounds, and is found in blueberries, red chicory, beetroot, black currant, Brussels sprouts, and red cabbage. These compounds, along with sulfites added as food preservative, can enhance the cleavage of thiamine, thus inactivating it.

Signs of Deficiency

Signs of deficiency depend on the duration and severity of the defect, but all degrees of deficiency affect muscle and nerve function. Mild deficiency may result in anorexia, weakness, paresthesias, edema, and lowered blood pressure and body temperature. The infant with acute onset of thiamine deficiency presents with abdominal distension and tenderness, colicky pain and vomiting, and a decreased appetite.

Usual Presentation

The usual presentation of chronic deficiency in the Western world is associated with alcoholism or malabsorption. In these cases, multiple deficiencies may be present that can alter the signs and symptoms of pure thiamine deficiency. The features of thiamine deficiency are cardiac failure, peripheral neuropathy, subacute necrotizing encephalomyelopathy, cerebellar signs, and Wernicke encephalopathy (35). This presentation can accompany any condition with persistent vomiting, malnutrition, or severe gastrointestinal or liver disease, as well as those with decreased dietary intake and reduced thiamine stores (35). Although the triad of oculomotor abnormalities, cerebellar dysfunction, and confusion is "classical" for Wernicke's encephalopathy, only about 16% of patients present with all three signs. Confusion is the most common presenting sign, and high suspicion for thiamine deficiency is justified in patients at risk, especially among alcoholics. Some evidence suggests that thiamine deficiency is not sufficient by itself to cause Wernicke–Korsakoff encephalopathy, but that alcohol is necessary for the pathogenesis of this syndrome.

Thiamine deficiency is also common in critically ill patients, and in this setting it is associated with a 50% increase in mortality (36). Thiamine deficiency should be suspected in patients with severe sepsis, burns, congestive heart failure (CHF), lactic acidosis, or neurological symptoms, especially on a background of alcoholism, starvation, chronic malnutrition, chronic parenteral nutrition, hyperemesis gravidarum, or bariatric surgery.

Severe deficiency (beriberi) is characterized by neuritis and heart failure (acute mixed type), congestive failure and emaciation (wet type), or polyneuritis and paralysis (dry type). Signs of deficiency may worsen if glucose is administered without thiamine. If lactic acidosis accompanies thiamine deficiency, acute and severe cardiac failure can occur (37). Thiamine deficiency often is neglected as a cause of lactic acidosis, especially in the setting of cardiac failure (dyspnea, palpitations, cardiomegaly, gallop, increased venous pressure, and a prolonged QT interval). Neuropathy and myelopathy are accompanied by aching and burning and decreased muscle strength, more so in the legs than in the arms. Alcoholic myopathy may complicate the effects of thiamine deficiency. There is no recognized syndrome of marginal thiamine deficiency.

Treatment

Deficiency

Thiamine hydrochloride is available in tablets (5 to 1,000 mg), in injectable form (100 or 200 mg per mL), and as an elixir (2.25 mg per 5 mL). Mild deficiency may be treated with 15 mg per day parenterally (or 25 to 50 mg orally) for 1 week, followed by a maintenance oral dose. Benfotiamine (S-benzoylthiamine-O-monophosphate) is a lipid-soluble thiamine analogue that reaches plasma levels 5 times those of comparable thiamine doses (38). There is no known clinical benefit derived from these higher plasma levels. Severe deficiency may require somewhat larger doses, up to 100 mg twice daily for 3 days, followed by oral supplementation of 5 to 30 mg per day until a normal diet is resumed. The amount of thiamine that enters the cerebrospinal fluid is limited; thus, larger doses must be given when the central nervous system (CNS) is involved. When Wernicke's encephalopathy is suspected, oral thiamine cannot be relied upon for adequate treatment. In such cases, 500 mg should be given intravenously for 2 to 3 days, followed by 250 mg per day for the next 3 to 5 days (39). Because thiamine deficiency is often associated with deficiencies of other B vitamins, it is reasonable to provide thiamine as part of a multivitamin preparation.

Inborn Errors

A few, rare thiamine-responsive inborn errors of metabolism have been described in which the enzyme involved uses thiamine pyrophosphate as a cofactor. The defective enzymes/transporters implicated include branched chain α-ketoacid dehydrogenase (maple syrup urine disease), pyruvate decarboxylase (Leigh disease), and α-ketoglutarate dehydrogenase, thiamine pyrophosphokinase, or thiamine transporter SLC19A2 (megaloblastic anemia, diabetes mellitus, and deafness) (40). These disorders require pharmacologic doses for therapy (50 mg per day or more), as do the disorders of thiamine transport, TRMA, and thiamine-responsive Wernicke's type encephalopathy.

Preventive Therapy

Preventive therapy should be given to patients whose intake is limited and to those with malabsorption or increased requirements lasting more than 2 weeks. The dose required depends on need, but is usually 1 to 2 mg per day.

Nondeficiency States

It has been suggested that thiamine improves energy levels during exercise and in the elderly, and increases cognition in patients with Alzheimer-type dementia, but the small number of studies do not support these uses (41). Low levels of thiamine have been reported in patients with recurrent aphthous mouth ulcers, and in a single trial, replacement therapy with vitamins B_1, B_2, and B_6 led to sustained improvement, but only in those patients with detectable deficiency (41).

Toxicity

Excess thiamine is rapidly cleared from the circulation by the kidneys. The UL has not been set because of a lack of suitable data (3). Reported side effects have included headache, irritability, insomnia, tachycardia, and weakness (42). Occasionally, an anaphylactic reaction has been noted after thiamine injection, probably a consequence of hypersensitivity in patients who received the vitamin previously.

Riboflavin (Vitamin B_2)

Requirement

Riboflavin is the 10-D-ribityl derivative of the 3-ring polyphenolic red pigment, flavin. Other dietary flavonoids result from reduction of C-C double bonds (flavanones), reduction of ketones (flavonols), or hydroxylation of various points on the ring structure (43). The color of the pigment depends on pH, so riboflavin and flavonoids are components of foods that are red, blue, or purple. Riboflavin forms the active portion of the coenzymes involved in biologic oxidation reactions. Therefore, requirements have been linked to protein or energy intake. Requirements have been determined by following the urinary excretion of riboflavin and by monitoring the signs of deficiency. Table 6-7 lists the daily allowances at all ages. In contrast to thiamine requirements, those for riboflavin do not seem to change as energy requirements are increased at any given age. For adults older than 51 years with a low caloric intake, a minimum riboflavin requirement of 1.2 mg per day (women) or 1.4 mg per day (men) is suggested. Otherwise, allowances for all ages have been computed as 0.6 mg per 1,000 kcal. For persons engaged in strenuous exercise,

TABLE 6-7 Recommended Riboflavin Intakes

Life Stage Group	Riboflavin (mg/day)
Child	
0–0.5 year	0.3[a]
0.5–1.0 year	0.4[a]
1–3 years	0.5
4–8 years	0.6
Males	
9–13 years	0.9
14–>70 years	1.3
Females	
9–13 years	0.9
14–18 years	1.0
19–>70 years	1.1
Pregnant	1.4
Lactating	1.6

[a]Estimate based on adequate intake (AI). All others based on recommended dietary allowance (RDA).
Data from Standing Committee on the Scientific Evaluation of Dietary Reference Intakes, Food and Nutrition Board, Institute of Medicine. *Dietary Reference Intakes for Thiamine, Riboflavin, Niacin, Vitamin B6, Folate, Vitamin B12, Pantothenic Acid, Biotin, and Choline.* Washington, DC: National Academies Press, 1998.

the allowance has been estimated as high as 1 to 6 mg per 1,000 kcal. The requirement to avoid deficiency symptoms is probably 0.4 to 0.5 mg per 1,000 kcal.

Food Sources

Riboflavin is widely distributed, especially in all leafy vegetables and in the flesh of mammals. The best sources are yeast, milk, egg whites, kidney, liver, and leafy vegetables. Fish, meat, and poultry are good sources. Other vegetables and legumes are not as good. Milk, eggs, meat, grains, and green leafy vegetables are the usual dietary sources in Western countries. Table 6-8 lists the riboflavin content of specific foods. Enrichment accounts for much of the riboflavin in dairy products and grains. Flavonoids are also prominent in a large variety of foods, flavonols (in teas, red grapes, and many foods), flavanones (citrus foods), flavones (green leafy spices), isoflavones (soybeans, legumes), and anthocyanidins (red, purple, and blue berries) (43). Intake of flavonoids varies from less than 1 mg per day for flavones to approximately 30 mg per day for flavonols. The role of flavonoids (other than riboflavin) in health is uncertain, but they have been linked to cancer prevention (see Chapters 15).

Effects of Processing

Much riboflavin in milk and grains is free, but in other sources, it is conjugated to protein. It is heat-stable but unstable in UV light. It leaches out into cooking water, with average losses of 15% to 20%. If food is exposed to light during cooking, losses can be as great as 50% of the amount in uncooked food. However, exposure of processed milk to light does not affect its riboflavin content. Little riboflavin is lost during the pasteurization of milk, but canning of foods can cause up to 30% of the vitamin content to be lost into the water. The riboflavin values listed in Table 6-8 are those of the unprocessed foods in most cases. Riboflavin is lost during the processing of grain and is added back to white flour, corn meal, and rice. The average Western diet contains about 2.7 mg per day, in excess of the RDA. Decaffeination decreases the flavonol levels of teas. Storage and cooking reduces some, but not all flavonoids.

Colonic Bacteria

Colonic bacteria produce riboflavin. Although the transport system for riboflavin is present in colonic mucosa, it is not clear whether bacterial riboflavin is available for absorption in sufficient quantity to fulfill daily needs.

TABLE 6-8 Approximate Riboflavin Content of Selected Foods

Food	Portion	Riboflavin[a] (mg)	Percentage of RDI[b]
Grain Products			
White bread	Slice	0.087	5–12
Whole-wheat bread	Slice	0.059	1–5
Frankfurter rolls	Roll	0.132	5–12
Spaghetti, cooked	1 cup	0.137	5–12
Rice, cooked	1 cup	0.027	1–5
Meats			
Beef, ground, lean	3 oz	0.176	10–24
Beef liver	3 oz	3.52	100
Chicken, light meat, roasted	3 oz	0.098	5–12
Hot dog, beef	One	0.058	1–5
Pork, center loin chop, broiled	4 oz	0.217	10–24
Tuna, canned, water	4-oz can	0.194	10–24
Bacon, cooked	3 pieces	0.054	1–5
Vegetables			
Asparagus, cooked from fresh	1/2 cup	0.104	5–12
Spinach, cooked from fresh	1 cup	0.425	10–24
Cabbage, raw	1 cup	0.022	1–5
Corn on cob, boiled	1 in	0.08	1–5
Potato, baked	4.75 × 2.3 in	0.067	1–5
Tomatoes	2.4 in	0.059	1–5
Dairy Products and Eggs			
Milk, whole	1 cup	0.395	10–24
Eggs, large	One	0.265	10–24
Cheese, cheddar	1 oz	0.106	5–12
Cheese, cottage, low fat <2%	1 cup	0.416	10–24
Ice cream	1 cup	0.329	10–24

[a]Data from Hands ES. *Food Finder.* 2nd ed. Salem, OR: ESHA Research, 1990.
[b]Recommended dietary intake is 1.7 mg.

Assessment

Intake

Riboflavin is unique among vitamins in that it is minimally metabolized or stored by the body. Thus, urinary excretion correlates well with intake during normal conditions. Urinary levels of riboflavin are measured by means of HPLC with fluorometric detection (32). During fasting or prolonged bed rest, urinary excretion can be falsely elevated. Because urinary levels reflect the recent dietary intake of riboflavin, variations can be considerable. The values are reported as micrograms of riboflavin per gram of creatinine to correct for body size and allow random sampling in 2-hour collections. Samples are usually obtained in the fasting state to avoid the variations caused when the subject consumes a meal near the time of collection. However, a deficient patient retains most of the ingested vitamin, and such variations are minimal in patients whose body stores are depleted. Table 6-9 provides guidelines for the interpretation of this measurement.

Body Stores

The riboflavin-dependent enzyme erythrocyte glutathione reductase catalyzes the following reaction:

$$NADPH + H^1 + GSSG \rightarrow NADP^1 + 2GSH$$

where GSSG = oxidized glutathione and GSH = reduced glutathione.

This assay is performed on whole blood with and without the addition of flavin adenine dinucleotide (FAD). Normally, no stimulation is noted, but when body stores of the vitamin are decreased, activity is markedly stimulated. The activity coefficient value is independent of

TABLE 6-9 Guidelines for Interpretation of Assessment of Riboflavin Status

Age (years)	Marginal (moderate risk)	Deficient (high risk)
Riboflavin Excretion (μg/g creatinine)		
All adults	40–119	<40
Erythrocyte Glutathione Reductase (activity coefficient)		
All ages	1.2–1.4 (20%–40% ↑)	>1.4 (>40% ↑)

Data from Sauberlich HE. *Laboratory Tests for the Assessment of Nutritional Status*. 2nd ed. Boca Raton, FL: CRC Press, 1999.

age and sex. An activity coefficient above 1.40 is diagnostic of severe deficiency. This sensitive assay is the procedure of choice (32).

Physiology
Coenzyme Function
Riboflavin forms a part of the two coenzymes flavin mononucleotide (FMN) and FAD. The prosthetic group is bound to the enzyme, accepts an H+ ion, and then is reoxidized by interacting with another H+ acceptor, usually a cytochrome of the mitochondrial electron transport chain (44). Flavins participate in both one- and two-electron transfers. Enzymes that require these coenzymes include succinic dehydrogenase; oxidases of fatty acids, glucose, and glycine; and xanthine oxidases. Thus, the richest sources of the vitamin are metabolically active tissues, not storage tissues. The highest concentrations of the vitamin are in the liver, heart, and kidneys. Riboflavin circulates in the blood largely bound to proteins (75%). The mean concentration in blood is 32 μg per L.

Absorption and Excretion
Dietary riboflavin occurs in the free form, and as FMN and FAD, the latter two forms requiring conversion to the free form before absorption. This conversion occurs by luminal and intestinal phosphatases. Riboflavin is absorbed rapidly in the intestine by a site-specific and saturable system that is energy- and sodium-dependent; however, the capacity for absorption is limited to approximately 30 mg per day. Two transporters, RFT-1 and RFT-2, are present in both small bowel and colon, although much more in small bowel (33). Human RFT-2 (hRFT-2) is more efficient than RFT-1; a third transporter, RFT-3, is brain specific. Mutations in hRFT-2 cause a rare neurologic syndrome, Brown–Vialetto–Van Laere, that presents with low plasma riboflavin. Intestinal transporters are induced during deficiency states, and are downregulated in the presence of excessive substrate. In vitro studies demonstrate down-regulation by certain drugs (amiloride, chlorpromazine), although the clinical significance of this regulation is unknown. The intestine, along with liver and other tissues, also phosphorylates the vitamin. The vitamin enters plasma as free FMN, is bound to albumin and immunoglobulins, and is then excreted as riboflavin or its metabolites (45). Urinary excretion is increased by a negative nitrogen balance and by large amounts of thiamine. Excretion is decreased by low-carbohydrate diets, exercise, and pregnancy. Riboflavin is excreted in milk, up to about 10% of the daily intake (i.e., 300 μg per day). Excretion in sweat is much lower.

Deficiency
Signs and Symptoms
Early symptoms are related to oral and ocular lesions. Soreness and burning of the lips, mouth, and tongue develop along with photophobia, tearing, burning, and itching of the eyes. Angular stomatitis is characteristic but not specific. This lesion is characterized by maceration and bilateral transverse fissures of the mucocutaneous junction at the angle of the mouth. Lesions of the vermilion of the lips, termed *cheilosis,* frequently occur along the line of closure in riboflavin deficiency. Geographic tongue and denudation of papillae may occur. Desquamation of the skin and seborrheic dermatitis may be seen, especially in the nasolabial fold and scrotum. Corneal vascularization develops around the entire circumference. Hypochromic anemia is associated

with erythroid hypoplasia. Growth and appetite are poor. Some of these symptoms also occur in vitamin B_6 deficiency because the oxidase required to produce the functional form of vitamin B_6 is riboflavin-dependent (34). Thus, the range of symptoms specifically caused by riboflavin deficiency is not known with certainty. Patients at risk include pregnant or lactating women, infants and schoolchildren, and groups that have high utilization and partially depleted stores.

The association with neurological symptoms of riboflavin deficiency has been clarified by the description of the Brown–Viatletto–Van Laere syndrome, a rare neurodegenerative disease that presents with sensorineural hearing loss, bulbar palsy, and respiratory symptoms. This syndrome responds to riboflavin supplementation.

Associated Deficiencies

Riboflavin-containing foods often contain other B vitamins. Moreover, riboflavin is required for the metabolism of vitamin B_6, folate, niacin, and vitamin K. Thus, multiple other deficiencies often accompany riboflavin deficiency (Table 6-3). The usual settings in which deficiency develops are conditions characterized by poor intake, such as alcoholism or malabsorption. Hemodialysis can lead to losses of water-soluble vitamins, and deficiency can develop if they are not replaced. Drugs can prevent conversion to the active coenzyme; chlorpromazine, imipramine, amitriptyline, and quinacrine have been implicated.

Differential Diagnosis

The differential diagnosis of lip lesions includes poorly fitting dentures with malocclusion; sensitivity to lipsticks, toothpaste, and similar substances; and iron-deficiency anemia. Similar tongue lesions can be seen with iron deficiency, smoking, pernicious anemia, pellagra, and antibiotic therapy.

Treatment

Deficiency States

Deficiency states should be treated with 5 to 10 mg per day by mouth. Often, other B-complex vitamin deficiencies accompany riboflavin deficiency, and some (e.g., niacin deficiency) cannot be distinguished easily on clinical grounds. When malabsorption is present, prophylactic use of the vitamin at a dose of about 3 mg per day is useful. Tablets are available in doses of 5 to 100 mg, and an injectable solution is available at a concentration of 35 mg per mL.

Nondeficiency States

Riboflavin is used in rare genetic disorders in which the formation of specific flavoproteins is deficient and as a supplement during phototherapy for neonatal jaundice. During the photosensitized oxidation of bilirubin to more polar derivatives that can be excreted, riboflavin is destroyed, and additional vitamin needs to be provided. Migraine-like headaches occur in the syndrome of mitochondrial encephalopathy, in which riboflavin therapy appears to be effective. In a randomized, double-blinded, placebo-controlled trial of high-dose (400 mg per day) riboflavin, the frequency of migraine attacks was reduced during a period of 3 months (46). However, the severity of the attacks was not affected, and the benefit of riboflavin was apparent only at the end of the study. More such trials are needed to demonstrate the effectiveness of riboflavin therapy in this condition.

Toxicity

Up to 10 mg per kg can be given without any apparent toxic effects. However, insufficient data are available to recommend an UL (3). Riboflavin may cause a yellow-orange discoloration of the urine.

Niacin (Vitamin B_3)

Requirement

The term *niacin* is used for both nicotinic acid and nicotinamide. Estimates of requirement are complicated by the fact that some tryptophan is converted to nicotinic acid in humans. On the basis of three studies in adults, a Food and Nutrition Board Task Force estimated that 60 mg of ingested tryptophan is equivalent to 1 mg of niacin—that is, from 60 mg of tryptophan enough is oxidized to provide about 1 mg of niacin. Niacin is required for the function of respiratory enzymes, and therefore allowances are based on energy expenditures. Estimates of the requirement are usually reported in terms of niacin equivalents (NE) (i.e., 1 mg of niacin or 60 mg of

TABLE 6-10 Recommended Dietary Intakes of Niacin

Life Stage Group	Niacin Equivalent (mg/day)
Infants	
0–6 months	2[a]
7–12 months	4[a]
Children	
1–3 years	6
4–8 years	
Males	
9–13 years	12
14–>70 years	16
Females	
9–13 years	12
14–>70 years	14
Pregnancy	
≤18–>50 years	18
Lactation	
≤18–>50 years	17

[a]Estimate based on adequate intake (AI). All others based on recommended dietary allowance (RDA).
Data from Standing Committee on the Scientific Evaluation of Dietary Reference Intakes, Food and Nutrition Board, Institute of Medicine. *Dietary Reference Intakes for Thiamine, Riboflavin, Niacin, Vitamin B6, Folate, Vitamin B12, Pantothenic Acid, Biotin, and Choline.* Washington, DC: National Academies Press, 1998.

tryptophan). The availability of tryptophan for niacin synthesis also depends on the presence of other essential amino acids. Table 6-10 gives the daily requirements and allowances for adults and children.

Most data on deficiency are for adults, but estimates have been made for children. Daily allowances are based on an intake of 6.6 mg NE per 1,000 kcal. A minimum for adults over the age of 18 years is 15 (women) or 19 (men) mg NE per day. During lactation, about 1.6 mg of niacin is lost daily in 850 mL of milk.

Food Sources

Nicotinic acid is present in most foods except fats and oils, mainly as the pyridine nucleotides NAD and NADP. It is removed during grain processing, but is added back during enrichment. It is particularly abundant in meat, fish, and grain products. It is sometimes present in a form that is not absorbable (e.g., in corn). It is stable in foods and can survive a reasonable amount of heating, cooking, and storage. Average diets in the United States supply 6 and 24 mg of niacin and 700 and 1,100 mg of tryptophan per day for women and men, respectively. This intake amounts to a total of 16 to 24 mg NE per day. Animal proteins provide more tryptophan than vegetable proteins (1.4% on average vs. 1.0%). Human milk contains about 0.17 mg of niacin and 22 mg of tryptophan per deciliter and is adequate to supply the needs of an infant. Table 6-11 lists the niacin content of various foods. However, food tables based on niacin content alone are not helpful unless the content is linked to energy, ingested tryptophan, or both.

Assessment

Intake or Absorption Measured by Urinary Excretion

Normally, adults excrete 20% to 30% of niacin as N'-methylnicotinamide and 40% to 60% as the 2-pyridone metabolite. Values for these metabolites fall as intake decreases. HPLC procedures provide a rapid and sensitive method for determining the levels of both metabolites. The level is usually reported per gram of creatinine to allow for random sampling; however, this method is available only for adults. In children, the level of creatinine excretion is more variable, and good guidelines for the interpretation of excretion have not been worked out. The measurement of

TABLE 6-11 Approximate Niacin Content of Selected Foods

Food	Portion	Niacin Content (mg)	Percentage of RDI[a]
Grain Products			
White or whole-wheat bread	Slice	1.05	5–12
Corn bread	Muffin	0.850	1–5
Frankfurter roll	One	1.58	5–12
40% bran flakes[b]	1/2 cup	2.1	5–12
Puffed wheat	1 cup	1.2	5–12
Rice, cooked	1 cup	3.03	10–24
Meats			
Beef, ground, lean	3 oz	4.23	10–24
Pork, center loin chop	4 oz	4.35	>40
Chicken, light meat, roasted	3 oz	10.6	25–39
Fish (e.g., halibut), broiled	3 oz	6.06	>40
Liver, beef	3 oz	12.3	>40
Tuna in water	4-oz can	12.3	10–24
Vegetables and Fruits			
Green beans, cooked fresh	1 cup	0.768	1–5
Cauliflower, cooked	1/2 cup	0.342	1–5
Peas, frozen, cooked	1/2 cup	1.18	5–12
Potato, baked	4.75 × 2.3 in	3.32	10–24
Tomato, fresh	2.6 in	0.772	1–5
Apple	2.75 in	0.106	<1
Banana	8.75 in	0.616	1–5
Peanuts	1 cup	20.6	100
Peanut butter	2 tbs	4.23	10–24
Milk and Eggs			
Milk, whole	1 cup	0.205	1–5
Egg, large	One	0.033	<1

[a]Recommended dietary intake is 20 mg.
[b]Most cold cereals are enriched; check labels.
Data from Hands ES. *Food Finder.* 2nd ed. Salem, OR: ESHA Research, 1990.

2-pyridone in plasma may be a more reliable assay than the ratio of the two niacin metabolites in the urine (32). Table 6-12 provides guidelines for interpreting urinary excretion data.

Body Stores

The levels of 2-pyridone and N'-methylnicotinamide in plasma have been reported in a few small studies to be a more reliable indicator of these metabolites than their urinary concentrations. In addition, the measurement of pyridine metabolites in red cells may be useful and more reliable (Table 6-12). Thus, it is possible that as HPLC methods become more widely available, one of these plasma or red cell measurements may identify patients with low body stores of niacin.

Physiology

The precise mechanism by which niacin is absorbed in the intestine is not known, although a high affinity uptake system that is acid pH-dependent and sodium-independent has been described in vitro in Caco-2 cells (33). A role for the organic acid transporter 10 has been suggested but not proven. Once absorbed, nicotinic acid is an essential component of the coenzyme nicotinamide adenine dinucleotide and its phosphate (NAD+ and NADP+). These coenzymes function to carry hydrogen from a substrate through the mitochondrial electron transport system. They are really cosubstrates rather than coenzymes because they join and leave the enzyme along with the substrate. Many dehydrogenases are NAD- and NADP-dependent. Perhaps the most important

TABLE 6-12 Guidelines for Interpretation of Niacin Status

Patient	Acceptable	Deficient Intake	Low Intake
	Urinary Excretion: Ratio of mg N′-Methylnicotinamide/g Creatinine to 2-Pyridone-N′-Methylnicotinamide		
Males and nonpregnant, nonlactating females	1.6–4.29	<0.5	0.5–1.50
Women, pregnant			
1st trimester	1.6–4.29	<0.5	0.5–1.59
2nd trimester	2.0–4.99	<0.6	0.6–1.99
3rd trimester	2.5–6.49	<0.8	0.8–2.49
	Plasma N′-Methylnicotinamide-2-Pyridone (µg/dL)		
Young men[a]	16.3 ± 5.9 (28 NE/day)	3.7 ± 0.9 (10 NE/day)	1.2 ± 2.3 (6 NE/day)
	Erythrocyte NAD/Erythrocyte NADP Ratio		
Young men[a]	<1.0		

NE, niacin equivalent; NAD, nicotinamide adenine dinucleotide; NADP, nicotinamide adenine dinucleotide phosphate.
[a]Based on a single study of niacin-deficient diets.
Data from Sauberlich HE. *Laboratory Tests for the Assessment of Nutritional Status*. 2nd ed. Boca Raton, FL: CRC Press, 1999.

pathway is that of oxidation of glucose-6-phosphate. The products of oxidation, NADH and NADPH, are then used for other metabolic processes, such as fatty acid synthesis. Nicotinic acid is produced from tryptophan in the liver by a series of enzymes. NAD+ and NADP+ inhibit the first enzyme of this synthetic pathway, tryptophan oxygenase, thus regulating the production of nicotinic acid. The fourth enzyme in this pathway, kynureninase, requires pyridoxal phosphate, so that deficiencies of these two vitamins are linked. NAD+-dependent protein deacetylases (sirtuins or Sir2-like proteins) are important regulators of many biological processes, including deacetylation of histones (47). The NADPH complex includes NADPH oxidase that produces superoxide, and may be implicated in vasculopathy in humans (48). A granulocyte colony stimulating factor (G-CSF)-mediated pathway to increase the production of neutrophils has been described, that involves the intracellular phosphorylation of nicotinamide (49). This pathway raises the possibility that vitamin B_3 might be useful in the future in treating neutropenia.

Nicotinic acid, but not nicotinamide, exhibits two pharmacologic properties—peripheral vasodilation and a plasma lipid-lowering effect. The latter effect is more marked when cholesterol levels are high. Nicotinic acid is used to decrease levels of triglycerides and of total and low-density lipoprotein (LDL) cholesterol, and to increase levels of high-density lipoprotein (HDL) cholesterol. The receptor for nicotinic acid has been identified as the G_i-coupled receptor HM74A (also known as GPR109A and hydroxyl carboxylic acid receptor 2), present on adipocytes, dermal dendritic cells and macrophages, and immune cells in other organs (50). Activation of this receptor on adipocytes may account for the antilipolytic effects of nicotinic acid by decreasing cAMP production and thus lipolysis. Activation of immune cells in the skin probably accounts for the flushing response, probably related to mobilization of arachidonic acid and production of vasodilatory prostaglandins PGD_2 and PGE_2.

Deficiency
Pellagra
The classic deficiency syndrome, pellagra, is associated with skin, gastrointestinal, and CNS changes. Dermatitis, which occurs in exposed areas, is symmetric and exacerbated by trauma. Cracking and crusting develop over thickened areas of skin. Soreness is common in the mouth,

with a red, swollen, and painful tongue, and mucous membranes. Angular stomatitis is often seen, but is probably caused by associated riboflavin deficiency. Diarrhea is a common feature of niacin deficiency and may be related to mucosal atrophy. Early neurologic symptoms include headache, sleep disturbances, anxiety, depression, and thought disorders. The peripheral neuropathy seen with pellagra cannot be distinguished from thiamine deficiency, and does not respond to niacin alone, so is likely due to multiple vitamin deficiencies (35). Psychomotor retardation and stupor may ensue. As the deficiency progresses, confusion, hallucinations, and agitation develop, and finally seizures or catatonia alternating with lucid spells.

Associated with Vitamin B_6 Deficiency

Tryptophan and niacin deficiencies are often compounded by vitamin B_6 deficiency because B_6 is required in the conversion of tryptophan to nicotinic acid. Isoniazid therapy can lead to pellagra because hydrazine drugs form adducts with pyridoxal phosphate. If vitamin B_6 is provided and tryptophan is available, exogenous niacin is not needed. Isoniazid resembles nicotinic acid chemically and acts as an inhibitor. However, other hydrazine drugs that are more potent inhibitors than isoniazid do not cause pellagra. Thus, inhibition of the vitamin alone may not explain the clinical deficiency.

Hartnup Disease

Hartnup disease is a rare inherited condition of neutral amino acid malabsorption that produces a clinical syndrome mimicking pellagra. Dermatitis with photosensitivity, ataxia, and psychiatric changes are common. Decreased intestinal and renal tubular absorption of tryptophan may explain in part the relative tryptophan deficiency associated with this condition. Protein synthesis seems adequate, but sufficient extra tryptophan is not available for nicotinic acid synthesis. The fact that the disorder responds to oral niacin confirms the role of tryptophan in daily niacin production.

Carcinoid Syndrome

Carcinoid syndrome often presents with low blood levels of tryptophan, probably a result of increased synthesis of serotonin from tryptophan. Rarely, pellagra occurs in the carcinoid syndrome and may be overcome by oral niacin.

Treatment

Deficiency

Isolated niacin deficiency is uncommon, and usually other B-complex vitamins must also be given. Niacin (nicotinic acid) is available in immediate-release tablets (20 to 500 mg), as sustained-release/long-acting (100, 500, and 750 mg), as extended-release (Niaspan or Slo-Niacin) capsules (500, 750, and 1,000 mg), and as an injectable solution (10, 50, and 100 mg per mL). Nicotinamide is also available in comparable doses. Nicotinamide does not have hypolipidemic or vasodilating effects. The glossitis, dermatitis, diarrhea, and mental symptoms of pellagra respond to oral doses of 100 to 500 mg per day, depending on the severity of symptoms. The peripheral neuritis seen in pellagra responds to niacin or B_6 replacement, depending on the vitamin deficiency responsible for the syndrome.

Pharmacologic Effects

Cardiovascular Disease

Nicotinic acid (1 to 3 g per day in three or four divided doses), but not nicotinamide, lowers serum levels of triglyceride, total cholesterol, and LDL cholesterol (51). Most randomized, placebo-controlled trials show significant decreases in recurrent myocardial infarction, cerebrovascular events, total mortality, and angiographic progression of atherosclerosis in patients on nicotinic acid monotherapy (3 g per day) (52). Combination therapy with a statin appears to be more potent for lowering LDL cholesterol than monotherapy alone in one study, but a subsequent trial (AIM-HIGH), adding niacin to simvastatin in patients with mild hypertriglyceridemia, showed no benefit on cardiovascular events (53,54).

Diabetes Mellitus

Despite a protective effect on beta cells in animals and an increase in C-peptide levels as a measure of beta-cell function in humans, C-peptide secretion is not altered in humans, but intensive insulin therapy with nicotinamide added appears to improve diabetic control in patients with type I diabetes (55).

Hair and Skin Conditioners

Both nicotinamide and niacin are present in cosmetics (shampoos, hair tonics, skin moisturizers, cleansing preparations) at concentrations from 0.0001% to 3% (56). They appear to be safe to the skin at these low concentrations.

Toxicity

The UL for niacin intake has been set at 35 mg per day for subjects over 18 years of age. Large doses of nicotinic acid (>1 g per day) cause flushing secondary to histamine release, with burning of the hands and face. This effect may wear off with time. Taking the drug with meals in divided doses or with aspirin may diminish the flushing (57). At doses of 3 g per day or more, nausea, vomiting, diarrhea, and arrhythmias may occur. Symptoms of dyspepsia can be aggravated by the large acid load. Hyperuricemia secondary to competition for excretion occurs in about 40% of patients. Gout occurs less frequently (7%). Cardiac arrhythmias occur uncommonly. About one-fourth of patients develop rash, pruritus, hyperkeratosis (especially at higher doses of >3 g per day), and glucose intolerance. Laboratory evidence of hepatic injury may be found. Elevations of aspartate aminotransferase and bilirubin are common (30% to 50%), even at doses as low as 750 mg per day. These elevations are more likely with the use of long-acting or sustained-release niacin, as these form the active metabolite nicotinamide (58). The dose of 2 g per day should not be exceeded. Cholestatic jaundice and submassive necrosis have been reported, again at high doses. Rarely, acanthosis nigricans can be seen that is not associated with occult neoplasm. Toxicity is more common with timed-release preparations taken at high doses. A new timed-release preparation delivering up to 2,000 mg per day was thought to be safer than immediate-release niacin (59), but in the HPS2-THRIVE trial, using this formulation in addition to simvastatin, with ezetimibe when needed, a 26% increase in myopathy was found in patients taking extended-release niacin (60). Moreover about the same increased percentage of patients developed serious infections, serious bleeding into the brain and gut, and new onset diabetes, with even more patients presenting with serious rash and other skin lesions (61). These increased adverse events are currently attributed to the extended-release niacin, and have raised questions about whether to continue to use niacin for lowering serum triglyceride levels.

Pyridoxine (Vitamin B_6)

Requirement

The term *vitamin B6* encompasses three naturally occurring pyridines—pyridoxine, pyridoxal, and pyridoxamine. These are all interrelated functionally, and a quantitative requirement would depend on knowledge of the intake and activity of all three. Such data are not readily available in humans. The estimates of requirement are based on production or cure of clinical signs of deficiency or, more often, on production or reversal of abnormal biochemical test results (e.g., excretion of tryptophan metabolites after a tryptophan load). Requirements are increased during intake of large amounts of protein.

The vitamin B_6 allowance has been estimated according to a ratio of 0.016 mg of the vitamin per gram of protein ingested. Thus, the estimates for women and men are based on the lower rates of protein intake in women than in men (Table 6-13). These figures slightly exceed the estimated requirement based on repletion studies. In the elderly, the incidence of biochemical pyridoxine deficiency was nearly 50% (62), but there is little evidence to indicate that this deficiency is based on differences in energy intake (63). Thus, the recommendations are higher in the older-aged population. The protein requirements of pregnant and lactating women are increased; in addition, they must supply the fetus or newborn with vitamin B_6. The additional allowances suggested for these stresses have been made without much quantitative data to support the recommendations. The vitamin B_6 content of human milk is low in the first few weeks. Oral contraceptive intake for more than 30 months before pregnancy can decrease vitamin B_6 levels.

Food Sources

Dietary intake of the vitamin comes from vegetables as pyridoxine, and from meat in the form of pyridoxamine. These forms are oxidized to pyridoxal-5-phosphate by pyridoxamine oxidase. Vitamin B_6 is produced by intestinal microorganisms, but it is not known how much of this is absorbed. The three forms of the vitamin are present in low concentrations in all plant and

TABLE 6-13 — Recommended Daily Dietary Intakes of Vitamin B_6

Life Stage Group	Vitamin B_6 (mg/day)
Infants	
0–6 months	0.1[a]
7–12 months	0.3[a]
Children	
1–3 years	0.5
4–8 years	0.6
Males	
9–13 years	1.0
14–50 years	1.3
51–>70 years	1.7
Females	
9–13 years	1.0
14–18 years	1.2
19–50 years	1.3
50–>70 years	1.5
Pregnancy	
≤18–50 years	1.9
Lactation	
≤18–50 years	2.0

[a]Estimate based on adequate intake (AI). All others based on recommended dietary allowance (RDA).

Data from Standing Committee on the Scientific Evaluation of Dietary Reference Intakes, Food and Nutrition Board, Institute of Medicine. *Dietary Reference Intakes for Thiamine, Riboflavin, Niacin, Vitamin B6, Folate, Vitamin B12, Pantothenic Acid, Biotin, and Choline.* Washington, DC: National Academies Press, 1998.

animal tissues. For this reason, dietary deficiency is uncommon. Bound forms of the vitamin are found as β-D-glucosides in plants; about 60% of this is bioavailable. Most vitamin B_6 is associated with glycogen phosphorylase, and this source accounts for much of the storage pool of the vitamin. Table 6-14 lists the content of the vitamin in various foods. Pyridoxal represents 80% of the B_6 vitamins in human milk. This abundance of pyridoxal is needed because the premature infant (<29 weeks) cannot utilize pyridoxine to any extent. Losses of vitamin B_6 have been observed during the heating and storage of some foods, as Schiff base forms between pyridoxal phosphate and the ε-amino lysines in proteins. Bioavailability can be as low as 40% but usually ranges from 60% to 80%. Losses occur during processing, often exceeding 50%. Sometimes, the availability of vitamin B_6 is increased during food processing.

Assessment

Intake or Absorption

The vitamin is excreted in the urine mainly as pyridoxal and to a lesser extent as pyridoxamine. About 20% to 50% is excreted as the metabolite *4-pyridoxic acid*. The excretion of free vitamin B_6 correlates closely with intake. Dietary protein does not affect urinary excretion. Urinary excretion reflects recent dietary intake but may not reflect the degree of deficiency. Random samples provide as good data as do 24-hour excretion studies. Chromatographic (HPLC) methods are very reliable for all metabolites, especially 4-pyridoxic acid. Low intake correlates with excretion of less than 5.0 μg of 4-pyridoxic acid per day. Urinary excretion is probably not a reliable measure of pyridoxine status in patients being treated with vitamin B_6 antagonists, such as isoniazid. Table 6-15 provides guidelines for the interpretation of urinary levels. Measurement of plasma 4-pyridoxic acid has been suggested as a marker of short-term status, but this requires the use of sensitive liquid chromatography (LC) (64).

TABLE 6-14 Approximate Vitamin B₆ Content in Selected Foods

Food	Portion	Vitamin B₆ Content (mg)	Percentage of RDI (2.0 mg)
Grain Products[a]			
Bread			
White	1 piece	0.009	<1
Whole wheat	1 piece	0.052	1–5
Rice, cooked	1 cup	0.283	10–24
Spaghetti, enriched	1 cup	0.049	1–5
Cornflakes	3 oz	0.060	1–5
Meats			
Beef, ground, lean	3 oz	0.210	10–24
Pork, center loin chop	4 oz	0.348	10–24
Salmon	3 oz	0.186	5–12
Chicken			
Dark meat, roasted	3 oz	0.304	10–24
White meat, roasted	3 oz	0.510	25–39
Fruits and Vegetables			
Banana	8.75 in	0.659	25–39
Apples	2.75 in	0.066	1–5
Grapes	10 each	0.060	1–5
Cauliflower, cooked	1/2 cup	0.125	5–12
Peas, green, cooked	1 cup	0.250	5–12
Potatoes, baked	1 each	0.701	25–39
Tomatoes, fresh	1 each	0.098	5–12
Peanuts	1 cup	0.367	10–24
Peanut butter	2 tbs	0.124	5–12
Dairy Products and Eggs			
Milk, whole	1 cup	0.102	5–12
Cheese, cottage, 27% fat	1 cup	0.172	5–12
Egg	One	0.060	1–5

RDI, recommended dietary intake.
[a]Cereals are sometimes fortified with B₆; check label.
Data from Hands ES. *Food Finder.* 2nd ed. Salem, OR: ESHA Research, 1990.

Body Stores

Transaminases

Transaminases are enzymes requiring vitamin B_6. Because the level of transaminase activity is greater in red cells than in serum and is less variable, erythrocyte transaminases are used for this determination. The assay is performed with and without the addition of pyridoxal phosphate. However, in contrast to what occurs in the stimulatory tests for thiamine and riboflavin, transaminase activity in normal subjects is increased by the addition of pyridoxal. Activity is reported as a ratio of stimulated to unstimulated activity, termed the *erythrocyte transaminase (E-AST or E-ALT) index*. Normal subjects have an E-AST index of less than 1.7 and an E-ALT index of less than 1.25. Deficiency is correlated with an E-AST index of more than 2.2. Ratios between 1.8 and 2.2 are marginal. This test remains the best readily available functional assessment of vitamin B_6 status.

Pyridoxal-5′-phosphate

Pyridoxal-5′-phosphate (PLP) is also a sensitive measure of vitamin status and correlates with body stores. However, plasma levels can be modified by physical exercise, pregnancy, and by plasma alkaline phosphatase activity. PLP can be measured in whole blood (50 to 120 nmol per L) and in plasma (17 ± 7 μg per L), with ranges of 30 to 134 nmol per L and 5 to 33 μg per L, respectively

(32). If the 95% reference limits for PLP derived from white populations are used, many African Americans have low levels of pyridoxine. Thus, low PLP levels in African Americans do not necessarily indicate deficiency (65). The assay has been performed in an enzymatic assay with tyrosine apodecarboxylase as the apoenzyme. HPLC is now more widely available, and is more accurate. Using HPLC, deficiency is defined as a plasma concentration of less than 20 nmol per L, with marginal status identified as 20 to 30 nmol per L, and adequate levels over 30 nmol per L (64). The most sensitive assay available involves LC with fluorescence or with mass spectroscopy, although these are the least available. The advantage of this method is that it allows simultaneous measurement of PLP, pyridoxal, and 4-pyridoxine. In some situations, stores are not correctly assessed by PLP measurement. Patients with cirrhosis metabolize PLP more rapidly than normal persons do. However, metabolism is not to pyridoxic acid, so excretion of that metabolite does not assess depletion. PLP is also elevated in hypophosphatasia (66). Thus, its level may vary with alkaline phosphatase activity. The difficulty with assessing body stores is that multiple forms of the vitamin exist and must be measured (32).

Xanthurenic Acid Excretion

Xanthurenic acid excretion following a 2- or 4-g tryptophan load is also a sensitive functional assay of vitamin B_6 status, perhaps even more sensitive than the transaminase ratio (32). The HPLC assay is reproducible, but because of the convenience of sampling blood or plasma, it has not been used as much as the transaminase ratio and PLP concentrations.

Homocysteine

Vitamin B_6 is one of three vitamins important in the metabolism of Hcy (along with folate and vitamin B_{12}), and levels of this metabolite are elevated when the vitamin is deficient. Detection is very accurate by HPLC. Hcy is elevated to ≥ 12 μmol per L fasting and ≥ 38 μmol per L after methionine load. When Hcy is elevated, plasma levels of PLP are significantly lower than in people with normal levels. However, elevation of Hcy is not specific for pyridoxine deficiency (Table 6-15). Folic acid is probably the main determinant of the Hcy increase associated with coronary artery disease (see sections on folic acid and vitamin B_{12}).

Cystathionine

Plasma cystathionine has been suggested as a functional assay for B_6 deficiency, as the enzyme cystathionine-γ-lyase that converts cystathionine to cysteine is dependent only on B_6 and not

TABLE 6-15 Guidelines for Assessment of Vitamin B_6 Status

Parameter	Acceptable Values	Plasma (homocysteine)[a]	
		<16.3 μmol/L	>16.3 μmol/L
Plasma pyridoxal-5′-phosphate	>30 nmol/L		
Urinary 4-pyridoxic acid	>3.0 μmol/day		
Erythrocyte AST activity coefficient	<1.80		
Erythrocyte ALT activity coefficient	<1.25		
Urinary xanthurenic acid excretion	<65 μmol/day (2 g L-tryptophan load)		
Pyridoxal-5′-phosphate	≥30 nmol/L	83 ± 76	56 ± 50
Plasma folate	≥5 nmol/L	6.7 ± 3.6	5.5 ± 2.9
Plasma cobalamin	±200 pmol/L	275 ± 148	202 ± 61

AST, aspartate aminotransferase; ALT, alanine aminotransferase.
[a]Values from reference 46.
Data from Standing Committee on the Scientific Evaluation of Dietary Reference Intakes, Food and Nutrition Board, Institute of Medicine. *Dietary Reference Intakes for Thiamine, Riboflavin, Niacin, Vitamin B6, Folate, Vitamin B12, Pantothenic Acid, Biotin, and Choline.* Washington, DC: National Academies Press, 1998.

on folate or B_{12}. This measurement requires the use of one of the methods using advanced spectroscopy, and its clinical usefulness is not yet established (67).

Physiology

The phosphorylated forms of vitamin B_6 must be dephosphorylated before absorption. The forms of vitamin B_6 are rapidly absorbed in the small intestine by a pH-dependent, sodium-independent carrier-mediated mechanism (68). The precise system for absorption has not yet been identified. The colonic mucosa appears to contain some absorption capacity, but the amount of absorption relative to the small bowel is not known (33). The absorbed vitamin is distributed among enzyme proteins as the coenzyme pyridoxal phosphate. Most enzymes use this form, although transaminase can also use pyridoxamine. The ability of the human fetus (up to 30 weeks of age) to convert pyridoxine phosphate to pyridoxal phosphate via pyridoxine oxidase is limited. Enzymes that require vitamin B_6 are involved in the synthesis and catabolism of all amino acids. Thus, the requirement is linked to protein intake. Most of the transaminases require vitamin B_6, as do many amino acid decarboxylases. Important among this latter group are the enzymes that convert histidine to histamine, ornithine to polyamines, aromatic amino acids to dopamine, and serotonin and glutamate to γ-aminobutyric acid. The enzymes serine deaminase, which produces pyruvic acid, and threonine deaminase, which produces 2-oxybutyrate, both require vitamin B_6. The synthesis of CoA, which is the first step in porphyrin (heme) synthesis, the conversion of linoleic to arachidonic acid, and the production of nicotinic acid from tryptophan via kynurenine are all B6-dependent steps. The vitamin binds to a nuclear steroid hormone receptor and thus acts as a negative control of steroid hormone action.

Deficiency

Because the vitamin is widely distributed in food and is also made by intestinal bacteria, dietary restriction rarely leads to deficiency. The usual clinical situations in which deficiency arises include malabsorption, old age, alcoholism, and treatment with vitamin B_6 antagonists. The deficiency syndrome is not well defined in humans. The major findings include seborrhea-like lesions about the eyes, nose, and mouth; cheilosis; glossitis; hypochromic anemia; and peripheral neuropathy (35). Nausea, vomiting, dizziness, irritability, insomnia, and convulsions can occur. Vitamin B_6 deficiency can impair interleukin-2 production and lymphocyte proliferation in elderly adults. Most of these symptoms are induced by the use of vitamin B_6 antagonists and may not reflect symptoms of the true deficiency state. Deficiency of pyridoxamine oxidase produces fetal distress with intractable seizures by preventing production of the active form of the vitamin, pyridoxal-5-phosphate (69).

Hyperhomocysteinuria

Hyperhomocysteinuria has been identified as an independent risk factor for vascular disease and may be associated with a deficiency of cystathionine synthase, the B_6-dependent enzyme that catalyzes the conversion of Hcy to cystathionine. Significantly lower levels of PLP, cobalamin, and folic acid were found in patients with moderately elevated levels of Hcy (≥ 16.3 μmol per L) (70). Most studies implicate folic acid as the major factor related to hyperhomocysteinemia (see section on folic acid in this chapter). However, when pyridoxine alone has been used to lower Hcy levels, rather low doses were used (2–10 mg per day) (71). These are doses in the range of the DRI for vitamin B_6, but most patients with hyperhomocysteinemia do not have plasma pyridoxine levels in a range that would be considered deficient, so the implication of the vitamin's role in Hcy levels in humans is still unresolved. It is premature at present to recommend the widespread use of these supplements to alter atherogenesis in this subset of patients with hyperhomocysteinemia.

Vitamin B_6 Antagonists

The most common antagonists are isoniazid, hydralazine and other hydrazines, oral contraceptives, dopamine, and penicillamine. Cycloserine also can act in this way. These compounds increase urinary excretion (e.g., isoniazid) or combine with pyridoxal or pyridoxal phosphate to form inactive drugs (e.g., hydrazones are derived from hydrazines and a thiazolidine derivative from penicillamine). These effects can be reversed with vitamin B_6 supplements, usually in the range of 2 to 5 mg per day (72).

Cyclooxygenase inhibitors used long term (>6 months) can lower circulating pyridoxal-5-phosphate serum levels, although long-term clinical effects of this different B_6 status are not clear (73). Large doses of the vitamin have also been used to treat Gyromitra mushroom (monomethylhydrazine) poisoning. Some experts advocate prophylaxis for all patients on isoniazid; others suggest supplements only for those at risk for neuropathy. Large doses (600 mg bid) have been used to treat neuroleptic-induced akathisia (restlessness) and tardive dyskinesia, presumably due to its effects on neural transmission (74).

Pyridoxine-Dependent Syndromes

These syndromes have been reported, in which tissue levels of the vitamin are normal but binding of the cofactor to the enzyme is impaired. These inherited disorders respond to larger doses of vitamin B_6 than are required to treat deficiency states (40). Table 6-16 lists the syndromes.

Venous Thromboembolism

An association of low serum vitamin B_6 levels with increased risk of venous thromboembolism has been reported (75). This risk was not associated with serum Hcy levels. The results of intervention studies are not sufficiently clear to allow a recommendation for routine use.

Colorectal Cancer

An association between plasma PLP levels and the risk of colorectal cancer (CRC) has been demonstrated, although there was no correlation with vitamin B_6 intake (76). In the Nurses'

TABLE 6-16 Pyridoxine-dependent Errors of Metabolism

Disorder	Enzyme	Clinical Findings	Laboratory Findings
Infantile seizures, B_6-dependent	Glutamic acid decarboxylase	Convulsions	None
Chronic anemia, B_6-dependent	δ-aminolevulinic acid (ALA) synthase	Hypochromic anemia	Increased serum iron
Homocystinuria	Cystathionine β-synthase	Mental retardation, severe collagen disease involving vessels, eye problems, osteoporosis	Homocystinemia, homocystinuria, hypermethioninemia
Cystathioninuria	γ-cystathionase	Mental retardation, blood dyscrasia, heart disease	Cystathionuria
Xanthurenic aciduria	Kynureninase	Urticaria, mental retardation	Xanthurenic aciduria
Gyrate atrophy of choroids and retina	Ornithine aminotransferase	Chorioretinal degeneration, blindness	None diagnostic
X-linked sideroblastic anemia	Erythroid specific δ-ALA synthase	Anemia	Ringed sideroblasts
Primary hyperoxaluria	Alanine-glyoxylate aminotransferase	Renal stones	Hyperoxaluria
Developmental delay	Aromatic-L-aminoacid decarboxylase	Hypotonia, oculogyric crises	Elevated 5-hydroxytryptophan in CSF, plasma, and urine
Cohen syndrome	β-alanine α-ketoglutarate transaminase	Hypotonia, obesity, mental retardation, facial/oral/ocular/limb anomalies	None diagnostic

CSF, cerebrospinal fluid.
Data from Frank T, Bitsch R, Maiwald J, et al. High thiamine phosphate concentrations in erythrocytes can be achieved in dialysis patients by oral administration of benfotiamine. *Eur J Clin Pharmacol.* 2000;56:251.

Health Study and the Health Professionals Follow-Up Study cohort, vitamin B_6 intake was followed every 4 years using food frequency questionnaires (77). Although initially a 20% to 30% lower risk of CRC was associated with a higher B_6 intake, this effect was attenuated with time, making it less likely that the vitamin played a role in CRC pathogenesis in adults. It is not known whether supplemental B_6 will protect against CRC.

Therapy
Deficiency
Pyridoxine hydrochloride is available as 5-, 10-, 25-, 50-, 100-, 200-, 250-, and 500-mg tablets and as a solution for injection containing 50 or 100 mg per mL. It is a component of many multivitamin tablets at doses of about 2 mg. In treating deficiencies, it is often advisable also to give other B-complex vitamins because multiple deficiencies frequently occur simultaneously. For *prophylactic* use with isoniazid to prevent peripheral neuropathy, 5 mg per day is probably sufficient, but doses up to 25 mg are used. Treatment of established neuropathy requires 50 to 300 mg per day. Pyridoxine is sometimes given to patients with sideroblastic anemia, dystonia, or Parkinson disease treated with L-dopa, and to newborns with seizure disorders.

Pharmacologic Doses
The vitamin has been used to treat a variety of disorders that may or may not be associated with decreased intake, but little evidence of efficacy has been provided by properly conducted trials (78). Pyridoxine has been used in carpal tunnel syndrome (79), asthma, and autism, with no clear evidence of efficacy from available studies (15). A meta-analysis of 10 RCTs of premenstrual syndrome found efficacy in doses of 50 mg once or twice a day (80), although the quality of the studies was questioned and was considered relatively poor. In fact, dietary intake of B_6 was not correlated with incident premenstrual syndrome, although thiamine and riboflavin intakes were inversely related (81). Depressive symptoms were helped more than others, and no side effects were noted. However, a systematic review of double-blinded placebo-controlled trials using vitamin B_6 supplements found no evidence for short-term benefit in improving mood (depression, fatigue, tension) or cognitive function (82).

Toxicity
When pyridoxine is ingested in large amounts (0.5 to 6 g per day), a peripheral sensory neuropathy can occur (83) that is completely reversible when treatment is stopped. Possible explanations include neurotoxicity directly caused by pyridoxine, neurotoxicity caused by a minor contaminant, or inhibition of the formation of pyridoxal phosphate by unconverted pyridoxine. The UL for adults has been established at 100 mg per day (3).

Folate (Folic Acid, Folacin, Pteroylglutamic Acid)

Requirement
Difficulty of Estimation
Estimating the folate requirement is complex. *Folacin* is a generic term denoting compounds with a structure and function similar to those of folic acid (pteroylglutamic acid), and more than 150 forms are known to exist in foods. The forms differ in the degree of reduction of the double bonds in the ring structure (e.g., tetrahydrofolate), the presence of 1-carbon groups (e.g., methyltetrahydrofolate), and the number of glutamyl residues in the peptide chain (e.g., folate pentaglutamate). Moreover, individual compounds are variably absorbed and retained by the body. Dietary folates are mostly in the polyglutamate form, which is not quite as available as the unconjugated vitamin. Absorption does not necessarily correlate with retention in the body because more of the monoglutamate form of pteroylglutamic acid is excreted in the urine after ingestion than of other forms.

Folacin is variably available in foods because of the presence of binders, inhibitors, and other factors. Enterohepatic recirculation of 5-methyltetrahydrofolic acid (5-MeTHF) is important in the retention of body stores, but the relative importance of this factor in individuals can only be guessed at. An exact determination of total body pools of folacin is not available because the data are based on too few determinations. The form of folate used commercially, pteroylglutamic acid, is a relatively poor substrate for dihydrofolate reductase; consequently, the rates of tissue utilization and retention for this form are much lower than those for the natural methylated or reduced folates found in food. However, folacin requirements have been assessed by replacement with pteroylglutamic acid.

A meta-analysis of 11 trials found that folate biomarkers in plasma and red cells increased in response to dose, but only up to 400 µg per day (84). Doses above that level showed no dose–response relationship, and thus cannot provide information on requirements in humans.

Dietary References Intakes

The recommendations for folate intake have been modified dramatically (3) since the RDA of 200 µg per day for adults was offered in 1989 in the 10th edition of *Recommended Dietary Allowances*. Subsequently, the need for extra folate to reduce the incidence of neural tube defects was recognized (85), as was the role of folate intake and elevated serum Hcy concentrations in cardiovascular disease (86). The report of the Institute of Medicine (IOM) expresses dietary folate as folate equivalents, adjusted for the apparently greater bioavailability of synthetic folic acid in comparison with naturally occurring folate, and for the estimated amount of ingested folate needed to maintain folate levels in RBCs (i.e., body stores) in long-term metabolic studies (3). The resulting recommendations are all higher by 100 to 200 µg per day than previous estimates (Table 6-17). Pregnant and lactating women require extra folate to build RBCs and produce milk, respectively. African American women have lower serum folate levels compared with white American women both pre- and post-folic acid administration (87). This difference is likely to be biologically based.

Food Sources

The folacin content of selected foods is given in Table 6-18. Major sources are orange and other citrus juices, white bread, dried beans, green salads, liver, eggs, and enriched breakfast cereals. However, much dietary folate comes from food sources that are frequently consumed but in which the vitamin is not especially concentrated, and from cereals and grain foods (flour, pasta, rice, cornmeal) that are fortified with folate.

TABLE 6-17 Dietary Reference Intakes for Folate

Life Stage Group	Folate (µg/day)
Infants	
0–6 months	65[a]
7–12 months	80[a]
Children	
1–3 years	150
4–6 years	200
Males	
9–13 years	300
14–>70 years	400
Females	
9–13 years	300
14–50 years	400 SFA + diet
51–>70 years	400
Pregnancy	
≤18–50 years	600 (400 as SGA)
Lactation	
≤18–50 years	500

SFA, synthetic folic acid. Because it is more readily available than dietary folate and is the form shown to prevent some neural tube defects, this form is recommended during the childbearing years and pregnancy.
[a]Estimate based on adequate intake (AI). All others based on recommended dietary allowance (RDA).
Data from Standing Committee on the Scientific Evaluation of Dietary Reference Intakes, Food and Nutrition Board, Institute of Medicine. *Dietary Reference Intakes for Thiamine, Riboflavin, Niacin, Vitamin B6, Folate, Vitamin B12, Pantothenic Acid, Biotin, and Choline.* Washington, DC: National Academies Press, 1998.

TABLE 6-18 Approximate Folacin Content of Selected Foods

Food	Portion	Total Folacin (µg)	Percentage of RDI (400 µg)
Meat			
Beef or pork, cooked	3 oz	3–4	1–5
Liver, beef, cooked	3 oz	123	25–39
Liver, chicken, cooked	1 each	204	>40
Vegetables			
Asparagus	1 cup	86	10–24
Spinach, cooked	1 cup	164	25–39
Beans, green, cooked	1 cup	41	10–24
Cauliflower	1 cup	42	10–24
Turnip greens	1 cup	52	10–24
Lettuce, head or leaf	1 cup	20	5–12
Lettuce, romaine	1 cup	98	10–24
Nuts			
Walnuts	1 cup	66	10–24
Peanuts	1 cup	153	25–39
Peanut butter	1 tbs	13	1–5
Almonds	1 cup	136	25–39
Breads and Cereals			
Bread			
White	1 slice	10	1–5
Whole wheat	1 slice	16	1–5
Rice	1 cup	20	1–5
Eggs			
Egg	1 each	29	5–12
Beverages			
Wine, spirits	8 oz	None	0
Beer	12 oz	21	5–12
Milk, whole	1 cup	12	1–5
Orange juice, fresh or frozen	1 cup	136	25–39

RDI, recommended dietary intake.
Source: An extensive list of folacin content of foods is given by Perloff BP, Britrum RR. Folacin in selected foods. *J Am Diet Assoc.* 1977;70:161.

Polyglutamate Versus Monoglutamate Forms

Folacins occur in food largely as polyglutamates. The pentaglutamate form predominates, although forms with four and six residues also are common. The assessment of polyglutamate forms in foods is difficult because of rapid breakdown to the monoglutamate form in mammalian tissues. This problem is relevant to estimates of the availability of folacins in foods because they must be deconjugated to the monoglutamate form for absorption. Moreover, the microorganisms used to assay folacin content differ in how they use the monoglutamate and oligoglutamate forms. In situ deconjugation in the tissues affects the assessment of nutritional folacin availability. Estimates of folacin available as the monoglutamate form vary from 30% in orange juice to 60% in cow's milk.

Folacin Availability

Most dietary folacins are reduced and methylated forms; 5-methyl pteroylglutamic acid accounts for 60% to 95% of dietary folacin, 10-formyl pteroylglutamic acid for 14% to 40%, and other reduced forms for 10% to 20%. The 5-methyl and *N*-10-formyl folacins are heat-stable, whereas unsubstituted, reduced pteroylglutamic acids are unstable. Some dietary folates are bound to specific binding proteins (e.g., in milk). In steaming and frying, as much as 90% of the food content can be lost. Boiling for 8 minutes causes a loss of about 80% of folacin activity from most vegetables. Boiling destroys heat-labile folacin in cow's milk; during boiling, the folacin content of milk falls from about 54 μg per L to less than 10 μg per L. Thus, infants fed with boiled milk formulas must receive supplements. Some foods are judged to contain highly bioavailable folacins, such as bananas, lima beans, liver, and yeast. Foods in which the folacin bioavailability is low include orange juice, lettuce, egg yolk, cabbage, soybean, and wheat germ. It seems unlikely that a single figure for folate bioavailability will be found that is applicable to every diet for every person, However, in general, food folate is less bioavailable than folic acid by 35% to 40% (87).

Folacin Content of Average Diets

The new DRIs use the concept of dietary folate equivalents (DFEs) to calculate estimates, and DFEs are used to estimate dietary content. The DFE converts all forms of dietary folate, including synthetic folate in fortified foods, to an equivalent of food folate (88). The estimated equivalent of food folate for synthetic folate is 50%, and the estimated equivalent for synthetic folate added to food, as opposed to synthetic folate by itself, is 85%. Thus, synthetic folic acid added to food is 85/50 or 1.7 times more available than synthetic folate alone. Alternatively, the DFE equation described general folate bioavailability as $50/85 \times 100 = 59\%$, but the range is from approximately 44% to 80%. The diets of adults in the United States and Canada contained 262 to 2,807 μg of DFEs per day, with mean daily intakes of 708 and 718 μg for adult men and women, respectively (in the second National Health and Nutrition Examination Survey [NHANES II], 1988–1994), and of 718 and 644 μg, respectively (in the Continuing Surveys of Food Intakes by Individuals, 1994–1996) (89). With allowances made for the increased availability of foods fortified with folate and the increased use of supplements, it was estimated that 67% to 95% of the US population was meeting the new estimated average requirement (88). However, 68% to 87% of women of childbearing age still had intakes of synthetic folate below the recommended level of 400 μg per day, and about 20% of children under the age of 8 had intakes over the newly established UL of 400 μg per day for that age group (1,000 μg per day for adults).

Assessment

Intake or Absorption

Only small amounts of folacin are excreted in the urine (about 1% of dietary intake) (32). Moreover, not all dietary forms are excreted in the same proportions. Thus, urinary excretion is not useful in assessing intake. Oral folic acid tolerance tests have been described, but they do not clearly distinguish between folate and vitamin B_{12} deficiencies because folate utilization is decreased in vitamin B_{12} deficiency. The serum folate level is quite sensitive to changes in dietary folate intake and is a measure of the status at the time of assay (90). A low serum level (2 or 3 to 6 ng per mL) reflects only a recent low dietary intake and may not reflect tissue stores (Table 6-19). Continued low levels (<2 or 3 ng per mL) are usually associated with megaloblastic anemia and decreased tissue reserves. Folate is assayed microbiologically with *Lactobacillus casei*, which uses the 5-methyl vitamers, the only circulating form of folacin. Alternatively, measurements based on binding assays or radioimmunoassays (RIAs) are used. Although the microbiologic assay is the reference method, binding assays are simpler and faster, avoid interference from antibiotics in serum samples, and allow simultaneous measurement of serum B_{12} levels. Results are quite variable with the microbiologic assay, especially as different pH extraction methods are used (91). Variability was only 9% to 11% for folic acid–fortified foods, but much more so (>45%) for natural foods. As a result of this variation, the Association of Official Analytical Chemists recommends using a trienzyme extraction to recover folic acid from food (92). In addition, the results of radioassays are quite variable between laboratories, and the radioassays require more expensive reagents and equipment. Single-stage (competitive) and two-stage (noncompetitive) assay kits are available, with the latter providing slightly better sensitivity. A roundtable dialogue to discuss the NHANES monitoring of biomarkers of folate and vitamin B_{12} status concluded that the microbiological assay was the gold standard for measuring serum and red cell folate (93). Clinical laboratories often use automated competitive protein-binding (SPB) assays, with folate-binding protein (FBP) to capture the vitamer (94). The FBP usually used is β-lactoglobulin from cow's

TABLE 6-19 Guidelines for Interpreting Folate Status

Test	Folate Deficiency	Low Recent Folate Intake[a]	Normal	Vitamin B$_{12}$ Deficiency
Serum folate (ng/mL)	<4[b]	3–6	>6	High
Red cell folate (ng/mL)	<151[b]	150–160	>160	<150
Bone marrow	Megaloblasts	Normocytic, normochromic	Normocytic, normochromic	Megaloblasts
Peripheral blood smear	Multilobed polymorphonuclear leukocytes,[c] macrocytosis	Normal	Normal	Multilobed polymorphonuclear leukocytes, macrocytosis
	Moderate/Severe Risk	**Low Risk**	**Normal**	
Serum homocysteine (μmol/L)	>30	>16	<12–15 (40+ years M)	
			<10–12 (40+ years F)	

[a] Low serum levels also may reflect hypoproteinemia or the ingestion of drugs that alter folic acid metabolism or binding, such as folate antagonists, phenytoin, alcohol, and oral contraceptives. Hemolysis may falsely elevate the serum values.
[b] de Benoist B. Conclusions of a WHO Technical Consultation on folate and vitamin B$_{12}$ deficiencies. *Food Nutr Bull.* 2008;29:S238.
[c] Multilobed: >3.5 lobes per cell on average, or >5% of cells have five lobes, or >1 six-lobed leukocyte per 100 cells.

milk, and captures 5-MeTHF as well as other folate forms, depending on the pH. Some labs use chemiluminescent immunoassays (CLIA). The microbiological assay method correlates well with the CLIA for both serum and RBC folate, although the absolute numbers are different (95).

Most circulating folacin is in the form of 5-MeTHF acid. About 90% is loosely attached to albumin and 10% to specific binding proteins. Therefore, hypoalbuminemia can lead to a low total serum folic acid level, and this result does not necessarily imply a deficiency of the vitamin. Aspirin, at a dose of 650 mg every 9 hours, can produce a reversible decrease in total and bound folate (96). Other albumin-binding drugs produce the same effect. Low values are also associated with decreased intake, malabsorption, or ingestion of drugs that affect folate absorption or utilization. These drugs include folate antagonists, phenytoin, prednisone, alcohol, and oral contraceptive agents. Alcohol lowers serum folate levels by increasing urinary folate excretion (97). Because both red and white cells contain much larger amounts of folacin than serum does, hemolysis or a very high white blood cell count, especially when the white cells are abnormal, falsely elevates serum folate levels. One-third of hospitalized patients may have low folate levels, which implies a recent negative folic acid balance. However, few of these patients require long-term supplementation.

Tissue Stores

Although serum and red cell folate levels decline in parallel, the red cell folate level is a more accurate reflection of tissue stores. It is less variable and reflects the folate status at the time of red cell formation. However, the red cell contains monoglutamate and polyglutamate forms of folic acid, so that the dose–response curves are altered in binding assays. Because RBC folate requires sample pretreatment, introducing variability, and because the C677T polymorphism of methylenetetrahydrofolate reductase alters the distribution of folate forms in red cells, serum folate is still preferred as an assessment of folate status (98). Folate is measured in both serum and whole blood, and the folate level in red cells is calculated on the basis of the hematocrit. In primary vitamin B_{12} deficiency, folate is not well utilized. Thus, in 15% to 25% of cases of vitamin B_{12} deficiency, serum folate levels rise and red cell levels fall. When both the serum and red cell levels are low, folate deficiency is the cause, although the red cell folate level falls after the serum folate level. Table 6-19 outlines the guidelines used for interpreting folate levels.

Other Assays

The presence of hypersegmented lobes can be helpful, but the determination is somewhat subjective. Macrocytosis (mean corpuscular volume > 97) may be present but is not specific. Urinary excretion of formiminoglutamic acid after an oral 20-g load of histidine (normal rate, >50 mg per 12 h) is a functional assay, as is the deoxyuridine suppression test. These tests are not routinely available and are not clearly more discriminating than the red cell folate level in detecting deficiency.

Serum Homocysteine

Serum Hcy (but not methylmalonic acid [MMA]) levels are elevated in folate deficiency (see section on vitamin B_{12}). However, they also reflect inadequacies of vitamins B_6 and B_{12}. Other causes of elevated serum Hcy concentrations include renal insufficiency, hypovolemia, hypothyroidism, psoriasis, and inherited metabolic defects (99). A common cause of hyperhomocysteinemia is a genetic predisposition secondary to a polymorphic substitution in the methylenetetrahydrofolate reductase gene. In interpreting elevated Hcy levels, it is best to obtain serum MMA levels simultaneously (Table 6-20). Part of the problem in identifying hyperhomocysteinemia is the variability in assay results and normal values. This variability is partly a consequence of the multiple forms of Hcy in serum (reduced, oxidized, protein-bound), and partly a consequence of the different and noninterchangeable results of HPLC, enzyme immunoassay, and fluorescence polarization immunoassay (100). Reference values for total serum Hcy increase with age and are higher for men than for women at all ages (101).

Physiology

Absorption

Absorption takes place through a pH-dependent active process in the proximal intestine, with maximum transport occurring after deconjugation to the monoglutamate form. Some, but not

TABLE 6-20	Interpretation of Serum Methionine Metabolite Assays	
Metabolite(s)	Folate Deficiency (% in patients with deficiency)	Vitamin B_{12} Deficiency
Methylmalonic acid (MMA) ↑	12	98
Homocysteine (Hcy) ↑	91	96
MMA ↑, Hcy normal	2	4
Hcy ↑, MMA normal	80	1
MMA, Hcy normal	7	0.2

Data from Savage DG, Lindenbaum J, Stabler SP, et al. Sensitivity of serum methylmalonic acid and total homocysteine determinations for diagnosing cobalamin and folate deficiencies. *Am J Med*. 1994;96:239.

all, dietary folate is nutritionally available. Polyglutamate forms of folate in food are hydrolyzed by folylpoly-γ-glutamate carboxypeptidase; the products of hydrolysis, which contain decreased numbers of glutamate residues, include the monoglutamate form, found in small amounts in human salivary, gastric, pancreatic, and jejunal juice. The activity of this ubiquitous carboxypeptidase is also increased in intestinal mucosa, liver, pancreas, kidney, and placenta. Both brush border and lysosomal sites of folate conjugase activity have been reported in human jejunum. The brush border enzyme is necessary for the hydrolysis of dietary folates.

The intestinal transporter for folate is the same as the reduced folate carrier (RFC) found in red cells, the *SLC19A1* sodium/folate cotransporter, which acts as an anion exchanger, linking the downhill flow of organic phosphates with the uphill transport of folate substrates (102). The RFC is expressed in all human cells, and is the major uptake pathway at neutral pH. The proton-coupled folate transporter (PCFT; *SLC46A1*) is widely expressed but is active only at low pH, as in the microenvironment of the brush border membrane of the proximal intestine and renal tubule (pH ~5 to 6). Thus, PCFT is considered the major transporter for intestinal absorption of dietary folates (103). This is the protein that is mutated in hereditary folate malabsorption, and it is also expressed abundantly in human tumors. Thus, it has become a target for delivery of drugs to tumor cells. RFC and PCFT probably mediate folate transport across the choroid plexus and the placental syncytiotrophoblast. ATP-binding cassette transporters are expressed in all mammalian cells, and as one of their functions export folate monoglutamates, thus countering the role of the RFC and PCFT.

Folate receptors (FR) bind folic acid, reduced folates, many antifolates, and folate conjugates. These FRs exist as α and β isoforms with different tissue distribution, and a soluble form exists in plasma and milk (103). The folate receptor-α is encoded by the *FOLR1* gene, and is present in the apical membrane of epithelium of the intestine, kidney, choroid plexus, and epididymis, where it is not exposed to circulating folate. FRβ is restricted to placenta and hematopoietic cells. FRs are bound to the membrane by a glycosylphosphatidylinositol structure, and mediate uptake by endocytosis. Thus, they have become targets for delivery of drugs to tumor cells (102). Deficiency of the receptor in mice leads to decreased reabsorption of folate in the renal tubule, and confirms the importance of this receptor in folate uptake in vivo (104). Megalin, a large member of the LDL receptor family, mediates soluble folate-receptor uptake in the renal tubule, but its role in regulating uptake of the membrane-bound receptor is still unclear (103).

Reduced folates are better absorbed than oxidized forms. Pteroylglutamic acid, used in tablets, is not as good a substrate for dihydrofolate reductase and must be reduced before it can be maximally utilized. Methyltetrahydrofolic acid is absorbed rapidly and not changed. Other forms are converted in enterocytes to reduced formylated and methylated derivatives. Some vitamin escapes unreduced and is metabolized in the liver. The reduced methylated form is delivered to all tissues. Folate absorption may be decreased in elderly patients with gastric atrophy, a situation that can be corrected by administering hydrochloric acid to lower the gastric and intestinal pH.

Reabsorption

After conversion in the liver to 5-MeTHF, the vitamin can enter the plasma as the monoglutamate, be stored in tissue as the polyglutamate, or be reexcreted in bile and reabsorbed. The rate of enterohepatic circulation is estimated to be 100 µg per day. This figure is comparable with the amount of daily tissue folate utilized (50 to 100 µg). Thus, folate deficiency develops more rapidly in malabsorption than in dietary deficiency alone. During deficiency states, the concentration of folate in the bile decreases, so the enterohepatic circulation does not contribute to losses at a constant rate. The large intestine contains an efficient carrier-mediated transport mechanism for folate (presumably the reduced folate receptor-α), raising the possibility that the colon might participate in folate reabsorption (105).

Intracellular Metabolism

Natural forms of folic acid are converted to coenzymes by reduction of the pyrazine ring (two possible sites), elongation of the peptide chain with glutamyl residues (six possible additions), and addition of a one-carbon fragment in position 5 or 10 (six possible fragments). Thus, a large variety of folate coenzymes exist. The tetrahydrofolate form is frequently involved, and it is thought that a polyglutamate form is the active coenzyme. These coenzymes function in many reactions involving one-carbon transfers, including purine and thymidylate synthesis, metabolism of several amino acids (especially serine and Hcy), methylation of biogenic amines, and initiation of protein synthesis by formylation of methionine (106). The coenzymes are quite unstable in cells because peptidases degrade the polyglutamyl chain. For mobilization of the storage form in the liver and release into the blood, hydrolysis to the monoglutamate form is required. One-carbon metabolism in the mitochondria is essential for the catabolism of choline, purines, and histidine, and the biosynthesis of serine and glycine.

The folate cycle of one-carbon metabolism via tetrahydrofolate form interfaces with the methionine cycle, driven by the regeneration of methionine from Hcy, a process facilitated by vitamin B_{12}. This process produces S-adenosylmethionine (SAM), a very important methyl donor for methylation of DNA and RNA, as well as synthesis of neurotransmitters. The balance between these two systems allows methylation to be allocated between DNA synthesis and repair for cell growth, and epigenetic processes for cellular regulation. Evidence is increasing that folates and folate cofactors are compartmentalized within the cell, making understanding the multiple pathways of one-carbon metabolism even more complicated (107). Thus intracellular partitioning and trafficking of folate cofactors must be added to the factors involved in folate metabolism and human disease.

Protein Binding

Two-thirds of plasma folate is protein-bound because it is negatively charged at physiologic pH. This binding, largely to α2-macroglobulin and albumin, is loose. In addition, folate is tightly bound to a specific binder that recognizes reduced folates. The role of this binder is unclear.

Deficiency

"Classic" Deficiency

Because folate coenzymes are active in RNA, DNA, and protein synthesis, conditions of rapid growth or metabolic utilization (pregnancy, lactation) are associated with a high risk for deficiency. Acute symptoms of folate deficiency have been noted after the administration of antagonists. These include anorexia, nausea, diarrhea, mouth ulcers, and hair loss. Thrombocytopenia occurs frequently. Chronic deficiency is characterized by fatigue, a sore tongue, and anemia, with few neurologic signs. If folate stores are normal at the start, deficiency takes about 4 months to develop. If stores are depleted initially, the symptoms of deficiency can develop in 2 to 3 months. Not all clinical deficiency can be defined by serum folate levels, because 10% to 20% of populations in Western nations may have low levels. Some of these are related to low recent intake. If prolonged, a decreased intake leads to deficiency (decreased body stores). Malabsorption of any cause can lead to deficiency. Diseases that are frequent causes of folate deficiency include tropical sprue, gluten-sensitive enteropathy, and alcoholism (108). In this setting isolated folate deficiency is rarely seen, but is associated with other vitamin deficiencies. Neurologic manifestations are rare and mild, so any attribution of these presentations should encourage a search for other causes, for example vitamin B_{12} or B_6 deficiency (35).

Neural Tube Defects
The results of randomized trials show that at least half of neural tube defects could be prevented if women consumed adequate amounts of folic acid early in pregnancy (83,109,110). The data have been repeated in areas with a high and low incidence of neural tube defects (3,111). Based on the results of these trials and on uncontrolled observations of the effects of lower doses of folic acid, the US Department of Health and Human Services published *Recommendations for the Use of Folic Acid to Reduce the Number of Cases of Spina Bifida and Other Neural Tube Defects*, with the suggestion that 400 µg of folic acid be ingested daily by all women capable of becoming pregnant. High doses were not recommended because of the concern that such doses might mask B_{12} deficiency. These recommendations have been confirmed by the Standing Committee on the Scientific Evaluation of Dietary Reference Intakes (3). Not all neural tube defects can be prevented, and folate should be ingested before conception as well as after. Some experts advise women who have had a prior pregnancy in which the fetus had a neural tube defect to take 4.0 mg of folic acid per day. At this dose, folic acid may interfere with anticonvulsant therapy in epilepsy. The synthetic form of folate is recommended. To derive an equivalent intake from the diet, about 10 servings of fruits and vegetables a day would be required, and the folate in foods is less bioavailable.

Folic acid is clearly a vitamin essential for reproductive health. Despite the evidence that supplementation has been beneficial, the amount of folate in commercial breads in the United States declined after 2001 (112). Moreover, educational efforts to promote daily folic acid supplementation by women of reproductive age have not led to increased supplement use (113). The groups most vulnerable to not following the recommendations are women who are young, poor, or have unplanned pregnancies (114). In addition, some countries have not yet decided to mandate folic acid fortification.

Bottle-fed Infants
Bottle-fed infants are susceptible to folate deficiency because heating can destroy milk folacins. Total serum Hcy level appears to be a sensitive indicator of folate deficiency in children on a poor diet, with HIV infection, and with antifolate drug treatment (115).

Pregnancy
Pregnancy is associated with low serum folate levels because of hemodilution and increased requirements. Anemia is often secondary to iron deficiency also. One-third of pregnant women have low serum folate levels at delivery (see Chapter 4).

Cerebral Folate Deficiency
Two separate hereditary disorders lead to folate deficiency in the brain. Mutations in the *SLC46A1* gene encoding the PCFT leads to severe folate deficiency from birth, with decreased brain folate, exacerbated by the location of PCFT on the choroid plexus that supplies folate across the blood–brain barrier (116). Treatment with large doses of folinic acid (5-formylTHF) can normalize folate levels in the blood, but much larger doses are needed to correct cerebrospinal fluid folate. Mutations in the FRα gene, *FOLR1*, also cause low brain folate, as this receptor is present on the choroid plexus (but not the intestine), where it mediates folate transport. Folinic acid is also useful for treatment. Cerebral folate deficiency is also found in the presence of folate-receptor antibodies that block choroid plexus transport of folate (117). These antibodies can produce a cerebral folate-deficiency syndrome in infants, older children, and occasionally in adults, resulting from blocked folate transport into the brain (118). Serum and RBC folate and serum Hcy levels are normal, but 5-methyltetrahydrofolate in the cerebrospinal fluid is low, consistent with the regional (brain) folate deficiency. If folate stores are normal in the mother and infant, symptoms will appear initially at about 4 months.

Anticonvulsant Drugs
Anticonvulsant drugs (especially phenobarbital, phenytoin, and primidone) cause macrocytosis in 40% of patients, but only half of these patients have low serum and RBC levels of folate. Most patients have normal levels of vitamin B_{12}. Thus, the mechanism is not entirely clear. Some alteration in absorption of folates is postulated.

Increased Utilization
Folate deficiency occurs in disorders in which utilization is increased, such as hemolytic anemia, chronic myelofibrosis, leukemia, sideroblastic anemia, and chronic exfoliative dermatitis.

Alcohol Ingestion
Alcohol ingestion in excess of 80 g of ethanol per day is associated with macrocytosis (>80%) and low serum levels of folate. Alcohol reduces expression of folate transporters in both intestine and kidney, thus decreasing absorption and increasing excretion (119).

Sulfasalazine
Sulfasalazine can cause deficiency by decreasing folate absorption. The same effect is not caused by 5-aminosalicylic acid.

Inhibition of Dihydrofolate Reductase
Inhibition of dihydrofolate reductase impairs the conversion of folates to the active coenzyme. Dihydrofolate reductase inhibitors include methotrexate, trimethoprim, pyrimethamine, and triamterene. The frequency of clinical deficiency is greatest with methotrexate.

Hyperhomocysteinemia
Hyperhomocysteinemia can be the result of folate deficiency when there is no elevation of MMA, a feature of vitamin B_{12} deficiency. Other conditions that can elevate serum Hcy include hypothyroidism, vitamin B_6 deficiency, and renal failure, the latter also elevating MMA (120). Vegans generally support normal serum concentrations of thiamine and folate, but have low vitamin B_{12} and B_6 levels associated with hyperhomocysteinemia (121). Three inborn errors of metabolism can produce elevated Hcy levels associated with atherosclerosis: deficiency of cystathionine synthase, methionine synthase, and methylenetetrahydrofolate reductase (122). These cases, along with data in animals, led to the proposal that Hcy was a significant risk factor for atherosclerosis in the general population. Hcy levels are correlated with an increased risk of myocardial infarction in about 10% of patients (86). It is not clear whether the metabolite itself is sufficient or whether it is a cofactor. Folate levels are usually normal, but feeding supplemental folate can reduce the hyperhomocysteinemia. A 400 μg per day dose provides a maximal effect (~20% to 25%) (123). Other factors, including vitamins B_2, B_6, betaine, and choline, may have some effect, the latter two particularly in the presence of high methionine intake (124). Other dietary factors, such as tea, coffee, high-protein meal, and methionine, elevate Hcy levels, but these postprandial rises can be transient. It is generally felt that folate intake has the largest effect in reducing these elevations, postprandial or otherwise, but it is not clear whether lowering Hcy levels reduces the risk of cardiovascular disease or risk for stroke (123).

Hyperhomocysteinemia is considered by many to be an independent risk factor for cardiovascular disease and mortality (125), including the large prospective Women's Health Study (126). However, there are other factors that are associated with an increased risk of vascular disease, including C-reactive protein, lipoprotein(a), and fibrinogen (127). Where these factors fit into a screening and risk-stratification strategy along with Hcy is not clear. Strong epidemiological associations implicating Hcy as a risk factor for heart disease continue to appear (128,129), but folate status is not always associated with elevated total Hcy levels, perhaps due to the presence of other confounding risk factors (130). Another reason for the lack of confirmation of epidemiologically determined risk factors is the accrual of larger numbers. For example, the risk possibly related to the C677T polymorphism of the gene for methylenetetrahydrofolate reductase appeared to be less well supported when 26,000 cases are analyzed (131).

Data from prospective studies with folate (and vitamins B_6 and B_{12}) supplementation have not yet provided consistent support for Hcy as a significant risk factor for heart disease in the general population. The Homocysteine Lowering Trialists' Collaboration has attempted to estimate by meta-analysis the size of the reduction in Hcy levels due to different doses of folic acid with or without the other vitamins, all in RCTs. One meta-analysis showed an approximately 25% reduction in Hcy with doses of folic acid ranging from 0.5 to 3 mg per day (132). A second meta-analysis that included additional studies showed that 0.8 mg of folate could lower Hcy by approximately 23%, with only a 7% increased effect on addition of vitamin B_{12}, and no change after addition of vitamin B_6 (133). For recurrent cardiovascular events it was estimated that the risk increases for each 5 μmol per L increase in serum Hcy concentration.

The Trialists' Collaboration is currently following 12 randomized trials that involve 52,000 participants, 32,000 with vascular disease in unfortified populations, and 14,000 with vascular disease and 6,000 with renal disease in fortified populations (134). A meta-analysis of 37,485 individuals at risk for cardiovascular disease found no significant effects of folate supplementation to lower homocysteine levels for any vascular outcomes or overall vascular or cancer mortality over 5 years of follow-up (135). Another trial of secondary prevention of myocardial infarction using all three vitamins including 0.8 mg folic acid showed a possible harmful effect on the rate of acute myocardial infarction (136). Both studies showed an approximately 25% reduction in plasma Hcy concentrations. A similar negative result has been shown with prevention of ischemic stroke (137). Thus, the strength of association of Hcy with risk of vascular disease is probably weaker than suggested by the epidemiologic data, and may not exist at all (138).

The studies thus far continue to be consistent with the recommendations of the American Heart Association (AHA) to screen for hyperhomocysteinemia only in those patients at high risk (e.g., premature arteriosclerosis, renal failure) (139). The AHA and the Canadian Task Force on Preventive Health Care recommend a well-balanced diet without supplemental vitamins. Any change in these recommendations should await the results of studies that confirm a role of folate and/or other vitamins in altering the risk of cardiovascular disease in high-risk populations (140). The AHA and American Stroke Association guidelines for stroke prevention note that the use of vitamins (folate, B_6, and B_{12}) has not been effective in lowering the risk of stroke in most studies, yet recommend that the use of such a vitamin complex "might be considered for prevention of ischemic stroke in patients with hyperhomocysteinemia, but its effectiveness is not well established" (141). Hyperhomocysteinemia has been found in patients with IBD, but not associated with thromboembolic complications (142).

Cognitive Decline

Low levels of folate and cobalamin are seen in aged patients with cognitive decline. The low vitamin status is likely secondary to decreased intake. Many poorly controlled trials have suggested a role for folate supplementation in improving cognition, but the severity of cognitive decline is not correlated with the degree of folate deficiency (143). Although folic acid (0.75 mg per day) lowers serum Hcy levels, a systematic review of double-blind, placebo-controlled intervention trials revealed that no benefit was seen in measures of cognition or mood in older, healthy women or in patients with mild to moderate cognitive decline (144). At least one study subsequently demonstrated a modest improvement in immediate and delayed memory performance, following 2-year supplements with 400 μg of folate and 100 μg of vitamin B_{12} (145). It is not clear whether such a modest change is clinically significant, but the change was detected only at 24 months; so longer treatment might improve the effect. Epidemiologic studies continue to record that high Hcy and low B-vitamin levels predict cognitive decline, but whether this is merely an indicator of another process or a causative link will need to be determined by further studies (146).

Depression

An association between folate and serotonin metabolism has been suggested, in that folate-mediated methylation of Hcy produces SAM, a metabolite that alters serotonin metabolism. This suggestion has led to RCTs of folate in treatment of depression. Analysis of two such trials provided a suggestion that an active form of folate in large doses (15 or 50 mg of methyltetrahydrofolate) might be useful as adjunctive therapy with other antidepressant drugs (147). In addition there is an association between depression and low folate levels (148). However, a review of available studies, both epidemiological and supplement-based, found inadequate data to justify the uses of folate in severe or chronic depression (149). It remains uncertain whether folate should be added to patients with folate deficiency who have not responded to other treatment.

Cancer

The evidence for protective effects of folate in cancer first came from epidemiological studies showing associations between foods rich in folate (vegetables and some fruits) and lower cancer rates. Plasma levels of folate are decreased in smokers who have bronchial metaplasia in comparison with smokers who do not have metaplasia. There is a suggestion from Howe epidemiological data that higher folate intake can protect against lung cancer risk (150). The issue of whether folate deficiency can develop and cause tissue damage is not resolved.

The Nurses' Health Study found that the risk of the development of CRC was lower in women who had used vitamin supplements containing folate for more than 15 years than in women who had used such preparations for shorter periods (151). This association has been repeated in the Swedish Mammography Cohort (152). Moreover, in the large (519,978 patients) cohort that is the European Prospective Investigation of Cancer and Nutrition from 10 countries, folate in food may be protective of CRC, but there is no effect of added supplements (153). This modest effect of higher folate intake on reducing the risk of CRC is supported by many prospective studies (154). Folate supplements have been shown to decrease mucosal proliferation (155) and to reverse DNA hypomethylation (156) in high-risk groups of patients with recurrent colonic adenomas. However, supplemental folate has not yet been shown prospectively to have a protective effect on the rate of CRC or adenoma formation. Epidemiologic studies also provide some support for a modulating role of folate in breast and pancreatic cancer; however, the findings are only suggestive, despite the prospective nature of some of the studies (153).

On the other hand, rodent models of CRC and some clinical trials have shown an acceleration in the development of CRC from premalignant adenomas (157). However, a meta-analysis of many trials showed only a 5% increase in total cancer risk, which was within the 95% confidence intervals (158). There are two theoretical reasons by which folate might promote cancer growth: (a) supporting the high requirement for DNA synthesis via pyrimidine synthesis, and (b) hypermethylation of DNA to switch off tumor suppressors, via the methylation cycle. However, a large study of American Association of Retired Persons confirmed the decreased association of CRC with higher dietary or total folate intake (159). What is not resolved is the possibility that elderly subjects with premalignant lesions now exposed to higher folate doses (from fortification and supplements) might still be at risk for accelerated development of CRC.

Treatment

Medication

The form of folacin used therapeutically is the unreduced pteroylglutamic acid. Tablets of 0.1, 0.4, 0.8, and 1.0 mg are available, and quantities of 0.2 to 1.0 mg are included in some multivitamin preparations; 200 to 500 µg per day is needed to treat most deficiency states. Oral replacement is preferred, except in severe malabsorption, in which parenteral (intramuscular, intravenous, or subcutaneous) folate (5 mg per mL) can be used. At the concentrations used for total parenteral nutrition, folate is stable if the pH of the solution is above 5.0. 5-methyltetrahydrofolate (levomefolic acid) is available as OTC supplements or by prescription, at doses of 1 to 15 mg. Indicated uses are for many of the questionable indications (e.g., depression). Leucovorin calcium (5-CHOH-tetrahydrofolic acid) is available as solutions (3 mg per ampule or 10 mg per mL in 5-mL vials). This compound is used after methotrexate therapy to avoid toxicity, and in large doses for treatment of cerebral folate deficiency. In the large doses offered, it is not meant as vitamin replacement therapy for deficiency states, especially because the large doses might mask vitamin B_{12} deficiency.

Fortification

The US Food and Drug Administration (FDA) specified in 1996 that certain grain products (especially most enriched breads, flours, cornmeal, rice, noodles, and macaroni) be fortified with 0.14 mg of folic acid per pound of product. The FDA estimated that this practice would raise the folate intake of women of childbearing age by 100 µg per day yet avoid exceeding the UL of 1,000 µg per day in nontarget populations (160). This UL was selected so as to avoid the possible masking of vitamin B_{12} deficiency and allow neurologic progression. Considerable debate regarding all aspects of the fortification program continues, including the dose added, the effect on nontarget populations, and the risk for masking pernicious anemia. The use of a higher level of cereal-based folate supplementation (499 to 665 µg per day) than that recommended by the FDA (127 µg per day) produced a greater rise in serum folate and a significant fall (11%) in serum Hcy levels; these findings suggest that more folate should be added to foods (161). However, in a study of a cohort before and after folate fortification was approved, the percentage of subjects with low serum levels of folate fell from 22% to 1.7%, and the percentage of those with high serum Hcy levels fell from 18.7% to 9.8% (162). The ability of folate to lower serum Hcy may be related to the intake of other vitamins (e.g., >500 mg of vitamin C per day) that can interfere with vitamin B_{12} metabolism (163). Mandatory folate fortification has nearly eliminated the incidence of folate-deficiency anemia in older adults in the United States (164). Additional studies show that only a small percentage of the population developed folate levels above the UL (165). Moreover, the current fortification dose (140 μ per day) is adequate to achieve the full effect in preventing neural tube defects, when 36 weeks is allowed for red cell folate levels to plateau (166). This conclusion is confirmed by the use of a 200 μg per day dose to decrease plasma total Hcy levels over 6 months (167).

The safety of fortification has been questioned by some. For example, the increase in incidence of autism phenotypes increased after 1970, following the increase in 1973 in the limit of folic acid in OTC daily vitamins to 400 μg, and the onset of grain fortification in 1996 (168). However, periconceptual folate supplements were associated with a lower rate of autistic disorder in Norway (169)

The UL of 1,000 μg per day has been challenged on the grounds that all but eight cases of masked neurologic progression in vitamin B_{12} deficiency occurred in patients taking more than 5 mg of folate per day (89). This concern does not affect most patients on supplemental folic acid. Since folate supplementation of grain in the United States began, there has not been an increase in low vitamin B_{12} levels seen in a large Veterans Affairs center (170). In addition, analysis of more than 60,000 blood samples showed no correlation between vitamin B_{12} deficiency (the presence of low cobalamin levels and macrocytosis [elevated MCV]) and whether the serum folate was low or high (171). In a young adult population high folate concentrations from supplements and fortified foods did not lead to increased biochemical abnormalities related to vitamin B_{12} deficiency (172). Thus, the putative risk of high folate exposure to create a conditional vitamin B_{12} deficiency has yet to be demonstrated.

Toxicity

Folic acid and phenytoin compete for intestinal transport and possibly uptake in the brain. Thus, very large doses of folate (>100 times the RDA) may precipitate convulsions in patients treated with phenytoin (173). A few cases of hypersensitivity have been documented at doses of 1 to 10 mg. Fever, urticaria, pruritus, and respiratory distress have been reported (174).

Cobalamin (Vitamin B_{12})

Dietary Reference Intake

The total body content of cobalamin is approximately 2 to 2.5 mg, most of which is in the liver. Estimates of half-life vary from 480 to 1,284 days. Thus, daily losses of cobalamin average about 1.3 μg. Because absorption is about 70% efficient at low levels of intake, the RDA for adults of approximately 2 μg per day was formerly considered sufficient to maintain the body pool. In response to findings that 10% to 30% of people more than 51 years old may have protein-bound vitamin B_{12} malabsorption, the new DRI for this age group has been set at 2.4 μg per day (3). Malabsorption in the elderly is probably a consequence of reduced secretion of pepsin and gastric acid, perhaps related to *Helicobacter pylori* infection. Because intrinsic factor is present, these people can absorb free (synthetic) vitamin B_{12}. Thus, it is recommended that the vitamin be ingested mostly in the form of a dietary supplement to ensure that intake is adequate (175). Table 6-21 gives the DRIs for adults and children.

Food Sources

The term *cobalamin* refers to cobalt-containing corrinoids with biologic activity in humans. The average diet in the United States provides 5 to 15 μg per day. Cobalamin is produced by bacteria and enters animal tissues during the ingestion of contaminated foods or after production in the rumen. Microorganisms in the colon synthesize cobalamin, but the vitamin is not absorbed at that site. Thus, cobalamin deficiency develops in strict vegetarians. Most of the cobalamin in normal feces arises from bacterial synthesis in the colon and does not represent unabsorbed vitamin, so that fecal excretion is unrelated to dietary intake. The usual dietary sources are seafood, meat and meat products, fish, eggs, and, to a lesser extent, milk and milk products. The vitamin is now added to many grain products, including cereals, breads, pasta, and enriched rice. Most cooking

TABLE 6-21 Dietary Reference Intakes for Cobalamin

Life Stage Group	Cobalamin (µg/day)
Infants	
0–6 months	0.4[a]
7–12 months	0.5[a]
Children	
1–3 years	0.9
4–8 years	1.2
9–13 years	1.8
Adolescents and Adults	
(M/F) 14–>70 years	2.4
Pregnancy	
≤18–50 years	2.6
Lactation	
≤18–50 years	2.8

[a]Estimate based on adequate intake (AI). All others based on recommended dietary allowance (RDA).
Data from Standing Committee on the Scientific Evaluation of Dietary Reference Intakes, Food and Nutrition Board, Institute of Medicine. *Dietary Reference Intakes for Thiamine, Riboflavin, Niacin, Vitamin B6, Folate, Vitamin B12, Pantothenic Acid, Biotin, and Choline.* Washington, DC: National Academies Press, 1998.

methods do not destroy cobalamin. Boiling meat can lead to losses of up to 30% into the water. However, during drying, the cobalamin in some food is converted to inactive analogues (176). Evidence that ingesting megadoses of vitamin C (500 to 1,000 mg) destroys some of the cobalamin in food is conflicting. It is not clear how frequently, if ever, cobalamin deficiency occurs in persons who take megadoses of vitamin C. Table 6-22 lists selected foods containing cobalamin.

Assessment
Intake or Absorption
No reliable method is available to assess intake of cobalamin, but the Schilling test accurately reflects absorption. Free cobalamin does not occur in plasma or elsewhere until all binding proteins are saturated, after which free cobalamin is filtered through the glomerulus. A parenteral injection of 1,000 µg of unlabeled cyanocobalamin is given to saturate binding proteins in tissue and serum. Any serum to be drawn for assessment of body stores must be obtained beforehand. An oral dose of [^{57}Co]B_{12} linked to intrinsic factor is then given. Excretion of the labeled cobalamin in urine for 24 hours should exceed 8% of the administered dose if absorption is normal. In cases of possible bacterial overgrowth, absorption can be tested after the administration of 1 g of tetracycline per day.

A value greater than 8% and less than 10% is an indeterminate result and accounts for about 25% of test results (177). Problems with the test involve the collection of urine and intertest variability (as much as 30% to 50%). When urine collection is incomplete or renal disease is present, a low rate of cobalamin excretion is unreliable. It is a mistake to attach too much importance to an arbitrary normal limit of 10% excretion. Stimulation of urinary excretion by twofold or more with the addition of intrinsic factor is suggestive of intrinsic factor deficiency, even if the excretion without intrinsic factor is in the 8% to 10% range. In 30% to 40% of cases, low serum cobalamin levels cannot be explained by the decreased absorption of free vitamin B_{12}. The multiple causes of a "falsely" normal Schilling test result include the following: (a) erroneous value; (b) dietary insufficiency of cobalamin; (c) metabolic disorder of cobalamin metabolism, such as an inborn error; (d) malabsorption of cobalamin that has been corrected by the use of antibiotics; (e) "falsely" low serum cobalamin level, which occurs much less often than formerly assumed (see section on body stores); and (f) malabsorption of food-bound cobalamin. The absorption of cobalamin in food requires the liberation of free cobalamin by gastric proteases. Therefore, the Schilling test result may not always correlate with physiologic alterations in cobalamin absorption, especially when gastric physiology is altered.

TABLE 6-22 Approximate Cobalamin Content of Selected Foods

Food	Portion	Cobalamin (µg)	Percentage of RDI (6 µg)
Beef, ground	3 oz	2.4	>40
Liver, beef	3 oz	95	>100
Liver, chicken	1 each	1.87	25–39
Oysters, raw	1 cup	40–48	>100
Crab	1 cup	9.9	>100
Salmon	3 oz	4.93	>40
Egg	1 each	0.59	5–12
Lamb chop	3 oz	1.58	25–39
Pork, center loin chop	4 oz	0.62	5–12
Chicken, light meat, roasted	3 oz	0.291	1–5
Cheese	1 oz	0.2–0.45	5–12
Milk, whole/skim	1 cup	0.871/0.93	10–24
Yogurt, whole/low-fat, plain	1 cup	0.84/0.9	10–24
Soy products/meat substitutes[a]	1 patty/link	1.49–1.72	~25
Cereals (Total/Bran flakes)[a]	1 cup	7.0/2.49	50–100

RDI, recommended dietary intake.
[a] Amounts refer to fortified products. Check label to make certain the product is fortified. Soy milk by itself contains no cobalamin.
Data from Hands ES. *Food Finder*. 2nd ed. Salem, OR: ESHA Research, 1990.

Commercial production of ^{57}[Co]cobalamin was discontinued in the late 1990s, and use of the Schilling test was abandoned. It is possible to perform a Schilling test using unlabeled hydroxycobalamin, but the assay for the vitamin would require more sophisticated analysis than is available in commercial laboratories (178). Two other tests for absorption have been developed, one following the increase in transcobalamin–cyanocobalamin (TC–Cbl) in blood by TC immunoprecipitation, enzymatic release of Cbl, and HPLC separation (179), and the other measuring holotranscobalamin (holoTC) by immunosorbent assay for 24 hours after ingestion of three 9 µg doses of vitamin B_{12} (180). Both of these methods require complex analyses that have made it difficult for the test to be widely available. But, the holoTC test has reliable endpoints (holoTC increase > 10 pmol per L) and is >22%, and a reliable enzyme-linked immunoassay kit has been developed (181). However, with the availability of more sensitive and convenient assessment of body stores, there is very limited need to perform absorption tests. When dealing with a population at risk for developing cobalamin deficiency, the first step is to assess body stores, and if low, assume that the mechanism whereby deficiency develops is consistent with that seen in the population at risk. If the diagnosis of vitamin B_{12} deficiency can be made with assurance from the results, one can assume that malabsorption is the underlying cause in most cases.

Body Stores

Serum Vitamin B_{12} (Cobalamin)

This parameter usually correlates with body stores. Unlike the folacins, cobalamin is not more concentrated in blood cells than in serum. Thus, hemolysis is not a major factor in producing false results. Transcobalamin II (TCII), the serum carrier protein that delivers cobalamin to tissues, accounts for 30% to 40% of total serum cobalamin (182). The rest is bound to haptocorrin. Therefore, in TCII deficiency, serum levels of cobalamin can be normal, but the vitamin is not delivered to tissues, and body stores are low. However, it is clear that marginally low levels (150 to 200, or even up to 350 pg per mL) can be associated with neurologic defects.

For decades microbiological assays were used, but they are tedious and time consuming. These have been replaced by and large by assays that are more sensitive, but require small amounts of cobalamin-binding proteins, usually gastric intrinsic factor (183). Competitive binding luminescent assays (CBLA) are now preferred by many clinical laboratories. This assay is based on competition of cobalamin in serum with cobalamin labeled with a chemiluminescent marker for binding to intrinsic factor. The assay has good sensitivity and reproducibility, and is quite specific. Radioisotope dilution assays are based on the principle that endogenous serum cobalamin competes with radioactive cobalamin for binding to a limited amount of cobalamin-binding protein (32). These assays are also simple and reliable. Some commercial kits make it possible to measure cobalamin and folate simultaneously. Heparinized samples cannot be used because heparin interferes with the assay. A number of studies have found that the results of the radioisotope dilution assay compare well with those of the older microbiologic assay.

A serum cobalamin level of less than 150 pg per mL is always associated with low body stores if dilution, protein deficiency, folate deficiency, or altered cobalamin-binding protein levels are not present (Table 6-23). Cobalamin deficiency should be suspected in patients with levels from 150 to 200 pg per mL. Such patients should undergo further testing (MMA, Hcy levels), or the results should be correlated with abnormal hematologic or neurologic findings. Evidence of cobalamin deficiency will not be found in all patients with marginal serum cobalamin levels. However, in doubtful cases, a therapeutic trial with cobalamin replacement is safe, and reversal of the abnormal findings is diagnostic. Thirty percent of patients with folate deficiency have low serum cobalamin levels, although the reason is not clear. Protein deficiency lowers the amount of total serum cobalamin without having as much effect on delivery of cobalamin to tissues because about 10% to 30% of the cobalamin-binding protein in serum is TCI. Up to 75% of strict vegetarians have low serum cobalamin levels without evidence of deficiency. Signs of anemia are likely to develop in patients with continued inadequate dietary intake. In patients with HIV infection,

TABLE 6-23 Guidelines for Interpretation of Serum Cobalamin Levels

Range	WHO	Lindenbaum et al.	Comments
Deficient	<110 pmol/L <150 pg/mL		
Low	110–147 pmol/L 150–200 pg/mL		Falsely low: folate deficiency, pregnancy, oral contraceptives, multiple myeloma, haptocorrin deficiency
Acceptable	≥147 pmol/L ≥201 pg/mL	≥258 pmol/L ≥350 pg/mL	Falsely normal: myeloproliferative disorders (PV, CML), liver disease, TCII deficiency, intestinal bacterial overgrowth, treatment with cobalamin

PV, polycythemia vera; CML, chronic myelogenous leukemia; TCII, transcobalamin II; WHO, World Health Organization.

Data from Sauberlich HE. *Laboratory Tests for the Assessment of Nutritional Status.* 2nd ed. Boca Raton, FL: CRC Press, 1999; Lewis CJ, Crane NT, Wilson DB, et al. Estimated folate intakes: data updated to reflect food fortification, increased bioavailability, and dietary supplement use. *Am J Clin Nutr.* 1999;70:198; Lindenbaum J, Rosenberg IH, Wilson PW, et al. Prevalence of cobalamin deficiency in the Framingham elderly population. *Am J Clin Nutr* 1994;60:2; de Benoist B. Conclusions of a WHO Technical consultation on folate and vitamin B12 deficiencies. *Food Nutr Bull.* 2008;29:S238.

cobalamin deficiency may create cognitive changes when clinically acquired immunodeficiency syndrome (AIDS) is not present. Pregnant women have low cobalamin levels secondary to dilution and redistribution of the binding proteins. Transcobalamin I (haptocorrin) deficiency is uncommon, but can present with low cobalamin levels, because at least half of the serum cobalamin is carried on this protein. The condition may be more common than has been suspected (184).

Standard competitive binding assays for cobalamin do not always accurately detect low levels, especially in pernicious anemia. In this condition making the diagnosis is essential, but the presence of anti-intrinsic factor antibodies interferes with the competitive binding assays that use intrinsic factor as the binding protein (185). However, the problem goes beyond the presence of intrinsic factor antibodies when three different luminescent assays are used, as many samples with normal binding by radioisotope dilution assay (also dependent upon binding) showed normal B_{12} levels, and one sample without intrinsic factor antibodies had nearly normal levels in all three CBLAs (186). When suspicion is high for deficiency and serum cobalamin is normal or near normal by competitive binding assays, holoTC and/or MMA levels should be obtained.

For elderly patients, a cutoff of 200 pg per mL may be too low to detect all cases of deficiency. A level of 258 pmol per L (350 pg per mL) has been suggested for patients older than 67 years because serum MMA was found to be markedly elevated in 11% of patients with cobalamin levels below that threshold (187). Between 8% and 20% of elderly patients and a smaller percentage of others present with a serum cobalamin level of less than 180 pg per mL, yet they do not exhibit anemia, macrocytosis, clinical deterioration, or a RBC response to cobalamin treatment, and their Schilling test result for cobalamin absorption is normal. These patients need to be further evaluated in all cases because subclinical cobalamin deficiency (SCCD) may be present and lead to neurologic damage. Workup should include (a) a careful neurologic examination and (b) measurement of serum metabolites.

Concentrations greater than 1,000 pg per mL are seen in acute liver disease because of the release from hepatocytes, and in leukocytosis because white blood cells produce haptocorrin, which increases the total cobalamin-binding capacity. These disorders can also raise the levels of serum cobalamin in patients with cobalamin deficiency to normal values. A high level (up to $10\times$ ULN) can be seen in patients with acute or chronic myelogenous leukemia, and in hypereosinophilic syndrome, as haptocorrin is secreted from the abnormal white cells (188). Less striking elevations can be seen in patients with polycythemia vera, myelofibrosis, and chronic myelomonocytic leukemia. More commonly, a high level is due to parenteral injection of the vitamin. Lymphoproliferative diseases almost never present with elevated serum cobalamin.

Serum Methylmalonic Acid and Total Homocysteine

Levels of these metabolites increase when the two cobalamin-dependent enzymes, methylmalonyl CoA mutase (MMA, increased) and methionine synthetase (Hcy, increased), are impaired. Other metabolites that can be assayed include cystathionine (produced from Hcy by a vitamin B_6-dependent enzyme) and 2-methyl citric acid, a methyl acceptor metabolite derived from methionine via *SAM*. These metabolites can be used to differentiate the effects of vitamin B_6 deficiency (increased Hcy, decreased D-cystathionine) and folate deficiency (increased Hcy, decreased 2-methyl citric acid) from those of cobalamin deficiency alone (increased Hcy, increased MMA) (Table 6-20). Definitive reference values are not available, because many factors influence the concentration in serum, including age, gender, and test method. The range of normal serum values for MMA is 70 to 270 nmol per L (189). The cutoff value for MMA to diagnose vitamin B_{12} deficiency is 376 nmol per L. The level of serum MMA that should detect all cases of vitamin B_{12} deficiency is less than 638 nmol per L, to correspond with the cutoff of serum cobalamin (350 pg per mL or 258 pmol per L) that detects nearly all cases of cobalamin deficiency (187). Causes of elevated serum MMA, besides cobalamin deficiency, include renal insufficiency (GFR <20), hypovolemia, and inherited metabolic defects, although the elevations are relatively modest. Commonly used cutpoints for serum cobalamin had a greater effect on prevalence estimates in an NHANES sample (3% to 27%, and did different cutpoints for MMA (2% to 6%) (190). Cutpoints greater than 148 pmol per L for B_{12} and less than 210 nmol per L for MMA led to significant misclassifications. Using the combination of low B_{12} and elevated MMA, about 1% of adults had a definite deficiency of vitamin B_{12}, and 92% had adequate status, leaving a significant number of adults whose status must be further investigated.

"Normal" values for Hcy are 2.2 to 13.2 µmol per L (191). Levels of Hcy in "typical" Western populations are approximately 12 µmol per L (132). There is still uncertainty whether this level of Hcy carries a risk for chronic disease. The significance of serum Hcy levels for chronic disease risk is discussed in this chapter in the section on folate.

HoloTCII

The measurement of holoTCII has been suggested to be the most sensitive method to detect cobalamin deficiency and to detect deficiency earlier than other tests (192) (Table 6-24). The half-life of holoTCII is only 6 minutes, so levels are low within a week of cessation of oral cobalamin intake. HoloTCII (i e., cobalamin bound to TCII) is measured by separating TCII from haptocorrin–cobalamin in serum by a monoclonal antibody capture method (HoloTC RIA, Axis-Shield) (193). Because TCII delivers cobalamin to all tissues, a fall in the TCII–cobalamin complex (i.e., holoTCII) may detect early stages of deficiency, even when serum cobalamin levels are normal. HoloTCII levels, in parallel with red cell folate and total serum cobalamin levels, are inversely related to serum Hcy concentrations (192). Values below 35 pmol per L (<46 pg per mL) are considered deficient, with borderline low values ranging from 35 to 44 pmol per mL (46 to 60 pg per mL). The new assays are more accurate than the original ones, and reference values are available from laboratories in both the United Kingdom (192) and the United States (129). Values are different in men and women and also vary with age. Measurement of holoTC explained more of the observed variance in methymalonic acid and Hcy levels than did total vitamin B_{12}, but ROC curve analysis showed that serum vitamin B_{12} and holoTC were essentially equivalent in their ability to diagnose deficiency (193). Because holoTC may become abnormal at an earlier time, it may be used together with serum vitamin B_{12} as a screening test for deficiency. HoloTC appears to function better than total serum vitamin B_{12}, although the test has not been used for population-based assessments (194). The test also performs better than MMA in patients with normal renal function, and the combination of low holoTC with elevated MMA can detect deficiency in patients with normal serum cobalamin (195). These data fit with the recommendation of the consensus roundtable that for population-based studies, vitamin B_{12}

TABLE 6-24 Criteria and Biomarkers that Define Clinical and Subclinical Cobalamin Deficiency (SCCD)

Criterion	Clinical Deficiency	SCCD
Serum cbl (<148 pmol/L)	sensitivity 95%–97%; specificity uncertain, but <80%	sensitivity ~38%, 55%–84% with higher cutoffs, less specificity
↑ serum MMA or homocysteine	sensitivity >95%; sensitivity < for MMA	sensitivity unknown, as abnormal tests are required for Dx of SCCD
Low serum holoTC	sensitivity/specificity > for cbl	sensitivity/specificity 2%–6% > cbl
Clinical signs	present	Absent
Cbl malabsorption	causative	mild (<40% of cases); no role
Prognosis	usually progressive	unknown progression; static/fluctuating
Need for therapy	always	Unknown
Frequency	0.1% adult, 1%–2% elderly	higher, incidence unknown

Data from Bailey RL, Carmel R, Green R, et al. Monitoring of vitamin B12 nutritional status in the United States using plasma methylmalonic acid and serum vitamin B12. *Am J Clin Nutr.* 2011;74:552; Carmel R. Biomarkers of cobalamin (vitamin B-12) status in the epidemiologic setting: a critical overview of context, applications, and performance characteristics of cobalamin, methylmalonic acid, and holotranscobalamin. *Am J Clin Nutr.* 2011;94:348S.

status should be measured by one circulating vitamin B_{12} level and one functional assay (93). When compared with RBC cobalamin concentration as the gold standard for deficiency, serum holoTC was the best predictor, with the area under the ROC curve of 0.9 compared with 0.8 for serum cobalamin and 0.78 for MMA (196). Thus, it is possible in future that holoTC alone may supplant serum cobalamin as the screening test of choice.

Screening

Because abnormal serum parameters of cobalamin metabolism precede manifestations of tissue damage, screening populations who are at risk for deficiency is recommended. Persons at risk include strict vegetarians; those older than 65 years (especially if institutionalized or with a history of decreased food intake); patients with unexplained neurologic or psychiatric symptoms; those with anemia, *H. pylori* infection (or taking proton-pump inhibitors on a long-term basis), thyroid or autoimmune disease, HIV disease, Crohn disease, chronic pancreatitis, multiple sclerosis, or malabsorption of any cause; and persons who have undergone gastric or small-bowel surgery. Serum holoTC measurements are available routinely now, and they can be used initially or in conjunction with serum cobalamin levels. If serum cobalamin is used alone, values less than 350 pg per mL (Lindenbaum Criteria, Table 6-23) should be investigated further if cobalamin deficiency is suspected clinically. Tests to confirm deficiency include measurements of serum MMA, Hcy, and serum holoTCII, depending on availability and cost. When a serum cobalamin level below 350 pg per mL (268 pmol per mL) is used, an elevated MMA concentration has a diagnostic sensitivity of 0.4 and a specificity of 0.98, certainly enough to recommend the measurement of MMA to detect deficiency (189). If anemia is present, the status of folate, iron, and copper must also be considered. Table 6-25 summarizes the relative value of the three tests used for determining vitamin B_{12} status.

Subclinical Cobalamin Deficiency

Physicians commonly encounter asymptomatic patients with mild biochemical abnormalities suggesting cobalamin deficiency, much more often than patients with the clinical syndrome of cobalamin deficiency. Because this "condition," called SCCD, is defined solely by its laboratory findings, it has not been clear exactly who has the condition, if or when to treat it, and how long to follow it. The roundtable consensus panel gathered by NHANES to discuss population-based cobalamin screening did not endorse SCCD as a distinct entity (93). However, when faced with an individual patient, the problem does not disappear, and must be dealt with, especially if the patient is elderly, and the issue of cognitive decline has been raised (197). Table 6-24 outlines the characteristics of SCCD compared with clinical deficiency (198). Two major uncertainties surround this entity: (a) What is the most appropriate cutoff value for serum cobalamin?

TABLE 6-25 Comparison of Markers of Vitamin B_{12} Status

Parameter	Serum Vitamin B_{12}	Serum HoloTC	Serum MMA
Body stores	good sensitivity, poor specificity, better when combined	good sensitivity and specificity	good sensitivity in combination
Short vs long term status	better for long term	short + long term	short + long term
Function	not useful	reflects MMA, good for absorption	excellent when no confounders
Confounders	age (lower intake), pregnancy, renal/liver disease, high WBC	renal disease?, pregnancy	renal disease, pregnancy, bacterial overgrowth
Cutoff values	<150 ng/mL but not sensitive at that level	<35 pmol/L	> 260 nmol/L

Data from Green R. Indicators for assessing folate and vitamin B_{12} status and for monitoring the efficacy of intervention strategies. *Am J Clin Nutr.* 2011;94(suppl):666S.

(b) What is the natural history of the abnormalities, that is, do they progress and/or lead to symptomatic deficiency? Unfortunately, no answers to these questions are known. When presented with the problem, the clinician should obtain at least one functional test (MMA or holoTC), and, depending on the results, follow at intervals with repeated tests.

Physiology

Conversion to Coenzymes

The stable cyanocobalamin must be converted to active coenzymes in the body. Adenosyl cobalamin is the form of 70% of the vitamin stored in liver, whereas methyl cobalamin is the major form in plasma (60% to 80%). The addition of the adenosyl moiety to cobalamin (AdoCbl) occurs in a complex series of steps. First, an adenosyltransferase adds the deoxyadenosine group from ATP to inactive cobalamin, and the ATP ejects a second-bound AdoCbl in a mechanism like a rotary engine (199). The second nucleotide-driven step is regulated by MeaB, a G-protein chaperone, which mediates an exchange between the adenosyl transferase and MMA. Indeed, mutation in MeaB leads to methylmalonic aciduria. Cobalamin forms the coenzyme for two enzymes, methylmalonyl CoA mutase and 5-methyltetrahydrofolate-homocysteine methyltransferase (methionine synthetase). Methionine synthetase links cobalamin to folate metabolism by transferring the methyl group from methylfolate to regenerating tetrahydrofolate. Therefore, in cobalamin deficiency, the movement of plasma methyltetrahydrofolate into cells is decreased. Serum folate levels are normal or high, whereas red cell folate levels are low (200).

Cobalamin Absorption

Cobalamin is bound to enzymes in food and must first be liberated by gastric proteases. The free vitamin is then bound to haptocorrin (nonintrinsic factor–binding protein) in the stomach; haptocorrin has a tenfold greater affinity for cobalamin than does intrinsic factor. In the upper small bowel, pancreatic enzymes hydrolyze haptocorrin to produce free cobalamin (201). Intrinsic factor is not protease-sensitive and now binds cobalamin. The intrinsic factor–cobalamin complex attaches to its specific receptor, cubilin, in the ileal mucosa and is taken up by the cell via receptor-mediated endocytosis (103). Cubilin is attached to the membrane by binding to the product of the amnionless gene. This complex mediates the uptake of intrinsic factor, utilizing CUB domains 5 to 8 and calcium binding sites (202). Megalin, a 600 kD member of the LDL receptor family, participates in the uptake of intrinsic factor–cobalamin complexes in the renal tubule, a function not yet demonstrated in the intestine. In the kidney the cubilin–amnionless complex also mediates the uptake of albumin, apolipoprotein A–I, and transferring (203). Thus, patients with a defect in amnionless gene (many Imerslund-Grasbeck patients) also have proteinuria. In the absence of ileal receptors, only about 1% of the vitamin is absorbed passively. Cathepsin L degrades intrinsic factor within lysosomes, liberating cobalamin to bind to TC in another compartment of the enterocyte, from which it is released and carried to tissues where it is needed. The crystal structure of TC has been discovered, consisting of two domains with the cobalamin buried inside the domain interface (204). The receptor for TC (CD320) mediates uptake into all cells of the body, and is relatively small membrane-bound protein with two LDL receptor-like domains and an EGF sequence (205). In the liver, cobalamin is bound again to haptocorrin and excreted in the bile. In the intestine, the biliary haptocorrin–cobalamin complex is digested and absorbed in the same manner as the dietary vitamin. The enterohepatic circulation delivers approximately 5 to 10 μg of cobalamin per day to the intestine, an amount nearly equal to daily dietary intake. Potential daily losses without malabsorption are 1 to 2 μg. With malabsorption, estimated daily losses can approach 10 μg. Therefore, depletion of the 4 to 5 mg of body stores occurs slowly in dietary deficiency, but much more rapidly in malabsorption.

Deficiency

Deficiency occurs in a variety of clinical situations (Table 6-26). Symptoms are insidious and develop during 2 to 3 years. Weakness, fatigue, and dyspnea are related to anemia. However, fatigue is a very nonspecific symptom, and cobalamin supplementation is widely overused for this indication. Sore tongue, paresthesias, anorexia, loss of taste, and dyspepsia are seen, along with diarrhea, hair loss, impotence, irritability, and memory disturbances. Numbness and tingling due to peripheral neuropathy are noted first in the lower limbs, but deficiency can be associated with myelopathy or myeloneuropathy as well (35). Some patients present with a psychiatric

TABLE 6-26 Patient Populations at Increased Risk for Cobalamin Deficiency

Disorder	Prevalence	Pathophysiology
Decreased intake	High	Elderly, strict vegans, alcoholism
Pernicious anemia	Near 100%	Autoimmune gastritis, lack of IF
Helicobacter pylori gastritis	Variable	Chronic gastritis, some ↓ in IF
Age >65 years	~10%	Atrophic gastritis, malabsorption of food-bound CBL
Crohn disease	↑ With resection	Ileal disease or resection, loss of IF receptor
HIV disease	~15%	↓ Acid/IF secretion, ↓ ileal absorption
Gastric surgery	High	Loss of parietal cells producing IF
Bacterial overgrowth	Variable	Organisms compete for CBL in bowel
Chronic pancreatitis	Low	Lack of pancreatic enzymes to transfer CBL to IF
Malabsorption	Variable	Loss of IF-CBL receptor, if ileum involved
Zollinger–Ellison syndrome	Moderate	Prolonged inhibition of gastric (and IF) secretion
Hyperhomocysteinemia	Moderate	↓ Activity of methionine synthase; r/o folate, B_6 deficiency
Dementia	Moderate	↓ Myelin formation

IF, intrinsic factor; CBL, cobalamin.
Data from Oh RC, Brown JL. Vitamin B_{12} deficiency. *Am Fam. Physician.* 2003;67:979.

illness, often depression. Macrocytosis is a feature in many cases. This anemia must be differentiated from the macrocytosis of alcoholism and hypothyroidism, or that seen in patients with IBD who are treated with 6-mercaptopurine or azathioprine.

Dietary deficiency occurs exclusively in persons on a strict vegetarian diet. Cheese, milk, and eggs have low levels of cobalamin, but can provide the needed amounts when they are major sources of calories. Increased utilization can occasionally lead to low serum cobalamin levels, as in bone marrow cells in multiple myeloma (206). Patients taking metformin have decreased cobalamin absorption and low serum cobalamin and holoTCII levels, thought due to the effect of the drug on a calcium-dependent ileal membrane system (207). HIV-infected patients can have low serum levels of vitamin B_{12} without clinical AIDS. The clinical significance is uncertain; not all patients with decreased cobalamin absorption improve when intrinsic factor is replaced. The mechanisms of these changes require clarification. Deficiency can develop during the prolonged use of proton-pump inhibitors, particularly when doses greater than 1.5 PPI pills per day are used for 2 or more years (208). The same risk occurs with prolonged use of H2-receptor antagonists.

Pernicious anemia was at one time the most common cause of Cbl deficiency. This disease (also called Biermer's disease and Addisonian anemia) is an autoimmune disorder characterized by antibodies against intrinsic factor and parietal cells, leading to chronic gastritis, gastric atrophy, and Cbl malabsorption due to intrinsic factor deficiency (209). Patients are usually elderly, and other autoimmune disorders (thyroiditis, type II diabetes mellitus) can be comorbid conditions. Low gastric acid results from loss of parietal cells, leading to enterochromaffin cell-like hyperplasia and hypergastrinemia, risk factors for gastric cancer, but an increased risk of gastric cancer is still uncertain. More recently, subtle clinical presentations without anemia and especially with neuropsychiatric findings have been the most common presenting picture, especially in the elderly (210). Food-cobalamin malabsorption as well as decreased Cbl intake may contribute to the increase in deficiency in the elderly (211). In addition, because the total body pool of Cbl is very large (~2 mg) compared with the maximal daily loss in patients without overt malabsorption (5 to 10 μg per day), loss of body stores is very gradual, and increased longevity may then dispose to Cbl deficiency, when accompanied by other risk factors such as mild food malabsorption and/or decreased intake.

"Subclinical" Neuropsychiatric Disease

Patients with multiple sclerosis can have low serum cobalamin levels and high Hcy levels (212). The problem is complicated by the fact that the presentation of the two conditions can be confused. The neuropathology of cobalamin deficiency involves the myelin sheath and white matter. MRI of the brain and spinal cord can show, in some cases, a pattern of white matter degeneration similar to multiple sclerosis, including a hyperintensity on the T2 image in the cord and periventricular white matter (213). It has been proposed that SCCD aggravates underlying multiple sclerosis, but this association remains to be confirmed. One study has shown that in patients with biochemical cobalamin deficiency, unexplained chronic cough improved, presumed due to sensory neuropathy (214). This study suggests that peripheral nerve function may be impaired in diseases other than "classical" vitamin B_{12} deficiency, and perhaps by mechanisms different from spinal cord involvement.

The neurologic manifestations of cobalamin deficiency occur in about 75% of patients (215) (Table 6-27). Moreover, they often develop in the absence of anemia and may thus not be suspected, but can be the major presentation in elderly patients. This is the sense in which they are subclinical, as distinguished from the condition of SCCD, which is only detected by laboratory abnormalities. Both folate and cobalamin have been linked to psychiatric disease, especially depression. Although the evidence for folate deficiency is unresolved, there is no evidence that cobalamin deficiency is related to depression (216). The evidence for B_{12} deficiency and impaired cognition is variable. Some studies are negative, with or without folate (144). Other studies show improvement when given with other B vitamins (145), or with a complete multivitamin and mineral mix (217). One study showed very modest improvement in elderly patients in a dementia scale, giving 1 mg of vitamin B_{12} subcutaneous monthly for 6 months, but only the mildest cases responded (218). Other studies showed no benefit (219). Possible associations of low serum Cbl have been reported in Alzheimer's disease (AD), but the association has not been consistent; it is possible that Cbl deficiency in the elderly was coexistent with AD. Theoretical reasons for linking vitamin B_{12} metabolism with AD include the role of the

TABLE 6-27   Neuropsychiatric Presentations of Cobalamin Deficiency

Clinical Syndrome	% of Cases	Symptoms	Signs	Localization
Myeloneuropathy	54%	Paresthesias, numbness, weakness, incontinence	↓ Vibration, touch, position, ↓ reflexes	Peripheral/ autonomic nerves
Peripheral neuropathy	9%			
		Gait ataxia	Romberg sign, ↑ reflexes, Babinski sign, spasticity	Spinal cord
Neuropsychiatric and dementia	38%	Aphasia, hemiparesis, impaired visual fields	Lateralized signs, optic atrophy	CNS (r/o stroke)
Cognitive dysfunction	34%	↓ Memory, concentration, depression, confusion, ↓ processing speed	Abnormal symptom scales	CNS (r/o Alzheimer)

Prevalence of neurologic syndromes adapted from Aaron S, Sudhir K, Vijayan J, et al. Clinical and laboratory features and response to treatment in patients presenting with vitamin B12 deficiency-related neurological syndromes. *Neurol India.* 2005;53:55.

vitamin in maintaining Hcy metabolism via methionine synthase activity and maintenance of S-adenosylmethionine levels (219). A similar rationale has been offered for using high-dose cobalamin in patients in the ICU (220). However, no interventional studies have convincingly shown benefit (221). Biochemical measurements are corrected, but no improvement in cognition has been found. Perhaps the studies were too short (6 months usually), or the dose was insufficient to produce changes in the CNS. In patients suspected of subtle cobalamin deficiency, even 1,000 μg per day was not sufficient to maintain markers of normal Cbl status (222). In some studies, lower doses (25 μg per day) lowered but did not normalize MMA levels (223), although other studies show that many subjects achieved normal levels (224). It seems best, therefore, to make certain that elderly patients, especially those with cognitive impairment, have a normal cobalamin status, but it is not known whether that is associated with improved neuropsychiatric function.

Hyperhomocysteinemia

Hcy is regulated by folate, vitamin B_6, and cobalamin. Serum concentrations are also related to age, sex, renal function, drug ingestion, genetic polymorphism, and other factors as yet unknown. The variable rates of prevalence and the still uncertain upper limit of normal values may be associated with the need to use freshly separated plasma so as to avoid Hcy synthesis by RBCs in vitro. The implications of this finding in regard to cardiovascular disease are still unclear (see section on folate). Even when folate and cobalamin levels are found to be below average, it is not clear whether this represents a clinically significant deficiency state and whether supplemental vitamins will either correct the plasma abnormality or prevent any clinical disorders, particularly cardiovascular disease (225). The fact that an increase in cardiovascular disease has not been detected in pernicious anemia, the most common cause of cobalamin deficiency, raises a question about the nature of the association with hyperhomocysteinemia.

Treatment

Cobalamin is available in four different chemical forms (cyanocobalamin, methylcobalamin, adenosylcobalamin, and hydroxocobalamin), and at least three different formulations (oral, parenteral, and nasal). The forms and formulations available vary from country to country. In the United States, the major form is cyanocobalamin, whereas in the United Kingdom, only hydroxocobalamin is available. Absorption data are very limited, but oral absorption is probably not the same for all forms (226). Thus, equivalent doses cannot be estimated. There is no evidence that the active forms of the vitamin (adenosyl-, methyl-) are preferable to cyanocobalamin, as within a short time after administration of cyano- or hydroxocobalamin orally, conversion to the active forms occurs in mammalian cells. After uptake into a cell, cobalamin of any form binds to the MMACHC (methylmalonic aciduria and C type Hcy) protein, which catalyzes removal of the upper axial ligand by dealkylation (AdoCbl, MeCbl) or decyanation (CNCbl) before formation of the active intracellular forms, AdoCbl or MeCbl (227). Thus, there is no convincing theoretical rationale for ingestion of cobalamin forms with different axial ligands. Indications for adenosyl- and methylcobalamin that are offered in much larger oral doses include conditions for which no efficacy data are available. These include polyneuritis, neuralgia, liver disease, peripheral nerve injury, etc. Available preparation of vitamin B_{12} include:

Cyanocobalamin: oral doses in μg, 100, 250, 500, 1,000
    Parenteral in μg per mL, 100, 1,000
    Nasal (Nascobal), 500 μg in one nostril per week
Hydroxocobalamin: parenteral 25 mg per mL
Adenosylcobalamin (cobamamide): oral in mg, 1, 3, 5
    Parenteral, 25 mg per mL
Methylcobalamin (dibenzocide): oral in mg, 2, 3, 5
    Parenteral, 1,000 μg per mL

Dietary deficiency responds to as little as 1 to 3 μg per day taken orally. Malabsorption requires additional supplementation (150 to 300 μg per month) because the enterohepatic circulation is interrupted. A single injection of 100 μg produces a complete remission of symptoms in most cases. An increased sense of well-being is noted within 24 hours, painful tongue improves in 48 hours, and reticulocytosis begins in 5 to 7 days. Serum folate falls rapidly. Neurologic findings may take 6 months to reverse. Monthly injections of 100 to 200 μg sustain the remission, although 1,000 μg is often used. Patients with rare inborn errors of metabolism, such as vitamin B_{12}-responsive methylmalonic acidemia, require treatment with large amounts of the vitamin because they are resistant to normal levels of cobalamin.

Elderly subjects are advised to meet daily needs by taking synthetic cobalamin in enriched foods or supplements (3). The amount of cobalamin found in most multivitamins ($\leq$6 μg) is not sufficient to treat cobalamin deficiency, which is more prevalent in the elderly. Healthy people under age 50 consuming a diet that contains animal products do not require cobalamin supplements. Some healthy people over the age of 50 may require supplements, but it is not clear how many. Thus, it seems reasonable to screen this population, but the best approach to population screening and the best dose to prevent deficiency are still uncertain. If elevated levels of MMA or holoTCII are found, treatment with cobalamin in deficiency doses can normalize them.

No studies have tested whether Alzheimer-type dementia responds to cobalamin. Because these patients are elderly, they should be screened and treated if deficiency is present. Some data support the use of cobalamin to treat painful uremic neuropathy (228). Elevated Hcy levels are seen in patients with stroke, and in a study of 628 Japanese patients with poststroke hemiplegia, combined therapy with folate and methylcobalamin reduced the risk of fractures by approximately 80%, without improving bone mass or reducing falls (229). The effect was so striking that it needs repeating, but this may not be easy to do in countries with folate supplementation. Cobalamin injections have been used for years to treat fatigue, because of the striking response to replacement therapy in patients with clinical vitamin B_{12} deficiency. But evidence of its efficacy has not been found in controlled trials in patients with chronic fatigue syndrome (230).

Parenteral cobalamin is supplied in solutions of 1,000, 100, and 30 μg per mL. Oral cobalamin can be used for treatment in most patients with an adequate gastrointestinal tract, although the response is slightly slower than when an injectable vitamin is used (231,232). A systematic review revealed two RCTs of oral versus parenteral cobalamin treatment for cobalamin deficiency, and concluded that 2 mg per day initially and then weekly or monthly for life were as effective as parenteral vitamin in patients with an intact intestine (233). Nasal cobalamin is available (Nascobal, 500 μg per 0.1 mL) for maintenance use once a week. It appears to be well tolerated and can even be used more frequently for the initial treatment of mild deficiencies (234).

Fortification?

Mandatory fortification of foods is currently not being done, but arguments have been raised in its favor. These include the increased prevalence of cobalamin deficiency in the elderly, and the presumed prevalence of SCCD (235). But cobalamin is not the same as folate, in that the turnover of the vitamin is so much slower, so effects of fortification will be felt over a longer time. In addition, the physiology of absorption is more complex, so the two major problems causing deficiency, malabsorption, or decreased intake, might have limited bioavailability of a fortified product (236). There are still too many issues that are unresolved to recommend fortification, so treatment of Cbl deficiency will have to be done one patient at a time.

Toxicity

Cobalamin causes no toxic effects, so no UL has been suggested (3).

Vitamin C (Ascorbic Acid)

Requirement

A daily intake of 10 mg of ascorbic acid cures clinical signs of scurvy, but does not maintain body stores. When the daily intake is above 200 mg, most of the ingested vitamin is excreted. Between these extremes, body stores vary with intake. Age and sex have only minor effects on the vitamin C requirement. The requirement is compounded by the fact that vitamin C has been proposed to have a chemoprotective effect in many disorders, at doses far in excess of those necessary to prevent scurvy. These include cancers, heart disease, and cataracts. A well-designed study has identified the vitamin C intake and tissue saturation levels that allow maximal protective effects of the vitamin (237). With the ingestion of 60 mg of vitamin C per day (the previous RDA), wide fluctuations

TABLE 6-28 Dietary Reference Intakes for Vitamin C

Life Stage Group	Vitamin C (mg/day)
Infants	
0–6 months	40[a]
7–12 months	50[a]
Children	
1–3 years	15
4–9 years	25
Males	
9–13 years	45
14–18 years	75
19–>70 years	90
Females	
9–13 years	45
14–18 years	65
19–>70 years	75
Pregnancy	
≤18 years	80
19–50 years	85
Lactation	
≤18 years	115
19–50 years	120

[a]Evidence sufficient to suggest a DRI based only on adequate intake (AI).
All others based on recommended dietary allowance (RDA).
Data from Standing Committee on the Scientific Evaluation of Dietary Reference Intakes, Food and Nutrition Board, Institute of Medicine. *Dietary Reference Intakes for Vitamin C, Vitamin E, Selenium, and Beta-Carotene and Other Carotenoids.* Washington, DC: National Academies Press, 2000.

in plasma vitamin C were associated with small changes in the amount consumed. The first intake dose at which plasma levels were beyond the first sigmoid part of the saturation curve was 200 mg per day. Saturation did not occur until intake levels were at 1,000 mg per day. These data fit with the estimated vitamin C content of diets (~225 mg per day) that appears to be of chemoprotective value (238). The DRI values represent a compromise between the old RDA value of 60 mg per day and the value needed for possible efficacy in chemoprevention (Table 6-28). This compromise also takes into account dietary availability, bioavailability, urinary excretion, potential adverse effects, and biochemical and molecular function in relation to vitamin concentration.

Needs are increased at some life stages. Premature infants have low body pools. Newborn infants ingest about 35 mg from breast milk, and the DRI for them is set to at least equal that source. During pregnancy, about 10 mg of vitamin is added to the fetus each day, which must be added to the DRI for pregnant women. The vitamin C concentration in human milk is about 30 mg per L for a volume of 750 mL (first 6 months), which creates an additional need of 22 mg per day. Vitamin C is not produced by colonic microflora, unlike the situation with many other water-soluble vitamins.

Food Sources

Ascorbic acid is widely distributed in foods in high concentrations, especially in green vegetables and citrus fruits. However, the content is quite variable from one food to another and within each type, even for foods from the same region and source, depending on species and degree of ripeness (239). Table 6-29 lists the ascorbic acid content of some common foods. Grain products do not contain ascorbic acid unless they have been enriched. Nuts and sweets contain little or no ascorbic acid. The DRI for adult men (90 mg) can be achieved with one and a half glasses of freshly squeezed orange juice, or three-fourth cup of raw broccoli. Consumption of five servings of fruits/vegetables

TABLE 6-29 Ascorbic Acid Content of Foods

Food	Serving	Ascorbic Acid Per Portion (mg)	Percentage of RDI (60 mg)
Fruits			
Banana	One (9 in)	10	10–24
Cantaloupe	1 cup	68	>100
Orange	Whole (2 1/2 in)	70	>100
Grapefruit	Half, red	47	>40
Strawberries	1 cup	85	>100
Pear	One Bartlett	7	10–24
Apple	One (2.75 in)	8	10–24
Fruit Juices			
Orange, fresh	1 cup	124	>100
Orange, frozen	1 cup	97	>100
Grapefruit, canned	1 cup	72	>100
Pineapple, frozen	1 cup	30	>40
Grape drink[a]	1 cup	250	>100
Vegetables			
Green beans, fresh uncooked	1 cup	18	25–39
Spinach, cooked from fresh	1 cup	40	>40
Cabbage, cooked	1 cup	36	>40
Broccoli, cooked from fresh	1 cup	116	>100
Peas, frozen fresh, cooked	1/2 cup 1 cup	8 23	10–24 25–39
Potato, baked	1 each	26	>40
Lettuce, iceberg	1 cup	2.2	1–5
Tomato, fresh	1 each (2.2 in)	22	25–39
Green pepper, fresh cooked	1/2 cup 1/2 cup	44 50	>40 >40
Dairy Products			
Milk, cow's, whole	1 cup	2.3	1–5
Milk, human	1 cup	7–12	10–24
Cheese	1 oz	0	0
Egg	1 each	0	0
Meats			
Beef liver, fried	3 oz	19	25–39
Bacon, lunch meat	2 pieces	10	10–24
Fish	3 oz	4	5–12

RDI, recommended dietary intake.
[a]Vitamin C is fortified in some drinks; check label.
Data from Hands ES. *Food Finder.* 2nd ed. Salem, OR: ESHA Research, 1990.

each day can provide from 200 to 280 mg per day. However, in the third NHANES (NHANES III), vitamin C intake for adults was only 70 to 80 mg per day (240). Furthermore, ascorbic acid is heat-labile and easily destroyed by oxidation. Prolonged exposure to oxygen, iron, or copper destroys the vitamin. In addition, like other water-soluble vitamins, ascorbic acid can be lost in cooking water. Often, only 50% of the content of the raw food survives processing and cooking.

Assessment

Intake or Absorption

In general, plasma or serum ascorbate levels reflect intake. Low levels do not necessarily indicate scurvy, but scurvy is invariably associated with low levels. Plasma levels may not always reflect

TABLE 6-30 Guidelines for Interpreting Vitamin C Status

Test	Deficient (high risk)	Low (moderate risk)	Acceptable (low risk)
Serum ascorbic acid (µmol/L)	<11	11–23	>23
Leukocyte ascorbate (µmol/L)	<150	<200	300–600

From second National Health and Nutrition Examination Survey, Canada Nutrition Survey, and adapted from Sauberlich HE. *Laboratory Tests for the Assessment of Nutritional Status.* 2nd ed. Boca Raton, FL: CRC Press, 1999.

intake. Levels of ascorbate may be reduced in patients with chronic inflammatory diseases, cigarette smokers, persons experiencing acute emotional or environmental stress, and women taking oral contraceptives. The nutritional meaning of these changes is obscure. This test is readily available, and its value is that a normal result rules out scurvy. Vitamin C is stable in plasma when collected in metaphosphoric acid. The method of choice for plasma or blood vitamin C measurement is HPLC, according to the recommendations of the WHO (32). Levels less than 23 µmol per L indicate deficient intake or absorption (Table 6-30). Seasonal changes occur, with the highest levels seen in summer, when large amounts of fresh fruits and vegetables are consumed. Levels are very high in the first 3 days of life. When intake is decreased, deficiency develops within 3 to 5 months. Severe infections and acute illness can lower serum levels in the absence of deficiency. Levels should be measured in patients at risk, including those with a poor diet (elderly, alcohol or drug abusers, patients with chronic disease or cancer), patients on dialysis, and smokers.

Body Stores

Ascorbate concentrations in leukocytes are more closely related to body stores than concentrations in plasma. Red cell levels of ascorbate do not fall with depleted stores. Separation of cells on a Ficoll density gradient followed by HPLC analysis has made accurate measurement possible in blood samples of 2 mL or less. Both ascorbic acid and the oxidized form, dehydroascorbate, can be measured. Because a fivefold variation in vitamin C content (µg per 10^8 cells) is seen between mononuclear cells (higher) and polymorphonuclear cells (lower) (32), vitamin C levels vary with differing degrees of leukocytosis. Because the diagnosis of scurvy must be made quickly, a test must be rapid and readily available to be of any use at all. For these reasons, when an assessment is obtained, plasma ascorbate is preferred, even though it does not measure tissue stores. Guidelines for the interpretation of the results of these tests are listed in Table 6-30.

Physiology

Absorption

The absorption of ascorbic acid is carrier-mediated, active, and sodium-dependent. Two sodium-dependent vitamin C cotransporters have been cloned, *SLC23A1* (SVCT1) and *SLC23A2* (SVCT2) (241). SVCT1 is found in kidney, intestine, and liver. Loss of SVCT1 in the knockout mouse kidney leads to massive loss of vitamin in the urine, suggesting an important role for this transporter in humans incapable of synthesizing ascorbate. A single nucleotide polymorphism of SVCT1, rs33982313, was associated with a reduction in plasma vitamin C concentration, although it has not been correlated with gastric or CRC (242). SVCT2 is in choroid plexus and pigmented epithelium of the retina, and is more widely distributed, accounting for ascorbate accumulation against its concentration gradient in many tissues. Efflux across the basolateral membrane is mediated by an unknown sodium-independent mechanism. Neither cotransporter recognizes oxidized ascorbic acid (dehydroascorbate). This metabolite crosses the blood–brain barrier via the GLUT1 glucose transporter, and ascorbic acid is regenerated in the brain and thus trapped in that tissue. Most tumor cells cannot transport ascorbate in the reduced form, but use glucose transporters (GLUT 1,3 and 4) to take up the oxidized dehydroascorbate (243). Ascorbic acid efflux occurs by exocytosis and by volume-sensitive pathways, triggered by glutamate.

The efficiency of ascorbic acid absorption decreases with a daily intake above 180 mg. In such cases, 55% to 90% of the ingested vitamin appears in the urine. The stool contains the rest, with the proportion increasing as the oral dose increases. When excessive ascorbate is ingested, osmotic diarrhea ensues (244). Plasma concentrations are tightly controlled, so the concentration needed for antitumor activity in vitro (>100 μmol per L) cannot be achieved in humans by oral dosing (245). This finding, and the inability of most tumor cells to transport reduced ascorbate, may explain the negative results of studies trying to link vitamin C intake or plasma levels to cancer prevention. Ascorbic acid is catabolized to oxalate and accounts for 20% to 30% of urinary oxalate under normal conditions. Ingestion of more than 4 g per day increases urine oxalate excretion. Large doses of vitamin C increase oxalate excretion to 60 to 100 mg per day. The range of molar conversion varies from 2.5% to 3.0%. Average stores are about 900 mg, and the mean daily excretion of dietary vitamin C is 2.7%. At higher doses, the vitamin is uricosuric.

Metabolic Functions

Metabolic functions of ascorbic acid are not completely understood (246). It is important in the hydroxylation of proline and lysine and affects collagen formation. It enhances the hydroxylation of lysine to hydroxylysine, and of proline to hydroxyproline. The collagen matrix produced under stimulation by ascorbic acid may potentiate differentiation. Ascorbic acid influences tyrosine metabolism when large amounts of tyrosine are ingested. It is involved in the formation of norepinephrine from dopamine and in converting tryptophan to 5-hydrotryptophan and subsequently to serotonin. Vitamin C also aids in the synthesis of carnitine and adrenal hormones, and enhances microsomal drug metabolism, wound healing, and leukocyte functions. Ascorbic acid is an excellent antioxidant, scavenging free radicals. The half-life in the body is 10 to 20 days. By its reducing power, the vitamin enhances the absorption of inorganic iron and the transfer of iron from transferrin to ferritin, and it may function as an antioxidant for vitamins A and E. The formylation of tetrahydrofolic acid is enhanced by vitamin C.

Deficiency

Scurvy is manifested by weakness, irritability, bleeding gums, gingivitis, joint pains, and loosening of teeth. Musculoskeletal problems dominate the clinical picture, including arthralgia, myalgia, hemarthrosis, and hematomas in the muscle (247). Trabecular and cortical loss of bone mass is common. Interference with neurotransmitter synthesis may explain the fatigue, weakness, and vasomotor instability associated with scurvy. Hemorrhaging occurs in the skin, especially in the perifollicular regions, conjunctivae, nose, and gastrointestinal and genitourinary tracts. Anemia and hyperkeratosis of hair follicles are common. The condition can present as leukocytoclastic vasculitis (248). Infants are subject to weight loss and subperiosteal hemorrhage. Cessation of the growth of long bones is a prominent feature of infantile scurvy. Scurvy is a rare disorder in the United States because of the wide availability of fresh fruits and vegetables and the common supplementation of packaged foods with vitamin C. When scurvy occurs, it is usually in alcoholics. Because the assessment of vitamin C stores is difficult, information is lacking about other possible deficiency syndromes. Despite many claims to the contrary, no deficiency state for vitamin C other than scurvy has been definitively documented.

As in the case of other nutrients, "conditional" vitamin C deficiency has been reported in surgical patients in the ICU (249). Vitamin C requirement is assumed to increase, as blood levels fall after uncomplicated surgery, and more than 500 mg per day intravenously may be required to return blood levels toward normal. However, clinical benefits and the dose required to achieve such benefits have not been established. Vitamin C deficiency as defined by the load needed to restore urinary excretion to normal has been associated with peptic ulcer disease, and perhaps this is related to the conversion of ascorbic acid to its oxidized form at pH > 2 in the gastric lumen (250). This deficiency has been thought to contribute to oxidative damage to the gastric mucosa. However, vitamin C sufficiency is restored by eradication of *H. pylori* and produced by chronic proton-pump inhibitor therapy, so the primacy of vitamin C deficiency in these conditions is questionable.

Therapy

Scurvy

Scurvy responds to as little as 10 mg of vitamin C per day. A dose of 60 to 100 mg per day is recommended for replenishing body stores. Tablets are available in doses of 25, 50, 100, 250,

500, 1,000, and 1,500 mg. It is available as a syrup at a dose of 500 mg per 5 mL. Parenteral preparations offer 500 mg per mL.

Low Serum Levels of Vitamin C
Persons at risk include the elderly (older than 65 years), smokers (especially men), diabetics, and oral contraceptive users. They should be encouraged to increase their vitamin C intake, most likely via a supplement, because 5 to 10 servings of fruits/vegetables are needed to fulfill their increased requirement.

Prevention of Chronic Disease
In addition to its antiscorbutic role, many potential benefits of vitamin C have been suggested, so that vitamin C supplements are now more widely used than any other supplement in the United States. Evidence exists for a role of vitamin C in the prevention of cataracts, diabetes, hypertension, coronary heart disease, cancer, asthma, and the common cold (40,246). Vitamin C concentration in cells is high and falls rapidly during stress and infection, leading to the concept that ascorbate plays a role in immune responses (251). The data on the prevention of rhinovirus infection are still equivocal. A systematic review of vitamin C prophylaxis for the common cold found no benefit in the general population at doses of up to 8 g per day (252). However, in six trials involving marathon runners, skiers, and soldiers on sub-Arctic exercise, there was a 50% reduction in colds. Similarly, the evidence for a role in relieving asthma or allergy is equivocal (253).

Vitamin C has an effect on endothelial function through effects on nitric acid production, and modest effects on systolic and diastolic blood pressure have been noted, but the effects are modest (-−4.5 and 1.5 mm Hg, respectively), and have not been demonstrated long term (254).

The role of vitamin C as an antioxidant has been extensively examined in humans, often in combination with other potential antioxidants, especially vitamin E, but no change in markers of oxidation or clinical benefit have been found in general (255) (see also the section on vitamin E in this chapter). Evidence in small numbers of subjects suggests a possible role for vitamin C in enhancing immune function, but none in exercise-induced oxidative stress. Many epidemiologic studies show an inverse correlation between vitamin C levels and coronary artery disease and also between vitamin C levels and hypertension (256,257), but prospective trials have not been performed. An epidemiologic study in 83,639 male physicians showed no correlation of vitamin C (or E) use with changes in cardiovascular mortality over 5 years (258). On the other hand, another study of 85,118 women showed a 28% reduced risk in those who took vitamin C supplements, but not in those with the highest intake of dietary vitamin C (259). Another large study showed an inverse association between cardiovascular mortality and vitamin C plasma levels and vitamin C intake (mostly due to supplements) (260). The same correlations and lack of prospective interventional studies have been noted for cataracts (40) and gastric, esophageal, oral, and pharyngeal cancers (261). It is reasonable to suggest an increased dietary vitamin C intake for these patients, but it is premature to recommend supplements. If supplements were given, there are no data on the necessary dose, whether vitamin C alone would be effective, whether primary or secondary prevention would be affected, or which population might respond the best (262).

On the other hand, prospective interventional trials in high-risk populations for precancerous gastric lesions (263) or precancerous colonic adenomas (264) have not demonstrated benefit, either as single agents or in combination with other antioxidant vitamins A, E, and β-carotene. The use of high-dose (up to 18 g per day) intravenous vitamin C has been promoted on the basis of isolated case studies (265,266). The basis for such treatment is that unlike oral administration where the Cmax is regulated by increased urinary and fecal excretion, ascorbic acid concentrations continue to risk linearly when given linearly, thus possibly driving the reduced form into tumor cells in the absence of specific transporters (267). However, neither a phase 1 (268) nor a phase 2 clinical trial (269) in patients with advanced malignancy showed an objective anticancer response in any of 24 patients in each study. Despite claims about efficacy from complementary and alternative practitioners (270), there is no evidence that high-dose ascorbic acid has a place in current therapy (271).

Iron Absorption
The addition of ascorbate to inorganic iron preparations enhances absorption. The effectiveness of ascorbate in improving ferrous sulfate absorption is greater when used with meals that contain

inhibitors of iron absorption, requiring a molar ratio of ascorbate:iron of 4:1, or approximately 10 mg per mg of iron (272),

Industrial Uses

Industrial uses of ascorbic acid include prevention of food spoilage, maintenance of the red color of canned meat, prevention of rancidity of fats, and stabilization of milk.

Toxicity

Earlier reports of adverse effects with supplemental vitamin C have largely not been substantiated in normal healthy populations (273). However, a UL for adults has been set at 2,000 mg per day (3). Although the urinary excretion of oxalate increases with high doses of the vitamin, a relationship with kidney stones in normal persons has not been demonstrated conclusively. Large cohort studies have shown that doses of ascorbic acid greater than 1,000 mg per day is associated with the risk of symptomatic kidney stones in men (274). Another large cohort study of Swedish males confirmed an association of increased risk for developing stones with ascorbic acid supplements, but not other vitamins, even after accounting for many other confounding factors (275). Similar results have not been found in women. Likewise, the inorganic iron-enhancing feature of the vitamin does not affect serum ferritin. High doses of vitamin C do not appear to destroy cobalamin. Nonetheless, it would be well to remember that this lack of toxicity applies only to normal populations, and that high doses of supplemental vitamin C have not been shown to be beneficial. Moderation of intake can be suggested for any patients considered at risk for iron overload or renal oxalate stones.

The pH of chewable vitamin C tablets (500 mg) is less than 2.0. Because vitamin C acidifies the urine, it can decrease the excretion of acidic drugs such as aspirin and increase the excretion of basic drugs such as tricyclic antidepressants. Large doses (>500 mg) can also interfere with the laboratory measurement of levels of serum bilirubin, glucose, lactic dehydrogenase, and transaminases, and with chemical tests to detect fecal occult blood. Such doses can cause false-negative determinations of urine glucose with glucose oxidase and false-positive determinations with copper reduction or Benedict's solution.

Biotin

Requirement

Biotin is synthesized by many microorganisms, and it is felt that colonic flora contribute to the available biotin in humans. Moreover, colonocytes contain the transport mechanism for biotin. Thus, estimation of the requirement is difficult. It has been suggested that a biotin intake of 60 μg per 1,000 kcal prevents deficiency. The estimated safe dietary intake ranges from 30 to 100 μg per day in adults because data on the availability in foods and the intestinal contribution are incomplete. The DRIs for biotin are 5 to 12 μg per day in infants and children, 20 to 25 μg per day in adolescents, and 30 μg per day in adults (3).

Food Sources

The average diet in the United States contains 100 to 300 μg of biotin. It is present in free and bound forms. In egg yolks, biotin is bound by the protein avidin. Biotin is liberated in the intestine by enzymatic hydrolysis. The vitamin is heat-labile, but much of it is retained in processed foods. Rich sources (600 to 2,000 μg per 100 g) include yeast extracts, liver and other organ meats, fish, soybeans, dairy products, and egg yolks (276). Poor sources (<10 μg per 100 g) include muscle meats, dairy products, grains, fruits, and vegetables. Many of the values in foods are likely to be inaccurate, as the results show marked variability compared to a sensitive avidin-binding assay (276).

Assessment

Biotin is measured with *Lactobacillus plantarium* as the assay organism. Values for plasma and whole blood in the literature are variable. Normal whole blood levels are 244 ± 61 pmol per L. Mean urinary excretion is 35 ± 14 nmol per 24 hours (32). Values well below these have been reported in biotin deficiency (277). Expression of mRNA for biotin-related genes may be relatively sensitive indicators of marginal biotin deficiency (278). These genes include methylcrotonyl-CoA carboxylase chains A and B, propionyl-CoA carboxylase isoforms A and B, holocarboxylase synthetase, biotinidase, and the biotin transporter, sodium-dependent multivitamin transporter (SMVT).

Physiology

Biotin in the diet is present as the free vitamin and protein-bound. After the action of luminal proteases, biocytin (biotinyl-lysine) and biotin-peptides remain, and are converted to the free vitamin by biotinidase (33). Biotin uptake is sodium-dependent and is mediated by the SMVT that also transports pantothenic acid and lipoate, and is the product of the *SLC5a6* gene (279). When that gene is knocked out in mice, carrier-mediated biotin uptake in the intestine is completely inhibited; thus, SMVT is solely responsible for biotin transport (280). Biotin transport is upregulated when biotin is limiting, and is downregulated by excessive intake or by alcohol, carbamazepine, and primidone. Biotin deficiency has been reported in patients taking either of those antiepileptic drugs (33).

Biotin is a cofactor for carboxylating enzymes. Biotin accepts carbon dioxide to form an intermediate compound and then transfers carbon dioxide to the substrate. It is thus essential as an intermediary in the metabolism of carbohydrate, protein, and fat. Colonic and small-bowel absorption explains the rarity of human deficiency states. Fecal synthesis by bacteria is prominent but can be inhibited by broad-spectrum antibiotics.

Deficiency

Dietary Biotin Deficiency

Dietary biotin deficiency is rare in humans (281). High levels of phenylpyruvate, seen in phenylketonuria, inhibit pyruvate carboxylase and lead to a functional biotin deficiency. In experimental deficiency, a maculopapular dermatitis (along with lingual atrophy) and pallor are noted after many weeks. Lassitude, muscle pain, paresthesias, and anorexia with nausea occur. In some children with seborrheic dermatitis, biotin levels are low. Ingestion of large amounts of raw egg has produced a deficiency as a result of an excess of avidin, which binds biotin. Biotin deficiency as a complication of long-term total parenteral nutrition can produce alopecia and dermatitis (282). Dermatitis and alopecia are also seen in deficiencies of essential fatty acids and zinc. Biotin deficiency produces a scaly dermatitis, whereas in zinc deficiency, the dermatitis is wetter. A correlation between marginal biotin status and teratogenicity has been reported during pregnancy (283).

Biotin-Responsive Carboxylase Deficiencies

These types of deficiencies have been rarely reported. Affected children present with an erythematous rash, alopecia, and keratoconjunctivitis. It is not clear that the syndrome is caused by biotin deficiency, but at least one case has responded to biotin supplements of 10 mg per day (284). Single cases of biotin deficiency have been reported due to deficiency in 3-methylcrotonyl-CoA carboxylase (285) and to a defect in cellular transport of biotin (286).

Biotinidase Deficiency

Biotinidase deficiency is an autosomal recessive disorder in which biotin cannot be cleaved from peptides and recycled. Patients may become biotin-deficient during early childhood, with seizures, rash, alopecia, ataxia, hearing loss, delayed development, coma, and death. A simple screening test is available for blood in neonates, and the symptoms are reversed by pharmacologic doses (10 mg) of biotin provided they are given early in the course (287).

Therapy

The addition of 200 to 1,000 μg of biotin daily reverses the symptoms of deficiency. The vitamin is available in multivitamin preparations and as 1-, 5-, and 10-mg tablets.

Toxicity

No toxic effects have been reported, and no UL has been established.

Pantothenic Acid (Vitamin B$_5$)

Requirement

When consuming 5 to 7 mg of pantothenic acid daily, normal subjects excrete 2 to 7 mg per day in the urine and 1 to 2 mg per day in the stool. The data are insufficient to base the DRIs for pantothenic acid on RDAs. The AI-based recommendations are 4 mg for adolescents 9 to 13 years old, and 5 mg per day for older adolescents and adults (3). The AI for children is 1.7 to 3 mg per day. During pregnancy and lactation, deficiency has not been reported, but increments of 1 and 2 mg per day are suggested, respectively.

Food Sources

Animals and some microbes cannot synthesize pantothenate, and are dependent on exogenous vitamin. Pantothenic acid is widely distributed in foods (the term *pantothenate* is derived from the Greek "pantothen" meaning "from all sides"), especially in animal tissues, whole-grain cereals, and legumes. Cow's milk contains 3.5 mg per L. An egg contains 1 mg, and liver contains about 8 mg per 100 g. Beef and pork contain about 0.3 to 0.6 mg per 100 g; vegetables and fruits contain less vitamin. Microflora may produce some vitamin, although this has not been clearly demonstrated in humans. Some vitamin is lost during the heating and processing of foods.

Assessment

Urinary excretion correlates with intake, and excretion of more than 1.0 mg per day is probably normal. No good method exists to determine body stores of pantothenic acid.

Physiology

Pantothenate is available in the intestine from the diet and from bacteria. It is transported in the small and large intestine by the SMVT system shared with biotin and lipoate (279). Pantothenic acid is the "backbone" of CoA, which is needed to activate acetate for its many functions in the synthesis of fatty acids, cholesterol, and sterols, and in acetylation reactions. In addition, it is a key participant in the formation of citric acid, which enters the Krebs cycle. The rate-limiting step in CoA synthesis is pantothenate kinase, and is controlled by the end-products of the pathway (288). This is the enzyme that when mutated causes a neurodegenerative disease.

Deficiency

Because of the wide availability of pantothenate in foods, a syndrome of spontaneous human deficiency is not clearly recognized. Experimental deficiency induced by an antagonist, ω-methylpantothenic acid, leads to tenderness of the heels and feet, fatigue, paresthesias, weakness, sleep disturbances, irascibility, and leg cramps. The "burning feet" syndrome seen in malnourished persons responds to pantothenic acid and may represent a specific deficiency. The disease, formerly known as Hallervorden–Spatz syndrome and now known as neurodegeneration with brain iron accumulation (NBIA), is due to mutations in the *PANK2* gene, one of four genes encoding pantothenate kinase (289). Thus, it is clear that severe pantothenate deficiency can cause disease in humans.

Treatment

If deficiency is suspected, it is treated by the oral administration of 10 mg per day. The vitamin has been used to treat paralytic ileus, with 50 to 100 mg per day given parenterally. No evidence for its effectiveness has been noted. Tablets of 25 and 500 mg are available as calcium pantothenate. Pantethine is a somewhat less stable disulfate form of pantetheine, the metabolic component that constitutes the active part of coenzyme A. Pantethine contains the active SH component that is needed for the activity of coenzyme A and acyl carrier proteins, but degrades with time and must be refrigerated. Pantethine has been studied for its effects on hypercholesterolemia. Studies in hyperlipidemic subjects (mostly from Italy) with cholesterol levels greater than 200 mg per dL or TG levels greater than 150 mg per dL showed a fall of 15% and 33%, respectively, after 5 months on a mean dose of 900 mg pantethine per day (290). In patients in North America with only modest cardiovascular risk, the same dose was also effective, but very modestly, lowering serum LDL cholesterol by a mean of 4 mg per dL (291). The mechanism for the effect is not clear, as the doses used are in great excess of the AI level (~5 mg). The vitamin is marketed as an "antistress" treatment, but no evidence supports this claim.

Toxicity

Daily administration of as little as 10 to 20 mg of the calcium salt has been reported to produce diarrhea. Ordinarily, larger doses are required before this complication is seen. As a result, no UL has been established.

Coenzyme Q

Requirement
Coenzyme Q is a fat-soluble, vitamin-like quinone, with 10 repeated isoprenyl units in the side chain of a benzoquinone core, known otherwise as ubiquinone and vitamin Q_{10}. It is associated with a number of deficiency syndromes in humans, and so it is included in the vitamin section, even though it can be synthesized de novo by mammalian cells. No exogenous requirement is known for coenzyme Q.

Food Sources
Coenzyme Q_{10} was isolated first from beef mitochondria, and is found in all tissues, but more concentrated in those with high-energy turnover, such as heart, brain, liver, muscle, and kidney (292). Humans get about 3 to 5 mg per day from the diet in addition to their endogenous synthesis (293).

Assessment
Heparinized blood must be collected on ice and frozen until analyzed by high-performance LC (294). Total coenzyme Q is the sum of ubiquinone and ubiquinol. Reference mean values (95% CI) for adults are 1.04 µmol per L (0.5 to 1.77 µmol per L), and for older children 0.88 µmol per L (0.37 to 1.54 µmol per L). Because coenzyme Q is carried on lipoproteins, concentration is referenced to LDL. For adults total CoQ/LDL is 0.33 µmol per L (0.17 to 0.53); for older children it is 0.37 (0.21 to 0.58). Levels tend to decrease after the age of 40.

Physiology
Coenzyme Q is an obligatory factor in transfer of electrons in the mitochondrial respiratory chain, the final product of which is ATP. Coenzyme Q increases ATP levels, prevents lipid peroxidation, and stabilizes calcium channels to prevent calcium overload (292). It also provides an antioxidant action by its presence in mitochondria, lysosomes, Golgi, and plasma membranes. Levels appear to decrease as CHF worsens in animals and in humans. Coenzyme Q_{10} supplements have protected animals from perfusion–reperfusion injury.

Deficiency
Deficiency of coenzyme Q (CoQ_{10}) was established by recognition of a rare autosomal recessive disorder with five major phenotypes: an encephalomyopathic form (exercise intolerance, myopathy, myoglobinuria, seizures, ataxia); a multisystem infantile form (encephalopathy, cardiomyopathy, ataxia, optic nerve atrophy, deafness, nephritic syndrome); a cerebellar form (ataxia, cerebellar atrophy); Leigh syndrome (growth retardation, ataxia, deafness); and isolated myopathy (295,296).

A state of relative deficiency of coenzyme Q has been proposed for a number of conditions. One RCT of 1,200 mg per day showed less functional decline in patients with Parkinson disease (292). Another study showed improvement on high-dose coenzyme Q10/vitamin E supplements, and the response correlated with lower baseline serum coenzyme Q10 levels (293). Some mitochondrial encephalomyopathies tend to respond, but maximum effect can take 6 months or more, blurring the relationship between dosing and improvement (297). A number of RCTs found several parameters of CHF improved, but the data are not clearly supportive. The Agency for Healthcare Research and Quality (AHRQ) report of studies with more than 60 participants followed for 6 months concluded that the value of coenzyme Q supplements is still unresolved (http://www.ahrq.gov/clinic/epcsums/antioxsum.htm). Plasma coenzyme Q10 levels may predict survival in patients with chronic congestive failure, however (298). Supplementation with coenzyme Q10 appears to lower blood pressure, although its role relative to other drugs is unknown (299). Its efficacy may be due to an effect on endothelial function (300). One placebo-controlled study using 3 × 100 mg per day for 3 months showed an effect on prevention of migraine (301).

Treatment
Most commercial sources of coenzyme Q are produced in Japan from fermentation of yeast strains. They are available in many forms, but absorption is erratic, and maximum serum concentrations are not reached for several weeks (293). The need for higher bioavailability is to

facilitate better tissue uptake, especially in the brain. The many forms of "soluble" coenzyme Q10 when used in high doses appear to increase plasma concentrations in a roughly dose-related fashion (302). One form, UbiQGel, was granted orphan status by the FDA for treatment of mitochondrial cytopathies. Doses range from 150 mg per day up to 3,000 mg per day after titration. Claims for treatment of CHF for coenzyme Q10 have been allowed in Japan for 3 decades. Doses for CHF have usually been 50 to 200 mg per day. Doses available range usually from 100 to 300 mg per soft gel, which is the usual form. A full list of brands is available at http://www.consumerlab.org/results/CoQ10.asp (292).

Toxicity
Despite one report of warfarin interaction, that issue has not been confirmed. Several studies showed coenzyme Q10 depletion following statin treatment, particularly at higher doses. Depletion tends to occur more in the elderly and those with heart failure (patients possibly with lower pretreatment levels), and the laboratory evidence of depletion can be prevented by supplementation with doses of up to 200 to 300 mg per day (303). The American College of Cardiology feels that the value of coenzyme Q10 supplements with statin use has not been established, and that more studies are needed (304).

FAT-SOLUBLE VITAMINS

The functions, symptoms of deficiency, and common food sources of the fat-soluble vitamins are summarized in Table 6-3.

Vitamin A
Requirement
Dietary Reference Intakes
The estimated average requirement on which the current RDAs are based is intended to ensure adequate stores of vitamin A (305). The term *vitamin A* refers to retinoids with the biologic activity of retinol, and also includes retinal, the aldehyde, and retinoic acid. The infant AI is derived from the average retinol content of human milk (485 μg per L). If 780 mL of milk is ingested, breast-feeding supplies about 385 μg of retinol. Because of the large body stores in the liver and the lack of functional criteria for vitamin A status in infants, a precise daily requirement for infants is not known. The allowance for adults is based on many experimental nutritional studies and amounts to 900 μg of retinol per day for men and 700 μg for women. The allowance for children and adolescents is extrapolated to fall between the values for infants and those for adults. The allowance is increased only slightly in pregnancy, on the basis of the small fetal hepatic content. The increase during lactation is based on the vitamin A content of milk.

The determination of dietary vitamin A is complex, and the determination of β-carotene is even more so. Dietary provitamins (of which carotene is the major one) are used much less efficiently than retinol or its esters. No reproducible biologic activities in humans are available to use in establishing the AI. Epidemiologic studies show a correlation between low (but within normal range) serum levels and a variety of chronic diseases, but intervention trials have not produced positive results (306). In addition, some carotenoids (e.g., lutein and zeaxanthin) are preferentially accumulated in the retina and other ocular tissues (307), whereas others lack provitamin A activity but exhibit other biologic activities (e.g., lycopene) (308). Although many observational studies suggest that higher blood levels of β-carotenes and other active carotenoids are associated with a lower risk for several chronic diseases, evidence is not currently convincing that a certain percentage of dietary vitamin A must be derived from provitamin A carotenoids as part of the RDA for vitamin A. However, recommendations to increase the consumption of fruits and vegetables rich in carotenoids for their health-promoting benefits are supported strongly by the Standing Committee on the Scientific Evaluation of Dietary Reference Intakes (4). The DRIs for vitamin A are included in Table 6-31.

Retinol Equivalents
Most often, vitamin A activity in foods is expressed in international units (IUs); 1 IU is the equivalent of 0.3 μg of all-*trans*-retinol or of 0.6 μg of β-carotene. Since 1969, the RDAs have been expressed as retinol equivalents (REs). This change was considered desirable because

TABLE 6-31 Recommended Daily Dietary Intakes of Vitamin A

Life Stage Group	Vitamin A (µg/day)
Infants[a]	
0–6 months	400
7–12 months	500
Children	
1–3 years	300
4–8 years	400
Males	
9–13 years	600
14–18 years	900
19–>70 years	900
Females	
9–13 years	600
14–18 years	700
19–>70 years	700
Pregnancy	
14–18 years	750
19–50 years	770
Lactation	
14–18 years	1,200
19–50 years	1,300

[a]Estimate based on adequate intake (AI). All others based on recommended daily allowance (RDA).

Data from Standing Committee on the Scientific Evaluation of Dietary Reference Intakes, Food and Nutrition Board, Institute of Medicine. *Dietary Reference Intakes for Vitamin A, Vitamin K, Arsenic, Boron, Chromium, Copper, Iodine, Iron, Manganese, Molybdenum, Nickel, Silicon, Vanadium, and Zinc*. Washington, DC: National Academies Press, 2001.

of the poorer utilization of dietary provitamins in comparison with retinol. The Committee currently uses retinol activity equivalents (RAEs) to measure dietary provitamin A carotenoids, mainly β-carotene, α-carotene, and β-cryptoxanthin (305). The RAE values of these nutrients have been set at 12, 24, and 24 µg, respectively. The RAE has been estimated as one-half of the vitamin A activity in comparison with the RE. This change in equivalence was made because of the observation that β-carotene activity in oil is twice that of dietary β-carotene (309). As a result of the change, more darkly colored, carotene-rich fruits and vegetables are needed to meet the vitamin A requirement; the change also means that vitamin A intake was overestimated in the past. When the RAE is used, approximately 26% and 34% of vitamin A consumed by men and women, respectively, is derived from provitamin A carotenoids. Ripe or cooked colored fruits and yellow tubers contain more readily converted carotenoids than do equal weights of dark-green, leafy vegetables. By the 2001 definition:

1 REA = 1 µg of all-*trans*-retinol
= 12 µg of all-*trans*-β-carotene
= 24 µg of other provitamin A carotenoids
= 10.8 IU of activity from β-carotene

The previously accepted 6:1 equivalence of β-carotene to vitamin A has been questioned, also because of the inefficient bioconversion of plant carotenoids (310). There is wide variation in the conversion factors reported, however, not only between different studies, but also between individuals in a particular study (311). Conversion efficiency of dietary β-carotene to retinol varies from 3.6 to 28.1 by weight.

Until 10 years ago, the provitamin A content of foods was measured by extinction at 450 nm of a nonpolar organic extract. However, this measurement included carotenoids with no vitamin

A activity. Food content is now measured with HPLC, which correctly identifies the provitamin A content. The equivalence from the older measurements may vary from 1:2 in orange fruits to 1:26 in green plants. β-Carotene in red palm oil has an equivalence of 1:2 to 1:3. Thus, with vegetarian diets and in areas where intake from animal sources is poor, a conversion of 21 µg of β-carotene per microgram of retinol has been proposed, which reduces retinol intake to well below the RDA (305). In many regions in Africa, South America, and Asia, supplementation with preformed vitamin A should be considered.

Food Sources

Synthesis is limited to plants and microorganisms. Median daily intake in the United States is about 624 RE. Vitamin A as retinyl esters is found only in animal foods, whereas provitamin or vitamin A precursors are found in the vegetable kingdom. Knowledge of the content of retinol or β-carotene in many foods is incomplete. Grains and flours are not sources of vitamin A unless egg, milk, or fruit is added to baked goods. More than 600 carotenoids are found in food among the 5 to 10,000 bioactive plant compounds, only about 50 of which have provitamin A activity and 40 of which are part of the usual diet in the United States. Only about 20 carotenoids are found in human blood and tissues, the most abundant of which (in the United States) are β-carotene, lycopene, α-carotene, lutein, and zeaxanthin. Table 6-32 lists the vitamin A content and RE values of selected foods. Enriched foods account for much of the vitamin A intake, including ready-to-eat cereals (0.7 to 2.5 mg per 100 g), instant powdered breakfast foods (3 to 6 mg per 100 g), and margarines (0.8 mg per 100 g) (312). Liver content varies from 4 to 20 mg per 100 g, and carotenoids in carrots, sweet potatoes, pumpkin, kale, spinach, collards, and squash contain approximately 5 to 10 RE per 100 g. Losses of vitamin A during cooking are small. Many food lists are still given in IUs. When IUs are given for vegetable sources, the total must be divided by 6 to estimate the REs because of poor absorption and conversion to retinol. The Committee on Dietary Allowances of the Food and Nutrition Board recommends that food tables list retinol and provitamin carotenoids separately so that the total REs (µg) can be calculated.

In many countries, including the United States, dairy products and margarines are supplemented with retinyl esters, which are the main dietary source (313). Factors that affect bioavailability include fiber intake (314), cholesterol-lowering drugs (315), and fat-free foods. Human milk contains 400 to 600 RE per L. A linear decline in levels is seen during the first 6 weeks after childbirth. Esters (85% of the total) are split by milk lipase, which is activated by bile salts (316). Richer sources among animal foods are liver and enriched dairy products. Many factors affect the absorption of vitamin A and carotenoids, and therefore their bioavailability. These factors are generally more significant for carotenoids. In general, pigmented vegetables and fruits, especially the yellow ones, contain large amounts of β-carotene. Dried fruits are concentrated sources. Table 6-33 provides an estimate of carotenoid sources in foods.

Assessment

Intake or Absorption

Carotene is not stored in the body. Thus, persons with only preformed vitamin A in their diet will have vitamin A in their serum without carotene. The intake of both carotene and vitamin A is reflected in the serum levels. Total and individual carotenoids are easily determined by HPLC methods; when this test is performed, it is important to determine whether carotene has been ingested recently. When intake is persistently low, the serum vitamin A level falls. This result reflects both low intake and marginal body stores. With continued low intake, serum levels fall further and more accurately reflect decreased body stores. Low carotene levels are meaningful only if carotene is being ingested in the diet. Furthermore, low levels do not distinguish low intake from poor absorption. Therefore, spot vitamin A and carotene levels by themselves are poor screening tests for malabsorption.

Body Stores

The stellate (Ito) cells contain stores of vitamin A as esters, which are hydrolyzed and taken up by hepatocytes or parenchymal cells when needed. These stores turn over at a rate of 0.5% per day in adults. The storage efficiency of dietary vitamin A is about 50% in the repleted state. The liver produces retinol-binding protein, which is secreted into the serum and metabolized by the

TABLE 6-32 Approximate Vitamin A Content of Selected Foods

Food	Portion	RE As Retinol	As Provitamins	Percentage of RDI (1,000 RE)
Grains				
Corn bread	1 muffin	16	16	1–5
Wheat bread	1 slice	0	0	0
Meats				
Salmon	3 oz	43		1–5
Liver, beef	3 oz	9,119		>100
Chicken, roasted	1 cup	22		1–5
Shrimp	1 oz	6		>1
Tuna, fresh broiled	3 oz	642		>40
Tuna, canned, water	4 oz	62		5–12
Fruits and Vegetables				
Apple	2.75 in		7	1–5
Orange	2.6 in		27	<1
Strawberries	1 cup		5	>40
Cantaloupe	1 cup		516	>40
Watermelon	1 cup		59	5–12
Green beans, fresh	1 cup		83	5–12
Spinach, cooked, fresh	1 cup		1,750	>100
Corn, cooked, fresh	1/2 cup		18	1–5
Potatoes, white	8.75 in		0	0
Potatoes, sweet	1 each		2,450	>100
Carrots, cooked	1/2 cup		1,292	>100
Tomatoes	1 each		139	10–24
Dried apricots	16 halves		676	>40
Dried prunes	7 halves		187	10–24
Dairy				
Milk				
Whole	1 cup	76		5–12
Skim, enriched	1 cup	149		10–24
Eggs, large	1 each	97		5–12
Butter	1 tbs	106		5–12
Ice cream	1 cup	133		10–24

RE, retinol equivalents; RDI, recommended dietary intake.
Data from Hands ES. *Food Finder*. 2nd ed. Salem, OR: ESHA Research, 1990.

kidney. Serum/plasma retinol concentrations, serum retinol-binding protein levels, and the relative dose–response assay are used to assess vitamin A status (32).

Retinol. Retinol can be measured by fluorometric, spectrophotometric, or HPLC methods, and retinol measurement is the most commonly used method to determine vitamin A status. The WHO recommends HPLC methods for population surveys. The vitamin is stable in serum or plasma for up to 2 years. Breast milk retinol has been proposed as a good population measure of vitamin A status, as the samples do not have to be processed in the field (317). However, the secretion of vitamin A in chylomicrons is not highly regulated, and thus milk concentrations of vitamin A reflect the mother's current vitamin A status. Serum vitamin A levels reflect body stores, but only when the level is very low is the interpretation clear (Table 6-34). Serum vitamin A levels increase somewhat with age, but usually do not exceed 65 µg per dL. Samples should be obtained in the fasting state to avoid the fluctuations that follow meals. Retinol levels can

TABLE 6-33   Relative Content of Carotenoids in Food Sources

Food	β-Carotene	α-Carotene	Lutein/Zeaxanthin	Lycopene
Apricots	4+	—	—	1+
Beet greens	1+	tr	—	—
Broccoli, cooked	1+	—	1+	—
Carrot, cooked	3+	2+	—	—
Corn	tr	—	—	1+
Mango	1+	tr	—	—
Spinach, raw	2+	—	3+	—
Tomato juice, canned	1+	—	—	1+

1+, 8–25 mg/3.5 oz; 2+, 25–60 mg/3.5 oz; 3+, 60–110 mg/3.5 oz; 4+, >110 mg/3.5 oz; tr, trace.
Data from Sauberlich HE. *Laboratory Tests for the Assessment of Nutritional Status*. 2nd ed. Boca Raton, FL: CRC Press, 1999. Other good sources of β-carotene include red palm oil, herbs and greens, peaches, sweet potatoes, pumpkin, squash, and tomato ketchup; of α-carotene, pumpkin and banana; of lutein, beets, egg yolk, and kiwi fruit; of zeazanthin, egg yolk and potato; and of lycopene, watermelon.

TABLE 6-34   Guidelines in Interpreting Serum Vitamin A and Carotene Levels

	Vitamin A		Carotene	
Interpretation	(µg/dL)	(µmol/L)	(µg/dL)	(µmol/L)
Normal	>20	>0.7	>40	>1.4
Normal, not ingesting vegetables	>20	>0.7	<40	<1.4
Low intake, marginal stores	10–19	0.35–0.66	20–39	0.7–1.34
Deficient stores	<10	<0.35	Variable	
Severe liver disease	<20	<0.7	>40	>1.4
Excess vitamin A ingestion	>65	>2.28	>40	>1.4
Excess carotene ingestion (also, hypothyroidism, hyperlipidemia, anorexia nervosa, hypercholesterolemia of diabetes)	>20	>0.7	>300	>10.5

Data from Sauberlich HE. *Laboratory Tests for the Assessment of Nutritional Status*. 2nd ed. Boca Raton, FL: CRC Press, 1999.

decline with fever, physical exercise, and prolonged exposure to the sun. There is not complete agreement on cutoff levels for deficiency in different age groups (318). Occasionally, the serum level of vitamin A may be normal in the face of depleted hepatic stores. This situation may be seen in alcoholic liver disease—either fatty liver or alcoholic hepatitis. The therapeutic implications of such a discrepancy are not clear because an adequate serum level would imply adequate tissue delivery. In well-nourished young adults, on the other hand, liver reserves of vitamin A were consistent with intake, as determined by stable isotope techniques (319).

Low levels of vitamin A can be unrelated to decreased intake or absorption, as in chronic infection and liver disease. In severe liver disease, the vitamin A level falls because retinol-binding protein is not produced. However, carotene is not converted to vitamin A, and carotene levels tend to rise. Dose–response tests to detect deficiency assume that aporetinol-binding protein accumulates in the liver as liver reserves become depleted, and in response to a challenge dose of vitamin A, serum concentrations increase within a few hours if liver stores are low (320). Moreover, plasma retinol falls 11% to 24% in the presence of subclinical infection (321). Such infection might be suggested by a rise in acute-phase proteins. This finding complicates the use of serum retinol as an indicator of vitamin A stores. It is unclear whether the fall in serum retinol occurs only in patients who have a marginally sufficient vitamin A status and whether they require therapy. Levels of vitamin A can be elevated (>100 µg per dL) in patients on hemodialysis because of impaired conversion of retinol to retinoic acid in the kidney. Elevated carotene levels with low vitamin A levels are sometimes seen in anorexia nervosa. Pregnancy and the use of oral contraceptives raise vitamin A levels by increasing serum retinol-binding protein. Because retinol-binding protein is catabolized in kidney, vitamin A levels rise in renal disease.

Retinol-Binding Protein and Transthyretin (Prealbumin). Retinol-binding protein circulates as a 1:1 molar complex; filtration and loss from the kidney are prevented by prealbumin. The normal concentrations in plasma are 40 to 50 µg per mL (1.9 to 2.4 µmol per L) for retinol-binding protein and 200 to 300 µg per mL for prealbumin. Radial immunodiffusion assay kits are commercially available. Retinol and retinol-binding protein levels are lowered in diabetes, zinc deficiency, and protein–calorie malnutrition, and in response to trauma and infection. Levels of both parameters are elevated in women taking oral contraceptive pills. Liver disease lowers the levels of retinol-binding protein and transthyretin, whereas renal disease raises them. In these situations, the serum levels of vitamin A do not correlate with body stores.

Relative Dose–Response Assay. This test is based on the fact that when vitamin A stores are low, aporetinol-binding protein accumulates in the liver (206,206a). Thus, the test measures the changes in retinol concentration in serum following the administration of a small oral dose (450 to 1,000 µg) of retinol. An increase of more than 20% implies low hepatic stores of retinol. Because the test depends on hepatic synthesis of the binding protein, a false-negative result can be obtained in the presence of liver disease, protein malnutrition, infection, inflammation, or trauma.

Functional Assays. The conjunctival impression cytology assay provides an early measure of histologic ocular changes. Examination for night blindness also can be sensitive in establishing vitamin A deficiency (322). The clinical demonstration of night blindness also provides evidence of inadequate body stores. Impaired dark adaptation is an early sign of vitamin A deficiency in patients with cirrhosis. However, this finding is not specific, resulting also from zinc and protein deficiency.

Physiology
Absorption
Vitamin A is usually ingested as the ester or as carotene, and is hydrolyzed by pancreatic retinol ester hydrolase and brush border phospholipase B before absorption (312)_. Pancreatic retinol ester hydrolase does not require bile salts as a cofactor for activity. The retinol transporter has not yet been identified. Carotenes in food are bound to macromolecules and are more poorly absorbed than either dietary or synthetic vitamin A. Factors that influence vitamin A or carotenoid release from food and its inclusion in lipid droplets in the intestinal lumen include heating (increased), ingestion of lipid-rich foods (increased), and lipid malabsorption or ingestion of lipid drugs or additives (decreased). Such compounds include mineral oil, cholestyramine (which causes fat malabsorption), and olestra. In addition, some carotenoids are more lipophilic (carotenes, lycopene) than others (lutein, zeaxanthin), affecting their relative rates of absorption. Lycopene is absorbed more slowly in cigarette smokers.

Metabolism of Retinol and Carotene
Inside the enterocyte, retinol is converted back to a retinyl ester by the action of acyl CoA:retinol acyltransferase or lecithin CoA:retinol acyltransferase and is incorporated into chylomicrons (323). Carotene is either hydrolyzed in the enterocyte to two retinol molecules or absorbed intact. In the former case, it is handled like dietary retinol; in the latter, it is transported intact in the lymphatics. About 10% of the carotene cleaved in the gut is converted to retinoic acid, a metabolite that supports cell growth but does not function in the visual cycle or in reproduction. Most absorbed retinol arrives at the liver in chylomicron remnants, and uptake is mediated by LDL receptors on hepatocytes. Retinol bound to retinol-binding protein is released and taken up by stellate (Ito) cells. The retinyl esters are stored in lipid droplets in Ito cells in the liver (~80% of liver content) or are converted to retinol for transport to the tissues (324). Absorbed carotene

is also converted to retinol in the liver. A small percentage (~10%) of hepatic retinol is converted to retinoic acid via the aldehyde retinal. Vitamin A induces expression of fibroblast growth factor 15 (Fgf15) via the retinoid X receptor/farnesoid X receptor heterodimer, and is independent of bile acids. Vitamin A replacement reverses the effect on Fgf15 (325). Thus, this receptor may function as a vitamin A status sensor.

Enterohepatic Circulation of Retinoic Acid

Retinoic acid is conjugated with glucuronide and excreted in the bile to be reabsorbed by the intestine via the portal vein. This enterohepatic circulation retains retinoic acid, which is not helpful for visual functions. The concentration of vitamin A metabolites in bile is low when liver stores are low, but the excretion rate increases proportionally as hepatic reserves enlarge (326). However, in malabsorptive states, those metabolites are lost from the body. Because body stores of retinol are converted in part to retinoic acid, this loss can lead to a further depletion of the body pool of retinol, but the significance of the loss is unknown. In vitamin A deficiency, little of the incoming vitamin is deposited in the liver, but is delivered to depleted tissues.

Function of Retinol

Retinol maintains normal epithelia by aiding in glycoprotein synthesis. It (but not retinoic acid) also forms an essential part of the visual cycle and is required for normal reproductive function. Vitamin A is felt to play a role in cell growth. It suppresses malignant transformation of cell lines, prevents chemical induction of some animal tumors in vivo, and has been reported to induce regression of basal cell carcinomas. Vitamin A plays a major role in cell differentiation and morphogenesis. Thus, it is important in reproduction, bone development, skin integrity, and immunity. Retinoic acid, transported to the nucleus, interacts with one or more retinoic acid receptors, which are members of the superfamily of secosteroid receptors. The effect of retinoic acid is not limited to embryonic tissues, but the precise mechanism by which it mediates differentiation is not known.

Function of Carotenoids

Carotenoids mediate many functions, including antioxidation, intercellular communication, immune response, neoplastic transformation, and modification of detoxifying enzymes (327). These effects can be mediated by the parent carotenoid or by retinoid metabolites, and are influenced by other carotenoids and metabolic products. Thus, it is not possible to estimate the overall effect of carotenoids in humans, and no reproducible effect has been identified other than their provitamin A activity.

The evidence that carotenes are antioxidants is crucial to their use in nondeficiency states, but in fact, it is not clear that they are general antioxidants. They are good scavengers of singlet oxygen, but they are neither generalized reducing agents (like vitamin C) nor universal antioxidants (like vitamin E). β-Carotene differs greatly in potency from system to system in comparison with vitamin E (327). Moreover, its antioxidant properties are unpredictable in humans. Although β-carotene has been approved as an antioxidant in foods and supplements, the FDA has noted that no direct scientific evidence exists for such activity in humans and has based its decision to allow the antioxidant label on the antioxidant properties of β-carotene demonstrated in vitro.

Deficiency

The only unequivocal clinical signs of deficiency in humans occur in the eye. These changes have been classified in five stages, listed in order of increasing severity:

X0—Effect on the retina: poor dark adaptation.
X1—Effect on the conjunctiva: xerosis (dryness) detected by dullness of the conjunctiva in bright light; frequent presence of Bitot spots, an accumulation of foamy white debris and fatty material near the limits of the eye, especially laterally.
X2—Effect on the cornea: xerosis along with superficial erosion.
X3—Effect on the cornea: irreversible corneal ulceration.
X4—Effect on the cornea: scarring and softening.

In the United States, only night blindness is usually encountered, most frequently in chronic alcoholics. Persons with malabsorptive states are the other major group at risk for vitamin A deficiency. When zinc deficiency is also present, the effect on visual adaptation may be magnified.

In a chronically undernourished population, repleting maternal stores with recommended dietary intakes before, during, and after pregnancy improved lung function in the offspring (328). All-*trans*-retinoic acid is important in the formation of fetal bronchi and bronchioles in rodents, and may provide an explanation of an effect of vitamin A on lung function (329).

The major carotenoids (β-carotene, lutein, β-cryptoxanthin, lycopene, α-carotene, and zeaxanthin) comprise about 90% of the forms in human serum, but none of these is considered an essential nutrient, or is rate-limiting for a critical metabolic pathway. Thus, they are rarely used in therapy by themselves (330). Studies using β-carotene in combination with vitamin E will be discussed in the section on that vitamin.

Therapy

When vitamin A is used for therapy, it is provided entirely in the form of retinol, and its biologic potency is expressed in IUs. In this use, therefore, 1 IU and 1 RE are identical. Because of continued frequent use, the doses are listed here in IUs.

Deficiency

Deficiency states respond to daily doses of vitamin A from 5,000 to 30,000 IU. The higher doses should be used when severe malabsorption is the cause of the deficiency. A dose of 5,000 IU three times weekly has been effective in treating vitamin A deficiency in extremely low-birth-weight infants, and in slightly decreasing the risk for lung disease (331). Loading doses of vitamin A supplements recommended for patients with severe malnutrition (on day 1), measles (days 1 and 2), and xerophthalmia (days 1, 2, and 14) are the following: young infants (0 to 5 months) 50,000 IU, older infants (6 to 11 months) 100,000 IU, and children (>12 months) 200,000 IU (332). These schedules are also recommended by the WHO as single doses for prevention of disease in high-risk populations. However, when to give vitamin A supplementation is not firmly established, although many studies support treating infants immediately after birth (332). Vitamin A is available in liquid form (5,000 IU per 0.1 mL); an emulsifier solubilizes the vitamin but probably does not enhance absorption when bile acids are deficient in the intestinal lumen. The vitamin is also available as capsules of 5,000 to 50,000 IU and in injectable forms (50,000 IU per mL).

Therapeutic doses of vitamin A are available as retinol, whereas the RDA of 5,000 IU (1,000 μg RE) per day assumes an intake that is half retinol and half β-carotene. Thus, 5,000 IU of retinol, the "standard" replacement dose, is in fact excessive (333). This is one of the reasons why vitamin A toxicity develops in some persons when it is taken in large doses.

Vitamin A Derivatives

13-*cis*-Retinoic acid and etretinate, an aromatic analogue, have been used to treat severe acne, rosacea, fulminant psoriasis, and Darier disease. Etretinate has been reported to decrease bronchial metaplasia in heavy smokers, but serum levels of vitamin A are normal in patients with cancer. ATRA is effective in the treatment of acute promyelocytic leukemia by causing blast cells to differentiate (334). ATRA combined with anthracycline-based chemotherapy achieves a 90% to 95% response rate, and 5-year survival approaches 75%. However, no other differentiating agents have been useful in other forms of leukemias. Fenretinide [4-hydroxy(phenyl) retinamide] is a proapoptotic and pro-oxidant vitamin A derivative that accumulates in breast tissue, and is being studied as a potential preventive therapy for patients at very high risk for breast cancer (335).

Prevention of Chronic Disease

Because of their antioxidant properties in vitro, carotenoids have been implicated in many chronic diseases often linked with vitamins E and C, the other vitamin antioxidants (40,306,327). This topic is also discussed under the section for vitamin E in this chapter, and in Chapter 15.

Epidemiologic studies showed an inverse association between intake of total vitamin A (retinol plus carotenes) and the risk of certain cancers (306). Moreover, laboratory studies in animals showed that β-carotene was protective against cancers and was antiproliferative in cell culture studies. The World Cancer Research Fund evaluation in 1997 by a panel of experts concluded that carotenoid intake was indeed effective against lung cancer. However, more recent reviews, especially that of the National Research Council's Dietary Reference Intake Panel on Antioxidants concluded that the data were insufficient to make a recommendation regarding the relationship of any carotenoid to any chronic disease, including lung and prostate cancer, and age-related macular degeneration (305). A review of carotenoid intake and lung cancer in seven cohort studies in North America and Europe reached the same conclusion that there was no evidence for an association (336). No relationship was found between intake of β-carotene and cancers of the gastrointestinal tract, even when combined with vitamin A, C, or E (337). Greater intake of fruit and vegetables appears protective against chronic cardiovascular disease, but there are no convincing data implicating individual components of these foods. None of the main dietary carotenoids (lycopene, β-carotene, α-carotene, β-cryptoxanthin, lutein, and zeaxanthin have been found to have consistent associations as risk factors for cardiovascular disease (338).

Prevention of Infection

Vitamin A has been used to treat children severely ill with measles (339) and at doses of 8,333 IU per day to prevent mortality from infection in children less than 3 years old in areas where deficiency is endemic (340). Current evidence suggests that two doses of vitamin A reduced mortality and pneumonia-specific mortality in children under the age of 2 years, but no benefit was found when a single dose was used (339).

Toxicity

Amount of Intake

Because vitamin A is readily stored in the body, toxic levels can accumulate if intake is excessive. At levels of daily intake above 4,000 IU per kg (especially >500,000 IU per day), toxic symptoms can develop (341). These levels can easily be achieved by the use of supplements that offer the vitamin in capsules of 50,000 IU. Unfortunately, these higher doses of vitamin A can be obtained without a prescription. Toxicity is correlated with serum levels of more than 1,000 µg per dL, with intake of 18,000 IU per day for 1 to 3 months in infants less than 6 months old, and with intake of 1 million IU for 3 days, 50,000 IU per day for more than 18 months, or 500,000 IU per day for 2 months in adults. UL values have been set for adults at 3,000 µg of retinol per day (~10,000 IU) (305).

Manifestations

In children with acute hypervitaminosis A (>10 times the RDA), vomiting and bulging fontanelles are noted. In older children, growth failure, pseudotumor cerebri, sixth nerve paresis, and optic atrophy develop. At all ages, nonspecific findings such as irritability, skin dryness, desquamation of the skin over the palms and soles, myalgia, arthralgia, abdominal pain, and hypoplastic anemia may be present. Hepatosplenomegaly also occurs. In chronic hypervitaminosis, cortical thickening of bones of the hands and feet develops, with tenderness and weakness. Premature closure of the epiphyses has been observed.

In adults, early symptoms of overdose include nausea, vomiting, anorexia, malaise, cracking of skin and lips, headache, and irritability. Long-term use of vitamin A by the elderly can lead to increased plasma levels of retinol and biochemical evidence of liver damage (32). Hepatic fibrosis has been associated with excessive ingestion of vitamin A in a few cases. In adults receiving 50,000 to 100,000 IU per day, nausea, vomiting, skin desquamation, fatigue, hair loss, bone pain, and hepatomegaly can occur (342). One case-control study has shown that a high intake of dietary retinol is associated with an increased risk for osteoporosis (343).

Teratogenicity

Doses of 15,000 IU per day ingested between days 14 and 40 of gestation can cause microcephaly, dilated ventricles, and aqueduct stenosis. Spontaneous abortions have been reported with isotretinoin. Microphthalmos and atresia of the external auditory meatus have been reported. The risk of a malformation in the newborn was 1 in 57 for mothers who ingested more than 10,000 IU of preformed vitamin A as a supplement during pregnancy (344). However, mothers ingesting supplemental vitamin A in current multivitamin preparations (up to 6,000 IU per day) were not found to be at increased risk for delivering infants with birth defects. Thus, it is probably safe for mothers to ingest an amount of vitamin A not in excess of the RDA (800 RE, or 2,640 IU of vitamin A as retinol). Because folate supplementation, needed to prevent neural tube defects, is most readily available in multivitamin preparations, it is important that mothers not shun both supplements for fear of excessive vitamin A ingestion.

Retinoic Acid Syndrome

Retinoic acid syndrome is the main adverse event resulting from tretinoin therapy for promyelocytic leukemia. It is characterized by elevated and rising leukocyte counts, weight gain, respiratory distress, serous effusions, and cardiac and renal failure (345). The average time of onset is 7 to 12 days, but it can begin after 1 day of treatment. It can be reversed or controlled with dexamethasone.

Osteoporosis

Four large prospective observational studies have been reported from the United States and Scandinavia, regions with a high prevalence of osteoporosis (341). These studies found an association between preformed vitamin A intake and hip fracture or osteoporosis, with doses as low as 1,500 RE per day, much lower than the tolerable UL of 3,000 RE. These reports do contradict earlier studies. The UK-based Expert Group on Vitamins and Minerals concluded that the effect is a graded one and for that reason did not establish a safe upper level for intake (http://www.food.gov.uk/multimedia/pdfs/vitamin2003.pdf).

Inflammatory Bowel Disease

The manufacturer's insert for isotretinoin states that the drug has been associated with IBD, but a population-based cohort study showed no significant association (346). Such a link has biological plausibility, as retinoids inhibit white cell chemotaxis, regulate peripheral immune tolerance, and prevent formation of IL-17 CD4+ cells (347). However, awareness of a possible association is all that is indicated, in the absence of convincing evidence.

Vitamin D

Requirement

Types of Vitamin D

Vitamin D_2 is produced during ultraviolet (UV) irradiation of ergosterol, a fungal and yeast sterol. Small amounts can be found in plants contaminated with fungi or yeasts (348). Vitamin D_3, cholecalciferol, is formed from 7-dehydrocholesterol in the skin of mammals and in small amounts in the leaves of several plant species mostly belonging to the species *Solanaceae* (potatoes, tomatoes, peppers) by the action of UV light. Vitamin D_3 occurs in fish, but there is no evidence that fish contain a synthetic pathway, and they are exposed to limited UV light. There are some data supporting the production of D_3 in algae, which might provide a source for the vitamin in fish (348). However, the data are too fragmentary to be certain about the role of algae in vitamin D_3 production.

About 100 IU of vitamin D_3 is produced per day from endogenous sources in persons living in temperate zones. The maximum amount of previtamin converted to vitamin D_3 is increased by an elevated skin temperature and is limited to 15% to 20% daily regardless of the amount of light. This limitation is a consequence of photoisomerization to other compounds. 7-Dehydrocholesterol in membranes after sunlight is converted to the 5,6-*cis,cis* (cZc) conformer of previtamin D_3 that is rapidly converted to vitamin D_3, and cannot rotate to the more stable 5,6-trans,cis (tZc) form (349). Other photoproducts include lumisterols, tachysterols, suprasterols, and toxisterols. Thus, the skin cannot generate toxic levels of D_3 after sunlight. Sunscreens (protection 15) can reduce production of D_3 by more than 95%. If tanning occurs, then vitamin D is being produced. When melanin is abundant in the skin, 10 to 50 times more sunlight is needed to equal the amounts of vitamin D produced in the skin without melanin pigment.

Estimating the amount of sunlight needed for producing adequate vitamin D have been developed, assuming exposure without sunscreen 3 times a week in a swimsuit or shorts and a T-shirt. The estimates are based on the UV index and skin type (350). UV index is an international scale that assesses the UV radiation at any site at maximum for that day, usually about noon. Exposure times vary from 1 to 15 min for skin that always burns (type I) at a UV index of 3 to 5, to 40 to 60 min for dark skin types V and VI that never burn. Not surprisingly, 25-OH vitamin D levels fall with distance from the equator, as skin darkness declines, and bone density is not abnormal in dark-skinned people (351).

Because in the past it was estimated that more than 90% of circulating 25-hydroxycholecalciferol (25(OH)D_3) in the plasma is derived from vitamin D_3 and thus is endogenously produced, the daily requirement has not been established. Moreover, intake becomes important in persons with normal absorption only when exposure to sunlight is limited. However, all-source inputs to basal serum vitamin D levels are an order of magnitude higher than can be estimated from natural foods, and cutaneous sources account for only 10% to 25% of unsupplemented input even in the summer (352). Thus, other input must come from unknown food sources, possibly as preformed 25(OH)D.

Foods of animal origin contain not only vitamin D_3, but also 25(OH)D. In muscle meat, fish, or eggs, the content of 25(OH)D can equal or surpass that of the provitamin D_3, but in organs (liver, kidney), the provitamin is usually in great excess. In nonenriched milk, vitamin D content is low, but is present mostly as vitamin D_2. When cows are supplemented with vitamin D_3 in their feed, the content of their milk reflects that (353).

Pharmacology of D3 vs 25(OH)D: The current food-composition database for the United States does not include 25(OH)D data. Thus, data for meat, fish, and poultry are probably underestimated. Supplementing with 25(OH)D found that this form was approximately 5 times more effective in raising serum 25(OH)D more than comparable doses of vitamin D_3, at least up to a dose of 20 mcg (354). Moreover, these forms of vitamin D differ in their pharmacology. Although vitamin D_3 is stored mainly in adipose tissue, 25(OH)D in humans (and some animals) is stored mainly in skeletal muscle, probably bound to tissue proteins (355). The oral absorption of D_3 and 25(OH)D are comparable, although 25(OH)D is absorbed somewhat faster, because of its greater water solubility and absorption in the proximal intestine (353). However, the variability in response between individuals is much less for 25(OH)D (354,355). This may be due to the lower need for fat in the diet and formation of mixed micelles, and the longer plasma half-life (12 h) for 25(OH)D compared with D_3 (2 to 3 h). In addition, the distribution volume (Vd) for 25(OH)D is 0.1 to 0.2, and oral bioavailability is 60% to 90% (355). In contrast, vitamin D_3 has a Vd of 4, owing to its segregation into adipose tissue, and its variable release from that tissue. 25(OH)D also binds to a second site on the vitamin D receptor in tissues, and has a dissociation constant much lower than vitamin D_3, making it more designed for rapid nongenomic actions. Clinical trials are needed to establish whether 25(OH)D also has clinical advantages for supplementation. Obese subjects have lower serum 25(OH)D concentrations and higher parathormone concentrations than age-matched controls, and the increase in 25(OH)D was 37% lower after irradiation of the skin, correlating also with a lower rise in serum 25(OH)D after oral D_3 supplements (356). These differences in bioavailability may be due to decreased release of vitamin D forms from adipose tissue and/or muscle. It is not clear whether obese subjects would benefit more from 25(OH)D supplements.

D3 vs D2 preference: Currently in the United States all vitamin D supplements are either D_3 (cholecalciferol) or D_2 (ergocalciferol), and the advertised content of the commercially available products appears reliable (357). There has been much debate about the relative value of each of these forms for human supplementation. A systematic review of 10 RCTs found that D_3 produced a mean increase of 15 nmol per L (6 ng per mL) at doses of 25 to 100 μg (358). Moreover, large bolus doses also favored D_3. The debate about selection of the "best" form of vitamin D has been sharpened by the availability of vitamin D_3 in higher dose strengths (1,000 and 2,000 IU, 25 to 50 μg) for OTC use. Thus, preference for D_3 has been shifted in part due to availability.

Food fortification: The preferred form of vitamin D becomes an issue also for vitamin D food fortification, a program that is voluntary in the United States and Canada, and not carried out in the United Kingdom and many other countries. If the target serum 25(OH)D concentration is 50 nmol per L (20 μg per mL), the combination of sunlight and natural food is not sufficient to achieve that level (359). Foods are fortified with both forms, but probably primarily with D_3. Milk is a commonly fortified food, as it is low in natural vitamin D. Novel approaches to fortification include animal feed fortification with vitamin D rich foods, or manipulation of foods postharvest or preprocessing (360). These various methods will lead to wide variability in efficacy for use of fortified foods. Trials of the efficacy of food fortification show an increase in serum 25(OH)D varying from 10 to 51 nmol per L, in the range needed to achieve the target concentration (361). The efficacy of fortified foods and supplements depends upon the target 25(OH)D concentration. 75 nmol per L (30 μg per mL) has been promoted by many experts as the level needed to achieve prevention of chronic diseases (362). To achieve such levels would require supplements of 1,600 IU (41 μg) per day, outside the range of most fortified foods by themselves (363). Moreover, the need for such high supplementation is still controversial, and lies behind the reluctance of the United Kingdom (and other nations) to embark on fortification. The controversy regarding target 25(OH)D concentrations will be discussed in the next section.

Dietary Reference Intake

Estimated allowances were previously given in IUs, but now are usually expressed as micrograms of cholecalciferol (10 μg of cholecalciferol = 400 IU of vitamin D). Vitamin D in a dose of 2.5 μg (100 IU) prevents rickets, but 10 μg (400 IU) was recommended previously as the RDA for growing children. This recommendation represented in part the underdeveloped 25-hydroxylase activity in the liver of newborns. After the age of 24 years, 5 μg (200 IU) was considered adequate. After a careful review of the literature in 1997, the IOM concluded that it is not possible to determine an RDA for vitamin D, but suggested an AI of 5 μg for infants, older children, and young adults (2). This AI recommendation was based on the literature and assumed some exposure to sunlight. In some elderly patients (>70 years), calcium intake and exposure to the sun may be decreased, and they may convert less of the dietary previtamin to the active form and produce less active metabolites of vitamin D in response to calcium depletion. Vitamin D deficiency is more prevalent in persons over the age of 50 than in younger adults. Thus, the recommended AI of vitamin D for adults older than 50 years was set at twice that of younger adults, and for adults older than 70 years, it is three times greater (15 μg or 600 IU per day). A UL for infants 0 to 12 months of age has been set at 25 μg per day (1,000 IU), and for older children and adults it has been set at 50 μg per day (2,000 IU).

Because of continued concern about conflicting messages on the benefits of calcium and vitamin D, and because these nutrients were among the first to be reviewed by the IOM, The US and Canadian governments asked the IOM to reassess the data on these nutrients. The resulting 2011 report set new DRIs for vitamin D (364) (Table 6-35). Estimates were made for lifestyle groups according to estimated average requirement that would satisfy the needs of 50% of persons in each group, or to RDA that would satisfy the needs of 97.5% of persons in each group. These recommendations were matched with those for calcium (see Chapter 7), for which current intake was judged adequate, except for girls aged 9 to 18, and for postmenopausal women, who were taking excessive supplements. Vitamin D intake was judged to be insufficient, but the Committee relied on national surveys that found average blood levels of 25(OH)D above the 20 ng per mL (50 nmol per L) level felt to be needed for all individuals for bone health (365). Thus, the IOM felt that sunlight was contributing meaningful amounts of vitamin D and that the majority of the population was meeting its need for vitamin D. Some subgroups (e.g., older patients, those in institutions not exposed to sunlight, and those with darker skin) might have increased needs. For disease outcomes other than bone health (e.g., cancer, cardiovascular disease, diabetes, falls, autoimmune disorders), the Committee found the evidence to be inconsistent and its role in causality uncertain, and thus insufficient

TABLE 6-35 Dietary Reference Intakes for Vitamin D

Life Stage group	Estimated Avg Requirement (EAR) (IU/day)	Recommended Dietary Intake (DRI) (IU/day)	Upper Level Intake (UL) (IU/day)
Infants 0–12 months	—	—	1,000
1–3 years old	400	600	2,500
4–8 years old	400	600	3,000
9–50 years old	400	600	4,000
51–70 years old male/female	400	600	4,000
>70 years old	400	800	4,000
14–50 years old pregnant/lactating	400	600	4,000

Data from Ross AC, Manson JE, Abrams SA, et al. The 2011 report on dietary reference intakes for calcium and vitamin D from the Institute of Medicine: what clinicians need to know. *J Clin Endocrinol Metabl.* 2011;96:53.

on which to base a DRI recommendation. In particular, there were few randomized trials in which nonskeletal outcomes were the primary prescribed outcomes. Moreover, the evidence suggested that, while moderate 25(OH)D levels were associated with a lower risk of chronic disease, both higher and lower levels were associated with increased risk. Limited data on the requirements for growing children and adolescents suggest that perhaps the RDA of 600 µg is a bit too low, and should be 750 µg per day (366). While admitting that data from adults should not be relied upon to make recommendations for children and adolescents, in the face of limited data, it seems reasonable to recommend the use of small supplements to reach somewhat higher intake levels (367).

The 2011 IOM conclusions were similar to those of the 2009 AHRQ systematic review (368). They have also been echoed by European experts harmonizing DRIs for vitamin D across Europe (369). These experts noted the consensus on defining cutoff values for vitamin D deficiency for extraskeletal health effects, but used the same cutoff value of 20 ng per mL for bone health, and suggested that older adults should ingest 20 µg of vitamin D (800 IU), but differed from the IOM report by noting that this level was best reached by taking supplements. The European Food Safety Authority was asked to evaluate the ULs of vitamin D for all population groups, and decided on the same ULs as the IOM report (Table 6-35). This is twice the 1997 recommendation, but accords with the more recent data that vitamin D taken without excessive calcium is safe at higher levels than previously considered (370).

The recommendations of the IOM Committee are well supported by the literature, but are conservative, as befits recommendations aimed at an entire population. They acknowledge the need for maintaining a 25(OH)D level higher than that associated with the detection of vitamin D deficiency (10 to 15 ng per mL) and the safety of larger daily intakes of vitamin D. The recommendations have produced a large volume of protest from vitamin D experts, who feel that the target concentration of serum 25(OH)D has been set too low. Their view is that 30 ng per mL (75 nmol per L) is more realistic, a value based on that which turns off secretion of parathormone, and fits with the epidemiological/observational data linking vitamin D levels below that cutoff value to nonskeletal chronic disease (371). The IOM Committee felt that correlation does not prove causation, that prospective randomized trials will be needed. Moreover, much of the information used by both groups is included in the full IOM and AHRQ reviews, so the data on chronic disease associations are not ignored. Time will tell whether vitamin D intake should be increased above the 2011 RDAs, but these do set a new and higher goal for the US (and Canadian and European) populations, and their implementation on a population-wide basis will surely improve the average level of bone health.

The argument about RDAs revolves around which cutoff value to use for defining vitamin D deficiency, and whether a subclinical vitamin D deficiency state in fact exists. This issue is still unresolved, as it is for many other micronutrients, such as cobalamin, vitamin K, and zinc (13). The fact that in none of these cases has the clinical importance of a subclinical deficiency state been shown to predict chronic health problems makes caution in assigning one to vitamin D seem reasonable. Moreover, the IOM recommendations do not prevent other groups from making recommendations for specialized populations as needed, and this has been and will continue to be done. For example, Osteoporosis Canada has placed more emphasis on the epidemiological data suggesting that musculoskeletal benefits are maximized at 75 nmol per L of serum 25(OH)D, and have thus recommended routine supplementation of 400 to 1,000 IU for healthy adults at low risk for osteoporosis (372). For adults over age 50 or with moderate risk of osteoporosis, supplementation should be perhaps higher, with 75 nmol per L serum level of 25(OH)D as the target. Trials of larger doses of vitamin D (e.g., 2,000 and 4,000 IU) have been used in special populations (during pregnancy) and found to increase 25(OH)D levels in the mothers, although 4,000 IU was not superior to 2,000 IU, and was associated with fewer maternal complications, although none reached statistical significance (373). Whether studies like this will lead to recommendations for increased level of supplementation in pregnant women is unclear at this time.

Food Sources

Endogenous production is the most important source. The usual dietary intake in the United States is 1.25 to 1.75 µg per day (US Department of Agriculture, *National Food Consumption*

Survey, 1977–1978). The major natural food sources are fatty fish (e.g., mackerel, salmon), fish liver and oils, egg yolk, and beef liver. Fortified foods now provide the major dietary source. Milk and breakfast cereals are the major fortified foods in the United States, whereas in Canada, milk and margarine are fortified (374). Fortification occurs in countries in Northern Europe as well, but the level of fortification is under evaluation, as 25(OH)D levels are low during the long winters above the 51.9o latitude (Ireland, Denmark, Finland) (375). In countries without staple food fortification, vitamin D levels are too low (376).

The reason for the high vitamin D content of fish liver is not apparent. It has been speculated that fish liver contains a nonphotochemical system for making vitamin D, but no real evidence for such a system has been found. Most likely, the source is from algae (377). Table 6-36 lists the major dietary sources of vitamin D. The content in cow's milk varies with the seasons from 4 IU per quart in winter to 40 IU per quart in summer, unless supplements are added. The mean concentration of vitamin D in human milk is 0.5 µg per L and is proportional to maternal intake. This is well below the level needed to prevent rickets, yet rickets occurs only when milk is not given and sunshine is not provided. Thus, vitamin D in milk may be more biologically available than that from other dietary sources.

Assessment

Assessment of vitamin D status may include measurement of serum 25(OH)D (body stores), serum 1,25-dihydroxyvitamin D (1,25(OH)$_2$D) (renal metabolism), or serum levels of total and ionized calcium, inorganic phosphate, and alkaline phosphatase (late-stage tissue damage) (32).

25-Hydroxyvitamin D

The 25(OH)D level is low when body stores, intake, or endogenous production is low, and measurement of this level is a satisfactory (but not sensitive) method for assessing deficiency of the vitamin D body pool. Of all the possible markers of vitamin D status, the serum 25(OH)D concentration has proved the most robust (377). This measurement has been validated as a biomarker of nutrient status even for populations (378). The available methods include HPLC, competitive protein binding, and RIA. HPLC methods are good for determining both vitamin D metabolites in a single serum sample. Commercial RIA kits are also available that are equally sensitive and practical, but they measure only one metabolite at a time. The cutoff values for vitamin D deficiency based on Gaussian distribution of population levels are below 30 nmol per L (Table 6-37). Competitive protein-binding assays give values that are 20% to 30% higher than for RIA (379). When measurements for 25(OH)D were compared using either RIA, HPLC, or chemiluminescent protein-binding assays, the variability of results produced

TABLE 6-36 Foods Sources of Vitamin D

Food	Portion	Vitamin D Content (IU)
Milk, whole or nonfat	1 cup	100
Butter	1 tsp	1.4
Cheese, cottage	1 cup	5
Egg yolk	1 each	23
Egg white	1 each	0
Cereals (e.g., corn flakes, raisin bran)	1 cup	40–50
Beef liver	3 oz	11.9
Oysters, raw	4 each	2.9
Canned sardines	1 oz	85
Canned salmon	1 oz	142
Lunch meats	1 piece	8–12
Margarine	1 tsp	15–20
Cod liver	1 tsp	400

Data from Hands ES. *Food Finder.* 2nd ed. Salem, OR: ESHA Research, 1990.

TABLE 6-37 Suggested Guidelines for Evaluating Vitamin D Status

Test	Deficient	Low	Acceptable	High
25-Hydroxyvitamin D				
(nmol/L)	≤12	<25	≥30	>200
(ng/mL)	≤4.8	<10	≥12	>80
1,25-Dihydroxyvitamin D				
(pmol/L)			48–100	
(pg/mL)			20–42	
24-Hour urinary calcium (mg/kg)	<2		>2	
Bone density (SD from mean)	>2.5	>2	1–1.5	

Data derived in part from Sauberlich HE. *Laboratory Tests for the Assessment of Nutritional Status.* 2nd ed. Boca Raton, FL: CRC Press, 1999. Estimates by some experts, based on the vitamin D level necessary to prevent secondary hyperparathyroidism, put the acceptable range as >80 nmol/L or >32 ng/mL (365).

problems with making the diagnosis of vitamin D deficiency, even when the same method was used (380). However, immunoassays usually provide values that are lower than those with liquid chromatography/tandem mass spectroscopy (LC-MS/MS) (381). Because of more widespread availability of this more sophisticated methodology, LC-MS/MS is now the method preferred by many experts (382).

Because assay variation confounds the diagnosis of vitamin D deficiency, there is a great need for standardization (380), and concerns have been raised about the inability of some 25(OH)D assays to measure 25(OH)D$_2$, when ergocalciferol is the supplement used. The international Vitamin D Quality Assessment Scheme has been established since 1989 (http://www.deqas.org), and there are now more than 100 participating laboratories in 18 countries (383). This group has compared values for 25(OH)D$_2$ obtained from the DiaSorin RIA, the IDS RIA, the IDS EIA, the competitive protein-binding assay, HPLC, and the Nichols automated chemiluminescence assay. Most commercial methods were found to give results close to the standard value, but results were highly operator dependent. Moreover, the Nichols method consistently produces higher values than the other methods. In the United States many commercial supplements have converted to the use of the 25(OH)D$_3$ form, making this source of variation somewhat less critical. A program has been developed to apply standard protocols to existing 25(OH)D ELISAs, using reference standards assessed by LC-MS/MS. The Vitamin D Standardization Program was established in 2010 to promote accurate and comparable measurements of 25(OH)D. This program involves using results from a comparison study to develop an equation that would convert values to the reference measurement. Such an approach has been used with success for the Irish National Adult Nutrition Survey (384). More than 90% of plasma 25(OH)D is derived from cholecalciferol produced by the skin. However, the production of this vitamin is not closely regulated—levels rise or fall as its precursor is made available. The mitochondrial 25-hydroxylase is not regulated by vitamin D, unlike the microsomal enzyme, which is regulated by its substrate. Concentration in plasma is 5 to 10 times greater than in other tissues, except for adipose tissue. 25(OH)D in plasma is bound to a protein that binds all metabolites and is less than 5% saturated. Finally, the plasma half-life of 25(OH)D is long (24 hours). Thus, the level reflects recent intake or exposure to sunlight, so that the sensitivity of this measurement in the assessment of vitamin D deficiency is limited.

The binding capacity of the plasma for excess 25(OH)D is very great, and levels rise as intake increases. Moreover, levels remain elevated for some time. Therefore, 25(OH)D levels reflect vitamin D intake or production only in a general way but do correlate with body stores until they become depleted. Levels of 25(OH)D are low in states of dietary deficiency, decreased absorption, deficiency of UV light, prematurity, and severe liver disease, and when drugs are ingested that alter its metabolism (e.g., anticonvulsants). Levels are low when plasma-binding capacity is decreased. Although levels are low in dark-skinned people, this is due to a lower plasma vitamin D-binding protein content (385). The free 25(OH)D levels and bone density content are normal in such peoples.

Levels are high in growing children, conditions associated with hyperparathyroidism, sarcoidosis, and certain forms of idiopathic hypercalciuria (386). Factors other than intake affect plasma levels of 25(OH)D. The amount of UV irradiation reaching the skin is dependent upon the intensity of sunlight, thickness of the ozone layer, and pigmentation of the skin. Thus, the 25(OH)D levels rise in summer and fall in winter. Pregnancy, ovulation, and the use of oral contraceptives increase the plasma level of vitamin D–binding protein. Because this protein is normally unsaturated, the capacity of the plasma to retain vitamin D metabolites is increased, not necessarily the steady-state levels of the metabolites. Despite these confounding factors, the 25(OH)D concentration is the best available test for determining vitamin D status. The level is almost always low when deficiency is present. The 25(OH)D level is an accurate parameter of vitamin D intoxication (levels above 150 ng per mL or 375 nmol per L) because the level rises progressively as intake is increased.

1,25-Dihydroxyvitamin D_3

The production of this vitamin is regulated, but not by vitamin D stores unless they are extremely low. The metabolite is assayed by HPLC or by RIA with use of a nuclear receptor. The normal concentration of 20 to 42 pg per mL (48 to 100 pmol per L) cannot be increased by feeding $1,25(OH)_2D_3$. Normal ranges differ with the age and calcium intake of the population studied. Fluctuations occur during the ovulation cycle and also diurnally. Levels are higher during periods of growth and decline during growth retardation. The serum concentration responds to calcium and phosphate levels and is part of the endocrine system of vitamin D metabolism. The production rate and concentration of this vitamin are altered rapidly and inversely by high (3 g per day) and low (0.5 g per day) intakes of phosphorus (387). The plasma half-life is 4 to 6 hours; hence the rapid functional changes. The level of this form of vitamin D correlates with certain functions of vitamin D but not with intake, absorption, or body stores until deficiency is apparent. Values of $25(OH)D_3$ fall in the winter and are lower in patients over 60 years of age.

Various conditions are associated with abnormal values. $1,25(OH)_2D_3$ levels are low in profound vitamin D deficiency, and in chronic renal disease (if serum phosphorus levels are high and renal enzyme activity is decreased despite elevated parathyroid hormone levels), hypoparathyroidism, vitamin D–resistant rickets type I, and osteolytic states not related to parathyroid hormone (cancer, hyperthyroidism, and possibly osteoporosis of the elderly). However, $1,25(OH)_2D_3$ levels do not always reflect total body stores. In primary biliary cirrhosis, this metabolite is not excreted in bile, so that synthesis is decreased and plasma levels are normal, yet malabsorption of vitamin D and osteopenia develop (388). Primary hyperparathyroidism, vitamin D–resistant rickets type II, and pregnancy are conditions in which $1,25(OH)_2D_3$ levels are elevated. In hypervitaminosis D, the $25(OH)D_3$ level is markedly elevated, but the $1,25(OH)_2D_3$ level is altered only slightly.

Twenty-Four-Hour Urinary Calcium Excretion

Because of problems with the interpretation or availability of vitamin D metabolite levels, the state of vitamin D repletion is often assessed by functional measurements. This is best accomplished in patients with a normal intestine by measuring the 24-hour urinary calcium excretion as an estimate of calcium absorption. At steady state, urinary calcium excretion equals net intestinal absorption. If no intestinal disease is present and the serum parathyroid hormone level is normal, calcium absorption depends in large part on the active vitamin D metabolites. Patients should be kept on a constant calcium intake of 800 to 1,200 mg per day for 4 to 5 days before a 24-hour urine sample is collected. Normal urinary calcium levels range from 100 to 300 mg (about 2 to 4 mg per kg of body weight). Although urinary calcium excretion may be useful when low, it is an insensitive measure of vitamin D status. In fact, at 25(OH)D concentrations from 40 to 130 nmol per L, calcium absorption rises without reaching a threshold (389). Thus, calcium excretion is not a useful measure for determining any degree of nutrient status other than deficiency.

Serum Alkaline Phosphatase

Serum alkaline phosphatase levels become elevated in osteomalacia secondary to vitamin D deficiency. However, the increase develops late in deficiency states, and elevations of phosphatase occur for a large number of other reasons. Thus, the usefulness of this test is limited. It is clear that the value of serum calcium, phosphate, and alkaline phosphatase are not reliable in detecting vitamin D deficiency, even when 25(OH)D levels were sufficiently low to elicit a response of elevated PTH levels (390).

Bone Densitometry

Single-photon absorptiometry of the forearm and os calcis is rapid (15 minutes) and relatively inexpensive. However, in patients under the age of 60 years, it does not assess risk for vertebral fracture. Computed tomography and dual-photon absorptiometry of the spine are better predictors of vertebral fracture (see section on assessment of calcium deficiency in Chapter 7). For patients at risk for vitamin D deficiency, these screening tests are very useful. Their role in screening postmenopausal women for osteoporosis is much less clear. 25(OH)D_3 levels vary directly with vertebral bone density in some studies of postmenopausal women (391). Thus, vitamin D deficiency may be more common than appreciated in this group of patients.

Physiology

Calcium and Phosphate Absorption

Calcium and phosphate absorption is increased by 1,25(OH)$_2$$D_3$ to maintain blood levels of calcium and phosphorus (392,393). Bone mineralization results because the plasma is supersaturated with both minerals. In addition, the vitamin mobilizes calcium (and phosphate) from bone and increases the renal reabsorption of calcium. A decline in calcium concentration leads to reduction of calcium binding to the calcium-sensing G-protein coupled transporter system found in the parathyroid gland (394). All these effects result in increased serum levels of calcium and phosphate and normal mineralization. Evidence for an independent effect of the vitamin (especially 25(OH)D) on bone mineralization is limited. 1,25(OH)$_2$D produced in the kidney under regulation by PTH plays an important role in mobilizing calcium from bone to maintain serum calcium and phosphorus levels within a normal range. PTH also binds to receptors on the osteoblast, stimulating increased bone turnover and calcium/phosphorus mobilization (395). Both PTH and 1,25(OH)$_2$$D_3$ enhance distal tubular calcium reabsorption, retaining most of the 7 g of calcium filtered each day.

Other Functions

Vitamin D improves muscle function and corrects decreased phosphate concentrations in muscle in deficiency states. Some vitamin D metabolites, especially 25(OH)D, may have a direct effect on bone to improve calcium deposition. Insertion of a 24-hydroxyl group into 1,25(OH)$_2$D reduces the affinity of the vitamin for the nuclear vitamin D receptor (VDR) and thus its classic activity. Other hydroxylations (C23 and C26) may lead to various selective activities on growth and differentiation via effects on the nuclear receptor.

The VDR contains two overlapping ligand binding sites. When the genomic pocket site (VDR-GP) is occupied by 1,25(OH)2D, it forms a heterodimer with the retinoid X receptor to bind vitamin D responsive elements (VDREs) that mediate gene transcription of functions controlling "traditional" roles, such as calcium and phosphate absorption (249a). Examples of such gene products include TRPV6 (calcium transport), LRP5 (bone anabolism), RANKL (bone resorption), PTH (calcium homeostasis), and FGF23 and klotho (renal phosphate reabsorption). Expression of CYP24A1 regulates 1,25(OH)2D detoxification, and CYP3A4 mediates xenobiotic detoxification. Occupancy of the alternative VDR binding site (VDR-AP) controls gene expression of rapid nongenomic responses and metabolic steps, some of which have been implicated in delaying chronic diseases, such as cancer, diabetes, and cardiovascular disease (396). Examples of rapid responses include an alternative route of calcium absorption, insulin secretion, smooth muscle cell migration, and opening of calcium and chloride channels in osteoblasts.

Vitamin D has been implicated in many general cellular functions, such as cell proliferation and myocardial function. 1,25(OH)$_2$$D_3$ downregulates hyperproliferative cell growth (349). Cancer cells have 1-hydroxylase activity, and low exposure to sunlight is associated with increased mortality from breast cancer. Vitamin D also induces 24-hydroxylase activity, which acts on 1,25(OH)$_2$$D_3$ to form the inert metabolite calcitroic acid. Other examples of vitamin D–induced gene regulation perhaps related to chronic disease include p21, p53, and FOX1 (cell cycle control), CBS (Hcy clearance), cathelicidin (innate immunity), IL-17 (adaptive immunity), NFκB and COX2 (inflammation), and FOXO3 (oxidative damage) (376). Demonstration of these genes in modifying autoimmunity, inflammation, neurodegenerative disorders of aging, or heart disease or cancer have been obtained in cell systems and/or animal models. Their translation to human disease is the subject of ongoing research and debate.

Regulation of phosphate reabsorption in the kidney is closely linked to the role of 1,25(OH)2D and its occupancy of the VDR. 1,25(OH)2D, along with phosphate and leptin, regulate FGF23 production in osteocytes as a phosphate regulator (397). Also regulated is production of α-klotho, a longevity factor and coreceptor for FGF23. FGF23 regulates 1,25(OH)D production by repressing CYP27B1 and inducing CYP24A1 to enhance degradation of the vitamin. 1,25(OH)2D also represses Npt2a/c, the phosphate transporter, thus enhancing phosphate excretion by the kidney. This 1,25(OH)2D/VDR-FGF23-klotho-CYP24A1-phosphate system for phosphate excretion balances the better known 1,25(OH)2D/VDR-PTH-CYP27B1-calcium system (397).

$1,25(OH)_2D_3$ is produced from the 1-hydroxylated intermediate (made in the liver) by the action of 25(OH)D-1 α-hydroxylase (CYP27B1), an enzyme that is present in many extrarenal sites (398). These sites include osteoblasts, colonocytes and other epithelial cells, macrophages, synovial cells, keratinocytes, pancreatic islets, and vascular endothelial cells. In these extrarenal sites, regulation is not tightly linked to $1,25(OH)_2D_3$ levels as it is in the kidney. Thus, the possibility exists for intracellular deficiency of the active $1,25(OH)_2D_3$, predisposing to multiple chronic diseases. Thus, patients with chronic renal or cardiac disease, cancer, diabetes, musculoskeletal disorders, or infectious, inflammatory, or autoimmune diseases in theory could be relatively deficient in vitamin D. See the section on vitamin D deficiency below for possible functions of vitamin D in specific disorders.

Metabolism

Vitamin D from the skin is bound to a plasma-binding protein, so that its uptake by the liver is limited. Dietary vitamin D is absorbed by incorporation into mixed micelles and enters very-low-density lipoproteins or chylomicrons, which are taken up by the liver. Thus, hepatic uptake is not limited by the plasma-binding protein, and toxic levels of metabolites can be reached after oral ingestion. The liver adds a 25-hydroxyl group, whereas the kidney adds hydroxyl groups at positions 1 and 24. Adipose tissue is the major storage site of vitamin D metabolites. Both $1,25(OH)_2D_3$ and other polar metabolites of vitamin D are excreted in bile and participate in an enterohepatic circulation, although the quantitative importance of this in humans is not clear. In deficiency of either calcium or phosphorus, the formation of $1,25(OH)_2D_3$ is increased. Parathyroid hormone, calcitonin, estrogens, prolactin, and growth hormone enhance the formation of active dihydroxyvitamin D. Many of these factors also regulate (reciprocally) the formation of $1,25(OH)_2D_3$, but some other metabolites are also functional. The production of $24,25(OH)_2D_3$ in the kidney is not closely regulated. The biologic importance of this metabolite is not established, but it may alleviate bone disease in uremic patients.

Deficiency

Several syndromes result from vitamin D deficiency, all related to decreased body stores of calcium or phosphorus. However, consideration of deficiency states depends upon the cutoff value used for serum 25(OH)D, the most reliable biomarker of vitamin D status. The IOM cutoff value of greater than 20 ng per mL (50 nmol per L) will cover the requirements of 97.5% of the population. The Endocrine Society's recommendations, however, suggest somewhat higher values (30 ng per mL, 75 nmol per L), a level that will take more supplementation to achieve (600 to 1,000 IU per day for children > 1 year and 1,000 to 2,000 IU per day for adults) (399). Although the data are still somewhat conflicting and controversial regarding the role of vitamin D in prevention/treatment of diseases not related to bone health, the concept of a subclinical state of relative vitamin D deficiency has been proposed (400). This state is, by definition, asymptomatic and defined by serum 25(OH)D concentrations, but the cutoff value to define this state is based in large part on association of the 25(OH)D levels with fractures and chronic disease states (401). Moreover, not all studies agree with this higher level. In an 11-year follow-up of the Cardiovascular Health Study, the threshold concentration associated with increased risk for relevant clinical disease events was approximately 20 ng per mL (50 nmol per L) (402).

Treating vitamin D deficiency, therefore, is not yet completely evidence-based for all levels of deficiency. Moreover, the results of interventions with vitamin D, calcium, or a combination of the two nutrients have been inconsistent, making recommendations for supplementation very complex and uncertain regarding subclinical vitamin D deficiency (403). We will discuss first those conditions generally agreed to require and respond to vitamin D (rickets, osteomalacia), followed by osteoporosis and the extraskeletal indications. In general, for every 100 IU of vitamin D ingested, serum 25(OH)D concentration increases by approximately 1 ng per L (~2.5 nmol per L) (404). The response is greater when the baseline values are lower. Thus, the chronic dose needed may not be the same for all persons. The evidence for many of the proposed uses in subclinical vitamin D deficiency has been reviewed (405).

Rickets

Rickets, the major deficiency syndrome, is caused by poor bone mineralization. The newborn infant is at high risk because the vitamin D content of unfortified milk (<1 μg per L) is low and 25-hydroxylase activity in the liver is not fully developed. The incidence seems to be increasing in children, most of whom do not ingest the recommended intake of vitamin D. Reasons for increased incidence in children in North America include dark pigmented skin, little exposure to sunlight, limited vitamin D supplementation, and breast-feeding as the only source of nutrition (379). A minimum of 400 IU of vitamin D per day has been recommended throughout childhood and adolescence to prevent rickets.

In rickets, or childhood osteomalacia, the calcification of newly formed bone and epiphyseal cartilage is decreased. Decreased amounts of calcium are deposited in the collagen elaborated by cartilage cells. Wide osteoid seams are found most often in the long bones because they grow the fastest. Craniotabes, chest deformity, bending of long bones, enlarged epiphyses of long bones, greenstick fractures, swollen wrists, muscle weakness, seizures, tetany, inability to initiate walking, and decreased growth are all noted. Serum calcium levels may be normal or low. The tetany associated with vitamin D deficiency results from hypocalcemia. Muscle weakness is probably caused by a decrease in muscle phosphate.

Adult Osteomalacia

Vitamin D deficiency (defined as 25(OH)D levels of less than 15 ng per mL (<37.5 nmol per L) affected 42% of African American women and only 4.2% of white women aged 15 to 49 years, in the NHANES III database (406). In adults, the endochondral growth of long bones has ceased; consequently, decreased calcification of cartilage is not a factor. Osteoblast-mediated mineralization is affected by vitamin D deficiency, but changes occur over a longer period of time, and the clinical presentation is not as fulminant as in children. Subclinical bone disease occurs with normal blood calcium levels. By the time bone disease has become severe, hypocalcemia and hypophosphatemia are often present. Skeletal pain and muscle weakness occur anywhere in the body, but the long bones are less affected than are bones in the shoulders, hips, and spine. Adult osteomalacia is associated with aging, renal disease (lack of 1-α-hydroxylase), severe hepatic disease (decreased 25-hydroxylase activity), and intestinal resection and celiac disease (decreased absorption); it is also seen after gastric surgery (possibly because of decreased uptake), in IBD (multifactorial), pancreatic insufficiency/cystic fibrosis (malabsorption due to steatorrhea with calcium–fatty acid complex formation), and after use of anticonvulsant medication (which may cause inactive metabolites to form) (407). Vitamin D–resistant rickets is the cause of osteomalacia in a few patients.

Malabsorption

Although "deficiency" of vitamin D is considered important in the pathogenesis of mucosal disease in IBD, benefit from vitamin D in prospective trials has been difficult to validate (408). The contribution of an interrupted enterohepatic circulation to vitamin D deficiency in malabsorption is probably small. Fewer than one-third of highly polar metabolites are excreted in bile, and virtually no 25(OH)D$_3$. It has been suggested that a loss of bile salts alters the hepatic metabolism of vitamin D and leads to the rapid half-life of the vitamin in malabsorption. During chronic liver disease, vitamin D is malabsorbed, and these patients also may have decreased sunlight exposure and dietary intake. Moreover, production of 25(OH)D may be decreased when hepatic function is severely impaired in cirrhotic patients (409). Supplementation of 1,000 to 2,000 IU (25 to 50 μg) per day is recommended for such patients, although higher doses may be required when malabsorption is the cause of deficiency. Patients with Crohn disease are more likely to have low bone mineral density than those with ulcerative colitis (410). This finding is probably related to many factors, including malabsorption, chronic inflammation, smoking, and chronic steroid use.

Involutional Osteoporosis

This disorder is defined by a low bone mass. Although vitamin D and calcium (e.g., via PTH and RANKL) are the primary nutrients involved, other vitamins (K, C, and B_6) also play a role in bone formation (411). Moreover, factors unrelated to vitamin regulation contribute to osteoclast function (e.g., Scr kinase, cathepsin K) and osteoblast function (e.g., Wnt/β-catenin pathway and its inhibitors dickkopf-1 and sclerostin) (412). Three etiologic categories of osteoporosis are recognized: early postmenopausal, late postmenopausal (after 70 years of age), and drug-induced. A decline in renal 1-α-hydroxylase activity with age may result in decreased calcium absorption and increased secretion of parathyroid hormone. Chronic vitamin D deficiency may be a factor in osteoporosis in elderly patients in nursing homes. In about 15% of elderly people, dietary intake is poor or outdoor activity is decreased. Vitamin D deficiency develops because of decreased skin production, decreased metabolism of vitamin D to the 1,25-dihydroxylated form, and decreased oral intake (413). Chronic abuse of alcohol is a frequently overlooked cause of osteoporosis in men (414). The cause(s) are probably multifactorial and include vitamin D deficiency. Chronic pancreatitis and small-bowel injury resulting from alcohol abuse may impair calcium and amino acid absorption. Elevated blood levels of cortisol and parathyroid hormone may contribute to bone destruction. Decreased intake of vitamin D, lack of sunlight, and altered vitamin D metabolism (in cirrhotics) are probably important. The hypomagnesemia seen in many alcoholics may play a role. Reversal of important factors in individual patients may retard the otherwise progressive bone loss.

Osteoporosis is the most common bone disease relevant to the DRIs for calcium and vitamin D, so screening for osteoporosis should be part of the evaluation of calcium and vitamin D intake in an attempt to prevent osteoporosis. The US Preventive Services Task Force (USPSTF) report recommended screening for women aged ≥ 65 years and in younger women with additional risk factors, using the Fracture Risk Assessment tool, FRAX, developed by the WHO (http://www.shef.ac.uk/FRAX) (415). FRAX estimates a 10 year risk for fracture, based on clinical information, age, BMI, parental fracture history, and tobacco and alcohol use. FRAX has been validated in many countries, but there is debate about whether it provides better prediction of osteoporotic fracture above that found with age and bone mineral density (BMD) alone (416). Also, FRAX is not widely available, although the calculation may become more available from downloadable apps.

The screening test used most for BMD is dual energy x-ray absorptiometry. Screening intervals are uncertain, but at least 2 years of follow-up are needed to see a significant change in BMD in most patients with age as the only risk factor (415). Once fractures or low BMD are detected, treatment is recommended. Because BMD is not the only factor associated with fracture risk, widespread use of BMD is not yet recommended beyond women *older than age 65*. However, patients with known previous fractures and/or secondary causes of osteoporosis (e.g., Crohn disease) or a BMD value consistent with osteoporosis (T score −2.5 or less) should be followed.

Deficiency in the Elderly and Hospitalized Patients

Oral vitamin D maintains vitamin D status less effectively than skin-derived vitamin D; with the latter, release is more constant and the rate of hepatic metabolism to less active isomers slower. Nevertheless, oral supplements are sometimes needed. Dietary deficiency still occurs, especially in hospitalized patients (417). The prevalence of vitamin D deficiency using a cutoff point of 20 ng per mL has increased markedly worldwide (418). Indications for supplementation also include breast feeding in infancy, fat malabsorption, advanced age, institutionalization (especially if the patient is not exposed to the sun), uremia, and long-term use of corticosteroids. Many forms of vitamin D are available. Some vitamin D products contain tartrazine, which may cause allergic reactions in susceptible persons. Use of 800 IU per day improved vitamin D levels to greater than 20 ng per mL in postmenopausal women (419). Although this treatment increases absorption of calcium at lower baseline levels of serum 25(OH)D, other factors in improving bone health may result from treatment (420).

Baseline serum 25(OH)D levels fall after 3 days in the ICU, and remain low (421). Although low vitamin D levels are not correlated with 28 day mortality in these patients, there was a suggestion that they were associated with higher infection rates. Moreover, those surviving patients with the highest 25(OH)D levels had a shorter time to ICU discharge.

Both vitamin D insufficiency and cognitive decline occur in the elderly population. Observational studies and a meta-analysis of RCTs suggested a possible effect of vitamin D supplements on the symptoms of depression and altered cognition, but the quality of the studies was limited (422). Two prospective studies showed that the relative risk of cognitive decline was 40% to 60% greater in adults with very low 25(OH)D levels (<25 nmol per L) compared with patients with sufficient levels ($\geq$ 75 nmol per L) (423). Longitudinal cognitive change has been correlated with polymorphisms in the VDR gene (424). Moreover, in patients with Parkinson's disease, vitamin D supplementation (1,200 IU per day for 1 year) showed that in patients more likely to have persisting vitamin D deficiency, disease outcome was worse, suggesting that low vitamin D status worsens disease progression (425). Also, there was evidence of interaction with VDR polymorphisms, suggesting that this might be a mechanism for a vitamin D effect. Clearly, when vitamin D deficiency (<20 ng per mL) or insufficiency (<30 ng per mL) is recognized in the elderly, vitamin D should be supplemented to increase the level. It remains to be seen if this will have a reproducible effect on cognition or other chronic neurological conditions.

Bone Health and Fractures

When taken with calcium, vitamin D increases serum 25(OH)D levels, minimizes bone loss observed on bone density testing, and may reduce the incidence of fractures (399). Calcium absorption is only about one-third of normal (10% vs. 33%) when vitamin D is deficient (426). An analysis of 137 studies (6 trials received special attention) was performed on behalf of the US Preventive Services Task Force, and concluded that for noninstitutionalized adults without a history of fractures there was insufficient evidence to assess the balance of the benefits and harms for primary prevention of fractures in premenopausal women or men (427). Thus, the Task Force recommends against daily supplementation with 400 IU (or less) of vitamin D and 1,000 mg (or less) of calcium. The Task Force relied on two systematic reviews and one meta-analysis, as well as the European DIPART (vitamin D Individual Patient Analysis of Randomized Trials), and a patient-level meta-analysis (428). The effect of vitamin D on BMD has been studied in 17 RCTs. At low doses (300 to 400 IU per day) no effect was found, but at doses of over 700 IU per day given with calcium (500 to 1,200 mg per day), bone loss in the lumbar spine and femoral neck was prevented. Fifteen RCTs in postmenopausal women and older men, using vitamin D doses of 300 to 800 IU per day, showed no reduction in fractures, although the effect was heterogeneous (427). An analysis of 11 RCTs with or without calcium showed reduction in the risk of fracture only at the highest vitamin D intake level (800 IU or greater), with a 30% reduction in fracture (429). These results were consistent with the IOM recommendation of 800 IU per day for persons over 65 years of age, but a vitamin D level of 24 ng per mL (60 nmol per L) may be needed for reducing the risk of fracture. As not all the studies used calcium supplementation, it is possible that the calcium-sparing effect of vitamin D may allow a lower calcium intake when vitamin D is provided in adequate amounts (430). It is still unclear whether higher doses of vitamin D and/or calcium might be useful in fracture prevention. The more conservative recommendation would be to identify patients who are deficient in vitamin D and provide adequate replacement to raise their 25(OH)D levels above 20 ng per mL, the level recommended by the IOM for bone health.

Muscle Function and Falls

Concentrations of 25(OH)D are lower in elderly patients with less handgrip strength, those who had recently fallen, or those who could not climb stairs or participate in outdoor activity (431). Muscle cells express a VDR, and the vitamin alters cellular metabolism via interaction with transcription factors and genes to alter calcium and phosphate uptake and cellular differentiation into mature muscle fibers. In addition, muscle cells in culture demonstrate rapid changes in calcium metabolism that cannot be explained by the slower effects on the genes. Fourteen RCTs evaluating the effect of vitamin D on falls in postmenopausal women and older men showed a small benefit, but the extent of the benefit was inconsistent between trials (427). In patients with symptomatic knee osteoarthritis, vitamin D supplementation improved the 25(OH)D levels to greater than 36 ng per mL, but did not reduce knee pain or loss of cartilage volume (432). Plasma concentrations of 25(OH)D decrease after an inflammatory insult such as primary knee arthroplasty, and so the level is not likely to be a reliable measure of vitamin D status in patients with a significant systemic inflammatory response (433). This caveat raises questions about the association of 25(OH)D levels in patients with chronic inflammatory conditions, such as cancer or cardiovascular/metabolic disorder.

Mortality

In 14 progressive cohort studies, a nonlinear decrease in mortality risk was associated with increasing 25(OH)D concentrations, with the optimal concentration reached at approximately 75 nmol per L (434). However, observational studies cannot prove whether vitamin D is a causative vector or just a marker of other underlying risk factors. A review of 24 RCTs of vitamin D supplementation found a 7% reduction in mortality when vitamin D was provided with calcium, but not alone (435). But the primary aim of the RCTs reviewed was not to assess mortality, so the possibility of a reporting bias exists in those trials that reported mortality as an endpoint (436).

Cancer

The theory that vitamin D can help to prevent cancer and other chronic diseases is biologically plausible. Data from observational studies suggested that for each 10 nmol per L increase in blood 25(OH)D concentration, there was a 6% reduced risk for CRC, but not for breast or prostate cancer (429). Among never smoking postmenopausal women, intake of more than 800 IU per day was associated with lower risk of lung adenocarcinoma (437). However, the three largest interventional trials found no clear indication of reduction of risk of cancer (438). Limited data from 3 RCTs suggest that higher dose supplementation (1,000 IU per day) might reduce the risk for total cancer. However, cancer risk was not the primary endpoint for these studies, and the ranges of 25(OH)D varied between studies. The largest study from the Women's Health Initiative used only 400 IU per day, and 8 years of follow-up may not have been long enough to detect enough new onset cases of CRC. Smaller intervention trials in various cancers have provided inconsistent results (439). It is possible that the doses shown to be effective in cell cultures cannot be achieved in vivo in the tumor cells themselves, and that targeted delivery of vitamin D may be needed. Nonetheless, the hypothesis that vitamin D prevents cancer has yet to be proven. It is sensible to maintain adequate levels of vitamin D in adults and in elderly patients without being able to recommend this policy for cancer prevention based on current evidence. The issue then becomes one of determining an "adequate" vitamin D level, whether the current DRI values (Table 6-35) or the higher ones currently suggested by some experts.

Cardiovascular Disease (CVD)

In epidemiological studies low levels of 25(OH)D are associated with an increased risk of CVD and mortality (440). Low vitamin D levels have been associated with many individual CVD risk factors, such as hypertension, diabetes, and metabolic syndrome (441). A stronger association was found with studies with less than 10 years of follow-up, and the whole range of 25(OH)D concentrations has not been noted in the observational studies to conclude that higher levels are protective (442). Prospective trials of vitamin D supplementation have not shown a significant effect on hypertension, CV outcomes, or diabetes risk or control (443). Doses of vitamin D varied widely from 400 to greater than 5,000 IU per day. Moreover, five trials of vitamin D plus calcium intervention showed no significant decrease in CVD risk (444). One RCT of paricalcitol (1α-24(OH)2-19-nor-D_3, Zemplar™) for 48 weeks found no effect on left ventricular mass index or diastolic function in patients with chronic renal disease (445). In healthy obese patients in a voluntary weight loss program, supplemental vitamin D at 83 μg per day did lower PTH and TNF-α levels, both of which are CVD risk factors (446).

Most of the evidence supporting a role for vitamin D in CVD comes from laboratory or observational studies. A role for comorbid conditions such as obesity or behavioral factors cannot be excluded. Moreover, as in the case of cancer, it may be the intracellular concentration of the vitamin that determines the biological role, not the serum concentration of the precursor, 25(OH)D. Biological plausibility is supported by the fact that 1,25(OH)2D does inhibit vascular smooth muscle cell proliferation, regulates the renin–angiotensin system, and exhibits anti-inflammatory properties. However, no large-scale studies have been performed with CVD as the primary endpoint. The current evidence is not sufficient to support a recommendation for CVD prevention.

Diabetes Mellitus

Observational studies have found an association between lower serum 25(OH)D concentrations and obesity-related chronic diseases, including diabetes mellitus, and metabolic syndrome (447). Vitamin D concentration was inversely associated with HbA1c levels in US adults in one study (448). In another study, however, 25(OH)D concentrations did not vary with insulin sensitivity, or with blood glucose levels, when matched for degree of obesity (449). In one RCT using high-dose replacement (4,000 IU) in diabetic patients with deficiency of vitamin D (mean baseline 25(OH)D levels of 21 nmol per L), improvement was seen in calculated insulin resistance (HOMA) but not in insulin secretion (450). In another RCT of deficient patients, supplementation with 500 IU per day improved glycemic status (451). Supplementation of 2,000 IU to sufficient diabetic patients improved insulin secretion, with no effect on HbA1c levels (452). The data suggest that vitamin D deficiency should be treated when recognized, but it is not clear whether there is a therapeutic role for vitamin D supplementation in the management of diabetes mellitus.

Liver Disease

The immune regulation mediated potentially by vitamin D includes induction of antimicrobial peptides, suppression of the innate immune response, induction of Th2 cytokines, and stimulation of T regulatory cells (453). Prospective trials of vitamin D supplementation suggest improved efficacy of interferon plus ribavirin for hepatitis C response. One trial shows that 25(OH)D can suppress hepatitis C viral assembly. Higher 25(OH)D concentrations are associated with less inflammation and liver fibrosis in patients with hepatitis C (454), but lower concentrations are associated with patients who have nonalcoholic fatty liver disease (455). It is not clear whether these changes are related to disease severity or are causative. One suggestion that there might be a causal relationship is the observation that vitamin D concentration was inversely associated (in a single study) with elevated serum alanine aminotransferase levels (456). The available studies are too few to make any conclusions at this time.

Lung Disease

Vitamin D deficiency has been linked to an accelerated decline in lung function, owing to increased inflammation and reduced immunity in chronic lung diseases (457). However, supplementation with 100,000 IU of vitamin D every 4 weeks for a year did not reduce exacerbations of COPD (458). Nor did large doses of vitamin D improve response to treatment for tuberculosis (459). Whether vitamin D in pharmacological doses has a role in chronic lung disease is not clear.

Vitamin D Preparations

Cholecalciferol (Vitamin D3). Cholecalciferol (Vitamin D_3) is the natural form of the mammalian vitamin. In the past it was not the major source available in supplements in the United States, but now it is the form routinely added to multivitamin and to vitamin D + calcium preparations. This is the most effective form of vitamin D to elevate the serum $25(OH)D_3$ level (460), as it is more efficient than ergocalciferol (vitamin D_2) (358). The best source of cholecalciferol as a single ingredient is BioTech Pharmacal, Inc., an FDA-approved source that makes capsules of 1,000, 5,000, and 50,000 IU (Table 6-38). Many health food stores sell capsules from other providers of 1,000 IU. Many more preparations can be expected to contain 1,000 or 2,000 IU of cholecalciferol as the publicity for increasing vitamin D intake increases. 2,000 IU per day will ensure that approximately 80% of Americans will achieve a vitamin D level of approximately 35 ng per mL or higher without toxicity (461). For breast-fed children, a safe and inexpensive preparation containing vitamin D is Tri-Vi-Sol. An appropriate mixture of preparations might be one multivitamin containing 400 IU of cholecalciferol and one vitamin D supplement containing 400 to 1,000 IU of cholecalciferol (349). Taking too many multivitamin tablets would lead to excessive vitamin A being ingested (>5,000 IU of

TABLE 6-38 Available Forms of Vitamin D and its Metabolites

Compound Name	Generic Name	Commercial Name	Daily Dose (µg)
Activated 7-dehydrocholesterol cholecalciferol	Vitamin D		10–50
(5Z,7E,22E)-(3S)-9, 10-ergosta-5,7,10(19), 22-tetraen-3-ol	Ergocalciferol	Drisdol, Calciferol	5–25
10,19-dihydrotachysterol	Dihydrotachysterol	Hytakerol[b]	125–1,000
$1\alpha,25(OH)_2D_3$	Calcitriol	Rocaltrol[b]	0.5–1.0
$1\alpha,25(OH)_2D$	Calcitriol	Calcijex (IV)[b]	0.5 (IV)
$1\alpha(OH)D_2$	Doxercalciferol	Hectorol[b]	10, 3×/week
$1\alpha(OH)D_3$	Alfacalcidol	One-alfa, Alpha-D_3[a]	0.25–1.0
$1\alpha,24(OH)_2$-19-nor-D_3	Paricalcitol	Zemplar[b]	2.8–7 qod
$1\alpha,24(OH)_2D_3$	Tacalcitol	Bonalfa[a,c]+	40–80 (topical)
$1\alpha,24S(OH)_2$-22-ene-24-cyclopropyl-D_3	Calcipotriene	Dovonex[c]	40–80 (topical)

[a]Available in Japan (Onealfa, Bonalfa), in Denmark (One-alfa), and Israel (Alpha-D_3), but not in the United States.
[b]Indicated for renal osteodystrophy, or for renal osteodystrophy with secondary hyperparathyroidism (Zemplar).
[c]Indicated for plaque psoriasis.

all-*trans*-retinol per tablet). Vitamin A antagonizes the actions of vitamin D in some way and the vitamin A content in one serving of liver (10,000 to 20,000 IU) can antagonize the rapid calcium response (nongene mediated) to vitamin D in humans (462). The fastest way to replete a patient with vitamin D deficiency and normal intestinal absorption is to give 50,000 IU of cholecalciferol once a week for up to 8 weeks, checking to ensure that the serum vitamin D level exceeds 35 ng per mL (349).

Vitamin D2 (Ergosterol, Ergocalciferol). Vitamin D_2 is available in large doses of 600 or 1,200 µg (25,000 or 50,000 IU per capsule) for daily replacement. These large doses are used for patients with refractory rickets or malabsorption. In liquid form, ergosterol is available solubilized with polysorbate 80 or polyethylene glycol at a concentration of 200 µg (8,000 IU) per milliliter (Drisdol, Sanofi Winthrop Pharm; Calciferol, Schwarz Pharma). These preparations contain 200 IU (5 µg) per drop, if it is assumed that a milliliter contains 40 drops. The liquid form, which is adequate for most needs, provides the greatest flexibility.

Dihydrotachysterol. Dihydrotachysterol (DHT), a vitamin D_2 derivative that is active without 1-α-hydroxylation, is available in tablets or capsules of 0.125 mg, and in tablets of 0.2 or 0.4 mg and in oral solution (0.2 mg per mL). It is used to treat postoperative tetany; 1 mg is equivalent to 3 mg of vitamin D_2.

1,25-Dihydroxyvitamin D_3 (Calcitriol). $1,25(OH)_2D_3$ (Calcitriol) is marketed as 0.25- and 0.5-µg tablets, in oral solution of 1 µg per mL, and in injectable (IV) form (1 or 2 µg per mL). The usual IV dosage is 0.01 to 0.05 µg per kg 3 times per week. This form is indicated for renal osteodystrophy with hypocalcemia. It is most often given to patients undergoing renal dialysis, for whom such frequent IV dosing is possible. This form of vitamin D does not alter serum levels of 25(OH)D or $1,25(OH)_2D$, so repletion should be monitored by measurement of serum or 24-hour urinary calcium. Daily oral requirements are met by 0.5 to 1.0 µg per day, with indications for renal osteodystrophy, hyperparathyroidism and associated hypocalcemia, and postmenopausal osteoporosis.

No good information exists to estimate dose when malabsorption is present. To avoid toxicity, serum and urinary calcium levels should be followed, although toxicity is unlikely in the presence of malabsorption. Although $1,25(OH)_2D_3$ is more water-soluble than the parent compound and does not require incorporation into bile acid micelles for solubility, its advantages in the treatment of malabsorption have yet to be demonstrated, and it is more expensive. Its use should be confined mostly to patients who cannot form $1,25(OH)_2D_3$ (e.g., those with renal failure) when the aim is rapid reversal of hypocalcemia. It is often used to induce the mild hypercalcemia required to offset excess calcium secretion in renal failure. $1,25(OH)_2D_3$ is degraded in the gut (463). Thus, the oral drug is not delivered to tissues as efficiently as the IV drug. Parenteral calcitriol is available for IV use. It is used to normalize plasma ionized calcium in some uremic patients. The recommended dose is 1 to 2 µg 2 to 3 times weekly in predialysis patients greater than 3 years of age. Parenteral use suppresses parathyroid hormone levels more effectively than oral dosing. This formulation is not suitable for replacement of vitamin D in deficient patients.

25-Hydroxyvitamin D_3 (Calcifediol, Calderol). $25(OH)D_3$ (calcifediol, Calderol) is no longer available, as the product has been discontinued by West Orange, Organon (NJ). The rationale for this decision was likely that maintenance of $25(OH)D$ levels is achieved as well by providing cholecalciferol that is now more regularly available.

Synthetic Analogues. Other analogues (Table 6-38) have been synthesized primarily for the indication of renal osteodystrophy, as the active vitamin, $1,25(OH)_2D_3$, cannot be made by patients with this condition. Paricalcitol (Zemplar) decreases PTH in patients with ESRD, without an effect on serum calcium or phosphate levels (464,465). Moreover, the drug improved survival from cardiovascular and infectious causes of death. The rationale for improvement in cardiovascular disease, based on cell system and animal in vivo data, includes anti-inflammation, protection against blood vessel injury, inhibition of cardiac hypertrophy, and regulation of the renin-angiotensin system (466). Paricalcitol is available as a parenteral preparation, given at doses from 0.04 to 1 µg every other day. Paricalcitol and doxercalciferol (Hectorol) are available in the United States. Other analogues (tacalcitol, alfalcalcidol) are available only in Japan (Table 6-38). The value of these preparations over calcitriol is not clear, although they have been designed to produce less hypercalcemia.

Toxicity

Hypervitaminosis D occurs because the plasma-binding capacity for $25(OH)D_3$ is relatively unlimited. Although serum $1,25(OH)_2D$ concentrations are regulated by calcium levels, $25(OH)D$ levels are not. Because $25(OH)D_3$ itself has physiologic effects, albeit less potent than those of $1,25(OH)_2D$, hypercalcemia and hypercalciuria can ensue. Toxicity is caused by excessive oral ingestion rather than UV irradiation because skin production of the active vitamin is limited to 15% to 20% of the provitamin content per day. In trials of vitamin D supplementation doses from 400 to 4,000 IU per day did not produce any significant symptoms of toxicity (427). Total body sun exposure potentially provides up to the equivalent of 250 µg (10,000 IU) of vitamin D per day (467). A UL of 100 µg per day has been recommended for adults (370).

Acute hypercalcemia causes nausea, anorexia, itching, polyuria, abdominal pain, constipation, bone pain, metallic taste, and dehydration. In chronic cases, nephrocalcinosis, metastatic calcification, renal failure, and kidney stones may develop. Weight loss, irritability, psychosis, pancreatitis, photophobia, hypertension, cardiac arrhythmias, and elevated levels of blood urea nitrogen, cholesterol, aspartate aminotransferase, and alanine aminotransferase have been reported. For treatment, prednisone, diuresis, and a low calcium diet may be required, along with withdrawal of vitamin D. Periodic measurement of $25(OH)D$ is essential, as levels below 140 nmol per L are not associated with adverse effects (467). The 24-hour urine calcium excretion provides a functional assay because it reflects excessive absorption of calcium. If this method is used to assess vitamin D toxicity, measurement should be frequent, perhaps monthly, during the initiation of therapy if malabsorption is not the cause of deficiency, and should be repeated every 3 to 6 months for patients on long-term replacement. The product of serum calcium and phosphate ($CA \times P$) should not exceed 70 to prevent precipitation of calcium phosphate.

Vitamin E

Requirement

Chemical Forms

It is not possible to determine vitamin E requirements accurately for several reasons: (a) the vitamin is heterogeneous chemically; (b) the requirements depend on the intake of natural oxidants, such as polyunsaturated fatty acids (PUFAs) and selenium; and (c) evidence of vitamin E deficiency develops uncommonly (468). The term *vitamin E* refers to all tocopherols showing biologic activity of D-α-tocopherol. The natural vitamin E produced by plants includes at least eight different forms (α, β, γ, and δ plus the corresponding tocotrienols). Tocopherols contain a phytyl tail with three places where they could be either L or R isomers. D-α-tocopherol is now called *RRR*-α-tocopherol to designate the orientation of the three chiral centers in the molecule (469). The synthetic form contains eight stereoisomers in equal amounts, and so is called *all-rac*-α-tocopherol acetate (all racemers). It is the form used in food fortification. In mixed diets, the non–α-tocopherols account for about 20% of the total activity, although they are less potent than α-tocopherol. γ-Tocopherol is the major form of vitamin E in the US diet (470). It is a more effective trap for lipophilic electrophiles than is the α isomer, but it is largely metabolized and does not accumulate. The γ form and its major metabolite inhibit cyclo-oxygenase activity. There is no evidence that α-tocopherol supplements can block the antioxidant effect of vitamin E in food, but it is not known whether the pro-oxidant effect of α-tocopherol has any biological importance (471).

One IU of vitamin E equals 1 mg of DL-α-tocopherol acetate. The natural form of the vitamin, D-α-tocopherol, has a biopotency of 1.36 IU (acetate) and 1.21 IU (succinate). Commercial vitamin E is made from a mixture of many stereoisomeric synthetic forms of α-tocopherol acetate or succinate. The synthetic DL-α-tocopherol succinate has a potency of 1.49 IU. The requirement for vitamin E increases as PUFA intake increases, but dietary fats also contain vitamin E, so that dietary deficiency is unlikely. About 0.4 to 0.8 mg of vitamin is needed for each gram of PUFA, and possibly more than 1.5 mg per g in diets containing high numbers of long-chain PUFAs. Variability in requirement can be related both to dietary PUFA intake and to tissue composition, depending on prior dietary habits.

Dietary Reference Intake

The RDA was based previously on assumptions of a diet containing no more than 0.1 parts per million of selenium, average amounts of sulfur amino acids, 0.4 mg of vitamin E for each gram of PUFA, and less than 1.5% linoleic acid in 1,800 to 3,000 kcal. Current recommendations take into consideration the possible role of vitamin E as an antioxidant in preventing chronic disease and the increased intake of PUFAs in the US diet, in addition to serum vitamin E concentrations from NHANES III. However, these levels were not corrected for serum lipid or cholesterol, which might exaggerate the prevalence of low vitamin E body stores. The new DRIs are set at levels about 50% higher than the RDAs of 1989 (Table 6-39). Cigarette smoke alters the human vitamin E requirement by leading to faster formation of a major metabolite (472). The hepatic enzymes involved in this metabolism are not known.

Food Sources

Vitamin E is found in lipids of green leafy plants and in oils or seeds. Animal sources derive most of the vitamin from alfalfa, corn, and soybean foods. The richest sources for humans are salad oils, shortenings, and margarines, especially those derived from soybean, cottonseed, peanut, corn, and safflower oils, and wheat germ and nuts. Some of these oils contain more γ-tocopherol than α-tocopherol. Animal sources containing the highest amounts include eggs, liver, and muscle meats.

Vitamin E Content in Foods

Vitamin E content in foods (Table 6-40) is greatly affected by processing, storage, and preparation, especially if cooking in oil is followed by storage. Freezing does not prevent peroxide formation and the destruction of biologic activity. Many foods (e.g., milk) show a seasonal variation in vitamin E content, which is highest in summer. A 2,000- to 3,000-kcal diet in the United States contains 8 to 11 mg equivalents of tocopherol, just barely sufficient for the average adult.

TABLE 6-39 Dietary Reference Intakes for Vitamin E[a]

Life Stage Group	Vitamin E (mg/day)
Infants[b]	
0–6 months	4
7–12 months	6
Children	
1–3 years	6
4–8 years	7
Adults (M/F)	
9–13 years	11
14–>70 years	15
Pregnancy	
≤18–50 years	15
Lactation	
≤18–50 years	19

[a]Values refer to α-tocopherol forms occurring naturally, and to the synthetic isomers with comparable biologic activity that occur in fortified foods and supplements.
[b]Estimate based on adequate intake (AI). Other values based on recommended dietary allowance (RDA).
Data from Standing Committee on the Scientific Evaluation of Dietary Reference Intakes, Food and Nutrition Board, Institute of Medicine. *Dietary Reference Intakes for Vitamin C, Vitamin E, Selenium, and Beta-Carotene and Other Carotenoids*. Washington, DC: National Academies Press, 2000.

An extensive summary of the food content of vitamin E has been published (473). Nuts are high in fat, but are an excellent source of α-tocopherol, as well as monounsaturated fatty acid, squalene, and phytosterols (474).

Ratio of Vitamin E to PUFAs

The ratio of vitamin E to PUFAs is lower in vegetable oils than in animal products, and the proportion of non–α-tocopherols is often much greater. Olive oil, however, contains much less vitamin E than other vegetable oils (475). Its ability to retard LDL oxidation is attributed to polyphenol compounds. Fish oils are higher in PUFAs but lower in vitamin E; fortunately, the vitamin is ubiquitous in foods. The tocopherol–linoleic acid ratio in milk is 0.79 mg per g, more than the 0.5 mg per g recommended for newborns. Tocopherol levels are higher in colostrum than in milk.

Intake

Median intake in the United States is less than the RDA, 7.3 and 5.4 mg per day in men and women, respectively (NHANES II), and only about half of the current DRI for adults over the age of 19 years. Data from NHANES 1999–2000 showed that the use of vitamin E supplements ≥400 IU per day was common (476). Increased use of supplements is occurring more widely in the world, and both men and women appear to take vitamin E supplements (477). NHANES III data show that serum concentrations of vitamin E are below 20 µmol per L (low normal) in 20% of whites and 41% of African Americans (478). The vitamin E–PUFA ratio is more than 0.4 mg per g, which is acceptable. About 20% of intake is derived from fruits and vegetables and 20% from fats and oils. Fortunately, most foods high in vitamin E are also high in PUFAs.

Assessment

No measures are available that reflect recent intake because absorption is poor and the tocopherols are carried as part of the lipoprotein complex. Thus, all available assays correlate with body stores (Table 6-41).

Erythrocyte Hemolysis

Serum tocopherol levels and the erythrocyte hemolysis test correlate well, but the latter is a functional assay. It is based on the ability of hydrogen peroxide to liberate hemoglobin from red cells. In

TABLE 6-40	Approximate Vitamin E Content of Selected Foods	
Food	β-Tocopherol (mg/100 g)	Non-β-Tocopherol (mg/100 g)
Grains		
Bread		
White	0.1	0.13
Whole wheat	0.45	1.75
Oatmeal	2.27	1.7
Meat		
Bacon	0.53	0.06
Beef	0.3	0.3
Beef liver	0.6	1.0
Chicken	0.4	1
Pork chops, fried	0.16	0.44
Salmon	1.35	0.46
Shrimp	0.6	6
Vegetables		
Carrots	0.11	0.1
Celery	0.38	0.19
Onion	0.22	0.12
Peas		
Fresh	0.55	1.2
Frozen	0.23	0.4
Canned	0.02	0.02
Peanuts	7	5
Potatoes, French fried	0.3	1
Fruits		
Apple	0.31	0.2
Banana	0.22	0.2
Orange juice	0.04	0.16
Dairy		
Milk, whole	0.036	0.057
Butter	1	0
Margarine	13	48
Eggs	0.46	1
Fats		
Corn oil	12	53
Olive oil	4	—
Peanut oil	19	14
Safflower oil	34	7
Sesame oil	—	53
Soybean oil	10	85

the absence of the natural antioxidant, vitamin E, the reaction proceeds more rapidly. Erythrocyte hemolysis above 10% or a serum α-tocopherol level below 0.5 mg per dL is often associated with vitamin E deficiency. The test result is affected by circulating PUFA levels, and is positive only at very low serum levels of vitamin E. Unfortunately, it is not clear that this assay (or serum tocopherol itself) indicates α-tocopherol status in body tissues other than blood, especially the major storage pool in adipose tissue. Thus, the exact usefulness of this test has not yet been determined.

Serum Vitamin E

The vitamin E levels of infants and children are lower than those of adults, in fact below 0.5 μg per mL. Therefore, both serum α-tocopherol levels and the erythrocyte hemolysis test should be

TABLE 6-41 Guidelines for Interpreting Vitamin E Status

Test	Vitamin E Status Category		
	Deficient	Low	Acceptable
Plasma α-tocopherol			
µmol/L	<11.6	11.6–16.2	≥16.2
µg/ml	<5.0	5.0–7.0	≥7.0
Erythrocyte hemolysis (%)	>20	10–20	≤10
α-Tocopherol/lipid ratios			
Plasma α-tocopherol/total lipid (µg/mg)			$>0.8 \times 10^{-3}$
Plasma α-tocopherol/cholesterol (µg/mg)			$>2.22 \times 10^{-3}$
Serum/plasma α-tocopherol (µmol/L)			≥11.6

Data from Sauberlich HE. *Laboratory tests for the assessment of nutritional status*, 2nd ed. Boca Raton, FL: CRC Press, 1999.

performed to see whether both suggest a deficiency state. Earlier methods for assessing vitamin E levels have been largely replaced by HPLC procedures (32). The levels are highly correlated with total lipid, and the ratio of vitamin E to total lipid is considered a better indicator of vitamin E stores. This is because vitamin E is carried in plasma exclusively on lipoproteins. Thus, in hypolipidemic states (e.g., malabsorption), vitamin E levels are characteristically low. Premature infants are at special risk for vitamin E deficiency because their levels fall after birth. The ratio of α-tocopherol to cholesterol is the one most conveniently obtained (479). All the samples must be taken in a fasting state, and total lipids can be the sum of triglyceride and cholesterol because the phospholipid concentrations are much lower.

Tissue Damage in Vitamin E Deficiency
End-organ damage is more common than once thought, but detection requires sophisticated techniques in some instances. Neurologic examination may disclose ataxia or peripheral neuropathy. Examination of the fundus may reveal retinal pigment degeneration, and examination of the visual fields can disclose central scotomata. The electroretinogram shows delayed and reduced potentials. Sensory evoked potentials are delayed in the lower limb.

Breath Ethane and Pentane
Ethane and pentane are generated though peroxidation of n-3 and n-6 fatty acids, respectively. Breath ethane has been used to evaluate vitamin E status in children, in whom it correlates negatively with vitamin E serum levels. This test may be useful to screen children and assess response to therapy (480). High doses of vitamin E decrease breath pentane in heavy smokers. A modification of the method uses purified air, which avoids the problem that ambient air contains considerable amounts of ethane (481). Breath pentane and ethane levels are also elevated in vitamin C deficiency, β-carotene deficiency, and low glutathione levels.

Physiology
Function
Vitamin E is localized in membranes and provides a defense against lipid peroxidation of PUFAs. Selenium in glutathione peroxidase is located in the cytosol and provides another defense system. Other antioxidant defense mechanisms include the enzymes catalase, glucose-6-phosphate dehydrogenase, and glutathione reductase; the plasma proteins ceruloplasmin and transferrin; sulfhydryl-containing amino acids; and zinc, copper, and riboflavin. Vitamin E protects the membranes of intracellular organelles from damage. If all the peroxide formed by superoxide dismutase is not destroyed, then singlet oxygen is formed in the presence of ferric ions. Vitamin E acts to destroy these peroxides, which promote peroxidation of LDL in the subendothelial space. Oxidized LDL in turn can induce cytokine production in endothelial cells, which leads

to recruitment of macrophages, proliferation of smooth muscle, vasoconstriction, and platelet aggregation. Vitamin E delays these effects, providing a theoretical basis for a role in preventing cardiovascular disease (482).

Platelet adhesion is impaired by an antioxidant-independent action of vitamin E, although a daily dose of 400 IU is required to show an effect *in vivo*. Fewer platelet pseudopods are produced during vitamin E-induced inhibition of protein kinase C (483), which is likely to be the basis of the effect of the vitamin in ischemic damage and the rationale for conjoint therapy with inhibitors of platelet aggregation.

Absorption

Absorption requires biliary (bile salt micelles) and pancreatic (esterase) secretions. Less than 40% of an oral dose is absorbed, and this amount is decreased by excess unsaturated fatty acids in the lumen. The natural form ingested is D-α-tocopherol acetate, which must be hydrolyzed in the intestine by a bile salt-dependent pancreatic esterase. Esterases on the brush border membrane of the enterocyte can also hydrolyze tocopherol esters, and γ-tocopherol esters in food are similarly handled (484). Vitamin E forms are secreted with chylomicrons or HDL particles via an ATP-binding cassette A1. Mostly free α-tocopherol is found in the intestinal lymph. In serum, two-thirds of the vitamin is bound to and hydrolyzed on LDL, and the remnants are transferred to HDL (485). Some vitamin is transferred to extrahepatic tissues (adipose and muscle), with the rest taken up by the liver via three receptors, for LDL, for the LDL-related protein, and by the scavenger receptor B type II (SR-B1). Absorption is inefficient; 70% absorption requires 6 to 7 hours. The ratio of RRR-α-tocopherol absorption from the free form or from esters is relatively consistent, with a ratio of approximately 1.0, although the absolute absorption is quite variable (486). Cmax in plasma does not occur until 12 hours, and peak concentrations in red cells are further delayed (27 h). One study showed that vitamin E bioavailability was greater from fortified cereal than from encapsulated vitamin taken as a supplement (487). No carrier is specific for vitamin E; therefore, its serum level is proportional to the total lipid level. The percentage of vitamin E that is absorbed decreases at doses above 30 mg because the vitamin is passively absorbed. Most is deposited initially in liver as lipoprotein lipase acts on lipoproteins, and vitamin E is then distributed to adipose tissue. The α-tocopherol transfer protein in hepatic and cardiac cytosol transfers the vitamin to mitochondria, but the mechanism of transfer is not known (485). Plasma and tissue α-tocopherol are exchanged rapidly. Excess vitamin E is excreted in bile or metabolized by β- or ω-oxidation by P450-dependent hydroxylases. The vitamin is excreted largely in feces, where it is mostly degraded (488). It is not known whether an enterohepatic circulation exists or whether all fecal vitamin derives from oral sources. Less than 1% is excreted in urine.

Antioxidant Theory

The theory that a relative deficiency of antioxidant molecules (especially vitamins A/carotenoids, C, and E) is a factor in production of cancer and other chronic diseases (diabetes, cardiovascular, cataracts, etc.) has driven much of the use of vitamin supplements. Because vitamin E is the vitamin most often associated with this theory, the concept will be discussed here (see sections on vitamins A and C and Chapter 15 for other implications of this theory). The theory has been supported largely by experimental studies in animals, and by cell culture data. The animal data are conflicting. Genetic manipulation of the antioxidant defense system components in mice has not prolonged lifespan, but when transgenic/knockout animals are used with models of age-related pathology (e.g., diabetes, chronic inflammation), alterations in disease progression or severity have been found, consistent with the antioxidant theory (489). The concept has arisen that antioxidants may play a role under the right environmental background of chronic "stress." In humans epidemiologic cohort and some longitudinal studies have shown inverse correlations between chronic disease and vitamin intake and/or serum levels. The strongest evidence links specific foods (fruits, vegetables, whole grains) to decreased risk of certain cancers (490). These results have led to the current dietary recommendations to prevent cancer (see also Table 15-1).

Among the groups of fruits and vegetables found to be associated with a lower incidence of chronic diseases, the cruciferous (i.e., brassica) and green leafy vegetables have shown more effect than for specific nutrients such as antioxidants. The brassica group includes broccoli, cauliflower, kale, Brussels sprouts, cabbage, and bok choi. In addition to showing a protective relationship against epithelial cancers in cross-sectional studies, the same protection has now been demonstrated for lymphoma (491). Perhaps one reason for the failure of individual antioxidants is that they might be the wrong component of cruciferous vegetables. Glucosinolates and glucarates are other components that show anticarcinogenic activity. These components activate "phase 1" and "phase 2" enzyme systems that degrade carcinogens and other toxins (492). Another finding that suggests that factors other than antioxidants might be active ingredients is that there is great variation in the antioxidant content of food products (493).

Another potential confounder to assessing the role of antioxidant vitamins is the large number of natural compounds identified in foods with potential activity for cancer treatment and prevention (494). These include tubulin-binding agents (e.g., taxanes), topoisomerase inhibitors (e.g., camptothecins), and plant products (e.g., flavones, glucans, lycopenes). Many "nutraceuticals" contain some of these products, and these are ingested along with supplemental vitamins, possibly confounding retrospective epidemiologic studies of vitamin ingestion and risk of cancer or chronic disease.

More convincingly, the addition of supplements in double-blind RCTs has not confirmed the antioxidant theory. Most studies used a combination of antioxidant vitamins (E, C, β-carotene) plus selenium and/or zinc, so the role of each component cannot be judged. Many reasons have been given for these negative results, including the use of monotherapy when multiple factors are involved, the time lag to develop chronic disease, the use of older adults as the populations for these studies, and the use of nutritionally repleted subjects. Nonetheless, it is possible that too much has been expected from the antioxidant theory, and that vitamin supplementation on an individual patient level has little to recommend it other than ensuring adequate nutritional status, a worthwhile goal in itself. The antioxidant theory has been questioned for lipoprotein oxidation in cardiovascular disease (495). That the relationship of antioxidant to chronic disease is still an unproven theory needs to be kept in mind when reviewing the data (see below) and deciding on intervention with supplements.

Deficiency

Persons at Risk

Persons at risk include newborns and premature infants, food faddists, and patients with fat malabsorption or biliary obstruction. Vitamin E crosses the placenta poorly, and adipose tissue stores are small in the fetus *in utero*. The antioxidant properties of the vitamin cannot explain all manifestations of the uncommon deficiency state. Moreover, in most cases, no symptoms have been noted that respond to vitamin E when serum α-tocopherol levels are low. Low serum concentrations of vitamin E, ranging from 0.5% to 24%, were found in a variety of populations, but these were not correlated with serum lipid content, and the significance in regard to risk for disease is uncertain (496).

Deficiency as Part of Medical Conditions

In some muscular dystrophies, the pathologic features are similar to those of experimental vitamin E deficiency in animals, but no relationship of human dystrophies to the vitamin is known. Hemolytic anemia can occur in the premature infant with low body stores, especially if supplementation with linoleic acid and iron is given. Edema, tachypnea, and restlessness are noted. In adult malabsorption syndromes, especially in association with biliary obstruction, α-tocopherol levels decline, and red cell hemolysis and creatinuria have been reported. When serum levels are very low, a ceroid pigment has been found in smooth and skeletal muscle. In short-bowel syndrome and abetalipoproteinemia, unsteady gait, tremor, weakness, ophthalmoplegia, pigmentary retinopathy, and proprioceptive impairment have been noted (35). It is rare for vitamin E deficiency to present as an isolated neuropathy. Patients with hereditary abetalipoproteinemia also can present with myopathy and cerebellar dysfunction. In cystic fibrosis, changes in posterior column axons and nuclei and sensory nuclei of the fifth cranial nerve in the medulla have been observed, but without clinical neurologic defects. A progressive neurologic syndrome associated with low serum vitamin E concentrations has been described in children with cholestatic liver disease. The syndrome includes areflexia, gait disturbance, decreased proprioceptive and vibratory sensation, and paresis of gaze (497). Lipofuscin pigment accumulates in neurons but has no obvious harmful effect.

Isolated Vitamin E Deficiency
A genetic defect in hepatic α-tocopherol transfer protein that prevents vitamin E from reaching tissues results in ataxia and peripheral neuropathy (498).

Cardiovascular Disease
Patients with these conditions have been noted to have serum levels of vitamin E lower than those of control groups. In nearly all such studies, the serum tocopherol levels were not corrected for lipid content. There are theoretical reasons for a response to antioxidants, and many studies have examined the effect of supplemental vitamin E (sometimes given together with β-carotene). Table 6-42 lists some of the prospective, double-blinded, randomized studies that have been performed. The results are more negative than positive for heart disease, whether given alone or combined with β-carotene or other antioxidant vitamins or minerals (499,500). Vitamin E supplements (600 IU per day) with aspirin (100 mg qod) did not affect the overall risk of heart failure in healthy women over age 45 (501). In the Physicians' Health Study of US male physicians over age 50, vitamin E (400 IU) and vitamin C (500 mg) had no effect on the risk of major cardiovascular disease (502). The AHA consensus statement on vitamin E does not consider that vitamin E can yet be recommended for routine use (503). The Health Professionals Follow-up Study of Males showed no correlations between vitamin E, vitamin C, or β-carotene intake and the risk for stroke (504). The failure of vitamin E in these trials could be due to the fact that supplementation with α-tocopherol decreases serum levels of γ-tocopherol, a potent anti-inflammatory compound (505).

Cancer Prevention
The SU.VI.MAX study found a benefit in cancer incidence and mortality in men only, perhaps due to the low serum baseline levels of β-carotene, but vitamin E was combined with other antioxidant vitamins and minerals (506). The Linxian study in China found a decreased mortality from gastric cancer, but again multiple vitamins or minerals were provided (507). Most studies, however, find little evidence to support an association of either vitamin E or β-carotene and the risk of gastric cancer (508). The ATBC study gave only vitamin E and showed no effect on cancer incidence, a finding confirmed by the HOPE-TOO trial (509). After controlling for smoking, no effect on the incidence of lung cancer was found in eight prospective studies using vitamins A, C, and E (510), or in 14 trials of antioxidant vitamin supplements for prevention of gastrointestinal cancer (337).

The SELenium and vitamin E Cancer prevention Trial (SELECT) treated 35,533 men for a mean of 5 years with vitamin E (400 IU) and selenium (200 µg) daily to prevent prostate cancer. This trial was expected to be positive because secondary analyses of the Nutritional Prevention Cancer trial (NPC) showed a 53% reduction in prostate cancer risk with selenium supplements. However, the SELECT trial was stopped because of no evidence for efficacy (511). In a dose–response meta-analysis of all trials in prostate cancer, higher (135 to 170 ng per mL) plasma selenium levels were associated with 15% to 25% reduction in risk of prostate cancer compared to lower levels (60 ng per mL) (512). Yet, with further follow-up of the SELECT cohort, dietary supplementation with vitamin E was found to significantly increase the risk of prostate cancer (513). Both the meta-analysis and the NPC trial focused on the risk of advanced prostate cancer, and the mean plasma selenium level in the SELECT cohort was 135 ng per mL, already in the protective range, according to the meta-analysis by Hurst et al. Perhaps the reported increased risk with vitamin E is related to its pro-oxidant capacity. Another trial of supplementation of women with vitamins E, C, and β-carotene found no effect on cancer incidence or mortality (514), and the Physicians' Health Trial found no effect of supplements on risk of prostate cancer of greater than 14,000 men (515). Thus, there continues to be very little evidence to support the role of supplemental α-tocopherol in cancer prevention.

Nonalcoholic Fatty Liver Disease (NAFLD)
NAFLD covers a spectrum of disorders ranging from triglyceride accumulation in the liver to inflammation (steatohepatitis) with or without fibrosis or cirrhosis (516). Oxidative stress resulting from an imbalance between pro-oxidant and antioxidant systems is one of the theories for the pathogenesis of NAFLD. Treatment of NAFLD includes weight loss; improvement of insulin resistance (metformin, rosiglitazone, pioglitazone); use of cytoprotective agents such as

TABLE 6-42 Randomized Double-blinded Controlled Studies of Vitamin E Supplementation to Prevent Cardiovascular Disease and Cancer

Study	Population	No.	Intervention (dose of vitamin/day)	Outcome
ASAP (2003)	Men and postmenopausal women, cholesterol ≥193 mg/dL	488	D-α-tocopherol 272 IU + vitamin C 500 mg	Intima-media thickness ↓ only in male smokers
ATBC[1] (1994, 2004)	Finnish M smokers, no MI, 50–69 years	27,271	α-tocopherol 50 mg, β-carotene 20 mg or both, 5–8 years	No ↓ fatal, nonfatal MI, cancer rates
ATBC[2]	Male smokers, Hx of MI	1,862	"	↑ Deaths on β-carotene
ATBC[3]	Male smokers, angina	1,795	"	No benefit
CHAOS[4] (1996)	Angiogram-positive atherosclerosis	2,002	α-tocopherol 400 or 800 IU, ~2 years	72% ↓ Nonfatal MI, no Δ death
GISSI (1999)	Post-MI adults	11,324	Vitamin E 300 mg (synthetic) + 3-n PUFA	No effect on MI, CVD death, stroke
HATS (2001)	Patients with CVD	160	α-tocopherol 800 IU, + 1 g vitamin C + 25 mg natural β-carotene, + 0.1 mg selenium	Progression of stenosis with antioxidant cocktail
HOPE[7] (2000)	>55 years with CV risk factors	9,541	Natural source E 400 mg, 4.5 years	No Δ in CV outcomes
HPS (2002)	High risk for coronary disease, DM, PVD	20,536	Synthetic vitamin E 600 IU + vitamin C 250 mg + β-carotene 20 mg	No Δ in any CV outcome
IVUS (2002)	After cardiac transplantation	40	α-tocopherol 400 IU + vitamin C 500 mg	No ↑ in intimal index
Linxian (1993)	General population (Chinese)	29,584	Group D, β-carotene 15 mg, vitamin E 33 IU, selenium 0.05 mg	21% ↓ in gastric cancer mortality, 5% ↓ in overall mortality, no ↓ in CV mortality
MICRO-HOPE (2002)	Male and female diabetics	3,654	Natural source vitamin E, 400 IU, 4.5 years	No effect on MI, CVD death, stroke
PPP (2001)	Subjects at risk for CVD	4,495	Synthetic vitamin E 300 mg	No effect on IM, CVD death, stroke
SPACE (2000)	Hemodialysis patients with CVD	196	" + natural α-tocopherol 800 IU	2.2 fold ↓ in primary endpoint, a composite of MI, ischemic stroke, unstable angina. No ↓ in CVD mortality

Study	Population	N	Intervention	Outcome
SU.VI. MAX	Healthy men and women	12,741	Vitamin E (unspecified) 33 IU, β-carotene 6 mg, selenium 0.1 mg, zinc 20 mg for 7.2 years	No ↓ in CVD mortality or cancer incidence in whole study ↓ cancer incidence and all-cause mortality in men, not women
VEAPS (2002)	Elevated LDL-C	353	dl-α-tocopherol 400 IU	No effect on intima-media thickness or clinical events
WAVE (2002)	Postmenopausal women with CVD	423	Vitamin E 800 IU + vitamin C 500 mg + hormone replacement therapy	↑ all-cause mortality in antioxidant + HRT group
SELECT (2009)	Men ≥ 55 yrs (AA ≥ 50 y) at risk of prostate cancer	35,533	Vitamin E 400 IU + selenium 200 μg	No reduction in prostate cancer rate for E or selenium
SELECT (2011)	Final follow-up 7–12 yrs	54,464	Vitamin E + selenium	1.6× increase in prostate cancer risk with vitamin E
Physicians Health II '09	Male physicians ≥ 50 yrs	14,641	Vit E 400 IU qod, vit C 500 mg qd	Neither vitamin reduced risk of prostate cancer
Women's Antioxidant CV Study '09	Women at high risk for cardiovascular disease	8,171	Vit E 600 IU qod, vit C 500 mg qd, β-carotene 50 mg qod	No overall benefit in total cancer incidence or related mortality
Physicians Health II '09	Male physicians ≥ 50 yrs	14,641	Vit E 400 IU qod, vit C 500 mg qd	Neither vitamin reduced risk of cardiovascular events
Women's Health Study (2012)	Healthy women ≥ 45 yrs	39,815	Vit E 600 IU qod	No altered risk of heart failure
TONIC (2011)	Age 8–17 with biopsy-confirmed NAFLD	173	Vit E, 800 IU, or metformin 1,000 mg	No improved sustained reduction in ALT levels
SU.VI.MAX Subgroup '09	Post hoc analysis on patients with MetS variables	5,220	Vit E 30 mg, vit C 160 mg, β-carotene 6 mg	No benefit on serum MetS markers (glucose, chol, lipid)

MI, myocardial infarction; DM, diabetes mellitus; LDL-C, low density lipoprotein cholesterol; PVD, peripheral vascular disease; PUFA, polyunsaturated fatty acid. ASAP, Antioxidant Supplementation in Atherosclerosis Prevention study; ATBC, Alpha Tocopherol Beta Carotene cancer prevention study; CHAOS, Cambridge Heart Antioxidant Study; GISSI, Gruppo Italiano per lo Studio della Sopravivenza nell'Infarto miocardico-prevenzione study; HATS, HDL-Atherosclerosis Treatment study; HOPES, Heart Outcomes Prevention Evaluation Study; HPS, Health Protection Study; IVUS, Intravascular Ultrasonography Study; MICRO-HOPE, Microalbuminuria Cardiovascular Renal Outcomes-Heart Outcomes Prevention Evaluation trial; SELECT, SELenium and vitamin E prostate Cancer prevention Trial; SPACE, Secondary Prevention with Antioxidants of Cardiovascular Disease in End-Stage Renal Disease; SU.VI.MAX, Supplémentation en Vitamines et Mineraux Antioxydants; TONIC, Treatment of Nonalcoholic liver disease In Children; VEAPS, Vitamin E Atherosclerosis Prevention Study; WAVE, Women's Angiographic Vitamin and Estrogen Study. Individual references are included in Kris-Etherton PM, Lichtenstein AH, Howard BV, et al, for the Nutrition Committee of the American Heart Association Council on Nutrition, Physical Activity, and Metabolism. Antioxidant vitamin supplements and cardiovascular disease. *Circulation* 2004;110:637; Pham DQ, Plakogiannis R. Vitamin E supplementation in cardiovascular disease and cancer prevention: part 1. *Ann Pharmacother.* 2005;39:1870.

ursodeoxycholic acid; lipid-lowering agents (e.g., clofibrate); and antioxidants (e.g., vitamin E, betaine) (517). A few randomized, prospective trials of vitamin E have been carried out, one with 1,000 IU per day along with vitamin C (518), and one with 800 IU of vitamin E along with a weight-reducing diet and metformin (519). The study with E and C showed improvement in fibrosis but not inflammation scores. The trial with vitamin E alone showed less effect than the use of metformin. No effect of vitamin E or metformin was found in children and adolescents with NAFLD (520). Moreover, in a subgroup of the SU.VI.MAX study, there was no effect on the risk of developing metabolic syndrome, diagnosed by blood sugar and lipid levels (but not by liver enzymes) (521). More studies will be needed to know whether vitamin E or other antioxidants are useful in patients (either ambulatory or in ICUs) with NAFLD where mitochondrial dysfunction is felt to be more prevalent (522).

Other Conditions (Alzheimer Disease, Parkinson Disease, Tardive Dyskinesia, Cataract) (523)

Because of its antioxidant properties, supplements or intake of vitamin E have been examined in a variety of other conditions. Preliminary evidence in small numbers of patients suggests that vitamin E may play a role in immune function, Alzheimer disease, tardive dyskinesia, lung function, diabetes, and exercise performance in highly trained athletes, but the data are contradictory. Vitamin E alone had no benefit on patients with mild cognitive impairment or the rate of progression to Alzheimer disease (524). Although there are no clear answers as to the use of vitamin E in Alzheimer disease, current practice often favors its use, because there are few other options (525). A large trial (PREADVISE) as an ancillary trial to SELECT (the prostate cancer prevention trial) is in progress (526). Data from large, well-designed studies in Parkinson disease and cataract do not support the use of vitamin E (523). Some data suggest prevention of tardive dyskinesia in the first 6 months of therapy with antipsychotic drugs, but more data are needed to make a firm recommendation. Supplementation with vitamins C and E do not reduce the risk of preeclampsia in nulliparous women (527). A subset of the ATBC study identified 50 patients with amyotrophic lateral sclerosis, and found that higher serum α-tocopherol was associated with a lower risk of disease (528). A small trial of 411 patients on vitamins E, C, A, and selenium found a lower risk of recurrent colonic adenomas (529). All of these possible indications need much larger patient groups to know if these results will be verified.

Patients with cholestasis malabsorb vitamin E, but clinical signs of deficiency are usually present only in children whose neural development is immature. Oral vitamin E supplementation with 50 IU per day could normalize serum vitamin E levels, if the serum bilirubin were less than 4 mg per dL, indicative of less than severe cholestasis (530). Vitamin E 600 IU per day has been provided to 16 patients and 15 controls with chemotherapy-induced peripheral neuropathy, with lower mean neuropathy scores (531). This finding will require confirmation. Vitamin E has been used topically in cosmetics and is safe, but real clinical benefit in atopic dermatitis and protection from sunlight-induced malignancy will require prospective controlled studies (532).

Therapy

The premature infant absorbs vitamin E poorly, and large doses are required orally (30 to 60 mg or 45 to 90 IU). Larger doses may be needed for malabsorption syndromes. Vitamin E is available in tablets or capsules of 100, 200, 400, 500, 800, and 1,000 IU and in aqueous suspension at 50 mg per mL (Aquavit-E, Cypress). The therapeutic use of vitamin E falls into three categories (533).

Correction of Deficiency States

Examples include the hemolytic anemia of premature infants and the malabsorption syndromes of patients with cystic fibrosis, cholestatic liver disease, and hereditary abetalipoproteinemia. Large doses may be needed for a response. Up to 100 to 200 IU per kg per day can be given as a liquid emulsion with breakfast or 2 hours after medication that can interfere with absorption (e.g., cholestyramine, vitamin A, antacids). Parenteral (IM) vitamin E has been used as an investigational drug (Ephynal, Hoffman-La Roche, Nutley, NJ) at a dose of 1 to 2 IU per kg (534), but is not currently available. A truly water-soluble form, such as D-α-tocopheryl polyethylene glycol 1,000 succinate (535), is available over the counter as Liqui-E (Twin Lab, Hauppauge,

NY). This compound forms micelles when given at doses of 25 mg per kg per day. Blood levels of vitamin E may rise with replacement in 2 to 3 weeks unless hypolipidemia persists, as in abetalipoproteinemia. It is not clear what this means in terms of transfer of vitamin E to peripheral tissues. Oral vitamin E emulsion (1,000 to 2,000 IU per day) was reported to reverse a deficiency state when given orally three times a week with 0.7 to 3.0 mmol of desiccated ox bile (536).

Countering Effects of Pro-oxidants

Large doses have been used in conditions in which no deficiency exists but large amounts of oxygen or other oxidants are administered. Examples of such use include the prevention or partial relief of retrolental fibroplasia in premature infants, to whom 100 mg of vitamin has been given per kilogram of body weight per day (537). Large doses of the vitamin have been given to lessen the severity of pulmonary dysplasia in infants exposed to prolonged oxygen treatment for respiratory distress syndrome and also to prevent the cardiotoxic effects of the chemotherapeutic drug doxorubicin. Data to support efficacy in such conditions have not been sufficient to recommend the use of vitamin E on a routine basis.

Compensation for Preexisting Defects in the Antioxidant Systems of the Body

Large doses of vitamin E have been used in the absence of defined vitamin E deficiency to treat hemolytic anemia secondary to deficiencies in glutathione synthetase and in glucose-6-phosphate dehydrogenase (538). A decrease in the percentage of sickled cells in sickle cell anemia has been reported with 450 IU per day for 6 to 35 months (539). Of all the conditions associated with vitamin E listed in Table 6-42, cardiovascular disease is the most prevalent, and prevention of cardiovascular disease has the most support. Although no routine recommendations can be made for this use of vitamin E, doses between 100 and 400 IU per day might be considered for patients with or at high risk for cardiovascular disease, with the higher doses given to patients with documented disease (540). If vitamin E is used, it must be understood that the optimal dosage, duration of use, and appropriate source of the vitamin (diet or supplements) are not known.

Toxicity

No consistent ill effects are noted after ingestion of up to 2,112 mg (3,200 IU) per day in healthy volunteers or in patients with a variety of disorders (541). Occasionally, muscle weakness, fatigue, headaches, and nausea have been reported with these doses. High doses may impair the absorption of other fat-soluble vitamins by displacing them from the mixed bile acid–fatty acid micelle. At doses of 100 to 1,100 mg per day, vitamin E can block the oxidation of vitamin K to its active form, mimicking the action of warfarin; therefore, high-dose vitamin E may be contraindicated in patients with disorders of bleeding. However, no changes in prothrombin time have been noted in patients taking 800 to 1,200 IU per day while on Coumadin therapy. Thus, the UL for adults has been set at 1,000 mg per day (3) (Appendix B). Multiple organ toxicity has been reported in premature infants receiving IV vitamin E with polysorbate 80 as an emulsifier.

Some of the studies on vitamin E supplementation have suggested that the vitamin may actually increase mortality or morbidity (503). A systematic review of 19 RCTs showed that vitamin E supplementation either alone or combined with other micronutrients in doses ≥400 IU per day increased the risk for all-cause mortality (542). The largest systematic review of antioxidant trials found that vitamin E, given singly or in combination with other antioxidants, increases the risk of death (543). Because in many studies (10 of 19 studies) vitamin E was not the only supplement provided, it is not possible to know the effects of vitamin E alone. However, it does suggest that for safety the dose of vitamin E should be kept at less than 400 IU per day.

Vitamin K

Requirement

Two forms of vitamin K occur naturally—K_1 (phylloquinones) in green plants and K_2 (menaquinones) in bacteria and animals. Menaquinones are classified according to the length of their side chain. Menadione (vitamin K_3) is a compound without a side chain that is activated by conversion in the body to MK-4. MK-4 is found in the highest concentrations in the brain, kidney, and pancreas, but the vitamin side chain is removed during intestinal absorption, and menadione is transferred to tissues. Conversion from dietary vitamin K forms can occur in tissues either directly by side-chain cleavage of phylloquinone and subsequent geranylgeranylation, or by conversion of menadione with subsequent prenylation to MK-4. The enzyme that accomplishes this prenylation is UbiA prenyltransferase containing 1 (UBIAD1), and it is not inhibited by warfarin (544). The most common menaquinone found in food is a short-chain vitamer, MK-4 (545). Colonic bacterial synthesis provides an unknown amount of vitamin K, mostly the longer-chain menaquinones (MK-7 to MK-10) that has been estimated to be about 2 µg per kg of body weight. Because of the bacterial synthesis, dietary requirements are uncertain. The role of intestinal bacteria in providing any vitamin K in humans has been questioned, and its overall contribution to vitamin K status is felt to be fairly small (545). When antibiotics are given to alter intestinal flora, a vitamin K intake of 1 µg per kg per day prevents deficiency and is presumably adequate. Body stores of vitamin K are limited (~1 µg per kg body weight) and turnover time is about 1 to 2 days (546).

The RDAs of 1989 were based on the function of the vitamin for the coagulation proteins, but the requirement may be greater for the nonhepatic vitamin K–dependent proteins, including those in bone (547). Because of the lack of data to estimate an average requirement, an AI is based on representative dietary intake data from healthy persons (305). The lower limit of the AI for vitamin K is set at 120 µg for adult men and 90 µg for adult women (Table 6-43). The RDA for other age groups is based on the need for 1 µg per kg of body weight in infants and children. Because human milk contains low levels of vitamin K (2 µg per L) and intestinal flora are underdeveloped, breast-fed infants receiving no other food source are at risk for deficiency and intracranial hemorrhage. Vitamin K (150 µg per day) is now included in the recommendations for vitamin provision in the new FDA guidelines for TPN for adults (548).

Food Sources

Phylloquinone concentrations of plant leaves are proportional to their chlorophyll content. Thus, the best dietary sources are green leafy vegetables (spinach, kale, collards) and broccoli, although whole wheat and green tea are also sources. Although the food content varies widely, the

TABLE 6-43 Recommended Dietary Allowances for Vitamin K

Life Stage Group	Vitamin K (µg/day)
Infants	
0–6 months	2
7–12 months	2.5
Children	
1–3 years	30
4–8 years	55
Males	
9–13 years	60
14–18 years	75
19–>70 years	120
Females	
9–13 years	60
14–18 years	75
19–>70 years	90
Pregnancy, Lactation	
14–18 years	75
19–50 years	90

All estimates are based on adequate intake (AI).
Data from Standing Committee on the Scientific Evaluation of Dietary Reference Intakes, Food and Nutrition Board, Institute of Medicine. *Dietary Reference Intakes for Vitamin A, Vitamin K, Arsenic, Boron, Chromium, Copper, Iodine, Iron, Manganese, Molybdenum, Nickel, Silicon, Vanadium, and Zinc.* Washington, DC: National Academies Press, 2001. Available online at *http://www.nap.edu/books*, Crawler list *0309072794*. Accessed May 30, 2006.

vitamin is associated with chloroplasts, and bioavailability is also variable. Other primary dietary sources are certain plant oils, namely soybean, canola, cottonseed, and olive (549,550). However, other commonly used oils (peanut, corn, safflower, and sesame) have a very low content. Fruits, cereals, dairy products, and meat contain less vitamin K. The average diet in the United States contains 60 to 200 μg per day (547). Dihydrophylloquinone is formed during the hydrogenation of plant oils. Menaquinones, in particular MK-4, are found mostly in meat, fermented products, eggs, and dairy products (551). MK-4 is the major form of vitamin K in human brain. Menadione (synthetic vitamin K_3) is commonly added to chicken feed, and the MK-4 found in chicken products may be formed from this source. No single food item is especially rich in MK-4, but these foods are consumed in large amounts in a Western diet (including fast foods) and are probably important in the overall contribution of vitamin K intake. Some vitamin K in the body is derived from bacteria, but this is poorly absorbed, and diet is the major source. The content of representative foods is listed in Table 6-44. Only a small number of vegetables contribute substantially to dietary phylloquinones. Oral phylloquinone at a dose of 500 μg can overcome therapeutic doses of warfarin, but some reports have suggested that a much lower content in enteral products can cause dietary resistance to warfarin (552). If the dietary intake of green vegetables or high-content oils is reasonably constant, there is no need to be concerned with a dietary cause of unstable warfarin effect. High vitamin K intake can blunt the effect of warfarin, and low vitamin K stores can increase sensitivity to warfarin. Typical servings of vegetables (containing <100 μg of the vitamin) have little effect on the international normalized ratio (INR), but large intake of vegetables (e.g., 400 g containing 0.7 to 1.5 mg of vitamin K) can alter the INR transiently (553). The 2005 *Dietary Guidelines for Americans* suggests 3 cups per week of dark-green vegetables, which contain approximately 100 to 570 μg of vitamin K per serving. Thus, it seems that only excessive ingestion of dietary vitamin K will have an effect on the INR (see also Chapter 12, vitamin K–restricted diet).

Assessment
Intake: Plasma Phylloquinone
HPLC methods have made this a straightforward measurement. Normal plasma concentrations range from 1.04 nmol per L ± 0.13 in younger adults to 1.45 nmol per L ± 0.22 (150 to

TABLE 6-44 Vitamin K Content of Selected Foods

Food	Portion	Vitamin K Content (μg per serving)
Vegetables		
Broccoli	1/2 cup	88
Brussels sprouts	1/2 cup	225
Cabbage	1/2 cup	73
Collard greens	1/2 cup	374
Nuts, mixed (no peanuts)	1 oz	3.2
Potato, baked with skin	1 medium	1.5
Spinach	1/2 cup	324
Dairy		
Milk, 2%	8 oz	0.5
Meat		
Beef, ground	3 oz	2.0
Chicken breast, roasted	3 oz	<0.01
Chicken breast, home fried	3 oz	3.8
Oils		
Cottonseed, olive	1 oz	15
Corn	1 oz	1.5

Data from Booth SL, Suttie JW. Dietary intake and adequacy of vitamin K. *J Nutr.* 1998;128:785.

200 pg per mL) in older (70 years) adults (32). The recent dietary intake of vitamin K correlates best with the plasma level and is subject to wide variation. However, a single measurement of circulating phylloquinone is adequate to estimate long-term exposure to the dietary vitamin in older adults (554). Vitamin K is carried in lipoproteins, so levels should be measured after an overnight fast. Plasma levels are elevated most by dietary vitamin K_1, but levels rise more rapidly after ingestion of MK-4, and the plasma half-life of MK-9 is longer than that of other forms (555). The usual assay of phylloquinone does not directly measure menaquinones (551). However, menaquinones can contribute significantly to body stores. An alternative assessment of vitamin K is to measure urinary vitamin K metabolites, as both K_1 and K_2 are excreted as two side-chain shortened metabolites (555). The clinical value of this determination is still unclear.

Body Stores
Prothrombin Time
Because vitamin K stimulates the production of clotting factors II, VII, IX, and X, and of protein Z, protein S, and protein C in the liver, the one-stage prothrombin time is used to assess its presence indirectly. For this test, sources of tissue factor (thromboplastin) and calcium are added in excess. Under these conditions, all the clotting factors tested (II, V, VII, X) are responsive to vitamin K except for factor V. The rate of formation of clot is an indirect measure of the amount of factors II, VII, and X. In practice, factor VII is the usual rate-limiting factor. Factor V has a longer half-life than the vitamin K–dependent proteins and is not rate-limiting in the reaction. Normally, the test sample clots within 1.5 seconds of the control (INR of 1.0 to 1.1). The prothrombin time does not test vitamin K stores and is abnormal only when deficiency is present, synthesis of clotting factors is impaired by hepatic disease, or clotting factors are consumed in intravascular coagulation. Therefore, the test is nonspecific. It is most helpful when acute serious illness or liver disease is not present. In these situations, the interpretation regarding vitamin K is simple. If parenteral administration of vitamin K (5 to 10 mg) restores the prothrombin time to normal, deficiency in vitamin K becomes evident.

γ-Carboxyglutamic acid (Gla)-modified proteins
Because vitamin K mediates the addition of Gla to proteins, detection of these proteins has been examined to evaluate vitamin K status, particularly as applies to extrahepatic tissues. These assays are still not widely available, and more studies are needed before they can become clinically valuable. The assays used, and their "normal" values in adults, include plasma undercarboxylated prothrombin, protein induced by vitamin K absence (PIVKA)-II (1.58 μg per L), plasma undercarboxylated osteocalcin, (ucOC, 2 to 3.3 μg per L), plasma carboxylated osteocalcin (cOC, 7 to 10 μg per L), and urine Gla–creatinine ratio (3.16 in women, 3.83 in men) (32). Population studies show a correlation between vitamin K levels and those of ucOC and cOC. The most sensitive measure of vitamin K status for bone may be the ucOC/cOC ratio (555). Matrix Gla protein (MGP) is not made in the liver or bone, but in chondrocytes and vascular smooth muscle, and may reflect vitamin K status of those tissues.

Physiology
Absorption and Metabolism
Vitamin K absorption requires bile acids and is passive, occurring largely in the small bowel. If coprophagy is prevented, rats on a vitamin K–free diet develop deficiency within a few weeks, so colonic absorption of vitamin K is probably minimal (556). Other fat-soluble vitamins in very large amounts can displace vitamin K from the bile acid micelle and limit absorption. After absorption in the lymphatics, vitamin K_1 is taken up and metabolized in the liver and retained there, but vitamin K_2 appears to accumulate preferentially in extrahepatic locations (557). The vitamin is reduced and converted to the epoxide before the original vitamin is re-formed, all by microsomal enzymes.

Tissue Stores
Unlike other fat-soluble vitamins, vitamin K is not stored in large quantities in adipose tissue, and the total body pool is small. The amount in tissue is low, but the vitamin is found in adrenals, lungs, marrow, kidney, cartilage, vascular smooth muscle, and lymph nodes after it leaves the liver. The storage form differs from the plasma form, which is carried in lipoproteins.

Long-chain menaquinones are the predominant hepatic form. Phylloquinones account for only 10% of liver reserves, do not cross the placenta, and are depleted first in cases of deficiency.

Function

Vitamin K acts by carboxylating selected glutamic acid residues of proteins (α-Gla) so that they bind calcium. The Gla reaction is catalyzed by a microsomal enzyme, vitamin K–dependent gamma glutamyl carboxylase (GGCX), and requires four substrates: reduced vitamin K, oxygen, carbon dioxide, and the Gla-containing peptide. A microsomal electron transport system is coupled with carbon dioxide fixation during the reaction. This vitamin K cycle oxidizes vitamin K hydroquinone to vitamin K-2,3-epoxide in a process that provides the energy for carboxylation of glutamic acid residues (557). The epoxide is converted back to reduced vitamin K by the warfarin-sensitive vitamin K epoxide reductase (VKOR), acting either alone or with some other enzyme as yet unidentified (558). The endoplasmic reticulum chaperone protein calumenin appears to regulate the activity of the vitamin K–dependent carboxylation system. Vitamin K_2 may also play an independent regulatory role, as it regulates transcription of bone-specific genes by a different mechanism from that involved in the carboxylation of Gla residues (555).

Warfarin blocks the reduction of the epoxide to the quinone and the subsequent hydroxylation to the hydroquinone. The coagulation function of hepatic proteins is proportional to the degree of carboxylation. Variability in the VKOR gene and/or variation in the intake of dietary vitamin K may account for some of the variable effects of warfarin. Vitamin K–dependent procoagulants include prothrombin and factors VII, IX, and X. Vitamin K–dependent anticoagulants include proteins C and S. The half-life of activated protein C is quite short, and the pool of circulating protein C is depleted very quickly when severe septicemia occurs. It is not clear whether providing parenteral vitamin K to septic patients can restore protein C levels. Osteocalcin (bone Gla protein) is important in the extracellular matrix of bone, and MGPs in the extracellular matrix of other tissues. Other vitamin K–dependent proteins of unknown function include protein Z, nephrocalcin, plaque Gla protein, Gas-6, PRGP-1, and PRGP-2 (556).

Deficiency

To avoid deficiency, a person must have adequate intraluminal vitamin K, a normal concentration of bile acids, and a normal small bowel, colon, and liver. Deficiency is manifested by easy bruising and clotting abnormalities. Subjects at risk for deficiency include newborn infants, whose intestinal flora is not established; others are patients with malabsorption resulting from loss of intestine or bile acid insufficiency, patients with liver disease, and persons receiving no oral intake while on broad-spectrum antibiotics. Subclinical deficiency occurs not uncommonly, as it has no clinical phenotype. Elevation of PIKVA-II is relatively common in cholestatic liver disease, even with vitamin K supplementation (559). Suboptimal vitamin K (and D) status can be found in patients with chronic kidney disease, and manifested by low phylloquinone and high PIKVA-II concentrations (560). Patients with advanced cancer are at high risk for vitamin K deficiency because of decreased intake and use of antibiotics. Monitoring for plasma phylloquinone and PIKVA-II can detect subclinical deficiency before bleeding occurs (561).

Hemorrhagic Disease of the Newborn

Hemorrhagic disease of the newborn occurs because the placenta transports lipids poorly so body stores are low, the intestine is sterile in the first days of life, turnover of the vitamin is rapid, and human milk is a poor source of vitamin K. Premature infants are at highest risk. Thus, the fall in prothrombin time at birth could lead to bleeding, particularly intracranially. It was routine to give 1 mg of vitamin K by injection routinely (562). It became clear that the problem was seen only in infants fed entirely by breast milk, and the condition was renamed "vitamin K deficiency bleeding." It is not very common now, and occurs only in the first few weeks of life. Late bleeding (after week 2 of life) occurs only about 1 in every 6,000 breast-fed infants. Bottle-fed babies have almost no risk, because formula feeds are fortified with vitamins. Oral supplementation of newborns is effective, so that injectable vitamin K need not always be indicated (562).

Drug Interference

Drugs interfere with vitamin K metabolism as well as with production in the intestine. Warfarin inhibits vitamin K epoxide formation, hydantoins antagonize vitamin K in some way, certain antibiotics (e.g., moxalactam, cefamandole) decrease peptide carboxylation, salicylates inhibit vitamin K reductase, and the diuretic ticrynafen inhibits part of the microsomal electron transport system.

Bone and Vascular Health

Epidemiologic studies suggest that vitamin K deficiency can cause reductions in BMD, and a few intervention studies suggest further that supplementation with vitamin K can increase bone density and reduce fracture rates (545,555). In postmenopausal women, bone calcification is decreased but arterial calcification is increased. Population studies have suggested an inverse relationship between dietary intake of menaquinones and aortic calcification and cardiovascular death, but no prospective interventional studies have been reported. Two dose–response studies show that the amount of vitamin K needed for maximal γ-carboxylation of osteocalcin is much higher than what is needed to maintain synthesis of hepatic clotting factors, and is probably greater than can be provided by the diet (545). Some data suggest that vitamin K supplements should also contain calcium and vitamin D to have optimal bone effects. A purely dietary deficiency of vitamin K is rare, but expert opinion has begun to question the adequacy of the DRI recommendations for vitamin K intake, due to the possible need for larger intake for bone health and possibly for cardiovascular disease. Vitamin K is essential for the biosynthesis of some bone proteins, and hip fractures (but not bone density) are associated with intakes of less than 109 µg per day (563). Vitamin K in the form of MK-4 was administered to postmenopausal Japanese women for 2 years and increased bone mass (564), but the link between vitamin K deficiency, if it occurs, and hip fracture in elderly women is not clear (565). Two studies of warfarin use and the risk of fractures reached opposite conclusions, one showing no increase (566) and one showing no overall increase but more rib and vertebral fractures (567). The overall dataset provides some support for the hypothesis that vitamin K might be useful for osteoporosis, but use of the vitamin is not well accepted. Most of the prospective studies and use come from Japan, where MK-4 supplements (menaquinone) are commonly prescribed. However, Canadian guidelines do not recommend vitamin K for osteoporosis (568). Vitamin K status is lower in patients with Crohn disease than in healthy controls, and the rate of bone resorption was higher, suggesting a protective role of the vitamin in reducing bone turnover (569). Perhaps the most compelling data that link vitamin K with bone health is the observation of low osteocalcin and BMD in an infant with inherited deficiency of vitamin K–dependent coagulation factors, and the return to normal of the bone parameters following vitamin K supplementation (570).

Therapy

The only synthetic forms of vitamin K available for human consumption are K_1 and MK-4. Both forms are well absorbed, so that parenteral administration is not necessary in most cases. K_1 is the analogue used in virtually all the food supplements and multivitamin preparations in Western nations, but MK-4 is becoming available in health food stores. There are no data providing comparisons for efficacy of the two forms, but present formulations permit much larger doses of MK-4 (45 to 90 mg per day). The bioavailability of vitamin K is probably greater from supplements than from natural sources (555). Vitamin K is available in solutions of 2 mg per mL in 0.5 mL ampules or prefilled syringes for parenteral use. Injection should be subcutaneous or intramuscular when possible. For anticoagulant-induced or other deficiency of prothrombin in adults, use 2.5 to 10 mg initially or up to 25 mg. If the prothrombin time has not shortened satisfactorily within 6 to 8 hours, repeat the dose. Use blood replacement when it is hemodynamically necessary. For hemorrhagic disease of the newborn, prophylactic therapy consists of a single intramuscular dose of 0.5 to 1 mg within 1 hour of birth or 1 to 5 mg to the mother 12 to 24 hours before delivery. Hemolytic anemia and hepatotoxicity have been reported with high doses. Long-term use should be limited to patients with malabsorption. Vitamin K_1 is not a component of many multivitamin preparations, but can be prescribed individually as 5-mg tablets of phytonadione (Mephyton).

Toxicity

More than 500 times the RDA can be given without toxicity. Thus, no UL has been recommended (305). Large amounts of vitamin K given during pregnancy or to the newborn (>10 mg) can produce jaundice in the infant. It has been suggested that phylloquinone in infant formulas not exceed 20 µg per 100 kcal. Hydantoin antagonizes vitamin K and can produce hemorrhagic disease in the newborn when taken by the mother during pregnancy. IV use in adults has occasionally produced anaphylaxis, even when given at low dose and by slow dilute infusion (571). It is unclear whether this reaction is related to the drug itself or to the solubilizing vehicle, but should be a reminder that IV vitamin K should be used only when absolutely necessary. The newer formulations of the vitamin are well absorbed orally (562).

EFFECT OF DRUGS ON ASSESSMENT OF VITAMIN STATUS

Many drugs can alter the results of tests used to assess vitamin status. These are listed in Table 6-45. Many of the drugs listed alter only the laboratory assessment of nutrient status, and a clear clinical deficiency state is not always described. Therefore, unless treatment is prolonged, replacement therapy is usually not required.

TABLE 6-45 Drugs that Affect Vitamin Utilization and Plasma Concentrations.

Drug class	Drug	Vitamin Affected	Mechanism
Antibacterial	Isoniazid	Niacin, B_6	Competition with active coenzyme
	PAS	B_{12}	↓ Absorption
	Neomycin	B_{12}, K	↓ Absorption (bile salt sequestration)
	Pyrimethamine	Folate	Inhibits folate reductase
	Tetracycline	C	↑ Excretion
	Trimethoprim	Folate	Inhibits folate reductase
	Broad-spectrum	K	↓ Endogenous production
Anticoagulant	Warfarin	K	Blocks Gla formation
Anticonvulsant	Phenytoin	Folate	↓ Absorption
		D	↓ Hepatic metabolism to 1,25-$(OH)_2$D
		K	Induction of hepatic inactivating enzyme
Antihypertensive	Hydralazine	B_6	Competition with active coenzyme
Anti-inflammatory	Aspirin	C	↑ Excretion (competes with binding)
	Sulfasalazine	Folate	↓ Absorption
	Colchicine	B_{12}	↓ Absorption (intestinal damage)
	Phenylbutazone	Niacin, K	Displacement from albumin binding
Antineoplastic	Methotrexate	Folate	Inhibits folate reductase
Bile salt sequestrants	Cholestyramine	A, B_{12}, folate	↓ Absorption (binding
	Cholestipol	A, D, K	of water-soluble, luminal sequestration of fat-soluble)
Chelating	Penicillamine	B_6	↑ Urinary excretion (adduct formed)
Hormones	Birth-control pills	B_1, B_2	↑ Function
		B_6	↓ Plasma binding
		Folate	↓ Absorption, ↑ plasma binding
		B_{12}	↓ Plasma binding

Gla, Carboxy-glutamic acid; PAS, *para*-aminosalicylate.

REFERENCES

1. National Research Council. *Recommended Dietary Allowances*, 10th ed. Washington, DC: National Academies Press, 1989.
2. Standing Committee on the Scientific Evaluation of Dietary Reference Intakes, Food and Nutrition Board, Institute of Medicine. *Dietary Reference Intakes for Calcium, Phosphorus, Magnesium, Vitamin D, and Fluoride*. Washington, DC: National Academies Press, 1997.
3. Standing Committee on the Scientific Evaluation of Dietary Reference Intakes, Food and Nutrition Board, Institute of Medicine. *Dietary Reference Intakes for Thiamine, Riboflavin, Niacin, Vitamin B6, Folate, Vitamin B12, Pantothenic Acid, Biotin, and Choline*. Washington, DC: National Academies Press, 1998.
4. Standing Committee on the Scientific Evaluation of Dietary Reference Intakes, Food and Nutrition Board, Institute of Medicine. *Dietary Reference Intakes for Vitamin C, Vitamin E, Selenium, and Beta-Carotene and Other Carotenoids*. Washington, DC: National Academies Press, 2000.
5. Anonymous. Who should take vitamin supplements? *Med Lett Drugs Ther*. 2011;53:101.
6. Macpherson H, Pipingas A, Pase MP. Multivitamin-multimineral supplementation and mortality: a meta-analysis of randomized controlled trials. *Am J Clin Nutr*. 2013;97:427.
7. US Department of Agriculture and US Department of Health and Human Services. *Report of the Dietary Guidelines Advisory Committee on the Dietary Guidelines for Americans*, 2010. http://www.cnpp.usda.gov/DGAs2010-DGACReport.htm.
8. Fortmann SP, Burda BU, Sanger CA, et al. Vitamin, mineral, and multivitamin supplements for the primary prevention of cardiovascular disease and cancer: a systematic evidence review for the U.S. Preventive Services Task Force. Report No: 14-05199-EF-1. Agency for Healthcare Research and Quality, November 2013. http://www.ncbi.nlm.nih.gov/books/NBK173987/pdf/TOC.pdf.
9. Alexander DD, Weed DL, Change ET, et al. A systematic review of multivitamin-multimineral use and cardiovascular disease and cancer incidence and total mortality. *J Am Coll Nutr*. 2013;32:339.
10. Lamas GA, Boineau R, Goertz C, et al. Oral high-dose multivitamins and minerals after myocardial infarction. *Ann Intern Med*. 2013;159:797.
11. Kesse-Guyot E, Fezeu L, Jeandel C, et al. French adults' cognitive performance after daily supplementation with antioxidant vitamins and minerals at nutritional doses: a post hoc analysis of the Supplementation in Vitamins and Mineral Antioxidants (SU.VI.MAX) trial. *Am J Clin Nutr*. 2011;94:892.
12. Goldstein F, O'Brien J, Kang JH, et al. Long-term multivitamin supplementation and cognitive function in men: a randomized trial. *Ann Intern Med*. 2013;159:806.
13. Alpers DH. Subclinical micronutrient deficiency: a problem in recognition. *Curr Opin Gastroenterol*. 2012;28:135.
14. Haymes EM. Trace minerals and exercise. In: Wolinsky I, Hickson JF Jr, eds. *Nutrition in Exercise and Sport*. 2nd ed. Boca Raton, FL: CRC Press, 1994:224.
15. Lukaski HC. Vitamin and mineral status: effects on physical performance. *Nutrition*. 2004;20:632.
16. Russell RM. New views on the RDAs for older adults. *J Am Diet Assoc*. 1997;97:515.
17. Haller J. The vitamin status and its adequacy in the elderly: an international overview. *Int J Vitam Nutr Res*. 1999;69:160.
18. Selhub J, Bagley LC, Miller C, et al. B vitamins, homocysteine, and neurocognitive function in the elderly. *Am J Clin Nutr*. 2000;71:614S.
19. Smith AD, Smith SM, de Jager CA, et al. Homocysteine-lowering by B vitamins slows the rate of accelerated brain atrophy in mild cognitive impairment: a randomized controlled trial. *PLoS ONE* 2010;5:e12244.
20. Stroke and prevention—B vitamins. Arbor Clinical Nutrition Updates, Issue 318. http://www.nutrocencia.com.br/upload_files/antigos_download/acidente%20vascular%20cerebral%20%20e%20preven%C3%A7%C3%A3o%20--.pdf
21. Skarupski KA, Tangney C, Li H, et al. Longitudinal association of vitamin B-6, folate, and vitamin B-12 with depressive symptoms among older adults over time. *Am J Clin Nutr*. 2010;92:330.
22. Lyle BJ, Mares-Perlman JA, Klein BEK, et al. Serum carotenoids and tocopherols and incidence of age-related nuclear cataracts. *Am J Clin Nutr*. 1999;69:272.
23. US Preventive Services Task Force. Routine vitamin supplementation to prevent cancer and cardiovascular disease: recommendations and rationale. *Ann Intern Med*. 2003;139:51.

24. Fairfield KM, Fletcher RH. Vitamins for chronic disease prevention in adults: scientific review. *JAMA.* 2002;287:3116.
25. de Jong N, Chin AP, de Groot LC, et al. Nutrient-dense foods and exercise in frail elderly: effects on B vitamins, homocysteine, methylmalonic acid, and neuropsychological functioning. *Am J Clin Nutr.* 2001;73:338.
26. Vavricka SR, Rogler G. Intestinal absorption and vitamin levels: is a new focus needed? *Dig Dis.* 2012;30(Suppl 3):73.
27. O'Donnell K. Small but mighty: selected micronutrient issues in gastric bypass patients. *Pract Gastroenterol.* 2008;33:37.
28. Vieth R. The role of vitamin D in the prevention of osteoporosis. *Ann Med.* 2005;37:278.
29. Fawzi WW, Msamanga GI, Spiegelman D, et al. A randomized trial of multivitamin supplements and HIV disease progression and mortality. *N Engl J Med.* 2004;351:23.
30. Irlam JH, Visser ME, Rollins N, et al. Micronutrient supplementation in children and adults with HIV infection. *Cochrane Database Syst Rev.* 2005;(4):CD003650.
31. Alpers DH. Vitamins as drugs: the importance of pharmacokinetics in oral dosing. *Curr Opin Gastroenterol.* 2011;27:146.
32. Sauberlich HE. *Laboratory Tests for the Assessment of Nutritional Status.* 2nd ed. Boca Raton, FL: CRC Press, 1999.
33. Said HM. Intestinal absorption of water soluble vitamins in health and disease. *Biochem J.* 2011;437:357.
34. Ganapathy V, Smith SB, Prasad PD. SLC19: the folate/thiamine transporter family. *Pflugers Arch-Eur J Physiol.* 2004;447:641.
35. Kumar N. Nutritional neuropathies. *Neurol Clin.* 2007;25:209.
36. Manzanares W, Hardy G. Thiamine supplementation in the critically ill. *Curr Opin Clin Nutr Metab Care.* 2011;14:610.
37. Oriot D, Wood C, Gottesman R, et al. Severe lactic acidosis related to acute thiamine deficiency. *JPEN J Parenter Enteral Nutr.* 1991;15:105.
38. Frank T, Bitsch R, Maiwald J, et al. High thiamine phosphate concentrations in erythrocytes can be achieved in dialysis patients by oral administration of benfotiamine. *Eur J Clin Pharmacol.* 2000;56:251.
39. Thomson AD, Guerrini I, Marshall EJ. Wernicke's encephalopathy: role of thiamine. *Pract Gastroenterol.* 2009;34:21.
40. Ames BN, Elson-Schwab I, Silver EA. High-dose vitamin therapy stimulates variant enzymes with decreased coenzyme binding affinity (increased K_m): relevance to genetic disease and polymorphisms. *Am J Clin Nutr.* 2002;75:616.
41. Fragakis AS. *The professional's Guide to Popular Dietary Supplements.* 2nd ed. Hoboken NJ: JohnWiley & Sons Inc, 2002.
42. Alhadeff L, Gueltieri CT, Lipton M. Toxic effects of water-soluble vitamins. *Nutr Rev.* 1984;42:33.
43. Beecher GR. Overview of dietary flavonoids: nomenclature, occurrence, and intake. *J Nutr.* 2003;133:3248S.
44. McCormick D. Riboflavin. In: Shils M, Shike M, Ross AC, et al., eds. *Modern Nutrition in Health and Disease.* 10th ed. Philadelphia: Lippincott Williams & Wilkins, 2006:434.
45. Powers HJ. Riboflavin (vitamin B-2) and health. *Am J Clin Nutr.* 2003;77:1352.
46. Schoenen J, Jacquy J, Lenaerts M. Effectiveness of high-dose riboflavin in migraine prophylaxis. A randomized controlled trial. *Neurology.* 1998;50:466.
47. Denu JM. The Sir2 family of protein deacetylases. *Curr Opin Chem Biol.* 2005;9:431.
48. Muzaffar S, Shukla N, Jeremy JY. Nicotinamide adenine dinucleotide phosphate oxidase: a promiscuous therapeutic target for cardiovascular drugs? *Trends Cardiovasc Med.* 2005;15:278.
49. Khanna-Gupta A, Berliner N. Vitamin B3 boosts neutrophil counts. *Nat Med.* 2009;15:139.
50. Pike NB. Flushing out the role of GPR109A (HM74A) in the clinical efficacy of nicotinic acid. *J Clin Invest.* 2005;115:3400.
51. Bourgeois C, Cervantes-Laurean D, Moss J. Niacin. In: Shils ME, Shike M, Ross CA, et al., eds. *Modern Nutrition in Health and Disease.* 10th ed. Philadelphia: Lippincott Williams & Wilkins, 2006:442.
52. Meyers CD, Kamanna VS, Kashyap ML. Niacin therapy in atherosclerosis. *Curr Opin Lipidol.* 2004;15:659.
53. Anonymous. Drugs for hypertriglyceridemia. *Med Lett Drugs Ther.* 2013;55:17.

54. Giugliano RP. Niacin at 56 years of age—time for an early retirement? *N Eng J Med.* 2011;365:24.
55. Crino A, Schiaffini R, Ciampalini P, et al. A two year observational study of nicotinamide and intensive insulin therapy in patients with recent onset type 1 diabetes mellitus. *J Pediatr Endocrinol Metab.* 2005;18:749.
56. Cosmetic Ingredient Review Expert Panel. Final report of the safety assessment of niacinamide and niacin. *Int J Toxicol.* 2005;24(Suppl 5):1.
57. Jungnickel PW, Maloney PA, van der Tuin EL, et al. Effect of two aspirin pretreatment regimens on niacin-induced cutaneous reactions. *J Gen Intern Med.* 1997;12:591.
58. Rizkallah GS, Mertens MK, Brown ML. Should liver enzymes be checked in a patient taking niacin? *J Fam Pract.* 2005;54:265.
59. McCormack PL, Keating GM. Prolonged-release nicotinic acid: a review of its use in the treatment of dyslipidemia. *Drugs.* 2005;65:2719.
60. HPS2-THRIVE collaborative group. HPS2-THRIVE randomized placebo controlled trial in 25,673 high risk patients of ER niacin/laropiprant: trial design, pre-specified muscle and liver outcomes, and reasons for stopping study treatment. *Eur Heart J.* 2012;34:1279.
61. Jancin B. HPS2-THRIVE drives another nail in niacin's coffin. http://www.ecardiologynews.com/index.php?id=8736&type=98&tx_ttnews[tt_news]=141797&cHash=da03e20e36.
62. Bailey AL, Maisey S, Southon S, et al. Relationships between micronutrient intake and biochemical indicators of nutrient adequacy in a "free-living" elderly U.K. population. *Br J Nutr.* 1997;77:225.
63. de Groot CP, van den Broek T, van Staveren W. Energy intake and micronutrient intake in elderly Europeans: seeking the minimum requirement in the SENECA study. *Age Ageing.* 1999;28:469.
64. Lamers Y. Indicators and methods for folate, vitamin B-12, and vitamin B-6 status assessment in humans. *Curr Opin Clin Nutr Metab Care.* 2011;14:445.
65. Stabler SP, Allen RH, Fried LP, et al. Racial differences in prevalence of cobalamin and folate deficiency in disabled elderly women. *Am J Clin Nutr.* 1999;70:911.
66. Whyte M, Mahuren JD, Vrabel LA, et al. Markedly increased circulating pyridoxal-5′-phosphate levels in hypophosphatasia. Alkaline phosphatase acts in vitamin B_6 metabolism. *J Clin Invest.* 1985;76:752.
67. Gergory JF, Park Y, Lamers Y, et al. Metabolomic analysis reveals extended metabolic consequences of marginal vitamin B-6 deficiency in healthy human subjects. *PLoS ONE.* 2013;8:e63544.
68. Said HM, Ortiz A, Ma TY. A carrier-mediated mechanism for pyridoxine uptake by human intestinal epithelial Caco-2 cells: regulation by a PKA-mediated pathway. *Am J Physiol Cell Physiol.* 2003;285:C1219.
69. Mills PB, Surtees RA, Champion MP, et al. Neonatal epileptic encephalopathy caused by mutations in the PNPO gene encoding pyridox(am)ine-5′-phosphate oxidase. *Hum Mol Genet.* 2005;60:1413.
70. Selhub J, Jacques PF, Wilson PW, et al. Vitamin status and intake as primary determinants of homocysteinemia in an elderly population. *JAMA.* 1993;270:2693.
71. Anonymous. Vitamin B6 (pyridoxine; pyridoxal-5′-phosphate). *Altern Med Rev.* 2001;6:87.
72. Lheureux P, Penaloza A, Gris M. Pyridoxine in clinical toxicology: a review. *Eur J Emerg Med.* 2005;12:78.
73. Chang HY, Tang FY, Chen DY, et al. Clinical use of cyclooxygenase inhibitors impair vitamin B6 metabolism. *Am J Clin Nutr.* 2013;98:1440.
74. Lerner V, Bergman J, Statsendko N, et al. Vitamin B6 treatment in acute neuroleptic-induced akathisia: a randomized, double-blind, placebo-controlled study. *J Clin Psychiatry.* 2004;65:1550.
75. Eichinger S. Are B vitamins a risk factor for venous thromboembolism? Yes. *J Thromb Haemost.* 2006;4:307.
76. Larsson SC, Orsini N, Wolk A. Vitamin B6 and risk of colorectal cancer. *JAMA.* 2010;303:1077.
77. Zhang X, Lee JE, Ma J, et al. Prospective cohort studies of vitamin B-6 status and colorectal cancer incidence: modification by time? *Am J Clin Nutr.* 2012;96:874.
78. Bender DA. Non-nutritional uses of vitamin B_6. *Br J Nutr.* 1999;81:7.
79. Aufiero E, Stitik TP, Foye PM, et al. Pyridoxine hydrochloride treatment of carpal tunnel syndrome: a review. *Nutr Rev.* 2004;62:96.
80. Wyatt KM, Dimmock PW, Jones PW, et al. Efficacy of vitamin B-6 in the treatment of premenstrual syndrome: systematic review. *BMJ.* 1999;318:1375.

81. Chocano-Bedoya PO, Manson JE, Henkinson SE, et al. Dietary vitamin B intake and incident premenstrual syndrome. *Am J Clin Nutr.* 2011;93:1080.
82. Malouf R, Grimley Evans J. The effect of vitamin B6 on cognition. *Cochrane Database Syst Rev.* 2003;(4):CD004393.
83. Schaumberg H, Kaplan J, Windebank A, et al. Sensory neuropathy from pyridoxine abuse. A new megavitamin syndrome. *N Engl J Med.* 1983;309:445.
84. Duffy ME, Hoey L, Hughes CF, et al. Biomarker response to folic acid intervention in healthy adults: a meta-analysis of randomized controlled trials. *Am J Clin Nutr.* 2014;99:96.
85. Botto LD, Moore CA, Khoury MJ, et al. Neural-tube defects. *N Engl J Med.* 1999;341:1509.
86. Cesari M, Rossi GP, Sticchi D, et al. Is homocysteine important as risk factor for coronary artery disease? *Nutr Metab Cardiovasc Dis.* 2005;15:140.
87. Caudill MA. Folate bioavailability: implications for establishing dietary recommendations and optimizing status. *Am J Clin Nutr.* 2010;91(Suppl):1455S.
88. Bailey LB. Dietary reference intakes for folate: the debut of dietary folate equivalents. *Nutr Rev.* 1998;56:294.
89. Lewis CJ, Crane NT, Wilson DB, et al. Estimated folate intakes: data updated to reflect food fortification, increased bioavailability, and dietary supplement use. *Am J Clin Nutr.* 1999;70:198.
90. Snow CF. Laboratory diagnosis of vitamin B12 and folate deficiency: a guide for the primary care physician. *Arch Intern Med.* 1999;159:1289.
91. Koontz JL, Phillips KM, Wunderlich KM, et al. Comparison of total folate concentrations in foods determined by microbiological assay at several experienced U.S. commercial laboratories. *J AOAC Int.* 2005;88:805.
92. DeVries JW, Rader JI, Keagy PM, et al. Microbiological assay-trienzyme procedure for total folates in cereals and cereal foods: collaborative study. *J AOAC Int.* 2005;88:5.
93. Yetley EA, Coates PM, Johnson CL. Overview of a roundtable on NHANES monitoring of biomarkers of folate and vitamin B-12 status: measurement procedure issues. *Am J Clin Nutr.* 2011;94(Suppl):297S.
94. Pfeiffer CM, Fazili Z, Zhang M. Folate analytical methodology. In: Bailey LB, ed. *Folate in Health and Disease.* 2nd ed. Boca Raton, FL: CRC Press, 2010:517.
95. Nakazato M, Maeda T, Emura K, et al. Blood folate concentrations analyzed by microbiological assay and chemiluninescent immunoassay methods. *J Nutr Sci Vitaminol.* 2012;58:59.
96. Laurence VA, Loewenstein JE, Eichner ER. Aspirin and folate binding: *in vivo* and *in vitro* studies of serum binding and urinary excretion of endogenous folate. *J Lab Clin Med.* 1984;103:944.
97. Weir DG, McGing PG, Scott JM. Folate metabolism, the enterohepatic circulation and alcohol. *Biochem Pharmacol.* 1985;34:1.
98. Jarrell CJ, Kirsch SH, Herrmann M. Red cell or serum folate: what to do in clinical practice? *Clin Chem Lab Med.* 2013;51:555.
99. Klee GG. Cobalamin and folate evaluation: measurement of methylmalonic acid and homocysteine vs vitamin B(12) and folate. *Clin Chem.* 2000;46:1277.
100. Ubbink JB, Delport R, Riezler R, et al. Comparison of three different plasma homocysteine assays with gas chromatography-mass spectrometry. *Clin Chem.* 1999;45:670.
101. Selhub J, Jacques PF, Rosenberg IH, et al. Serum total homocysteine concentrations in the Third National Health and Nutrition Examination Survey (1991–1994): population reference ranges and contribution of vitamin status to high serum concentrations. *Ann Intern Med.* 1999;131:331.
102. Zhao R, Goldman ID. Folate and thiamine transporters mediated by facilitative carriers (SLC19A1-3 and SLC46A1) and folate receptors. *Mol Aspects Med.* 2013;34:373.
103. Desmoulin SK, Hou Z, Gangjee A, et al. The human proton-coupled folate transporter: biology and therapeutic applications to cancer. *Cancer Biol Ther.* 2012;14:1355.
104. Birn H, Spiegelstein O, Christensen EI, et al. Renal tubular reabsorption of folate mediated by folate binding protein 1. *J Am Soc Nephrol.* 2005;16:608.
105. Said HM, Mohammed ZM. Intestinal absorption of water-soluble vitamins: an update. *Curr Opin Gastroenterol.* 2006;22:140.
106. Fox JT, Stover PJ. Folate-mediated one-carbon metabolism. *Vit Horm.* 2008;79;1.
107. Stover PJ, Field MS. Trafficking of intracellular folates. *Adv Nutr.* 2011;2:325.
108. Davis RE. Clinical chemistry of folic acid. *Adv Clin Chem.* 1986;25:233.
109. MRC Vitamin Study Research Group. Prevention of neural tube defects: results of the Medical Research Council Vitamin Study. *Lancet.* 1991;338:131.

110. Czeizel AE, Dudas I. Prevention of the first occurrence of neural-tube defects by periconceptional vitamin supplementation. *N Engl J Med.* 1992;327:1832.
111. Berry RJ, Li Z, Erickson JD, et al. Prevention of neural-tube defects with folic acid in China. *N Engl J Med.* 1999;341:1485.
112. Tamura T, Picciano MF. Folate and human reproduction. *Am J Clin Nutr.* 2006;83:993.
113. Bailey LB, Rampersaud GC, Kauwell GP. Folic acid supplements and fortification affect the risk for neural tube defects, vascular disease and cancer: evolving science. *J Nutr.* 2003;133:1961S.
114. Eichholzer M, Tonz O, Zimmerman R. Folic acid: a public-health challenge. *Lancet.* 2006;22:1352.
115. Ueland PM, Monsen AL. Hyperhomocysteinemia and B-vitamin deficiencies in infants and children. *Clin Chem Lab Med.* 2003;41:1418.
116. Kirsch SH, HermannW, Obeid R. Genetic defects in folate and cobalamin pathways affecting the brain. *Clin Chem Lab Med.* 2013;51:339.
117. Gordon N. Cerebral folate deficiency. *Dev Med Child Neurol.* 2009;51:180.
118. Ramaekers VT, Rothenberg SP, Sequira JM, et al. Autoantibodies to folate receptors in the cerebral folate deficiency syndrome. *N Engl J Med.* 2005;352:1985.
119. Hamid A, Wani NA, Kaur J. New perspectives on folate transport in relation to alcoholism-induced folate malabsorption—association with epigenome stability and cancer development. *FEBS J.* 2009;276:2175.
120. Green R. Indicators for assessing folate and vitamin B-12 status and for monitoring the efficacy of intervention strategies. *Am J Clin Nutr.* 2011;94(Suppl):666S.
121. Majchrzak D, Singer I, Manner M, et al. B-vitamin status and concentrations of homocysteine in Austrian omnivores. *Ann Nutr Metab.* 2006;50:485.
122. McCully KS. Hyperhomocysteinemia and arteriosclerosis: historical perspectives. *Clin Chem Lab Med.* 2005;43:980.
123. Verhoef P, de Groot LC. Dietary determinants of plasma homocysteine concentrations. *Semin Vasc Med.* 2005;5:110.
124. Olthof MR, van Vliet T, Verhoef P, et al. Effect of homocysteine-lowering nutrients on blood lipids: results from four randomized, placebo-controlled studies in healthy humans. *PLoS Med.* 2005;2:e135.
125. Bostom AG, Silbershatz H, Rosenberg IH, et al. Nonfasting plasma total homocysteine levels and all-cause and cardiovascular mortality in elderly Framingham men and women. *Arch Intern Med.* 1999;159:1077.
126. Ridker PM, Manson JE, Buring JE, et al. Homocysteine and risk of cardiovascular disease among postmenopausal women. *JAMA.* 1999;281:1817.
127. Hackam DG, Anand SS. Emerging risk factors for atherosclerotic vascular disease: a critical review of the evidence. *JAMA.* 2003;290:932.
128. Voutilainen S, Jirtanen JK, Rissanen TH, et al. Serum folate and homocysteine and the incidence of acute coronary events: the Kuopio Ischaemic Heart Disease Risk Factor Study. *Am J Clin Nutr.* 2004;80:317.
129. Soinio M, Marniemi J, Laakso M, et al. Elevated plasma homocysteine level is an independent predictor of coronary heart disease events in patients with type 2 diabetes mellitus. *Ann Intern Med.* 2004;140:94.
130. Ganji V, Kafai MR. Demographic, health, lifestyle, and blood vitamin determinants of serum total homocysteine concentration in the Third National Health & Nutrition Survey 1988–1994. *Am J Clin Nutr.* 2003;77:826.
131. Lewis SJ, Ebrahim S, Davey Smith G. Meta-analysis of MTHFR 677C $\rightarrow$ T polymorphism and coronary heart disease: does totality of evidence support causal role for homocysteine and preventive potential of folate? *BMJ.* 2005;331:1053.
132. The Homocysteine Studies Collaboration. Homocysteine and risk of ischemic heart disease and stroke: a meta-analysis. *JAMA.* 2002;288:2015.
133. Homocysteine Lowering Trialists' Collaboration. Dose-dependent effects of folic acid on blood concentrations of homocysteine: a meta-analysis of the randomized trials. *Am J Clin Nutr.* 2005;82:806.
134. B-vitamin treatment Trialists' Collaboration. Homocysteine-lowering trials for prevention of cardiovascular events: a review of the design and power of the large randomized trials. *Am Heart J.* 2006;151:282.

135. Clarke R, Halsey J, Lweington S, et al. Effects of lowering homocysteine levels with B vitamins on cardiovascular disease, cancer, and cause-specific mortality: meta-analysis of 8 randomized trials involving 37,485 individuals. *Arch Intern Med.* 2010;170:1622.
136. Bonaa KH, Njolstad I, Ueland PM, et al. Homocysteine lowering and cardiovascular events after acute myocardial infarction. *N Engl J Med.* 2006;354:1578.
137. Schwammental Y, Tanne D. Homocysteine, B-vitamin supplementation and stroke prevention: from observational status to interventional trials. *Lancet Neurol.* 2004;3:493.
138. Bazzano LA, Reynolds K, Holder KN, et al. Effect of folic acid supplementation on risk of cardiovascular diseases: a meta-analysis of randomized controlled trials. *JAMA.* 2006; 296:2720.
139. Malinow MR, Bostom AG, Krauss RM. Homocysteine, diet, and cardiovascular diseases: a statement for healthcare professionals from the nutrition committee, American Heart Association. *Circulation.* 1999;99:178.
140. Chamberlain KL. Homocysteine and cardiovascular disease: a review of current recommendations for screening and treatment. *J Am Acad Nurse Pract.* 2005;17:90.
141. Goldstein LB, Bushnell CD, Adams RJ, et al. Guidelines for the primary prevention of stroke: a guideline for healthcare professionals from the American Heart Association/American Stroke Association. *Stroke.* 2011;42:517.
142. Oussalah A, Gueant JL, Peyrin-Biroulet L. Meta-analysis: hyperhomocysteinaemia in inflammatory bowel disease. *Aliment Pharmacol ther.* 2011;34:1173.
143. Mooijaart SP, Gussekloo J, Frolich M, et al. Homocysteine, vitamin B-12, and folic acid and the risk of cognitive decline in old age: the Leiden 80-plus study. *Am J Clin Nutr.* 2005; 82:866.
144. Malouf R, Evans JG. Folic acid with or without vitamin B12 for the prevention and treatment of healthy elderly and demented people. *Cochrane Database Syst Rev.* 2008;(4):CD004514.
145. Walker JG, Batterham PJ, Mackinnon AJ, et al. Oral folic acid and vitamin B-12 supplementation to prevent cognitive decline in community-dwelling older adults with depressive symptoms—the Beyond Ageing Project: a randomized controlled trial. *Am J Clin Nutr.* 2012;95:194.
146. Tucker KL, Qiao N, Scott T, et al. High homocysteine and low B vitamins predict cognitive decline in aging men: the Veterans Affairs Normative Aging Study. *Am J Clin Nutr.* 2005; 82:627.
147. Taylor MJ, Carney SM, Goodwin GM, et al. Folate for depressive disorders: systematic review and meta-analysis of randomized controlled trials. *J Psychopharmacol.* 2004;18:251.
148. Bottiglieri T. Homocysteine and folate metabolism in depression. *Prog Neuropsychopharmacol Biol Psychiatry.* 2005;29:1103.
149. Lazarou C, Kapsou M. The role of folic acid in prevention and treatment of depression: an overview of existing evidence and implications for practice. *Complement Ther Clin Pract.* 2010;16:161.
150. Dai WM, Yang B, Chu XY, et al. Association between folate intake, serum folate levels and the risk of lung cancer: a systematic review and meta-analysis. *Chin Med J.* 2013;126:1957.
151. Lee JE, Willett WC, Fuchs CS, et al. Folate intake and risk of colorectal cancer and adenoma: modification by time. *Am J Clin Nutr.* 2011;93:817.
152. Larsson SC, Giovannucci E, Wolk A. A prospective study of dietary folate intake and risk of colorectal cancer: modification by caffeine intake and cigarette smoking. *Cancer Epidemiol Biomarkers Prev.* 2005;14:740.
153. Bingham S. The fibre-folate debate in colo-rectal cancer. *Proc Nutr Soc.* 2006;65:19.
154. Kim DH, Smith-Warner SA, Speigelman D, et al. Pooled analyses of 13 prospective cohort studies on folate intake and colon cancer. *Cancer Causes Control.* 2010;21:1919.
155. Khosraviani K, Weir HP, Hamilton P, et al. Effect of folate supplementation on mucosal cell proliferation in high risk patients for colon cancer. *Gut.* 2002;51:195.
156. Pufulete M, Al-Ghnaniem R, Khushal A, et al. Effect of folic acid supplementation on genomic DNA methylation in patients with colorectal adenoma. *Gut.* 2005;54:648.
157. Kim YI. Folate: a mega-bullet or a double-edged sword for colorectal cancer promotion? *Gut.* 2006;55:1387.
158. Qin X, Cui Y, Shen L, et al. Folic acid supplementation and cancer risk: a meta-analysis of randomized controlled trials. *Int J Cancer.* 2013;133:1033.
159. Gibson TM, Weinstein SJ, Pfeiffer RM, et al. Pre- and post-fortification intake of folate and risk of colorectal cancer in a large prospective cohort study in the United States. *Am J Clin Nutr.* 2011;94:1053.

160. Mills JL. Fortification of foods with folic acid—how much is enough? *N Engl J Med.* 2000;342:1442.
161. Malinow MR, Duell PB, Hess DL, et al. Reduction of plasma homocysteine levels by breakfast cereal fortified with folic acid in patients with coronary artery disease. *N Engl J Med.* 1998;338:1009.
162. Jacques PF, Selhub J, Bostom AG, et al. The effect of folic acid fortification on plasma folate and total homocysteine concentrations. *N Engl J Med.* 1999;340:1449.
163. Mix JA. Do megadoses of vitamin C compromise folic acid's role in the metabolism of plasma homocysteine? *Nutr Res.* 1999;19:161.
164. Odewole OA, Williamson RS, Zakai NA, et al. Near elimination of folate deficiency anemia by mandatory folic acid fortification in older US adults: reasons for geographic and racial differences in stroke study. *Am J Clin Nutr.* 2013;98:1042.
165. Rosenberg I. Getting folic acid nutrition right. *Am J Clin Nutr.* 2010;91:3.
166. Houghton LA, Gray AR, Rose MC, et al. Long-term effect of low-dose folic acid intake: potential effect of mandatory fortification on the prevention of neural tube defects. *Am J Clin Nutr.* 2011;94:136.
167. Tighe P, Ward M, McNulty H, et al. A dose-finding trial of the effect of long-term folic acid intakes: implications for food fortification policy. *Am J Clin Nutr.* 2010;93:11.
168. Beaudet AI, Goin-Kochel RP. Some, but not complete, reassurance on the safety of folic acid fortification. *Am J clin Nutr.* 2010;92:1287.
169. Suren P, Roth C, Bresnahan M, et al. Association between maternal use of folic acid supplements and risk of autism spectrum disorders in children. *JAMA.* 2013;309:570.
170. Mills JL, Von Kohorn I, Conley MR, et al. Low vitamin B-12 concentrations in patients without anemia: the effect of folic acid fortification of grain. *Am J Clin Nutr.* 2003;77:1474.
171. Metz J, McNeil AR, Levin M. The relationship between serum cobalamin concentration and mean red cell volume at varying concentrations of serum folate. *Clin Lab Haematol.* 2004;26:323.
172. Mills JL, Carter TC, Scott JM, et al. Do high blood folate concentrations exacerbate metabolic abnormalities in people with low vitamin B-12 status? *Am J clin Nutr.* 2011;94:495.
173. Herbert V. Recommended dietary intakes (RDI) of folate in humans. *Am J Clin Nutr.* 1987;45:661.
174. Sesin GP, Kirschenbaum H. Folic acid hypersensitivity and fever: a case report. *Am J Hosp Pharm.* 1979;36:1565.
175. Ho C, Kauwell GPA, Bailey LB. Practitioners' guide to meeting the vitamin B-12 recommended dietary allowance for people aged 61 years and older. *J Am Diet Assoc.* 1999;99:725.
176. Yamada K, Yamada Y, Fukuda M, et al. Bioavailability of dried asakusanori (Porphyra tenera) as a source of cobalamin (vitamin B-12). *Int J Vitam Nutr Res.* 1999;69:412.
177. Fairbanks VF, Wahner HW, Phyliky RL. Tests for pernicious anemia: the "Schilling test." *Mayo Clin Proc.* 1983;58:541.
178. Wallis J, Clark DM, Bain BJ. The use of hydroxocobalamin in the Schilling test. *Scand J Haematol.* 1986;37:337.
179. Hardlei TF, Morkbak AL, Bor MV, et al. Assessment of vitamin B12 absorption based on the accumulation of orally administered cyanocobalamin on transcobalamin. *Clin Chem.* 2010;56:432.
180. von Castel-Roberts KM, Morkbak AL, Nexo E, et al. Holo-transcobalamin is an indicator of vitamin B-12 absorption in healthy adults with adequate vitamin B-12 status. *Am J Clin Nutr.* 2007;85:1057.
181. Greibe E, Nexo E. Vitamin B12 absorption judged by measurement of holotranscobalamin, active vitamin B12: evaluation of a commercially available EIA kit. *Clin Chem Lab Med.* 2011;49:1883.
182. Obeid R, Morkbak AL, Munz W, et al. The cobalamin-binding proteins transcobalamin and haptocorrin in maternal and cord blood sera at birth. *Clin Chem.* 2006;52:263.
183. Karmi O, Zayed A, Baraghethi S, et al. Measurement of vitamin B12 concentration: a review of available methods. *IIOAB J.* 2011;2:23.
184. Carmel R. Mild transcobalamin I (haptocorrin) deficiency and low serum cobalamin concentrations. *Clin Chem.* 2003;49:1367.
185. Yang DT, Cook RJ. Spurious elevations of vitamin B12 with pernicious anemia. *N Eng J Med.* 2012;368:1742.
186. Carmel R, Agrawal YP. Failures of cobalamin assays in pernicious anemia. *N Eng J Med.* 2012;367:385.
187. Lindenbaum J, Rosenberg IH, Wilson PW, et al. Prevalence of cobalamin deficiency in the Framingham elderly population. *Am J Clin Nutr.* 1994;60:2.

188. Ermens AAM, Vlasveld LT, Lindemans J. Significance of elevated cobalamin (vitamin B12) levels in blood. *Clin Biochem.* 2003;36:585.
189. Holleland G, Schneede J, Ueland PM, et al. Cobalamin deficiency in general practice. Assessment of the diagnostic utility and cost–benefit analysis of methylmalonic acid determination in relation to current diagnostic strategies. *Clin Chem.* 1999;45:189.
190. Bailey RL, Carmel R, Green R, et al. Monitoring of vitamin B12 nutritional status in the United States using plasma methylmalonic acid and serum vitamin B12. *Am J Clin Nutr.* 2011; 74:552.
191. Loehrer FM, Schwab R, Angst CP, et al. Influence of oral S-adenosylmethionine on plasma 5-methyltetrahydrofolate, S-adenosylhomocysteine, homocysteine and methionine in healthy humans. *J Pharmacol Exp Ther.* 1997;282:845.
192. Refsum H, Johnston C, Guttormsen AB, et al. Holotranscobalamin and total transcobalamin in human plasma: determination, determinants, and reference values in healthy adults. *Clin Chem.* 2006;52:129.
193. Miller JW, Garrod MG, Rockwood AL, et al. Measurement of total vitamin B12 and holotranscobalamin, singly and in combination, in screening for metabolic vitamin B12 deficiency. *Clin Chem.* 2006;52:2.
194. Nexo E, Hoffmann-Lucke E. Holotranscobalamin: a marker of vitamin B-12 status: analytical aspects and clinical utility. *Am J Clin Nutr.* 2011;94(Suppl):359S.
195. Obeid R, Hermann W. Holotranscobalamin in laboratory diagnosis of cobalamin deficiency compared to total cobalamin and methylmalonic acid. *Clin Chem Lab Med.* 2007;45:1746.
196. Valente E, Scott JM, Ueland PM, et al. Diagnostic accuracy of holotranscobalamin, methylmalonicacid, serum cobalamin, and other indicators of tissue vitamin B12 status in the elderly. *Clin Chem.* 2011;57:856.
197. Carmel R. Subclinical cobalamin deficiency. *Curr Opin Gastroenterol.* 2012;28:51.
198. Carmel R. Biomarkers of cobalamin (vitamin B-12) status in the epidemiologic setting: a critical overviewof context, applications, and performance characteristics of cobalamin, methylmalonic acid, and holotranscobalamin. *Am J Clin Nutr.* 2011;94:348S.
199. Padovani D, Banerjee R. A rotary mechanism for coenzyme B12 synthesis by adenosyltransferase. *Biochemistry.* 2009;48:5350.
200. Shane B, Stokstad EL. Vitamin B12–folate interrelationship. *Annu Rev Nutr.* 1985;5:115.
201. Seetharam B, Alpers DH. Cobalamin absorption. In: Field M, Frizzell RA, eds. *Handbook of Physiology, Section 6: The Gastrointestinal System.* Vol IV. Bethesda, MD: American Physiological Society, 1991:437.
202. Andersen CB, Madsen M, Storm T, et al. Structural basis for receptor recognition of vitamin B12-intrinsic factor complexes. *Nature.* 2010;464:445.
203. Nielsen MJ, Mie R, Rasmussen CB, et al. Vitamin B12 transport from food to the body's cells—a sophisticated multistep pathway. *Nat Rev Gastroenterol Hepatol.* 2012;9:345.
204. Wuerges J, Garau G, Geremia S, et al. Structural basis for mammalian vitamin B12 transport by transcobalamin. *Proc Natl Acad Sci U S A.* 2006;103:4386.
205. Quadros EV, Sequeira JM. Cellular uptake of cobalamin: transcobalamin and the TCb1R/CD320 receptor. *Biochimie.* 2013;95:1008.
206. Ermens AA, Sonneveld P, Michiels JJ, et al. Increased uptake and accumulation of cobalamin by multiple myeloma bone marrow cells as a possible cause of low serum cobalamin. *Eur J Haematol.* 1993;50:57.
206a. Tanumihadjo SA. Assessing Vitamin A status: past, present and future. *J Nutr* 2004;134:290S
207. Bauman WA, Shaw S, Jayatilleke E, et al. Increased intake of calcium reverses vitamin B12 malabsorption induced by metformin. *Diabetes Care.* 2000;23:1227.
208. Lahner E, Annibale B. Pernicious anemia: new insights from a gastroenterological point of view. *World J Gastroenterol.* 2009;15:5121.
209. Lam JR, Schneider JL, Zjao W, et al. Proton pump inhibitor and histamine 2 receptor antagonist use and vitamin B12 deficiency. *JAMA.* 2013;310:2435.
210. Stabler SP. Vitamin B12 deficiency. *N Eng J Med.* 2013;368:149.
211. Dali-Youcef N, Andres E. An update on cobalamin deficiency in adults. *Q J Med.* 2009;102:17.
212. Miller A, Korem M, Almog R, et al. Vitamin B12, demyelination, remyelination and repair in multiple sclerosis. *J Neurol Sci.* 2005;233:93.
213. Krishna KK, Arafat M, Ichaporia NR, et al. MRI findings in cobalamin deficiency. *J Clin Neurosci.* 2003;10:84.

214. Bucca CB, Culla B, Guida G, et al. Unexplained chronic cough and vitamin B-12 deficiency. *Am J Clin Nutr*. 2011;93:542.
215. Healton EB, Savage DG, Grust JC, et al. Neurologic aspects of cobalamin deficiency. *Medicine (Baltimore)*. 1991;70:229.
216. Hutto BR. Folate and cobalamin in psychiatric illness. *Compr Psychiatry*. 1997;38:305.
217. Harris E, MacPherson H, Vitetta L, et al. Effects of a multivitamin, mineral and herbal supplement on cognition and blood biomarkers in older men: a randomized placebo-controlled trial. *Hum Psychopharmacol Clin Exp*. 2012;27:370.
218. McCaddon A. Vitamin B12 in neurology and aging: clinical and genetic aspects. *Biochimie*. 2013;95:1066.
219. Celik M, Barkut IK, Oncel C, et al. Involuntary movements associated with vitamin B12 deficiency. *Parkinsonsim Relat Disord*. 2003;10:55.
220. Manzanares W, Hardy G. Vitamin B12: the forgotten micronutrient for critical care. *CurrOpin Clin Nutr Metab Care*. 2010;13:662.
221. McCracken C. Challenges of long-term nutrition intervention studies on cognition: discordance between observational and intervention studies of vitamin B12 and cognition. *Nutr Rev*. 2010;68(Suppl 1):511.
222. Favrat B, Vaucher P, Herzig L, et al. Oral vitamin B12 for patients suspected of subtle cobalamin deficiency: a multicenter pragmatic randomized controlled trial. *BMC Fam Pract*. 2011;12:2.
223. Rajan S, Wallace JI, Brodkin KI, et al. Response of elevated methylmalonic acid to three dose levels of oral cobalamin in older adults. *J Am Geriatr Soc*. 2002;50:1789.
224. Garcia A, Paris-Pombo A, Evans L, et al. Is low-dose oral cobalamin enough to normalize cobalamin function in older people? *J Am Geriatr Soc*. 2002;50:1401.
225. Langman LJ, Cole DEC. Homocysteine: cholesterol of the 90s? *Clin Chim Acta*. 1999;286:63
226. Adams JF, Ross SK, Mervyn L, et al. Absorption of cobalamin, coenzyme B12, methylcobalamin, and hydroxocobalamin at different dose levels. *Scand J Gastroenterol*. 1971;6:249.
227. Watkins D, Rosenblatt DS. Lessons in biology from patients with inborn errors of vitamin B12 metabolism. *Biochimie*. 2013;95:1019.
228. Kuwabara S, Nakazawa R, Azuma N, et al. Intravenous methylcobalamin treatment for uremic and diabetic neuropathy in chronic hemodialysis patients. *Intern Med*. 1999;38:472.
229. Sato Y, Honda Y, Iwamoto J, et al. Effect of folate and mecobalamin on hip fractures in patients with stroke: a randomized controlled trial. *JAMA*. 2005;293:1082.
230. Sease JM. Does vitamin B12 help relieve fatigue? *Medscape Pharmacists*. 2009. http://medscape.com/viewarticle/585589.
231. Lederle FA. Oral cobalamin for pernicious anemia. Medicine's best kept secret? *JAMA*. 1991;265:94.
232. Kuzminski AM, Giacco EJD, Allen RH, et al. Effective treatment of cobalamin deficiency with oral cobalamin. *Blood*. 1998;92:1191.
233. Butler CC, Vidal-Alaball J, Cannings-John R, et al. Oral vitamin B12 versus intramuscular vitamin B12 for vitamin B12 deficiency: a systematic review of randomized controlled trials. *Fam Pract*. 2006;23:279.
234. Anonymous. Vitamin B12 nasal spray. *Med Lett Drugs Ther*. 2005;47:64.
235. Allen LH. How common is vitamin B12 deficiency? *Am J Clin Nutr*. 2009;89(Suppl):693S.
236. Carmel R. Mandatory fortification of the food supply with cobalamin: an idea whose time has not yet come. *J Inherit Metab Dis*. 2011;34:67.
237. Levine M, Conry-Cantilena C, Wang Y, et al. Vitamin C pharmacokinetics in healthy volunteers: evidence for a recommended dietary allowance. *Proc Natl Acad Sci U S A*. 1996;93:3704.
238. Lachance P, Langseth L. The RDA concept: time for a change? *Nutr Rev*. 1994;52:266.
239. Vanderslice JT, Higgs DJ. Vitamin C content of foods: ample variability. *Am J Clin Nutr*. 1991;54:1323S.
240. Ausman LM. Criteria and recommendations for vitamin C intake. *Nutr Rev*. 1999;57:222.
241. Wilson JX. Regulation of vitamin C transport. *Annu Rev Nutr*. 2005;25:105.
242. Timpson NJ, Forouhi NG, Brian MJ, et al. Genetic variation at the SLC23A1 locus is associated with circulating concentrations of L-ascorbic acid (vitamin C): evidence from 5 independent studies with >15,000 participants. *Am J Clin Nutr*. 2010;92:375.
243. Rivas CI, Zuniga FA, Salas-Burgos A, et al. Vitamin C transporters. *J Physiol Biochem*. 2008;64:357.

244. Levine M, Padayatty SJ, Espey MG. Vitamin C: a concentration-function approach yields pharmacology and therapeutic discoveries. *Adv Nutr.* 2011;2:78.
245. Padayatty SJ, Sun H, Wang Y, et al. Vitamin C pharmacokinetics: evaluation of its role in disease prevention. *J Am Coll Nutr.* 2003;22:18.
246. Packer L, Fuchs J, eds. *Vitamin C in Health and Disease.* New York: Marcel Dekker Inc, 1997.
247. Fain O. Musculoskeletal manifestations of scurvy. *Joint Bone Spine.* 2005;72:124.
248. Francescone MA, Levitt J. Scurvy masquerading as leukocytoclastic vasculitis: a case report and review of the literature. *Cutis.* 2005;76:261.
249. Fukushima R, Yamazaki E. Vitamin C requirement in surgical patients. *Curr Opin Clin Nutr Metab Care.* 2010;13:669.
250. Aditi A, Graham DY. Vitamin C, gastritis, and gastric disease: a historical review and update. *Dig Dis Sci.* 2012;57:2504.
251. Wintergerst ES, Maggini S, Hornig DH. Immune-enhancing role of vitamin C and zinc and effects on clinical conditions. *Ann Nutr Metab.* 2006;50:85.
252. Douglas RM, Hemila H, D'Souza R, et al. Vitamin C for preventing and treating the common cold. *Cochrane Database Syst Rev.* 2004;18(4):CD000980.
253. Bielory L, Gandhi R. Asthma and vitamin C. *Ann Allergy.* 1994;73:89.
254. Juraschek SP, Guallar E, Appel LJ, et al. Effects of vitamin C supplementation on blood pressure: a meta-analysis of randomized controlled trials. *Am J Clin Nutr.* 2012;95:1079.
255. Padayatty SJ, Katz A, Wang Y, et al. Vitamin C as an antioxidant: evaluation of its role in disease prevention. *J Am Coll Nutr.* 2003;22:18.
256. Ness AR, Powles JW, Khaw KT. Vitamin C and cardiovascular disease: a systematic review. *J Cardiovasc Risk.* 1996;3:513.
257. Czernichow S, Blacher J, Hercberg S. Antioxidant vitamins and blood pressure. *Curr Hypertens Rep.* 2004;6:27.
258. Muntwyler J, Hennekens CH, Manson JE, et al. Vitamin supplement use in a low-risk population of US male physicians and subsequent cardiovascular mortality. *Arch Intern Med.* 2002;162:1472.
259. Osganian SK, Stampfer MJ, Rimm E, et al. Vitamin C and risk of coronary heart disease in women. *J Am Coll Cardiol.* 2003;42:246.
260. Khaw KT, Bingham S, Welch A, et al. Relation between plasma ascorbic acid and mortality in men and women in EPIC-Norfolk prospective study: a prospective population study. *Lancet.* 2001;357:657.
261. Weber P, Bendich A, Shcalch W. Vitamin C and human health—a review of recent data relevant to human requirements. *Int J Vitam Nutr Res.* 1996;66:19.
262. Frei B. To C or not to C, that is the question. *J Am Coll Cardiol.* 2003;42:253.
263. Plummer M, Vivas J, Lopez G, et al. Chemoprevention of precancerous gastric lesions with antioxidant vitamin supplementation: a randomized trial in a high-risk population. *J Natl Cancer Inst.* 2007;99:137.
264. Papaioannou D, Cooper KL, Carroll C, et al. Antioxidants in the chemoprevention of colorectal cancer and colorectal adenomas in the general population: a systematic review and meta-analysis. *Colorectal Dis.* 2011;13:1985.
265. Padayatty SJ, Riordan HD, Hewitt SM, et al. Intravenously administered vitamin C as cancer therapy: three cases. *CMAJ.* 2006;174:937.
266. Ohno S, Ohno Y, Suzuki N, et al. High-dose vitamin C (ascorbic acid) therapy in the treatment of patients with advanced cancer. *Anticancer Res.* 2009;29:809.
267. Padayatty SJ, Sun H, Wang Y, et al. Vitamin C pharmacokinetics: implications for oral and intravenous use. *Ann Intern Med.* 2004;140:533.
268. Hoffer LJ, Levine M, Assouline S, et al. Phase 1 clinical trial of i.v. ascorbic acid in advanced malignancy. *Ann Oncol.* 2008;19:1969.
269. Riordan HD, Casciari JJ, Gonzalez NJ, et al. A pilot clinical study of continuous intravenous ascorbate in terminal cancer patients. *PR Health Sci J.* 2005;524:269.
270. Padayatty SJ, Sun AY, Chen QI, et al. Vitamin C: intravenous use by complementary and alternative medicine practitioners and adverse effects. *PLoS ONE.* 2010;5:e11414.
271. Cabanillas F. Vitamin C and cancer: what can we conclude1,600 patients and 33 years later? *P R Health Sci J.* 2010;29:215.
272. Teucher B, Olivares M, Cori H. Enhancers of iron absorption: ascorbic acid and other organic acids. *Int J Vitam Nutr Res.* 2004;74:403.

273. Johnston CS. Biomarkers for establishing a tolerable upper intake level for vitamin C. *Nutr Rev.* 1999;57:71.
274. Taylor EN, Stampfer MJ, Curhan GC. Dietary factors and the risk of incident kidney stones in men: new insights after 14 years of follow-up. *J Am Soc Nephrol.* 2004;15:3225.
275. Thomas LDK, Elinder CG, Tiselius HG, et al. Ascorbic acid supplements and kidney stone incidence among men: a prospective study. *JAMA Intern Med.* 2013;173:386.
276. Staggs CG, Sealey WM, McCabe BJ, et al. Determination of the biotin content of select foods using accurate and sensitive HPLC/avidin binding. *J Food Compost Anal.* 2004;17:767.
277. Zempleni J, Mock DM. Biotin biochemistry and human requirements. *J Nutr Biochem.* 1999;10:128.
278. Vlasova TI, Tratton SL, Wells AM, et al. Biotin deficiency reduces expression of SLC19A3, a potential biotin transporter, in leukocytes from human blood. *J Nutr.* 2005;135:42.
279. Said HM. Cell and molecular aspects of human intestinal biotin absorption. *J Nutr.* 2009;129:158.
280. Ghosal A, Lambrecht N, Subramanya SB, et al. Conditional knockout of the Slc5a6 gene in mouse intestine impairs biotin absorption. *Am J Physiol Gastrointest Liver Physiol.* 2011;304:G64.
281. Said HM. Biotin: the forgotten vitamin. *Am J Clin Nutr.* 2002;75:179.
282. Mock DM, de Lorimer AA, Liebman WM, et al. Biotin deficiency: an unusual complication of parenteral alimentation. *N Engl J Med.* 1981;304:820.
283. Zempleni J, Mock DM. Marginal biotin deficiency is teratogenic. *Proc Soc Exp Biol Med.* 2000;223:14.
284. Thoene J, Baker H, Yoshino M, et al. Biotin-responsive carboxylase deficiency associated with subnormal plasma and urinary biotin. *N Engl J Med.* 1981;304:817.
285. Friebel D, von der Hagen M, Baumgartner ER, et al. The first case of 3-methylcorotonyl-CoA carboxylase (MCC) deficiency responsive to biotin. *Neuropediatrics.* 2006;37:72.
286. Mardach R, Zempleni J, Wolf B, et al. Biotin dependency due to a defect in biotin transport. *J Clin Invest.* 2002;109:1617.
287. Wolf B, Heard G, Jefferson LG, et al. Clinical finding in four children with biotinidase deficiency detected through a statewide neonatal screening program. *N Engl J Med.* 1985;313:16.
288. Leonardi R, Zhang YM, Rock CO, et al. Coenzyme A: back in action. *Prog Lipid Res.* 2005;44:125.
289. Gregory A, Hayflick SJ. Neurodegeneration with brain iron accumulation. *Folia Neuropathol.* 2005;43:286.
290. McRae MP. Treatment of hyperlipoproteinemia with pantethine: a review and anlaysis of efficacy and tolerability. *Nutr Res.* 2005;25:319.
291. Rumberger JA, Napolitano J, Azmano I, et al. Pantethine, a derivative of vitamin B(5) used as a nutritional supplement, favorably alters low-density lipoprotein cholesterol metabolism in low- to moderate-cardiovascular risk North American subjects: a triple-blind placebo and diet-controlled investigation. *Nutr Res.* 2011;31:608.
292. Anonymous, Coenzyme Q10. *Med Lett Drugs Ther.* 2006;48:19.
293. Henchcliffe C, Beal MF. Mitochondrial biology and oxidative stress in Parkinson disease pathogenesis. *Nat Clin Pract Neurol.* 2008;4:600.
294. Miles MV, Horn PS, Tang PH, et al. Age-related changes in plasma coenzyme Q10 concentrations and redox state in apparently healthy children and adults. *Clin Chim Acta.* 2004; 347:139.
295. Horvath R, Schneiderat P, Schoser BGH, et al. Coenzyme Q10 deficiency and isolated myopathy. *Neurology* 2006;66:253.
296. Lamperti C, Naini A, Hirano M, et al. Cerebellar ataxia and coenzyme Q10 deficiency. *Neurology.* 2003;60:1206.
297. Schapira AHV. Mitochondrial disease. *Lancet.* 2006;368:70.
298. Littarru GP, Tiano L. Clinical aspects of coenzyme Q10: an update. *Nutrition.* 2010;26:250.
299. Rosenfeldt FL, Haas SJ, Krum H, et al. Coenzyme Q10 in the treatment of hypertension: a meta-analysis of the clinical trials. *J Hum Hypertens.* 2007;21:297.
300. Gao L, Mao Q, Cao J, et al. Effect of coenzyme Q10 on vascular endothelial function in humans: a meta-analysis of randomized controlled trials. *Atherosclerosis.* 2012;22:311.
301. Sandor PS, Di Clemente L, Coppola G, et al. Efficacy of coenzyme Q10 in migraine prophylaxis: a randomised controlled trial. *Neurology.* 2005;64:713.
302. Bhagavan HN, Chopra RK. Plasma coenzyme Q10 response to oral ingestion of coenzyme Q10 formulations. *Mitochondrion.* 2007;78:S78.

303. Langsjoen PH, Langsjoen AM. The clinical use of HMG CoA-reductase inhibitors and the associated depletion of coenzyme Q10. A review of animal and human publications. *Biofactors.* 2003;18:101.
304. Vogel JH, Bolling SF, Costello RB, et al. Integrating complementary medicine into cardiovascular medicine. *J Am Coll Cardiol.* 2005;46:184.
305. Standing Committee on the Scientific Evaluation of Dietary Reference Intakes, Food and Nutrition Board, Institute of Medicine. *Dietary Reference Intakes for Vitamin A, Vitamin K, Arsenic, Boron, Chromium, Copper, Iodine, Iron, Manganese, Molybdenum, Nickel, Silicon, Vanadium, and Zinc.* Washington, DC: National Academies Press, 2001. Available on line at http://www.nap.edu/books, *Crawler list 0309072794*. Accessed May 30, 2001.
306. Cooper DA. Carotenoids in health and disease: recent scientific evaluation, research recommendations and the consumer. *J Nutr.* 2004;134:221S.
307. Brown L, Rimm EB, Seddon JM, et al. A prospective study of carotenoid intake and risk of cataract extraction in U.S. men. *Am J Clin Nutr.* 1999;70:517.
308. Aggarwal BB, Shishodia S. Molecular targets of dietary agents for prevention and therapy of cancer. *Biochem Pharmacol.* 2006;71:1397.
309. Tang G. Techiques for measuring vitamin A activity from β-carotene. *Am J Clin Nutr.* 2012;96(Suppl):1185S.
310. West CE, Eilander A, van Lieshout M. Letter to editor. *Am J Clin Nutr.* 2003;133:2917.
311. Tang G. Bioconversion of dietary provitamin A carotenoids to vitamin A in humans. *Am J Clin Nutr.* 2010;91(Suppl):1468S.
312. Harrison EH. Mechanisms of digestion and absorption of dietary vitamin A. *Annu Rev Nutr.* 2005;25:87.
313. Dimitrov NV, Meyer C, Ullrey DE, et al. Bioavailability of beta-carotene in humans. *Am J Clin Nutr.* 1988;48:298.
314. Rock CL, Swendseid ME. Plasma β-carotene response in humans after meals supplemented with dietary pectin. *Am J Clin Nutr.* 1992;55:96.
315. Elinder L, Hadell K, Johansson J, et al. Probucol treatment decreases serum concentrations of diet-derived antioxidants. *Arterioscler Thromb Vasc Biol.* 1995;15:1057.
316. Fredrikzon B, Hernell O, Blackberg L, et al. Bile salt-stimulated lipase in human milk: evidence of activity *in vivo* and of a role in the digestion of milk retinol esters. *Pediatr Res.* 1978;12:1048.
317. Tanumihardjo SA. Assessing vitamin A status: past, present and future. *J Nutr.* 2004;134:290S.
318. Valtuena J, Breidenassel C, Folle J, et al. Retinol, β-carotene, and vitamin D status in European adolescents; regional differences and variability: a review. *Nutr Hosp.* 2011;26:280.
319. Valentine AR, David CR, Tanumihardjo SA. Vitamin A isotope dilution predicts liver stones in line with long-term vitamin A intake above the current Recommended Dietary Allowance for young adult women. *Am J Clin Nutr.* 2013;98:1192.
320. Tanumihardjo SA. Vitamin A: biomarkers of nutrition for development. *Am J Clin Nutr.* 2011;94(Suppl):658S.
321. Thurnham DI, McCabe GP. Northrop-Clewes CA, et al. Effects of subclinical infection on plasma retinol concentrations and assessment of prevalence of vitamin A deficiency: meta-analysis. *Lancet.* 2003;362:2052.
322. Underwood BA. Method for assessment of vitamin A status. *J Nutr.* 1990;120(Suppl 11):1459.
323. Blomhoff R, Green MH, Norum KR. Vitamin A: physiological and biochemical processing. *Annu Rev Nutr.* 1992;12:37.
324. Senoo H, Kojima N, Sato M. Vitamin A-storing cells (stellate cells). *Vitam Horm.* 2007;75:131.
325. Schmidt DR, Homstrom SR, Tacer KF, et al. Regulation of bile acid synthesis by fat-soluble vitamins A and D. *J Biol Chem.* 2010;285:14486.
326. Hicks VA, Gunning DB, Olson JA. Metabolism, plasma transport and biliary excretion of radioactive vitamin A and its metabolites as a function of liver reserves of vitamin A in the rat. *J Nutr.* 1984;114:1327.
327. Pryor WA, Stahl W, Rock CL. Beta carotene: from biochemistry to clinical trials. *Nutr Rev* 2000;58:39.
328. Checkley W, West KP, Wise RA, et al. Maternal vitamin A supplementation and lung function in offspring. *N Engl J Med.* 2010;362:1784.
329. Massaro D, Massaro GD. Lung development, lung function, and retinoids. *N Eng J Med.* 2010;362:1829.
330. Anonymous. Carotenoids. *Adv Nutr.* 2013;4:474.

331. Tyson JE, Wright LL, Oh W, et al. Vitamin A supplementation for extremely low-birth-weight infants. *N Engl J Med.* 1999;340:1962.
332. Ross DA. Recommendations for vitamin A supplementation. *J Nutr.* 2002;131:2902S.
333. Latham M. The great vitamin A fiasco. *World Nutr.* 2010;1:12.
334. Zhou GB, Zhao WL, Wang ZY, et al. Retinoic acid and arsenic for treating acute promyelocytic leukemia. *PLoS Med.* 2005;2:33.
335. Lazzaroni M, Gandini S, Puntoni M, et al. The science behind vitamins and natural compounds for breast cancer prevention. Getting the most prevention out of it. *Breast.* 2011;20(Suppl 3):S36.
336. Mannisto S, Smith-Warner SA, Spiegelman D, et al. Dietary carotenoids and risk of lung cancer in a pooled analysis of seven cohort studies. *Cancer Epidemiol Biomarkers Prev.* 2004;13:40.
337. Bjelakovic G, Nikolova D, Simonetti RG, Gluud C. Antioxidant supplements for prevention of gastrointestinal cancers: a systematic review and meta-analysis. *Lancet.* 2004;364:1219.
338. Voutilainen S, Narmi T, Mursu J, et al. Carotenoids and cardiovascular health. *Am J Clin Nutr.* 2006;83:1265.
339. Huiming Y, Chaomin W, Meng M. Vitamin A for treating measles in children. *Cochrane Database Syst Rev.* 2005;19:CD001479.
340. Rahmathullah L, Underwood BA, Thulasiraj R, et al. Reduced mortality among children in Southern India receiving a small weekly dose of vitamin A. *N Engl J Med.* 1990;323:929.
341. Penniston KL, Tanumihardjo SA. The acute and chronic toxic effects of vitamin A. *Am J Clin Nutr.* 2006;83:191.
342. Ovesen L. Vitamin therapy in the absence of obvious deficiency. What is the evidence? *Drugs.* 1984;27:148.
343. Melhus H, Michaelsson K, Kindmark A, et al. Excessive dietary intake of vitamin A is associated with reduced bone mineral density and increased risk for hip fracture. *Ann Intern Med.* 1998;129:770.
344. Oakley GP, Erickson JD. Vitamin A and birth defects: continuing caution is needed. *N Engl J Med.* 1995;333:1414.
345. Fenaux P, DeBooton S. Retinoic acid syndrome: recognition, prevention and management. *Drug Saf.* 1998;18:273.
346. Anonymous. Absorica for Acne. *Med Lett Drugs Ther.* 2013;55:8.
347. Shale M, Kaplan G, Panaccione R, et al. Isotretinoin and intestinal inflammation: what gastroenterologists need to know. *Gut.* 2009;58:737.
348. Japelt RB, Jackobsen J. Vitamin D in plants: a review of occurrence, analysis, and biosynthesis. *Front Plant Sci.* 2013;4:1.
349. Holick MF. Vitamin D: importance in the prevention of cancers, type 1 diabetes, heart disease, and osteoporosis. *Am J Clin Nutr.* 2004;79:362
350. GB HealthWatch. http://gbhealthwatch.com/Did-you-know-Get-VitD-Sun-Exposure.php.
351. Durazo-Arvizu RA, Camacho P, Bovet P, et al. 25-Hydroxyvitamin D in Afro-origin populations at varying latitudes challenge the construct of a physiologic norm. *Am J Clin Nutr.* 2014;100:908.
352. Heaney RP, Arnas LA, French C. All-source basal vitamin D inputs are greater than previously thought and cutaneous inputs are smaller. *J Nutr.* 2013;143:571.
353. Schmid A, Walther B. Natural vitamin D content in animal products. *Adv Nutr.* 2013;4:453.
354. Cashman KD, Seamans KM, Lucey AJ, et al. Relative effectiveness of oral 25-hydroxyvitamin D3 and vitamin D3 in raising wintertime serum 25-hydroxyvitamin D in older adults. *Am J Clin Nutr.* 2012;95:1350.
355. Glossmann HH. Pharmacology of vitamin D: anything new? *Osteologie.* 2011;20:299.
356. Wortsman J, Matsuoka LY, Chen TC, et al. Decreased bioavailability of vitamin D in obesity. *Am J Clin Nutr.* 2000;72:690.
357. Arnas LA, Gregory P, Horst RL. Content of commercially available, single-ingredient vitamin D dietary supplements. *J EvidBased Complementary Altern Med.* 2012;17:54.
358. Tripkovic L, Lambert H, Hart K, et al. Comparison of vitamin D2 and vitamin D3 supplementation in raising serum 25-hydroxyvitamin D status: a systematic review and meta-analysis. *Am J Clin Nutr.* 2012;95:1357.
359. Vieth R. Implications for 25-hydroxyvitamin D testing of public policies about the benefits and risks of vitamin D fortification and supplementation. *Scand J Clin Lab Invest.* 2012;243(Suppl):144.

360. Calvo M, Whiting SJ. Survey of current vitamin D food fortification practices in the United States and Canada. *J Steroid Biochem Mol Biol*. 2013;136:211.
361. O'Donnell S, Cranney A, Horsley T, et al. Efficacy of food fortification on serum 25-hydroxyvitamin D concentrations: systematic review. *Am J Clin Nutr*. 2008;88:1528.
362. Bischoff-Ferrari H. Vitamin D: what is an adequate vitamin D level and how much supplementation is necessary? *Best Pract Res Clin Rheumatol*. 2009;23:789.
363. National Institute for Health and Care Excellence (NICE). Vitamin D Expert Review, Cancer Research UK. http://www.nice.org.uk/nicemedia/live/11871/49665/49665.pdf.
364. Institute of Medicine of the National Academy. *Dietary Reference Intakes for Calcium and Vitamin D*. Washington, DC: National Academies Press, 2011.
365. Ross AC, Manson JE, Abrams SA, et al. The 2011 report on dietary reference intakes for calcium and vitamin D from the Institute of Medicine: what clinicians need to know. *J Clin Endocrinol Metab*. 2011;96:53.
366. Cashman KD, FitzGerald AP, Viljakainen HT, et al. Estimation of the dietary requirements for vitamin D in healthy white adolescent girls. *Am J Clin Nutr*. 2011;93:549.
367. Abrams SA. Vitamin D requirements in adolescents: what is the target? *Am J Clin Nutr*. 2011;93:483.
368. Chung M, Balk EM, Brendel M, et al. Vitamin D and calcium: a systematic review of health outcomes. Evidence Report/Technology Assessments No. 183. AHRQ Publication No. 09-E015, Rockville, MD, 2009. http://www.ahrq.gov/downloads/pub/evidence/pdf/vitadcal/pdf.
369. Brouwer-Brolsma EM, Bischoff-Ferrari HA, Bouillon R, et al. Vitamin D: do we get enough? A discussion between vitamin D experts in order to make a step towards the harmonization of dietary reference intakes for vitamin D across Europe. *Osteoporosis Int*. 2013;24:1567.
370. EFSA Panel on Dietetic Products, Nutrition, and Allergies (NDA). Scientific opinion on the tolerable upper intake level of vitamin D. *EFSA J*. 2012;10:2813.
371. Heaney RP, Holick MF. Why the IOM recommendations for vitamin D are deficient. *J Bone Miner Res*. 2011;26:455.
372. Hanley DA, Cranney A, Jones G, et al. Vitamin D in adult health and disease: a review and guideline statement from Osteoporosis Canada. *CMAJ*. 2010;182:E610.
373. Wagner CL, McNeill RB, Johnson DD, et al. Health characteristics of two randomized vitamin D supplementation trials during pregnancy: a combined analysis. *J Steroid Biochem Mol Biol* 2013;136:313.
374. Calvo MS, Whiting SJ, Barton CN. Vitamin D fortification in the United States and Canada: current status and data needs. *Am J Clin Nutr*. 2004;80:1710S.
375. Tylavsky FA, Cheng S, Lyytikainen A, et al. Strategies to improve vitamin D status in Northern European children: exploring the merits of vitamin D fortification and supplementation. *J Nutr*. 2006;136:1130.
376. Calvo MS, Whiting SJ, Barton CN. Vitamin D intake: a global perspective of current status. *J Nutr*. 2005;135:310.
377. Seamans KM, Cashman KD. Existing and potentially novel functional markers of vitamin D status: a systematic survey. *Am J Clin Nutr*. 2009;89(suppl):1997S.
378. Taylor CL, Carriquiry AL, Bailey RL, et al. Appropriateness of the probability approach with a nutrient status biomarker to assess population inadequacy. *Am J Clin Nutr*. 2013;97:72
379. Hanley DA, Davison KS. Vitamin D insufficiency in North America. *J Nutr*. 2005;135:332.
380. Binkley N, Krueger D, Cowgill CS, et al. Assay variation confounds the diagnosis of hypovitaminosis D: a call for standardization. *J Clin Endocrinol Metab*. 2004;89:3152.
381. Lai JK, Lucas RM, Banks E, et al. Variability in vitamin D assays impairs clinical assessment of vitamin D status. *Intern Med J*. 2012;42:43.
382. Vogeser M. Quantification of circulating 25-hydroxyvitamin D3 by liquid chromatography-tandem mass spectroscopy. *J Steroid Biochem, Mol Biol*. 2010;20:565.
383. Carter GD, Carter R, Jones J, et al. How accurate are assays for 25-hydroxyvitamin D? Data from the International Vitamin D External Quality Assessment Scheme. *Clin Chem*. 2004; 50:2195.
384. Cashman KD, Kiely M, Kinsetta A, et al. Evaluation for the Vitamin D stardardization protocols for standardizing serum 25-hydroxyvitamin D data: a case study of the program's potential for National Nutrition/Health Survey. *Am J Clin Nutr*. 2013;97:1235.

385. Martins D, Wolf M, Pan D, et al. Prevalence of cardiovascular risk factors and the serum levels of 25-hydroxyvitamin D in the United States: data from the Third National Health and Nutrition Examination Survey. *Arch Intern Med.* 2007;167:1159.
386. Avioli L, Haddad JG. The vitamin D family revisited. *N Engl J Med.* 1984;311:47.
387. Portale AA, Halloran BP, Murphy MM, et al. Oral intake of phosphorus can determine the serum concentration of 1,25-dihydroxyvitamin D by determining its production rate in humans. *J Clin Invest.* 1986;77:7.
388. Kumar R. Hepatic and intestinal osteodystrophy and the hepatobiliary metabolism of vitamin D. *Ann Intern Med.* 1983;98:662.
389. Aloia JF, Dhaliwal R, Shieh A, et al. Vitamin D supplementation increases calcium absorption without a threshold effect. *Am J Clin Nutr.* 2013;99:624.
390. Smith GR, Collinson PO, Kiely PDW. Diagnosing hypovitaminosis D: serum measurements of calcium, phosphate, and alkaline phosphatase are unreliable, even in the presence of secondary hyperparathyroidism. *J Rheumatol.* 2005;32:684.
391. Sahota O, Masud T, San P, et al. Vitamin D insufficiency increases bone turnover markers and enhances bone loss at the hip in patients with established vertebral osteoporosis. *Clin Endocrinol.* 1999;51:217.
392. Jones G, Strugnell SA, DeLuca HF. Current understanding of the molecular actions of vitamin D. *Physiol Rev.* 1998;78:1193.
393. DeLuca HF. Overview of general physiologic features and functions of vitamin D. *Am J Clin Nutr.* 2004;80:1698S.
394. Breitwieser GE. Calcium sensing receptors and calcium oscillations: calcium as a first messenger. *Curr Top Dev Biol.* 2006;73:85
395. Suda T, Ueno Y, Fujii K, et al. Vitamin D and bone. *J Cell Biochem.* 2002;88:259.
396. Haussler MR, Jurutka P, Mizwicki M, et al. Vitamin D receptor (VDR)-mediated actions of 1α,25(OH)$_2$vitamin D3: genomic and non-genomic mechanisms. *Best Pract Res Clin Endocrinol Metab.* 2011;25:543.
397. Haussler MR, Whitfield GK, Keneko I, et al. The role of vitamin D in the FGF23, Klotho, and phosphate bone-kidney endocrine axis. *Rev Endocr Metab Disord.* 2012;13:57.
398. Peterlik M, Cross HS. Vitamin D and calcium deficits predispose for multiple chronic diseases. *Eur J Clin Invest.* 2005;35:290.
399. Holick MF, Binkley NC, Bischoff-Ferrari HA, et al. Evaluation, treatment, and prevention of vitamin D deficiency: an endocrine society clinical practice guideline. *J Clin Endocrinol Metab.* 2011;96:1911.
400. Pramyothin P, Holick MF. Vitamin D supplementation: guidelines and evidence for subclinical deficiency. *Curr Opin Gastroenterol.* 2012;28:139.
401. Bischoff-Ferrari HA. Optimal serum 25-hydroxyvitamin D levels for multiple health outcomes. In: Reichrath J, ed. *Sunlight, Vitamin D and Skin Cancer.* Austin, TX: Landes Bioscience; 2008: 55.
402. de Boer IH, Levin G, Robinson-Cohen C, et al. Serum 25-hydroxyvitamin D concentrations and risk for major clinical disease events in a community-based population of older adults. *Ann Intern Med.* 2012;156:627.
403. Chung M, Balk EM, Brendel M, et al. Vitamin D and calcium: a systematic review of health outcomes. *Evid Rep Technol Assess (Full Open).* 2009;183:1.
404. Rosen CJ. Vitamin D insufficiency. *N Eng J Med.* 2011;364:248.
405. Pludowski P, Holick MF, Pilz S, et al. Vitamin D effect on musculoskeletal health, immunity, autoimmunity, cardiovascular disease, cancer, fertility, pregnancy, dementia, & mortality—a review of recent evidence. *Autoimmun Rev.* 2013;12:976.
406. Nesby-O'Dell S, Scanlon KS, Cogswell ME, et al. Hypovitaminosis D prevalence and determinants among African Americans and white women of reproductive age: third National Health and Nutrition Examination Survey, 1988–1994. *Am J Clin Nutr.* 2002;76:187.
407. Javorsky BR, Maybee N, Padia SH, et al. Vitamin D deficiency in gastrointestinal disease. *Pract Gastroenterol.* 2006;19:52.
408. Palmer MT, Weaver CT. Linking vitamin D deficiency to inflammatory bowel disease. *Inflamm Bowel Dis.* 2013;19:2245.
409. Henkel AS, Buchman AL. Nutritional support in patients with chronic liver disease. *Nat Clin Pract Gastroenterol Hepatol.* 2006;3:202.

410. Udall JN, Jr. Crohn disease early in life and hypovitaminosis D: where do we go from here? *Am J Clin Nutr.* 2002;76:909.
411. Weber P. The role of vitamins in the prevention of osteoporosis—a brief status report. *Int J Vitam Nutr Res.* 1999;69:194.
412. Rachner TD, Khosla S, Hofbauer LC. New horizons in osteoporosis. *Lancet.* 2011;377:1276.
413. MacLaughlin J, Holick MF. Aging decreases the capacity of human skin to produce vitamin D_3. *J Clin Invest.* 1985;76:1536.
414. Spencer H, Rubio N, Rubio E, et al. Chronic alcoholism. Frequently overlooked cause of osteoporosis in men. *Am J Med.* 1986;80:393.
415. U.S. Preventive Services Task Force. Screening for osteoporosis: U.S preventive services task force recommendation statement. *Ann Intern Med.* 2011;154:356.
416. Das S, Crockett JC. Osteoporosis—a current view of pharmacological prevention and treatment. *Drug Des Devel Ther.* 2013;7:435.
417. Thomas MK, Lloyd-Jones DM, Thadhani RJ, et al. Hypovitaminosis D in medical inpatients. *N Engl J Med.* 1998;338:777.
418. Bandeira F, Griz L, Dreyer P, et al. Vitamin D deficiency: a global perspective. *Arq Bras Endocrinol Metab.* 2006;50:640.
419. Gallagher JC, Sai A, Templin T, et al. Dose response to vitamin D supplementation in postmenopausal women. *Ann Intern Med.* 2012;156:425.
420. Aloia JF, Chen DG, Yeh JK, et al. Serum vitamin D metabolites and intestinal calcium absorption efficiency in women. *Am J Clin Nutr.* 2010;92:835.
421. Higgins DM, Wischmeyer PE, Queensland KM, et al. Relationship of vitamin D deficiency to clinical outcomes in critically ill patients. *JPEN J Parenter Enteral Nutr.* 2012;36:713.
422. Barnard K, Colón-Emeric C. Extraskeletal effects of vitamin D in older adults: cardiovascular disease, mortality, mood, and cognition. *Am J Geriatr Pharmacother.* 2010;8:3.
423. Dickens AP, Lang IA, Langa KM, et al. Vitamin D, cognitive dysfunction and dementia in older adults. *CNS Drugs.* 2011;25:629.
424. Beydown MA, Ding EL, Beydown HA, et al. Vitamin D receptor and megalin gene polymorphisms and their associations with longitudinal cognitive change in US adults. *Am J Clin Nutr.* 2012;95:163.
425. Suzuki M, Yoshioka M, Hasimoto M, et al. Randomized, double-blind, placebo-controlled trial of vitamin D supplementation in Parkinson disease. *Am J Clin Nutr.* 2013;97:1004.
426. NIH Consensus Statement. Optimal calcium intake. 1994;12:1. http://consensus.nih.gov/1994/1994OptimalCalcium097html.htm.
427. Moyer VA, Vitamin D and calcium supplementation to prevent fractures in adults: U.S. Preventive Services Task Force recommendation statement. *Ann Intern Med.* 2013;158:691.
428. Moyer VA, LeFevre ML, Siu AL. Comments and responses. Vitamin D and calcium supplementation to prevent fractures in adults. *Ann Intern Med.* 2013;159:856.
429. Bischoff-Ferrari HA, Willett WC, Oray EJ, et al. A pooled analysis of vitamin D dose requirements for fracture prevention. *N Eng J Med.* 2012;367:40.
430. Bischoff-Ferrari H. Health effects of vitamin D. *Dermatol Ther.* 2010;23:23.
431. Janssen HCJP, Samson MM, Verhaar HJJ. Vitamin D deficiency, muscle function, and falls in elderly people. *Am J Clin Nutr.* 2002;75:611.
432. McAlindon T, La Valley M, Schneider E, et al. Effects of vitamin D supplementation on progression of knee pain and cartilage volume loss in patients with symptomatic osteoarthritis: a randomized controlled trial. *JAMA.* 2013;300:155.
433. Reid D, Toole BJ, Knox S, et al. The relation between acute changes in the systemic inflammatory response and plasma 25-hydroxyvitamin D concentrations after elective knee arthroplasty. *Am J Clin Nutr.* 2011;93:1006.
434. Zitterman A, Iodice S, Pilz S, et al. Vitamin D deficiency and mortality risk in the general population: a meta-analysis of prospective cohort studies. *Am J Clin Nutr.* 2012;95:91.
435. Rejnmark L, Avenell A, Masud T, et al. Vitamin D with calcium reduces mortality: patient level pooled analysis of 70,528 patients from eight major vitamin D trials. *J Clin Endocrinol Metab.* 2012;97:2670.
436. Thachek TD, Clarke BL. Vitamin D insufficiency. *Mayo Clin Proc.* 2011;86:50.
437. Chang TY, LaCroix AZ, Beresford SA, et al. Vitamin D intake and lung cancer risk in the Women's Health Initiative (WHI). *Am J Clin Nutr.* 2013;98:1002.

438. Manson JE, Mayne ST, Clinton SK. Vitamin D and prevention of cancer—ready for prime time? *N Eng J Med.* 2011;364:1385.
439. Plum LA, DeLuca HF. Vitamin D, disease and therapeutic opportunities. *Nat Rev Drug Discov.* 2010;9:941.
440. Pilz S, Tomaschitz A, Marz W, et al. Vitamin D, cardiovascular disease and mortality. *Clin Endocrinol (Oxf).* 2011;75:575.
441. Wang C. Role of vitamin D in cardiometabolic diseases. *J Diabetes Res.* 2013;2013:243934.
442. Wang L, Song Y, Manson JE, et al. Circulating 25-hydroxy-vitamin D and risk of cardiovascular disease: a meta-analysis of prospective studies. *Circ Cardiovasc Qual Outcomes.* 2012;5:819.
443. Pittas AG, Chung M, Trikalinos T, et al. Systematic review: vitamin D and cardiometabolic outcomes. *Ann Intern Med.* 2010;152:307.
444. Wang L, Manson JE, Song Y, et al. Systematic review: vitamin D and calcium supplementation in prevention of cardiovascular events. *Ann Intern Med.* 2010;152:315.
445. Thadhani R, Appelbaum E, Pritchett Y, et al. Vitamin D therapy and cardiac structure and function in patients with chronic kidney disease: the PRIMO randomized controlled trial. *JAMA.* 2012;307:674.
446. Zitterman A, Frisch S, Berthold HK, et al. Vitamin D supplementation enhances the beneficial effects of weight loss on cardiovascular disease risk markers. *Am J Clin Nutr.* 2009;89:1321.
447. Renzaho AM, Halliday JA, Nowson C. Vitamin D, obesity, and obesity-related chronic disease among ethnic minorities: a systematic review. *Nutrition.* 2011;27:868.
448. Kositsawat J, Freeman VL, Gerber BS, et al. Association of A1c levels with vitamin D status in US adults: data from the National Health and Nutrition Examination Survey. *Diabetes Care.* 2010;33:1236.
449. Lamendola CA, Ariel D, Feldman D, et al. Relations between obesity, insulin resistance, and 25-hydroxyvitamin D. *Am J Clin Nutr.* 2012;95:1055.
450. von Hurst PR, Stonehouse W, Coad J. Vitamin D supplementation reduces insulin resistance in South Asian women living in New Zealand who are insulin resistant and vitamin D deficient—a randomised, placebo-controlled trial. *Br J Nutr.* 2010;103:549.
451. Nikooyeh B, Neyestani TR, Farcid M, et al. Daily consumption of vitamin D- or vitamin D + calcium-fortified yogurt drink improved glycemic control in patients with type 2 diabetes: a randomized clinical trial. *Am J Clin Nutr.* 2011;93:764.
452. Mitri J, Dawson-Hughes B, Hu FB, et al. Effects of vitamin D and calcium supplementation on pancreatic β cell function, insulin sensitivity, and glycemia in adults at high risk of diabetes: the Calcium and Vitamin D for Diabetes Mellitus (CaDDM) randomized controlled trial. *Am J Clin Nutr.* 2011;94:486.
453. Han YP, Kongf M, Zheng S, et al. Vitamin D in liver diseases: from mechanisms to clinical trials. *J Gastroenterol Hepatol.* 2013;28(Suppl 1):49.
454. Gutierrez JA, Parikh N, Branch AD. Classical and emerging roles of vitamin D in hepatitis C virus infection. *Semin Liver Dis.* 2011;31:387.
455. Eliades M, Spyrou E, Agrawal N, et al. Meta-analysis: vitamin D and non-alcoholic fatty liver disease. *Aliment Pharmacol Ther.* 2013;38:246.
456. Liangpunksakul S, Chalasani N. Serum vitamin D concentration and unexplained elevations in ALT among US adults. *Dig Dis Sci.* 2011;56:2124.
457. Sundar IK, Rahman I. Vitamin D and susceptibility of chronic lung diseases: role of epigenetics. *Front Pharmacol.* 2011;2:50.
458. Lehouck A, Mathieu C, Carremans C, et al. High doses of vitamin D to reduce exacerbations in chronic obstructive pulmonary disease. *Ann Intern Med.* 2012;156:105.
459. Wejse C, Gomes VF, Rebona P, et al. Vitamin D as supplementary treatment for tuberculosis: a double-blind, randomized, placebo-controlled trial. *Am J Respir Crit Care Med.* 2009;179:843.
460. Cooper L, Clifton-Bligh PB, Nery ML, et al. Vitamin D supplementation and bone mineral density in early postmenopausal women. *Am J Clin Nutr.* 2003;77:1324.
461. Heaney RP. The vitamin D requirement in health and disease. *J Steroid Biochem Mol Biol.* 2005;97:13.
462. Rhode CM, DeLuca HF. All-trans retinoic acid antagonizes the action of calciferol and its active metabolite, 1,25-dihydroxycalciferol in rats. *J Nutr.* 2005;135:1647.
463. Slatopolsky E, Weerts C, Thielan J, et al. Marked suppression of secondary hyperparathyroidism by intravenous administration of 1,25-dihydroxy-cholecalciferol in uremic patients. *J Clin Invest.* 1984;74:2136.

464. Wu-Wong JR, Tian J, Goltzman D. Vitamin D analogs as therapeutic agents: a clinical study update. *Curr Opin Investig Drugs.* 2004;5:320.
465. Brown AJ, Dusso S, Slatopolsky E. Vitamin D analogues for secondary hyperparathyroidism. *Nephrol Dial Transplant.* 2002;17 (Suppl 10):10.
466. Levin A, Li YC. Vitamin D and its analogues: Do they protect against cardiovascular disease in patients with kidney disease? *Kidney Int.* 2005;68:1973.
467. Vieth R. Vitamin D supplementation, 25-hydroxyvitamin D concentrations, and safety. *Am J Clin Nutr.* 1999;69:842.
468. Weber P, Bendich A, Machlin LJ. Vitamin E and human health: rationale for determining recommended intake levels. *Nutrition.* 1997;13:450.
469. Brigelius-Flohe R, Kelly FJ, Salonen JT, et al. The European perspective on vitamin E: current knowledge and future research. *Am J Clin Nutr.* 2002;76:703.
470. Jiang Q, Christen S, Shegenaga MK, et al. γ-tocopherol, the major form of vitamin E in the US diet, deserves more attention. *Am J Clin Nutr.* 2001;74:714.
471. Bowry VW, Ingold KU, Stocker R. Vitamin E in human low-density lipoprotein. When and how this antioxidant becomes a pro-oxidant. *Biochem J.* 1992;288:341.
472. Bruno RS, Traber MG. Cigarette smoke alters human vitamin E requirement. *J Nutr.* 2005;135:671.
473. Bauernfeind JC. The tocopherol content of food and influencing factors. *Crit Rev Food Sci Nutr.* 1977;8:337.
474. Maguire LS, O'Sullivan SM, Galvin K, et al. Fatty acid profile, tocopherol, squalene and phytosterol content of walnuts, almonds, peanuts, hazelnuts and the macadamia nut. *Int J Food Sci Nutr.* 2004;55:171.
475. McLaughlin PJ, Weihrauch JL. Vitamin E content of foods. *J Am Diet Assoc.* 1979;75:647.
476. Ford ES, Ajani UA, Mokdad AH. Brief communication: The prevalence of high intake of vitamin E from the use of supplements among U.S. adults. *Ann Intern Med.* 2005;143:116.
477. Schwarzpaul S, Strassburg A, Luhrmann PM, et al. Intake of vitamin and mineral supplements in an elderly German population. *Ann Nutr Metab.* 2006;50:155.
478. Ford ES, Sowell A. Serum alpha-tocopherol status in the United States population: findings from the Third National Health and Nutrition Examination Survey. *Am J Epidemiol.* 1999;150:290.
479. Thurnham DI, Davies JA, Crump BJ, et al. The use of different lipids to express serum tocopherol:lipid ratios for the measurement of vitamin E status. *Ann Clin Biochem.* 1986;23:514.
480. Refat M, Moore TJ, Kazui M, et al. Utility of breath ethane as a noninvasive biomarker of vitamin E status in children. *Pediatr Res.* 1991;30:396.
481. Knutson MD, Handelman GJ, Viteri FE. Methods for measuring ethane and pentane in expired air from rats and humans. *Free Radic Biol Med.* 2000;28:514.
482. Chan AC. Vitamin E and atherosclerosis. *J Nutr.* 1998;128:1593.
483. Steiner M. Vitamin E, a modifier of platelet function: rationale and use in cardiovascular and cerebrovascular disease. *Nutr Rev.* 1999;57:306.
484. Brisson L, Castan S, Fontbonne H, et al. Alpha-tocopheryl acetate is absorbed and hydrolyzed by Caco-2 cells comparative studies with alpha-tocopherol. *Chem Phys Lipids.* 2008;154:33.
485. Hacquebard M, Carpentier YA. Vitamin E: absorption, plasma transport and cell uptake. *Curr Opin Clin Nutr Metab Care.* 2005;8:133.
486. Cheeseman KH, Holley AE, Kelly FJ, et al. Biokinetics in humans of RRR-α-tocopherol, the free phenol, acetate ester, and succinate ester forms of vitamin E. *Free Radic Biol Med.* 1995;19:591.
487. Leonard SW, Good CK, Gugger ET, et al. Vitamin E bioavailability from fortified breakfast cereal is greater than that from encapsulated supplements. *Am J Clin Nutr.* 2004;79:86.
488. Berdanier CD. *Advanced Nutrition: Micronutrients.* Boca Raton, FL: CRC Press, 1998.
489. Salmon AB, Richardson A, Perez VI. Update on the oxidative stress theory of aging: does oxidative stress play a role in aging or healthy aging? *Free Radic Biol Med.* 2010;48:642.
490. Williams MT, Hord NG. The role of dietary factors in cancer prevention: beyond fruits and vegetables. *Nutr Clin Pract.* 2005;20:451.
491. Kelemen LE, Cerhan JR, Lim U, et al. Vegetables, fruit, and antioxidant-related nutrients and risk of non-Hodgkin lymphoma: a National Cancer Institute-Surveillance, Epidemiology, and End Results population-based case-control study. *Am J Clin Nutr.* 2006;83:1401.
492. Park EJ, Pezzuto JM. Botanicals in cancer chemoprevention. *Cancer Metastasis Rev.* 2002;21:231.

493. Halvorsen BL, Carlsen MH, Phillips KM, et al. Content of redox-active compounds (i.e., antioxidants) in foods consumed in the United States. *Am J Clin Nutr.* 2006;84:95.
494. Heinecke JW. Lipoprotein oxidation in cardiovascular disease: chief culprit or innocent bystander? *J Exp Med.* 2006;203:813.
495. Nobili S, Lippi D, Witort E, et al. Natural compounds for cancer treatment and prevention. *Pharm Res.* 2009;59:365.
496. Haller J, Löwik MR, Ferry M, et al. Nutritional status: blood vitamins A, E, B_6, B_{12}, folic acid, and carotene. Euronut SENECA investigators. *Eur J Clin Nutr.* 1991;45:63.
497. Rosenblum JL, Keating JP, Prensky AL, et al. A progressive neurologic syndrome in children with chronic liver disease. *N Engl J Med.* 1981;304:503.
498. Tanyel MC, Mancano LD. Neurologic findings in vitamin E deficiency. *Am Fam Physician.* 1997;55:197.
499. Jialal I, Devaraj S. Scientific evidence to support a vitamin E and heart disease health claim: research needs. *J Nutr.* 2005;135:348.
500. Knekt P, Ritz J, Pereira MA, et al. Antioxidant vitamins and coronary heart disease risk: a pooled analysis of 9 cohorts. *Am J Clin Nutr.* 2004;80:1508.
501. Chae CU, Albert CM, Moorthy MV, et al. Vitamin E supplementation and the risk of heart failure in women. *Circ Heart Fail.* 2012;5:176.
502. Sesso HD, Burling JE, Christen WG, et al. Vitamins E and C in the prevention of cardiovascular disease in men: the Physicians' Health Study II randomized trial. *JAMA.* 2008;300:2123.
503. Kris-Etherton PM, Lichtenstein AH, Howard BV, et al; for the Nutrition Committee of the American Heart Association Council on Nutrition, Physical Activity, and Metabolism. Antioxidant vitamin supplements and cardiovascular disease. *Circulation.* 2004;110:637.
504. Ascherio A, Rimm EB, Hernan MA, et al. Relation of consumption of vitamin E, vitamin C, and carotenoids to risk for stroke among men in the United States. *Ann Intern Med.* 1999;130:963.
505. Devaraj S, Jialal I. Failure of vitamin E in clinical trials: is gamma-tocopherol the answer? *Nutr Rev.* 2005;63:290.
506. Hercberg S, Galan P, Preziosi P, et al. The SU.VI.MAX Study: a randomized, placebo-controlled trial of the health effects of antioxidant vitamins and minerals. *Arch Intern Med.* 2004;164:2335.
507. Pham DQ, Plakogiannis R. Vitamin E supplementation in cardiovascular disease and cancer prevention: part 1. *Ann Pharmacother.* 2005;39:1870.
508. Liu C, Russell RM. Nutrition and gastric cancer risk: an update. *Nutr Rev.* 2008;66:237.
509. Lonn E, Bosch J, Yusuf S; HOPE and HOPE-TOO Trial Investigators. Effects of long-term vitamin E supplementation on cardiovascular events and cancer: a randomized controlled trial. *JAMA.* 2005;293:1338.
510. Cho E, Hunter DJ, Spiegelman D, et al. Intakes of vitamins A, C and E and folate and multivitamins and lung cancer: a pooled analysis of 8 prospective studies. *Int J Cancer.* 2006;118:970.
511. Lippman SM, Klein EA, Goodman PJ, et al. Effect of selenium and vitamin E on risk of prostate cancer and other cancers: the Selenium and Vitamin E Cancer Prevention Trial (SELECT). *JAMA.* 2009;301:39.
512. Hurst R, Hooper L, Norat T, et al. Selenium and prostate cancer: systematic review and meta-analysis. *Am J Clin Nutr.* 2012;96:111.
513. Klein EA, Thompson IM, Tangen CM, et al. Vitamin E and the risk of prostate cancer: the Selenium and Vitamin E Cancer Prevention Trial (SELECT). *JAMA.* 2011;306:1549.
514. Lin J, Cook NR, Albert C, et al. Vitamins C and E and beta carotene supplementation and cancer risk: a randomized controlled trial. *J Natl Cancer Inst.* 2009;101:14.
515. Gaziano JM, Glynn RJ, Christen WG, et al. Vitamins E and C in the prevention of prostate and total cancer in men: the Physicians' Health Study II, a randomized controlled trial. *JAMA.* 2009;301:52.
516. Browning JD, Horton JD. Molecular mediators of hepatic steatosis and liver injury. *J Clin Invest.* 2004;114:147.
517. Bugianesi E, Marzocchi R, Villanova N, et al. Non-alcoholic fatty liver disease/non-alcoholic steatohepatitis (NAFLD/NASH): treatment. *Best Pract & Res Clin Gastroenterol.* 2004;18:1105.
518. Harrison SA, Torgerson S, Hayashi P, et al. Vitamin E and vitamin C treatment improves fibrosis in patients with nonalcoholic steatohepatitis. *Am J Gastroenterol.* 2003;98:2485.
519. Bugianesi E, Gentilcore E, Manini R, et al. A randomized controlled trial of metformin versus vitamin E or prescriptive diet in nonalcoholic fatty liver disease. *Am J Gastroenterol.* 2005;100:1082.

520. Lavine JE, Schwimmer JB, Van Natta ML, et al. Effect of vitamin E or metformin for treatment of nonalcoholic fatty liver disease in children and adolescents. The TONIC randomized controlled trial. *JAMA*. 2011;305:1659.
521. Czernichow S, Vergnaud AC, Galan P, et al. Effects of long-term antioxidant supplementation and association of serum antioxidant concentrations with risk of metabolic syndrome in adults. *Am J Clin Nutr*. 2009;90:329.
522. Paquot N, Delwaide J. Fatty liver in the intensive care unit. *Curr Opin Nutr Metab Care*. 2005;8:183.
523. Pham DQ, Plakogiannis R. Vitamin E supplementation in Alzheimer's disease, Parkinson's disease, tardive dyskinesia, and cataract: part 2. *Ann Pharmacother*. 2005;39:2065.
524. Petersib RC, Thomas RG, Grundman M, et al. Vitamin E and donepezil for the treatment of mild cognitive impairment. *N Engl J Med*. 2005;352:23.
525. Berman K, Brodaty H. Tocopherol (vitamin E) in Alzheimer's disease and other neurodegenerative disorders. *CNS Drugs*. 2004;18:807.
526. Kryscio RJ, Abner EL, Schmitt FA, et al. A randomized controlled Alzheimer's disease prevention trial's evolution into an exposure trial: the PREADVISE trial. *J Nutr Health Aging*. 2013;17:72.
527. Rumbold AR, Crowther CA, Haslam RR, et al. Vitamins C and E and the risks of preeclampsia and perinatal complications. *N Engl J Med*. 2006;354:17.
528. Freedman DM, Kunci RW, Weinstein SJ, et al. Vitamin E serum levels and controlled supplementation and risk of amyotrophic lateral sclerosis. *Amyotroph Lateral Scler Frontotemporal Degener*. 2013;14:246.
529. Bonelli L, Puntoni M, Gatteschi B, et al. Antioxidant supplement and long-term reduction of recurrent adenomas of the large bowel. A double-blind randomized trial. *J Gastroenterol*. 2013;48:698.
530. Roonpraiwan R, Suthutvoravut U, Feungpean B, et al. Effect of oral vitamin E supplementation in children with cholestasis. *J Med Assoc Thai*. 2002;85(Suppl 4):S1199.
531. Argyriou AA, Chroni E, Koutras A, et al. Vitamin E for prophylaxis against chemotherapy-induced neuropathy: a randomized controlled trial. *Neurology*. 2005;64:26.
532. Thiele JJ, Hsieh SN, Ekanayake-Mudiyanselage S. Vitamin E: critical review of its current use in cosmetic and clinical dermatology. *Dermatol Surg*. 2005;31:805.
533. Horwitt MK. Therapeutic uses of vitamin E in medicine. *Nutr Rev*. 1980;38:105.
534. Sokol RJ, Guggenheim MA, Iannaccone ST, et al. Improved neurologic function after long-term correction of vitamin E deficiency in children with chronic cholestasis. *N Engl J Med*. 1985;313:1580.
535. Sokol RJ, Butler-Simon N, Conner C, et al. Multicenter trial of d-alpha-tocopheryl polyethylene glycol 1000 succinate for treatment of vitamin E deficiency in children with chronic cholestasis. *Gastroenterology*. 1993;104:1727.
536. Sitrin MD, Lieberman F, Jensen WE, et al. Vitamin E deficiency and neurologic disease in adults with cystic fibrosis. *Ann Intern Med*. 1987;107:51.
537. Hittner HM, Godio LB, Rudolph AJ, et al. Retrolental fibroplasia: efficacy of vitamin E in a double-blind clinical study of preterm infants. *N Engl J Med*. 1981;305:1365.
538. Corash L, Spielberg S, Bartsocass C, et al. Reduced chronic hemolysis during high-dose vitamin E administration in Mediterranean-type glucose-6-phosphate dehydrogenase deficiency. *N Engl J Med*. 1980;303:416.
539. Natta CL, Machlin LJ, Brin M. A decrease in irreversibly sickled erythrocytes in sickle cell anemia patients given vitamin E. *Am J Clin Nutr*. 1980;33:968.
540. Spencer AP, Carson DS, Crouch MA. Vitamin E and coronary artery disease. *Arch Intern Med*. 1999;159:1313.
541. Bendich A. Safety issues regarding the use of vitamin supplements. *Ann N Y Acad Sci*. 1992;669:300.
542. Miller ER III, Pastor-Barriuso R, Dalal D, et al. Meta-analysis: high-dosage vitamin E supplementation may increase all-cause mortality. *Ann Intern Med*. 2005;142:37.
543. Bjelakovic G, Nikolova D, Gluud LL, et al. Mortality in randomized trials of antioxidant supplements for primary and secondary prevention: systematic review and meta-analysis. *JAMA*. 2007;297:842.
544. Nakagawa K, Hirota Y, Sawada N, et al. Identification of UBIAD1 as a novel human menaquinone-4 biosynthetic enzyme. *Nature*. 2010;468:117.

545. Adams J, Pepping J. Vitamin K in the treatment and prevention of osteoporosis and arterial calcification. *Am J HealthSyst Pharm.* 2005;62:1574.
546. Olson RE, Chao J, Graham D, et al. Total body phylloquinone and its turnover in human subjects at two levels of vitamin K intake. *Br J Nutr.* 2002;87:543.
547. Booth SL, Suttie JW. Dietary intake and adequacy of vitamin K. *J Nutr* 1998;128:785.
548. Helphingstine CJ, Bistrian BR. New Food and Drug Administration requirements for inclusion of vitamin K in adult parenteral multivitamins. *JPEN J Parenter Enteral Nutr.* 2003;27:220.
549. Bolton-Smith C, Price RJG, Fenton ST, et al. Compilation of a provisional UK database for the phylloquinone (vitamin K_1) content of foods. *Br J Nutr.* 2000;83:389.
550. Booth SL, Pennington JA, Sadowski JA. Food sources and dietary intakes of vitamin K-1 (phylloquinone) in the American diet: data from the FDA Total Diet Study. *J Am Diet Assoc.* 1996;96:149.
551. Elder SJ, Haytowitz DB, Howe J, et al. Vitamin K contents of meat, dairy, and fast food in the U.S. diet. *J Agric Food Chem.* 2006;54:463.
552. Booth SL, Centurelli MA. Vitamin K: a practical guide to the dietary management of patients on warfarin. *Nutr Rev.* 1999;57:288.
553. Johnson MA. Influence of vitamin K on anticoagulant therapy depends on vitamin K status and the source and chemical forms of vitamin K. *Nutr Rev.* 2005;63:91.
554. Presse N, Gaudreau P, Greenwood CE, et al. A single measurement of serum phylloquinone is an adequate indicator of long-term phylloquinone exposure in healthy older adults. *J Nutr.* 2012;142:1910.
555. Vermeer C, Shearer MJ, Zittermann A, et al. Beyond deficiency: potential benefits of increased intakes of vitamin K for bone and vascular health. *Eur J Nutr.* 2004;43:325.
556. Stafford DW. The vitamin K cycle. *J Thromb Haemost.* 2005;3:1873.
557. Spronk HM, Sourte BA, Schurgers LJ, et al. Tissue-specific utilization of menaquinone-4 results in the prevention of arterial calcification in warfarin-treated rats. *J Vasc Res.* 2003;40:531.
558. Wallin R, Hutson SM. Warfarin and the vitamin K-dependent γ-carboxylation system. *Trends Mol Med.* 2004;7:299.
559. Strople J, Lovell G, Heubi J. Prevalence of subclinical vitamin K deficiency in cholestatis liver disease. *J Pediatr Gastroenterol Nutr.* 2009;49:78.
560. Holdern RM, Morton AR, Garland JS, et al. Vitamins K and D status in stages 3–5 chronic kidney disease. *Clin J Am Soc Nephrol.* 2010;5:590.
561. Harrington DJ, Western H, Seton-Jones C, et al. A study of the prevalence of vitamin K deficiency in patients with cancer referred to a hospital palliative care team and its association with abnormal haemostasis. *J Clin Pathol.* 2008;61:537.
562. Hey E. Vitamin K—what, why, and when. *Arch Dis Child Fetal Neonatal Ed.* 2003;88:F80.
563. Booth SL, Tucker KL, Chen H, et al. Dietary vitamin K intakes are associated with hip fracture but not with bone mineral density in elderly men and women. *Am J Clin Nutr.* 2000;71:1201.
564. Ishida Y, Kawai S. Comparative efficacy of hormone replacement therapy, etidronate, calcitonin, alfacalcidol, and vitamin K in postmenopausal women with osteoporosis: the Yamaguchi Osteoporosis Prevention Study. *Am J Med.* 2004;117:549.
565. Feskanich D, Willett WW, Rockett H, et al. Vitamin K intake and hip fractures in women: a prospective study. *Am J Clin Nutr.* 1999;69:74.
566. Jamal SA, Browner WS, Bauer DC, et al. Warfarin use and risk for osteoporosis in elderly women. *Ann Intern Med.* 1998;128:829.
567. Caraballo PJ, Heit JA, Atkinson EJ, et al. Long-term use of oral anticoagulants and the risk of fracture. *Arch Intern Med.* 1999;159;1750.
568. Brown JP, Josse RG; for the Scientific Advisory Council of the Osteoporosis Society of Canada. 2002 clinical practice guidelines for the diagnosis and management of osteoporosis in Canada. *CMAJ.* 2002;167(10 Suppl):S1.
569. Duggan P, O'Brien M, Kiely M, et al. Vitamin K status in patients with Crohn's disease and relationship to bone turnover. *Am J Gastroenterol.* 2004;99:2178.
570. Orbak Z, Selimoglu A, Doneray H. Inherited vitamin K deficiency: case report and review of literature. *Yonsei Med J.* 2003;44:923.
571. Fiore LD, Scola MA, Cantillon CE, et al. Anaphylactoid reactions to vitamin K. *J Thromb Thrombolysis.* 2001;11:175.

7 Minerals

FACTORS INVOLVED IN MINERAL DEFICIENCY AND OVERLOAD

The minerals important in human nutrition can be classified into three groups: those stored in the body in large quantities (Na, K, Ca, Mg, P); those present in trace amounts whose role in human nutrition has been determined (Fe, Zn, Cu, I, F, Se, Cr); and those present in trace amounts (Co, Mo, Mn, Cd, As, Si, V, Ni) that are clearly important in laboratory animals but whose role in human nutrition is uncertain. Of this last group, only manganese is discussed in detail in this chapter because some deficiency of that element has been demonstrated in humans.

Intestinal Absorption and Secretion

Divalent Cations

The major divalent cations (Ca, Mg, Zn, Cu) are not absorbed efficiently. They are ingested in forms that are poorly soluble and must be converted to more soluble salts, and transport across the apical membrane is relatively slow. Moreover, significant amounts of these ions are secreted into the intestinal lumen each day via intestinal, pancreatic, and biliary juices. Thus, deficiency develops in the setting of either diarrhea or malabsorption. Iron is absorbed best in its divalent form and is lost mainly through bleeding into the gastrointestinal tract or from the uterus.

Monovalent Cations

The major monovalent cations (Na, K) are also secreted in digestive juices, but they are very efficiently reabsorbed. Nonetheless, their concentrations are so high that deficiency can develop when large amounts of body fluids are lost. Therefore, intestinal diseases often lead to decreases in the body stores of many minerals. Many minerals are reabsorbed by renal (Na, K, Ca, Mg, P) as well as intestinal cells. Thus, the potential for loss is great when these organs are diseased.

Effect of Diet on Acid–Base Balance and Renal Acid Excretion

Foods that contain an excess of fixed anions (Cl, P, S) over fixed cations (Na, K, Ca, Mg) can promote acidification of body fluids. Such acidic diets have developed over time as the plant:animal ratios in the diet have decreased (1). The intestine can exchange chloride for bicarbonate, and so modify the effect of ingested anions. Moreover, the liver can produce sulfate from sulfur-containing amino acids, or produce bicarbonate from citrate. Thus, the effect of diet on overall acid–base status is complex. A potential renal acid load of foods has been calculated. Fruits and vegetables reduce renal acid secretion; milk and yogurt provide mild acid loads; and meat, fish, poultry, cheese, and some grain products with higher P and S content can provide more than 3.5 mEq per 100 g of serving (2). Total net acid excretion and urinary pH can be influenced by the diet and can account for much of the variability in acid excretion in normal subjects.

Evaluation of Deficiency

Body Stores

Only in the case of iron do blood levels correlate with body stores. Bone is the major storage site of several minerals (Ca, P, Mg, F), and levels of these minerals in bone do not equilibrate rapidly with blood levels. In the case of some minerals (Na, K, Ca), many compensatory mechanisms exist to maintain blood levels within the normal range. These mechanisms are designed to regulate extracellular fluid (ECF) concentrations rather than body stores. Because blood levels do not usually correlate well with body stores, deficiencies of many minerals are difficult to assess from a practical point of view. The diagnosis of mineral deficiency should be suspected first by the presence of appropriate symptoms or signs in a high-risk setting. Table 7-1 outlines these general features. The details of each deficiency state are described in the sections on each mineral.

TABLE 7-1 Clinical Manifestations of Mineral Deficiency and Toxicity States

Mineral	Major Functions	Major Causes of Deficiency	Clinical Signs Deficiency	Clinical Signs Toxicity
Na	ECF volume, muscle and nerve function, nutrient absorption	GI, renal, and skin losses	Hypovolemia, weakness, nausea	Confusion, stupor
K	Acid-base balance, membrane transport, muscle contraction, protein synthesis	GI (nausea, diarrhea), renal (diuretics) losses	Arrhythmias, muscle weakness, nausea, irritability	Paresthesias, confusion, cardiac depression
Cl	Acid-base balance, osmotic pressure, HCl in stomach	GI (vomiting, diarrhea), renal (diuretics) losses	Alkalosis, muscle cramps, anorexia	Acidosis with renal failure
Ca	Bone/tooth formation, blood clotting, nerve transmission, muscle contraction,	↓ Intake, malabsorption, ↑ PTH secretion	Tetany, arrhythmia, osteomalacia	Anorexia, constipation, vomiting, coma
Mg	Cell metabolism, enzyme activation, nerve/muscle action	Malabsorption, renal tubular leak, EtOH	Muscle twitching, arrhythmia, nausea, weakness, confusion	Nausea, ↓ BP, confusion, ↓ reflexes
P	Bone/tooth formation, metabolic functions, nucleic	↑ renal excretion, wasting diseases	Weakness, bone pain, rhabdomyolysis,	Secondary ↑ parathyroidism acid formation
Fe	Heme formation, enzyme cofactor	Blood loss (GI, gynecologic); ↑ needs (pregnancy), ↓ intake (infants)	Anemia, increased infection (children)	Cirrhosis, heart failure, skin pigmentation
Zn	Enzyme cofactor, CO_2 transfer, DNA function, wound healing	Diarrhea, malabsorption	Stunted growth, skin changes, anorexia, lethargy, alopecia, photophobia	Cu deficiency, ↓ immunity, gastric erosions
Cu	Enzyme cofactor, function of nerves, vascular/bone structure	Malnutrition, prematurity	Anemia, neutropenia, skeletal defects, nerve degeneration	Vomiting, cardiomyopathy, congestive heart failure
I	Thyroxine synthesis	↓ Intake	Goiter, hypothyroidism	Hyperthyroidism
Mn	Enzyme cofactor	One case reported	↑ Cholesterol, weight loss, dermatitis, change in hair color	Neural damage (e.g., Wilson disease)
Cr	Insulin cofactor	TPN	Glucose intolerance, ↑ lipids, peripheral neuropathy	None for trivalent Cr
F	Bone/tooth formation	↓ Intake	Dental caries	Brittle bones, thickened cortex, mouth numbness, salty taste, diarrhea
Se	GSH peroxidase cofactor	↓ Intake, TPN	Cardiomyopathy, locomotor disturbance	Hair loss, fatigue, polyneuritis, gastroenteritis
Mo	Cofactor for oxidases (sulfite, xanthine, aldehyde)	Metabolic defect in Mo cofactor	Neurologic abnormalities	None

BP, blood pressure; ECF, extracellular fluid; EtOH, ethyl alcohol; GI, gastrointestinal; GSH, reduced glutathione; PTH, parathyroid hormone; TPN, total parenteral nutrition.

Subclinical Mineral Deficiency

The concept of subclinical deficiency refers to a condition in which the measurements of body stores are not yet low, but tissue concentrations are low enough to lead to altered cellular function without clinical signs or symptoms. This concept has arisen in part because the measurements to assess body stores are either insensitive (e.g., serum zinc), or have low specificity (e.g., serum ferritin) (3). Both serum iron and transferrin saturation can be altered by non–iron-related factors, making it difficult at times to detect deficient iron stores. Similarly, serum zinc can be falsely elevated by inflammation or acute-phase reaction, or simply be too insensitive to assess all cases of zinc deficiency, since serum zinc is a transit compartment and is only slowly in equilibrium with a large part of the zinc body pool.

Water Balance

In normal adults total body water accounts for approximately 60% of body weight, being somewhat lower in women and in the elderly, who can have smaller muscle mass and larger fat stores. Two-thirds of the water is intracellular, and only approximately 7% is intravascular, and water moves freely between body compartments according to the effective osmotic pressure (4). The major extracellular ions are sodium, potassium, chloride, and bicarbonate. Thus, changes in volume status can lead to changes in ion concentrations, most rapidly in the plasma. Weight gain is the best measure of volume overload, but edema may not be apparent until 2 to 4 kg of water have been retained (5). Other features of water overload may be anxiety or agitation, but if sodium overload is the cause of increased fluid retention, then signs of congestive heart failure or dependent edema may develop. The best measure of volume depletion in adults is postural hypotension, manifested by a fall in systolic blood pressure of greater than 15 mm Hg and/or an increase in pulse of greater than 15 beats per minute immediately after a shift in position. Other features of volume depletion include decreased skin turgor, dry mouth, thirst, and oliguria. When severe, weakness, lethargy or coma, and anuria may develop.

Water Requirements

Total water intake includes water in beverages (including drinking water), and water in food. On average, water in beverages accounts for approximately 80% of water intake in adults (4). The "requirement" for water is established in the form of an adequate intake (AI), set to prevent the acute effects of dehydration. The amount of water required may increase over the AI owing to physical activity and environmental conditions. Whether sodium and other minerals are needed along with water to maintain plasma osmolality depends upon whether fluid is lost from the lungs (mostly water), sweat (low sodium content), or gastrointestinal tract from vomiting (half isosmolar sodium and chloride) or from diarrhea (isosmolar sodium along with potassium and some bicarbonate). The AI for total water intake is based on median intake from the US Third National Health and Nutrition Examination Survey (NHANES III). AI for men and women age 19 to 70 is 3.7 and 2.7 L per day, respectively (4). The amount needed to achieve this AI from total beverages should be approximately 3.0 L (~13 cups) and 2.2 L (~9 cups) per day for men and women, respectively.

Mineral/Metal Overload and Toxicity

Many minerals are widely available in foods; moreover, they are easily provided as supplements. For these reasons, and because it is difficult to assess body stores, it is not surprising that overload syndromes occur more frequently in the case of minerals than of vitamins. Sodium, potassium, calcium, iron, and fluoride are the minerals most commonly involved in overload syndromes. Table 7-1 outlines the general features of overload syndromes.

There are some metals that cause toxicity in humans, but are not required nutrients, yet toxic amounts can be ingested in foods (4). Organic arsenic can be found in fish, meat and poultry, dairy products, grains and cereals, and fats and oil; inorganic arsenic is found in rice, flour, and grape juice. Arsenic toxicity is manifested by vomiting, colic, diarrhea, and renal failure. Boron is found most concentrated in fruit-based beverages, tubers, and legumes, but toxic amounts could only be ingested as boric tartrate, used for epilepsy at doses greater than 20 mg/kg/day. Nickel is most abundant in nuts and legumes, sweeteners, and chocolates, but toxicity (nausea, abdominal pain, diarrhea, vomiting) has occurred only after ingestion of water contaminated with nickel sulfate. Vanadium content is highest in mushrooms, shellfish, some spices including black pepper, and some processed foods, but vanadyl sulfate (up to 100 mg per day) and sodium metavanadate (up to 125 mg per day) have been used as supplements for diabetics and by weight-training athletes, with possible effects on renal morphology and serum urea concentration.

Toxicity from other heavy metals in food includes syndromes due to ingestion of cadmium (Cd), mercury (Hg), thallium (Tl), tin (Sn), and lead (Pb) occurring due to contamination with industrial waste (Cd, Hg, Tl), fungicides (Hg), elution from metal containers (Sn), or from calcium supplements derived from limestone (Pb) (6). Cd can be ingested in shellfish, grains, and peanuts, and causes nausea, vomiting, myalgia, abdominal pain, and renal failure. Mg is found in contaminated fish and in grains treated with fungicide, causing numbness, weakness, spastic paralysis, blindness, and coma. Tl can be transferred from soil to food crops, and excessive intake from crops grown on contaminated land can cause nausea, vomiting, diarrhea, parasthesias, hair loss, and polyneuropathy. Sn can contaminate foods stored in tin cans, but the decreased use of these has led to falling levels of ingestion. Sn toxicity can cause nausea, vomiting, and diarrhea. Pb used to contaminate some wines by elution at acid pH from brass tubing, but such tubing has been removed from commercial wine production. The only significant source of dietary Pb in the US diet is from calcium-supplemented food where the calcium is derived from limestone (7). Chronic Pb toxicity in children can cause weight loss, weakness, and anemia.

Treatment of Mineral Deficiency

Oral therapy is discussed in detail in this chapter. Parenteral therapy with major minerals (Na, K, Ca, Mg, P) is discussed in Chapter 11. Most healthy people do not require mineral supplements. However, certain groups of patients at high risk for deficiency of individual minerals should receive supplements. In infancy, iron may be needed at 6 to 8 weeks of life, especially if the mother has been deficient. Low-birth-weight infants require zinc. Iron supplements are often required by women after menarche and before menopause. More iron and calcium are needed during pregnancy because requirements are increased (see also Chapter 3). Persons who consume little or no milk require calcium; those on vegetable diets require iron. Patients with malabsorption may require calcium, magnesium, and zinc. In acute disorders characterized by severe vomiting or diarrhea, sodium and potassium must be replaced. Patients with chronic gastrointestinal bleeding may require iron replacement. Elderly patients whose calcium intake is decreased or who have osteopenia may require calcium supplements. The sections on the individual minerals should be consulted for details.

MAJOR MINERALS
Sodium (and Chloride)
Requirements

Sodium and chloride are found together in most foods, and the requirements are therefore considered together (4). There are examples in which one or the other mineral can be lost in excess of the other, or where the physiology of transport differs, and these differences will be discussed. Total body sodium levels range from 52 to 60 mmol per kg in male adults and from 48 to 55 mmol per kg in female adults. The body of a 70-kg man may contain between 3,600 and 4,200 mmol of sodium (83 and 97 g). About one-fourth of this, largely in the skeleton, is not exchangeable. Exchangeable sodium averages 40 mmol per kg in males and 37 mmol per kg in females. Changes in sodium concentration are corrected even at the expense of volume distribution. The kidney regulates sodium excretion by producing aldosterone. When sodium intake decreases, aldosterone levels increase, and urinary excretion of sodium falls. When sodium intake is high, urinary excretion rises. Thus, obligatory sodium losses are small in comparison with body stores. Minimal urinary and fecal losses are each about 23 mg (1 mmol) daily. Total body water losses contain from 46 to 92 mg of sodium (2 to 4 mmol) daily.

Adequate Intake

Minimal sodium needs in normal persons, when adaptation is maximal and sweating is minimal, can be met by an intake of 4 to no more than 8 mmol (92 to 184 mg) daily. The requirement increases when the production of sweat (containing 25 mmol of sodium per L) increases or losses in the urine or stool increase in disease states. Because of wide variations in physical activity and ambient temperatures, the AI is set for young adults, age 19 to 50, at 1.5 g (65 mmol) per day

(4). For children and adolescents age 9 to 18, the AI is the same, based on extrapolation from the adult AI, based on energy intake. The sodium requirement in children is set somewhat below that for adults: 120 mg for infants ages 0 to 6 months, 370 mg for infants ages 7 to 12 months, 1.0 g for children 1 to 3 years old, and 1.2 g for children 4 to 8 years old. The requirement in infants is largely provided by human milk (7 mmol per L) or cow's milk (21 mmol per L). In pregnancy, another 11 kg is added to the mother's body weight, of which 35% to 40% is ECF. This amounts to an additional 700 mmol of sodium, or 3 mmol (69 mg) per day, throughout the pregnancy. However, the AI for healthy adults is considered adequate to cover these needs during pregnancy and lactation. The AI for sodium (and chloride) for older adults and for the elderly is somewhat less, being 1.3 g (55 mmol) per day for adults aged 50 to 70 years, and 1.2 g (50 mmol) per day for men and women greater than 71 years old. The AI for chloride is set at a molar equivalent to that of sodium, so the AI for chloride for adults age 19 to 50 is 2.3 g (65 mmol) per day, equivalent to 3.8 g of sodium chloride. Although this value is not a recommended dietary intake, there are no data to suggest that more is needed.

Tolerable Upper Intake Level

The dietary reference intake (DRI) committee (2005) used the adverse effects of high sodium intake on blood pressure to establish the rationale for setting the UL for salt intake. Review of 10 meta-analyses of studies on salt intake and blood pressure determined that there was a direct and dose-related relationship between these factors throughout the whole spectrum of salt intake (4). Below an intake of 2.3 g (100 mmol) of sodium per day (3.8 g of salt), the effect of sodium restriction was larger. However, many of these interventional trials were for periods of less than 6 months. Patients with idiopathic hypertension, diabetes, and chronic renal disease, and older persons or African Americans are more sensitive to the effects of increased salt intake. The situation is further confounded by the observation that this rise in blood pressure can be altered by diets low in fat, or high in potassium or other minerals. Other factors, such as weight, level of exercise, genetic differences, and alcohol intake also affect the response to salt. Although the DRI Committee recognized the imprecision behind the estimate, they set the UL at 2.3 g (100 mmol) of sodium per day (3.8 g of salt). The comparable molar UL for chloride is 3.5 g per day. The Dietary Approaches to Stop Hypertension (DASH) diet also has similar properties to the Mediterranean diet associated with lower cancer risks, and in fact adherence to the DASH diet has been associated with a lower risk of colorectal cancer (8).

One view states that sodium is only one of many factors in hypertension, and that even randomized interventions (30% to 50% decrease in sodium intake) produce very modest changes (decrease of ~1 mm Hg in systolic pressure) (9). The DASH study compared a typical American diet (high in fat, low in fiber, low in potassium and calcium) with a diet rich in fruits and vegetables, both without and with low-fat dairy products (DASH diet); sodium intake and weight were kept stable throughout the 8-week trial in patients with systolic pressures below 160 mm Hg and diastolic pressures between 80 and 95 mm Hg (10). The DASH diet lowered systolic blood pressure by 11.4 mm Hg and diastolic blood pressure by 5.5 mm, much better results than those obtained with low-sodium diets. The National Heart, Lung, and Blood Institute 1999 Workshop on Sodium and Blood Pressure agreed that sodium restriction is most beneficial for older persons with established hypertension, but that only a small percentage of the US population is sensitive to the hypertensive effect of sodium (6). Moreover, much of the effect may represent a lower intake of potassium, calcium, and other minerals, rather than an excessive intake of sodium. In the DASH-sodium diet, the average intake was 1.5 g (65 mmol), estimated by mean urinary excretion (10). A later study by the DASH-Sodium Collaborative Research Group studied 412 subjects who ate low, medium, and high sodium foods for 30 days in random order, both with the DASH and control diets (11). At each sodium level, systolic blood pressure was lower with the DASH diet group, the drop being 11.5 mm Hg in patients with hypertension, and 7.1 mm Hg in those without. The decrease in sodium intake associated with a fall in systolic blood pressure was weakly correlated with a decrease in plasma sodium, suggesting a mechanism (decreased ECF volume) that could explain the blood pressure findings (12).

Proponents of the other point of view discount the small effects of randomized low-sodium trials because of their short time frame and cite data suggesting a high prevalence of sodium sensitivity (13). This argument has received support from the Cochrane systematic review that analyzed 11 trials (three in normotensives and eight in hypertensives) with follow-up from 6 months to 7 years, and found only a modest reduction in blood pressure (1.1 mm Hg systolic) that was not related to reduction in sodium intake (14). However, another systematic review accepting trials of a minimum of 4 weeks' duration (17 normotensive, 11 hypertensive) found a correlation between the magnitude of salt reduction and that of blood pressure (15). Studies of other factors, such as loss of weight, increased physical activity, and moderation of alcohol intake show that blood-pressure-lowering effects can be as low as those found using medications (16).

The 2010 Dietary Guidelines for Americans (DGA) agreed that sodium intake was responsible at least in part for the increase in cardiovascular (CV) events and recommended a sodium intake of less than 2,300 mg per day for those older than 2 years, and less than 1,500 mg per day for certain high-risk subgroups, including African Americans, individuals with hypertension, diabetes, or chronic kidney disease, or those greater than 50 years (17). The 2005 IOM (Institute of Medicine) Panel for DRIs on water, potassium, sodium, chloride, and sulfate did not feel that the evidence was sufficient to make such restrictive recommendations (4), but it is clear that even their more modest recommendations were not being followed. Twenty-four-hour urinary sodium excretion is the "gold standard" for assessing sodium intake, and by this standard, sodium intake in the US adult population in 38 studies was approximately 3,500 mg per day, and had not decreased from 1957 to 2003 (18). Because the DGA did not alter the potassium recommendation of 4,700 mg per day, the estimated Na/K ratio for intake should be 1,500/4,700 or 0.32. Foods that are common in Western diets (e.g., grains, breads, pastas, cereals, meats, poultry and fish, cheese, eggs, and dishes made from them had Na/K ratios greater than 1 (19). Citrus and fruit juices, white potatoes, and milk were the most common American foods eaten with ratios less than 1, but dark green and deep yellow vegetables, nuts, and dried fruits also had low ratios, but were eaten less often.

Despite acknowledging the high sodium ingestion of the adult US population, the IOM report of 2013 reiterated the conclusion that the data were insufficient to recommend a lower sodium intake of 1,500 mg per day and kept the suggested intake at 2,300 mg per day (20). The IOM Committee noted that no studies have examined the effects on CV outcomes of sodium intake from 1,500 to 2,300 mg per day. It also noted that, with the exception of heart failure where more sodium restriction may be helpful, not enough information was available to benefit and harm from sodium intakes less than 2,300 mg per day in other patient subgroups, such as diabetes or prior cardiac disease.

One key study that influenced the IOM report showed that sodium excretion greater than 7 g per day was associated with an increase in all CV events, but intake of less than 3 g per day was associated with increased CV mortality and hospitalization for heart failure (21). It is clear that those patients on low sodium intakes might have been placed on such diets because of preexisting heart failure. Many experts have felt that the recommended sodium intake should have been decreased in the IOM report, as was the case with the DGA (22). The argument is complicated by the conclusion that reduction of sodium intake of 1.2 g per day (3 g salt) from the current level of 4.12 g for men and 2.92 g for women would reduce CV events at a great savings in cost, but still not reach the recommended level of 2.3 g sodium intake per day for males and many females (23). Moreover, because 75% of the sodium intake in the United States comes from processed foods and not the addition of salt to food, it is difficult for the individual to modify sodium intake (24). Strategies to collaborate with industry to reduce sodium in prepared foods by approximately 10% have been suggested (25). Population-wide campaigns to decrease sodium intake in Finland have led to decreased urinary sodium excretion, lower blood pressure, and decreased rate of death from stroke and CV disease (26). It is still unclear, however, whether the apparently paradoxical CV outcomes with low sodium intake are causative, thus justifying a lower recommendation of 1,500 mg per day for populations on Western style diets.

Food Sources

In Western societies, an adult with free access to salt consumes from 2.3 to 6.9 g (100 to 300 mmol) of sodium per day, or from 8 to 12 g (140 to 250 mmol) of sodium chloride. Daily sodium intake alone can increase to 12 g (250 mmol) in very hot climates when hard work increases sweating (27). Most of the sodium is added to foods as salt (NaCl). Of total dietary sodium, about one-third comes from the shaker, one-third from processing, and one-third from the food itself. Cheese, milk, and shellfish, in addition to meat, fish, and eggs, are good natural sources of sodium. Cereals, fruits, and vegetables are low in salt unless it is added during processing. The amount of salt added in processing can be considerable and now approaches 75% of total intake in the United States (24). In processed foods, the food groups that are highest in sodium include processed meats, sauces and spreads, and, surprisingly, breads (28). Lowest sodium-containing foods include fresh fruits and vegetables, grains, and fresh meat, fish, or eggs (29). A sample moderate-cost menu with approximately 2,000 calories and approximately 1,800 mg sodium per day can be found at http://www.choosemyplate.gov/healthy-eating-tips/sample-menus-recipes.html.

Salt is added to foods to extract moisture from the food, in order to prevent spoiling. High salt concentrations may also prevent growth of some bacteria. In addition, salt adds flavor to processed foods, and adds texture to dried foods, such as crackers. Table 7-2 lists the sodium content of some foods at different stages of preparation and preservation.

Normally, sodium must be added to some cereals, such as those containing bran or fiber, to increase palatability. In other cereals (e.g., wheat cereals), the range of sodium content is very wide. The sodium content of some natural foods is listed in Table 7-3.

Much sodium can be added to foods in the form of condiments, fats, and salad dressings. Some of the most commonly used products are listed in Table 7-4.

A list of the sodium content of foods is presented in the US Department of Agriculture (USDA) booklet entitled *The Sodium Content of Your Food* (Home and Garden Bulletin No. 233, US Government Printing Office, Washington, DC). Some labels express sodium content in grams or milligrams. Some diets list salt content or milliequivalents of sodium. To convert salt to sodium content, multiply milligrams of salt by 0.4, the fraction of sodium chloride weight

TABLE 7-2 Effect of Food Processing on Sodium Content

Food	State	Portion	Na Content (mg)[a]
Corn	Fresh kernels	1/2 cup	12
	Canned kernels	1/2 cup	190
	Canned, creamed	1/2 cup	365
Potato	Baked	1 each	16
	Mashed, instant	1 cup	733
	Chips	14 chips	133
Tomato	Fresh chopped	1 cup	11
	Canned whole	1 cup	390
	Juice	1 cup	881

[a]These are representative figures, not brand-specific.

TABLE 7-3 Approximate Sodium Content of Natural Foods

Negligible	2–5 mg	5–9 mg	25–60 mg	≥120 mg
Butter, unsalted	Fruits (1/2 cup)	Bread without salt (slice)	Muscle or organ meat (1 oz)	Milk (1 cup)
Cream (tbs)	Corn, potato, peas, beans (1/2 cup)	Selected dry cereals (puffed rice, puffed wheat, shredded wheat) (1 cup)	1 egg	Salted butter (1 oz)
	Nuts (raw)		Fish (1 oz)	Vegetable margarines (1 oz)
			Root vegetables (celery, beets, turnip)	Processed meats (1 oz)
Cooking fat (tsp)		Most vegetables (1/2 cup)	Artichoke	

TABLE 7-4 Representative Sodium Content of Condiments

Product	Portion	Na Content (mg)	(mmol)
Baking powder	1 tsp	339	15
Baking soda	1 tsp	821	36
Catsup	1 tbs	202	9
Chili powder	1 tsp	25	1
Garlic salt	1 tsp	1,620	70
Meat tenderizer	1 tsp	1,750	76
Monosodium glutamate	1 tsp	492	21
Mustard, prepared	1 tsp	65	3
Onion salt	1 tsp	1,650	72
Olives, green	10 ea	936	41
Pickle, dill	1 medium	928	41
Pickle, sweet	1 tbs	107	40
Table salt	1 tsp	1,938	84
A-1 sauce	1 tbs	275	12
Barbecue sauce	1 tbs	130	6
Soy sauce, regular	1 tbs	1,029	45
Soy sauce, low-sodium	1 tbs	300	13
Worcestershire sauce	1 tbs	206	9
Butter, regular	1 tbs	116	5
Margarine	1 tbs	140	6
Salad dressing, bottled	1 tbs	109–224	5–10

that represents sodium. To convert sodium in milligrams to milliequivalents, divide milligrams by 23, the atomic weight of sodium. 1 tsp of salt = 2,325 mg of sodium.

Sodium in Prepared Foods

In food preparation, a number of compounds are added besides sodium chloride to increase the sodium content. These are listed below as they appear on labels:

Monosodium glutamate (MSG)—in packaged and frozen foods
Baking powder—in breads and cakes
Baking soda (sodium bicarbonate)—in breads and cakes. 1 tsp = 1,000 mg of sodium
Brine—in processed foods (e.g., pickles)
Disodium phosphate—in quick-cooking cereals and cheeses
Sodium alginate or caseinate—as thickener and binder
Sodium benzoate or nitrite—as preservative
Sodium hydroxide—to soften skins of fruits and olives
Sodium propionate—to inhibit mold in cheeses
Sodium sulfite—as preservative in dried fruit
Sodium citrate—as buffer for canned and bottled citrus drinks

For practical advice on following a low-sodium diet, see Chapter 12.

Sodium in Water and Medications

In addition to food, sodium is present in drinking water and in medications. Water may contain very little sodium or as much as 1,500 mg per L, depending on the degree of softening, a process that raises the sodium content of water. The various departments of public health can usually supply information on the sodium content of local water supplies. Bottled mineral water also varies widely in sodium content, depending on the source. Perrier contains only 12 mg per L, whereas Vichy water has 1,110 mg per L.

Most medications do not contain enough sodium to present a problem, but a few are very high in sodium. Table 7-5 lists some of these. In general, liquid formulas contain more sodium than do capsules or tablets.

TABLE 7-5 Sodium Content in Selected Medications (Sodium Per Therapeutic Unit[a])

<5 mg	5–25 mg	25–100 mg	>100 mg
Penicillin, potassium	Phenytoin	Penicillin, sodium	Alka-Seltzer (521 per tablet)
Analgesics (most)	Maalox liquid	Synthetic penicillins, sodium	Sal Hepatica (1,000 per tsp)
Nonpenicillin antibiotic tablets	Amphojel suspension	Antibiotic suspensions	Oral phosphate for colonoscopy
Titralac liquid[a]	Synthetic penicillins, sodium	Colace	Sodium bicarbonate
Dramamine	Bromo-Seltzer (717 per tablet)		Oral phosphate for colonoscopy
Vitamin tablets	Kaopectate		Sodium bicarbonate
Metamucil	Milk of magnesia		
Diuretics	Metamucil instant mix		
Antihypertensives	Endocrine agents		
Antihistamines	Cold syrups		
Mg/Al(OH)$_3$ antacid tablets (many)	Sedative elixirs		
Liquid vitamins	Di-Gel liquid		
Mylanta liquid			
Riopan liquid			
Laxatives (many)			
Psychoactive drugs			
Sedative capsules			

[a]The therapeutic unit of antacids is considered to be 30 mL of liquid or 2 tablets. The therapeutic dose of Titralac is 5 mL.

Assessment

Clinical

The signs of total body sodium excess are weight gain and edema. The signs of total body sodium deficiency are manifestations of hypovolemia and can include decreased skin turgor, hypotension, tachycardia, dry tongue or axillae, sunken eyes, and weight loss. In older adults, other explanations are often present for all these signs (30). Orthostatic hypotension is often used, defined in the American Academy of Neurology consensus statement as a decrease in systolic blood pressure of 20 mm Hg or in diastolic blood pressure of 10 mm Hg within 3 minutes of standing (31). Some clinicians prefer an increase in the pulse rate of 5 to 12 beats per minute (32). An increase of 20 beats per minute has greater specificity (33). However, postprandial hypotension resulting from splanchnic blood pooling is common in older patients, and blood loss is a common cause of postural hypotension. Usually, the decision to proceed with hydration therapy depends on a consideration of all the findings of the clinical and laboratory evaluation.

Serum Sodium and Chloride

Sodium and chloride are measured by ion-selective electrodes in either clotted blood or anticoagulated blood (not ethylenediaminetetraacetic acid, or EDTA). The serum sodium level (normal, 135 to 145 mmol per L) and chloride level (normal, 99 to 110 mmol per L) does not reflect the total body sodium but rather the relationship between total body sodium and ECF volume. A patient with excess total body sodium, manifested by edema, may have a low, normal, or high serum level of sodium depending on whether ECF volume is increased to a level in excess of, even with, or less than that of the total body sodium. Thus, a patient with edema and a serum sodium level of 125 mmol per L has a total body excess of sodium, but the serum sodium level is low because of retained water in excess of sodium. The serum sodium level can be high in hyperadrenalism, severe dehydration, diabetic coma, or treatment with sodium salts. Serum values greater than 160 mmol per L or less than 120 mmol per L are usually associated with symptoms and must be verified and corrected. Serum chloride levels fall when chloride is lost in excess of sodium, e.g., following extensive vomiting. Serum chloride levels rise when the anion cannot be excreted, as in chronic renal failure, or when chloride is reabsorbed in excess, in some patients with ureteroileal anastomoses in ileal bladders.

Other Laboratory Evaluation
Laboratory findings associated with hypovolemia include a high urine specific gravity, elevated hematocrit, and a blood urea nitrogen (BUN) elevated in excess of the serum creatinine level. The urinary sodium level does not correlate with intake or body stores except in the normal condition when excess sodium is excreted. The normal range is 27 to 287 mmol per 24 hours. In sodium retention syndromes, the urinary sodium level can be low when stores are high; in renal salt wasting, the urinary sodium level can be elevated when body stores are low. For acute assessment, the body weight provides a better measure of extracellular volume. When the glomerular filtration rate (GFR) per nephron ratio is decreased, as in prerenal azotemia, the urinary–plasma (U/P) creatinine ratio is greater than 20 (range, 20 to 50) and the urine sodium concentration is greater than 20 mEq per L. The fractional excretion of sodium is defined as $100 \times (U/P_{sodium} \div U/P_{creatinine})$ and is less than 1% in prerenal azotemia or total body sodium deficiency. In acute renal failure, the fractional excretion of sodium is more than 4%, the U/P creatinine ratio is less than 10, and the urinary sodium level is greater than 40 mmol per L. Plasma and urinary osmolarity have been used to detect dehydration, but these measures are confounded by many factors. Nonetheless, a single atypical P_{osm} of 301 ± 5 mosm per kg has been suggested as a starting assessment of dehydration (33).

For evaluation of sodium intake in population studies, 24 h urinary sodium excretion is the best available standard (34). Although 24 h urine samples are preferred, casual specimens are useful and practical, although correlations between intake and excretion are only 0.5 for individuals in contrast with approximately 0.75 for populations.

Physiology

Osmotic Responses to Dehydration

Osmotic constancy is maintained by secretion of arginine vasopressin (AVP), the antidiuretic hormone. The kidney responds to AVP by altering water excretion in response to shifts in intravascular volume. Loss of greater than 10% in blood volume is usually needed to trigger secretion of AVP from the hypothalamus (33). The usual causes of isotonic hypovolemia are secretory diarrhea and vomiting or diuretic use. In these cases where large losses of solute occur from circulating blood volume, water is not recruited from the larger extracellular space, and losses of less than 10% in blood volume may cause symptoms.

Sodium and Chloride Transport and Absorption

Transport of sodium and chloride across epithelium generates membrane potentials and osmotic gradients that drive transmembranous and paracellular fluid movement. Sodium uptake occurs in the small intestine through transporters that are coupled to sodium movement, including cotransporters for glucose-galactose (SGLT1 and 2), for amino acids (B0AT/SLC6 family of transporters), and bile salts (ASBT/SLC10A2) (35). Much of the apical sodium transport not linked to solute occurs via the amiloride-sensitive epithelial sodium channel (EnaC) that is electrogenically coupled to Na+/K+-ATPase (36). The rest of the sodium moves through the sodium–hydrogen exchange (NHE) gene family that includes exchangers located apically (NH2), basolaterally (NH1), and recycling (NH3), as well as intracellular isoforms (NH6,7,9) (37). These latter two mechanisms are dominant in the colon where solute-coupled sodium absorption is minimal. In the proximal colon, sodium is reabsorbed mainly via the NHE family, and in the distal colon via EnaC sodium channels.

Sodium appetite increases after a prolonged period of sodium deficiency, but is not caused by a decrease in plasma sodium concentration. This appetite is probably due in part to a simultaneous increase in circulating aldosterone and angiotensin II (38). It is not clear whether baroreceptor signaling is involved in this response, but intracerebral sodium concentration may be. There is no evidence that the absorptive capacity for sodium increases in response to states of deficiency.

Chloride transport across the apical membrane is mediated by a series of mechanisms, including the cAMP-dependent cystic fibrosis transmembrane conductance regulator (CFTR) channel (39), voltage-dependent Cl channels, the ClC family of chloride channels (40), calcium-activated Cl channels, CaCC and outward rectifying channels (ORCC) (20,22), ligand-gated (e.g., glycine) Cl channels (41), and SLC4 and SLC26 family of multifunctional anion exchangers, mostly Cl^-/HCO_3^- (42,43). This bewildering array is likely to grow larger, as there seems to be no common structure for chloride channels. Because mutations in many of these channels cause disease, it is not clear whether any of them are dominant in function in a given cell. CFTR modulates ATP release and regulates the calcium-dependent channels, CaCC and ORCC, and inhibits sodium absorption via EnaC (39). The CFTR potentiator VX-770 opens the dysfunctional channel gate of mutant CFTR, but does not require ATP to do so, and so works through a yet unknown mechanism (44). The ClC channels move H^+ and Cl^- ions in opposite directions, as do the Cl^-/HCO_3^- exchangers. Mutations in chloride channels produce cystic fibrosis (CFTR), but also many myopathies (ClC-1), epilepsy (ClC-2), Bartter syndrome (ClC-Kb), Dent disease (X-linked nephrolithiasis) (ClC-5), osteopetrosis (ClC-7), and hereditary hyperekplexia or startle disease (glycine-Cl channel) (40,41). All of these channels are located on the plasma membrane of cells, except for ClC-5 and -7 that are on endosomal membranes. The most important chloride channels for intestinal absorption are probably CFTR, NHE2, and SLC26A3. Mutated SLC26A3 produces congenital chloride diarrhea (35). One of the voltage-dependent chloride channels, ClC-2, is located apically and is activated by a bicyclic fatty acid, lubiprostone, an orally administered drug that increases intestinal secretion in patients with constipation (45). The significance of this channel in normal fluid secretion is not known. The Na/K-2Cl-symporter channel permits cotransport of sodium, potassium, and chloride bilaterally across the basolateral membrane. The Na+/K+ ATPase provides the energy for active Cl- secretion. Chloride secretion is regulated by the second messengers cAMP, cGMP, and free cytosolic calcium (46). Water follows passively along the osmotic gradients produced by sodium and chloride movement, either via paracellular or transcellular (via aquaporins) pathways.

Ion Excretion

Sodium and anions, usually chloride or bicarbonate, are present in most body secretions. Excessive loss of sodium can occur when any of these secretions is lost in large amounts from the body. The secretions and their ion contents are listed in Table 7-6. Only the kidney (and the colon and terminal ileum to a limited extent) is able to restrict or increase its loss of sodium. Because the urinary sodium level is so variable, it is not included in the list. Renal conservation involves a balance between filtration and reabsorption. The urinary sodium level reflects the sodium that escapes reabsorption in the nephron; therefore, sodium excretion depends on the GFR. Thus, renal regulation is well adapted to conserving the major extracellular cation.

Intestinal Reabsorption

The small bowel reabsorbs most of the electrolytes and water from luminal secretions under normal circumstances. Most of the sodium is absorbed from the jejunum and ileum by solute-dependent sodium cotransport along with sugars and amino acids. Non–nutrient-dependent sodium absorption in the proximal small intestine occurs mainly by Na/H exchange. The ileum and colon absorb sodium actively by a coupled Na/Cl cotransport and also secrete bicarbonate in exchange for chloride. The colon retains sodium most avidly and secretes potassium into the lumen. In small-bowel malabsorption, the colon is presented with an increased sodium load, which it reabsorbs at least partially. The colon and terminal ileum can respond to aldosterone, but are not able to retain sodium as efficiently as the kidney. Sodium absorption in the rectum occurs mainly through apically located sodium channels.

When diarrhea is mild or moderate and the colon is intact, sodium losses are moderate and proportional to the stool volume (Table 7-7). Potassium losses are also proportional to the stool volume when it is not excessive (<3 L per day). Chloride is lost as the predominant anion, and systemic alkalosis develops, so that the potassium loss is exacerbated through increased urinary

TABLE 7-6 Electrolyte Concentrations in Gastrointestinal Fluids and Sweat

Fluid Source	Na (mmol/L)	Na (mmol/d)	K (mmol/L)	K (mmol/d)	Cl (mmol/L)	Cl (mmol/d)	HCO$_3$ (mmol/L)	HCO$_3$ (mmol/d)
Sweat	30–50	15–25	5	2.5	45–55	25	—	—
Saliva	45	35–55	20	15–25	45	35–55	60	45–75
Stomach[a]	40–65	40–100	10	10–15	100–140	140–200	—	—
Bile	135–150	150–170	4	5	80–110	100–140	35–50	40–60
Pancreas[b]	135–150	120–130	7	6	60–80	55–70	70–90	80–100
Duodenum	90	180	15	30	90	180	90	180
Mid-small bowel	140	280	6	12	100	200	20	40
Terminal ileum	140	70	8	4	60	30	70	35
Rectum/stool	40	10	90	23	15	4	30	8
Diarrhea, moderate	50–100		20–30		50–100		<20	
Diarrhea, severe	100–140		20–40		80–100		30–50	

[a]Na and Cl vary inversely according to the rate of H$^+$ secretion.
[b]Cl and HCO$_3$ vary inversely according to the rate of secretion.

TABLE 7-7	Common Metabolic Consequences of Electrolyte Depletion Syndromes				
Syndrome	Major Ions Lost	Acid–Base Status	ECF Volume	Renal Response	[K]
Vomiting	H, Cl, K > Na	Alkalosis	↓	Na, HCO$_3$ retained, K lost	↓
Pancreatic fistula	Na, HCO$_3$	Acidosis	↓↓	Na, Cl retained	NL
Malabsorption	Na, Cl, K All > HCO$_3$	NL, alkalosis	↓	Na, Cl retained, K lost	↓
Ileostomy	Na, Cl > HCO$_3$	Alkalosis	↓	Na, HCO$_3$ retained, K lost	NL, ↓
Diarrhea, moderate	Na, K	NL	NL	K retained	NL, ↓
Diarrhea, severe	Na, HCO$_3$, K, Cl	Acidosis	↓↓	Na, Cl retained	↓
Salt wasting	Na, Cl	Alkalosis	↓	None	NL, ↑
↓ Sweating	Na, Cl	Alkalosis	↓	Na, Cl retained	NL, ↓
↓ Diuretics	Na, K, Cl	Alkalosis	↓	None	↓

ECF, extracellular fluid; NL, normal.

excretion. In secretory diarrheas, stool sodium is less than 70 mEq per L; in osmotic diarrhea, sodium is usually less than 70 mEq per L.

When diarrhea is severe, the colon is maximally stimulated to conserve sodium chloride. In the process, it secretes more potassium and bicarbonate. The result is greater loss of sodium (because the colonic capacity is exceeded) and greater loss of potassium. Sodium loss can increase without limit, depending on fecal volume. Large amounts of sodium can be lost in a short time whenever intestinal secretions are lost in large quantities. Sodium is the major extracellular cation and is involved in the maintenance of electrogenic potentials across the cell membrane. Because the body preserves serum sodium concentration at the expense of extravascular volume, early sodium deficiency is accompanied by signs of volume depletion rather than by hyponatremia.

Potassium loss is limited somewhat by the degree of sodium exchange, and the potassium concentration tends to plateau when fecal volumes are greater than 3 L per day. Bicarbonate losses can be large in severe diarrhea, and metabolic acidosis may result.

Deficiency

Sodium deficiency is nearly always the result of excessive losses and results in hypovolemia and dehydration (see the section on Assessment). Hyponatremia may accompany signs of dehydration. These signs (seen especially in children) include dry mucous membranes when dehydration is mild, sunken eyes and loss of skin turgor (moderate dehydration), and rapid faint pulse, cyanosis, rapid breathing, and lethargy (severe dehydration). The differential diagnosis of hyponatremia with contracted ECF volumes is aided by determining the urinary sodium levels. When the urinary sodium concentration is less than 10 mmol per L, sodium intake may be inadequate, but hypovolemia resulting from excessive sodium loss (sweating, diarrhea) is a more likely cause. When the urinary sodium concentration is more than 10 mmol per L, vomiting or excessive urinary loss of sodium may be the likely cause. When the cause of hyponatremia is not clear, the serum osmolality should be measured. Normal osmolality can be associated with hyperlipidemia or markedly elevated glucose or urea levels *(pseudohyponatremia)*. To ascertain whether the serum sodium concentration is normal in the presence of hyperglycemia or an elevated BUN value, the serum osmolarity can be estimated (normal, 275 to 295 mOsmol per kg):

$$\text{Serum osmolality} = 2 \times [\text{Na}] + ([\text{glucose}] \div 18) + ([\text{BUN}]) \div 2.8$$

where [Na] is expressed in mmol per L and [glucose] and [BUN] are expressed in mg per dL.

TABLE 7-8 Causes of Dilutional Hyponatremia

Pathophysiology	ECF Volume	Causes
Renal sodium loss	↓	Diuretic drugs, adrenal insufficiency, nephropathy, osmotic diuresis
Intestinal sodium loss	↓	Diarrhea, vomiting, blood loss
Skin sodium loss	↓	Excessive sweating/climatic heat
Fluid sequestration	↓	Burns, pancreatitis, bowel obstruction
Renal sodium retention	↓	CHF, cirrhosis, renal failure, pregnancy
Inappropriate antidiuretic hormone	NL	Cancer, CNS lesions and disorders, medications, pulmonary conditions, postoperative, HIV
↓ Solute intake	NL	Beer potomania, tea-and-toast diet
Excessive water intake	NL	Primary polydipsia, dilute infant formula

CNS, central nervous system; CHF, congestive heart failure; ECF, extracellular fluid; NL, normal; HIV, human immunodeficiency virus.

Dilutional (hypotonic) hyponatremia occurs when water is retained in excess of existing sodium stores. Although sodium depletion is a major cause of this syndrome, any water-retaining disorder may present with a similar serum sodium profile, although signs of dehydration are not present. Both sodium depletion and retention syndromes are characterized by low urinary sodium levels and an impaired capacity for renal water excretion. The serum sodium level is not a guide for volume loss, but symptoms (confusion, anorexia, lethargy, vomiting, seizures) can develop when the serum sodium level falls below 120 to 125 mEq per L. Other metabolic consequences accompany clinical situations in which sodium depletion develops (Table 7-8). These situations largely involve losses from the gastrointestinal tract. Losses of sodium from the gastrointestinal tract are proportional to the volume lost. The other ions lost (K, Cl, HCO_3) are determined by the source of the fluid. The serum sodium level is normal or low in these syndromes depending on how rapidly the losses occur. With large losses of gastric secretions, hypochloremia and alkalosis ensue. With severe losses from diarrhea, metabolic acidosis can develop when the colon is intact to generate bicarbonate. In mild to moderate cases of diarrhea, chloride is lost in proportion to or in excess of bicarbonate, and alkalosis is present if any acid–base disturbance is noted. Despite extensive losses of sodium and other salts with diarrhea, fat losses are minimal, unless a condition causing steatorrhea is the reason for the diarrhea (47).

Therapy

In sodium replacement, the amount given depends on the salt administered. Because 1 g of sodium equals 43 mmol of sodium and 1 g of sodium chloride equals 17 mmol of sodium, a 4-g sodium diet is roughly equivalent to a 10-g salt (NaCl) diet. Each gram of sodium bicarbonate represents 12 mmol of sodium. Sodium preparations are listed in Table 7-9.

Parenteral Replacement

When hyponatremia causes symptoms (lethargy, seizures), intravenous (IV) treatment is needed with normal or hypertonic saline solution. If the urine osmolality is appropriately dilute (<100 mOsm per L) and correctable causes of hyponatremia are not identified (e.g., excess water or diuretic use), hypertonic saline should be administered (48). Correcting too rapidly can lead to more dehydration of the brain, and the osmotic demyelination syndrome can ensue (49). This is a known complication of too rapid correction of serum sodium, although the syndrome has other etiologies. Typical features include quadriparesis and neurocognitive changes, and are related to central pontine myelinolysis. A consensus panel suggests that serum sodium concentrations be raised no more than 10 to 12 mEq per L during the first 24 h, so serum sodium levels should be checked frequently (q 1 to 2 h) during this period, especially over the first 4 h when delivering 3% saline containing 513 mmol per L.

When IV fluid is needed, the choice of additive or solution used (Table 7-9) sometimes depends on the source of lost fluid (Tables 7-6 and 7-8). When signs of volume depletion are obviously present, at least a 10% reduction in the ECF volume has occurred. In a normal person, the ECF volume

TABLE 7-9 Sodium Supplements

Product	Anion	Na per Dose (mmol)	Na per Dose (mg)	ECF Distribution (%)
Oral Supplements				
NaCl	Cl	17/1-g tablet	391	100
NaHCO$_3$	HCO$_3$	7.8/0.650-g tablet	138	?
Parenteral Fluids				
Normal saline	Cl	154/L	3,541	100
3% Saline	Cl	513/L	11,891	100
NaHCO$_3$	HCO$_3$	44.6/50 mL or 50/50 mL		?
Lactated Ringer solution	Lactate	130/L	2,990	97
0.45% Saline in water	Cl	77/L	1,771	73

ECF, extracellular fluid.

is about 20% of body weight. Because the sodium concentration is 135 to 146 mmol per L of ECF fluid, the milliequivalents of sodium required can be estimated to replace 10% of the ECF volume or 20% if the signs of volume depletion are severe. The sodium deficit can be estimated as follows:

$$\text{Na deficit (mmol)} = ([\text{Na}]_{\text{desired}} - [\text{Na}]_{\text{observed}}) \times 0.6 \times \text{weight (kg)}$$

Alternatively, one can estimate the effect on the serum sodium concentration of adding 1 L of infusate:

$$\text{Change in }[\text{Na}]_{\text{serum}} = [\text{Na}]_{\text{infusate}} - [\text{Na}]_{\text{serum}} \div (\text{total body water} + 1)$$

where total body water is estimated in liters as a fraction of body weight (0.6 for children; 0.6 and 0.5 for nonelderly men and women, respectively; 0.5 and 0.45 for elderly men and women, respectively) (50). For example, to treat a 70-kg young male with impending cerebral edema and a [Na]s of 105 with 3% saline, the equation would estimate: $513 - 105 \div [(0.6 \times 70) + 1]$ or $408 \div 43 = 9.5$. Thus, only 1 L of 3% saline should be used in the first hour.

Oral Replacement

Oral replacement solutions. In general, oral therapy is effective, less costly, and as effective as parenteral therapy for dehydration. Many oral rehydration solutions are available, but they are often underutilized in young children and infants because of concern that they are not as efficient as IV solutions (51), and in adults because of the general availability of IV solutions in hospitals (52) (Table 7-10). The mechanism of oral substitution is to restore fluid and electrolyte content by driving water across intestinal mucosa following sodium-coupled glucose uptake via the sodium–glucose cotransporter, SGLT1. The exact composition of the oral replacement solution for infants is still being debated because diarrheal stool sodium concentration is lower in children than in adults. Thus, when dehydration is severe, too much sodium (90 mmol per L) in a short time can occasionally cause hypernatremia. In this situation, solutions with 40 to 60 mEq per L are recommended (51,53). However, for children with mild to moderate dehydration and for adults with a normal intestine, the World Health Organization (WHO) solution containing 90 mmol per L is probably just as good. The use of rice-based and other cereal-based (as a substitute for glucose) oral rehydration solutions (glucose, e.g., Ceralyte, Ricelyte) is thought to reduce diarrhea by providing glucose slowly in the gut lumen without increasing osmolarity. Fecal losses have been reduced by adding resistant starch to the oral rehydration solution in the form of high-amylose maize starch, which allows colonic fermentation to short-chain fatty acid and sodium and fluid absorption in the colon (54). Fructooligosaccharides have been used in some preparations (e.g., Equalyte) because they can be fermented to short-chain fatty acids by colonic bacteria, thus providing the metabolic fuel preferred by colonocytes (but not small-bowel epithelia).

TABLE 7-10 Composition of Selected Oral Rehydration Solutions

Solution	Sodium (mmol/L)	Potassium (mmol/L)	Chloride (mmol/L)	Base (mmol/L)	Glucose mmol/L (g/L)	Osmolality (mOsm/kg)
Rehydration						
WHO packet	90	20	80	30	111[a] (20)	310
Rehydralyte	75	20	65	30	139 (25)	310
CeraLyte 70/90	70/90	20	60	30	222 (40)[b]	260/275
EqualLyte	78	22	68	32	139 (25)[d]	305
Washington U[e]	102	3	75	10	101 (18)	230
Maintenance[f]						
ESPGHN	60	20	60	30	90 (16)	240
Pedialyte	45	20	35	30	139 (25)	269
Resol	50	20	50	34	111 (20)	265
Infalyte (former Ricelyte)	50	20	40	30	111 (20)	270
Lytren	50	25	45	30	111 (20)	?
Naturalyte	45	20	35	48	139 (25)	?
Diocalm Junior[c]	60	20	50	10	111 (20)	251
Dioralyte[c]	60	20	60	10	90 (16)	240
Electrolade[c]	50	20	40	30	111 (20)	251
Rapolyte[c]	60	20	50	10	111 (20)	251
Unsuitable						
Gatorade	20	3	27	3	278 (45)[c]	330–380
Colas	1.6	<1	—	13.4	(5–15)	550–750
Orange juice	<1	50	—	50	666 (12)	High
Apple juice	<1	44	45	—	666 (12)	730
Chicken broth	250	8	—	0	0	500

ESPGHN, European Society of Pediatric Gastroenterology, Hepatology, and Nutrition; WHO, World Health Organization.
[a]May contain glucose or sucrose.
[b]Rice-based carbohydrate.
[c]Available in the United Kingdom.
[d]Also contains fructo-oligosaccharides.
[e]Washington University formula: G2 Gatorade (low calorie) 32 oz + 3/4 tsp salt + 2 tsp (10 ml) sodium citrate/citric acid (avaiable as Cytra-2, Bicitra, Oracit, or Shohl's). Mix, refrigerate, and use within 24 h.
[f]Reduced-sodium ORS is indicated for maintenance in adults, in children with mild/moderate dehydration, or for replacement therapy in infants or children with severe dehydration.

Solutions with higher sodium and glucose concentrations are used for rehydration, although whether 75 or 90 mEq of sodium per L is better is unclear. The Washington University formula has been developed for patients with short-bowel syndrome who require IV rehydration. The higher sodium concentration has been shown to convert such patients from fluid secretors to fluid absorbers (55). The oral rehydration solutions with lower sodium and glucose contents are used for maintenance. The WHO oral rehydration solution can be bought in many countries in dried packets to be rehydrated at home, or can be made from ingredients readily available at home. Recent modifications of the WHO solution contain less glucose to avoid osmotic diarrhea, and less sodium (50 mEq per L) to avoid hypernatremia and convulsions. The standard recipe involves 3/4 tsp of salt, 1/2 tsp of baking soda (or 1 tsp of baking powder), 4 tbs of table sugar, and 8 oz of orange juice (to provide potassium), diluted in 1 L (4 1/4 cups) of water. A Crystal-Light packet (or other product without sugar or electrolytes) can be added for flavor if needed.

The daily dose for adults is 2 to 3 L, for children 1 L plus food, and for infants 0.5 L plus food. The more substrate present, the better the cotransport of sodium. For this reason and to replace deficits resulting from malnutrition, infants and children should also be fed the regular diets appropriate for their age.

Food-based solutions. Food-based solutions may be less practical because the sodium and fluid may not be so readily available for rapid absorption. Most sodas contain 1 to 4 mEq of sodium per L and 0.1 to 0.6 mEq of potassium per L along with about 10% carbohydrate usually supplied as fructose-rich carbohydrate derived from corn syrup. Because they do not contain enough sodium, and because fructose is not absorbed by the SGLT1 glucose-Na cotransporter, they are inadequate for the treatment of dehydration. Fluid replacement drinks are available in grocery stores. The characteristics of some of these preparations are listed in Table 7-10. Gatorade® was designed to provide energy and replace electrolytes lost in sweat, and, consequently, the sodium concentration is too low to treat significant dehydration. However, it is isotonic, and all therapeutic oral replacement solutions are isotonic or mildly hypotonic. When fluid loss from vomiting or diarrhea is not severe in adults, Gatorade or similar beverages may be well tolerated because of their near-isotonicity. These products are helpful in maintaining fluid volume but not in treating volume depletion because the sodium concentration is too low. If fluid loss is moderate to severe, one of the other solutions is indicated.

Vasopressin receptor antagonists (vaptans). When hyponatremia is chronic, the cause is usually due to an excess in total body water rather than loss of sodium (e.g., cirrhosis, heart failure, SIADH), and sodium replacement is often harmful in the long run. When serum sodium is less than 125 mEq per L, vasopressin repressor antagonists (e.g., tolvaptan) can elevate serum sodium by 1 to 5 mEq per L, and decrease the risk for the osmotic demyelination syndrome. However, there seems less need for urgent treatment with vaptans when the sodium concentration is greater than 125 mEq per L, especially when unaccompanied by symptoms (56).

Toxicity

Sodium toxicity presents in two clinical syndromes: hypernatremia (usually with decreased body water), and dilutional hyponatremia (always with increased body water due to excessive sodium retention).

Hypernatremia

Sodium may be ingested or provided in excess of water to cause hypernatremia. Hypertonic sodium gain can be caused by the use of hypertonic IV or feeding solutions, ingestion of sodium chloride tablets, or the administration of hypertonic dialysis or saline enemas (57). Much more commonly, hypernatremia develops during net water loss (usually renal) in diabetes insipidus, the use of loop diuretics, osmotic diuresis, postobstructive diuresis, the polyuric phase of acute tubular necrosis, and intrinsic renal disease. The loss of hyponatremic gastrointestinal fluids (e.g., in vomiting) can also cause hypernatremia. The major signs of hypernatremia are evidenced in the central nervous system by confusion, obtundation, stupor, and even coma. These signs are similar to those of other hyperosmolar syndromes (e.g., hyperglycemia). The effect on serum sodium of 1 L of any infusion can be estimated by using the formula presented in the section on parenteral replacement in sodium deficiency. When water loss is the cause of hypernatremia, the amount of water required to correct the loss can be calculated as follows:

$$\text{Water deficit} = [([Na]_{plasma} - 140)] \div 140 \times \text{total body water (L)}$$

where total body water is estimated as a fraction of body weight that is 0.6 for children, 0.6 and 0.5 for nonelderly men and women, respectively, and 0.5 and 0.45 for elderly men and women, respectively (50). However, this equation underestimates total body water loss by as much as 40% to 50%, under conditions when serum sodium is elevated only 5 to 10 mmol per L (58). Moreover, dehydration is not equivalent to hypernatremia, probably because salt is also lost in fluids like sweat that lead to dehydration.

The rapid correction or overcorrection of hypernatremia should be avoided because shifts in cerebral edema can have major clinical consequences (57). The deficit should be corrected over 2 to 3 days, and should not lower the serum sodium by greater than 12 mmol per L during the first day. To avoid rapid shifts in serum sodium, it is better to deliver the water orally or enterally rather than intravenously.

TABLE 7-11 Natural Low-sodium Seasonings That Can Be Substituted for Salt

Uses	Alternate Seasonings
General cooking	Lemon juice, garlic, onion, and sour cream the most useful; pepper and chili powder good if tolerated
Meat	Lemon, garlic, onion, pepper, oregano, curry powder, rosemary, thyme, paprika, ginger, sour cream
Fish and poultry	Lemon, garlic, onion, pepper, ginger, oregano, paprika, parsley, sesame seed, savory, tarragon, thyme
Egg dishes	Pepper (red or black), basil, marjoram, onion, oregano, tarragon, thyme
Vegetables	Pepper, basil (especially for tomatoes), dill, thyme, oregano, chervil, rosemary, sour cream (potatoes especially)
Soups	Garlic, onion, pepper, bay leaf, basil, thyme

Abnormal Sodium Retention

Abnormal sodium retention, as in conditions associated with edema, is the more common cause of sodium overload (toxicity). Signs and symptoms are related to fluid overload. Treatment involves decreasing dietary or infused sodium and the use of diuretics. Booklets with low-sodium diets are available from the dietary divisions of most hospitals. The principles involved in dietary management are discussed in Chapter 12 in the section on low-sodium diets. Seasoning food can be a problem. Salt substitutes can be used, and other spices can be very helpful in making food more palatable. Table 7-11 outlines alternative seasonings and their suggested uses. Many commercial products are available offering various combinations of these spices.

Potassium

Requirements

The requirements for potassium are not as clearly defined as those for sodium because of adjustments in urinary excretion that follow changes in intake. The DRI Committee recommended AI values for potassium, the observed average or experimentally determined intake that maintains a defined status in a specific population. It is not the same as a recommended dietary allowance (RDA). The AI is set at 4.7 (120 mmol) per day for adolescents aged 14 to 18 and for adults over age 18. This intake is based on evidence that it will lower blood pressure, perhaps by blocking the effect of sodium chloride, will reduce the risk of kidney stones, and may possibly reduce bone loss (4). These beneficial effects appear to be associated with forms of potassium found naturally in foods (e.g., fruits and vegetables), including anions that are bicarbonate precursors. This AI is not meant to be satisfied by preparations of potassium chloride. The AI for infants 0 to 6 months of age is 0.4 g per day, and for infants of 7 to 12 months is 0.7 g per day, based on the average consumption of human milk and other foods. The AI of children is derived from extrapolating the adult AI based on energy intake relative to adults, and is set at 3.0, 3.8, and 4.5 g per day for children age 1 to 3years, 4 to 8 years, and 9 to 13 years, respectively.

All but a small amount of potassium is normally absorbed by the gastrointestinal tract. The kidney is the major excretory organ for potassium and regulates output. The normal kidney can adjust the amount of potassium excretion from 5 to 1,000 mEq per day. Moreover, sodium intake determines, in part, the amount of potassium excreted, as both are affected by the action of aldosterone. Thus, the sodium–potassium ratio in the diet is a factor in defining the daily excretion rate and the AI.

Potassium excretion is affected by changes in recent dietary intake. Maximal values for potassium excretion occur early after a few days of adaptation to a high intake of potassium. On the other hand, sodium excretion increases within hours of a sodium load. With potassium restriction, maximal renal preservation occurs after 1 to 2 weeks, whereas sodium adaptation is more rapid. These considerations further confuse the determination of minimal daily requirements based on urinary excretion. Therefore, the DRI Committee elected not to set an estimated adequate requirement (EAR) because a dietary intake could not be calculated that would provide an AI for half of the population (4).

Food Sources

Intake of potassium in adults varies from 2,000 to 6,000 mg per day (50 to 150 mmol per day), but the median intake in the United States is well below the AI, being 2.8 to 3.3 g per day for men and 2.2 to 2.4 g per day for women (4). Hospitalized patients generally receive adequate dietary sources of potassium. The average hospital diet provides about 4,000 to 4,800 mg. Low-sodium diets provide 3,800 to 4,000 mg, and full-liquid diets supply the same amount. Because potassium is an intracellular ion, meat is a rich source. Therefore, low-protein and low-calorie diets provide somewhat less potassium (2,000 to 3,000 mg). A clear liquid diet is low in potassium (~750 mg) and in other essential nutrients.

In natural foods, potassium is available primarily in complexes with anions that generate bicarbonate, such as citrate, or with phosphate. In most supplements or foods to which potassium has been added, the form of the salt is potassium chloride. Table 7-12 lists some good sources of potassium. Meat, fluid milk, and fruits are good sources. The highest content of potassium (mg per 100 kcal) is in leafy greens such as spinach, cabbage, lettuce, and kale, but the caloric provision of these foods is low. It is more practical to consider the content of potassium and other nutrients per serving. In general, fruits and meats provide 200 to 400 mg of potassium per serving, vegetables slightly more, milk 370 mg per glass, and dried fruits, nuts, and juices somewhat more. However, high-protein foods, such as meat and dairy, and high-protein grains do not contain as much of the bicarbonate precursor anions as is present in fruits and vegetables, although the exact content is not known. Thus, it is possible that bioavailability of potassium from those sources may not be quite so high (4). Foods high in sodium, processed foods, and diets low in fruits, vegetables, dairy, and whole grains may not provide enough potassium to meet minimum requirements. Because many potassium-rich foods also contain fiber and other vitamins and minerals, the consumption of dietary fruits, vegetables, and dairy products should be encouraged, rather than the use of potassium supplements.

The effect of food processing on potassium content can be significant, as it is on sodium. Potassium content can increase or decrease with processing, but not so much as sodium content (Table 7-2). Water itself contains very little potassium and does not affect food content after cooking. Table 7-13 lists some examples of the effects of processing on potassium content.

Assessment

Ionic potassium is measured in serum or plasma with the use of ion-selective electrodes. Hemolysis elevates values through the release of intracellular potassium. Of all the potassium in the body (~54 mmol per kg of body weight), only about 10% is extracellular. Moreover, only about 0.4% (0.2 mEq per kg) is found in the plasma or serum. The distribution of potassium depends on an energy-consuming process in which sodium is extruded from cells and potassium enters. At normal rates of dietary intake, the transfer of ingested potassium into cells occurs so rapidly that extracellular concentrations do not change noticeably.

Body Stores

The serum potassium concentration (normal, 3.5 to 4.5 mmol per L) reflects both total body stores and availability of energy (glucose). Values from 3.0 to 3.5 mmol per L correspond to mild hypokalemia, and values less than 2.5 mmol per L define severe hypokalemia. The serum potassium level does reflect body stores in the absence of impaired energy utilization (e.g., diabetes mellitus). It does not reflect changes in recent or chronic intake because the plasma level is adjusted fairly rapidly. However, the serum potassium level, at best, provides only an approximation of total body stores. A serum level not below 3.3 mmol per L often corresponds to a loss of 10% of body potassium; a level below 3.0 mmol per L suggests a loss greater than 20%. Small shifts in the transport of potassium can rapidly shift the equilibrium between intracellular and extracellular compartments. Hypokalemia also may occur during acute alkalosis or acute attacks of familial periodic paralysis. Conversely, the serum potassium level may be normal when body stores are low (or high) as measured by isotope studies.

Losses from the Body

Urinary potassium levels reflect excretion on any given day (K^+ excretion = Uvol $\times$ [K^+]). However, the ability of the kidney to alter potassium excretion is great, and adults on an average diet excrete 25 to 125 mmol per day (59). Therefore, the urinary potassium level may be

TABLE 7-12 Food Sources of Potassium

Food	Portion	Potassium Content (mg)
Grains		
White bread	1 slice	28
Whole wheat bread	1 slice	62
Rice, cooked	1 cup	80
Spaghetti noodles, cooked	1 cup	43
Meats		
Muscle red meats, broiled	3 oz	250
Organ meats	3 oz	250–300
Bacon, cooked	3 slices	92
Fish, broiled	3 oz	340–400
Chicken, white meat roasted	3 oz	209
Vegetables		
Asparagus, fresh, cooked	1/2 cup	279
Avocado	1/2 medium	530
Broccoli, cooked	1 cup	456
Brussels sprouts	1/2 cup	250
Celery	1/2 cup	186
Cucumber, sliced	1/2 cup	80
Green beans, cooked	1 cup	373
Kidney beans	1 cup	713
Lentils, cooked	1 cup	731
Mushrooms	1 cup	550
Potato, baked with skin	1 cup	844
Potato without skin	1 cup	600
Tomato	1 each	273
Tomato juice	1 cup	537
Zucchini, cooked	1 cup	456
Fruits and Juices		
Applesauce, canned	1 cup	295
Apple juice	4 oz	148
Cantaloupe	1 cup	494
Banana	1 medium	451
Apricots	5 dried	482
Orange	1 medium	273
Orange juice, frozen	4 oz	252
Grapefruit, white	1/2 grapefruit	175
Grapefruit juice	4 oz	210
Prunes	5 dried	365
Prune juice	4 oz	301
Raisins	1/3 cup	373
Watermelon slice	1 cup	186
Dairy Products		
Milk, skim or whole	1 cup	350–370
Yogurt, low fat, plain	1 cup	531
Cheese	1 oz	25–40
Egg	1 each	63
Other		
Nuts (peanuts, almonds)	1 oz	180–220
Coffee, brewed	4 oz	80
Tea, brewed	4 oz	16

Data from: Potassium content of foods and salt substitutes. *Pharmacist's Letter/Prescriber's Letter.* 2008;24:240904; Food sources of selected nutrients, USDA, http://www.health.gov/dietaryguidelines/dga2005/document/html/appendixB.htm.

TABLE 7-13 Effect of Processing on Potassium Content of Food

Food	Portion	Potassium Content (mg)
Potato		
Fresh baked	1 each	844
Instant mashed	1 cup	428
Canned	2 each	160
Chips	14 (1 oz)	369
Tomato		
Sliced	1 cup	400
Canned	1 cup	529
Catsup	1 tbs	82
Peas, Green		
Fresh cooked	1 cup	434
Frozen, cooked	1 cup	268
Canned, without liquid	1 cup	194

useful in assessing losses from the body when potassium depletion is present. When the kidney is normal, potassium excretion should be low but still significant (10 to 20 mmol per day). When losses from the gastrointestinal tract occur, the measurement of potassium in the appropriate fluid provides an additional assessment of the requirement for that patient (see Table 7-6 for the average daily potassium content of gastrointestinal fluids). Once hypokalemia is detected, measurement of the urinary potassium level may be helpful in determining the source of loss. A low urinary potassium level (<15 mmol per L) implies near-maximal renal conservation and suggests an extrarenal source of depletion. This interpretation is correct only if the patient has not been treated recently with diuretics. After diuretics are discontinued, the kidney responds to induced hypokalemia with maximal potassium conservation. However, if the urinary potassium level is high (>30 mmol per L), then renal conservation is inadequate, and this result suggests that the kidney is the source of potassium loss.

To distinguish the mechanism for excessive potassium secretion, the transtubular K+ concentration gradient (TTKG) is used. TTKG calculates the ratio of potassium concentration in the lumen of the collecting duct compared with that in the plasma. To estimate the concentration in the lumen, a correction is made to account for the amount of water reabsorbed in the medullary collecting duct by dividing the urinary $[K^+]$ by the quotient of urine and plasma osmolality, since the osmolality of the fluid in the cortical collecting duct equals plasma osmolality when antidiuretic hormone is active (60). Thus,

$$TTKG = ([K^+]_u \div (U_{osm}/P_{osm}) \div [K^+]_p$$

Tests to measure potassium excretion when hypo- and hyperkalemia are present are shown in Table 7-14.

Physiology
Potassium is the major intracellular cation, maintained at an intracellular concentration of approximately 145 mmol per L. Along with sodium and calcium, it is responsible for the maintenance of normal electric potentials across cell membranes. The membrane depolarization needed for muscle contraction depends on an influx of sodium into the cell coupled with an efflux of potassium. Membrane repolarization involves the reverse process. Thus, potassium helps to regulate neuromuscular contraction in addition to glycogen formation, protein synthesis, and acid–base balance.

Absorption
Potassium must be absorbed from the diet and from gastrointestinal secretions, from which it must be reabsorbed (Table 7-6). More than 85 potassium channels have been identified in all tissue cells (http://www.genenames.org/genefamily/KCN.php). When sodium moves into the small intestinal cell with transporters coupled to glucose and amino acids, the entry of a positive net

TABLE 7-14 Tests for Determining K+ Excretion When Hypo- or Hyperkalemia Is Present

Test	Expected Values	Advantages	Disadvantages
24 h K^+ excretion or K^+/creatinine	60–80 mmol/d 6–8 mmol/mmol Cr Hypokalemia <10 mmol/d Hyperkalemia >150 mmol/d	Overall renal response	Mechanism-independent Need 24-hour collection
Spot urine [K^+]	Hypokalemia <20 mmol/L if due to K deprivation Hypokalemia >20 mmol/L if due to a renal cause	Convenience	Affected by K^+ secretion and water reabsorption so wide variability
TTKG	Nonrenal hypokalemia <2 Nonrenal hyperkalemia >10	Corrects for water reabsorption	Assumptions are made in the calculation

TTKG, transtubular [K^+] gradient.
Data from Halperin ML, Kamel KS. Potassium. *Lancet.* 1998;352:135.

charge depolarizes the apical membrane, leading to an electrogenic transport of chloride. Basolateral K^+ channels open to hyperpolarize the cell, and the K^+ is recycled by the Na^+/K^+ ATPase. The luminal membrane is then hyperpolarized and apical electrogenic transport is initiated across the apical and basolateral membranes in order to repolarize the membrane voltage (36). K^+ channels probably play a role in restoring the absorbing cell size to normal, after being swollen during solute and fluid absorption. The types of K^+ channels present in the small intestine are still incompletely understood, but probably include a large-conductance channel, voltage-gated channels, calcium-activated small-conductance channels, and inwardly rectifying KATP-like channels.

Excretion

The kidney is the major regulatory site of potassium excretion, through the action of aldosterone, accounting for 77% to 90% of dietary potassium (1). Potassium excretion by the kidney is regulated by a secretory process, largely independent of the GFR and the amount of filtered potassium. Most filtered potassium (70% to 80%) is reabsorbed in the proximal nephron. The amount in the urine is regulated by the potassium ion concentration in the cells of the distal tubule and is high when the intracellular concentration is high. Thus, excretion is regulated in part by the intracellular content of renal cells. The kidney responds rapidly to alterations in potassium intake.

In contrast to the small intestine, the colon secretes potassium, especially in response to a high potassium intake and/or high aldosterone concentrations. The overall mechanism involves electroneutral transcellular secretion of KCl, rather than the Cl^- absorption and paracellular sodium absorption seen in the small intestine. Apical channels active in the colonic mucosa include large-conductance channels, a pH-sensitive ROMK-type channel, maxi K^+ channels, and KCNQ1 (61). In the colon, potassium secretion is aided by the electronegativity of the intestinal lumen. Ordinarily, stool volumes are low, so the relatively high potassium concentrations in stool are not the cause of serious losses. In diarrhea, large potassium losses may occur. Changes in colonic secretion do not alter the overall potassium balance unless the colon is removed, when losses through the ileostomy can be significant.

Deficiency

If one assumes that no metabolic factors are altering the serum potassium level, each decrease of 1 mmol per L corresponds to a loss of body potassium of 200 to 300 mmol. The major causes of deficiency include increased renal excretion and extrarenal losses, largely intestinal. Because of the widespread presence of potassium in foods, decreased intake is an uncommon cause of deficiency. However, clear liquid diets are low in potassium and may lead to deficiency after prolonged use.

Increased renal excretion, one cause of deficiency, may be secondary to the use of potent diuretics, chronic metabolic alkalosis (e.g., chronic obstructive pulmonary disease), diabetic ketoacidosis (with osmotic diuresis), and states associated with the development of edema. Distal renal tubular acidosis also can lead to large losses of potassium. Potassium can be lost at the rate of 150 to 300 mmol per day in these situations. Major causes of extrarenal losses include gastric or biliary drainage and chronic diarrhea. Because potassium is secreted by the colon, moderate diarrhea can lead to hypokalemia before sodium or volume depletion is clinically evident. The concentration of potassium in sweat is low (5 to 10 mEq per L), so large losses are not common with increased sweating. Nondiuretic medications, such as steroids, digoxin, and excess natural licorice, may cause an increase in potassium excretion (62).

The loss of 5% to 10% of body stores (200 to 300 mmol) may occur without hypokalemia and is tolerated without many symptoms. Elevated blood pressure may occur, especially changes that are sensitive to changes in salt intake. Manifestations of hypokalemia usually appear at serum levels less than 2.5 to 3.0 mmol per L. If the loss of potassium is rapid, symptoms may develop at a higher serum level. Prominent symptoms include weakness, paresthesias, orthostatic hypotension, and CV abnormalities. With depletion, the membrane electrical potential gradient increases, and muscle contraction is impaired. Muscle weakness and delayed cardiac repolarization are early effects. Electrocardiographic abnormalities include depressed ST segments, low T waves, and the presence of U waves. However, these findings are neither constant nor specific and cannot be relied on for diagnosis. The effects of digitalis are exaggerated by potassium deficiency. If depletion is chronic, the concentrating ability of the kidneys is impaired and polyuria results. Glucose intolerance, polydipsia, constipation, ileus, and metabolic alkalosis can occur. Common causes of depletion are gastrointestinal (vomiting and diarrhea) and urinary (diuretics) losses, glucocorticoid excess, and inadequate intake in the face of obligatory urinary excretion.

Potassium supplementation is associated with a significant but small reduction in systolic (3 mm Hg) and diastolic (2 mm Hg) pressures (63,64). This effect is noted most in patients with a high intake of sodium. However, in the DASH study, in which the diet of participants was rich in fruits and vegetables (average potassium intake of 4,100 mg per d), blood pressures fell (6). This diet also included low-fat dairy foods and reduced amounts of saturated and unsaturated fat, so the role of potassium alone is not clear. It is usually not necessary to prescribe potassium supplements for hypertensive patients except when hypokalemia is present.

Treatment

Hypokalemia is treated by oral replacement if possible. The reason for choosing this route is to allow the serum potassium level to rise slowly in equilibrium with the intracellular component. For mild deficiency, table foods may be adequate (Table 7-12). Foods high in potassium are those with more than 300 mg per portion. A daily intake of 120 mEq per day (4.7 g) is safe for patients with normal kidneys, because excess body potassium is excreted in the urine. However, when renal function is impaired (CrCl < 60 mL per min), total potassium ingestion (diet + supplements) should be less than 4.7 g per day. This caveat also pertains to patients taking medications that can produce hyperkalemia, including K-sparing diuretics, nonsteroidal anti-inflammatory drugs (NSAIDs), and angiotensin-converting enzyme (ACE) inhibitors.

Supplements

The Food and Drug Administration (FDA) now allows manufacturers to claim on the labels of certain "foods that are good sources of potassium and low in sodium may reduce the risk of high blood pressure and stroke." To qualify, the food must contain more than 10% of the recommended dietary value of potassium (or 350 mg), be low in sodium (<140 mg), and also be low in fat, saturated fat, and cholesterol, as defined by the FDA.

Potassium salts (gluconate, aspartate, citrate, chloride) are available as liquid, tablets, and capsules. Individual doses of nonprescription preparations are limited by the FDA to less than 99 mg (~2.5 mmol) because of the dangers associated with self-dosing. The salt most often used to treat moderate deficiency is potassium chloride. However, it has a bitter taste, and if it is not well tolerated, other salts are available. If the source of the potassium loss is in the intestine, fixed base will also be lost, so that a basic salt of potassium (e.g., potassium gluconate) may be more appropriate as replacement therapy. Although the risk of mucosal damage in the gastrointestinal tract caused by potassium chloride, a sclerotic agent, is smaller with currently available slow-release, wax matrix, and microencapsulated forms than with liquid potassium chloride, esophageal and small-bowel damage does still occur when slow-release tablets containing high doses of potassium chloride are ingested. Such preparations should not be used by patients with any condition that may delay transit through the gastrointestinal tract. For such patients, the gluconate or citrate salt is more appropriate. Liquid or effervescent preparations are preferable if they are well tolerated and should be mixed in 3 to 8 oz of water or juice and drunk slowly. Potassium chloride can be given IV to severely depleted patients if the salt is diluted to 20 to 40 mmol per L of fluid, no more than 40 mmol is administered per hour, and electrocardiographic monitoring is provided. Without such monitoring, replacement should not exceed 20 mmol per hour. A partial list of oral potassium preparations available by prescription is given in Table 7-15.

Salt Substitutes

Many patients who require potassium supplements are also on a low-sodium diet. Using herbs and spices can substitute for sodium. Individual spices can be tried or used in combination; commercially available herb and spice blends include Mrs. Dash, Chef Paul Prudhomme's Magic Salt-free Seasoning, Salt-free Spike, Benson's Gourmet Salt-free Seasonings, and Penzeys Salt-free Spice Blends. In addition, lemon juice activates some of the same taste receptors as sodium, and can be an effective substitute. As part of a reduced sodium diet, however, patients may be using a salt substitute. The potassium content of salt substitutes is considerable. If significant amounts of these salts are used, they may constitute a major supplementary source of potassium and should be considered in the overall oral intake. In addition, potassium chloride in the form of commercial salt substitutes is 10 times less expensive than potassium chloride solutions and powders. Characteristics of the salt substitutes are listed in Table 7-16. "No salt" products are the only ones with a nutritionally significant potassium content and an acceptably low sodium content, but are poorly accepted by patients who find them unpalatable.

Toxicity

Toxicity occurs when hyperkalemia develops (serum level >5.0 to 5.5 mEq per L). Because of the largely intracellular distribution of potassium, toxicity can be manifested without significant changes in total body levels of potassium.

Causes

Impaired renal excretion. Impaired renal excretion is the major cause of hyperkalemia because this mechanism is so important for normal function. When diuretics are used, potassium often must be replaced. Potassium-sparing diuretics increase potassium retention and can cause hyperkalemia. The concurrent use of ACE inhibitors may lead to hyperkalemia in certain patients.

Increased potassium intake. Increased potassium intake may also produce hyperkalemia, especially the use of prescription supplements. An increase in oral intake of 50 to 100 mEq within a short period can raise the serum potassium level by 0.5–1 mEq per L, but the abnormality is transient once cellular redistribution occurs. The use of salt substitutes along with other potassium supplements can result in excessive intake. Many herbal medications now contain potassium, including alfalfa, dandelion, horsetail, nettle, milkweed, and hawthorne berries. Increased endogenous potassium load can occur during prolonged exercise and/or if hemolysis, rhabdomyolysis, and gastrointestinal bleeding occur.

Other causes. Potassium penicillin contains 1.7 mEq per million units and can provide a large dose of potassium. The sudden breakdown of cells with disruption of the transcellular gradients can acutely raise the serum potassium level and produce toxic effects in the absence of changes in total body potassium. Transcellular shifts in potassium may also occur during hyperglycemia and acute metabolic acidosis owing to addition of mineral acids, with the use of nonselective β-blockers or somatostatin, with mannitol infusion, and due to drugs or herbals that inhibit Na/K ATPase. Such inhibitors include digoxin, toad skin, oleander, yew berry, lily of the valley, dogbane, Siberian ginseng, and red squill (65).

Signs and Symptoms. Signs and symptoms of hyperkalemia include those associated with decreased membrane potential, rapid repolarization, and slowed conduction velocity.

TABLE 7-15   Potassium Supplement Preparations[a]

Usual Preparation[b]	Anion	K+ Content/Unit Dose (mmol/15 mL or Per Tablet)
Liquids		
Kaochlor 10%	Cl	20
Kaon Cl 20%	Cl	40
Kay Ciel	Cl	20
Klorvess 10%	Cl	20
Klor-Con 10%		20
Rum-K	Cl	20
Potassium chloride solution 5%, 10%, or 20%	Cl	20
Kaon Elixir	Gluconate	20
Kolyum	Gluconate/Cl	20
Potassium triplex (Tri-K)	Acetate, HCO_3, citrate	45
Twin-K	Gluconate, citrate	20
Polycitra-K	Citrate, citric acid	30
Tablets[c]		
Effer K	HCO_3, citrate	25
K+ Care	HCO_3	20, 25
Slow-K	Cl	8
Klotrix	Cl	10 in wax matrix
Klor-Con/EF	HCO_3, citrate	25
Klor-Con 10	Cl	10 in wax matrix
Micro-K Extencaps	Cl	8, 10 controlled-release
K-tab	Cl	10
Kaon	Gluconate	5
K-lyte Effervescent	HCO_3, citrate	25 (DS = 50)
Klorvess Effervescent	HCO_3, Cl	20
K-Dur	Cl	10, 20 microencapsulated
Potassium chloride	Cl	10 in wax matrix, controlled-release, or microencapsulated
Powder		
Effervescent Kaon-Cl	Cl	6, 7, 10
K+ Care	Cl	15, 20, 25
K-Lor	Cl	15, 20
Klor-Con	Cl	20, 25
K-Lyte/Cl	Cl	25 (DS = 50)
Kay Ciel	Cl	20
Kolyum	Gluconate/Cl	20
Klorvess Effervescent	HCO_3, Cl	20
Micro-K LS	Cl	20 (extended-release)
Potassium chloride	Cl	20

DS, double strength.
All liquid preparations should be diluted in juice or water (4 oz for each 20-mmol dose). All packets or effervescent tablets should be dissolved in the same amount of liquid. Tablets (slow release in wax matrix or microencapsulated) should be swallowed whole with 4 oz of liquid.
[a]The K content (mmol/g) of potassium salts is K gluconate, 4.3; K citrate, 9.8; K bicarbonate, 10; K acetate, 10.2; K chloride, 13.4.
[b]Many preparations are available in liquid, tablet, and powder forms.
[c]Most tablets are either covered by wax matrix, microencapsulated, or in controlled-release forms.

TABLE 7-16 Characteristics of Salt Substitutes[a]

Product	Na Content (mmol/g)	K Content (mmol/g)	Na:K Ratio
Table salt	16.6	0.004	4,150
Flavored salt	11.9	0.049	243
Monosodium glutamate	5.3	0.004	1,325
Seasonings and marinades	7.0	0.087	80
Lemon pepper	4.4	—	—
Marinades	1.4	—	—
Meat tenderizer	12.0	—	—
"Low salt" substitutes	9.45	5.29	1.8
"No salt" substitutes[b]	0.014	12.8	<0.01
Adolph's salt substitute	—	12.8	—
Adolph's seasoned salt substitute	—	7	—
Morton's salt substitute	—	12.8	—
Morton's seasoned salt substitute	—	11.2	—
Nosalt	—	12.8	—
Neocurtasal	—	12	—
Nu-salt	—	13.6	—
Lawry's seasoned salt-free	—	6	—

[a]Mean values for classes of products are listed.
[b]Data for salt substitutes adapted from Cannon-Babb ML, Schwartz AB. Drug-induced hyperkalemia. *Hosp Pract.* 1986;21:99, and from *Drugs: Facts and Comparisons.* St Louis: C.V. Mosby, 1998. Adapted from Greenfield H, McCullum D, Wills RB. Sodium and potassium contents of salts, salt substitutes, and other seasonings. *Med J Aust.* 1984;140:460 and from Hands ES. *Food Finder.* 2nd ed. Salem, OR: ESHA Research, 1990.

Neuromuscular effects include paresthesias, weakness, mental confusion, and paralysis. The CV effects are a decrease in blood pressure and direct cardiac effects. The electrocardiogram shows peaked T waves, loss of P waves, a depressed ST segment, widened QRS complex, and prolongation of the PR interval. If severe, these features lead to heart block, atrial arrest, and asystole. The rate of onset of hyperkalemia, accompanying acid–base disturbances, and use of other drugs modify the degree of cardiac toxicity. In general, cardiac toxicity is rare when the serum potassium level is below 6.5 mEq per L, and common when it is above 8.0 mEq per L.

Treatment

Treatment should be started immediately. For mild hyperkalemia, cessation of potassium intake may be enough if renal function is normal. With more severe toxicity, active intervention should be used.

Calcium gluconate. If ECG abnormalities are present, 10 to 30 mL of 10% calcium gluconate should be given IV over a few minutes, but the effect is transient (1 to 2 h).

Glucose and insulin. Glucose and insulin can be used to drive the potassium intracellularly and can be given at the same time as calcium gluconate. A dose of 10 to 20 U of insulin per 100 g of glucose can be given after the glucose is started, and the effect lasts 6 to 12 hours. The glucose is not needed initially if the patient is hyperglycemic.

Sodium bicarbonate. Sodium bicarbonate is used when systemic acidosis is present. Two ampules (90 to 100 mEq) can be given IV over 5 to 10 minutes.

Potassium removal from the body. Oral exchange can be accomplished by giving the resin sodium polystyrene sulfonate (Kayexalate) orally (20 to 30 g in 70% sorbitol) or by enema

(50 to 100 g in 200 mL), as indicated by the serum potassium level. This dose can be repeated every 2 hours as needed. However, adverse gastrointestinal events can occur with the use of such exchange resins, including constipation, fecal impaction, intestinal obstruction, and rarely even intestinal necrosis (66). In severe toxicity or renal failure, hemodialysis is used.

Calcium

Requirement

Calcium is the major cation of bone. Calcium, like iron, is a threshold nutrient. This means that below a critical value, the ability of calcium to increase bone mass is limited by available mineral, whereas above the threshold, no further increase in intake results in functional benefit. Three factors define the requirements for calcium and explain the discrepancy between the actual requirement and the larger DRI: (a) Calcium is needed in increased amounts during periods of growth or new bone formation. (b) Because absorption is not efficient (~30%), the amount ingested must exceed the actual requirement. (c) There is an obligatory daily loss of calcium in the stool and urine. Thus, the requirement is greatest during childhood, adolescence, pregnancy, and lactation. The fact that bone mass is measured so long after the critical periods of growth of bone mass, and that calcium is a nutrient that improves function only below a given threshold may account for the difficulty in demonstrating a role for calcium in modifying bone mass in adults.

Other factors can play a role in the amount of calcium required for positive balance. The role of fiber is quite variable and is generally small. Wheat bran, but not fiber in green, leafy vegetables, reduces absorption of calcium (67). A high intake of phytate may decrease calcium absorption by binding to calcium (68). Beans contain both phytate and oxalate, but in spinach and rhubarb the calcium is bound to oxalate. The calcium bound to oxalate is less available than that bound to phytate. Animal data suggest that the optimal dietary calcium–phosphorus ratio is from 2:1 to 1:2. The ratio of the average US diet is 1:1.5. Although phosphate is an additive in many processed foods, especially canned foods and soft drinks, the effect of the added phosphorus on calcium absorption is unclear. At a luminal pH above 6, calcium forms complexes with phosphorus and with other anions. Thus, fecal calcium and phosphorus are usually correlated. However, various calcium phosphate salts are absorbed at about the same (low) rate as other calcium salts. Calcium phosphate is one of the major calcium salts in milk, the food that has the most bioavailable source of calcium. Because calcium absorption is inefficient in adults, changes in the phosphorus intake increase the fecal output relatively little. There is no evidence that calcium absorption is altered by changing the Ca:P ratio from 0.2 to 2.0, providing that adequate calcium intake is maintained (67).

Urinary calcium excretion increases as protein intake increases, but the effect is not always proportional to the protein intake. In balance studies, when phosphorus intake was stable, 1 g of dietary protein increased urinary calcium excretion by 1 to 1.5 mg (69). Thus, diets high in protein but with limited calcium intake (e.g., high in meat, low in dairy products) may increase urinary calcium loss and alter daily requirements. Despite this effect on urinary calcium, short-term consumption of high-protein diets does not alter calcium homeostasis and is not a risk factor for modifying bone metabolism (70).

The source of calcium is assumed to be the skeleton, but some of the calcium may come from increased calcium absorption (71). Calcium and sodium share the same transport system in the proximal tubule. Every gram of sodium excreted carries about 8 to 25 mg of calcium with it. Sodium bicarbonate does not have the same effect on urinary calcium loss as sodium chloride (67). In addition, 1 mg of calcium is lost with each 1 g of protein metabolized in the body. This effect may be related to calcium binding to the sulfate derived from sulfur-containing amino acids. The practical significance of this effect in making diet recommendations is not clear because diets with low intakes of calcium should be avoided. However, at low salt and protein intake, the minimum calcium requirement may be as low as 450 mg per day for a small woman, and as large as 2 g per day if protein and sodium intake are high. Each gram of sodium leads to the urinary excretion of about 15 mg of calcium when calcium intake is high or moderate (69). This problem persists when Western diets are consumed, as they are high in sodium and low in available calcium.

Until puberty, calcium absorption is increased up to twofold (60%) in comparison with absorption in adults. In pregnancy, absorption and retention of calcium are increased. After the age of 60, calcium absorption decreases, and the ability of the intestine to respond to a low-calcium diet by increasing the rate of absorption is impaired. The bowel and kidney excrete about 160 mg of calcium daily even when calcium intake is low. In addition, about 40 mg is lost per day through the skin (72). Thus, an intake of 200 mg per day is needed to offset these obligatory losses in the adult. Net calcium absorption will not occur until these obligatory losses have been satisfied.

Dietary Reference Intake

Bone density increases during the first 25 to 30 years of life and decreases thereafter. The FDA has approved the claim that the use of calcium supplements reduces the risk for osteoporosis (73). Because of conflicting messages about the benefits of calcium and vitamin D, the IOM was asked by the US and Canadian governments to review and update the DRIs. The committee reviewed more than 1,000 studies, many of which were not available in 1997 when the previous DRIs were published (69). The report of their findings has been widely distributed (74). Recommendations about vitamin D are discussed in Chapter 6.

The recommendations in Table 7-17 are meant to be reflections of national policy. They are not intended to be nutrient requirements for individuals. This issue is particularly troublesome for calcium because a long time may elapse before the effects of calcium deficiency are noted. Thus, an optimal intake is better stated for populations than for individuals. The debate over calcium guidelines continues to stress the need for calcium intake versus the complex relationship between calcium intake and bone health (75a–c). The determination for DRIs, especially in children, has utilized data relating calcium intake and absorption/retention, using the dual-tracer method to determine bioavailability (76). The increased recommendation for adolescents is based on their rapid growth of bone. The increased recommendation for older persons is based on data showing that their rate of calcium absorption is decreased.

The IOM established UL with supplement use in mind, allowing for adverse side effects such as hypercalcemia, hypercalciuria, and nephrolithiasis. The report accepted the possibility of a U-shaped curve for efficacy and side effects for vitamin D, and by implication for calcium, thus lowering the UL for older subjects (77). This recommendation is counter to the idea that "more is better," but its validity will need to be tested with time.

The current recommendations imply that a single universal requirement exists for calcium, regardless of the intake of protein, sodium, and fiber/phytate. This view has been challenged because of the fact that calcium intake is low in parts of the world where fracture rates are low, and high where fracture rates are high (72). In fact, a review of 58 studies of dairy or dietary calcium intake in children and young adults found no relationship between dairy or dietary calcium

TABLE 7-17 Dietary Reference Intakes for Calcium

Life Stage Group	Estimated Average Requirement (mg/d)	Recommended Dietary Allowance (mg/d)	Upper Level Intake (mg/d)
Infants 0–6 months	200	200	1,000
Infants 6–12 months	260	260	1,500
1–3 years old	500	700	2,500
4–8 years old	800	1,000	2,500
9–18 years old	1,100	1,300	3,000
19–50 years old	800	1,000	2,500
51–70 years old male	800	1,000	2,000
51–70 years old female	1,000	1,200	2,000
>70 years old	1,000	1,200	2,000
14–18 years pregnant/lactating	1,100	1,300	3,000
19–50 years pregnant/lactating	800	1,000	2,500

Data from Dietary Reference Intakes for Calcium and Vitamin D. (http://www.iom.edu/~/media/Files/Report%20Files/2010/Dietary-Reference-Intakes-for-Calcium-and-Vitamin-D/Vitamin%20D%20and%20Calcium%202010%20Report%20Brief.pdf; accessed 4/18/14)

intake and bone mineralization or fracture rate (78). It has been estimated that a diet low in sodium and protein can reduce the calcium requirement by as much as 200 to 300 mg per day.

Food and Dietary Sources

Primitive diets containing vegetables, bones of small animals or fish, and possibly insects have a high calcium density that approaches 80 to 100 mg per 100 kcal (74). In contrast, the median calcium density of the diet of women in NHANES III was only about 36 mg per 100 kcal, and the DRIs assume about 50 mg of calcium per 100 kcal (72). Milk contains 350 mg of calcium per 100 kcal (~300 mg per cup), and thus, dairy products are the most calcium-dense foods in the diets of most countries. Shellfish contain much calcium, but calcium levels are low in most meats, fish, or poultry. Three hundred milligrams of calcium can be found in 1 ½ oz of cheese, 1 ¾ cup of ice cream, 6 oz of low-fat yogurt, 1 ½ cup of cooked greens (e.g., kale, spinach, bok choy), and 5 oz of canned salmon. Other foods that contribute to daily calcium intake include dried beans, broccoli, and tofu (chemically set with calcium). However, the calcium in beans is only about 50% as available as that from animal sources. In animal products, calcium is bound largely to protein, which must first be digested before calcium can be absorbed. Organic anions, such as phytates and oxalates, are found in many green, leafy vegetables and inhibit calcium absorption either partially (phytate) or nearly completely (oxalate), so bioavailability is variable. Table 7-18 lists the calcium content of selected foods.

Calcium-fortified foods (e.g., fortified orange juice) contain up to 350 mg of calcium per 8 oz and may constitute a major source of dietary calcium for persons who do not use dairy products. Other sources of fortified calcium include soft drinks and breakfast cereals. However, adding mineral salts to foods can possibly decrease the bioavailability of natural minerals in the food. Interactions between calcium, iron, and zinc have been documented in humans (79). If intake of zinc is limited, high calcium intake can decrease uptake of zinc, especially in children. Because 29% of the body content of zinc is in bones, zinc status may be as important as calcium

TABLE 7-18 Calcium Content of Selected Foods

Food	Serving Size	Calcium Content (mg)
Calcium-fortified orange juice	1 cup	up to 350
Milk, all types (liquid)	1 cup	280–300
Yogurt, plain	1 cup	274–315
Hard cheeses	1 oz	213–287
Soft cheeses	1 oz	159–219
Figs, dried	10	269
Tofu, raw, firm	1/2 cup	258
Calcium-fortified cereals	3/4 cup	250
Spinach, cooked	1 cup	244
Collards, cooked	1/2 cup	179
Cottage cheese	1 cup	126–180
Ice cream	1 cup	176
Peanuts, roasted	1 cup	126
Beans (navy, pinto)	1 cup	80–120
Salmon, canned with bones	1 oz	110
Sardines, in oil	Two	92
Vegetables (carrots, kale, broccoli)	1/2 cup	36–52
Fruits	1 cup/piece	18–25
Pasta, rice	1 cup	10–23
Bread, white	Slice	35
Meat, fish	3 oz	3–10

Data from Hands ES, *Food Finder*, 2nd ed. Salem, OR: ESHA Research, 1990; Pennington JAT. *Bowes and Church's Food Values of Portions Commonly Used*. 17th ed. Philadelphia: Lippincott-Raven, 1998.

status in overall bone health. There is also a small, but significant, inverse relationship between calcium intake and iron body stores (68).

Supplementation with calcium is the most widely available means to increase calcium intake. There are at least 22 forms of calcium approved for supplement use by the US FDA, and these differ in formulation and bioavailability (68). Factors that affect bioavailability include dissolution time, solubility, coingestion of food, and timing of dose. However, solubility and bioavailability are not proportionately related in the case of all salts. There are sparse data available to allow an informed choice about the proper salt to use for supplementation and how to dose it. Calcium carbonate is preferred by consumers because of its high content (40% mg per kg), but its absorption may not be optimal owing to potential variability in solubility in the gut lumen.

Assessment
Intake/absorption

Intake/absorption is best measured by 24-hour urinary calcium excretion. This varies from 100 to 240 mg per day, with much individual variation noted. In adults, the amount excreted correlates with calcium absorption above 2 mg/kg/day (i.e., intake >6 mg/kg/day) because only about 30% is absorbed. When calcium intake or absorption is low, urinary calcium does not decline proportionally. The range of values for urinary calcium found with an inadequate calcium intake of less than 200 mg per day (30 to 160 mg of urinary calcium per day) overlaps with the range of values found with a normal calcium intake (100 to 240 mg per day). Thus, the values for urinary calcium excretion should not be interpreted too rigorously. Even when net calcium absorption is zero, the obligatory loss of urinary calcium continues. This situation is in contrast to what is observed with other minerals, such as sodium, potassium, magnesium, and phosphorus, the urinary excretion of which is regulated at low levels of intake/absorption. Thus, urinary excretion is not a good test for calcium deficiency; it is better used to monitor the adequacy of calcium intake when supplemental calcium is prescribed. It should be measured only after 3 to 4 days on a constant calcium intake and when drugs that alter urinary calcium (e.g., thiazide diuretics, tetracycline, glucocorticoids) are not being taken. A high intake of protein or renal leak may increase calcium excretion. Treatment with 1,25-dihydroxyvitamin D_3 can cause bone resorption and an increased urinary calcium that is unrelated to calcium absorption. In patients with bone disease, urinary calcium excretion may be constant and independent of calcium absorption.

Calcium Determination

Serum calcium and alkaline phosphatase measurements are the conventionally used tests of calcium status, but are inadequate for this purpose. Ionized calcium is maintained within a very narrow range, as calcium is mobilized from the bones. The nonionized calcium is protein-bound and pH-dependent, increasing with alkalosis and decreasing with acidosis. Thus, alkalosis or hyperproteinemia can cause a false-positive result for hypercalcemia, and acidosis or hypoproteinemia a false-positive result for hypocalcemia.

Calcium is measured by rapid automated procedures; the o-cresolphthalein complexone method is used often, along with flame photometry or atomic absorption spectroscopy (59). Normal values for serum calcium are given in Table 7-19. Because of the tight metabolic regulation

TABLE 7-19 Serum Calcium Biochemical Parameters

Parameter	Young Men	Young Women	Adults	Elderly
Total calcium (mmol/L)	2.41 ± 0.2	2.40 ± 0.2	2.43 ± 0.02	2.28 ± 0.12
Ionized calcium (mmol/L)	1.48	1.21	1.25 ± 0.04	1.24 ± 0.07
Alkaline phosphatase (IU/L)	63 (21–155)		80 (43–110)	

Data from Sauberlich HE. *Laboratory Tests for the Assessment of Nutritional Status*. 2nd ed. Boca Raton, FL: CRC Press, 1999.

of serum calcium, values outside this range cannot be interpreted according to nutritional status; rather, they usually suggest a pathologic mechanism. Ionized calcium levels reflect calcium metabolism better than total calcium does. Correction equations to estimate ionized calcium concentration have not been successful, as such formulas are sensitive to variability in many confounding factors, such as pH, bicarbonate, protein, and phosphate levels (80). Serum levels of ionized calcium can be low when calcium (or vitamin D) deficiency is severe and skeletal pools of calcium are low, but this is a late finding. Hypocalcemia is defined as less than 2.18 mmol per L (<85 mg per L), and hypercalcemia as more than 2.6 mmol per L (>105 mg per L).

Ionized calcium levels are sensitive to differences in collection conditions, especially pH. They are very useful in clinical conditions such as following a major surgery, during critical illness, and in neonates, when acid–base balance is in flux. Total serum calcium, although insensitive to accurate assessment of ionized calcium, remains useful as a screening test for calcium abnormalities (80).

Alkaline Phosphatase

Activity in serum represents the sum of liver and bone isozyme activity. During active bone resorption, alkaline phosphatase activity in serum increases, but this result is neither sensitive nor specific, even in the presence of secondary hyperparathyroidism (81). Origin of the enzyme in bone can be suggested by heat inactivation at 56°C (<15% remaining indicates origin in bone), or by determination of γ-glutamyl transpeptidase, a bile canalicular enzyme present in liver and biliary tissue but not in bone. When calcium deficiency is advanced and osteomalacic bone disease is present, alkaline phosphatase is elevated. The enzyme level is high in any condition in which bone remodeling is taking place, so that it is elevated in children and adolescents and in patients with metastatic bone disease or Paget disease.

Bone Mineral Density Measurements

Changes in bone density (usually by dual-energy X-ray absorptiometry (DXA) are measured for several years to follow the effects of dietary calcium supplements and other interventions on bone density, especially in the prevention and treatment of postmenopausal osteoporosis in women. The measure is not recommended for routine screening but may be useful in guiding treatment decisions for selected postmenopausal women (82–84). The National Osteoporosis Foundation recommends testing for postmenopausal women age 65 or over, or age less than 65 with one or more clinical risk factors (e.g., smoking, weight less than 57 kg, and a personal or family history of fractures due to fragile bones) (83). The International Osteoporosis Foundation (IOF) recommends screening for postmenopausal women with one or more clinical risk factors, and includes height loss, or radiographic osteopenia, or the need for prolonged hormone replacement therapy. The International Society for Clinical Densitometry (ISCD) has similar recommendations, but includes diseases known to be associated with bone loss as a risk factor. The WHO study group has emphasized the differences that may occur depending on the site tested for bone density and warns against using density to assess fracture risk, although a low bone density is one of the strongest risk factors for fracture. For every decrease of 1 SD in bone mineral density (BMD) at the hip, there is an approximately 2.6 fold increased risk of hip fracture and an approximately 6-fold increase in any fracture (85). The T-score from DXA is calculated by subtracting the mean BMD of a young adult population from the BMD of the patient, and dividing by the SD of the reference population. The WHO has suggested that intervention be recommended for persons with a T-score value less than 2.5 SD below the age-adjusted mean, but the USDA has accepted a score less than 2.0 SD below the mean. The WHO criteria suggest that a T-score less than 2.5 at either the lumbar or the femoral site can be used to diagnose osteopenia, but some evidence suggests that the lumbar site is more sensitive for younger patients (men <60, women <70 years), and the femoral site for older patients (86). The WHO diagnostic classification for T-scores measured by DXA is: normal, greater than -1.0; Low bone index (osteopenia), less than -1 and greater than -2.5; osteoporosis, < –2.5; and severe osteoporosis, < –2.5 and 1 or more fragility fractures (85). It is worth remembering that calculation of a T-score involves three values (patient's BMD, population BMD, and population SD), only one of which is the patient's BMD. The ISCD recommends using T-scores from several skeletal sites for classification purposes, but the WHO recommends only the femoral neck for epidemiologic studies.

Because of the variability in T-scores in predicting fracture as a clinical outcome, FRAX was developed as a computer-based algorithm to estimate fracture probability after 10 years in untreated patients aged 40 to 90 (http://www.shef.ac.uk/FRAX). This calculation records clinical risk factors, including age, sex, height, weight, previous fracture, current tobacco smoking, glucocorticoid use, rheumatoid arthritis, other causes of secondary osteoporosis, and alcohol consumption of greater than 3 units per day. These risk factors are combined, when possible, with a BMD in g per cm^2 measured by DXA. Guidelines for the use of FRAX in predicting fracture risk have been agreed by consensus among the ISCD and the IOF (87). The calculation has been customized for each country on the basis of local epidemiology of fracture. The website most closely aligned with the US FRAX (version 3.0) is https://riskcalculator.fore.org/default.aspx.

Guidelines for the use of bone density measurement. In 1996, the American Association of Clinical Endocrinologists developed guidelines for the treatment of osteoporosis that included bone density measurement (88). They recommended bone density measurement to assess risk in perimenopausal or postmenopausal women concerned about osteoporosis. They also recommended testing for women with radiographic evidence of the diagnosis, undergoing treatment for osteoporosis, with asymptomatic primary hyperparathyroidism, or receiving long-term glucocorticoid therapy, situations in which evidence of skeletal loss might alter clinical strategy. In 1996, the European Foundation for Osteoporosis and Bone Disease also published practical guidelines for the use of bone density measurement (89). These guidelines were similar but did not include a recommendation to perform a baseline hip measurement. All these guidelines recommend the use of multiple skeletal sites, with the caveat that each site (e.g., spine, hip) best predicts fractures at that site but not at others (90). The USDA recommends bone density measurement if "it is reasonable and necessary for diagnosing, treating, or monitoring the condition of a beneficiary" as indicated in "estrogen deficiency . . . vertebral abnormalities . . . glucocorticoid (steroid) therapy . . . hyperparathyroidism" (91). Potentially modifiable features in postmenopausal women (and others) that might encourage testing include current cigarette smoking, low body weight, estrogen deficiency, low calcium intake (lifelong), alcoholism, recurrent falls, inadequate physical activity, and glucocorticoid therapy (92).

The ISCD holds Position Development Conferences on a regular basis to review the guidelines for indications and interpretation of bone density tests. The 2013 guidelines are the first revision since 2007 (93). There are new criteria for screening women less than 65 years and men less than 70 years (e.g., if they have low bone mass risk factors, history of prior fractures, high-risk medication use) (94). The reference population for T-scores will be based on NHANES II data for femoral neck and total hip values for Caucasian women aged 20 to 29. New criteria for obtaining vertebral fracture assessment for patients with T-scores of less than -1.0 include one or more of the following: women under age 70 and men under age 80, height loss greater than 4 cm, glucocorticoid use >5 mg per day for 3 months, and self-reported vertebral fracture. New guidelines for the use of DXA for body composition are now included. There are also guidelines for pediatrics, available on the ICSD website. The new guidelines confirmed that in healthy premenopausal women, young males less than 50 years, and especially in children, Z-scores (based on reference population for age, sex, and ethnicity) rather than T-scores should be used. Also confirmed was the preference for using the terms "low bone mass" or "low bone density" instead of "osteopenia."

Factors other than BMD alone are considered risk factors for fractures. Chief among these is body mass index, particularly at low values (95,96). Mineral crystallinity, which is not measured by BMD, rather than mineral content itself is thought to account for some of the discrepancy between fracture rate and BMD (97). Although peak bone mass was formerly felt to be an independent risk factor, it is now considered that bone mass is more related to bone size or muscle function (98). It is worth remembering that when a BMD is done for the first time in a menopausal woman, 50% of women will have a negative T-score, but this does not imply recent bone loss (99).

Method. Most centers now use DXA to assess trabecular bone in the vertebrae and hips. The X-ray source in DXA, which replaced the isotopic source of the original dual-photon absorptiometry, is preferable because of its wider range and shorter scanning speed. Precision standards for DEXA measurement have been published by the ICSD (100). Peripheral DXA (P-DXA) measures density in bones that are not at risk to fracture from fragility, but the machines are portable and units can be used in an office (http://www.webmd.com/hw/osteoporosis/hw3738.asp). If spine or hip DXA is available, P-DXA is not needed. Quantitative computed tomography (QCT) measures volumetric BMD (g per cm^3), and is also useful for the spine and peripheral QCT for the wrist (85). Peripheral QCT is promising for assessing bone mass in children, in whom DEXA is still the gold standard, but is not as predictive of future fracture risk as in adults (101). Bone mass values from DEXA or QCT are difficult to interpret if metal in the spine, contrast material in the gastrointestinal tract or spinal canal, or focal bone lesions are present. Aortic calcification and prior spinal bone surgery can affect the measurement, although QCT is more useful with aortic calcification. Accuracy is only about 90% because of variation in marrow fat content. More radiation is delivered by QCT than by DXA, about 250 mrad.

Other techniques have been used to improve the fracture predictability that is still a problem with DXA. Quantitative ultrasound is used mostly in the heel. Infrared imaging spectroscopy has been used in an attempt to assess mineral crystallinity as well as mineral content, although no variations in crystallinity were produced by raloxifene (97,102).

Bone Biopsy. Calcium (or vitamin D) deficiency can sometimes be diagnosed by bone biopsy, which can demonstrate increased osteoid seams. Tetracycline labeling allows a distinction to be made between delayed mineralization (osteomalacia) and increased osteoid synthesis (bone remodeling states) by revealing the calcification front. This technique is not often needed to make clinical decisions.

Physiology

Calcium provides part of the matrix structure of bone. It is necessary for blood coagulation and for controlling membrane potential and the excitability of nerves and muscles. The calcium content of the human adult body is about 1,000 mg. More than 99% of this is in the skeleton. Young adults typically retain about 68 mg of calcium per day, with average retention efficiency of about 7.6% (92). About half of circulating calcium is turning over in the bone. Through the protein calmodulin, it helps to control myocardial function and contractility. It supports membrane integrity and is a second messenger for many secretory processes. It helps to maintain intracellular integrity and intercellular tight junctions (92). Because of the importance of all these functions, serum levels are maintained with precision at the expense of bone matrix if exogenous calcium is not available. The major systems involved in regulating calcium homeostasis include the parathyroid hormone (PTH), vitamin D, and calcitonin (103). Apical calcium entry channels have been found in calcium transporting epithelia, CaT1 (ECaC2, TRPV6) in the intestine, and ECaC (ECaC1, TRPV5) as well as TRP6 and 7 in the kidney. The G-protein-coupled calcium-sensing receptor (CaR) is responsible for the tightly regulated secretion of parathormone from the parathyroid gland, responsive to small changes in serum calcium (104). The CaR also regulates calcium and magnesium excretion by the kidney, calcium reabsorption by the intestine, and bone remodeling. Cinacalcet (Sensipar) is a receptor positive allosteric modulator that stimulates the CaR to suppress PTH secretion in patients with chronic renal failure. Negative allosteric modulators are being developed that might increase PTH secretion and improve bone anabolism in patients with age-related osteoporosis (104).

Absorption

When calcium intake is adequate, differences in calcium bioavailability probably play little role (105). When dietary calcium is low, however, or ingested in poorly soluble forms (e.g., green vegetables), availability may be a problem. Absorption of vegetable calcium has proved to be quite variable because effective digestion is difficult to predict and assess (92). The high solubility of dairy calcium has been attributed to its presence as the citrate salt, and also to the presence of peptides, amino acids, and lactose. Milk substitutes lack many of these features and are not as good a source of available calcium and phosphorus as milk or milk products. Synthetic triglycerides improve calcium absorption (60). Gastric acid does not have much effect on the absorption of dietary calcium when the calcium is ingested with a meal (106). Data from knockout mouse models suggest that gastric acid secretion may be required for normal bone mineralization, when the osteoclasts are not able to mobilize calcium from bone (107). When calcium enters the relatively alkaline lumen of the duodenum, less calcium is solubilized, and calcium carbonate, when taken alone, is poorly absorbed.

Active calcium absorption (entry and secretion) depends on vitamin D intake and the presence of calbindin in duodenal enterocytes (92). Most calcium is absorbed passively in the jejunum and ileum because transit time through the duodenum is so short. The degree of passive ileal absorption depends on many factors, including luminal solubility, residence time in the lumen, and the rate of paracellular diffusion. However, no direct regulation of paracellular calcium movement has been identified (92). Only a small amount ($<$10%) of calcium is absorbed in the human colon, all of it passively; active transport of larger amounts occurs in rats and sheep. The two apical calcium channels show 75% homology, and belong to the superfamily of the transient receptor potential (TRP) channels. Entry across the apical intestinal membrane via CaT1 is driven by a favorable electrochemical gradient. Inside the cell, calcium is bound to calbindins, vitamin D-dependent proteins that deliver calcium to the basolateral membrane (103,108). Intracellular calcium is in the nanomolar range, whereas extracellular calcium is millimolar. Thus, extrusion from the cell is mediated against this electrochemical gradient by the calcium pump, consisting of an ATP-dependent Ca^+-ATPase, and a Na^+-Ca^{++} exchanger, NCX1. About 4 mmol (~140 mg) of calcium is absorbed each day into the ECF, a compartment that contains about 25 mmol of calcium (93). Fourteen millimoles of calcium enter bone and is mobilized from it each day, but the largest movement of calcium occurs in the kidney, where 270 mmol is filtered each day, and 266 mmol is reabsorbed, via CaT1 and ECaC and the active calcium pump in the proximal tubules (70%), the ascending limb (20%), the distal convoluted tubule and connecting tubule (103,108).

Data from calbindin or TRPV6 knockout mice show that duodenal calcium transport still responds to 1,25-diOH vitamin D, even in a double knockout (92). Thus, there may be some additional factors regulating calcium absorption, perhaps TRPV5, or unknown factors. It is not helpful to measure 25(OH)D in relation to calcium absorption as a reflection of vitamin D insufficiency, probably because the system is more finely tuned by 1,25-di(OH)D (109).

Enteroenteric Circulation

About 300 to 400 mg of calcium is absorbed each day in a normal adult, but 200 to 300 mg is re-excreted into the lumen via pancreatic, biliary, and intestinal secretions. The newly absorbed calcium in the blood mixes with an exchangeable pool of about 1 g. The calcium pool is filtered through the kidney many times, so that 10 g is filtered each day, of which 99% is absorbed secondary to the action of PTH and 100 mg is excreted in urine. When intestinal or urinary losses are excessive, the rate of bone resorption increases until it cannot compensate for the losses and hypocalcemia develops.

Bone Metabolism

Calcium metabolism is linked with that of vitamin D and with phosphate reabsorption in the kidney. While calcium and phosphate are tightly associated in bone formation and resorption, they are independently regulated in the kidney and intestine, although both are influenced by vitamin D (110). FGF-23 is secreted by osteoblasts and osteocytes, and targets its receptor in the kidney complexed with α-klotho, which in turn inhibits PTH secretion (111). In patients with chronic renal disease this feedback is lost, and PTH secretion increases, leading to bone disease and hypercalcemia. Because uptake of calcium and phosphorus is closely linked in bone, but availability of these elements is regulated separately in the body, nanoparticles of soluble calcium phosphate are being developed as therapeutic agents (112).

Deficiency

Incidence

Dietary deficiency of calcium is more common than magnesium or phosphorus deficiency; dietary sources of calcium are more limited than those of magnesium and phosphorus, absorption is not as good as that of phosphorus, and the obligatory daily excretion (300 mg in stool, 100 mg in urine) is large in comparison with the exchangeable pool size (1 g) and the daily flux from bone (200 to 300 mg). Dietary deficiency is most likely to develop during infancy, adolescence, and pregnancy (when requirements are large) and during old age (when absorption is decreased and bone mass is lower).

Hypocalcemia
The usual causes of hypocalcemia are not related to deficiency but to metabolism. Hypocalcemia leads to enhanced neuromuscular transmission, tetany, altered myocardial function and arrhythmias (prolonged QT interval), and altered nerve conduction. Severe weight loss (e.g., anorexia nervosa) can lead to a prolonged QT interval and arrhythmia by a mechanism that is not explained by hypocalcemia (113).

Chronic Deficiency
The body contains about 1,000 g of calcium. A net loss of 100 mg per day would lead to a 20% (detectable) loss of bone calcium in about 2,000 days, or 6 years. Because bone loss is a slow process, the state of calcium nutrition at the time of clinical presentation, such as fracture, may bear little relationship to an earlier cause of bone loss. Thus, calcium intake should aim to achieve a peak bone density at ages 25 to 30 as well as to alter the rate of bone loss with aging (114). The expected rate of bone loss with aging is 0.5% yearly after age 40, except for the 5 years after menopause, when it increases to 2% annually. The major mechanisms that lead to bone loss greater than expected for age include failure to achieve an optimal bone mass during growth and development, excessive bone resorption, and inadequate replacement of lost bone.

Osteopenia can occur unevenly in different bones, so the bone density analysis must be performed on those most at risk in a given patient. As a person ages, however, the bone loss from various sites tends to equalize. Thus, measurements of density in the spine, proximal femur, middle portion of the radius, and os calcis all reflect similar degrees of bone loss in the elderly. In women 20 to 45 years old, the site of measurement may be critical (90). The spine is most often followed in postmenopausal osteoporosis; the rate of bone turnover in trabecular bone, such as that of the spine, is high, and measurement with DXA is most precise in the spine.

Causes
Malabsorption of calcium usually occurs in short-bowel syndrome and untreated celiac disease, but malabsorption may be of many causes. Renal failure and vitamin D deficiency lead to hypocalcemia and bone disease. The factors most often associated with low bone mass (not necessarily calcium deficiency) are postmenopausal osteoporosis (especially if the patient or a first-degree relative has a history of fracture), Caucasian race, female sex, advanced age, dementia, low body weight, current cigarette smoking, low calcium intake (lifelong), alcoholism, and poor general health. Gastric bypass surgery for morbid obesity can lead to an increase in bone turnover and a decrease in bone mass that can occur within 9 months of surgery, despite an increase in dietary calcium and vitamin D (115).

Certain drugs increase the risk for osteoporosis, but the mechanism is not at all clear, and probably is not directly related to calcium deficiency. With glucocorticoids the risk of fracture increases with dose and duration of therapy (116). The minimal treatment period creating such a fracture risk is 3 months. However, calcium supplementation is not recommended for prevention of glucocorticoid-induced osteoporosis (117). Proton-pump inhibitors (PPIs) have also been implicated in a direct effect on bone, leading to increased fracture risk, although the data are less clear than in the case of glucocorticoids (118).

Treatment
Any patient with calcium deficiency should also be evaluated for vitamin D deficiency (see Chapter 6), and if this is present, it should be treated.

Hypocalcemia
Acute symptomatic hypocalcemia (ionized calcium <1.12 mmol per L) is a medical emergency (119). It should be treated with 10 to 20 mL of a 10% solution of calcium gluconate (90 to 180 mg of elemental calcium) administered IV over 10 to 15 minutes. When the initial [iCa]s is less than 1 mmol per L, twice that amount can be given. This initial therapy should be followed by more prolonged IV infusion (e.g., 6 to 8 10-mL ampules of 10% calcium gluconate per L in D5W) until serum calcium levels can be maintained with oral supplements. Frequent ionized calcium and phosphorus determinations should be made, and electrocardiographic monitoring is indicated until serum calcium returns toward normal.

Nutritional Deficiency

Nutritional rickets still occurs in Third World nations. When rickets was caused by a low intake of calcium (200 mg per day), it responded better to treatment with calcium alone (1,000 mg per day) or in combination with vitamin D than to vitamin D alone (120). When calcium intake was below recommended levels but not very low (e.g., 800 mg per day) in mothers who were lactating or postweaning, supplementation with calcium (1,000 mg per day) enhanced bone density only modestly (~5%) in 6 months (121).

Osteoporosis in Medical Disorders

In certain intestinal diseases, fecal calcium loss is increased by diarrhea or malabsorption; patients with such diseases should undergo bone density screening, and any osteoporosis should be treated. Clinical risk factors are not good predictors of bone mass in these patients, and the threshold for measuring bone density should be low. Patients with celiac disease and inflammatory bowel disease (IBD) should be given adequate dietary calcium and supplementation to 1,500 mg per day in the form of tablets if necessary, although evidence for efficacy is rather slight (122). Vitamin D deficiency should be sought and treated (see Chapter 6). If patients are on glucocorticoids, the dose taken should be the lowest required to obtain benefit, and it should be taken for the shortest possible time. Physical activity and adequate nutrition should be promoted, and cigarette smoking should be discouraged (123). Studies suggest that supplementation with calcium, vitamin D, or both may not prevent bone loss in patients with IBD, but should be used in the periods between flares of disease activity (124). If low bone density persists, drug therapy for osteoporosis should be provided, with the addition of hormone replacement therapy for postmenopausal women, testosterone for men with low testosterone levels, and biphosphonates or calcitonin for others as indicated.

Osteoporosis

Evidence is available to support the role of calcium supplementation in improving bone density in elderly and adolescent populations (64). This relationship has been supported by the FDA, the National Institutes of Health, and the National Academy of Sciences. The beneficial effect of 1,000 mg of supplemental calcium, with or without vitamin D, has been seen in early postmenopausal women, even those with good initial calcium and vitamin D status. Some studies also show a decrease in the fracture rate with calcium alone (1,200 mg per day for 4 years) (125). Studies assessing the efficacy of estrogen therapy in postmenopausal women showed improved bone density in those whose dietary calcium exceeded 1,000 mg per day, but not in those whose dietary calcium was only half that amount (67,126). When adequate calcium (>1,000 mg per day) and vitamin D (to maintain 25-hydroxyvitamin D levels ≥ 75 nmol per L) were taken, bone sparing with low-dose hormone replacement therapy was as good as that achieved with high-dose hormone replacement therapy (127). However, one cannot assume that routine supplementation of postmenopausal women with 1,000 mg of calcium and 800 IU of vitamin D will be effective in prevention of fractures, either as primary (128) or secondary (129) prevention. The possible reasons for such failure are many and incompletely understood, but the message is clear that routine supplementation in nonstratified elderly women is not likely to be successful (130). This conclusion is supported by the low incidence of osteopenia developing in postmenopausal women with normal bone density or mild osteopenia (131). Whether replacing vitamin D adequately (see Chapter 6) or treating only those with vitamin D deficiency is the answer is still unknown.

Hypertension and Cardiovascular Disease

A small decrease in systolic, but not diastolic, pressure was observed with calcium supplementation between 500 and 2,000 mg per day (132,133). However, use of the DASH diet, low in fat and rich in fruits, vegetables, whole grains, and low-fat dairy products that provide 1,265 mg of calcium per day, produced a greater fall in pressure (9). The major problem is the variable calcium excretion related to the high sodium intake and relatively low calcium intake that characterize Western diets (67). A small decrease (2 to 4 mm Hg) has been reported in pregnant and hypertensive patients taking calcium supplements (134). With many options for drug treatment of hypertension, calcium supplements are not often indicated for the treatment of hypertension.

There is no evidence that increasing calcium intake over the DRI recommendations leads to any change in health outcomes for CV disease or obesity (134). Moreover, it is possible that calcium supplementation to patients without prior CV disease increased the risk of myocardial infarction by 30%, but with no increase in mortality or stroke (135). The trials reviewed, however, included supplementation with both calcium and vitamin D, and CV events were not the major reason for conducting most of the studies. In the absence of biological plausibility for this adverse effect, it must be considered preliminary at this time. This same conclusion was reached by a separate panel of experts (136).

Colon Cancer
Controlled studies measuring the effect of calcium on colonic proliferative rates have provided mixed answers (137) (see also Chapter 14). One large study showed a modest effect of calcium supplementation (1,200 mg per day) for 4 years in preventing colorectal polyps (138). The Women's Health Initiative found that patients treated with calcium and vitamin D for 5 years prevented 5 breast and 1 colorectal cancers (139). Any effects on colorectal cancer may be more related to vitamin D supplementation, but the data do not allow a clear separation of calcium and vitamin D effects (140).

Premenstrual Syndrome
The use of 1,200 mg of calcium per day for three cycles led to fewer symptoms in women ages 18 to 45 years (141). The use of calcium for this condition should still be considered uncertain until more studies have been reported.

Oral Preparations
Calcium carbonate is given to most patients because it contains the largest amount of elemental calcium per unit weight (142). However, it is less soluble than some other salts (glubionate, gluconate, citrate), which may be useful in selected cases because they are better absorbed (143). Calcium carbonate contains 40% elemental calcium. Tricalcium phosphate contains 33% elemental calcium, acetate 25%, dibasic phosphate 23%, citrate 21%, lactate 13%, gluconate 9%, and glubionate 6.5%. Table 7-20 lists some of the available preparations.

Toxicity
The tolerable upper intake level (UL) for calcium has been set for adults less than 50 years at 2,500 mg per day, and for older adults at 2,000 mg (Table 7-17). When intake exceeds 4,000 mg per day, hypercalcemia can develop, along with renal damage and metastatic calcification.

Populations at Risk
In patients on thiazide diuretics or with renal disease, urinary calcium excretion may be decreased. Patients with absorptive or renal hypercalciuria are at an increased risk for kidney stones, although normal persons are not (144). In patients with a previous calcium stone, increased fluid intake decreased the stone recurrence rate (145). Patients with primary hyperthyroidism and sarcoidosis are at risk for hypercalcemia and should avoid calcium supplements. Patients with calcium oxalate stones, especially if they are secondary to malabsorption of fat, should be treated with oral calcium to precipitate the soluble sodium oxalate in the intestinal lumen.

Interference with Absorption
Oral calcium may interfere with the absorption of many drugs (e.g., salicylates, bisphosphonates, fluoride, tetracyclines, atenolol, iron). Calcium supplements should not be taken at the same time as iron and other medications. Calcium supplements do not interfere with magnesium absorption in normal persons but may do so in cases of magnesium depletion, as in patients with diabetes, malabsorption, or acute alcoholic intake. In such cases, 100 mg of magnesium should be provided for every 500 mg of supplemental calcium used (144).

Hypercalcemia
Serum calcium levels above 11 mg per dL can be associated with symptoms related to decreased neuromuscular transmission and muscle contraction. These include weakness, ileus, altered cardiac conductivity, anorexia, nausea, vomiting, constipation, dry mouth, polyuria, and thirst. Serum calcium levels above 12 mg per dL can produce confusion, delirium, stupor, and coma, especially in the elderly. Changes on the electrocardiogram include short PR, ST, and QT intervals, with a prolonged QRS complex. Arrhythmias can occur, especially at levels above 13 mg per dL. The treatment of severe exogenous hypercalcemia should begin with IV normal saline solution (500 to 750 mL per h or as tolerated) and furosemide (80 to 120 mg per h) if renal function is adequate. These measures are usually rapidly effective. Long-term management consists of adjusting the doses of exogenous calcium, vitamin D, or both.

TABLE 7-20 Selected Calcium-containing Products for Oral Use

Calcium Supplement	Elemental Calcium (mg per tablet)	Vitamin D (IU per tablet)
Calcium Carbonate		
Alka 2	200	—
Alka-Mints	340	—
Biocal	250, 500	—
Calburst	500	200
Calciday	667	—
Calsup	300, 600	200
Caltrate + D	600	200
Os-Cal + D	250, 500	200
Oystercal	250, 375, 500	—
Titralac	200 (405/5 mL)	—
Tums	200, 500	—
Viactiv	500	100
Calcium Citrate		
Citracal	200 (500 per effervescent tablet)	—
Citracal + D	315	200
Calcium citrate + D	315	200
Calcium Complex/Components		
Calcium acetate	167–668 mg	—
Calcet (carbonate, lactate, gluconate)	150	100
Calcium gluconate	45/500 mg	—
Calcium lactate	42/325 mg	—
Ca Plus (protein)	280	—
Calcium Glubionate		
Neo-Calglucon	115/5 mL)	—
Calcium Phosphate		
Dical-D	350	400
Posture-D	600	125

Magnesium

Requirement

Magnesium requirements have been determined by balance studies and urinary measurements because the kidney is the main excretory organ. With an average US dietary intake of 120 mg per 1,000 kcal per day and maintenance of the serum concentration at 2 mg per dL (~1.7 mEq per L), the mean urinary excretion is about 72 mg per day. Because average absorption is 30% to 40%, the daily requirement should be about 200 mg for an adult. However, the requirements for infants and children have not been accurately assessed. Estimates of net magnesium accretion over all of childhood are approximately 4 mg per day (69). Magnesium replacement for infants is still uncertain (146). Human milk contains 40 mg of magnesium per L, and the average infant ingests about 850 mL per day. The 1997 DRIs are noted in Table 7-21.

Food Sources

Magnesium is bound to protein and phosphate ions, and to porphyrin in green leafy plants and vegetables. Hard water and mineral waters can contain as much as 120 mg per L. The sources of magnesium are widespread. Good dietary sources include whole grains, legumes, dark green leafy vegetables, nuts, fish, and cocoa. Dairy products, meat, and eggs contain lesser amounts of magnesium. The use of calcium supplements without magnesium is controversial. There is a theoretical

TABLE 7-21   Dietary Reference Intakes of Magnesium

Life Stage Group	Magnesium (mg/d)	Life Stage Group	Magnesium (mg/d)
Infants		**Females**	
0–6 months	30[a]	9–13 years	240
7–12 months	75[a]	14–18 years	360
		19–30 years	310
Children		31–>70 years	320
1–3 years	80		
4–8 years	130	**Pregnancy**	
		≤18 years	400
Males		19–30 years	350
9–13 years	240	31–50 years	360
14–18 years	410		
19–30 years	400	**Lactation**	
31–>70 years	420	≤18 years	360
		19–30 years	310

[a]Adequate intake (AI) is estimated from ingestion of human milk content. Other values reflect recommended dietary allowance (RDA).
Standing Committee on the Scientific Evaluation of Dietary Reference Intakes, Food and Nutrition Board, Institute of Medicine. *Dietary Reference Intakes: Calcium, Phosphorus, Magnesium, Vitamin D, and Fluoride.* Washington, DC: National Academies Press, 1997.

interaction between the ions for absorption, but practically the risk of producing deficiency in humans (particularly children) is not demonstrated (79). In the United States, the FDA encourages the use of foods with a low sodium content and a high content of calcium, magnesium, or potassium (by allowing health claims to be used for such products) (147). Table 7-22 lists the magnesium content of selected foods. The USDA Nutrient Database Web site provides a comprehensive list of foods containing magnesium (148). This source can be used for any other micronutrient as well.

Assessment
Intake and Absorption
When dietary information is available, urinary magnesium can be helpful because dietary intake and urinary excretion are strongly correlated (59). The kidney avidly retains magnesium when

TABLE 7-22   Magnesium Content of Selected Foods

Food	Serving Size	Magnesium Content (mg)
Cereals	3 oz	90–120
Legumes	1 cup	80–120
Nuts	1/2 cup	130–210
Fish, cooked	3 oz	20–60
Baked potato with skin	One	55
Spinach, cooked	1/2 cup	80
Vegetables, cooked	1 cup	5–30
Fruit	1 cup	20–30
Meat, cooked	3 oz	10–20
Milk	1 cup	28–33
Yogurt	1 cup	27–40
Beer	12 oz	23

dietary intake is low, and urinary levels fall. However, dietary deficiency of magnesium is uncommon because the mineral is widely distributed among foods. Thus, low urinary levels of magnesium usually reflect disease (e.g., prolonged diarrhea). Elevated urinary levels of magnesium often reflect diuretic therapy, not high dietary intake.

Body Stores

Serum magnesium is measured by colorimetric or fluorometric methods, although atomic absorption spectroscopy is more reliable. Hemolysis falsely elevates serum magnesium levels because the mineral is an intracellular cation. Extracellular ionized magnesium (filterable magnesium) is the biologically active fraction, so that the total serum magnesium level does not reflect total stores in a reliable fashion. As with calcium, ionized magnesium cannot be estimated using a correction for albumin. Magnesium-selective electrodes are available and have been incorporated into commercially available instruments (59). About 70% of the total magnesium in plasma is ionized, but the usefulness of measuring ionized magnesium in disease states is not well studied (149). Studies differ on whether total serum magnesium can predict changes in ionized magnesium, or whether ionized magnesium can predict clinical outcomes (150). Current electrodes used for ionized magnesium do not adequately select for magnesium over calcium, so results have to be corrected for ionized calcium (151). Moreover, the life span of existing electrodes is variable, and further standardization is needed. Hypomagnesemia, defined as levels below 1.25 to 1.50 mEq per L or 0.62 to 0.75 mmol per L (Table 7-23), is often accompanied by hypokalemia and hypocalcemia. Low levels can occur with pregnancy, malabsorption, reduced intake, diabetes mellitus, severe illness, acute alcoholism, or renal leak (or diuretic use). A normal level does not rule out deficient stores because the serum level is corrected by the action of PTH and calcitonin. Hypermagnesemia is found in renal failure and with the use of magnesium-containing antacids or laxatives.

Tissue magnesium levels should be the best measure of body stores of this intracellular cation, but practical methods are not available. Red and white cells have been isolated for this purpose, but the results are not sufficiently consistent for general use (150). The magnesium loading test has been used to assess deficiency (59). Thirty millimoles of magnesium chloride is infused over 12 hours, and urine is collected for 24 hours. Magnesium status is based on the amount of magnesium retained in the body. Normally, only 5% to 6% is retained. Another paradigm infuses 2.4 mmol per kg of parenteral magnesium, and retention of greater than 20% suggests magnesium deficiency (150). However, the care required to perform the test has limited its clinical usefulness. Moreover, this test is valid only when renal function is normal, and when magnesium deficiency is not related to decreased renal excretion (152).

Fecal Excretion

Normally, the fecal excretion reflects dietary intake, with 2/3 of intake appearing in the stool. Usually, there is no reason to measure fecal magnesium. However, when factitious diarrhea is suspected,

TABLE 7-23 Reference Values for Magnesium Assessment

Parameter	Magnesium Levels (mmol/L)	(mEq/L)
Serum magnesium (adult)	0.75–1.25	1.5–2.5
NHANES I (18–74 years)	0.75–0.96	1.5–1.92
Hypomagnesemia	>0.62–0.75	<1.25–1.5
Hypermagnesemia	>1.25	>1.5
Serum ionized magnesium	0.58 ± 0.006	
Erythrocyte magnesium (adult)	1.88 ± 0.12	
	Magnesium Urinary Excretion Per Day	
Magnesium load test	94%–95% (normal)	33%–69% (deficient)

NHANES, National Health and Nutrition Examination Survey.
Data from Sauberlich HE. *Laboratory Tests for the Assessment of Nutritional Status.* 2nd ed. Boca Raton, FL: CRC Press, 1999.

a magnesium concentration of greater than 50 mM in the fecal supernatant can be diagnostic of a magnesium laxative, and concentrations of 25 to 49 mM can be very suggestive (153).

Physiology

Magnesium is the fourth most abundant cation in the body, after sodium, potassium, and calcium. The 70-kg adult body contains about 2,000 mEq of magnesium, or 21 to 28 g. About 60% is in the bone, with the rest distributed equally between muscle and other soft tissues. Less than 5% is in the ECF, and only 0.3% is present in serum (154). Magnesium in extra- and intracellular fluid exists in 3 states: a) free, ionized fraction that is physiologically active, b) complexed to ions (phosphate, bicarbonate, and citrate), and c) protein-bound, mostly to albumin in serum (149). These 3 fractions are in equilibrium with each other. The exchangeable magnesium pool is about 5 g, but extracellular magnesium is only about 250 mg. Magnesium flux from bone replenishes the exchangeable pool, but the daily rate of this flux is not precisely known.

Function

More than 300 enzymatic reactions require magnesium. These involve transfer of phosphate groups, acylation of coenzyme A, hydrolysis of phosphates and pyrophosphates, and nucleic acid synthesis. All enzymatic reactions in which adenosine triphosphate is involved require magnesium. In addition, the cation is necessary for ribosomal RNA and DNA stability, activation of amino acids, degradation of DNA, neurotransmission, regulation of smooth muscle tone, and immune function. Magnesium is a calcium antagonist in some reactions, and interacts with potassium, pyridoxine, and boron.

Absorption

Magnesium is absorbed by two processes: nonsaturable passive paracellular diffusion (90%) and saturable active transport (10%). Paracellular absorption is impaired in the rare autosomal recessive disorder, primary hypomagnesemia, associated with a defect in a tight junction protein called paracellin 1 (PCLN1) or claudin 16 (155). Active transport of magnesium is mediated by a member of the cation channel TRP family, TRPM6. Mutations in this protein are found in the inherited disorder of hypomagnesemia with secondary hypocalcemia (156). The TRPM6 transporter is located apically in all parts of the intestine and in cells of the distal renal tubule. A portion of magnesium is absorbed in the colon, by a mechanism as yet uncertain, but probably involves TRPM6/7 (157). Absorption varies from 30% to 70% of ingested magnesium, depending on how much magnesium is presented to the gut. At the usual intake levels of 300 mg per day, absorption is about 30% to 50%. Active magnesium absorption is more readily detected in magnesium-deficient states. At physiologic concentrations, the effect of 1,25-dihydroxyvitamin D_3 on magnesium absorption is very small and is probably related to changes in calcium or phosphorus uptake (158). Much of the magnesium ingested in medicinal form (oxide, hydroxide, chloride, citrate) is poorly soluble and is not absorbed to a great extent. However, the laxative action of $MgSO_4$ has been attributed to upregulation of aquaporin 3 in the colon through adenylate cyclase activation (159). Aquaporin 3 is predominantly expressed in the colon and skin. Phosphate and organic chelators (e.g., oxalate, phytate) can delay absorption. Transit time is a major factor in determining the efficiency of magnesium absorption.

Urinary Excretion

The kidney is the major excretory organ. More than two-thirds of absorbed magnesium is excreted in the urine each day. Urinary excretion is about 80 to 120 mg (3% to 5%) of the filtered load of 2.4 g per day, and is increased in conditions associated with proteinuria. The proximal tubule reabsorbs 15% to 20% of filtered magnesium, and the thick ascending limb of the tubule absorbs 50% to 75%, so that excretion is reduced to less than 1 mmol per day. The distal tubule reabsorbs 5% to 10% of the ion, and together with the thick ascending loop is the major site of magnesium regulation (156). The major regulator is the serum magnesium concentration, and regulation is mediated by Ca/Mg-sensing receptors located on the capillary side of cells of the thick ascending limb. Maximal excretion in response to magnesium loading can exceed 160 mmol per day. Magnesium excretion is increased by volume expansion, hypercalcemia, diuretics, alcohol, and phosphate depletion, and is decreased by the action of PTH. Because of this tight urinary regulation, magnesium deficiency occurs rarely except when excessive amounts are lost from the body, in intestinal or renal disease.

Parathyroid Hormone Response

When hypomagnesemia is mild, PTH is released and calcium is released from bone. However, the direct effect of hypomagnesemia on decreasing calcium mobilization from bone blunts this effect (160). When magnesium deficiency is severe and the serum concentration very low, PTH secretion is impaired. Along with the direct effect of the hypomagnesemia on bone, calcium flux is lowered and hypocalcemia develops. In this case, hypocalcemia is less a manifestation of depleted calcium stores than of low stores of exchangeable magnesium. Thus, when magnesium deficiency is severe (e.g., in malabsorption), magnesium is required to treat the hypocalcemia.

Deficiency

Clinical Manifestations

Magnesium deficiency may not be associated with symptoms. Many of the symptoms of moderate or severe deficiency are nonspecific or are caused by associated electrolyte abnormalities, such as hypocalcemia, hypokalemia, and metabolic alkalosis (Table 7-24). The most common symptoms are muscular twitching and tremor, numbness, and tingling. Less common are muscle weakness, convulsions, apathy, anorexia, depression, and delirium. Refractory hypokalemia can develop because magnesium plays a role in determining the intracellular–extracellular ratio of the two ions. If magnesium is deficient, potassium supplements can restore serum potassium, but not intracellular potassium (161). Common manifestations include Chvostek sign and premature ventricular beats. Ventricular premature complexes, and ventricular tachycardia or fibrillation are more serious complications. Magnesium therapy is recommended for treatment of torsades de pointes, but no randomized trials have proven its efficacy (162).

Serum and dietary magnesium are inversely associated with CV risk (163). This finding supports the observation that low urinary magnesium concentration was associated with an increased risk of coronary heart disease (164). However, no prospective intervention studies have been completed to see if the proposed risk can be reversed.

Hypomagnesemia has been associated uncommonly with the use of PPIs. All PPIs have been involved, the disorder develops usually in the first year of PPI treatment, and the degree of hypomagnesemia can be severe (165). Esomeprazole has the lowest risk, and pantoprazole the highest in the FDA database (166). Elderly males are also more at risk, and hypocalcemia and hypokalemia often coexisted. The cause of the hypomagnesemia is unknown, but it responds rapidly to withdrawal of the PPI (167).

Causes

Most cases of magnesium deficiency arise from gastrointestinal or renal losses (Table 7-25) (150,168). Patient groups at risk for magnesium inadequacy include those with type 2 diabetes from osmotic diuresis, alcohol dependency from both gastrointestinal and renal mechanisms, and the

TABLE 7-24 Clinical Manifestations of Moderate/Severe Magnesium Deficiency

Symptoms	Signs	Laboratory Abnormalities
Carpopedal spasm, tetany	Chvostek	Hypocalcemia
Seizures, tremor	Trousseau	Hypokalemia
Vertigo/ataxia	Arrhythmia, prolonged QT or PR interval wide QRS, peaked T wave, ST depression	Carbohydrate intolerance
Muscle weakness		ECG: wide QRS complex, prolonged PR interval, inverted T waves, U waves, ventricular arrhythmias Numbness, tingling Depression, psychosis

ECG, electrocardiogram.

TABLE 7-25 Causes of Magnesium Deficiency

Gastrointestinal	Renal
Malabsorption	Volume expansion
Diarrhea, especially chronic	Osmotic diuresis
Short-bowel syndrome	Metabolic acidosis
Enterocutaneous fistulae	Drugs (thiazides, loop diuretics, alcohol, aminoglycosides, cisplatin, amphotericin B, cyclosporine, foscarnet, pentamidine)
Nasogastric suction, long-term	
Primary intestinal hypomagnesemia	
Malnutrition, severe	Phosphate depletion
Pancreatitis, acute	Postobstructive nephropathy
Prematurity	Diuretic phase of acute renal failure
	Renal transplantation
	Hungry bone syndrome
	Hypercalcemia of any cause
	Renal tubular dysfunction

elderly with decreased absorption, increased renal loss, and drug interactions (169). Hypercalcemia of any cause produces a high filtered load of calcium that competes with magnesium for reabsorption. Any kind of diuresis can decrease the tubular reabsorption of magnesium. In patients with short-bowel syndrome, urinary magnesium levels fall before serum levels and are an early indicator of evolving deficiency (170). Although urinary magnesium is not often useful in diagnosing deficiency, the situation may be different in short-bowel syndrome, in which absorption is so limited.

Treatment
The choice of oral or parenteral magnesium depends on the severity of depletion. The extent of depletion cannot be predicted by laboratory findings, but may be as high as 1–2 mmol per kg of body weight (150). However, acute magnesium infusion decreases magnesium absorption in the loop of Henle, so much of the infused parenteral magnesium is excreted. Thus, oral replacement is preferred if the clinical presentation allows. The problem with oral therapy is that most of the salts of magnesium are only poorly soluble.

Parenteral
Moderate or severe deficiency should be treated parenterally, especially if tetany or ventricular arrhythmias are present, with 4 to 8 mmol given as an IV loading dose (8 mmol is contained in 1 g of heptahydrated magnesium sulfate), followed by 25 mmol per day thereafter until the plasma magnesium is above 0.4 mmol per L (159). In patients with normal renal function, up to 20 mmol (2.5 g) can be infused IV over 3 hours in 5% dextrose or 0.9% normal saline solution if deficiency is severe. Magnesium sulfate is incompatible with soluble phosphates, and with alkaline carbonates and bicarbonates, except in dilute solution. For mild deficiency, 1 g can be given intramuscularly (IM) every 6 hours for a total of four doses. Magnesium has been used parenterally in the absence of deficiency in patients with preeclampsia. The MAGPIE trial used 32 mmol initially, followed by 8 mmol per hour in women with preeclampsia (171). For torsade de pointes the Advanced Cardiac Life Support Guidelines suggest a loading dose of 16 mmol of magnesium given over 15 minutes, followed by 8 mmol per hour (172).

Oral
Magnesium oxide is commonly used, but it is poorly soluble and can act as a cathartic. Magnesium gluconate is preferred because it is more soluble and is available in a palatable liquid form (Table 7-26). Thus, large numbers of tablets can be avoided for long-term therapy. Magnesium chloride is absorbed poorly, less well than magnesium acetate or dietary magnesium (from nuts), and should not be relied on for replacement therapy (173). Magnesium salts can decrease the absorption of some drugs, such as aminoquinolones, digoxin, nitrofurantoin, penicillamine, and tetracyclines. Calcium supplementation of more than 2.6 g per day can lead to a negative magnesium balance. When malabsorption requires supplementation with both calcium and magnesium, they should be given at separate times.

TABLE 7-26 Selected Oral Magnesium Preparations

Preparation	Anion	Tablet Size (mg)	Elemental Magnesium Content (mg Per Tablet or Per 5 mL)[a]
Mag-200	Oxide	400	241
Mag-Ox 400	Oxide	140	83
Magnesium oxide	Oxide	250, 600	130, 360
Uro-Mag	Gluconate	500	29
Magtrate	Gluconate	500	29
Magonate	Gluconate	5 mL	54
Magonate, Almora	Gluconate	500	27
Chelated magnesium	Amino acids	500	100
Slow-Mag	Chloride	535	64
Mag-Tab SR	Lactate		84
Maginex DS	Mg-L-aspartate-Cl	1,230 mg powder	122

[a]Assumes equal bioavailability, which is not the case.

Supplements for Chronic Medical Diseases

Magnesium supplements have been used for a variety of medical conditions in which patients are felt to be at risk for deficiency (e.g., diabetes) or in which improved muscular performance is desired (e.g., heart disease). Observational studies in heart disease have provided only a hint that magnesium may be useful for patients with mitral valve prolapse (64). Of course, patients should consume enough magnesium-rich foods or take supplements if their intake is not adequate. Double-blinded placebo-controlled trials of magnesium supplements in hypertension have not demonstrated a reproducible effect, perhaps related to differences in sodium intake. If patients are taking loop or thiazide diuretics, some additional magnesium may be needed to replace that lost in the urine, if one assumes that renal function is normal. Magnesium supplements have not consistently improved glycemic control in either type I or type II diabetes (64), although a few randomized trials show benefit without a change in serum magnesium concentration (174). Likewise, evidence does not support magnesium supplements to treat migraine headaches or premenstrual symptoms or to improve exercise tolerance.

Toxicity

The UL for magnesium is 65 mg per day (children 1 to 3 years old), 110 mg per day (children 4 to 8 years old), and 350 mg per day (all adolescents and adults) (69). Magnesium supplements are usually not toxic if renal function is normal. Soft stools and diarrhea have been reported after ingestion of more than 500 mg of elemental magnesium (175).

Hypermagnesemia

Hypermagnesemia develops when renal excretion is decreased (as in renal failure and eclampsia), in severe diabetic ketoacidosis, and in Addison disease. Blocking of neuromuscular transmission leads to decreased tendon reflexes (at levels >4 mEq per L) and respiratory paralysis and heart block (at levels >10 mEq per L). Infants of mothers with eclampsia treated with magnesium are at risk, as are patients with renal failure receiving magnesium-containing antacids.

Hypermagnesemia does not usually develop until the GFR falls below 13 mL per minute. In renal failure, magnesium excretion relative to the GFR is lower than expected from the plasma level. Thus, plasma levels can rise rapidly. At levels of 3 to 5 mEq per L, symptoms include nausea, vomiting, cutaneous vasodilation, and hypertension. At higher levels (5 to 9 mEq per L), drowsiness, hyporeflexia, and muscular weakness occur, and above 10 mEq per L, respiratory arrest is noted, along with prolongation of the QTc interval and atrioventricular block.

Therapy of Hypermagnesemia

Therapy of hypermagnesemia involves withdrawal of any oral or parenteral magnesium compounds, hemodialysis or peritoneal dialysis if renal failure is the cause, or infusion of calcium to

Phosphorus

Requirement

Ratio of Phosphorus to Calcium

The recommended ratio of calcium to phosphorus in the diet is between 2:1 and 1:2. Because dietary phosphorus is so abundant and deficiency from decreased intake occurs so rarely, the recommended phosphorus intake is similar to that for calcium except in young infants. In the case of infants ingesting cow's milk with a calcium–phosphorus ratio of 1.2:1, the relative increase in phosphorus intake may contribute to hypocalcemia in early life. Thus, the AI for phosphorus is set at 100 mg, in comparison with 210 mg for calcium for the first 6 months of life, but nearly equal for the next 6 months (Table 7-27).

Dietary Reference Intake

Data to establish a requirement for phosphorus are not available because, similar to urinary magnesium excretion, urinary phosphorus excretion does not reflect dietary intake. In general, if the protein intake is adequate, so is the phosphorus intake. About 1 g of phosphorus is needed for each 17 g of nitrogen retained. The DRI exceeds this because of incomplete absorption and obligatory urinary excretion. The efficiency of absorption varies with the source of phosphorus and the ratio of calcium to phosphorus in the diet, so that the recommendation for dietary intake is further confused. The current DRI for adults is 700 mg per day, somewhat below the DRI for calcium (1,000 to 1,200 mg per day); for growing adolescents and pregnant or lactating women, the DRI is 1,250 mg per day, nearly the same as that for calcium (1,300 mg per day).

Food Sources

Phosphorus is a constituent of all cells and is thus present in all foods. The phosphorus content of some foods is listed in Table 7-28. Both organic and inorganic phosphorus (Pi) esters are handled alike by the alkaline phosphatase present in the intestinal tract. Milk and milk products provide approximately 20% to 30% of dietary phosphorus for adults, with the same amount

TABLE 7-27 Dietary Reference Intake for Phosphorus	
Life Stage Group	Phosphorus (mg/d)
Infants	
0–6 months	100[a]
7–12 months	275[a]
Children	
1–3 years	460
4–8 years	500
Males	
9–18 years	1,250
19–>70 years	700
Females	
9–13 years	1,250
14–18 years	1,250
19–>70 years	700
Pregnancy/Lactation	
≤18 years	1,250
19–50 years	700

[a]Estimate based on adequate intake (AI). Other values reflect recommended dietary allowance (RDA).
Standing Committee on the Scientific Evaluation of Dietary Reference Intakes, Food and Nutrition Board, Institute of Medicine. *Dietary Reference Intakes: Calcium, Phosphorus, Magnesium, Vitamin D, and Fluoride.* Washington, DC: National Academies Press, 1997.

TABLE 7-28 Phosphorus Content of Food

Food	Portion	Phosphorus (mg)
Grains and Cereals		
Bread, white	1 slice	30
Hamburger bun	1 each	44
Cornbread muffins	1 each	128
Rice, cooked	1 cup	74
Bran flakes, 40%	1/2 cup	63
Meat and Fish		
Beef, lamb, veal	3 oz	125–300
Beef liver	3 oz	392
Chicken, white meat, roasted	3 oz	183
Fish	3 oz	230–330
Fruits		
Apple, medium	1 each	10
Banana, medium	1 each	22
Cantaloupe	1 cup	27
Orange	1 each	19
Vegetables		
Potato, baked	1 each	115
Tomato	1 each	30
Green peas, frozen	1/2 cup	69
Dairy Products		
Milk, whole	1 cup	227
Cheese	1 oz	200–250
Egg, large	1 each	86
Nuts		
Peanuts, almonds, walnuts	1 cup	520–730
Peanut butter	2 tbs	103
Beverages		
Colas	1 can	44–62
Colas, diet	1 can	27–39

from meat, poultry, fish, grains, and legumes (176). However, the bioavailability of phosphorus from whole foods varies with the food source and meal content.

Beverages, Including Milk and Soda

The important, relatively low-phosphorus food of animal origin is human milk. In newborns, who cannot respond to the stimulus of low calcium levels by increasing PTH output, this is a perfect food. One liter of human milk contains 150 to 175 mg of phosphorus, or 25 mg per 100 kcal. In contrast, each liter of cow's milk provides 1,000 mg of phosphorus, or 150 mg per 100 kcal. This is an excessive load of phosphorus for a newborn and tends to reduce the serum calcium level by increasing the serum phosphorus level. Colas and diet colas contain approximately 30 to 60 mg of phosphorus per can, and it has been suggested that high phosphorus intake with low calcium intake can contribute to low bone mass and fractures, especially in children (79). However, soft drink intake is linked with lower BMD in girls only and just for non-cola and diet drinks, not the sodas with the highest phosphorus content (179). Thus, the outcome may be related to displacement of other beverages (e.g., milk), and not to phosphorus intake. A dietary calcium:phosphorus intake of approximately 1.5 to 2.0:1 on a molar basis is a common recommendation, but its clinical value is unproven (79).

Grains and Cereals

A major source of phosphorus in grains and cereals is inositol hexaphosphoric acid, or phytic acid. Calcium, zinc, and magnesium phytates are insoluble and are excreted in the stool. During leavening and baking of bread, some of the phosphorus from phytic acid is converted to orthophosphate by the action of phytases, so that some of the phosphorus is absorbed. However, in countries where unleavened wheat is used, the phytate content of grain products is increased. If the intake of calcium and vitamin D is also limited, calcium deficiency may develop partly as a consequence of excess dietary phytate.

Unseen Sources

Phosphorus is present in many dietary supplements or prescription or OTC medications, and in food additives as well (176). Phosphorus-containing additives are also used in processing of many foods, ranging from baked goods and reconstituted meats to cola beverages. The exact content varies as the processing of new products develops, so food lists do not contain fast foods, or if they do, the P content may not be accurate. Phosphate salts are a component of many medications for treating hypertension, diabetes, and anemia, and are included in others, such as Tums, Crestor, Vocodin, Zithromax, Viagra, and Zoloft (176).

Assessment

Phosphorus is well absorbed from the intestine, and the plasma level is carefully regulated by the tubular reabsorption of phosphate. In addition, the movement of phosphorus across cell membranes is rapid and responds to alterations in metabolic activity (e.g., glucose utilization). Thus, neither plasma phosphate nor urinary excretion of phosphate reflects intake or body stores. Abnormal plasma levels can reflect real changes in body stores, but more often they reflect altered renal or metabolic activity.

Plasma Phosphate

The usual serum assay measures the colored ammonium phosphomolybdate complex. Specimens collected with EDTA or citrate are not acceptable because these compounds interfere with the color reaction of the assay. Hemolysis must be avoided because red cells have a high phosphate content. The normal level is 0.81 to 1.29 mmol per L (25 to 45 mg per L) in adults, 1.2 to 2.23 mmol per L (37 to 69 mg per L) in children, and 1.6 to 2.1 mmol per L (50 to 65 mg per L) in infants (59). An assay of fasting serum inorganic phosphate levels is important for meaningful interpretation. The interpretation of serum levels is difficult because many factors influence the phosphorus concentration. The rapid infusion of glucose or insulin can lower levels. In starvation, tissue catabolism releases phosphate, and plasma levels are maintained. When the starving patient is refed, it is essential to provide adequate phosphorus because serum levels can fall precipitously. Table 7-29 lists the major causes of altered plasma phosphate concentrations.

Urinary Phosphate

The average phosphorus excretion rate in the United States is 600 to 800 mg per day, reflecting a mean intake of 1,500 mg per day for men and 1,000 mg per day for women (178). With phosphate depletion, urinary excretion falls to nearly zero. Urinary phosphate varies with intake, but cannot be used to estimate intake because it is regulated largely by PTH. However, in the appropriate setting, a low urinary excretion rate can confirm a clinically suspected low dietary intake. Levels above 1,300 mg per day are considered high and reflect high intake. A nomogram has been constructed based on the fasting serum phosphate concentration and the fractional excretion of urinary phosphate, normalized for the glomerular filtration (179). When hypophosphatemia is present, a TmP/GFR value less than 0.7 mmol per L suggests inadequate renal phosphate reabsorption. A normal PTH level rules out hyperparathyroidism of any cause.

Physiology

Absorption

Dietary phosphorus is absorbed as the inorganic form and as a component of phosphoproteins, phosphosugars, and phospholipids. In cow's milk, the phosphorus is 70% inorganic, but in cereals and soft tissues of animals, it is largely organic. All the phosphorus must be liberated by phosphatases on the enterocyte brush border and in biliary secretions before absorption can take place. Net absorption is 65% to 75% from cow's milk but exceeds 80% from human milk. In adults and older children ingesting a mixed diet, absorption varies from 58% to 70% and is proportional to intake at all levels of ingestion. Alkaline phosphatase is quite resistant to damage in most diseases of the small bowel; thus, phosphate maldigestion is uncommon. Fecal output

TABLE 7-29 Causes of Altered Plasma Phosphate Levels

Condition	Mechanism
Hypophosphatemia	
Increased urinary excretion	PTH-dependent causes: hyperparathyroidism FGF23-dependent causes: tumor-induced osteomalacia, X-linked autosomal dominant or recessive forms of hypophosphatemia PTH- and FGF23-independent causes: alcoholism, drugs or toxins, renal tubular acidosis, Fanconi syndrome, hereditary hypophosphatemic rickets, decreased replacement on IV therapy
Decreased intestinal absorption	Vitamin D deficiency, dietary phosphorus restriction (severe), antacid abuse (phosphate binding), chronic diarrhea
Phosphate compartmentalization	Rapid shift of phosphate between body compartments, TPN, recovery from diabetic ketoacidosis, respiratory alkalosis, sepsis, refeeding syndrome, hormonal therapy (insulin, glucagon, corticosteroids), carbohydrate infusion (glucose, fructose, lactate)
Hyperphosphatemia	
Increased exogenous load	Feeding cow's milk to premature infants, IV infusion, oral supplements, vitamin D toxicity, phosphate enemas
Increased endogenous load	Hemolysis, lactic acidosis, respiratory acidosis, rhabdomyolysis
Decreased urinary excretion	Renal failure, hypoparathyroidism, acromegaly, vitamin D toxicity, bisphosphonate therapy, magnesium deficiency
False (pseudo) hyperphosphatemia	Hemolysis in vitro, hypertriglyceridemia, multiple myeloma

IV, intravenous; TPN, total parenteral nutrition; PTH, parathormone; FGF, fibroblast growth factor.

of phosphorus is not greater than intake—that is, no obligatory loss occurs in the gut. Digestive juices provide about 200 mg per day in adults. However, because two-thirds of luminal phosphorus is absorbed and the kidney can adjust phosphate excretion over a wide range, deficiency of phosphate from malabsorption rarely occurs.

Absorption is predominantly by passive diffusion. At low levels of phosphorus intake, active sodium-dependent transport (via the NPT2b transporter) is controlled by 1,25-dihydroxyvitamin D_3 (178). Because of the negative charge on phosphate and paracellular channels, simple diffusion between cells is unlikely. Efflux of phosphate across the basolateral membrane of the enterocyte is probably passive. Absorption is probably stimulated to some extent by vitamin D and perhaps by PTH. Although malabsorption of phosphorus can occur in vitamin D deficiency, sufficient phosphorus is usually absorbed to satisfy daily needs because dietary intake is high and absorption is fairly high, even when somewhat impaired.

Urinary Excretion

Plasma phosphate is derived from input from the intestine and bone. Unlike that of calcium and magnesium, the daily flux of phosphorus to and from bone, the major store of body phosphorus (85%), is quite small. This flux approximates 200 mg per day (3 mg per kg). Plasma levels are regulated mainly via the kidney. There are at least five sodium-dependent phosphate cotransporters (Table 7-30) (180). The type 1 cotransporter is an anion carrier that is not specific for phosphate. The type 2 transporter (encoded by the *SLC34A1* gene) is the major regulator in the renal proximal tubule. The main factor influencing tubular reabsorption of phosphate is PTH.

TABLE 7-30 Sodium-Dependent Phosphate Cotransporters

Parameter	NPT1	NPT2a	NPT2b	NPT2c	NPT3
Pi affinity	5–10 nM	0.1–.2 mM	0.05 mM	0.1–0.2 mM	0.025 mM
Na$^+$ affinity	50–60 mM	50–70 mM	33 mM	50 mM	40–50 mM
Localization	Kidney, liver	Kidney, lung	Gut, lung	Kidney	Kidney, others
Regulators	Glucose,	[Pi]s, PTH, insulin, glucagon	[Pi]s GH, 1,25-(OH)$_2$ vitamin D	[Pi]s	[Pi]s

GH, growth hormone; Pi, inorganic phosphate; PTH, parathormone.
Data from Takeda E, Yamamoto H, Nashiki K, et al. Inorganic phosphate homeostasis and the role of dietary phosphorus. *J Cell Mol Med.* 2004;8:191.

However, plasma phosphate levels do not regulate the secretion of PTH, but rather FGF23 secretion (see below). It is the calcium level that secondarily regulates phosphate levels. Other hormones—for example, thyroid and growth hormone, estrogens, calcitonin, and vitamin D—all influence plasma phosphate, but much less so than PTH does. Finally, phosphorus moves rapidly across cell membranes via NPT1 in response to requirements for intracellular phosphorus and available energy to form high-energy phosphate bonds. During phosphate depletion, the kidney becomes relatively resistant to the phosphaturic effects of PTH (159).

The NPT2b and c cotransporters are encoded by the *SLC34A2* and *SLC34A3* genes, respectively (180). The type 3 cotransporter system is comprised of two transporters, sodium-dependent transporter 1 (PiT1) and PiT2, encoded by the genes *SLC20A1* and *SLC20A2*, respectively. In the kidney NPT2a, NPT2c, and PiT2 are expressed at the apical domain, but most phosphate is transported by NPT2a. The expression of these transporters is reduced by PTH and fibroblast growth factor 23 (FGF-23). The sodium–hydrogen exchanger regulatory factor 1 (HHERF1) binds to the PTH type 1 receptor (PTH1R) and to NPT2a, thus modifying cAMP production induced by PTH in the proximal tubule. FGF-23 binds to its own receptor (FGFR1) in a complex with α-KLOTHO, the latter expressed only in the distal tubular cells.

Studies of inherited disorders have led to the discovery of two genes that regulate the sodium-dependent phosphate transporters, PHEX (phosphate-regulating gene with homologies to endopeptidase-1 on the X chromosome) and DMP1 (dentin matrix protein1) that are expressed in bone, and stimulate FGF-23 from bone (116a). PHEX is mutated in X-linked hypophosphatemic rickets, and encodes an endopeptidase expressed in bone and teeth, but not in kidney (178).

Phosphate Homeostasis

Phosphate homeostasis is mainly regulated by the relationship between absorbed phosphorus, plasma inorganic phosphate, and urinary phosphate. Absorbed phosphorus and urinary phosphorus rise with increased intake. Thus, at any given phosphorus intake, the individual adjusts the plasma phosphate to the level at which phosphorus influx into plasma and excretion into the urine are equal. FGF-23 expression in bone is increased by an increase in dietary phosphate (Pi) intake, and by 1,25(OH)2D, and is downregulated by the phosphate-regulating gene, *PHEX* (181). FGF23 acts on the renal tubules by binding to its receptor (FGFR1) and the coreceptor klotho, to a) inhibit renal phosphate reabsorption, b) decrease 1,25(OH)2D production in response to phosphate levels and perhaps by inhibition of 1α-hydroxylase and/or 24-hydroxylase, and c) inhibit PTH secretion by the parathyroid glands. The net effect of these actions is to decrease serum phosphate levels and increase serum 1,25(OH)2D levels, actions that in turn will enhance intestinal absorption of phosphate and stimulate FGF23 synthesis and secretion. Polymorphisms in the tissue-nonspecific alkaline phosphatase gene (encoding liver AP) have been associated with BMD, suggesting that the rate limiting step in phosphate absorption may also play a role in this homeostatic system (182).

The workup of abnormal fasting serum phosphate levels (especially low levels) should include 25OHD, 1,25(OH)2D, and possible FGF23 levels, as the latter are becoming more widely available clinically (183). It is not clear yet whether measuring soluble α-klotho concentrations in serum will add to the differential diagnosis of hypophosphatemia.

Function

Phosphorus is important for all cells; 80% to 85% of phosphorus is in the bone. The rest is important for energy production (adenosine triphosphate), phospholipid formation, nucleotide formation, buffering systems, and calcium homeostasis.

Deficiency

Causes

Most patients who manifest clinical evidence of hypophosphatemia have an underlying wasting disease (184,185). Acute phosphate depletion results from rapid transfer of the ion from extra- to intracellular fluid, or from extensive gastrointestinal loss. Chronic phosphate depletion occurs both with high serum calcium (hyperparathyroidism) or normal serum calcium (increased bone avidity in metastatic disease, diuretic use, renal tubular disease, and hyperphosphaturia from other causes). The common wasting diseases include intestinal malabsorption, malnutrition, cancer, and chronic alcoholism. Recovery from severe burns is also associated with hypophosphatemia. Other causes are listed in Table 7-29.

Hypophosphatemia at the onset of ketoacidosis probably indicates severe depletion. Multiple genes have been related to renal phosphate reabsorption, and include phosphate-regulating genes with homologies to endopeptidases on the X chromosome (*PHEX*), with fibroblast growth factor 23 (FGF-23), and the overproduction of FGF-23 and other proteins (matrix extracellular phosphoglycoprotein, MEPE, and frizzled-related protein 4, FRP-4) that increase in tumor-induced osteomalacia (186).

Clinical Manifestations

Hypophosphatemia

Clinical manifestations occur when plasma phosphorus levels fall less than 0.32 mmol per L (10 mg per L). Proximal myopathy and ileus may be the initial symptoms. Severe depletion can be manifested by hemolytic anemia (Pi <0.5 mg per dL), rhabdomyolysis (Pi <1.0 mg per dL), and a variety of complications in less severe depletion (Pi, 1.0 to 1.5 mg per dL). These include impaired chemotaxis, platelet dysfunction, metabolic encephalopathy, metabolic acidosis, peripheral neuropathy, central nervous system dysfunction including seizures, cardiac failure, osteomalacia, and decreased glucose utilization (187). A decrease in Pi leads to decreased levels of 2,3-diphosphogluconate (2,3-DPG), an altered affinity of oxygen for hemoglobin, and tissue anoxia. Renal loss of phosphate is often responsible for clinical phosphate deficiency. In an adult with a plasma phosphate level of 3.5 mg per dL and a GFR of 125 mL per minute, filtered phosphate amounts to 6,300 mg per 24 hour. With an intake of 1,500 mg of phosphorus and 60% intestinal absorption (900 mg), reabsorption of 5,400 mg or 85% of the filtered load is required. In renal tubular disease, loss of phosphate can lead to depletion, evidenced by muscle weakness, malaise, and anorexia. Ingestion of large amounts of aluminum hydroxide or calcium salts can lead to phosphate depletion, even in patients with normal kidneys. Such ingestion causes depletion more rapidly when malabsorption is present.

Hyperphosphatemia

Excess phosphate has been linked to the production of tissue damage, leading to CV disease, osteoporosis, and aspects of renal failure (188). A high-phosphate diet can lead to increased PTH production via FGF23 secretion, and bone loss. This sequence has been postulated to produce vascular calcification, and endothelial dysfunction (189). Moreover, decreased 1,25(OH)2D levels resulting from elevated phosphate might produce decreased cardiac contractility and myocardial fibrosis. Elevated tissue Pi levels (and accompanying decreased calcium levels) can increase oxidative stress in cells, and is also associated with fatigue (190). It is important to recognize that casual serum Pi levels may not detect an increase, as the levels vary during the day, so AM fasting levels are usually used. In patients with chronic renal disease, higher levels of phosphorus and mortality have been linked (191). Because of this increased risk, as well as to maintain normal serum calcium levels, phosphate binders are used in patients with chronic renal failure and hyperphosphatemia. These binders include anion exchangers (Sevelmer), lanthanum, magnesium salts, and calcium salts (189). These are reasonably effective, but produce gastrointestinal side effects, as well as increasing the risk for hypercalcemia and hypermagnesemia.

Another cause of hyperphosphatemia is the tumor lysis syndrome that occurs during treatment of hematologic malignancies (sometimes spontaneously), most often in Hodgkin's lymphoma and acute leukemia. It is a potential emergency, and results from release of cell contents into the bloodstream (192). The hyperphosphatemia is not isolated, occurring with increases in uric acid and potassium, and with hypocalcemia. Adverse clinical results include renal failure, cardiac arrhythmias, seizures, and sometimes death from multiple organ failure. Treatment is mostly preventive for at-risk patients, providing low-intensity initial treatment, adequate hydration and limiting potassium intake, but phosphate removal by dialysis is sometimes needed.

Treatment

Mild to Moderate Hypophosphatemia

Mild to moderate hypophosphatemia (15 to 25 mg per L) can be managed without supplemental phosphorus by treating the underlying disorder. When levels fall to 0.32 to 0.48 mmol per L (10 to 15 mg per L) or risk factors for phosphorus depletion are present, replacement is advised with oral supplements—either milk or other oral preparations. Usually, a dosage of 1,000 mg per day corrects phosphorus depletion. Cow's milk contains about 1 mg of phosphorus per mL and is an excellent replacement fluid. Oral supplements as tablets of sodium or potassium phosphate can be given at a dosage of 2 to 3 g per day, and contain 8 mmol of phosphorus/packet (193). Neutrophos (250 mg of phosphorus with 7 mEq of sodium and potassium per capsule) or Phospho-Soda (129 mg of phosphorus with 4.8 mEq of sodium per mL) is used most commonly. Uro-KP-Neutral and K-Phos-Neutral tablets also contain 250 mg of phosphorus and only 1 mEq of potassium with 250 to 300 mg of sodium. The usual dose is two capsules of Neutrophos or 5 mL of Phospho-Soda given two or three times a day. Oral therapy is limited by the production of diarrhea. These supplements should be used with caution if sodium or potassium restriction is required, because they contain significant amounts of these cations.

Antacids that contain magnesium, calcium, or aluminum can bind phosphate and prevent its absorption. When hypophosphatemia is caused in this way, it can be corrected simply by stopping the antacids. Sometimes, the binding properties of phosphate itself can be used for treatment. Calcium phosphate binds unconjugated bilirubin and has been used to supplement phototherapy in patients with Crigler-Najjar type I disease (194).

Hypophosphatemia occurs commonly in patients receiving specialized nutrition support, and replacement with phosphate is often recommended for treatment. A weight-related protocol is safe and efficacious, especially in critically ill patients (195). For patients with serum phosphorus of 0.73 to 0.06 mmol per L, treatment consists of 0.32 mmol per kg (low dose) intravenously; with phosphorus of 0.51 to 0.72 mmol per L, 0.64 mmol per kg (moderate dose) is used, and with phosphorus of ≤0.5 mmol per L, 1 mmol per kg is used (high dose). Patients with serum potassium less than 4 mmol per L receive potassium phosphate, and with higher potassium levels, sodium phosphate is used.

Severe Hypophosphatemia

Severe hypophosphatemia (<0.32 mmol per L, or <1 mg per dL) with symptoms should always be treated with IV phosphorus. One cause of such severe hypophosphatemia is the refeeding syndrome, but other causes include systemic alkalosis, alcoholism, surgery, sepsis, diabetic ketoacidosis (especially after insulin therapy), cirrhosis, and chronic obstructive pulmonary disease (196). IV therapy carries a risk of hypocalcemia and should be used with caution. Commercial solutions are mixtures of monobasic and dibasic sodium or potassium salts and provide 3 mmol of phosphate per mL. To avoid confusion, one should always order in terms of millimoles (mmol) of phosphorus. Initially, the dose should be 0.3 mmol of elemental phosphorus per kg of body weight given over 4 to 6 hours in normal saline solution. If the creatinine clearance is below 50 mL per minute, this dose should be reduced by half. Other protocols suggest 0.08 mg per kg over 8 hours, or 15 mmol of sodium phosphate over 2 hours (196). After serum phosphate and calcium have been checked, subsequent therapy depends on the response. To avoid hypocalcemia or sodium or potassium overload, the dosage of 0.3 mmol per kg of body weight every 6 to 8 hours should not be exceeded. These values must be viewed only as rough guidelines because severe hypophosphatemia may develop with normal body stores of phosphorus. Because phosphate infusion can cause hypocalcemia, IV phosphate should not be used when hypocalcemia is present. Also, calcium and phosphate should not be used in the same IV infusion to avoid precipitation. When renal insufficiency is present, great caution must be exercised in administering Pi by any route. However, the growing shortage of available phosphate preparations for IV use should make the use of oral phosphate replacement the routine for all but the most severe cases of hypophosphatemia (193). IV fat emulsions contain 15 mmol per L of phosphorus as egg phospholipids, but these are not sufficient to treat severe symptomatic hypophosphatemia.

Toxicity

Hyperphosphatemia develops in patients with renal insufficiency and a marked decrease in GFR. Secondary hyperparathyroidism can ensue with skeletal demineralization. The UL has been set at 4 g per day for adults up to age 70, and at 3 g for those older than 70 years (69). Treatment entails a low intake of phosphate and ingestion of phosphate binders—aluminum hydroxide, calcium carbonate, or sevelamer hydrochloride (Renagel) (189). Calcium carbonate is preferred initially because it is more palatable and is a more effective antacid in treating the duodenal inflammation commonly associated with chronic renal failure. It is not possible to eliminate dietary phosphorus completely because it is ubiquitous. However, a low phosphorus intake can be achieved and is important in the successful management of chronic renal disease (see Chapter 13).

Oral phosphate preparations (e.g., Fleet Phospho-Soda, Visicol) are now widely used for bowel cleansing prior to colonoscopy (197). Hyperphosphatemia and hypocalcemia have been reported, leading to an FDA alert for increased risk in patients with congestive heart failure, colitis, ileus, and those with limited ability to take adequate liquid during the preparation (198). The FDA suggests checking baseline and posttreatment electrolytes, especially if greater than 45 mL of oral sodium phosphate is used per 24 hours. The FDA has also issued an alert for acute phosphate nephropathy, a form of acute renal failure, associated with the use of oral sodium phosphate preparations used for bowel cleansing, and these preparations now carry a black box warning (http://www.fda.gov/drugs/drugsafety/postmarketdrugsafetyinformationforpatientsandproviders/ucm126084.htm). Individuals at risk for this complication include those with advanced age, with kidney disease, with decreased intravascular volume, and those using medicines that might affect renal perfusion, such as diuretics, ACE inhibitors, angiotensin receptor blockers, and NSAIDs.

Sulfate

Sulfur is the eighth most abundant element by mass in the human body. Inorganic sulfate is present in foods and water, but the major source for human nutrition derives from biodegradation of body protein (4). Thus, the "requirement" is dependent upon the dietary availability and half-life in the body of sulfur-containing amino acids (methionine, cysteine). Daily intake is about 2.8 g per day of inorganic sulfate from these sources. Drinking water contains less than 500 mg per L, largely because concentrations greater than 250 mg per L have an intolerable odor. This source provides approximately 17% and food approximately 19% of daily intake (2). Sulfur-reducing bacteria are common colonic organisms, and the resulting hydrogen sulfide has been the subject of much debate in terms of its role in colonic health (199). In the body, 3'-phosphoadenosine-5'-phosphosulfate is a precursor for the biosynthesis of many sulfated compounds, including keratans, chondroitins, and heparans. Sulfate is absorbed from the intestine by a sodium-dependent active process; greater than 80% is bioavailable as sodium or potassium sulfate. The apical membrane anion transporter NaS1 (*SLC13A1*) and the basolateral membrane transporter Sat1 (*SLC26A1*) mediate sulfate absorption in the intestine and reabsorption in the proximal tubule, thus regulating blood sulfate levels (200). Knockout of NaS1 in mice produces hyposulfatemia, and altered metabolism, growth, reproductive capability, gut physiology, and liver detoxification. Sat1-null mice show abnormalities in sulfate and oxalate metabolism, leading to hyperoxalemia and calcium oxalate urolithiasis, as well as hyposulfatemia and hypersulfaturia (200). These animal models may allow recognition of a human deficiency state, but thus far no convincing phenotype for sulfate deficiency has been reported. A syndrome of relative sulfate deficiency has been reported in undernourished children with edema (201). These children have low plasma concentrations of methionine and cysteine, and reduced synthesis of glutathione. Whether these are findings related to sulfate deficiency or more reflect protein malnutrition is not clear. Other claims for an association of sulfate deficiency with coronary heart disease and other metabolic disorders have not been substantiated at this time.

TRACE MINERALS
Iron
Requirement
Iron is stored mostly in functional compartments, so negative iron balance creates physiologic deficits once the small storage forms are depleted. Iron in the body is found mostly in hemoglobin (62% for men, 70% for women), and in myoglobin (10%). The major storage form, ferritin, contains 16% of iron in men, and 10% in women, while hemosiderin accounts for 5% to 8% of total body iron (202). Smaller amounts of iron (<2% of the body's total) are found in heme and non-heme enzymes and on the transport iron protein, transferrin. Unlike those of other minerals, iron stores are not regulated by increased or decreased excretion. Moreover, approximately 90% of daily iron needs are supplied endogenously from the breakdown of circulating red blood cells (203). The major control mechanism is intestinal absorption, which increases during iron deficiency.

Daily Losses
In the normal person, iron requirements are determined by the limited and fixed amount of iron excreted. Daily losses are through the gastrointestinal tract, skin, and urine; additional iron is lost from the uterus in women. Fecal iron averages from 6 to 16 mg per day, most of which is unabsorbed dietary iron. Endogenous losses from cells amount to 0.1 to 0.2 mg, and blood loss accounts for 0.3 mg. Biliary secretion is 1 mg per day, but only about 0.20 mg is excreted in the stool. Urinary losses are 0.1 to 0.3 mg per day. Dermal losses in sweat, hair, and nails range from 0.2 to 0.4 mg per day. Total daily losses range from 0.9 to 1.4 mg in males. Additional menstrual losses in women amount to 0.5 to 1.0 mg per day when averaged over a whole month.

Rate of Absorption
Iron requirements are estimated from the daily losses, and an assumption is based on the amount absorbed from food. The Food and Nutrition Board of the National Research Council and the WHO assume absorption of 10% to 15% provided the percentage of calories from animal sources containing heme iron is high, as it is in industrialized nations.

Recommended Dietary Allowance
Requirements per kilogram of body weight are highest in infancy (because of low iron stores), during periods of rapid growth, and during menstruation and pregnancy. Table 7-31 outlines the requirements and recommended allowances for iron at various stages. The Standing Committee on the Scientific Evaluation of DRIs has now assigned an RDA for males of all age groups and for postmenopausal women of 8 mg per day, and for premenopausal women of 18 mg per day (204). During pregnancy, the recommended intake is 27 mg. At birth, the placental supply of iron is replaced by the diet. Even the infant of an iron-deficient mother has normal iron stores at birth. Iron treatment during pregnancy is most beneficial to the mother because the infant has priority for available iron. Milk is a poor source of iron, but the AI for infants 0 to 6 months of age is based on the daily amount in ingested milk (~ 0.35 mg per L). Because it is assumed that milk intake and requirements are correlated with body size, the AI may not be adequate for all infants, especially those with a lower intake. In the first 6 to 8 weeks of life, the hemoglobin level falls to 10 mg per dL because increased erythropoiesis is required for oxygen delivery to tissues. Extramedullary hematopoiesis also decreases in this period. During the second 6 to 8 weeks of life, erythropoiesis increases, and the hemoglobin level rises to 12.5 mg per dL. In the third 6 to 8 weeks after birth, the dependency on dietary iron increases secondary to growth. The RDA for infants 7 to 12 months of age assumes that by 6 months, feedings complementary to milk are in place. It is at this time during infancy that extra iron is most needed, so that iron deficiency usually occurs at ages 6 to 24 months rather than earlier. Premature infants have decreased stores at birth and use their reserves faster during the growth spurt at 3 to 6 months of age. During

TABLE 7-31 Dietary Reference Intakes of Iron for Individuals

Life Stage Group	Iron (mg/d)
Infants	
0–6 months	0.27[a]
7–12 months	11
Children	
1–3 years	7
4–8 years	11
Males	
9–13 years	8
14–18 years	11
19–>70 years	8
Females	
9–13 years	8
14–18 years	15
19–50 years	18
51–>70 years	8
Pregnancy	
14–50 years	27
Lactation	
14–18 years	10
19–50 years	9

[a]Estimates based on adequate intake (AI). Other values are recommended dietary allowances (RDAs).
Data from Standing Committee on the Scientific Evaluation of Dietary Reference Intakes, Food and Nutrition Board, Institute of Medicine. *Dietary Reference Intakes for Vitamin A, Vitamin K, Arsenic, Boron, Chromium, Copper, Iodine, Iron, Manganese, Molybdenum, Nickel, Silicon, Vanadium, and Zinc.* Washington, DC: National Academies Press, 2002.

adolescence, the hemoglobin level rises 0.5 to 1.0 mg per dL per year. For this reason, adolescents require 50 to 100 mg of iron per year, or a total of about 300 mg during adolescence.

Food Sources

The iron bioavailability from mixed diets in industrialized countries is approximately 14% to 18%, but from vegetarian diets somewhat less (5% to 12%) (205). However, it is not clear how these figures (derived from WHO/FAO recommendations) were determined. Dietary iron is available in a variety of nuts and seeds and in red meat and egg yolks (Table 7-32). About 40% of the iron from these sources is heme iron, absorbed with about 15% to 45% efficiency. This accounts for 7% to 12% of dietary iron in the United States. Milk products, along with potatoes and fresh fruit, are poor in iron. Nonheme iron is absorbed with only about 1% to 15% efficiency. Vegetable iron content varies greatly according to the growing conditions of plants. Many sources of iron, especially inorganic salts and vegetable iron, are not well absorbed without ascorbic acid to reduce ferric to ferrous iron. However, continual ingestion of grams of vitamin C daily can interfere with copper absorption. The sources of nonheme iron often contain unidentified ascorbic acid (e.g., in meat, poultry, and fish), often in the form of erythorbic acid, an ascorbic acid derivative, which is used as an antioxidant (205). Other food enhancers of iron absorption include a factor in meat (as yet unidentified), and possibly nondigestible dietary carbohydrates. Organic acids (malic, ascorbic, citric) are found widely in foods and enhance absorption. Amino acids from protein, particularly cysteine and histidine, also enhance absorption.

Inhibitors are also present in natural and processed foods (e.g., tannic acid in tea; phytates (inositol phosphates) in whole grains and legumes; polyphenols in tea, coffee, and red wine; calcium in dairy products or tofu; and zinc in multimineral preparations). Inositol phosphates with 3 or fewer phosphate groups are inactive as inhibitors, so removal of these phosphates by phytases is one approach to improving bioavailability (205). The phytate/iron molar ratio is

TABLE 7-32 Iron Content of Selected Foods

Food	Portion	Iron Content (mg)	% of RDI (18 mg for females)[a]
Breads and Cereals			
White bread	1 slice	0.7	1–5
Hamburger bun	1 each	0.8	1–5
Saltines	4 each	0.5	1–5
Rice, cooked	1 cup	2.26	10–24
Oatmeal, cooked	1 cup	1.59	5–10
Bran flakes, 40%	1/2 cup	6.2	25–39
Spaghetti noodles, cooked (enriched)	1 cup	1.96	5–10
Bagel, enriched	1	1.2	2–5
Meat and Fish			
Beef, lamb, veal	3 oz	2.4–2.6	10–24
Beef liver	3 oz	5.34	25–39
Chicken, white meat roasted	3 oz	0.91	1–5
Fish, cooked	3 oz	0.5–1.0	1–5
Pork, ham	3 oz	0.6–0.8	1–5
Shrimp, boiled	3 oz	2.6	10–24
Sliced meats	1 piece	0.32–0.46	1–5
Vegetables			
Spinach, cooked fresh	1 cup	6.42	25–39
Green beans, frozen	1 cup	1.11	5–12
Peas, frozen	1 cup	2.5	10–24
Potato, baked	1 each	2.75	10–24
Tomato	1 each	0.5	1–5
Dried legumes	1 cup	4–5	10–24
Other vegetables	1 cup	0.8–1.2	5–12
Fruits			
Strawberries	1 cup	0.57	1–5
Apples	1 each	0.25	1–5
Bananas	1 each	0.35	1–5
Orange, small	1 each	0.14	1–5
Apricots, dried	16 halves	2.6	10–24
Dairy Products			
Milk, whole	1 cup	0.12	1–5
Cheese	1 oz	0.3	1–5
Eggs, large	1 each	0.72	1–5
Nuts			
Peanuts, pecans, almonds	1 cup	3.3–5.0	25–39
Peanut butter	1 cup	4.3	25–39
Soy Products/Meat Substitutes			
Tofu, raw, regular	~4 oz	6.65	25–39
Veggie burger	~3.4 oz	3.89	10–24
Soy burger	~3.4 oz	1.44	5–10

RDI, recommended dietary intake.
[a] ~5% bioavailable from nonheme sources, but % is variable, so % of RDI is based on total iron content.

much more important than polyphenol content in determining bioavailability (206). Treatment of the grains by soaking will reduce phytate content, and drying will activate phytases (207). Thus, it is difficult to assess the iron bioavailability from individual sources of grains (in which phytate content is high), but high phytate content remains a source of iron deficiency in infants who ingest a cereal- or legume-based diet (208). Zinc absorption is also inhibited by phytates, but zinc itself decreases nonheme iron bioavailability in humans (209). This interaction further complicates the estimation of iron availability from grains and legumes. Other inhibitors include soy protein, egg, EDTA, and phosphate salts (210). Calcium is often added to bread products and orange juice. EDTA is added to many foods to prevent oxidation and color changes. In addition, the use of antacids, histamine$_2$ receptor antagonists, or proton pump inhibitors decreases gastric acid secretion and impairs the absorption of inorganic iron. Another potential mechanism for inhibition of food iron utilization from the intestinal lumen is competition with bacteria. Bacterial mechanisms for binding and using iron include uptake directly from heme, transferrin, or lactoferrin, or acquiring iron through small secreted ferric-specific chelators called siderophores (211). Presumably, most of this competition occurs in the colonic lumen, but may occur more proximally if bacteria are present in large enough numbers.

Food Preparation and Supplements

Food preparation is important, especially for nonheme iron. Boiling can decrease the iron content of vegetables by 20%, and milling can decrease the iron content of grains by 70% to 80%. Availability of heme iron is much less dependent upon food preparation, but intake of heme iron is relatively limited in many populations. For these reasons, iron supplements and/or fortification are used to improve iron supply in the diet. Many iron supplements are available commercially in the United States. Approved forms considered safe (GRAS) include ferric salts (phosphate, pyrophosphate), ferrous salts (gluconate, lactate, sulfate), and reduced iron. Forms that are allowed but are non-GRAS include sodium iron EDTA, iron amino acid chelates, and carbonyl iron (68). Supplement use comprises a considerable portion of iron intake in the United States, according to the NHANES III. It may be necessary to ingest a sufficient excess of supplemental iron (e.g., >4 × DRI of 8 mg for males) in order to increase body stores (212).

Food Fortification

The iron content of some foods (e.g., grain products) is enhanced by fortification. Compounds recommended for fortification by the WHO include ferrous sulfate or fumarate, ferric pyrophosphate, and electrolytic iron powder. Many cereal foods, however, are fortified with elemental iron powders, which are even less bioavailable sources of iron (207). Iron-fortified infant formulas and cereals have been widely used, usually with iron sulfate or gluconate. They should contain 4 to 12 mg of iron per L to prevent deficiency. However, some of the iron salts used for fortification (ferric orthophosphate and pyrophosphate) are absorbed less well than other forms of nonheme iron in the diet. Vegetarians are at risk for iron deficiency because of limited iron availability. Moreover, when the basic diet has low iron bioavailability, use of iron-fortified foods has a limited effect on iron status (213). Iron fortification is provided for staple cereals such as wheat, rice, and maize, especially in countries in which these grains form a major part of the diet (68). Many well-absorbed iron salts are reactive in foods, causing lipid peroxidation and color change, and thus cannot be used. The United States mandates iron fortification of wheat flour at the level of 44 mg per kg; in the United Kingdom, the level is 16.5 mg per kg.

Intake

Average intake in the United States is 15 mg on a 2,500-kcal diet. The iron content of foods is fairly constant, about 6 mg per 1,000 kcal. Heme iron is relatively well absorbed, and the absorption of heme iron is not affected by the composition of the diet. However, heme iron accounts for only 1 to 3 mg per day in the diet. Nonheme iron is less available, and its absorption is influenced by dietary components (e.g., ascorbic acid). Besides the "classical" factors that affect iron absorption noted above, other food additives (e.g., caseinophosphopeptides, fructooligosaccharides) also affect iron bioavailability (214). Baked goods account for 20% of iron intake in the United States, which is usually added in the form of ferric orthophosphate or sodium acid sulfate salts. The amount of iron in fortified cereals may exceed the amount listed in the label by

100%, although its bioavailability may be rather low (215). The USDA Food Consumption Survey (1989 to 1991) showed that average diets meet or exceed the RDAs for all life stage groups, except 1- to 2-year-old children (91% of RDA) and women ages 12 to 49 years (75% of RDA). It is not surprising that these two groups are most at risk for dietary iron deficiency.

Breast milk contains only 0.3 mg per L and cow's milk 0.5 mg per L. Thus, only about 0.25 to 0.85 mg of iron is supplied by milk. If this is the only food source for no more than 3 months, deficiency will not develop. About 50% of iron in breast milk is absorbed, compared with less than 10% of formula iron. Thus, breast milk can be an important source of iron even though the content is low. Iron is added to other infant foods. Electrolytic iron is added to dry cereal at 10 times the normal grain content (45 mg per 100 g). This form of iron has a small particle size with a large surface area, but it is not clear how much is absorbed. During the first year of life, it is wise also to provide a meat source of iron to ensure good absorption. Iron deficiency can occur if the iron in enriched foods is poorly absorbed (fortified cereals) and can be avoided if the iron in iron-poor foods is well absorbed (breast milk, vegetables with ascorbic acid). Table 7-32 lists the iron content of selected foods.

Estimated Iron Absorption

An average of 40% of total iron in animal tissues is heme iron; all the rest in the diet is nonheme iron. Thus, in any meal, one calculates the amount of iron from meat, poultry, or fish, multiplies that number by 0.4, and assumes 23% absorption for the heme iron. For the remainder of the iron, 8% absorption is assumed if adequate ascorbic acid (>75 mg per meal) is present. Otherwise, 5% absorption is assumed for an ascorbate intake of 25 to 75 mg, and 3% absorption if less ascorbic acid is ingested (204). On this basis, meals can be categorized according to whether the iron content is of low, medium, or high availability. A low-availability meal provides less than 30 g of meat, poultry, or fish and less than 25 mg of ascorbate. A medium-availability meal provides 30 to 90 g of meat or 25 to 75 mg of ascorbic acid with adequate nonheme iron. A high-availability meal provides more than 90 g of meat or more than 75 mg of ascorbic acid with adequate nonheme iron, or 30 to 90 g of meat plus 25 to 75 mg of ascorbate and nonheme iron.

Estimates of the available iron in average diets change with age. From infancy to adulthood, dietary iron increases from 3 to 18 mg for males and to 11 mg for females. The available dietary iron is 50 μg per kg of body weight in infancy, 72 μg per kg of body weight in childhood, and 45 μg per kg of body weight in adolescence, falling to 39 μg per kg of body weight for adult men and 27 μg per kg of body weight for adult women. Because of the many factors that influence iron absorption, it is not surprising that there is a poor correlation in elderly (nongrowing) patients and iron intake (216). In such situations, a search for gastrointestinal disease or other sources of iron depletion should be pursued.

Assessment

Because iron absorption is so inefficient and excretion is not regulated, none of the routinely available tests reflect intake but rather assess body stores. They are all used to determine whether iron deficiency or overload syndromes are present. However, the tests for iron deficiency can be especially difficult to interpret. The separation of iron deficiency from anemia of chronic disease is a troubling aspect of nutritional management. A major problem in diagnosis is that iron deficiency often develops slowly, so that the detection of deficiency depends on the stage of iron depletion (217). Moreover, when chronic inflammation is present, iron cannot be mobilized from stores, and the clinical and laboratory presentation can look very similar to that seen when body stores of iron are deficient. Thus, no single test is sufficient. In addition, the tests vary in sensitivity. Table 7-33 outlines the various tests available, and highlights the distinction between iron deficiency and the anemia of chronic inflammation (218,219).

Hemoglobin

About 60% to 65% of total body iron is in hemoglobin, 4.5% in myoglobin, 10% in nonheme enzymes, and about 30% in storage (ferritin, hemosiderin). Only a small amount (~0.15%) is in transport (transferrin) or in cytochromes and other heme enzymes (0.2%). Because the size of the iron pool is related largely to hemoglobin, the size of the total pool varies with body size (and blood volume) and sex, and males have more hemoglobin than females. Table 7-34 lists

TABLE 7-33   Assessment of Functional Body Iron Status

Measurement	Diagnostic Use	Reference Range (adults)
Functional Iron		
Hemoglobin	Assess severity of anemia	13–18 g/dL (M); 12–16 (F)
Red cell indices	Reduced when iron supply or incorporation into Hb is low	MCV 80–94 µm^3; MCH 27–32 g/L
RBC zinc protoporphyrin	↓ Protoporphyrin and ↓ RBC ferritin indicate low iron supply to marrow	<70 µg/dL RBC
RBC ferritin	"	
Serum transferrin receptor	↓ in early iron deficiency when erythropoiesis increases; especially useful when ferritin is normal. Can increase suspicion of anemia of chronic inflammation, when normal or somewhat low, but can be elevated when erythropoiesis is increased by factors other than iron stores	3–40 attograms/cell 4–8.5 mg/L
Tissue Iron Supply		
Serum iron	Transit compartment, change rapidly	10–30 µmol/L
Serum transferrin	↓ in iron deficiency	47–70 µmol/L
Transferrin saturation	↓ in deficiency if transferrin is high, ↓ in iron overload	16%–60%
Iron Stores		
Serum ferritin	↓ in deficiency, low normal value is indeterminate in anemia of chronic disease	15–300 µg/L
Response to EPO	If storage iron cannot be used, anemia will respond	NA
Tissue iron	↓ in deficiency, normal in anemia of chronic disease	3–33 µmol/g of dry weight of liver

EPO, erythropoietin; MCH, mean corpuscular hemoglobin; MCV, mean corpuscular volume; RBC, red blood cell.
Data from Wormwood M. The laboratory assessment of iron status—an update. *Clin Chim Acta.* 1997;259:3; Weiss G, Goodnough LT. Anemia of chronic disease. *N Engl J Med.* 2005;352:1011.

TABLE 7-34   Normal Values for Hemoglobin and Mean Corpuscular Volume

	Hemoglobin (mg/dL)		MCV (µm^3)	
Age (years)	Median	Lower Limit	Median	Lower Limit
0.5–1.9	12.5	11	77	70
2–4	12.5	11	79	73
5–7	13	11.5	81	75
8–11	13.5	12	83	76
12–14 (females)	13.5	12	85	78
12–14 (males)	14	12.5	84	77
15–17 (females)	14	12	86	79
Adults (females)	14.5	12	87	80
Adults (males)	15.5	14	88	80

the median values and lower limits for hemoglobin and mean corpuscular volume. Other causes of both a low hemoglobin level and a low mean corpuscular volume include anemia of chronic inflammation and heterozygous thalassemia trait. The red cell distribution width is usually high (>14.5%) in iron deficiency and tends to be normal in heterozygous thalassemia, but high values are also associated with other conditions, so that red cell distribution width is a poor diagnostic tool for iron deficiency. However, falling values are an early manifestation of a response to oral iron supplementation.

Serum Iron

Analysis is based on the formation of a colored complex of ferrous iron and dye (69). Hemolysis interferes with the assay, as does EDTA, citrate, or gross lipemia (>1,000 mg per dL). Serum iron is largely bound to transferrin, a β-globulin with a molecular weight of 80 kDa. Two iron molecules are bound per mole of protein. At any time, 4 to 6 mg of transferrin-bound iron is present in plasma, and transferrin in plasma has the capacity to bind 25 to 30 mg. However, 25 mg of iron passes each day from the reticuloendothelial cells to the plasma, where it is turned over at a rate of 50% hourly. Therefore, the measurement of serum iron is inherently unstable. The daily coefficient of variation can be 30% in the same person. A diurnal variation is seen, with morning values about 30% higher than those in the evening. The value decreases before the menstrual cycle and is increased by the use of oral contraceptives because of progesterone. By the seventh month of pregnancy, the serum iron level reaches a nadir because of dilution and the mobilization of storage iron to the fetus.

The normal serum iron level in newborns is 150 to 250 μg per dL. This falls in the first few days and then rises again to 130 μg per dL by 2 weeks. In the infant who is not given supplemental iron, the level falls to 80 μg per dL by 6 to 12 months and probably reflects iron deficiency. Normal adult levels range from 65 to 200 μg per dL, with values in men slightly higher than those in women. Mean values for males are 100 ± 35 μg per dL (mean ± SD); for females, they are 90 ± 40 μg per dL.

Low iron levels are associated with blood loss, chronic illness and infection, malignancy, and chronic skin disease. The serum iron level is high when outflow from the plasma is decreased, as in aplastic anemia, and when inflow into the plasma is increased, as in megaloblastic anemia with inefficient erythropoiesis. Lysis of cells (hemolytic anemia, acute hepatitis) raises the serum iron level. None of these causes is correlated with increases in body iron stores. In hemochromatosis, alcoholic liver disease, and porphyria cutanea tarda, the increase in body stores is reflected in an elevated serum iron level.

Transferrin

Transferrin is made in the liver and has a half-life of 8 days in plasma. The coefficient of variation is only 8%, less than that for iron. Normal levels for males are 350 ± 50 μg per dL; for females, they are 380 ± 70 μg per dL. Each 500 mL of whole blood contains about 250 μg of iron not incorporated into hemoglobin; most of this is bound to transferrin.

In pregnancy, levels of transferrin can rise to 400 μg per dL because of the action of progesterone. In infants, the transferrin level is lower, 250 μg per dL (range, 180 to 320 μg per dL). Thus, in infancy, the serum iron level is higher, but the transferrin level is lower than in the adult. Transferrin levels are increased during iron deficiency, also during pregnancy even in the absence of iron deficiency. Transferrin levels are decreased by chronic disease, protein deficiency, and hepatic impairment. The usual interpretation of iron and of transferrin levels is based on combined values and the percentage saturation noted, in addition to the individual values.

Other iron-binding proteins are also altered by acute and/or chronic inflammation, usually because they are acute-phase reactants (220). Ceruloplasmin increases 30% to 60%, and haptoglobin can increase 2 to 5 fold. Lactoferrin is elevated by a different mechanism (release from granulocytes in acute infection) and can increase 2 to 5 fold. Soluble transferrin receptors do not usually change unless iron deficiency is present, making this measurement a useful differentiating biomarker (see below).

Free Erythrocyte Protoporphyrin

When iron is deficient, protoporphyrins cannot be utilized for heme synthesis and gradually increase during 2 to 3 weeks. They are usually, but not always, elevated (221). Free erythrocyte protoporphyrin levels are often elevated early in iron deficiency, often before anemia develops (>1.24 µmol per L of red blood cells). However, levels rise in most disorders associated with inefficient heme synthesis (e.g., anemia of chronic disease, sideroblastic anemias), so that these increases are nonspecific.

Ferritin

Ferritin is the major storage form of iron in the liver, spleen, and bone marrow (222). It also protects cells from high concentrations of free iron, which can be toxic. Each molecule has 24 subunits, at least two of which are immunologically distinct. Each ferritin complex, with a molecular weight of 450 kDa, has a capacity to bind 2,000 iron molecules or release them in the presence of reducing agents. The source of serum ferritin is unknown but is probably the reticuloendothelial cells. Normally, only very small amounts of apoferritin leak into the serum. The distribution of normal ferritin is skewed to the higher values. Males have larger stores of iron, a finding reflected in their serum ferritin levels. Serum levels reflect reticuloendothelial stores, a compartment that is increased in infection or chronic disease.

Serum ferritin levels are proportional to marrow iron and inversely proportional to transferrin levels, suggesting that ferritin levels reflect iron stores. One microgram of ferritin is equivalent to about 8 mg of storage iron, or 120 µg per kg of body weight. Values rise after birth as the destruction of fetal hemoglobin increases stores. Ferritin levels fall later in childhood as adult hemoglobin is produced. Median concentrations of ferritin are about 40 and 170 ng per mL in young women and men, respectively. In anemic, iron-deficient patients, the mean level is less than 10 ng per mL (women) and 15 ng per mL (men).

Iron deficiency and decreased stores are associated with levels less than 15 ng per mL in adult men, and with levels below 10 ng per mL in women. However, these values are present only about half the time (Table 7-35). The value for diagnosis depends on the stage of iron deficiency, with values in later anemic states falling below 10 ng per mL. Iron overload in patients with hemochromatosis or undergoing transfusion is often associated with high ferritin levels. However, acute liver damage or endogenous ferritin production by tumors elevates ferritin levels without an increase in body iron stores.

Ferritin is a positive acute-phase protein that is elevated in the presence of inflammation, infectious or not. Moreover, cell damage in inflammatory diseases is also associated with falsely high ferritin values. When iron deficiency is combined with reticuloendothelial cell destruction in chronic inflammation, serum ferritin levels are normal and do not reflect true body stores. When iron deficiency is not yet accompanied by anemia (i.e., subclinical), but acute/subacute inflammatory conditions are present, the ferritin values can be "corrected" by examining the ratio of ferritin levels to those of two other acute-phase proteins, C-reactive protein (CRP) and α1-acid glycoprotein (AGP). Using cutoff values of greater than 5 mg per L for CRP and greater than 1 g per L for AGP, ferritin was 30%, 90%, and 36% higher in comparison during the incubation, early convalescence, and late convalescent periods (223). These data from 32 studies suggested a correction factor for ferritin of 0.77, 0.53, and 0.75 in those three clinical periods.

TABLE 7-35 Diagnostic Use of The Serum Ferritin Test

Serum Ferritin (ng/mL)	Interpretation	Iron-Deficiency Anemia Present (%)	Absent (%)	Likelihood Ratio (present/absent)
<15	Very positive	59	1.1	52
15–34	Moderately positive	22	4.5	4.8
35–64	Nondiagnostic	10	10	1.0
65–94	Moderately negative	3.7	9.5	0.39
>95	Very negative	0.9	75	0.08

Data from Sackett DL, Richardson WS, Rosenberg W, et al. *Evidence-based Medicine*. New York: Churchill Livingstone, 1997:124.

Whether the correction factor for late convalescence will be useful prospectively for patients with chronic inflammatory conditions is not yet clear.

Serum ferritin levels can be abnormal as soon as a lack of iron is detected in bone marrow, but a cutoff value of less than 15 ng per mL is not sufficiently sensitive (Table 7-35). The likelihood of iron deficiency in patients with values between 15 and 34 ng per mL is still nearly 5%, and iron deficiency can be present even with higher values. Patients with iron deficiency and ferritin values above 15 mmol per L may be at an early stage of deficiency, or they may have a chronic inflammatory condition that raises the level of serum ferritin, an acute-phase reactant protein. In such cases, values of serum ferritin about twice those in Table 7-35 may be of the same diagnostic significance. Because the "gray" area for serum ferritin is so large (between 15 and 100 mmol per L), it is logical to combine serum ferritin with other measures of the severity of disease. Several tests have been used, none with complete success. The most promising is the soluble plasma transferrin receptor (sTfR), or the ratio of soluble transferrin receptor to the log of serum ferritin (219).

Serum ferritin can be elevated in hereditary hemochromatosis, when transferrin saturation is high, but it can also be elevated when transferrin saturation is normal or only slightly modified (224). The L-ferritin gene is mutated in the hereditary hyperferritinemia cataract syndrome without iron overload presenting with congenital cataracts. The ferroportin I gene is mutated commonly with iron overload predominantly in endothelial cells, and is an important form of dominant hereditary iron overload that may explain the condition known as "African hemochromatosis," and was supposed to be associated with consumption of beer prepared in lead containers. The ceruloplasmin gene is mutated rarely in Japanese families, presenting with late onset of neurologic symptoms with hyperferritinemia and aceruloplasminemia (224).

Soluble Plasma Transferrin Receptor

The plasma protein is a truncated form of the membrane receptor (lacking its first 100 amino acids) that is present as a transferrin receptor (TfR)–transferrin complex (225). The TfR number on the cell surface is a reflection of the iron status, increasing as deficiency develops. Marrow erythropoietic activity in erythroblasts, not reticulocytes, is the most important determinant of sTfR concentrations, so levels are decreased when marrow activity is low (anemia of chronic inflammation) and high when erythropoiesis is stimulated (hemolysis, ineffective erythropoiesis). Normal values average 5.0 ± 1.0 mg per L, but because of the lack of an international standard, there is considerable variation from lab to lab. The sTfR levels correlate best with Hb levels among all the other tests of iron status. Iron status influences sTfR, in that iron deficiency elevates serum levels fivefold to eightfold. Iron overload lowers sTfR, but only by approximately 20%. Thus, the test can be very useful in the patient with iron deficiency with inflammation in whom the serum ferritin levels are normal and sTfR levels are high. The lack of elevation of sTfR suggests anemia of chronic inflammation, but this diagnosis cannot be made with quite the same degree of confidence. This is because sTfR is a marker of erythropoiesis only when iron stores are adequate and available, and is a marker of iron status only when there is tissue iron deficiency. The log transformation of the ferritin value has been suggested as part of a ratio of TfR/log ferritin (TfR–F index) to normalize TfR values in patients with chronic inflammation (225,226). This increases specificity but not sensitivity for the diagnosis of iron deficiency. sTfR can be normal when iron is deficient, if cytokine production suppresses erythropoiesis. Conversely, levels can be high if erythropoiesis is stimulated by factors other than iron status. sTfR is also a marker of erythroid response to recombinant human erythropoietin (rHuEPO), so it does not help identify the etiology of the anemia. Finally, sTfR can be elevated in erythroid and nonerythroid malignancies, and in myelofibrosis. It remains to be seen whether this (or any related) measure is robust in repeated studies.

Hepcidin

Hepcidin is a protein synthesized in the liver that inhibits iron export from enterocytes and macrophages (see Physiology section below). Thus, it has been considered a promising biomarker for iron status in difficult patient groups (infants, chronic renal disease). Serum hepcidin (as the mature form, hepcidin-25) can be measured reproducibly by mass spectrometry, radioimmunoassay (RIA), and enzyme-linked immunosorbent assays (ELISA) (227). However, method harmonization is needed between these methods. The major problem with the usefulness of hepcidin is that it, like ferritin, is an acute-phase reactant, so its value has thus far been limited

(228). In patients with IBD, serum hepcidin is low (<2 nM) when serum ferritin was indeterminate (100 to 200 ng per mL), thus allowing a diagnosis of iron deficiency (229). In other clinical settings (e.g., obesity) serum hepcidin is elevated in the face of iron deficiency, suggesting more response to chronic inflammation than to iron status (230). With time, serum hepcidin may become a useful biomarker for iron deficiency in selected populations, but it is too early to make recommendations about its usefulness.

Direct Methods for Assessing Iron Stores

Iron stores can be assessed directly by three means: phlebotomy, marrow staining, and liver biopsy.

Phlebotomy

If 500 mL is removed per week until the hemoglobin remains below 10 mg per dL for 2 weeks without further bleeding, it can be assumed that iron deficiency has been achieved. The red cell deficit can then be calculated from the hemoglobin content (each 1-g decrease in hemoglobin per dL corresponds to a total loss of about 100 mg of iron). Addition to the red cell deficit of 2 mg per day for absorbed iron gives an estimate of the mobilizable storage iron. Normal values in the United States range from 600 to 900 mg for males and from 200 to 300 mg for females. This method is used only when iron overload is present and treated by phlebotomy.

Marrow Staining

Marrow staining is a qualitative method that distinguishes low iron stores in iron deficiency from other conditions in which stores are normal. In such conditions, low serum measurements of iron deficiency can be caused by chronic disease or a decreased release of iron from the tissues. Marrow staining is not a reliable method for assessing iron overload in hemochromatosis, in which marrow iron is normal.

Liver Biopsy

The normal hepatic iron concentration is 70 to 100 µg per g of dry liver weight. In adults, values in hemochromatosis are consistently in excess of 5 g. With values below 70 µg of iron per g of liver, iron staining is scanty and stores are low.

Response to Therapy

The response to therapy is sometimes the best diagnostic approach when iron deficiency occurs in chronic inflammation and test results are indeterminate. Interpretation of the response can be complicated in patients with intestinal disease because oral iron may be poorly absorbed. In some cases, it is appropriate to use IV iron (see below) or erythropoietin (218,219).

The response to rHuEPO has revealed a new phenotype of iron deficiency in such patients. Iron stores and serum ferritin levels are often normal or elevated, transferrin saturation is often (but not always) below 20%, and mean red cell indices are normal. Such patients may have adequate storage iron, but cannot mobilize it rapidly enough to mount a sustained hemoglobin response. In these cases, IV iron may be needed to achieve a good response and reduce the amount of erythropoietin needed (226).

Summary of Assessment

Iron deficiency is usually suggested when anemia is present, although evidence for deficient stores can be found before anemia develops. Iron depletion is progressive, so that the test values diagnostic of deficiency may change during progression from depletion of iron stores without anemia to deficiency with anemia. The best screening test is the serum ferritin level because the only cause of a low value is a decrease in iron stores (2,319). Values less than 15 ng per mL confirm iron deficiency in the presence of anemia, but values between 15 and 100 ng per mL also can indicate deficiency in patients with chronic inflammation. Determinations of serum iron and binding capacity are often ordered at the same time, and if the results are consistent, these help to confirm inadequate iron stores. When iron-binding capacity was elevated, 78% of patients were iron-deficient, but only 26% were deficient when a low transferrin saturation was the parameter used (232). Low serum iron and low binding capacity are the best indicators of anemia associated with chronic inflammation. How to proceed when ferritin values are between 35 and 100 ng per mL is not certain, but the soluble TfR may be the next best test to perform (219). An elevated red cell distribution width may be helpful in monitoring response

TABLE 7-36	Summary of Changes in Serum Concentrations of Markers of Iron Status					
Iron Status	Serum Concentrations of					Ratio
	Hb	Iron	Transferrin	Ferritin	sTfR	sTfR/Log Ferritin
IDA	↓	↓	↑	↓	↑	↑↑ (>2)
AOI	↓	↓	↓-N	N-↑	N	N (<1)
IDA + AOI	↓	↓	↓-N	↑	N-↑	↑ (>2)

sTfR, soluble transferrin receptor; Hb, hemoglobin; IDA, iron deficiency anemia; AOI, anemia of inflammation
Data from Northrop-Clewes CA. The interpretation of indications of iron status during an acute phase response. http://www.who.int/nutrition/publications/micronutrient/anaemia-iron-deficiency/9789241596107.annex4.pdf.

to therapy but does not discriminate very well in detecting iron deficiency (233). If confusion still exists, because of the many factors that affect the results of these assays, staining of a bone marrow aspirate can provide a direct measure of iron stores. Histologic staining for iron is only semiquantitative, but is good enough to distinguish iron deficiency from disorders of iron metabolism in which tissue iron is normal. Sometimes, the iron status is not clear, even after all tests are completed, and the response to therapy must be used. Table 7-36 summarizes the changes in serum concentrations of biomarkers of iron status in iron-deficiency anemia (IDA), anemia of inflammation, or when both conditions are present.

Screening for Iron Deficiency and Overload
The tests available now for iron deficiency can also be used to screen for hereditary hemochromatosis (234,235). In addition, genotyping can be performed to detect the typical C282Y mutation of the hemochromatosis gene, *HFE*. Table 7-37 summarizes the strategies available for screening populations for iron-related disorders. Transferrin saturation and serum ferritin levels remain the "standard" approach, but genotyping for C282Y homozygosity is often performed, particularly in family members of probands, as the test can identify iron overload even in the absence of clinical disease. Adult genetic hemochromatosis is mostly related to mutations of the HFE gene (C282Y and H63D), but is rarely associated with mutations of the TFR2 gene (224). Juvenile hemochromatosis is rare, and related to mutations in the HJV gene for hemojuvelin and the HAMP gene encoding for hepcidin.

Physiology
Iron exchange functions as a closed system, moving from plasma transferrin to red blood and tissue cells, from red blood cells to macrophages, and from macrophages back to plasma transferrin (aspects of iron metabolism can be viewed at http://www.irontherapy.org). Iron is involved in many reactions: as a redox cofactor for nonheme enzymes (iron–sulfur protein and metalloflavoproteins); as a required cofactor for nonoxidative enzymes (aconitase, ribonucleotide reductase); as a component of heme enzymes involved in electron transport (cytochromes); and as a major constituent of heme as an oxygen-carrying cofactor (hemoglobin, myoglobin). Iron is absorbed differently depending on whether it is ingested as heme (1.5 to 3 mg per day) or in vegetables and nuts (15 to 20 mg per day). The inorganic or nonheme iron is affected by gastric pH and by other salts in the lumen. Heme iron is not affected by luminal factors and is absorbed intact, bound to a putative "heme receptor" on the brush border or intercalated directly into the membrane. Inside the mucosal cell, hydrolysis by heme oxygenase, a microsomal enzyme, liberates free iron. Iron absorption by this route is very efficient (20% to 40%), depending on the state of total body iron stores. When anemia is present, absorption rates are higher. Iron either enters the body or is deposited as ferritin in the mucosal cell. The signal for iron absorption is probably not mucosal ferritin itself, which is increased when the rate of absorption is low. Mucosal ferritin may provide a mechanism of iron excretion into the lumen when the cell is exfoliated.

Iron Loss
Although the term *iron stores* usually refers to those tissues that contain ferritin and hemosiderin (e.g., liver, spleen), most of the iron in the body is in tissues that require it for function (red blood cells, marrow, muscle). It is also from these functional tissues that iron is lost. Iron can be

TABLE 7-37 Screening Strategies for Iron Deficiency and Hemochromatosis

Parameter	Phenotypic	Phenotypic/ Genotypic	Genotypic/ Phenotypic
Iron Deficiency			
Initial tests	Hb, Tfr saturation, ferritin		
Secondary tests	RBC protoporphyrin, sTfR, marrow stain, response to therapy		
Genetic Hemochromatosis			
Initial test	Tfr saturation (>50 for men, >45 for women), ferritin (>300 µg/L for men, >200 for women)	Tfr saturation, ferritin	C282Y mutation
Secondary test	Repeat Tfr saturation and ferritin	C282Y mutation	Ferritin, Tfr saturation
Liver biopsy needed or phlebotomy needed	Yes, hepatic iron ≥ 5,000 µg/g dry weight, 3–4+ iron staining	No	No
	> 4 g of iron removed	No	No
Detects all genetic hemochromatosis	No	No	Yes
Detects noniron overloaded hemochromatosis	No	No	Yes

Tfr, transferrin; Hb, hemoglobin; sTfR, soluble transferrin receptor; RBC, red blood cell.
Data from Adams PC. Population screening for hemochromatosis. *Hepatology*. 1999;29:1324; Whitlock EP, Garlitz BA, Harris EL, et al. Screening for hereditary hemochromatosis: a systematic review for the U.S. Preventive Services Task Force. *Ann Intern Med*. 2006;145:209.

lost through bleeding because red blood cells contain most of the iron of the body (2,750 mg in 70-kg males and 2,180 mg in females). Bone marrow and muscle contain 610 and 520 mg, respectively, in the two sexes.

Red Blood Cell Production

Only 25 to 30 mg of iron (or 0.5% of a total store of 4 g) is needed for new red cell production each day (236). This iron comes from the marrow. Only about 5 mg of iron is mobilized per day from storage tissues (liver, spleen), and such mobilization does not provide a rapid buffering for when acute iron loss occurs due to bleeding (about 250 mg of hemoglobin iron per 500 mL of blood) (237).

Absorption and Body Stores

When the size of the iron body pool is decreased, iron absorption increases (238). As much as 5 mg of iron (20% to 30% of intake) can be absorbed each day. When stores are normal (~4 to 5 g in adults), absorption varies from 1 mg in males to 2 to 3 mg in premenopausal women and matches daily iron losses. Iron overload occurs because excretory capacity is limited. In hemochromatosis, iron absorption is paradoxically elevated. Alcoholics may absorb excess iron from iron complexes in alcoholic beverages and by both paracellular and normal mechanisms.

Factors Affecting Absorption

Iron is absorbed most efficiently in the upper small intestine, especially the duodenum. Gastric acid, hydrogen ions from a reducing agent such as ascorbic acid, or a brush border ferrireductase, Dcytb, is needed to reduce nonheme ferric ions to the ferrous form, which is much better absorbed (239,240). Organic acids (citric, lactic) and amino acids (histidine, lysine, cysteine) form chelates with iron that enhance absorption. Disease or bypass of the proximal small bowel decreases absorption of both heme and nonheme iron. The presence of phytates in grains and of phosphates decreases nonheme iron absorption (241). Inorganic zinc can inhibit the uptake of iron. Humans are unique among mammals in the relatively small amount of dietary iron that is available for absorption and the limited loss of iron from the body.

Heme iron is iron-protoporphyrin IX that is released by digestion from myoglobin. The heme is transported into enterocytes by PCFT/HCP1 (*SLC46A1*), a member of the solute carrier family of membrane proteins (242,243). This protein also functions as the folate transporter. Heme oxygenase releases iron from the absorbed heme, although the exact mechanism by which these components make contact is not known (244). There are two heme exporter proteins in the basolateral membrane, BCRP (breast cancer resistance protein) and FLVCR (feline leukemia virus, subgroup C receptor), providing a mechanism whereby heme may cross the enterocyte intact before being exported into the serum. The major transmembrane iron transporter for nonheme iron absorption is natural resistance-associated macrophage protein 2 (nramp2), now called *divalent metal ion transporter 1* (DMT1) (239). DMT1 is related to nramp1, which is involved in host resistance to intracellular pathogen. DMT1 is expressed mostly in the apical brush border of the duodenal epithelium, especially the crypts. Expression is markedly increased in diet-induced iron deficiency, which suggests that it is regulated by iron status. An inverse relationship has been found between DMT1 and serum ferritin in normal persons, but not in patients with hereditary hemochromatosis (245). DMT1 also distributes iron from the surface within the red cell cytoplasm, and thus loss of function leads to ineffective erythropoiesis and accumulation of hepatic iron. Ferric iron must be reduced to the ferrous form, either by luminal factors, such as ascorbic acid, or within the cell by duodenal cytochrome b (Dcytb). It is then transferred to the basolateral export protein, ferroportin-1 (FPN1), as is all intracellular free iron, regardless of its mode of entry (246).

The third major mechanism for iron absorption is via nonheme ferritin, found in legumes and meat. This large protein–iron complex is relatively resistant to proteolysis, and is absorbed by clathrin-dependent receptor endocytosis, although the receptor has not been identified (244). The protein in the absorbed complex is degraded inside the enterocyte, liberating the iron.

With such a complex system of absorption, it is not surprising that large variations have been observed in the mean absorption of nonheme iron, ranging from 0.7% to 22.9% (247). Absorption was higher when enhancers were used, but the variation was still considerable. Iron status was also a major confounding factor.

Oxidation and Transport of Absorbed Iron

The ferroxidase reaction converts ferrous to ferric ion. This conversion is catalyzed by ceruloplasmin in the serum or by its membrane-bound homologue, hephaestin (248). When the reaction occurs in serum, the ferric ion is incorporated into apotransferrin, although the mechanism for this capture is not clear. Another ferroxidase that is different from ceruloplasmin is also found in serum. This circulating form of iron is not toxic, as it is unable to generate free radicals. Iron is brought from storage forms as ferritin in the ferric (Fe^{+++}) form. The release of iron from ferritin occurs via a ferritin reductase system.

Transferrin delivers iron to the cells via two types of plasma membrane TfR (248). Both receptors bind diferric transferrin and deliver the complex via endocytosis in clathrin-coated pits into specialized endosomes. Inside the cell, iron regulatory proteins (IRPs) bind to iron regulatory elements (IREs) located in the untranslated portions of the TfR mRNA. The hemochromatosis protein HFE is a membrane protein that binds to TfR1 and reduces the affinity of transferrin to its receptor. Transferrins can bind two ferric ions with a high affinity. Although iron is the major metal bound with high affinity at neutral pH, 36 other metals have been shown to bind to one or both of the metal-binding sites of transferrin (248).

Transcellular Iron Transport

The mechanism by which iron is released from transferrin involves receptor-mediated endocytosis (239) and release in acidic vesicles when iron–transferrin complexes are involved. Once inside the red cell, ferrous iron is incorporated into the protoporphyrin of hemoglobin by a ferrochelatase. When the red cell dies after about 120 days, the iron in hemoglobin is oxidized and methemoglobin is formed. The iron is reused for hemoglobin synthesis or stored as the ferric ion. High intracellular iron levels downregulate ferritin synthesis via an iron-responsive element-binding protein (90 kDa) that depresses translation (249). The movement of iron across the basolateral membrane is mediated by ferroportin I along with the iron oxidase hephaestin (240,242). The activity of ferroportin I is regulated by the liver β-defensin-like peptide, hepcidin (250). Hepcidin has antimicrobial activity and regulates intestinal iron absorption and macrophage iron release negatively. Thus, it reduces the amount of iron available to bacteria, and it affects them directly. Its effect on reducing iron absorption and increasing macrophage stores is a secondary action that has a marked effect on iron homeostasis. The hemojuvelin (HJV), TfR2, and the hemochromatosis gene (HFE) are involved in regulating hepcidin synthesis, but the precise pathways are unclear (250). Hepcidin synthesis is downregulated by low iron concentration, by anemia, and by hypoxia. Hepcidin is correlated inversely with DMT1, Dcytb, and ferroportin I expression, and it causes internalization of ferroportin I, leading to decreased cellular iron efflux. When proinflammatory cytokines are elevated, hepcidin synthesis increases. Iron is kept within cells, helping to create the situation seen in anemia of chronic inflammation, when normal iron stores and decreased erythropoiesis are largely driven by inflammatory cytokines.

The sensing of iron status and downstream signaling is complex, but fairly well understood. Hepcidin is the major iron regulator that inhibits not only absorption, but also release from the liver and the macrophage system by interfering with iron export from cells by ferroportin (251). In fact, most forms of hereditary hemochromocytosis are due to hepcidin deficiency (252). In types 1,2, and 3 hepcidin upregulation does not occur, and so iron absorption continues. The binding capacity of Tf is then exceeded, and iron accumulates in the tissue. The expression of hepatic hepcidin is modulated by a variety of proteins, including HJV, bone morphogenetic protein 6 (BMP6), TfR2, hereditary hemochromatosis protein (HFE), and Tf (253). The sensing of iron deficiency also depends upon matriptase-2, which cleaves HJV, thereby decreasing hepcidin expression (254). In iron deficiency, hypoxia-inducible factor-2α (HIF-2α) in the enterocyte activates the transcription of DMT1 and Dcytb to increase nonheme iron absorption.

The cellular metabolism of iron utilizes a large number of proteins involved not only in uptake, export, and storage, but also in intracellular trafficking (251,255). The latter proteins include ATP binding cassette family members B6,7, and 10, but also mitoferrin-1, glutaredoxin 3, and frataxin. Mitochondrial activity is very important in the formation of iron–sulfur clusters that chaperone iron (251). IRPs (IRP1 and 2) alter mRNAs posttranscriptionally (255). Poly (rC)-binding proteins cal also act as iron chaperones to target protein–protein interactions involving nonheme enzymes (256).

The importance of HIF in iron regulation has been realized. When oxygen or iron levels are low, the prolyl hydroxylases that degrade HIF are inhibited, allowing HIF to transactivate target genes, among which are TfR1 and DMT1, which promote iron uptake (257). Moreover, ferrochelatase, which facilitates iron incorporation into heme, is also enhanced. Regulation of HIF degradation involves several proteins. The factor inhibiting HIF (FIH), itself an iron-dependent enzyme, hydroxylates HIF, reducing its transcriptional activity (258). The von Hippel-Lindau tumor suppressor protein (VHL) then binds to the hydroxylated HIF, which targets HIF for degradation by a multiprotein ubiquitin ligase complex.

Deficiency

Iron deficiency is characterized mainly by symptoms of anemia—weakness and pallor. In addition, other signs and symptoms are caused by iron deficiency alone: angular stomatitis, atrophic lingual papillae, and koilonychia. Iron deficiency in children is associated with anorexia, decreased resistance to infection, decreased growth, and reversible protein-losing enteropathy. In the absence of anemia in children, iron deficiency can have deleterious effects on behavior and cognitive functions (259). The tests used to diagnose iron deficiency vary according to the stage of the deficiency. Table 7-38 outlines the predictive value of such tests.

Increased Utilization

Iron deficiency is common in children 6 to 24 months old because of increased need and limited body stores. These patients are at risk for developing impaired intellect, although the degree of

TABLE 7-38 Predictive Values of Laboratory Tests in Different Stages of Iron Deficiency

	Stage of Iron Deficiency[a]			
	I	II	III	IV
Test	(Predictive value, %)			
Bone marrow iron stain	100	100	100	100
Serum ferritin (µg/L)	100	100	100	100
Zinc protoporphyrin (µmol/mol of heme)	0	100	100	100
Transferrin saturation (%)	0	71	78	96
Hemoglobin (g/L)	0	0	100	100
MCV (µm^3)	0	0	22	100
MCH (pg)	0	0	33	100

[a]The prevalence rates of patients presenting in each stage of deficiency are about 24%, 23%, 15%, and 38%, respectively, for stages I through IV.
Data from Hastka J, Lassere JJ, Schwarzbeck A, et al. Laboratory tests of iron status: correlation or common sense? *Clin Chem.* 1996;42:5.

impairment is not closely correlated with anemia (260). Thus, treatment with iron until body stores are fully repleted is often justified.

Blood Loss
In premenopausal women, anemia is caused by blood loss during menstruation. Iron deficiency in an adult or adolescent male or a postmenopausal woman frequently signifies blood loss from the body, usually from the gastrointestinal tract. Each unit of blood contains approximately 250 mg of elemental iron.

Inadequate Intake
Iron deficiency is often associated with ingestion of foods in which iron bioavailability is low. It is also associated with other vitamin and mineral deficiencies, most notably with folic acid deficiency in pregnancy and intestinal disease and with zinc deficiency in children that produces anemia, dwarfism, and hypogonadism (261). Iron is no longer included in home total parenteral nutrition (TPN) formulations, so IDA can develop in patients on long-term home TPN (262). Small regular amounts of iron (10 to 75 mg on any given day) are recommended according to estimated daily loss.

Malabsorption
Another significant cause of iron deficiency is malabsorption, either in mucosal disease (celiac disease, atrophic gastritis), or after bypass of the proximal bowel, as in subtotal gastrectomy with gastrojejunostomy, or in patients with short duodenal residence time, such as short-bowel syndrome (263).

Gastrointestinal Loss
The GI tract is the major site of extra-physiologic iron loss in men and in postmenopausal women. Increased blood loss can occur from any organ from mouth to anus. IBD can produce anemia either from blood loss or from marrow suppression due to chronic inflammation, or both (264). The use of PPIs does not necessarily prevent the development of IDA; anemia cannot be ruled out as a consequence of PPI use, although this explanation seems less likely (265).

In IBD, IV iron provides a more consistent response than oral iron, and is at least as well tolerated. It is indicated when there is intolerance to or failure of oral iron, severe anemia that requires rapid repletion of iron stores, and when erythropoietin is needed to overcome the anemia of chronic inflammation (266).

Iron Deficiency in Other Medical Conditions
Patients with chronic heart failure develop iron deficiency, presumably from slow blood loss, although IL-6 is elevated in this condition, and this cytokine stimulates hepcidin production,

while downregulating the expression of ferroprotein 1, preventing the release of iron from body stores (267). Iron deficiency in the elderly may be due to either decreased intake or increased slow GI loss, or both. Anemia in chronic renal failure is usually related to low production of erythropoietin and not to iron deficiency per se. Anemia is common in patients with cancer, although IDA accounts for only a portion of the total, and is usually related to blood loss. Response to erythropoiesis-stimulating agents often suggests iron deficiency, but detection of IDA before treatment can be difficult (268). Iron plays a role in learning and memory in early life, presumably by an effect on developing hippocampal neurons (269). It is not clear whether iron deficiency plays any role in memory loss late in life. The use of iron therapy to treat fatigue in nonanemic patients has been an area of controversy. However, at least one study shows that when evidence of iron deficiency was clear (ferritin concentration <15 ng per mL) in nonanemic women, fatigue responded to the use of IV iron (270).

Restless Leg Syndrome

Iron deficiency can occur with or without anemia, especially in elderly patients with this syndrome, a sleep disorder associated with unpleasant leg sensations (271). Brain acquisition of iron appears to be impaired, perhaps by neuromelanin cells (272). Local brain deficiency may be more important than total body stores of iron, however, because low CSF ferritin levels have been reported, and brain MRI studies have reported low iron levels in the substantia nigra and putamen in patients with severe restless leg syndrome (RLS) (273). An abnormality in brain iron metabolism may explain why the association with iron deficiency is not tight, and also why treatment is not persistently effective. The American Academy of Sleep Medicine Clinical Practice Guideline (2012) finds no evidence for iron supplementation in the treatment of RLS, except occasionally in patients with documented iron deficiency or RLS refractory to other treatments (274).

Iron-refractory Iron-deficiency Anemia

This condition is an autosomal recessive disorder in which patients are unresponsive to oral iron, but partially responsive to parenteral iron. Iron-refractory IDA (IRIDA) is due to mutations in the *TMPRSS6* gene, which encodes matriptase-2, a protease that cleaves HJV, thus downregulating hepcidin production (275). IRIDA shares features (low MCV, low Tf saturation, low ferritin) with other disorders associated with overproduction of hepcidin, such as the anemia of chronic inflammation. When there is no response to oral iron, and no evidence for a chronic inflammatory condition, and response to parenteral iron, one should consider the presence of malabsorption or request genetic testing.

Treatment

Oral Iron

Oral iron is available in a wide variety of preparations as the only nutrient (Table 7-39) or in combination with other vitamins, in doses ranging from 27 to 200 mg of elemental iron per multivitamin/mineral dose. The dose of iron given is not crucial provided that it is adequate because the amount absorbed is not linearly related to the dose ingested. In fact, above doses of 10 mg of elemental iron, the increase in milligrams of iron absorbed is rather limited. However, even at high doses of ingested elemental iron (100 mg), only 10–20% is absorbed by the anemic patient. The ferrous salt is absorbed about three times better than the ferric salt, and all ferrous salts are absorbed equally well. The side effects of iron preparations (nausea, indigestion, diarrhea, abdominal cramping) limit the amount that can be given. The oral route is preferred in virtually all situations, despite the frequency with which side effects occur. Gastrointestinal side effects may be less common with slow-release forms of oral preparations, but the response varies greatly. Some preparations contain tartrazine, which may cause allergic reactions in susceptible patients. Iron absorption may be decreased by antacids, coffee, tea, eggs, or milk. Iron interferes with the absorption of penicillamine and tetracyclines. Oral iron can be used with only slightly increased intolerance (25%) over control subjects (17%) (276).

Oral iron preparations should be used for 1 to 3 months until the hemoglobin level is restored to normal and then given for 1 to 3 months longer to allow tissue stores to be replenished. Hemoglobin contains only about 60% of body iron. Thus, it is usually necessary to treat during this second period for nearly as much time as is required to restore hemoglobin levels to normal.

Because iron is absorbed better when body stores are low, it is absorbed best during the first month of treatment. Absorption during the second period, when tissue stores are being repleted, is less efficient. The iron deficit can be determined roughly by calculating the amount of iron necessary to replace red blood cell hemoglobin, with 1,000 mg added for an average-sized male adult to replete stores:

$$\text{Iron deficit (mg)} = \text{Body weight (lb)} \times [15 - \text{Hemoglobin (g/dL)} \div 1,000]$$

One can use 13 g per dL as the figure for females. If one assumes an overall absorption rate of 10%, the total elemental iron needed can be estimated by multiplying the iron deficit by 10. The dose tolerated per day, once determined, allows the required duration of therapy to be estimated.

Oral iron causes nausea and epigastric distress, constipation or diarrhea, and darkened stools. It is taken on an empty stomach unless gastrointestinal side effects occur. In that case, it is usually given after meals 2 or 3 times a day. Side effects often dictate the dose that can be tolerated orally. Preparations coated with a wax matrix are available (e.g., Slow Fe, which contains 50 mg of Fe per 160-mg tablet) and may be better tolerated. Children should be given iron in a dose of 3 mg per kg per day. Complex vitamin and iron preparations should not be used for symptomatic iron deficiency because other additives can decrease iron availability (277).

It is important to recognize when laboratory tests are not specific for iron deficiency, and will not respond to oral iron. When iron is low after acute stress, such as surgery, but body stores are normal, iron supplements will not help (278). The anemia of chronic inflammation presents with low hemoglobin and iron, but ferritin is usually low, although it can be elevated from proinflammatory cytokines. These patients may need erythropoietin in addition to iron in order to respond (279). Iron therapy is often attempted in women who complain of fatigue but who are not anemic, and most of the time such therapy is unsuccessful. However, one study showed that using full doses of iron (80 mg per day) raised ferritin levels and improved fatigue in women who were not anemic, but had low or borderline ferritin levels (280). Thus, it is important to investigate possible iron deficiency in patients with unexplained fatigue.

Most products contain ample iron to treat iron deficiency, provided that absorption is reasonably normal (Table 7-39). During iron deficiency, net absorption is increased to about 15% to 20% of the ingested dose. Ascorbic acid is included in many preparations, but it is not certain that it enhances absorption to a clinically significant degree. In determining the dose of iron to be given, one should think of the total content of elemental iron, not iron salt. Because the amount of each salt in the tablets varies among manufacturers, one should calculate the elemental iron based on the percentage of iron in each individual salt (Table 7-40).

Parenteral Iron

Indications. When bleeding is recurrent and the rate of loss exceeds the capacity to absorb iron, when malabsorption is the cause of deficiency, or when oral iron cannot be tolerated, parenteral iron may be needed. In addition, other indications include a) when anemia is severe but chronic and rapid repletion is needed, b) when an erythropoiesis-stimulating agent is required and iron availability is needed to achieve maximal response, and c) when anemia of chronic inflammation is present and parenteral iron is needed to overcome the block to absorption of iron from the gut and the block in mobilization of iron from storage sites (both blocks mediated by increased hepcidin concentration) (281). Iron supplements are not included in standard parenteral nutrition (PN) therapy but can be safely given when iron deficiency is present (282). Parenteral iron is often given to dialysis patients with or without erythropoietin to prevent iron deficiency, treat iron deficiency, or enhance the response to erythropoietin when iron has been repleted (283). Suggested guidelines for initiating such therapy in dialysis patients include a serum ferritin level below 100 μg per L, a transferrin saturation below 20%, and the presence of more than 10% hypochromic red cells. A combination of IV iron and erythropoietin has also been used in chronic inflammatory conditions, such as Crohn disease or ulcerative colitis. Most patients with IBD respond to IV iron alone, but erythropoietin or the related darbepoetin-alfa (with a longer half-life) can enhance the response (284). There are six formulations available in the United States: iron dextran, sodium ferric gluconate, iron sucrose, iron carboxymaltose, ferumoxytol, and iron isomaltoside (285) (Table 7-41).

TABLE 7-39 Selected Iron-containing Prescription Products for Oral Use[a]

Product	Formulation	Dose Total mg (elemental mg)	Other Components
Ferrous Sulfate[b]			
Various brands	Tablet	325 (65)	None listed
Various brands	Elixir (5 mL)	220 (44)	5% Alcohol, sweeteners
Various brands	Drops (0.6 mL)	75 (15)	0.2% Alcohol, stabilizers, sweeteners
Ferrous Sulfate Exsiccated			
Feratab	Tablet	187 (60)	
Feosol	Tablet	200 (65)[c]	Glucose
Slow FE	Tablet, slow release	160 (50)	Cetostearyl, lactose
Ferrous Gluconate			
Various brands	Tablet	325 (36)	None listed
Fergon	Tablet	240 (27)	Sucrose
Ferrous Fumarate			
Various brands	Tablet	325 (106)	Polydextrose
Mission brand	Tablet	200 (66)	Sugar
Slow-release iron	Tablet, slow release	150 (50)	Maltodextrin
Nephro-Fer	Tablet	350 (115)	None listed
Feostat	Tablet, chewable	100 (33)	Chocolate flavor
Feostat	Suspension (5 mL)	100 (33)	Preservative, butterscotch flavor
Carbonyl Iron			
Feosol	Tablet	(50)	Lactose, sorbitol, PEG
Ircon	Tablet	(66)	None listed
Icar	Suspension (1.25 mL)	(15)	Sorbitol
Polysaccharide–Iron Complex			
Niferex	Tablet	(50)	Lactose
Various brands	Capsules	(150)	Sucrose
Niferex, Nu-Iron	Elixir (5 mL)	(100)	10% Alcohol, sorbitol
Iron with Vitamin C			
Ferrex 150 plus	Capsule	(150)	Polysaccharide iron, 50 mg AA
Vitelle Irospan	Tablet, timed release	(65)	Ferrous sulfate exsiccated, 150 mg AA
Fero-Grad-500	Tablet, timed release	(105)	Ferrous sulfate, 500 mg sodium ascorbate
Hemaspan	Tablet, timed release	(110)	Ferrous fumarate, 200 mg AA, sugar

[a]The content in milligrams is given as the iron salt, with the elemental iron content in parentheses. The percentage of elemental iron provided in salts is ferrous sulfate, 20%; ferrous sulfate exsiccated, 30%; ferrous gluconate, ~12%; ferrous fumarate, 33%. All forms listed are available over the counter. Data from *Drug Facts and Comparisons.* 59th ed. St Louis, MO: Facts & Comparisons, 2005:36.
[b]Available as elixir, 44 mg of iron per teaspoon.
[c]Preparations available with or without vitamin C.

TABLE 7-40 Elemental Iron Content of Therapeutic Iron Preparations

Iron Salt	Approximate Percentage as Elemental Iron
Sulfate anhydrous	30
Sulfate, 7·H_2O hydrated	20
Fumarate	33
Gluconate	11.6

Table 7-41   Preparations Available for Intravenous Iron Supplementation (Dec 2013)

Parameter	Iron Dextran[a] (LMW)[b]	Iron Gluconate	Iron Sucrose	Iron Carboxy-Maltose	Ferum-Oxytol	Iron Isomaltoside
USA	INFeD	Ferrlicit	Venofer	Injectafer	Feraheme	—
MW (kD)	165	37.5	43	150	730–50	150
Test dose required	yes	no	yes	no	no	no
Maximum dose approved	20 mg/kg BW	125 mg	200 mg × 5 within 14 d	1,000 mg	510 mg repeat 3–8 d	1,000 mg
Infusion Period	360 min	30 min	210 min	15 min	17 sec	15 min
Delivery	diluted	diluted	diluted	bolus	bolus	bolus
Hypersensitivity	moderate	low-mod	low-mod	low	low	low

[a]Also available as High MW iron dextran (Dexferrum)
[b]Can also be administered intramuscularly

Modified from Dignass AU, Stein J. Management of iron deficiency anaemia in inflammatory bowel disease with special emphasis on intravenous iron. *Pract Gastroenterol.* 2011;35:17.

Dose calculation. The total iron (in milligrams) needed to restore hemoglobin and replace stores can be delivered as iron dextran and iron isomaltoside, but is useful to calculate for all patients, regardless of the preparation to be used. The calculated dose is available on websites by providing patient gender, weight, height, and current Hb and target Hb concentrations. If calculated by hand, several formulas are in current use for patients greater than 33 kg:

1. 0.4442 (Target Hb – observed Hb) [g/L] × Lean Body Weight [kg] + (0.26 × LBW)
   LBW = 50 kg + 2.3 kg for every inch greater than 5 ft in height (males)
   LBW = 45.5 kg + 2.3 kg for every inch greater than 5 ft (females)
2. Ideal body weight × (Target Hb – Actual Hb0 [g/L] × 0.24 + iron stores [mg]
   Ideal body weight is calculated as for LBW above. Body stores are estimated at 500 mg for patients greater than 35 kg.

To calculate the dose in milliliters, divide the result by 50 for iron dextran, by 12.5 for ferric gluconate complex, and by 20 for iron sucrose. This formula is applicable only for patients with chronic IDA, not for those who require iron replacement after blood loss. When the patient weighs less than 30 lb, use 80% of the required dose to adjust for a normal hemoglobin value of 12 g per dL in that age group.

Iron dextran low-molecular weight (InFeD, Imferon, DexFerrum, Cosmofer, Dexiron). Parenteral iron can be given in the form of iron dextran, a complex of ferric hydroxide [$Fe(OH)_3$] and dextran in normal saline solution containing 50 mg iron per mL. The complex is dissociated by the reticuloendothelial system and the iron transferred to transferrin. A normal reticuloendothelial system is needed for iron dextran to be useful.

Intramuscular route. First inject a test dose of 0.5 mL IM. Although anaphylactic reactions usually occur within a few minutes, a waiting period of 1 hour is recommended before the treating dose is administered. Each day's dose should not exceed 0.5 mL (25 mg) for infants weighing less than 10 lb, 1 mL (50 mg) for children less than 20 lb, and 2 mL (100 mg) for all others. Injection should be only into the upper outer quadrant of the buttock, placed deeply with a 2- or 3-inch needle. If the patient is standing, inject into the buttock that is not bearing weight. If the patient is in bed, inject the uppermost buttock. To avoid leakage into subcutaneous tissues, a Z-track method, in which the skin is displaced laterally before injection, is recommended. IM injections can produce brown discoloration at the injection site, sterile abscesses, lymphadenopathy, and local soreness.

Intravenous route. The IV route of administration is preferred for parenteral iron because it is better tolerated than repeated IM injections. A test dose (0.5 mL) was previously recommended for some products, but there are no clear data that a test dose decreases the risk of subsequent hypersensitivity reactions, so it is no longer recommended. These reactions can be mild or serious, and may be due to true allergy (symptoms of milder reactions suggest this, including fever, urticaria, and arthralgias) or due to toxicity of free iron (more likely for serious anaphylactoid responses that are not IgE-mediated).

Iron dextran (many preparations). IV injections of 2 mL or less can be given slowly (<1 mL per min), or the full dose can be diluted in 250 or 500 mL of normal saline solution and infused slowly over 2 to 3 hours. Iron dextran is not very compatible with PN formulations and is best administered separately. If maintenance doses are added, they should be used with nonlipid formulations and added just before infusion. Twenty-five to 50 mg per month (0.5 to 1.0 mL) is usually adequate for patients on chronic PN.

The manufacturer recommends that no more than 2 mL be administered at any one time, but this is not always practical when large deficiencies are present. When great care is used and resuscitation equipment is available, full replacement can be provided with iron dextran. Iron can be provided in low-dose (up to 100 mg per infusion), medium-dose (100 to 400 mg per infusion), or high-dose (500 to 1,000 mg or up to full replacement per infusion) regimens. The total calculated dose of iron replacement can be given safely IV to patients with chronic illness (286) and to patients undergoing dialysis (287). Total dose replacement is more convenient, less expensive, and just as efficacious as divided doses, and it is safe when precautions and observation are adequate.

Anaphylaxis/anaphylactoid reactions are extremely rare when iron dextran is given in this way. When it occurs, the reaction is usually within the first few minutes after administration and is characterized by respiratory difficulty and CV collapse. Therefore, iron dextran injections should be administered only to patients with clear indications of iron deficiency who cannot take oral iron. The incidence of all acute hypersensitivity reactions other than anaphylaxis has been estimated to be 0.2% to 3.0% (288). Such reactions include dyspnea, urticaria, itching, arthralgias, myalgias, and fever. Severe (anaphylactic) reactions have been reported at 0.6% to 0.7% with the older IV iron preparation (289). Since the introduction of other preparations that appear to produce fewer severe reactions, the use of iron dextran has decreased, making it difficult to assess accurately the incidence of anaphylaxis with the newer iron dextran formulations (290). Local phlebitis, vascular flush with too rapid infusion, and hypotension can occur after IV injection. Because of these risks, all patients should be closely supervised. IV iron should be given cautiously to persons with a history of asthma or significant allergy. Epinephrine (0.5 mL of a 1:1,000 solution) should be available for acute hypersensitivity reactions. All iron preparations can induce reactions to what is thought to be "free iron" if the circulating plasma transferrin saturation is exceeded. When more than 2 mL is given IV at one time, patients can experience fever, malaise, arthralgias, headache, nausea, shivering, and flushing, reminiscent of a serum-sickness-like illness. Despite concerns about iron overload in patients with chronic diseases who require repeated injections of iron, no evidence of this has been found provided iron is used in conjunction with erythropoietin (283).

Sodium ferric gluconate (Ferrlecit, Nulicet) and iron sucrose (Venofer). Both preparations carry a warning about hypersensitivity, and life-threatening hypotension and collapse have been reported. Venofer requires a test dose of 25 mg given intravenously over 15 minute. If this does not lead to any signs or symptoms of hypersensitivity, then the remainder of the dose can be infused at a rate no greater than 50 mg per 15 minute. There is no known cross sensitivity between IV iron preparations. A number of nonallergic adverse reactions have been reported with all IV iron preparations, especially hypotension when the rate of infusion is rapid (283). Myalgia, arthralgia, backache, fever, headache, nausea, vomiting, and dizziness can occur. Although there is a wide experience using large replacement doses of iron dextran, experience with the newer products is limited, and they are usually given daily in smaller doses until full replacement is reached. The recommended dosage for sodium ferric gluconate is 125 mg per day and for iron sucrose 200 mg given up to 5 times over 14 days for a total dose of 1,000 mg. These preparations have been used most extensively for patients on chronic hemodialysis who are receiving erythropoietin.

Iron carboxymaltose (Ferinject, Injectafer). These preparations are iron complexes stabilized by a carbohydrate shell, and can provide up to 1,000 mg of iron during an administration time of 15 minute, thus offering some advantages in ease of administration (291). These preparations contain aluminum (up to 75 μg per mL), and might cause long-term concern in dialysis patients (281). Hypersensitivity reactions have been reported.

Ferumoxytol (Feraheme). This is an iron complex with superparamagnetic iron oxide, coated with polyglucose sorbitol carboxymethylether (292). It has a particle weight of approximately 730 kDa, larger than the other preparations. It can be given as a single dose of 510 mg. Hypersensitivity reactions do occur, and the package insert carries a black box warning about severe reactions.

Iron isomaltoside (Monofer). The carbohydrate structure of the iron complex differs from that of the other preparations, in that the linked glucose units are nonbranched, and the iron molecules interact with these small (1 kDa) linear oligomers (293). The final complex contains about 10 iron molecules per carbohydrate pentamer. Like other IV preparations, the iron is released slowly from the complex, limiting acute toxicity reactions. The complex can be delivered in doses from 200 to 1,000 mg over 15 minutes, and appears to be well tolerated. Its different structure may protect against severe hypersensitivity reactions, as no mild hypersensitivity has been reported, but more use will see if it offers unique properties.

Response to Iron Therapy
Reticulocytosis may be mild initially and usually peaks at 5 to 10 days after the start of therapy. The reticulocyte count or red cell distribution width need be checked only if there is concern

about obtaining a response, and then only until it is ascertained that an adequate response has occurred. The reticulocyte count should be corrected for the degree of anemia:

Corrected reticulocyte count = measured reticulocyte count × Hct/40

The hemoglobin level usually rises gradually over 1 to 2 months. Failure to respond suggests inadequate intake or absorption of iron, an incorrect diagnosis, or the simultaneous development or detection of folate or vitamin B_{12} deficiency. When erythropoietin (epoetins or darbepoetins) are used to treat anemia of chronic inflammation, iron deficiency will develop unless there is available iron, either from transfusions or from iron infusions. Body iron stores of 800 to 1,200 mg should be provided over any given year (~20 to 25 mg per week), if there are no excessive losses. The best way to monitor for iron therapy is with serum ferritin and transferrin iron saturation (226). The National Kidney Foundation guidelines for erythropoietin and iron use in chronic renal failure conclude that more iron supplements will not help if transferrin saturation is greater than 20% and serum ferritin is greater than 100 μg per dL (288). For renal patients, a target hemoglobin level of 11 to 12 g per dL is suggested.

Hypersensitivity Reactions

As each new iron complex is approved for IV use, the risk of hypersensitivity reactions at first appears less than with older preparations, but with increased use these have been reported. The package inserts contain highlighted warnings about hypersensitivity reactions. As with all these preparations, head-to-head comparisons about risk for anaphylaxis are lacking. Allergic reactions to all the IV iron products, mostly collected from postmarketing spontaneous reports, have been reviewed and summarized by the European Medicines Agency (EMA) Article 31 (http://www.ema.europa.eu/docs/en_GB/document_library/Referrals_document/iv_iron_31/WC500150771. The total number of allergic reactions reported is small, and the benefit/risk ratio was regarded as favorable. Dextran containing products (iron dextran, ferumoxytol, and isomaltoside 1,000) cross-react with dextran. Most people have antibodies against dextran, as dextran is produced by mouth and intestinal bacteria, but the role of these antibodies is unclear in allergic reactions to IV iron. These reactions can include anaphylactoid and other serious complications, including death. These serious complications are thought to be related to free plasma iron, either from oversaturation of ferritin, or from unstable preparations, leading to increased free radical formation and cellular toxicity.

If indeed the severe "hypersensitivity" reactions to IV iron are related to true allergy, then the preparation should not be used again in the same patient. However, if the reactions are due to toxicity, then decreasing the dose and/or decreasing the rate of administration may allow further use without discontinuing the therapy. Data are not available to choose between these options. After examination of the adverse events from all involved pharmaceutical companies, the EMA could not find significantly different rates of allergic reactions in the dextran-free products (iron sucrose, iron ferric gluconate, iron carboxymaltose). Thus, the recommendations for use are the same for all products: 1. use only in an environment with a staff trained to recognize and treat the allergic reactions. 2. The risk of hypersensitivity is increased in patients with a history of allergic reactions or with immune or inflammatory conditions. 3. Caution is needed for providing each dose of IV iron, even if that product has been well tolerated in the past.

Toxicity

Iron overload syndromes are seen when iron absorption exceeds excretion. This can occur when large doses are ingested or when massive transfusions are administered in diseases of red cell destruction in which iron is not lost in excess from the body. Acute ingestion of less than 20 mg of iron is generally nontoxic to adults. Ingestion of 20 to 50 mg per kg produces gastrointestinal symptoms such as nausea, vomiting, diarrhea, and abdominal pain. The UL is set at 45 mg per day (204). Doses above 60 mg per kg are potentially lethal. Shock, intestinal perforation, oliguria, coagulopathy, acidosis, and lethargy may occur. A serum iron level below 350 μg per dL is not associated with toxicity. Levels above 700 μg per dL are often (50%) associated with toxicity. Chronic overload also develops when iron absorption is excessive but intake is not. This situation arises in genetic hemochromatosis, cirrhosis of the liver, and porphyria cutanea tarda. Tissue damage to the liver, pancreas, heart, joints, and endocrine glands may occur.

Diagnosis

Diagnosis of iron overload is best suggested by a high ferritin level and an elevated transferrin saturation, and confirmed by liver biopsy (294).

Phlebotomy

Phlebotomy (500 mL per month) can remove 250 mg of iron at a time and reverse some of the tissue damage, especially to the heart and liver. This is the treatment of choice for hemochromatosis. Secondary iron overload after multiple transfusions (as in thalassemia) can be prevented by the use of deferoxamine, best administered subcutaneously by a pump capable of providing a continuous mini-infusion. The range of doses is 20 to 40 mg per kg per day. Adverse effects include local pain and itching, allergic reactions, blurred vision, diarrhea, and tachycardia. For acute symptomatic iron intoxication (serum Fe >350 μg per dL), deferoxamine should be administered IV at a dose of 10 to 15 mg per kg of body weight. Oral chelators related to deforoxamine are available, and are best used when the degree of overload is not severe (295). Deferasirox is used once daily at doses of 20 to 40 mg/kg/day. It can produce rash, gastrointestinal symptoms, and occasionally severe renal or hepatic impairment.

Zinc

Requirement

The body contains between 1.5 and 2.5 g of zinc (in females and males, respectively), so that it is the second most abundant "trace" mineral in the body, after iron. Nearly 60% of body zinc is in skeletal muscle, and approximately 30% in bone, explaining the sex difference in body content. Turnover of body zinc measured by radioisotope studies is about 6 mg per day in adults. Balance studies show that 12.5 mg of dietary zinc is needed per day to maintain a positive balance. Daily loss is estimated at 2.5 mg, mostly in feces. Absorption averages 30% to 40%, but has been estimated at 20% for diets containing the highest amounts of fiber. The Standing Committee on the Scientific Evaluation of DRIs has set the RDAs at 9 and 13 mg per day for adult women and men, respectively. The RDAs for various age groups are outlined in Table 7-42. Because of the relatively poor absorption of zinc,

TABLE 7-42 Dietary Reference Intakes of Zinc

Life Stage Group	Zinc (mg/d)
Infants	
0–6 months	2[a]
7–12 months	3
Children	
1–3 years	3
4–8 years	5
9–13 years	8
Males	
14–>70 years	11
Females	
14–18 years	9
19–>70 years	8
Pregnancy	
14–18 years	13
19–50 years	11
Lactation	
14–18 years	14
19–50 years	12

[a]Estimate based on adequate intake (AI). All others based on recommended dietary allowances (RDAs). Data from Standing Committee on the Scientific Evaluation of Dietary Reference Intakes, Food and Nutrition Board, Institute of Medicine. Dietary Reference Intakes for Vitamin A, Vitamin K, Arsenic, Boron, Chromium, Copper, Iodine, Iron, Manganese, Molybdenum, Nickel, Silicon, Vanadium, and Zinc. Washington, DC: National Academies Press, 2002.

subjects ingesting a vegetarian diet, especially with high phytate content, may require as much as 50% more than those ingesting animal foods as their major source of zinc (204).

The additional amount of zinc needed for fetal development is estimated to be 0.53 to 0.73 mg per day for the last half of gestation. Because zinc is important for the fetus, a liberal allowance of 3 mg of additional zinc is recommended during pregnancy, with the assumption that many diets do not contain much zinc. The rate of absorption of zinc increases during pregnancy, when the level of ingestion (9 mg per day) was marginal (296). Thus, there may be compensation in absorption during periods of marginal zinc intake. Zinc loss in milk is about 1.2 mg per day and 0.6 mg per day for the first and second 6 months of lactation, respectively (highest in the first month at 2.1 mg per day); the additional recommendation of 4 mg per day during lactation assumes a 20% availability and absorption. Zinc requirements may vary with dietary availability. Assuming that a Western-type diet is ingested with 35% to 40% availability, infants should need 5 mg per day, whereas children ages 1 to 10 years need 10 mg. These amounts may not be enough if a large amount of unrefined cereals containing phytates is ingested or if zinc is lost in sweat or in the intestinal tract.

Food Sources

The average zinc content of diets ingested by adults in the United States has been reported to range from 10 to 15 mg per day or from 6 to 12 mg per day. Whichever figures are correct, the amount of zinc ingested is probably adequate to provide the RDA because clinical zinc deficiency is not common in the United States when the losses of zinc are not excessive, and dietary inhibition by cereal or grain phytates is not extensive.

Zinc content of food varies with the content of the soil in which the food is grown and with the content of the fertilizer used. In general, the available zinc is proportional to protein intake because muscle meats and seafood have the highest content and vegetable sources contain zinc-binding anions. More than half of the zinc in US diets comes from animal foods, and half of that from beef (210). Lacto-ovo vegetarian diets with phytate-zinc ratios of 5:15 show only approximately 33% absorption of zinc, compared with approximately 50% from meat diets. Despite the low bioavailability of zinc from vegetarian diets, it is still usually adequate to use legumes and whole grains to supply zinc, because their high zinc content usually compensates for less efficient absorption, if other sources of zinc are included in the vegetarian diet (e.g., eggs, vegetables).

Zinc is lost during the process of milling cereals. Breast milk is low in zinc. The risk for zinc deficiency is greater in patients ingesting a lacto-ovo vegetarian diet, but this can be countered by increasing the ingestion of whole grains and legumes (297). An increased rate of growth has been documented in children given modest zinc supplementation in double-blinded, controlled conditions, which suggests a preexisting growth-limiting state of zinc deficiency (298). These findings led to zinc fortification of cow's milk formulas in the mid-1970s. Table 7-43 lists the zinc content of selected foods.

Zinc Content of Diets

The NHANES III estimated total nutrient intake, including that in beverages and dietary supplements. Mean intakes of zinc were 5.5 mg in infants and up to about 13 mg in adults, with higher values in male adolescents and adults and values 2.5 to 3.5 mg higher in adults than the mean dietary intake (299). This difference represented supplements taken by 20% of the adult population. Slightly more than half of the population was ingesting more than 77% of the RDA. Those most at risk for inadequate zinc intakes were children from 1 to 3 years old, female adolescents from 12 to 19 years old, and elderly persons more than 71 years old. A general hospital diet provides 13 to 14 mg of zinc daily. However, a low-protein diet (40 g) contains only 6 to 7 mg. Full-liquid diets are marginal in zinc content (8 to 9 mg), and clear liquid diets are quite inadequate (0.3 to 0.4 mg). Vegetarian diets may be limited in bioavailable zinc (300).

Assessment

None of the available methods reliably and accurately reflects intake and absorption or body stores. Daily losses can be estimated from fecal zinc, but this determination is not routinely available. The plasma zinc determination is the best screening test, but many factors can alter the level, unassociated with a change in body stores. Thus, it is a poor measure of marginal zinc

TABLE 7-43 Zinc Content of Selected Foods

Food	Portion	Zinc Content (mg)	Percentage of RDI (11 mg)
Grains			
Bread, white	1 piece	0.173	1–5
Bread, rye	1 piece	0.38	1–5
Spaghetti noodles, cooked	1 cup	0.742	1–5
Product 19 (Kellogg)	1 cup	15	100
Bran flakes	1 cup	5.15	30–40
Meat and Fish			
Beef, lamb	3 oz	4–6	25–39
Chicken, breast, roasted	1 each	1.05	5–12
Chicken, thigh	1 each	1.75	10–24
Turkey, dark meat	3 oz	3.80	25–39
Turkey, light meat	3 oz	1.73	10–24
Liver, beef	3 oz	4.2	25–39
Clams	1 each	0.5	1–5
Fish	3 oz	0.41–0.53	1–5
Oysters, eastern	1 cup	226	100
Oysters, Pacific	1 cup	41	100
Vegetables/Fruits/Nuts			
Vegetables, cooked	1 cup	0.45–0.6	1–5
Peas, green, cooked from fresh	1 cup	1.9	10–24
Lentils, cooked	1 cup	2.52	15–25
Kidney beans, red, cooked	1 cup	1.89	10–24
Fruits, fresh	1 each	0.05–0.09	1
Nuts	1 cup	4.1–4.8	25–39
Peanut butter	2 tbs	1.06	5–15
Dairy/Soy/Egg Products			
Milk, whole	1 cup	0.93	5–12
Yogurt, low-fat, plain	1 cup	2.02	10–24
Cheese	1 oz	0.7–0.93	5–12
Eggs	1 each	0.55	1–5
Soy milk	1 cup	2.90	20–30
Tofu, raw, firm	0.5 cup	1.98	10–24
Egg substitute	0.5 cup	1.6	10–20
Beverages			
Cola	1.5 cup	0.28	1–5
Orange juice	1 cup	0.128	1–5

RDI, recommended dietary intake.

deficiency (301). Plasma zinc does respond in a dose-dependent way to dietary manipulation, and urinary zinc excretion also reflects zinc status (302). Hair zinc reflects zinc status, but is not readily available. If zinc deficiency is suspected clinically, it is best diagnosed by a symptomatic response to zinc replacement.

Plasma

Plasma zinc is relatively insensitive to body status, and several weeks of severe dietary restriction are often needed to see any change in concentration (210). Changes in plasma zinc do not occur until tissue zinc has been reduced. Thus, plasma zinc is a measure of the exchangeable zinc pool, from which an initial loss of zinc produces deficiency (301). Because plasma zinc can decline after a meal, fasting samples should be used. Most of plasma zinc is bound either tightly to α_2-macroglobulins (30% to 40%) or loosely to albumin. The binding sites on albumin are interdependent with fatty acid binding site, providing yet another variable factor in the steady state concentration of plasma zinc (303). In red cells, 60% of the zinc is in hemoglobin and 20% in the enzyme carbonic anhydrase. About 80% of zinc in blood is in red cells—whole blood contains 8.8 μg per mL and plasma contains 0.7 to 1.4 μg per mL (59). Therefore, minor degrees of hemolysis alter plasma zinc levels. Hypoproteinemia and hyperproteinemia, whether caused by chronic illness or inflammation, stress, or altered protein nutrition, affect plasma zinc levels. Drugs (e.g., glucocorticoids, epinephrine) may alter zinc binding to plasma proteins. Although normal plasma levels (115 ± 12 μg per dL) do not rule out deficiency, low levels (<70 μg per dL) indicate deficiency when unaccompanied by hypoproteinemia, acute stress, or the ingestion of drugs that affect zinc levels. Levels less than 50 μg per mL are associated with an increased risk of the development of symptoms, and patients with levels less than 30 μg per mL nearly always manifest some aspect of the zinc deficiency syndrome. Marginal zinc deficiency is always difficult to assess with certainty. Table 7-44 outlines a suggested guide to interpretation of plasma zinc levels.

Neutrophil zinc is theoretically a better assessment of body stores, but because it has not been used frequently, it is not known how much better than plasma zinc it is (59). Normal values are 108 ± 11 μg per 1,000 neutrophils. Alkaline phosphatase is a zinc-requiring enzyme, and its activity correlates with plasma zinc levels before and after zinc treatment (304). Low levels can corroborate zinc deficiency.

Urine

Zinc excretion in urine is relatively low and fixed (i.e., it does not respond to changes in zinc stores). Moreover, it can be affected by altered protein binding in plasma. The major change in obligatory zinc loss in response to varying dietary loads occurs by altering endogenous fecal, not urinary, losses (305). Endogenous fecal excretion is about 1 to 2 mg per day when zinc intake is 5 mg per day. Urine is easily contaminated in some instances with stool; the concentration in stool is higher than that in urine, which ranges from 0.3 to 0.6 mg per day. Thus, urinary zinc levels are not helpful in determining zinc status.

Hair and Nails

Hair and nails contain 90 to 280 parts per million and may reflect zinc intake. Levels of less than 70 parts per million have been associated with poor growth and appetite in children. However, much individual variation is seen because the levels are affected by rate of hair growth and external contamination. Bleaching and cold waving decrease zinc content. Before it is collected, the hair must be washed with water, a nonionic detergent, and EDTA to remove all the easily extractable zinc. It is not clear whether some of the zinc loosely bound to hair is endogenous and should be considered in the total content of the hair. Because collections must be taken with such care, determinations of zinc levels in hair remain a research procedure despite their potential to reflect intake.

Zinc Status in Populations

Three indicators of zinc status have been recommended by the WHP/UNICEF at the population level: a) the prevalence of zinc intake below the EAR, b) the percentage of persons with low serum zinc concentrations, and c) the percentage of children age less than 3 who are stunted (306). While these parameters are useful, they are each imperfect. For example, serum zinc concentrations do

TABLE 7-44 A Suggested Guide to Interpretation of Plasma Zinc Concentrations

	[Zn]p	
Interpretation	(μg/dL)	(μmol/L)
Undesirable	<75	<11.5
Low/borderline	75–85	11.5–13
Acceptable	85–125	13–19
Elevated	>150	>23

Data from Malone AM. Supplemental zinc in wound healing: is it beneficial? *Nutr Clin Pract.* 2000;15:253.

not predict growth in response to zinc supplements. Thus, these parameters are better for defining populations at risk for zinc deficiency, but not for diagnosing deficiency itself (307).

Physiology

Zinc is not a redox active metal, and so it complexes readily with thiols, hydroxyl groups and ligands with electron-rich nitrogen donors. Most of the 1.4 to 2.3 g of zinc in the body is bound to zinc-containing enzymes. These include carbonic anhydrase, carboxypeptidases A and B, alcohol dehydrogenase, glutamate dehydrogenase, malate dehydrogenase, glyceraldehyde-3-phosphate dehydrogenase, alkaline phosphatase, RNA and DNA polymerase, and reverse transcriptase. Zinc is required for both catalytic and structural functions. Zinc may activate or inhibit enzymes, modify membrane function, and bind to transcription factors (zinc fingers). In addition, studies of experimental zinc deficiency in animals reveal that zinc regulates other proteins not known to require zinc for activity, including intestinal fatty acid binding protein, cholecystokinin, J chain of immunoglobulins, and ubiquinone oxidoreductases (308). Cells require zinc to be distributed into all the cellular compartments that contain these many proteins, thus necessitating a complex series of transport mechanisms (309).

Absorption

About 20% to 30% of ingested zinc is absorbed, particularly in the proximal bowel. The bioavailability of luminal zinc depends upon pH, other dissolved salts, and the presence of phytate, the single most important inhibitor of absorption, accounting for 80% of the variability of zinc absorbed (310). Between the dietary Ph/Zn ratios of 7:1 to 37:1 there is a negative relationship between zinc absorption and dietary phytate. Zinc interactions also occur between other ions, especially copper and iron, and zinc itself can interfere with iron absorption at dietary intake ratios as low as 2:1 (311).

The site of zinc absorption is primarily the small intestine. In rats, the colon may play a role, but data in humans suggest that colonic absorption is not significant (312). Both carrier-mediated and nonsaturable diffusion components have been reported, but the former is more active when zinc intake is low. The mammalian ZIP family of zinc transporters has been well described (there are 10 members of the ZnT family, and 14 members of the ZIP family of transporters), but the precise mechanism of transport in all tissues is not clear (305,313). It is not clear whether the free zinc ion or loosely associated zinc is the rate limiting factor in absorption from the lumen, although the data appear to favor the former hypothesis (311). ZIP4 is induced by low dietary zinc in mice, and becomes more localized to the apical membrane. With normal zinc intake, mucosal metallothionein increases, and ZIP5 is located in the basolateral membrane (313), but these effects appear to be secondary, perhaps to buffer intracellular zinc. Low zinc intake causes a fall in pancreatic cells in expression of zinc transporter genes, Znt1 and Znt2, along with a reduction in metallothionein and internalization of ZIP5. These changes are thought to represent an attempt to restore zinc homeostasis by increasing absorption and decreasing pancreatic secretion.

The great majority of body zinc is in target tissues (~1.2g), with only 2 to 3 mg in serum. This serum compartment is in slow equilibrium with target tissues, but in more rapid equilibrium with the intestinal lumen (4 to 15 mg per day), the combination of dietary and endogenously secreted zinc from pancreatic and biliary sources (314). Zinc homeostasis is maintained by alterations in the absorption rate of zinc and in the excretion rate of endogenous zinc into the intestinal lumen (315). When intake of zinc is near or below the optimal level, changes in endogenous excretion can occur rapidly, but it takes longer for absorption rates to adjust, at least in animals. Endogenous zinc absorption does not seem to be affected as much by dietary phytate as is dietary zinc intake (314). Loss of homeostatic regulation of endogenous fecal zinc excretion may be important in the pathogenesis of zinc deficiency in children with environmental enteropathy (316).

Copper binds to metallothionein more avidly than zinc does (317). Thus, when zinc is used to treat Wilson disease, the presumed mechanism involves induction of metallothionein with decreased transfer of copper to the body (318). Acrodermatitis enteropathica is a rare disorder of zinc deficiency due to impaired zinc absorption. Homozygosity mapping of genes from affected families led to identification of a gene, SLC39A4, designated hZIP4, a member of a larger family of zinc transport proteins. hZIP4 is located in apical membranes, and appears to be the transporter responsible for intestinal absorption of zinc (319). Moreover, zinc deficiency in cultured cells upregulates hZIP4, supporting a role for this protein in controlling dietary zinc absorption (320). However, acrodermatitis is a disease that affects infants but not adults, suggesting that other mechanisms (possibly ZIP1) take over during human development. Another member of the ZIP family, ZIP5, is located basolaterally on the enterocyte, and may supply zinc to the enterocyte from body stores and/or regulate the degree of zinc absorption (309).

Similar to calcium and magnesium, the absorption of zinc is decreased by phosphate and nonphosphate binders in the lumen (321). Phytates are particularly rich in whole grains and soy products. Calcium availability affects the zinc–phytate relationship because calcium forms a complex in foods such as cereals, corn, and rice. Inositol hexaphosphates and pentaphosphates are the compounds that inhibit zinc absorption the most. Release of zinc from the complex can be affected by trace metals (especially copper) and by amino acids. Moreover, the biopotency of phytate is affected by food processing. Thus, the availability of zinc from cereals cannot be predicted (322). Zinc absorption is decreased by a high intake of calcium, phosphate, or both. Zinc oxide, carbonate, and sulfate salts are equally well absorbed by animals, but comparable data are not available in humans. When inorganic zinc is ingested (as sulfate), its absorption is decreased by inorganic iron in the lumen, especially if taken as a separate supplement (323). If either zinc or iron is present as the organic form (food zinc or heme iron), such competition does not occur. Thus, the absorption of zinc from liquid formulas or mineral supplements may depend on the luminal content of iron (or even calcium and phosphate). Cd, increasingly found in foods, also inhibits absorption.

Zinc absorption is promoted by animal proteins and by low-molecular-weight organic compounds, such as sulfur-containing amino acids and hydroxy acids (324). Physiologic states that increase the demand for absorbed zinc, such as infancy, pregnancy, and lactation, may affect zinc absorption. Once absorbed, zinc enters a vascular compartment that rapidly turns over and that equilibrates slowly with two extravascular pools, located primarily in the liver, red blood cells, and kidney (296).

Binding and Cellular Uptake

In plasma, zinc is tightly bound to α_2-macroglobin and transferrin. About 60% to 75% of plasma zinc is loosely bound to albumin. Although this binding was thought to be nonspecific, a potential site requiring five coordinates has been identified, and this site is altered by high fatty acid binding (325). In the liver, zinc is bound in part to the metal-binding protein metallothionein. It is not clear if this represents a storage form of zinc separate from the functional enzymes, which contain most of the zinc in the body.

Within cells there are two families of eukaryotic zinc transporters (309,313,326). The ZIP family (Zrt- or Irt-like proteins) has been given the systematic name SLC39. These proteins transport zinc and other metals from the extracellular space (or from the lumen of an organelle) into the cytoplasm. This family is well preserved by all phyla. The mechanism of transport is not clear, but may involve a bicarbonate gradient. There are 14 known members of the ZIP family in the human genome. ZIP1 is directed to the plasma membrane of many tissues from a subcellular location, and is the major uptake system in some cells, for example, prostate. ZIP2 is present only in prostatic and uterine tissue. ZIP3 appears to mediate zinc uptake by mammary epithelial cells and may regulate zinc secretion into milk (326). ZIP4, as noted above, appears to mediate intestinal absorption of zinc in infants, but other mechanisms presumably develop by the time the intestine is fully mature. ZIP14 is involved in uptake of zinc into the liver in response to inflammation.

The second family of zinc transporters is called CDF (cation diffusion facilitator), also known as ZnT, or by the systematic name SLC30. This family supports movement of zinc in the opposite direction to that of the ZIP family proteins, i.e., it transports zinc and other metal ions from the cytoplasm in the lumen of organelles or across the plasma membrane to the outside of the cell. This family contains many members, but the role of four of them (ZnT 1 to 4) has been fairly well characterized. ZnT-1 is the major efflux transporter in the plasma membrane of eukaryotic cells. It may account for reabsorption of zinc in the renal tubule, and in intestinal absorption, as it is located in the duodenum and jejunum, although on the basolateral membrane (195). ZnT-2 is located on endosomal/lysosomal membranes and leads to accumulation of zinc in these structures. ZnT-3 is found only in the brain (in membranes of synaptic vesicles) and testis. Thus, it may facilitate neuronal transmission. ZnT-4 in mammary gland epithelium is responsible for zinc transport into milk, and in basolateral endosomes in the enterocyte may help to regulate transport of zinc across the cell (326).

Excretion

The major route of excretion is in the feces (2 to 3 mg per day). About 7.5 to 14 mg of zinc from body stores (1.5 to 2.0 g per 70-kg person) is secreted daily into the upper intestine. This amount is equal to ingested sources. During passage through the small intestine, an amount equivalent to endogenous loss is usually reabsorbed, but the margin of safety is small. The amount of zinc secreted with each meal is variable, and efficient absorption is required to maintain a normal zinc balance (321). The major normal source of endogenous fecal zinc may be pancreatic juice. Diarrheal fluid may contain more than 11 mg of zinc per L. Thus, the severity of diarrhea is a good indication of the risk for zinc depletion in patients with gastrointestinal diseases. Urinary excretion is not altered by changes in oral intake, whereas fecal zinc increases in proportion to intake. Another route of excretion is sweat, which has an average concentration of 1.15 mg per L. Thus, during profuse sweating, up to 4 mg can be lost daily. During menses, about 0.4 to 0.5 mg of zinc is lost with the blood. Seminal emissions contain an average of 0.6 mg of zinc per ejaculum. Urinary losses average 0.5 mg per day but are unregulated. Urinary losses can be increased in nephrosis, sickle cell disease, and cirrhosis, and after therapy with penicillamine. Daily loss in normal persons has been estimated at 2.2 to 2.8 mg.

Immune Function

Zinc deficiency causes a rapid decline in antibody- and cell-mediated immune responses in both humans and animals (327). Low zinc status alters cellular mediators of the innate immune system, affecting macrophage, neutrophil, and natural killer T cell activity (318). These defects contribute to the lymphopenia seen in patients with sickle cell anemia, HIV infection, acrodermatitis enteropathica, and chronic renal and gastrointestinal diseases. T cells and B cells are lost from the bone marrow. Because zinc deficiency often accompanies protein–calorie malnutrition, the cause of these defects may be multifactorial. Even in the healthy elderly person with low serum levels of zinc, Th-1 cytokine production by leukocytes may be diminished (328). Many of the features of zinc deficiency and aging are similar, including a shift toward a Th2 profile, and impaired function of the innate immune system. These similarities have suggested that perhaps marginal zinc deficiency, always difficult to assess, might be quite prevalent among the elderly population (329).

Deficiency

Zinc deficiency in humans is clearly associated with certain clinical syndromes and has been implicated in others (330).

Definite or Likely Syndromes

As a result of the documentation of these syndromes, the clinical manifestations of zinc deficiency are now better defined (Table 7-45). The symptoms are often nonspecific, but in the

TABLE 7-45 Clinical Manifestations of Zinc Deficiency

Degree of Deficiency	Cause	Manifestations
Moderate	Diet, alcohol, malabsorption, chronic renal disease, sickle cell disease	Growth retardation, hypogonadism (males), skin rashes, poor appetite, lethargy, taste abnormalities, abnormal dark adaptation
Severe	Acrodermatitis enteropathica, TPN, alcoholism, penicillamine therapy, malabsorption, or severe diarrhea	Bullous pustular dermatitis, alopecia, weight loss, neurosensory and psychiatric symptoms, depressed immune function, impaired reproduction

TPN, total parenteral nutrition.
Data from Prasad AS. Zinc deficiency in women, infants, and children. *J Am Coll Nutr.* 1996;15:113.

appropriate clinical setting, zinc deficiency can be suspected. Acrodermatitis enteropathica is a hereditary disorder that begins in early childhood. It is characterized by pustular and eczematous lesions on the skin and by diarrhea. Oral, anal, and genital ulcers also occur. Irritability and cerebellar ataxia may be present. Growth retardation, anorexia, lethargy, and hypogonadism have been reported, especially in young males in Iran and Egypt, where available dietary zinc is low. Acute zinc deficiency has been reported after weeks of TPN, penicillamine therapy, or severe alcoholism. The findings include a rash on the face and limbs; the rash can be pustular, vesicular, bullous, seborrheic, or acneiform. Moist, indolent skin ulcers, when associated with serum zinc levels below 1.0 µg per mL, have been reported to heal with zinc therapy. Alopecia, confusion, apathy, depression, and loss of taste are associated with zinc deficiency in uremia. Symptoms suggestive of zinc deficiency can be found in patients with gastrointestinal diseases who have documented or suspected increased fecal losses. Diarrheal disease in infants leads to low serum levels of zinc (331). The rapid transit exacerbates the zinc malabsorption that occurs in diseases of the intestine. These diseases include malabsorption syndromes, IBD, and other secretory diarrheas. Endogenous losses of up to 20 mg per day have been documented. Malabsorption can lead to a loss of more than 90% of dietary zinc because of decreased transport of zinc across the mucosa and malabsorption of zinc binders, which accumulate in the lumen. Zinc absorption is impaired after Roux-en-Y gastric bypass, and even with zinc supplementation, zinc deficiency can present 1 to 2 years after surgery (332). Zinc deficiency associated with protein losses occurs in patients with protein-losing enteropathy and nephrotic syndrome, burns, or trauma.

Twenty percent of the total body zinc resides in the skin, so that a severe burn is especially likely to cause zinc deficiency. Requirements for zinc are increased in periods of growth and during pregnancy, so that any superimposed increased losses accelerate the development of zinc deficiency.

Acute Diarrhea in Children at Risk for Zinc Deficiency

A clear beneficial effect has been found in treating acute diarrhea in children under the age of 5, but not in infants under the age of 6 months (333). The response is perhaps due to zinc deficiency, although a pharmacologic effect of supplemental zinc cannot be ruled out (334). This confusion arises as the patients treated have been in general at high risk for zinc deficiency, but definitely low serum zinc was not an entry criterion for entrance into the studies. Zinc supplements were associated with a 13% decrease in mortality, and a 15% decrease in mortality from pneumonia (335). One study has shown that zinc supplements reduce morbidity and mortality in very low-birth-weight preterm neonates, and in an industrialized country (Italy) (336).

Candidate Syndromes

Patients with cirrhosis excrete excess zinc in their urine; testicular dysfunction, anorexia, lethargy, and night blindness responsive to zinc may develop. One study showed improvement in encephalopathy grade with zinc supplements in patients with cirrhosis (337). Sickle cell anemia leads to urinary losses of zinc. Attributed to zinc deficiency are delayed puberty, hypogonadism, small stature, anorexia, decreased body hair, chronic leg ulcers, and hypogeusia. The gonadal function (potency, libido, sperm count) of patients on hemodialysis has been reported to improve after the administration of oral zinc at a dosage of 50 mg per day (330). However, a review of 24 studies of zinc on fertility showed no clear effect, as studies were small and most were not randomized (338).

Poor wound healing is said by some authors to respond to zinc sulfate replacement. However, others note no change. Zinc supplements may improve the innate immunity of the skin in inflammatory dermatoses, but the studies were all open label (339). Zinc deficiency can be associated with a diminished response of insulin to glucose, but it is not clear whether zinc plays a role in normal glucose homeostasis or in diabetes. Altered taste (dysgeusia) or smell as an isolated finding in nonuremic patients has been said to respond to oral zinc. Other possible causes of an abnormal sense of taste include iron deficiency, candidiasis, psychiatric disorders, and medications (341). A double-blinded study of the effect of zinc supplements on taste and smell dysfunction did not support a role for zinc (341). Acute or persistent diarrhea in children less than 5 years old is prolonged by low weight for age and by decreased cell-mediated immunity, both associated with zinc deficiency in developing countries (333,335). Zinc has been implicated in depression and other mood disorders, because of its putative role in neuronal transmission (342).

One study found an association of lower serum zinc in patients with Alzheimer and Parkinson disease, although urinary zinc was no different from controls (343). However, the mean values for serum zinc in the two disease conditions were still above the usual cutoff value (75 μg per dL) for serum zinc, and no treatment intervention trials have been reported. A small blinded study shows in post hoc analyses that 6 months of zinc therapy improved two cognitive measures in Alzheimer patients (344). This study needs confirmation. In addition, its action in oxidative stress suggests a possible role in degenerative disorders, such as CV disease, and its activity in regulation of bone metabolism suggests a role in osteoporosis. Elderly hospitalized patients may be at risk for lower serum zinc concentrations (345). However, the European ZENITH study (Zinc Effect in Nutrient/Nutrient Interactions and Trends on Health and Aging) found that total zinc intake (diet plus supplements) up to 40 mg per day did not have any long-term effects on immune status in healthy elderly subjects (342).

Treatment

Zinc is available as a component of many multivitamin and mineral preparations. It can better be provided as an individual oral supplement in the form of zinc sulfate or gluconate. The 67-mg zinc sulfate tablet provides 15 mg of elemental zinc, equivalent to the RDA, or roughly the amount contained per kilogram of stool. When estimated needs are greater, the patient can be given the 220-mg tablet, which contains 50 mg of elemental zinc. Treatment should continue until the symptoms prompting the use of zinc resolve. Then a maintenance dose (67 mg of zinc sulfate) can be given daily. Zinc sulfate (1 or 5 mg per mL) or zinc chloride (1 mg per mL) is available for IV administration but must be diluted first in saline solution.

It is difficult to choose a dose for zinc treatment. Zinc is widely available in a Western-type diet. Therefore, if zinc is given in certain disorders (e.g., malabsorption) to prevent the development of deficiency, it is not possible to determine whether the treatment is beneficial. It seems better to reserve treatment for those syndromes that respond to zinc therapy, and for conditions in which zinc has been shown to be beneficial.

Wilson Disease

In addition to a diet low in copper, 25 mg of zinc can be given every 4 hours from 7:00 A.M. to 7:00 P.M. and 50 mg at 11:00 P.M., or 50 mg can be given three times a day to decrease copper absorption.

Macular Degeneration

The use of antioxidant supplements (vitamin C, β-carotene, vitamin E, and zinc) for age-related macular degeneration has suggested some efficacy, but whether zinc plays a specific role is not known (346). Zinc supplements cannot be recommended at this time.

Decreased Dietary Intake

Supplements are indicated when the estimated intake is less than the RDA. However, long-term use of large doses (100 to 300 mg per day) can lead to copper deficiency and elevated levels of cholesterol (64). The results of studies of the effects of zinc supplements on calcium absorption and vice versa have been mixed, but there is no effect on iron status (347).

Common Cold

Trials of zinc supplementation for upper respiratory infection continue to provide contradictory results. A systematic review of randomized, controlled, double-blinded trials of rhinovirus infection showed no statistical benefit (348). The issue is still debated, although the data are not sufficient to warrant a recommendation of zinc supplementation. Other reviews concluded that zinc gluconate lozenges are useful, but that it is important to begin therapy within 48 hours and to have the patient suck the lozenges every 2 hours while awake (349). Using the delivery conditions outlined above, a prospective trial administered 12.8 mg of zinc acetate and showed a 40% reduction in the duration of cold symptoms (350). Zinc gluconate nasal gel might be preferable, although the data are mixed (351).

Prevention of Illness by Zinc Supplementation

The incidence, prevalence, duration, and severity of diarrhea and pneumonia may be reduced by zinc supplementation of children in the developing world, but the data are inconclusive for very young children less than 2 years (352,353). Although the data are not certain, it is likely that intake of bioavailable zinc is low in these populations. The problem again is the difficulty in identifying marginal zinc deficiency. Zinc supplementation has also been reported to relieve the diarrhea of acrodermatitis enteropathica, decrease the prevalence of malaria, and improve the neuropsychiatric performance of children at risk for zinc deficiency (354). Risk factors for zinc (and copper and iron) deficiency are present in patients following bariatric bypass surgery, and supplementation has been suggested with 8 to 15 mg per day of elemental zinc (355). Because the patients are also at risk for copper deficiency, and luminal zinc interferes with copper absorption, 1 mg of supplemental copper is recommended for patients postbariatric surgery who take supplemental zinc. Using the same strategy, in Wilson disease zinc supplements are used to interfere with copper absorption (see under 'Copper' in this chapter).

Toxicity

Zinc is relatively nontoxic. Because there is an incomplete correlation between plasma and tissue zinc, the level for elevated zinc (>23 µmol per L) is placed above the range of normal values (13 to 19 µmol per L), as the interpretation of the intermediate levels is not clear (Table 7-44). Because the zinc content of most foods is low, dietary excess is unlikely. Ingestion of more than 150 mg per day can interfere with copper or iron metabolism, but only if intake of these other ions is limited (356). Impaired immune function and an adverse effect on the ratio of low-density-lipoprotein to high-density-lipoprotein cholesterol have also been reported. All these effects have been reported less frequently with doses between 15 and 100 mg per day. However, the UL for adults is 40 mg per day, based on a reduction in erythrocyte copper/zinc superoxide dismutase activity (204). Very high doses (450 mg per day) have induced copper deficiency with sideroblastic anemia (354). Large acute overdoses (>200 mg) can produce nausea, vomiting, rash, dehydration, and gastric ulceration. Tetracycline absorption may be impaired by zinc.

There are rare examples of familial hyperzincemia (3 to 4 times normal) with a normal phenotype, as the excess zinc is bound to albumin (357). These cases show that elevated plasma zinc does not necessarily predict toxicity, and also show that excess zinc can bind to albumin, as normally only approximately 2% of albumin molecules have zinc bound to them. Two other spontaneous disorders of zinc overload have reinforced the concept that zinc can be toxic, however, if enough of the mineral enters the body. Myelopathy and pancytopenia can present with high zinc and low copper levels, in the absence of excessive zinc intake (358). The anemia was reversed with copper supplementation, and high copper intake (8 mg per day) partially reversed neurologic signs. More striking is the syndrome in children of hyperzincemia and hypercalprotectinemia, as the zinc levels reached 77 to 200 µmol per L, or greater than 300 µg per dL (359). Patients presented with recurrent infection, systemic inflammation, anemia, and growth failure. Iron and copper status was normal. Levels of serum calprotectin (a calcium-binding protein) were approximately 6,000-fold increased over normal (360). Zinc levels fell by half after treatment with cyclosporine A in a single case (361).

Copper

Requirement

Copper is a trace element that is essential for humans and many other animals. Estimates of copper requirements are based on balance studies of fecal and other losses and copper absorption for various age groups (204,362). Obligatory losses in adults are about 580 µg per day, and absorption averages about 25%. However, when intake is low, excretion falls, so the formerly recommended intake in excess of 35 µg per kg per day to avoid a negative balance is considered too high (363). Current recommendations for DRIs range from 400 to 900 µg per day for children greater than 4 years to elderly adults (Table 7-46). Premature infants are born with low copper reserves and may require more copper. Milk provides about 120 µg of copper per day. Infant formulas may contain copper in a poorly available form (e.g., bound to insoluble anions), and the copper requirement may be higher (~0.1 mg per kg of body weight daily) when these mixtures are used.

TABLE 7-46 Dietary Reference Intakes of Copper

Life Stage Group	Copper (μg/d)
Infants	
0–6 months	200[a]
7–12 months	220[a]
Children	
1–3 years	340
4–8 years	440
Adults (M/F)	
9–13 years	700
14–18 years	890
19–>70 years	900
Pregnancy-all ages	1,000
Lactation-all ages	1,300

[a]Estimates based on adequate intake (AI). Other values are recommended daily allowances (RDAs). Data from Standing Committee on the Scientific Evaluation of Dietary Reference Intakes, Food and Nutrition Board, Institute of Medicine. *Dietary Reference Intakes for Vitamin A, Vitamin K, Arsenic, Boron, Chromium, Copper, Iodine, Iron, Manganese, Molybdenum, Nickel, Silicon, Vanadium, and Zinc.* Washington, DC: National Academies Press, 2002.

Food Sources

The richest sources of copper, as of zinc, are crustaceans and shellfish (especially oysters and crabs), and also organ meats (364). The next richest sources are nuts and legumes, dried fruits, and cocoa. Poor sources include dairy products, sugar, and honey. Surveys show that most adults in the United States consume 1 mg of copper or less per day. A hospital diet may contain less than 1 mg of copper because it includes few copper-rich foods. Full-liquid diets provide less than 0.5 mg and clear liquid diets less than 0.1 mg. Table 7-47 lists the copper content of some common foods.

Assessment

Plasma Copper

Most of the copper in the body (80 mg) is in tissues. Red blood cells contain 60% of blood copper as erythrocuprein, a copper and zinc protein that functions as a superoxide dismutase. In plasma, copper is tightly bound to ceruloplasmin (molecular weight of 160 kDa), which binds 80% of the plasma copper at a ratio of seven copper molecules per molecule of protein. The rest of the copper is bound to transcuprein and albumin. The amount of copper exchanged from ceruloplasmin is small compared with the amount absorbed. Therefore, the plasma copper level does not correlate with intake; it only roughly reflects body stores because the plasma compartment comprises such a small percentage of body stores and the turnover of copper within the compartment is slow. Nonetheless, the plasma copper level is a better initial indicator of copper status than is the tissue copper level when deficiency is suspected because tissue copper levels are more stable.

Normal plasma copper levels for males are 0.91 to 1.0 ± 0.12 μg per mL, and for females they are 1.07 to 1.23 ± 0.16 μg per mL. Oral contraceptives increase the range to 2.16 to 3.0 ± 0.7; this is largely an estrogenic effect. Levels peak in pregnancy at 38 weeks and return to normal within 2 weeks postpartum. Plasma total copper levels can increase in acute and chronic infections and decrease in nephrosis, Wilson disease, kwashiorkor, or any condition that causes protein malnutrition. Free serum copper values are more instructive than total copper values because the latter are affected by factors that alter binding capacity. Bound copper is estimated to be three times ceruloplasmin levels (μg per dL) because each milligram of ceruloplasmin contains 3.3 μg of copper (365). Free (not bound to ceruloplasmin) copper equals total serum copper minus bound copper. Values below 25 μg per dL are considered within normal range. This calculation is designed to detect elevated levels of free copper, as in Wilson disease, rather than to detect copper deficiency. Because of the insensitivity of serum copper in detecting deficiency

TABLE 7-47 Copper Content of Foods

High (>0.2 mg/Portion)	Moderate (0.1–0.2 mg/Portion)	Low (0.1 mg/Portion)
Meat and Meat Substitutes		
Liver and other organ meats, shellfish, variety meats, lamb, pork, duck, tofu, nuts	Dark meat of chicken, fresh fish, turkey	Beef, veal, bologna, beef frankfurters, eggs
Dairy Products		
	Dried skim milk powder, sharp cheeses	Butter, margarine, milk, ice cream, most cheeses, cheese spreads
Vegetables		
Lentils, mushrooms, dried beans, pimentos, French fried potatoes, canned tomatoes	Spinach, sweet potato, squash, beets, asparagus, peas (fresh and canned), baked potato	Green beans, broccoli, cabbage, carrots, cauliflower, corn, Brussels sprouts, cucumber, lettuce, green pepper, turnip
Bread and Cereal		
Wheat germ and bran, English muffins, bran flakes	Whole wheat bread, pasta, sugar or vanilla wafers	White bread, white rice
Miscellaneous		
Curry powder, nuts, chocolate, molasses, cocoa, Ovaltine, licorice, soup mixes, syrup, canned soup	Pickles, ginger, black pepper, frozen pizza, popcorn, potato chips, pretzels, soda	Hard candy, Jell-O, honey, jelly, white sugar, lemonade, catsup, mayonnaise

Data from Pennington JT, Calloway DH. Copper content of foods. *J Am Diet Assoc.* 1973;63:143.

states, biomarkers of copper status have been sought, focused on a range of cuproenzymes, and copper chaperones (366). However, to date none of these has achieved any clinical usefulness.

Ceruloplasmin

Ceruloplasmin is a protein that is made in the liver. It functions as a ferroxidase, converting ferrous to ferric ion, and thus affects the flow of iron from cell to plasma. With copper deficiency, ceruloplasmin levels fall, to about 30% in severe deficiency. Iron mobilization is decreased, and a hypochromic, microcytic anemia develops. When ceruloplasmin levels are low in Wilson disease, other ferroxidases in plasma appear to be able to mobilize iron. Normal levels are 105 to 500 µg per dL. Estrogens increase the levels, and low levels are seen in patients with Wilson disease (including 10% to 20% of heterozygotes), uremia, and nephrosis and in persons with a low protein intake. Other forms of chronic liver disease associated with a decreased synthesis of plasma protein can produce a low level. In Wilson disease, ceruloplasmin levels are less than 23 µg per dL (367). This value provides an adequate screening test, but false-normal levels may occur in a small percentage of patients. The free serum copper concentration is probably a better measure in Wilson disease (368).

Hair

A determination of copper in hair entails the same problems as do the determinations for zinc and other trace metals—individual sex- and age-related variations, exogenous contamination, and strict requirements for sample preparation. It cannot be routinely recommended to test body stores.

Urinary Copper

From 0.01 to 0.06 mg is excreted daily in the urine. This amount does not usually vary much according to changes in copper intake and reflects free tissue copper and plasma copper loosely bound to albumin. Thus, it does not reflect body stores. In Wilson disease, free copper in tissues is increased, and urinary excretion can exceed 1.5 mg per day. However, this value is quite variable and can be within the normal range. Values below 50 µg per day, however, virtually exclude Wilson disease.

Physiology

About one-third of body copper is in the liver, with large amounts in the brain, heart, spleen, and kidneys. Newborns have three times the adult level in their liver, but this falls rapidly after birth and is probably related to immature excretory mechanisms. The newborn has ceruloplasmin in the liver but low levels in the plasma. Most copper is in the cytosol, bound to enzymes or other copper-binding proteins. The enzymes include cytochrome oxidase, amine oxidases, superoxide dismutase, ceruloplasmin, tyrosinase, dopamine-β-dehydrogenase, uricase, lysyl oxidase, and histaminase, among others (365,369). Copper is important for the enzymes mediating the absorption and release of iron from tissues, and thus it is important in hemoglobin production. It is needed for the development and maintenance of blood vessels, tendons, and bones, functioning of the central nervous system, pigmentation of hair, and normal fertility.

Copper Absorption and Organ Distribution

Dietary copper is absorbed from the stomach and the small intestine. The mechanism of absorption of dietary copper is not established with certainty. A protein with a high affinity for copper, hCtr1 (*SLC31A1*), may transport copper into enterocytes, although it is expressed in a wide range of other tissues (369). A second copper transporter, Ctr2, may mediate low-affinity copper uptake (370). The divalent metal transporter, DMT1, has a wide substrate range (copper, iron, manganese, cobalt) and may be involved as well (371). Intracellular transport of copper is better understood. hCtr1 delivers copper by acting as a permease or via endocytosis (372). There is no free copper inside cells, because copper is a prooxidant, but the metal is bound to various chaperones (370). CCS1 directs copper to superoxide mutase 1, a defense mechanism against oxidative stress. ATOX1 guides copper to the copper transporting ATPase, ATP7B (373). The gene for Wilson disease, ATP7B, is located on the long arm of chromosome 13, and has a cysteine-rich metal-binding region on the amino terminus that is critical for its intracellular distribution. Most mutations in Wilson disease are point missense mutations. After binding to ATP7B, copper is bound to glutathione and metallothionein and other peptides (372). Excess copper is taken up by hepatocytes and excreted from those cells into bile via the apical canalicular membrane. The copper transporting ATPase resides in the *trans*-Golgi, where it provides the copper for ceruloplasmin bound for export. When intracellular copper rises, the ATP7B protein is redistributed to endosomal vesicles for delivery to bile. This accounts for the basal rate of copper excretion in Wilson disease and probably prevents severe copper toxicity in neonates.

The Menkes gene protein, MNK (ATP7A), is another membrane-associated P-type adenosine triphosphatase that is required for secretion of copper excretion primarily in enterocytes and the placenta and cells of the central nervous system (374). The major function of this ATPase is in axonal growth, integrity of synapses, and neuronal activation. Thus, mutations in *ATP7A* produce two neurologic syndromes in addition to Menkes disease, namely occipital horn syndrome (OHS) and isolated distal motor neuropathy. The mechanism of excretion is now clearly understood, as the structure of a bacterial analogue of the Menkes P1B-type ATPase has been crystallized. Copper binds to three sites as it passes through the membrane-bound ATPase. It is delivered to the first of these sites by a mobile heavy metal–binding domain in the copper chaperone LpCopA (375). Mutations of both ATPases in Menkes syndrome and Wilson disease lead to impaired trafficking across the *trans*-Golgi membrane, and thus present with hypoceruloplasminemia. Hephaestin is a multicopper oxidase that is deficient in mice with sex-linked anemia. It is a membrane-bound analogue of ceruloplasmin required for iron (but not copper) export from the intestine. In the plasma, copper binds to albumin and perhaps histidine, and is taken up by hCtr1 on the liver membrane.

Intracellular Copper Metabolism

Once hCtr1 mediates copper uptake, a series of small cytoplasmic copper chaperones (e.g., hCOX17, HAH1, and CCS) distribute copper to various cellular compartments or mediate incorporation into proteins (369). In all tissues but liver, MNK transports copper into the Golgi apparatus for incorporation into secreted proteins. MNK then moves to the plasma membrane, where it may mediate copper efflux. In the liver, the protein that is deficient in Wilson disease, WND, is present in the Golgi and presumably serves a similar function. No chaperone has been isolated for delivering copper to metallothionein.

Metallothionein

Metallothionein, a small protein (molecular weight of 6 kDa) with tightly bound zinc and copper, is found in many tissues. The high level in fetal liver may allow safe storage of increased liver copper. It may be the initial hepatocyte acceptor for albumin-bound copper from the plasma and may play a role in detoxification. Finally, it has been suggested as a mechanism to block enterocyte absorption of copper. Normally, about 80% of hepatic copper is bound to metallothionein, which is polymerized and insoluble. In Wilson disease, only about half as much copper is in this form, so that free tissue copper levels rise.

Hepatic Copper Content in Disease

In many disorders, especially Wilson disease, hepatic copper is increased—prolonged cholestasis, Indian childhood cirrhosis, copper poisoning, thalassemia, hemochromatosis, and biliary cirrhosis. However, more stainable copper is demonstrated in the liver in these illnesses than in Wilson disease, and metallothionein levels may be normal. For this reason, these conditions may not be associated with the same degree of tissue toxicity, presumably secondary to free copper, as Wilson disease.

Excretion and Absorption

Copper from the liver is mainly excreted into bile. This is the major excretory route for copper from the body, and the rate of excretion is 0.5 to 1.3 mg per day. The amount excreted usually balances that absorbed each day from the upper small intestine. Absorption is relatively inefficient (~30%), allowing biliary excretion to remove excess copper from the body. The form of inorganic copper affects absorption. The carbonate and nitrate forms are better absorbed than the sulfate, chloride, or oxide. Phytates and ascorbic acid decrease absorption. Copper complexed to amino acids may be better absorbed. Other metals (e.g., Ca, Cd, Zn, Fe, Pb, Ag, Mo) decrease absorption (322).

Other Functions

Copper deficiency leads to low serum levels and high tissue levels of iron. This function of copper is carried out by the multicopper ferroxidases, of which ceruloplasmin was the first reported. Ceruloplasmin knockout mice show a severe impairment of iron efflux from reticuloendothelial cells and hepatocytes (376). The multicopper oxidases may bind to iron transport proteins or may be involved primarily in iron export, as is hephaestin. Copper is also necessary to prevent lipid peroxidation, perhaps by playing a role in selenium metabolism. Both humoral and cell-mediated immunity is impaired by copper deficiency in animals.

Deficiency

Dietary deficiency is uncommon but may occur in premature infants or in malnourished patients repleted with low-copper diets (377). Table 7-48 lists the manifestations of copper deficiency in humans.

TABLE 7-48 Signs and Symptoms Associated with Deficiency of Trace Metals

Mineral	Signs and Symptoms Infants and Children	Adults
Cu	Anemia, neutropenia, osteopenia, vascular aneurysms, kinky hair, hypothermia, impaired CNS development	Anemia, neutropenia
Mn	None reported	Hypercholesterolemia, weight loss, change in hair color (one case reported)
Cr	None reported	Glucose intolerance, peripheral neuropathy
Se	Cardiomyopathy, chondrodystrophy	Cardiomyopathy, myositis

CNS, central nervous system.
Data from Triplett WS. Clinical aspects of zinc, copper, manganese, chromium, and selenium. *Nutr Int.* 1985;1:60.

Premature Infants
When milk is the major food source, both copper and iron intakes are low. The copper content of the body increases markedly just before birth, so prematurity is associated with low body stores. Anemia secondary to either iron or copper deficiency can develop. Bone abnormalities have been reported. Copper deficiency is commonly seen in infants with cholestasis on PN (378). Despite the concern that cholestasis might lead to copper retention, these infants may need more copper replacement to prevent deficiency.

Malnutrition
When repletion is high in calories but low in copper content, neutropenia, anemia, diarrhea, and scurvy-like bone changes may occur that are all responsive to copper. Tissue copper levels are often, but not always, decreased. Osteoporosis has been reported in severe copper deficiency (379).

Menkes Kinky Hair Syndrome
Menkes kinky hair syndrome is an X-linked recessive inherited disorder caused by a defect in copper absorption (MIM #309400) (380). The tissue content of copper is always low. Characteristic features are failure to thrive, mental deterioration, hypothermia, defective keratinization of hair, metaphyseal lesions, degeneration of aortic elastin, and depigmentation of hair. Most children die early in infancy. Copper supplementation is not helpful, but a copper–histidine complex may delay the onset of some symptoms (381).

Cardiovascular Disease
The copper deficiency theory of ischemic heart disease was first proposed in the 1980s, suggested by sudden death in domestic animals with copper deficiency (e.g., "falling disease" of dairy cattle). The evidence is all indirect but nevertheless intriguing. Decreased activity of lysyl oxidase and superoxide dismutase may lead to a failure of collagen and elastin cross-linking (382). Copper deficiency can be associated with low levels of copper in cardiac muscle, increased levels of plasma cholesterol, and electrocardiographic abnormalities. Patients with ischemic heart disease have low cardiac and leukocyte copper concentrations. Short-term copper depletion experiments in humans have produced changes in lipid profiles, electrocardiographic changes, and impaired glucose tolerance (382). The data are not sufficient to recommend replacement therapy at present.

Myeloneuropathy and Anemia
Myeloneuropathy and anemia due to copper malabsorption is being increasingly recognized (383). The clinical presentation resembles that of cobalamin deficiency, with long tract signs and lower extremity weakness (384). Copper replacement parenterally reverses the neurologic symptoms. Most cases have had gastric resection (385). The duodenum is the primary site of copper absorption in animals, perhaps accounting for the role of gastrectomy in producing the syndrome. A similar syndrome has been reported in a patient taking 15 to 30 times the recommended daily intake of zinc (as gluconate) to prevent the common cold (383). Changes are associated with T2 hyperintense foci on MRI, seen in subcortical white matter, atrophy of the cerebrum and cerebellum, and in the dorsal cord (386). Although the neurologic symptoms are reversible if treated early, they can become chronic if copper deficiency is not recognized.

Therapy
Because copper deficiency is uncommon, supplementation is unnecessary with most diets. Despite this fact, copper is included in many multivitamin and mineral preparations. Copper sulfate, the form usually available, contains 0.4 mg of elemental copper per milligram of the anhydrous salt. A daily addition of about 1.0 to 1.5 mg of copper adequately treats deficiency states. However, if oral treatment is used, three times this amount should be given, or about 3 mg of copper as copper sulfate, to allow for the 30% absorption efficiency. For replacement in cases with myeloneuropathy, doses up to 10 mg per day for 1 to 2 months may be necessary to restore the serum copper level to normal (355).

Toxicity
Although deficiency is more of a public health problem than toxicity, copper intake may be sufficient to produce toxicity (387). The mechanisms of copper toxicity are related to its ability to generate reactive oxygen species (388).

Acute Toxicity

The UL for adults is 10 mg per day based on protection from liver damage, which is the critical toxic effect (204). Ingestion of more than 15 mg of elemental copper causes nausea, vomiting, diarrhea, and abdominal cramps resulting from direct mucosal toxicity (389). At larger doses, hemolysis results from inhibition of glucose-6-phosphate dehydrogenase. Gastrointestinal bleeding, azotemia, and hematuria may occur. When ingestion is potentially fatal, jaundice with acute hepatic necrosis and renal tubular swelling are seen. The treatment for acute overdose usually involves gastric lavage. If the dose ingested is very high, penicillamine (1 g per day in adults) can be added to remove excess copper from the body.

Chronic Toxicity

In Wilson disease, free tissue copper and total liver copper (>250 μg per g net weight of liver) are increased. Other diseases are associated with increases in hepatic copper (chronic active hepatitis, primary biliary cirrhosis), but tissue damage related to excess copper has not been seen to develop, perhaps because the level of free tissue copper is not increased. The initial treatment for Wilson disease consists of a low-copper diet and chelating therapy (penicillamine or trientine). It may be important to combine the diet with chelation therapy initially to reduce the excess copper stores. Zinc supplements also may be helpful for maintenance therapy (373).

Iodine

Requirement

Iodine is a nonmetallic halogen element required for the synthesis of thyroid hormone. About 1 μg of iodine is required per kilogram to prevent goiter in adults. The RDAs are currently based on balance studies (204). Studies of urinary excretion indicate that more than 50 μg is needed per gram of creatinine per day. Goitrogens in the diet (fluoride or rubidium) affect the requirement by decreasing thyroid uptake of iodine. To allow a margin of safety, the RDA for children aged 9 to 13 and for adults is set at 150 μg per day. For infants age 0 to 6 months, the recommended AI is set at 110 μg per day, for infants 7 to 12 months at 130 μg per day, and for children ages 1 to 8 at 90 mg per day. Because the iodine content of human milk is 30 to 100 μg per L, another 70 μg per day is needed during pregnancy, and an additional 70 μg per day (290 μg total) is needed during lactation. The AI for infants 0 to 6 months old is 110 μg per day; for infants 7 to 12 months old, it is 130 μg per day, and it is 90 μg per day for children ages 1 to 8 years. The RDA is 120 μg for children 9 to 13 years old and 150 μg per day for adolescents and children of both sexes 14 years of age or older. The RDA during pregnancy is 220 μg per day, and it is 290 μg per day during lactation.

Food Sources

The iodine content of food and water is closely related to the iodine content of the soil. Areas where the iodine content is likely to be low include glaciated and mountainous regions and areas with heavy rainfall. Seafood is an excellent and consistent source of iodine. The iodine content of dairy products, eggs, and meat depends on the iodine content of the animal feed. The water content varies from 0.1 to 2 μg per L in goitrogenic areas to 2 to 15 μg per L in nongoitrogenic areas. Fruits and vegetables in general are low in iodine. Except for seafood, the source is more important than the type of food in determining iodine content. Shellfish or saltwater fish contain about 70 μg per 4 oz. Eggs contain about 4 to 10 μg each, meats about 5 μg per oz, dairy products about 3 to 4 μg per oz, and fruits 1 μg per oz. Breads are low in iodine unless made by the continuous mix process, during which the dough absorbs atmospheric iodine. Some plants contain natural substances that interfere with iodine absorption. These include Brussels sprouts and legumes.

Average iodine intake in the United States is 250 and 170 μg per day for males and females, respectively. The usual supplement for dietary iodine in the United States is iodized table salt, which contains 76 μg of iodine per gram of salt. The use of 3.4 g of iodized salt per day on average adds 260 μg of iodine to the daily intake. In noncoastal regions, iodized salt should be used. In coastal regions, atmospheric iodine is much higher and provides an extra source of iodine.

Assessment

The body contains 15 to 20 mg of iodine, 60% to 80% of which is in the thyroid gland. The concentration of inorganic iodine is low, and organic compounds are the usual circulating form (thyroxine, triiodothyronine, diiodotyrosine, and monoiodotyrosine). Measurement of these compounds in blood is a measure of thyroid function, and this measurement correlates with iodine stores in the absence of other thyroid disease. Thyroid-stimulating hormone is regulated by circulating thyroid hormone levels. Because RIAs and immuno-chemiluminometric assays for thyroid-stimulating hormone are stable and easily used, this measurement is preferred (59).

The inorganic iodine concentration is only 0.08 to 0.6 µg per dL. About 3 mL of serum is required, and the assay depends on the catalytic effect on the reduction of ceric ion by arsenious acid. Thyroxine (T_4) is present at a level of 7 to 11 µg per dL. About 0.5% to 0.07% of this is not protein-bound. The level of free thyroxine, therefore, is 5.4 ± 1 ng per dL. Triiodothyronine (T_3) resin uptake is a measure of the protein-binding capacity for triiodothyronine and is not a determination of iodine content. Values of thyroid-stimulating hormone are 0.1 to 5.0 mU per L in euthyroid subjects (59). Under conditions of caloric restriction with adequate protein intake, the serum T3 concentration is reduced by 30%, an effect probably related to the caloric restriction (~1,800 kcal) (390).

Urinary iodine is the preferred test to detect iodine deficiency (391). Iodine concentration per L or per mole of creatinine is an acceptable substitute for 24-hour urinary collections. A urinary concentration of 788 nmol per L (100 µg per L) correlates with an intake of approximately 150 µg per day, the RDA for adolescents and adults. Optimal values are 100 to 200 µg per L (781 to 1,580 nmol per L) (Table 7-49) (392).

Physiology

Food contains mostly inorganic iodide, which is reduced in the gut lumen and nearly completely absorbed. Some iodinated compounds (e.g., thyroid hormones, amiodarone) are absorbed intact. Iodide is handled like chloride and passes easily across membranes, unlike other trace minerals (except for fluoride). It is concentrated in the thyroid and salivary glands by the action of the sodium/iodide cotransporter, SLCA5 (NIS), a member of the sodium/glucose cotransport family (393). This transporter also uses Br, NO3, SCN, and ClO4 as substrates. It is present in basolateral membranes of the thyroid, breast, colon, and ovary. It is secreted as inorganic iodine in saliva and milk but only as the organic form from the thyroid, probably via the apically located sodium/iodide cotransporter, AIT, another member of the SLC5 family. The iodide pool is replenished from the diet, saliva, gastric juice, and the breakdown of organic thyroxine derivatives. The thyroid gland, kidneys, and salivary and gastric glands all compete for free iodide. The thyroid must trap about 60 µg of iodide per day to maintain thyroxine levels. Iodide is concentrated by the sodium/iodide cotransporter, a member of the family of cotransporters that use electrochemical sodium gradients to drive coupled uphill transport of sugars, amino acids, vitamins, ions, and water. Iodide is also taken up by stomach, salivary glands, and mammary glands (394). The three pools of body iodide are the circulating inorganic, intrathyroid organic, and circulating organic pools. Iodide is excreted mostly in urine (>50 µg per day), with lesser losses in stool and sweat.

TABLE 7-49 Urinary Iodine Excretion as a Measure of Iodine Nutritional Status

	Urine Concentration	
Iodine Status	(µg/L)	(nmol/L)
Sufficient/optimal	100–200	781–1,580
Deficiency, mild	50–99	391–780
Deficiency, moderate	20–49	160–390
Deficiency, severe	<20	<160
More than adequate	201–300	1,581–2,360
Excessive/toxic	>300	>2,360

Data from Stanbury JB, Dunn JT. Iodine and iodine deficiency disorders. In: Bowman BA, Russell RM (eds.), *Present Knowledge in Nutrition*. 8th ed. Washington, DC ILSI, 2001:344.

Deficiency

Iodine deficiency is one cause of hypothyroidism. This deficiency in childhood can result in delayed growth. At all ages, it causes decreases in cellular oxidation and the basal metabolic rate and thus weakness, fatigue, and slow mental responses (395). Depending on the degree of deficiency and age at onset, mental changes can vary from mild intellectual impairment to severe retardation. Iodine deficiency is the most common form of preventable brain damage in the world (396). Hypotension and bradycardia, constipation, pretibial edema, and slow deep tendon reflexes are all seen. Thyromegaly often accompanies dietary iodine deficiency. Because iodide is easily absorbed, malabsorption syndromes do not cause deficiency. Because thyroid hormone production is decreased, the gland becomes hypertrophic in an attempt to compensate, and a goiter develops. Iodine requirement increases in pregnancy, and many women still do not maintain an AI without a supplement (397). The assessment of subclinical iodine deficiency in pregnant women can be difficult in the absence of gestation-specific values, and may consist only of an absence of the usual free T4 spike and a smaller than expected increase in total T4 during pregnancy (398). The maternal requirement for iodine increases by 50% during pregnancy, and if deficiency results it could have effects on cognitive function of the children (399).

Treatment

Iodine is a component of many multivitamin and mineral preparations. However, supplementation with 2 g of iodized salt per day provides the full RDA. In the United States, recent trends show a decline in iodine intake, especially among women of reproductive age (400). More than 90 countries currently iodize their salt products, at concentrations from 30 to 100 µg per g of salt. In countries without easily available iodized salt, iodized oil has been successfully used as a source of supplemental iodine to prevent goiter (410). Adult doses of supplemental iodine to treat suspected deficiency are usually 150 to 300 µg per day (399). When radioactive iodine therapy is administered, it may be necessary to place patients with a high intake of iodine on a low-iodine diet for 1 to 2 weeks so that the uptake of the radioactive element will be sufficient.

Toxicity

Excessive Dietary Intake

When intake exceeds 2,000 µg per day, iodide uptake by the thyroid gland is impaired and organic formation falls. These dietary levels can be reached by a large intake of iodine from iodized salt, vitamin and mineral preparations, or iodine-containing coloring dyes and dough conditioners. The margin of safety is great, and toxicity remains unusual at the present level of iodine supplementation. The tolerable ULs are 200 µg per day for children 1 to 3 years old, 300 µg per day for children 4 to 8 years old, 600 µg per day for children 9 to 13 years old, 900 µg per day for children 14 to 18 years old, and 1.1 mg per day for adults, based on serum thyroid-stimulating hormone concentrations during different levels of iodine intake (204). High intake in iodized salt, leading to a urinary excretion greater than 300 µg per L can produce hypothyroidism and autoimmune thyroiditis (402).

Excessive Therapeutic Iodine

Iodine-induced thyrotoxicosis may paradoxically result from excessive iodine therapy given to patients with multinodular goiter or quiescent Graves disease. Commonly used iodine-containing medications include expectorants and antithyroid medications. The iodine content of these medications far exceeds the normal dietary allowance, as listed in Table 7-50.

TABLE 7-50 Iodine Content of Medications

Drug	Iodine or Iodide Content Per Therapeutic Dose
Glycerol, iodinated	15 mg iodine per tablet or 30 mg per teaspoon of elixir
Calcidrine syrup	152 mg calcium iodide per teaspoon
Potassium iodide syrup	300 mg potassium iodide per teaspoon
Potassium iodide	
Solution	1 g potassium iodide per milliliter
Tablet	320 mg per tablet
Lugol solution	5% iodine in solution

Chapter 7 • Minerals | 337

The side effects of potassium iodide include rash, swelling of the salivary glands, a metallic taste in the mouth, stomach upset, allergic reactions, and headache. Iodinated glycerols are contraindicated in newborns and nursing mothers because of the possibility of producing hypothyroidism.

Fluoride

Fluoride is not considered an essential nutrient, because data defining its necessity for life are lacking. It does have a pharmacologic action on the enamel of teeth, by making hydroxyapatite of tooth enamel and dentin more resistant to attack by acid (403).

Requirement

The protective effect of fluoride on teeth is observed at intakes from 1.5 to 2.5 mg in adolescents. These levels are consistent with the range of fluoride intake in the United States. Therefore, the total AI recommended from food and drinking water is 3 mg per day for adult women and 4 mg per day for men (69). Because fluoride is required for the growth of bone and enamel, these recommendations are based on the prevention of dental caries, not on total body requirements. For children and adolescents, the primary beneficiaries of the prevention of dental caries with fluoride, the AI is 0.7 mg for ages 1 to 3 years, 1.0 mg for ages 4 to 8 years, 2 mg for ages 9 to 13 years, and 3 mg for ages 14 to 18 years. To avoid the danger of mottling of the teeth of infants and children, the UL for infants ages 0 to 6 months is 0.7 mg and 0.9 mg for ages 7 to 12 months. Comparable ULs for children are 1.3 mg for ages 1 to 3 years and 2.2 mg for ages 4 to 8 years. The UL for all others is 10 mg to avoid producing brittle bones.

Food Sources
Type of Food

Like other anionic trace elements (I, Se), the source of the food (where it is grown) is more important than the type. One exception is ocean fish, each gram of which contains 5 to 10 μg of fluoride. Other foods contain less than 0.5 parts per million (ppm). Tea is the other food naturally high in fluoride, containing 100 to 200 μg per g. The content of food can be decreased by cooking, during which water is lost, or increased by commercial processing, during which water is added. Cereals contain 1 to 3 μg per g of dry weight and are a major source of fluoride for infants. The availability of cereals for infants has raised the question of the need for water supplements (404). Daily intake in the United States averages about 0.4 mg from food; with water content added, the average is about 0.9 mg per day for boys.

Water

Water is the other major source of fluoride. Surface water contains about 1 ppm or less; deep water contains 4 to 8 ppm. The fluoride intake in cities with fluoridated water supplies is from 1.7 to 3.4 mg per day, with a mean of 2.6 mg, exclusive of water ingestion. In nonfluoridated areas, fluoride intake from food averages 0.9 mg per day. The difference represents food preparation. Water intake accounts for 1 to 1.5 mg daily in fluoridated areas and 0.1 to 0.6 mg in nonfluoridated areas. Thus, intake varies from 1 to greater than 4 mg per day. Because water supplies most dietary fluoride, either by itself or in foods, it is recommended that water supplies contain at least 1 mg per L, which ensures adequate fluoride intake to decrease the incidence of dental caries. Fluoride-containing dentifrice is ingested (~25%) by children less than 5 years old, who may ingest 0.3 mg fluoride per brushing. Thus, daily intake of young children brushing twice daily could be doubled.

Assessment
Body Stores

No fluorine deficiency state has been defined; thus, there is no basis for assessing a low body fluorine status (403). Because fluoride is required for the growth of bone and enamel, these recommendations are based on the prevention of dental caries, not total body requirement. Because most of the fluoride is in bone and enamel and not in extraosseous tissues, no practical method is available for assessing body stores. Bone content ranges from 300 to 600 ppm but is not usually measured.

Urine Levels

Urine levels are proportional to intake and average 0.5 to 0.6 ppm. Urine excretion reflects current ingestion or prior exposure to high levels. The efficient renal excretion mechanisms keep blood fluoride at a low narrow range independent of intake. Excretion of >15 mg per L suggests a daily exposure of 20 to 30 mg, a level at which more than 10 years of exposure could cause toxic fluorosis (403).

Physiology

Fluoride is concentrated in bones and teeth, where it is incorporated into the crystalline structure of hydroxyapatite. This results in increased resistance of the teeth to caries, especially in the preeruptive phase. Fluoride is completely absorbed (90% in the stomach) and is distributed like chloride in soft tissues. Uptake in bone depends on its growth and vascularity. Aluminum, iron, magnesium, and calcium salts can decrease the rate of absorption. About 50% of dietary fluoride is excreted in the urine each day (405).

Deficiency

Because fluoride is present in nearly all water supplies, plants, and animals, deficiency does not occur in humans. Fluoride is an essential element for growth in mice and rats, but has not been implicated in growth failure in humans.

Treatment

Over 40% of the water supplies in the United States are still not fluoridated (406). For children living in a nonfluoridated area, the daily addition of the AI for the appropriate age is adequate to prevent caries. Treatment in adults may prevent further caries. Each 2.2 mg of sodium fluoride contains 1 mg of fluoride. Sodium fluoride is available in chewable tablets (1 mg), lozenges (1 mg), drops (0.125 mg per drop), and solution (0.2 mg per mL). The use of slow-release fluoride formulations has largely prevented the gastritis that occurred with earlier preparations. Data showing the protective effect of fluoride via water fluoridation are solid, but evidence for caries protection from dietary or supplemental fluoride is lacking (407). Sodium fluoride has been used to treat osteoporosis (up to 60 mg of fluoride per day alternated in 6-month periods with calcium and vitamin D) in an attempt to stimulate the formation of new bone, which is then hardened by fluoride. No convincing evidence has been found that this treatment is beneficial in the prevention of osteoporosis. Currently, the FDA does not approve this form of therapy, because long-term safety has not been demonstrated, and the benefits have been limited to a reduction in vertebral fractures alone (406).

Toxicity

Fluoride is toxic when ingested in excess.

Mottled Teeth

Mottled teeth have been found in children ingesting water containing more than 8 ppm. The most common form of fluorosis is hypermineralization of tooth enamel from excessive systemic fluoride during the period of enamel development, but before tooth eruption. This is manifested by chalky white spots on the teeth (mottling). Mottling occurs only in permanent teeth and is usually not significant. Eczema, urticaria, gastric distress, and headache have been reported.

Systemic Fluorosis

With ingestion of 20 to 80 mg per day for years, a syndrome including osteosclerosis, genu valgum, kyphosis, and spine stiffness can occur. Systemic fluorosis has occurred in areas where a high fluoride intake is endemic (some parts of the Indian subcontinent and South Africa). The UL for adults has been set at 10 mg per day (69). The American Dental Association has recommended that no more than 120 mg of fluoride be dispensed at one time, to avoid the chance for severe fluorosis (406).

Manganese

Requirement

Manganese is a trace mineral essential to animals and probably humans. Many problems arise when balance methods are used to estimate trace minimal requirements, and no overt deficiency state exists in humans. Thus, data are insufficient to establish an EAR for manganese, and all the DRIs are based on median AIs (204). The AI for infants ages 0 to 6 months is 3 μg per day based on total estimated intake from milk. The estimated AIs for other life groups are as follows: 0.6 mg (infants 7 to 12 months old); 1.2 mg (children ages 1 to 3 years); 1.5 mg (children ages 4 to 8 years); 1.9 mg, 2.2 mg, and 2.3 mg (females ages 9 to 13 years, 14 to 18 years, and 19 to 70 years, respectively); 1.6

mg, 1.6 mg, and 1.8 mg (males ages 9 to 13 years, 14 to 18 years, and 19 to 70 years, respectively); 2 mg for pregnancy; and 2.6 mg during lactation. Because the current dietary intake seems adequate, an estimated safe and adequate dietary intake has been set at those levels, 2 to 5 mg for adults (204). Safe intakes are recommended for children and adolescents as follows: 1 to 1.5 mg for ages 1 to 3 years, 1.5 to 2.0 mg for ages 4 to 6 years, and 2 to 3 mg for ages 7 to 10 years. Safe intakes for formula-fed and breast-fed infants are 0.005 mg per day and 0.30 mg per day, respectively (408).

Food Sources

Nuts, dried fruit, cereals and unrefined grains, pineapple, pineapple juice, and tea are very rich in manganese (>1 mg per serving). Legumes, rice, spinach, sweet potatoes, pasta, and whole wheat bread are good sources of manganese (>0.5 mg per serving). Vegetables and fruits contain only moderate amounts, and dairy products, muscle meats, and seafood contain only small concentrations of the mineral. Drinking water contains approximately 10 µg per L of manganese from most sources (409). Human milk contains 3 to 10 µg per L, but soy formula has a much higher content (200 to 300 µg per L). The average daily intake for adults in the United States is 2.2 mg for women and 2.8 mg for men. Vegetarian diets or diets rich in whole grain products may provide as much as 8 to 10 mg per day. Hospital diets provide about 1 to 2 mg per day, and low-sodium and low-protein diets may supply less than 1 mg per day. Components of the diet can limit manganese absorption or increase excretion, including iron, phosphorus, calcium, copper, phytates, fiber, and polyphenols.

Assessment

As with other divalent cations, no measurement accurately assesses body stores. Like copper, manganese is excreted mainly in bile, not urine. Therefore, urine does not provide a good measure of recent intake. Red cells contain 13.6 to 16.9 µg per L, but serum/plasma contains only 0.59 to 1.3 µg per L (594). The usual assay is based on atomic absorption spectrometry, which measures total manganese. Radiochemical neutron activation analysis has also been used. Manganese is present in serum as the trivalent form, bound to β_2-globulin. Because this level does not change with altered intake and because deficiency in humans is not recognized, the usefulness of serum levels is small. Urine values vary little, are quite low, and are not useful in assessing manganese status. Hair content varies more among individuals and with such factors as exogenous contamination, color, and season than with manganese status.

Physiology

Function

The body contains about 12 to 20 mg of manganese. The liver and pancreas have the highest content. A few metalloenzymes (superoxide dismutase, pyruvate carboxylase) and many metal–enzyme complexes (hydrolases, kinases, decarboxylases, transferases) contain manganese.

Absorption

Absorption occurs in the small bowel but is very inefficient. Absorption efficiency is increased in animals when they are deficient. Like the absorption of other cationic metals, the absorption of manganese depends on its form; carbonate and silicate salts are poorly absorbed. Luminal calcium, phosphate, and iron decrease absorption. The most likely mechanism for iron competition is common use of the divalent metal transporter (DMT-1) (409). Manganese is bound largely to albumin and gamma globulin, but a small amount of trivalent (3+) ion is bound to transferrin. Tissues with high energy demand (brain) and high pigment content (retina, dark skin) contain the highest concentration of manganese. Excretion varies with bile output, which regulates body content. Manganese activates many enzymes, but is an absolute requirement for only a few; thus, deficiency states are rare.

Deficiency

In animals, neonatal ataxia, retarded skeletal growth, decreased reproductive function, and defects in lipid metabolism are seen. In humans, one case has been reported with weight loss, hypocholesterolemia, dementia, nausea, vomiting, and altered hair color (410). Manganese deficiency was induced in 39 days in young men and caused a fleeting dermatitis (411). Some epileptics have been reported with low blood levels of manganese. Manganese deficiency has not been reported in humans consuming a natural diet, and supplements are not indicated for healthy subjects. Men on experimental low manganese diets developed a rash on their torsos, and women on diets containing less than 1 mg of Mn per day developed altered mood during the premenstrual period (409).

Treatment

Manganese is a component of some multivitamin and mineral supplements. Therapy for specific deficiency symptoms is indicated very rarely. There is no good evidence for including manganese in trace element supplements to parenteral feeding regimens (412). As the intestine-biliary regulatory mechanisms for limiting body manganese are bypassed by parenteral administration, the risk of toxicity may be increased.

Toxicity

Manganese is relatively nontoxic when ingested, presumably because absorption is low. However, when inhaled as dust, it can produce psychiatric disorders and extrapyramidal signs. Manganese oxide is absorbed across the lungs and is a concern for miners. The UL, set at 11 mg per day, is based on no observable adverse effects on Western-type diets (204). Hypermanganesemia during treatment with TPN (usually 100 to 800 μg per day) can lead to increased signal density in the globus pallidus on magnetic resonance imaging (413). It can be seen in patients with cholestatic liver disease receiving TPN, but is not a risk when only the liver disease is present (414). Patients with cholestasis or neurologic symptoms or who are receiving prolonged TPN should be monitored for hypermanganesemia. If present, the infusion of manganese should be stopped or diminished. It is standard practice to supplement infants receiving TPN with a neonatal trace element solution containing 25 μg per mL of manganese. The *Pediatric Nutrition Handbook*, 5th edition, and the A.S.P.E.N. report of 2004 recommend 1 μg per kg per day for preterm infants, and 3 μg per kg per day for term infants weighing 3 to 10 kg (409). Whole blood measurement of manganese should be monitored to prevent accumulation.

Chromium

Requirement

Chromium is an essential trace mineral that potentiates the action of insulin in certain conditions. A safe intake of chromium would be based on the content of a varied diet that does not lead to deficiency, but deficiency is not readily identified in humans. Thus, the current dietary intake recommendations are based on the median intake of chromium at various ages (AI) (204). The adequate daily intake ranges are listed in Table 7-51. The lower recommendations for younger ages are based on extrapolations of expected food intake. However, the WHO has recommended lower intakes of 25 μg per day to prevent deficiency and 33 μg per day to maintain tissue stores (415) because earlier estimates were based on less accurate measurements of chromium.

Food Sources

Trivalent chromium is widely distributed as chromite in the soil. Plants contain between 100 and 500 μg per kg and foods between 20 and 590 μg per kg (416). The form or availability of chromium in specific foods is generally not known. A balanced diet provides chromium with an average availability of 1% to 2%. Spices (>10 μg per g) and brewer's yeast (>40 μg per g) contain the highest concentrations. Meat products (1 to 2 μg per g), dairy products (1 to 1.5 μg per g), and eggs (1 to 2 μg per g) are good sources. Leafy vegetables contain chromium in a relatively unavailable form. Rice and sugar are poor sources. Drinking water contains chromium from natural and man-made sources, and may be a risk factor for malignancy (417). Estimates of daily intake are complicated by the availability of more soluble chromium compounds (picolinate, nicotinic acid) available over the counter in supplements at doses from 50 to 600 μg (64). The best diet to maximize chromium status is one low in simple sugars and rich in unprocessed foods.

Assessment

Measurement of chromium in tissues is difficult because of the very low levels. Serum levels (2.5 to 5.2 nmol per L) are 10 times lower than tissue concentrations and are not in equilibrium with the body stores (59). Serum levels increase rapidly as insulin levels increase and decrease with infection. Urine excretion is 5 to 20 nmol per L, but it correlates poorly with intake because absorption is so poor. Graphite furnace atomic absorption spectrometry is the method most often used. Hair levels are better related to body stores, but still are affected by exogenous contamination, individual variations, and the other problems that beset this assay in the case of other trace minerals. Normal chromium levels in hair are about 990 ppm at birth; they fall to about 440 ppm after 2 or 3 years

TABLE 7-51 Dietary Reference Intakes of Chromium

Life Stage Group	Chromium (μg/d)
Infants	
0–6 months	0.029/kg
7–12 months	0.611/kg
Children	
1–3 years	11
4–8 years	15
Males	
9–13 years	21
14–18 years	24
19–50 years	25
51–>70 years	20
Females	
9–13 years	25
14–18 years	35
19–50 years	35
51–>70 years	30
Pregnancy	
14–18 years	29
19–50 years	30
Lactation	
14–18 years	44
19–50 years	45

Estimates based on adequate intake (AI).
Data from Standing Committee on the Scientific Evaluation of Dietary Reference Intakes, Food and Nutrition Board, Institute of Medicine. *Dietary Reference Intakes for Vitamin A, Vitamin K, Arsenic, Boron, Chromium, Copper, Iodine, Iron, Manganese, Molybdenum, Nickel, Silicon, Vanadium, and Zinc.* Washington, DC: National Academies Press, 2002.

of life. The best way to diagnose chromium deficiency is to observe whether symptoms or signs that appear during TPN (hyperglycemia, neuropathy) respond to chromium infusion (404).

Physiology

Chromium is poorly absorbed (~1% to 2%) regardless of the level of intake or body stores. Oxalates and vitamin C increase and phytates and antacids decrease absorption (418). The hexavalent ion is absorbed better than trivalent chromium. Chromium picolinate and organic complexes from brewer's yeast or with nicotinic acid are absorbed better than the chloride salt. After absorption, chromium is widely distributed in the body, with internal organs (liver, kidney, spleen) achieving the highest concentrations (419). Excretion occurs mainly in the urine. A glucose load or insulin injection increases excretion, especially in diabetics. Trivalent chromium is required for normal glucose metabolism in animals, probably acting as a cofactor for insulin. A low-molecular-weight chromium-binding substance (LMWCr) has been identified as an oligopeptide that binds four chromium ions and activates the insulin receptor (416,420).

Deficiency

Severe chromium deficiency in humans is very rare, but subclinical deficiency may occur, because average dietary intake is lower than the minimum recommended intake of 25 to 50 μg per day (421). Deficiency has been noted after prolonged TPN (see Chapter 11). Glucose intolerance and impaired release of free fatty acids have been noted, along with increased circulating levels of insulin, neuropathy, encephalopathy, and hypercholesterolemia and hypertriglyceridemia (422). Deficiency is hard to document because no good method is available to assess body stores. It is generally agreed that chromium is an essential element, but the data are largely supportive and not definitive (419,423).

Treatment

IV administration of 5 to 10 μg of chromium chloride daily for the first few days, followed by 10 μg weekly, is probably adequate therapy. Chromium has been marketed as a weight loss aid and a muscle builder, and as an aid in glucose assimilation. However, no studies have shown a definite benefit in controlling diabetes or blood lipids, increasing lean body mass or decreasing body fat, improving muscle mass in athletes, or improving osteoporosis (64,417,423).

Toxicity

The hexavalent salt is more toxic than the trivalent salt in animals and has been associated with the production of lung tumors. No well-recognized toxic syndrome in humans has been reported (424). Thus, a UL has not been set (204). Randomized, controlled trials of 175 to 1,000 μg of chromium per day given from 6 to 64 weeks have shown no toxic effects (416). The Environmental Protection Agency has assigned a safety factor of 1,000 to chromium because of no observed adverse effect. This translates to a safe upper limit of 1.47 mg per kg per day. Isolated adverse effects have been reported, but their significance is not clear. Renal failure has been associated with chromium picolinate in two cases (416). The Expert Group on Vitamins and Minerals of the UK Joint Food Standards and Safety Group recommended in 2003 that the health supplement industry voluntarily withdraw chromium picolinate-containing products (423). The FDA is considering possible regulation of the sale of this compound, because of continued evidence of some toxicity. Headaches, sleep disturbances, and mood swings have been reported (64).

Selenium

Requirement

Selenium is an essential trace mineral that is a component of the enzyme glutathione peroxidase. Safe selenium requirements for adult Chinese men to prevent deficiency (Keshan disease) have been estimated at 40 μg per day, and two small supplementation studies suggested 70 and 55 μg per day as the intake required to achieve plateau concentrations of plasma glutathione peroxidase (425). To adjust for differences in weight and individual variation, the DRI for adults has been set at 55 μg per day, between the highest and lowest estimates (Table 7-52).

TABLE 7-52 Selenium Dietary Reference Intakes and Tolerable Upper Intake Levels

Life Stage Group	DRI	UL
	μg/d	
Infants		
0–6 months	15[a]	45
7–12 months	20[a]	60
Children		
1–3 years	20	90
4–8 years	30	150
Males, Females		
9–13 years	40	280
14–>70 years	55	400
Pregnancy		
≤18–50 years	60	400
Lactation		
≤18–50 years	70	400

DRI, dietary reference intakes; UL, upper intake levels.
[a]Estimated on adequate intake. All other DRI values represent recommended dietary allowances (RDAs).
Data from Standing Committee on the Scientific Evaluation of Dietary Reference Intakes, Food and Nutrition Board, Institute of Medicine. *Dietary Reference Intakes for Vitamin C, Vitamin E, Selenium, and Beta-carotene and Other Carotenoids.* Washington, DC: National Academies Press, 2000.

Because selenium can be toxic, the ULs have been set not too far above the DRIs. The UL of 400 μg per day for adults is close to the reference dose of 5 μg per kg per day set by the Environmental Protection Agency.

Food Sources

Selenium is present in foods as selenomethionine or selenocysteine. Plant content varies with the soil content. Unlike in the United States, there are few selenium-rich food sources in the European diet. The development of deficiency syndromes in livestock in European countries led to measures to increase selenium intake, such as top dressing of pasture land with fertilizers to which selenium has been added, which may increase the soil content. Still, selenium intakes in many parts of Europe are lower than in the United States (426,427). Wheat is a good source of selenium in North America but not in Europe. Much of the selenium in grains is lost in the milling process. The selenium content of animal foods is affected by the selenium content of the animal feed. The best sources of selenium are Brazil nuts and kidney, neither a routine food. Moderately good sources include fish, shellfish, other organ meats, muscle meats, and whole grains. Fruits and vegetables are poor sources. Selenium intakes in the United States average 108 μg per day, with a range of 83 to 129 μg per day. In Europe, comparable values are lower, ranging from 29 to 70 μg per day (426). Food sources supply selenomethionine and selenocysteine, which are incorporated into proteins in place of methionine, but they must be catabolized to an inorganic precursor to form selenophosphate, the precursor for selenocysteine, the active form in selenoproteins. Supplements also provide selenomethionine; however, sometimes the more available selenate and selenite are provided, although they carry the risk for acute toxicity when taken in excess. The estimation of selenium in foods is hampered by the lack of methods that can extract the element reliably while maintaining its chemical form (428).

Assessment

Serum levels respond to changes in the diet but can be falsely lowered by any cause of hypoproteinemia. About half of the selenium in serum is incorporated into protein in selenoprotein P. After digestion of serum to remove organic material, a selenium complex is measured fluorometrically (59). Normal serum levels are 0.132 to 0.139 μg per mL. Selenium deficiency is defined as a plasma level ≤0.85 μg per mL (427). Red cells contain higher amounts (0.23 to 0.36 μg per mL of cells), and hemolysis can alter the serum levels. Low serum levels are not associated with decreased cellular selenium and thus do not reflect body stores. Blood levels range from 3.14 to 3.32 μmol per L. Biologically active selenium can be estimated by measuring glutathione peroxidase in red cells (429). The correlation between these variables (enzyme and serum levels) has been inconsistent. This inconsistency has been resolved by the discovery that another protein, selenoprotein P, contains more than 60% of serum selenium in the rat. Hair content correlates with body stores in animals, but the determination is subject to the same problems of contamination and individual variation that arise in measuring the hair content of other trace metals.

Physiology

Liver and kidney contain the most selenium, with muscle, skin, and nails having the next highest concentrations. Inorganic selenium is poorly absorbed; organic (food) selenium is assimilated best into the body. The absorption rate is not regulated and is highest in the duodenum, varying from 60% to 80% in humans. Feces and urine are the usual excretory routes. Selenium is present in bile in low concentrations. It forms complexes with heavy metals and protects against Cd and Mg toxicity. The metabolism of selenium depends upon the form in which it is present in the body. Selenomethionine, selenocysteine, selenate and selenite enter the pool of selenides (anions with an oxidation number of -2), and from there the element is used for biosynthesis or excretion (428). Selenomethionine can be used directly for protein synthesis, however. There are 25 known selenoproteins in humans with a variety of functions. Selenium provides a system for intracellular redox regulation. The best-known example of this is its role as a cofactor of glutathione peroxidase, which reduces hydrogen peroxide and protects membranes from oxidative damage. Glutathione peroxidase is now known to be a family of at least six various selenoproteins, in different cellular locations, both intra- and extracellular (427). Some peroxidases are localized only to specific tissues (e.g., sperm, gastrointestinal mucosa). Selenium also plays a role in electron transfer functions and affects drug-metabolizing enzymes. Selenium is included as the selenoamino acid, selenocysteine, in more than 35 proteins, including thioredoxin reductase and the iodothyronine deiodinases that produce active thyroid hormone (426). The exact functional significance of this amino acid is not clear. Other selenoproteins include selenoprotein P (protecting endothelial cells against peroxynitrite), selenoprotein W (an antioxidant for cardiac and striated muscle), selenoprotein 18kDa (preserving kidney selenium), and selenoprotein N (associated with muscle dystrophy) (427,430). A number of selenoproteins still have no known function.

Deficiency

Definite

Only a few descriptions of a disorder in humans caused by dietary selenium deficiency have been published, even in areas where selenium deficiency in livestock is widespread. A cardiomyopathy that affected children was described in China (Keshan disease); it can be eliminated with oral selenium (431). Plasma and red cell selenium levels can fall during TPN without causing symptoms for 1 month (432). Common symptoms in these patients have been those of cardiomyopathy and myositis (427). A similar syndrome has been reported in the Saudi population (433). A chondrodystrophy (Kashin-Beck disease) also occurs in selenium-deficient areas of China (434). Other causative factors are felt to be involved in both these conditions.

Possible

Deficiency of selenium is associated with loss of immunocompetency, and supplementation improves laboratory parameters of immune function; however, no clinical syndrome is associated with these changes (64). Patients in the ICU present with low serum selenium concentrations, but the clinical significance of this finding is uncertain (435). Deficiency has been linked to infection with some viruses, including HIV and coxsackievirus (426). Selenium is important for reproduction in animals, but the data on humans is inconclusive. Low selenium levels have been associated with depression, and high dietary levels of selenium seem to be associated with fewer such symptoms. Epidemiologic studies linking selenium deficiency to heart disease provide conflicting results. Evidence does not support a role for selenium in improving exercise function (64). Controlled interventions with supplements are needed to determine what role, if any, selenium has in these conditions. Perhaps the largest body of data on associated disorders comes from cancer prevention, particularly cancer of the prostate (427). An inverse relationship has been reported between plasma selenium concentration and risk of colorectal adenomas (436). However, no evidence in humans has shown that selenium supplements when used as adjunctive therapy improve survival in cancer patients (437).

Treatment

Deficiency

If dietary deficiency occurs, 100 to 200 µg daily should be adequate therapy. Areas in the United States rich in selenium are the Great Plains and Rocky Mountain states, especially the Dakotas and Wyoming. If dietary selenium (in the form of selenoamino acids) is not considered adequate, a multivitamin/mineral tablet supplying 55 to 70 µg of selenium can be used. Organic forms (selenocysteine and selenocystine) have been used in recent years, but earlier preparations contained inorganic salts, such as selenite, selenium dioxide, and selenate. Sodium selenite is the most efficacious IV form.

Gastrointestinal Diseases

In severe malabsorption, a low serum level of selenium was almost always noted (438). Epidemiologic evidence has been found that higher plasma levels of selenium are associated with a decreased prevalence of intrahepatic cholestasis of pregnancy (439).

Cancer Chemoprevention

Supplements of selenium given to patients in many regions with selenium-poor soil and foods have been shown to prevent liver and esophageal cancer in China, oral cancer in India, and colon cancer in Italy (440). However, the quality of many of these studies is uncertain, as studies used either mixed or single supplements, the form of selenium was often unknown, and the statistics were often not well described. The evidence for prevention of prostate cancer shows that apparent benefit is limited to those with low basal plasma selenium, and/or those who smoke (441).

The Nutritional Prevention of Cancer trial showed a lower rate of cancers of the skin, prostate, colon, and lung in those receiving 200 μg per day of selenium, but the greatest benefit was found in patients with the lowest basal selenium levels (442). This study has been extended as the Prevention of Cancer by Intervention with Selenium (PRECISE) treating with 200 μg or 400 μg per day for 5 years, to see if the results of the original study can be validated. The SELECT trial of selenium and vitamin E supplements in patients at risk for prostate cancer showed no differences in mortality in any form of cancer (443).

Toxicity

A UL for selenium intake has been set at 400 μg per day, and clinical toxicity resulting from much higher intakes in overly potent tablets (>20 mg per tablet) has been reported (425). Nausea, vomiting, fatigue, hair loss, diarrhea, irritability, paresthesias, and abdominal cramps have been reported. Ingestion of 5 mg per day in the diet in Enshi County, China, led to loss of hair and nails, skin lesions, tooth decay, and nervous system abnormalities (444). Toxic symptoms are found with blood selenium levels above 13.3 μmol per L, but urinary measurements are probably a better indicator of toxicity. Urinary levels should be less than 100 μg per L to avoid selenium toxicity (59).

DRUGS THAT AFFECT MINERAL STATUS

A number of drugs cause minerals to be lost from the body in either urine or feces. The use of such drugs may cause or intensify a deficiency of a given mineral. Table 7-53 lists some of these drugs and the changes in serum levels of the minerals affected. The use of laxatives can lead to sodium and water depletion and dehydration, usually with no change in the serum sodium level. Potassium is secreted from the colon under these conditions, and hypokalemia

TABLE 7-53 Drugs That Alter Status of Minerals

↓ [Na]s
Acetazolamide, carbamazepine, cyclophosphamide, chlorpropamide, furosemide, heparin, hydrochlorothiazide, morphine, oxytocin, pentamidine, selective serotonin reuptake inhibitors (SSRIs), spironolactone

↓ [Na]s
Colchicine, ethacrynic acid, foscarnet, furosemide, hypertonic sodium salts, lithium, phenytoin, vinblastine

↓ [K]s
Acetazolamide, amiloride, amphotericin B, ampicillin and derivatives, aspirin, beta-blockers, carboplatin, carmustine, corticosteroids, cytarabine, diuretics, intravenous dextrose, didanosine, dobutamine, dosorubicin, fluconazole, foscarnet, ganciclovir, gentamicin, insulin, itraconazole, levodopa, lithium, metolazone, nifedipine, ondansetron, pamidronate, phosphates, polymyxin B, rifampin, risperidone, salmeterol, sargramostim, sirolimus, sodium salts, sorbitol, SSRIs, tacrolimus, terbutaline, tobramycin, torsemide, vincristine

↓ [K]s
Amiloride, beta-blockers, captopril and related drugs, cotrimoxazole, cyclosporine, heparin, NSAIDs, pentamidine, potassium salts, spironolactone, tacrolimus, triamterene

↓ [Mg]s
Albuterol, amphotericin B, carboplatin, cholestyramine, cisplatin, corticosteroids, cyclosporine, didanosine, digoxin, diuretics, estrogen, ethanol, foscarnet, gentamicin, insulin, laxatives, oral contraceptives, penicillamine, pentamidine, phosphates, sargramostim, tacrolimus, tobramycin, torsemide, zoledronic acid

↓ [Mg]s
Lithium, magnesium salts

(continued)

TABLE 7-53	Drugs That Alter Status of Minerals *(continued)*

↓ [PO$_4$]s
Acetazolamide, Al-Mg antacids, bisphosphonates, calcitonin, calcium salts, carmustine, cefotan, cholestyramine, cisplatin, digoxin, ethanol, foscarnet, magnesium, osmotic diuretics, sevelamer, sirolimus/tacrolimus, zoledronic acid

↓ [PO$_4$]s
Phosphate salts

↓ [Ca]s
Antacids, bleomycin, calcitonin, carboplatin, cholestyramine, cisplatin, codeine, corticosteroids, cyclosporine, diuretics, doxorubicin, estrogens, fluoride, 5-fluorouracil, foscarnet, H$_2$-receptor antagonists, interferon, isoniazid, ketoconazole, macrolide antibiotics, magnesium, pentamidine, phenytoin, phosphates, rituximab, sargramostim, triamterene

↓ [Ca]s
Calcium salts, ganciclovir, lithium, thiazide diuretics, tamoxifen, theophylline

Data from Boullata JI, Influence of medication on nutritional status. In: Bendich A, Deckelbaum RJ, Sommer A (Eds.), *Preventive Nutrition: The Comprehensive Guide for Health Professionals*. 3rd ed. Totowa, NJ: Humana Press, 2006:833.

results. Sodium depletion presents clinically when diuretics are used in the absence of sodium overload syndrome. Diuretics can exacerbate hypomagnesemia, but usually do not cause it when body stores are normal. Some drugs cause changes in body stores without altering serum concentrations of the mineral. For example, glucocorticoids are associated with osteopenia, which is not a result of decreased calcium stores alone; abnormal vitamin D metabolism is probably also involved. Other drugs can alter serum concentrations without altering body stores. For example, Neutrophos treatment can cause hypocalcemia without a decrease in body calcium stores.

REFERENCES

1. Strohle A, Hahn A, Sebastian A. Estimation of the diet-dependent net acid load in 229 worldwide historically studied hunter-gatherer societies. *Am J Clin Nutr*. 2010;91:406.
2. Remer T. Influence of diet on acid–base balance. *Semin Dial*. 2000;13:221.
3. Alpers DH. Subclinical micronutrient deficiency: a problem in recognition. *Curr Opin Gastroenterol*. 2012;28:135.
4. Standing Committee on the Scientific Evaluation of Dietary Reference Intakes, Food and Nutrition Board, Institute of Medicine. *Dietary Reference Intakes for Water, Potassium, Sodium, Chloride, and Sulfate*. Washington DC: National Academies Press, 2005.
5. Elgart HN. Assessment of fluids and electrolytes. *AACN Clin Issues*. 2004;15:607.
6. Zalepuga R, Di Palma JA. Metals. *Pract Gastroenterol*. 2002;25:14.
7. Manton WI, Angle CR, Krogstrand KL. Origin of lead in the United States diet. *Environ Sci Technol*. 2005;39:8995.
8. Fung TT, Hu FB, Wu K, et al. The Mediterranean and Dietary approaches to stop hypertension (DASH) diets and colorectal cancer. *Am J Clin Nutr*. 2010;92:1429.
9. McCarron DA. The dietary guidelines for sodium: should we shake it up? Yes! *Am J Clin Nutr*. 2000;71:1013.
10. Craddick SR, Elmer PJ, Obarzanek E, et al. The DASH diet and blood pressure. *Curr Atheroscler Rep*. 2003;5:484.
11. Sacks FM, Svetkey LP, Vollmer WM, et al; DASH-Sodium Collaborative Research Group. Effects on blood pressure of reduced dietary sodium and the Dietary Approaches to Stop Hypertension (DASH) diet. *N Engl J Med*. 2001;344:3.
12. He FJ, Markandu ND, Sagnella GA, et al. Plasma sodium: ignored and underestimated. *Hypertension*. 2005;45:98.
13. Alderman MH. Dietary sodium and cardiovascular health in hypertensive patients: the case against universal sodium restriction. *J Am Soc Nephrol*. 2004;15:S47.

14. Hooper L, Bartlett C, Davey SG, et al. Advice to reduce dietary salt for prevention of cardiovascular disease. *Cochrane Database Syst Rev.* 2004;(1):CD003656.
15. He JF, MacGregor GA. Effect of longer-term modest salt reduction on blood pressure. *Cochrane Database Syst Rev.* 2004;(3):CD004937.
16. Krousel-Wood MA, Muntner P, He J, et al. Primary prevention of essential hypertension. *Med Clin North Am.* 2004;88:223.
17. US Department of Agriculture and US Department of Health and Human Services. *Dietary Guidelines for Americans, 2010,* 7th ed. Washington, DC: US Govt Printing Office, 2010.
18. Bernstein AM, Willett WC. Trends in 24-h urinary sodium excretion in the United States, 1957–2003: a systematic review. *Am J Clin Nutr.* 2010;92:1172.
19. Drewnowski A, Maillot M, Rehm CD. Reducing the sodium-potassium ratio in the US diet: a challenge for public health. *Am J Clin Nutr.* 2012:96:439.
20. Strom BL, Yaktine AL, Oria M (eds), Committee on the consequences of sodium reduction in populations, Food and Nutrition Board, Institute of Medicine. *Sodium Intake in Populations: Assessment of Evidence*, Washington, DC: National Academies Press,, 2013.
21. O'Donnell MJ, Yusuf S, Mente A, et al. Urinary sodium and potassium excretion and risk of cardiovascular events. *JAMA.* 2011;306:2229.
22. Whelton PK. Urinary sodium and cardiovascular disease risk: informing guidelines for sodium consumption. *JAMA.* 2011;306:2262.
23. Bibbins-Domingo K, Chertow GM, Coxson PG, et al. Projected effect of dietary salt reductions on future cardiovascular disease. *N Eng J Med.* 2010;362:590.
24. Appel LJ, Anderson CAM. Compelling evidence for public health action to reduce salt intake. *N Eng J Med.* 2010;362:650.
25. Smith-Spangler CM, Juusola JL, Enns EA, et al. Population strategies to decrease sodium intake and the burden of cardiovascular disease: a cost-effectiveness analysis. *Ann Intern Med.* 2010;152:481.
26. Kotchen TA, Cowley AW, Frohlich ED. Salt in health and disease—a delicate balance. *N Eng J Med.* 2013;368:1229.
27. Sawka MN, Montain SJ. Fluid and electrolyte balance: effects on thermoregulation and exercise in the heat. In: Bowman BA, Russell RM, eds. *Present Knowledge in Nutrition.* 8th ed. Washington DC: ILSI Press, 2001:115.
28. Webster JL, Danford EK, Neal BC. A systematic survey of the sodium contents of processed foods. *Am J Clin Nutr.* 2010;91:413.
29. Guenther PM, Lyon JM, Appel LJ. Modeling dietary patterns to assess sodium recommendations for nutrient adequacy. *Am J Clin Nutr.* 2011;97:842.
30. McGee S, Abernethy WB, Simel DL. Is this patient hypovolemic? *JAMA.* 1999;281:1022.
31. Consensus statement on the definition of orthostatic hypotension, pure autonomic failure, and multiple system atrophy. *Neurology.* 1996;46:1470.
32. Streeten DH. Variations in the clinical manifestations of orthostatic hypotension. *Mayo Clin Proc.* 1995;70:713.
33. Cheuvront SN, Kenefick RW, Charkoudian N,et al.Physiologic basis for understanding quantitative dehydration. *Am J Clin Nutr.* 2013;97:455.
34. Brown IJ, Dyer AR, Chan Q, et al. Estimating 24-hour urinary sodium excretion from casual urinary sodium concentrations in Western populations. *Am J Epidemiol.* 2013;177:1180.
35. Martin MG, Wright EM. Disorders of epithelial transport in the small intestine. In: Yamada T, Alpers DH, Kaplowitz N, et al. (eds.) *Textbook of Gastroenterology*, 5th ed. Oxford, UK: Blackwell Publishing, Ltd., 2007:2088.
36. Eisenhut M. Changes in ion transport in inflammatory diseases. *J Inflamm (Lond).* 2006;3:5.
37. Zachos NC, Tse M, Donowitz M. Molecular physiology of intestinal Na^+/H^+ exchange. *Annu Rev Physiol.* 2005;67:411.
38. Geerling JC, Loewy AD. Central regulation of sodium appetite. *Exp Physiol.* 2008;93:178.
39. Marcet B, Boeynaems JM. Relationships between cystic fibrosis transmembrane conductance regulator, extracellular nucleotides and cystic fibrosis. *Pharmacol Ther.* 2006;112:719.
40. Miller C. ClC chloride channels viewed through a transporter lens. *Nature.* 2006;440:484.
41. Puljak L, Kilic G. Emerging roles of chloride channels in human diseases. *Biochim Biophys Acta.* 2006;1762:404.
42. Alpers SL. Molecular physiology of SLC4 anion exchangers. *Exp Physiol.* 2006;91:153.
43. Mount DB, Romero MF. The SLC26 gene family of multifunctional anion exchangers. *Pflugers Arch.* 2004;447:710.

44. Eckford PD, Li C, Bamjeesingh M, et al. Cystic fibrosis transmembrane conductance regulator (CFTR) potentiator VX-770 (Ivacaftor) opens the defective channel gate of mutant CFTR in a phosphorylation-dependent but ATP-independent manner. *J Biol Chem.* 2012;387:36639.
45. Anonymous. Lubiprostone: RU 0211, SPI 0211. *Drugs R D.* 2005;6:245.
46. Murek M, Kopic S, Geibel J. Evidence for intestinal chloride secretion. *Exp Physiol.* 2009;95:471.
47. Hammer HF, Santa Ana CA, Schiller LR, et al. Studies of osmotic diarrhea induced in normal subjects by ingestion of polyethylene glycol and lactulose. *J Clin Invest.* 1989;84:1056.
48. Vaidya C, Ho W, Freda BJ. Management of hyponatremia: providing treatment and avoiding harm. *Cleveland Clin J Med.* 2010;77:715.
49. King JD, Rosner MH. Osmotic demyelination syndrome. *Am J Med Sci.* 2010;339:561.
50. Adrogue HJ, Madias N. Hyponatremia. *N Engl J Med.* 2000;342:1581.
51. Sentongo TA. The use of oral rehydration solutions in children and adults. *Curr Gastroenterol Rep.* 2004;6:307.
52. Alpers DH. Oral rehydration solutions for adults: an underutilized resource. *Curr Opin Gastroenterol.* 1998;14:143.
53. Hahn S, Kim S, Garner P. Reduced osmolarity oral rehydration solution for treating dehydration caused by acute diarrhea in children. *Cochrane Database Syst Rev.* 2002;(1):CD002847.
54. Ramakrishna RB, Venkataraman S, Srinivasan P, et al. Amylase-resistant starch plus oral rehydration solution for cholera. *N Engl J Med.* 2000;342:308.
55. Matarese LE, O'Keefe SJ, Kandil HM, et al. Short bowel syndrome: clinical guidelines for nutrition management. *Nutr Clin Pract.* 2005;20:493.
56. Borne RT, Krantz MJ. Lixivaptan for hyponatremia—the numbers game. *JAMA.* 2012;308:2345.
57. Sam R, Feizi I. Understanding hypernatremia. *Am J Nephrol.* 2012;36:97.
58. Cheuvront SN, Kenefick RW, Sollanek KJ, et al. Water-deficit equation: systematic analysis and improvement. *Am J Clin Nutr.* 2013;97:79.
59. Sauberlich HE. *Laboratory Tests for the Assessment of Nutritional Status.* 2nd ed. Boca Raton, FL: CRC Press, 1999.
60. Halperin ML, Kamel KS. Potassium. *Lancet.* 1998;352:135.
61. Warth R, Barhanin J. Function of K^+ channels in the intestinal epithelium. *J Memb Biol.* 2003;193:67.
62. Gennari FJ. Hypokalemia. *N Engl J Med.* 1998;339:451.
63. Whelton PK, He J, Cutler JA, et al. Effects of oral potassium on blood pressure: meta-analysis of randomized controlled clinical trials. *JAMA.* 1997;277:1624.
64. Fragakis AS. *The Health Professional's Guide to Popular Dietary Supplements.* 2nd ed. Hoboken NJ: Wiley, 2002.
65. Evans KJ, Greenberg A. Hyperkalemia: a review. *J Intensive Care Med.* 2005;20:272.
66. Erfani M, Akula Y, Zolgaghari T, et al. Sodium polystyrene sulfate (SPS): sorbitol-induced colonic necrosis. *Pract Gastroenterol.* 2010;34:47.
67. Heaney RP. Osteoporosis: protein, minerals, vitamins, and other micronutrients. In: Bendich A, Deckelbaum RJ, Sommer A (eds.), *Preventive Nutrition: The Comprehensive Guide for Health Professionals.* 3rd ed. Totowa, NJ: Humana Press, 2005:433.
68. Fairweather-Tait SJ, Teucher B. Iron and calcium bioavailability of fortified foods and dietary supplements. *Nutr Rev.* 2002;60:360.
69. Standing Committee on the Scientific Evaluation of Dietary Reference Intakes, Food and Nutrition Board, Institute of Medicine. *Dietary Reference Intakes: Calcium, Phosphorus, Magnesium, Vitamin D, and Fluoride.* Washington, DC: National Academies Press, 1997.
70. Cao JJ, Pasiakos SM, Margolis LM, et al. Calcium homeostasis and bone metabolic responses to high protein diets during energy deficit in healthy young adults: a randomized control trial. *Am J Clin Nutr.* 2014;99:400.
71. Kerstetter JE, O'Brien KO, Insogna KL. Low protein intake: the impact on calcium and bone homeostasis in humans. *J Nutr.* 2003;133:855S.
72. Nordin C. Calcium requirement is a sliding scale. *Am J Clin Nutr.* 2000;71:1381.
73. Food and Drug Administration. Food labeling: health claims, calcium and osteoporosis. *Fed Regist.* 1993;58:2665.
74. Ross AC, Manson JE, Abrams SA, et al. The 2011 report on dietary reference intakes for calcium and vitamin D from the Institute of Medicine: what clinicians need to know. *J Clin Endocrinol Metab.* 2011;96:53.
75a. Miller GD. Year 2000 dietary guidelines: new thoughts for a new millennium. *Am J Clin Nutr.* 2000;71:657.
75b. Heaney RP. There should be a dietary guideline for calcium. *Am J Clin Nutr.* 2000;71:658.

75c. Specker BL. Should there be a dietary guideline for calcium intake? No. *Am J Clin Nutr.* 2000;71:661.
76. Abrams SA. Setting dietary reference intakes with the use of bioavailability data: calcium. *Am J Clin Nutr.* 2010;91(Suppl):1474S.
77. Zhang V, Hang S, Faruckhi YZ, et al. Vitamin D and calcium: what do we need to know? *Clin Obstet Gynecol.* 2013;56:654.
78. Lanou AJ, Berkow SE, Barnard ND. Calcium, dairy products, and bone health in children and young adults: a reevaluation of the evidence. *Pediatrics.* 2005;115:736.
79. Abrams SA, Atkinson SA. Calcium, magnesium, phophorus and vitamin D fortification of complementary foods. *J Nutr.* 2003;133:2994S.
80. Toffaletti JG. Clinical Laboratory News. Calcium. 2011;37. http://www.aacc.org/publications/cln/archive/2011/September/Pages/calcium.aspx.
81. Smith GR, Collinson PO, Kiely PD. Diagnosing hypovitaminosis D: serum measurements of calcium, phosphate, and alkaline phosphatase are unreliable, even in the presence of secondary hyperparathyroidism. *J Rheumatol.* 2005;32:684.
82. Alexeera L, Burkhardt P, Christiansen C, et al. *Assessment of Fracture Risk and Application of Screening for Postmenopausal Osteoporosis.* World Health Organization Technical Report Series 843. Geneva: World Health Organization, 1994.
83. Baddiyra R, Awada H, Okais J, et al. An audit of bone densitometry practices with reference to ISCD, IOF, and NOF guidelines. *Osteoporos Int.* 2006;17:1111.
84. Raisz LG. Screening for osteoporosis. *N Engl J Med.* 2005;353:164.
85. Lewiecki EM. Bone density measurement and assessment of fracture risk. *Clin Obstet Gynecol.* 2013;56:667.
86. Moayyeri A, Soltani A, Bahrami H, et al. Preferred skeletal site for osteoporosis screening in high-risk populations. *Public Health.* 2006;120:863.
87. Hans DB, Kanis JA, Baim S, et al. Joint official positions of the International Society for Clinical Densitometry and International Osteoporosis Foundation on FRAX. *J Clin Densitom.* 2011;14:171.
88. Hodgson SF, Johnston CC. AACE clinical practice guidelines for the prevention and treatment of postmenopausal osteoporosis. *Endocr Pract.* 1996;2:155.
89. Kanis J, Devogelaer J, Gennari C. Practical guide for the use of bone mineral measurements in the assessment of treatment of osteoporosis: a position paper of the European Foundation for Osteoporosis and Bone Disease. *Osteoporos Int.* 1996;6:256.
90. Bonnick SL. *Bone Densitometry in Clinical Practice: Application and Interpretation.* Totowa, NJ: Humana Press, 1998.
91. Bone mass measurement act (BMMA). *Fed Regist.* 1998;63:34324.
92. Bronner F. Recent developments in intestinal calcium absorption. *Nutr Rev.* 2008;67:109.
93. ICSD indications for bone mineral density testing. 2013. http://www.iscd.org/documents/2013/07/2013-icsd-official-position-adult.pdf.
94. Malabanan AO, Rosen HN, Vokes TJ, et al. Indications of DXA in women younger than 65 yr and men younger than 70 yr: the 2013 official positions. *J Clin Densitom.* 2013;16:467.
95. De Laet C, Kanis JA, Oden A, et al. Body mass index as a predictor of fracture risk: a meta-analysis. *Osteoporosis Int.* 2005;16:1330.
96. Dargent-Molina P. Bone density measurement in older women: who and why? *Joint Bone Spine.* 2004;71:264.
97. Faibish D, Ott SM, Boskey AL. Mineral changes in osteoporosis: a review. *Clin Orthop Relat Res.* 2006;443:28.
98. Schonau E. The peak bone mass concept: is it still relevant? *Pediatr Nephrol.* 2004;19:825.
99. Kleerekoper M, Nelson DA. BMD testing appropriate for all menopausal women? *Int J Fertil Womens Med.* 2005;50:61.
100. Shepherd JA, Lu Y, Wilson K, et al. Cross-calibration and minimum precision standards for dual-energy X-ray absorptiometry: the 2005 ISCD official positions. *J Clin Densitom.* 2006;9:31.
101. Bachrach LK. Measuring bone mass in children: can we really do it? *Horm Res.* 2006;65 (Suppl 2):11.
102. Dennison E, Cole Z, Cooper C. Diagnosis and epidemiology of osteoporosis. *Curr Opin Rheumatol.* 2005;17:456.
103. Ramasamy I. Recent advances in physiological calcium homeostasis. *Clin Chem Lab Med.* 2006;44:237.
104. Ward DT, Riccardi D. New concepts in calcium-sensing receptor pharmacology and signaling. *Br J Pharmacol.* 2012;165:35.

105. Deroisy A, Zartarian M, Meurmans L, et al. Acute changes in serum calcium and parathyroid hormone circulating levels induced by the oral intake of five currently available calcium salts in healthy male volunteers. *Clin Rheumatol.* 1997;16:249.
106. Recker RR. Calcium absorption and achlorhydria. *N Engl J Med.* 1985;313:70.
107. Boyce BF. Stomaching calcium for bone health. *Nat Med.* 2009;15:610.
108. Hoenderop JGJ, Bindels RJM. Epithelial Ca^{2+} and Mg^{2+} channels in health and disease. *J Am Soc Nephrol.* 2005;16:15.
109. Aloia JF, Chen DG, Yeh JK, et al. Serum vitamin D metabolites and intestinal calcium absorption efficiency in women. *Am J Clin Nutr.* 2010;92:835.
110. Bonjour JP. Calcium and phosphate: a duet of ions playing for bone health. *J Am Coll Nutr.* 2011;30:438S.
111. Qualres JD. 'Dem bones' are made for more than walking. *Nat Med.* 2011;17:428.
112. Sun L, Chow LC, Frukhtbeyn SA, et al. Preparation and properties of nanoparticles of calcium phosphates with various Ca/P ratios. *J Res Natl Inst Stand Technol.* 2010;115:243.
113. Anonymous. Calcium deficiency. *Lancet.* 1985;1:1431
114. Raisz LG. Pathogenesis of osteoporosis: concepts, conflicts, and prospects. *J Clin Invest.* 2005;115:3318.
115. Coates PS, Fernstrom JD, Fernstrom MH, et al. Gastric bypass surgery for morbid obesity leads to an increase in bone turnover and a decrease in bone mass. *J Clin Endocrinol Metab.* 2004;89:1061.
116. Weinstein RS. Glucocorticoid-induced bone disease. *N Eng J Med.* 2011;365:62.
117. Hansen KE, Wilson HA, Zapalowski C, et al. Uncertainties in the prevention and treatment of glucocorticoid-induced osteoporosis. *J Bone Min Res.* 2011;26:1989.
118. Ito T, Jensen RT. Association of long-term proton pump inhibitor therapy with bone fractures and effects on absorption of calcium, vitamin B12, iron, and magnesium. *Curr Gastroenterol Rep.* 2010;12:448.
119. Dickerson RN, Morgan LG, Caughen AD, et al. Treatment of acute hypocalcemia in critically ill multiple-trauma patients. *JPEN J Parenter Enteral Nutr.* 2005;29:436.
120. Thacher TD, Fischer PR, Pettifor JM, et al. A comparison of calcium, vitamin D, or both for nutritional rickets in Nigerian children. *N Engl J Med.* 1999;341:563.
121. Kalkwarf HJ, Specker BL, Bianchi DC, et al. The effect of calcium supplementation on bone density during lactation and after weaning. *N Engl J Med.* 1997;337:523.
122. Scott EM, Gaywood I, Scott BB; British Society of Gastroenterology: Guidelines for osteoporosis in coeliac disease and inflammatory bowel disease. *Gut.* 2000;46(Suppl 1):1.
123. Compston JE. Management of bone disease in patients on long-term glucocorticoid therapy. *Gut.* 1999;44:770.
124. Ghishan FK, Kiela PR. Metabolic bone disease in inflammatory bowel disease. *Pract Gastroenterol.* 2012;36:16.
125. Storm D, Eslin R, Porter ES, et al. Calcium supplementation prevents seasonal bone loss and changes in biochemical markers of bone turnover in elderly New England women: a randomized placebo-controlled trial. *J Clin Endocrinol Metab.* 1998;83:3817.
126. Nieves JW, Komar L, Cosman F, et al. Calcium potentiates the effect of estrogen and calcitonin on bone mass: a review and analysis. *Am J Clin Nutr.* 1998;67:18.
127. Recker RR, Davies KM, Dowd RM, et al. The effect of low-dose continuous estrogen and progesterone therapy with calcium and vitamin D on bone in elderly women: a randomized, controlled trial. *Ann Intern Med.* 1999;130:897.
128. Porthouse J, Cockayne S, King C, et al. Randomized controlled trial of calcium and supplementation with cholecalciferol (vitamin D3) for prevention of fractures in primary care. *BMJ.* 2005;330:1003.
129. Grant AM, Avenell A, Campbell MK, et al; The RECORD trial group. Oral vitamin D3 and calcium for secondary prevention of low-trauma fractures in elderly people (Randomized Evaluation of Calcium OR vitamin D, RECORD): a randomized placebo-controlled trial. *Lancet.* 2005;365:1671.
130. Hamdy RC, Baim S, Brow SB, et al. Algorithm for the management of osteoporosis. *South Med J.* 2010;103:1009.
131. Gourlay ML, Fine JP, Preisser JS, et al. Bone-density testing interval and transition to osteoporosis in older women. *N Eng J Med.* 2012;366:225.
132. Allender PS, Cutler JA, Follman D, et al. Dietary calcium supplementation on blood pressure: a meta-analysis of randomized clinical trials. *Ann Intern Med.* 1996;124:825.

133. Bucher HC, Cook RJ, Gfuyatt GH, et al. Effects of dietary calcium supplementation on blood pressure. A meta-analysis of randomized controlled trials. *JAMA*. 1996;275:1016.
134. Uusi-Rasi K, Karkkainen UM, Lamberg-Allardt CJE. Calcium intake in health maintenance—a systematic review. *Food Nutr Res*. 2013;57:1082.
135. Bolland MJ, Avenell A, Baron JA, et al. Effect of calcium supplements on risk of myocardial infarction and cardiovascular events: meta-analysis. *BMJ*. 2010;341:c3691.
136. Heaney RP, Kopecky S, Maki KC, et al. A review of calcium supplements and cardiovascular disease risk. *Adv Nutr*. 2012;3:763.
137. Bostick RM. Human studies of calcium supplementation and colorectal epithelial cell proliferation. *Cancer Epidemiol Biomarkers Prev*. 1997;6:971.
138. Baron JA, Beach M, Mandel JS, et al. Calcium supplements for the prevention of colorectal adenomas. Calcium Polyp Prevention Study Group. *N Engl J Med*. 1999;341:101.
139. Bolland MJ, Grey A, Gamble GD, et al. Calcium and vitamin D supplements and health outcomes: a reanalysis of the Women's Health Initiative (WHI) limited-access data set. *Am J Clin Nutr*. 2011;94:1144.
140. Zhang X, Giovannucci E. Calcium, vitamin D and colorectal cancer chemoprevention. *Best Pract Res Clin Gastroenterol*. 2011;25:485.
141. Rhys-Jacobs S, Starkey P, Bernstein D, et al; Premenstrual Syndrome Study Group. Calcium carbonate and the premenstrual syndrome: effects on premenstrual and menstrual symptoms. *Am J Obstet Gynecol*. 1998;179:444.
142. Straub DA. Calcium supplementation in clinical practice: a review of forms, doses, and indications. *Nutr Clin Pract*. 2007;22:286.
143. Anonymous. Drugs for prevention and treatment of postmenopausal osteoporosis. *Med Lett*. 2002;1:13.
144. Heaney RP. Calcium supplements: practical considerations. *Osteoporos Int*. 1991;1:65.
145. Fink HA, Wilt TJ, Eidman KE, et al. Medical management to prevent recurrent nephrolithiasis in adults: a systematic review for an American College of Physicians clinical guideline. *Ann Intern Med*. 2013;158:535.
146. Durlach J, Pages N, Bac P, et al. New data on the importance of gestational Mg deficiency. *Magnes Res*. 2004;17:116.
147. Karppanen H, Karppanen P, Mervaala E. Why and how to implement sodium, potassium, calcium, and magnesium changes in food items and diets? *J Human Hypertens*. 2005;19:S10.
148. USDA Nutrient Database. Magnesium content of foods. http://www.ars.usda.gov/SP2UserFiles/Place/12354500/Data/SR25/nutrlist/sr25a304.pdf.
149. Zhang W. Point of care testing of ionized magnesium in blood with potentiometric sensors—opportunities and challenges. *Am J Biomed Sci*. 2011;3:301.
150. Tong GM, Rude RK. Magnesium deficiency in critical illness. *J Intensive Care Med*. 2005;20:3.
151. Dimeski G, Badrick T, St John A. Ion selective electrodes (ISEs) and interferences—a review. *Clin Chim Acta*. 2010;411:309.
152. Massry SG, Seelig MS. Hypomagnesemia and hypermagnesemia. Magnesium Online Library 2007; http://www.mgwater.com/hypomagnesemia.shtml.
153. Philips S, Donaldson L, Geisler K, et al. Stool composition in factitial diarrhea: a 6-year experience with stool analysis. *Ann Intern Med*. 1995;123:97.
154. Seelig MS, Altjura BM. The Magnesium Online Library 2007; http://www.mgwater.com/laboratory_test.shtml.
155. Simon DB, Lu Y, Choate KA, et al. Paracellin-1, a renal tight junction protein required for paracellular Mg2+ resorption. *Science*. 1999;285:103.
156. Chubanov V, Gudermann T, Schlingmann KP. Essential role for TRPM6 in epithelial magnesium transport and body magnesium homeostasis. *Pflugers Arch-Eur J Physiol*. 2005;451:228.
157. Schweigel M, Martens H. Magnesium transport in the gastrointestinal tract. *Front Biosci*. 2000;5:D666.
158. Weisinger JR. Magnesium and phosphorus. *Lancet*. 1998;352:391.
159. Ikarashi N. The elucidation of the function and the expression control mechanism of aquaporin-3 in the colon [in Japanese]. *Yakugaku Zasshi*. 2013;133:955.
160. Graber ML, Schulman G. Hypomagnesemic hypocalcemia independent of parathyroid hormone. *Ann Intern Med*. 1986;104:804.
161. Reinhart RA. Magnesium metabolism: a review with special reference to the relationship between intracellular content and serum levels. *Arch Intern Med*. 1988;148:2415.
162. Kudenchuk PJ. Advanced cardiac life support antiarrhythmic drugs. *Cardiol Clin*. 2002;20:79.

163. Joosten MM, Gansevoort RT, Mukamal KJ, et al; for the PREVEND Study Group. Urinary and plasma magnesium and risk of ischemic heart disease. *Am J Clin Nutr*. 2013;97:1299.
164. Hoorn EJ, van der Hoek J, de Man RA, et al. A case series of proton pump inhibitor-induced hypomagnesemia. *Am J Kidney Dis*. 2010;56:112.
165. Luk CP, Parsons R, Lee YP, et al. Proton pump inhibitor-induced hypomagnesemia—what do FDA data tell us? *Ann Pharmacother*. 2013;47:773.
166. Cundy T, Mackay J. Proton pump inhibitors and severe hypomagnesaemia. *Curr Opin Gastroenterol*. 2011;27:180.
167. Del Gobbo LC, Imamura F, Wu JH, et al. Circulating and dietary magnesium and risk of cardiovascular disease: a systematic review and meta-analysis of prospective studies. *Am J Clin Nutr*. 2013;98:160.
168. Mouw DR, Latessa RA, Sullo EJ. What are the causes of hypomagnesemia? *J Family Pract*. 2005;54:174.
169. Office of Dietary Supplements. Magnesium: dietary supplement fact sheet, 2013. https://ods.od.nih.gov/pdf/factsheets/Magnesium-HealthProfessional.pdf.
170. Fleming CR, George L, Stoner GL, et al. The importance of urinary magnesium values in patients with gut failure. *Mayo Clin Proc*. 1996;71:21.
171. Duley L, Farrell B, Spark P, et al; MAGPIE Trial Collaboration Group. Do women with preeclampsia and their babies, benefit from magnesium sulphate? The Magpie Trial: a randomized placebo controlled trial. *Lancet*. 2002;359:1877.
172. Cummins RO, Hazinski MF, Baskett PJ, et al; The American Heart Association and the International Liaison Committee on Resuscitation. Guidelines 2000 for Cardiopulmonary Resuscitation and Emergency Cardiovascular Care. *Circulation*. 2000;102(Suppl):1.
173. Fine KD, Santa Ana CA, Porter JL, et al. Intestinal absorption of magnesium from food and supplements. *J Clin Invest*. 1991;88:396.
174. Rodriguez-Moran M, Guerrero-Romero F. Oral magnesium supplementation improves insulin sensitivity and metabolic control in type 2 diabetic subjects: a randomized double-blind controlled trial. *Diabetes Care*. 2003;26:1147.
175. Shils ME. Magnesium. In: Shils ME, Olson JA, Shike M, et al. (eds.), *Modern Nutrition in Health and Disease*, 10th ed. Philadelphia: Lea & Febiger, 1999:169.
176. Calvo MS, Uribarri J. Contributions to total phosphorus intake: all sources considered. *Semin Dial*. 2013;26:54.
177. McGartland C, Robson PJ, Murray L, et al. Carbonated soft drink consumption and bone mineral density in adolescence: the Northern Ireland Young Hearts Project. *J Bone Miner Res*. 2003;18:1563.
178. Takeda E, Yamamoto H, Nashiki K, et al. Inorganic phosphate homeostasis and the role of dietary phosphorus. *J Cell Mol Med*. 2004;8:191.
179. Walton RJ, Bijvoet OL. Nomogram for derivation of renal threshold phosphate concentrations. *Lancet*. 1975;2:309.
180. Prie D, Friedlander G. Genetic disorders of renal phosphate transport. *N Eng J Med*. 2010;362:2399.
181. Bergwitz C, Collins MT, Kamath RS, et al. Case 33-2011: a 56-year-old man with hypophosphatemia. *N Eng J Med*. 2011;365:1625.
182. Goseki-Stone M, Sogabe N, Fukushi-Irie M, et al. Functional analysis of the single nucleotide polymorphism (787T>C) in the tissue-nonspecific alkaline phosphatase gene associated with BMD. *J Bone Miner Res*. 2005;20:773.
183. Lee R, Weber TJ. Disorders of phosphorus homeostasis. *Curr Opin Endocrinol Diabetes Obes*. 2010;17:561.
184. Knochel JP. The clinical status of hypophosphatemia: an update. *N Engl J Med*. 1985;313:447.
185. LaRoche M. Phosphate, the renal tubule, and the musculoskeletal system. *Joint Bone Spine*. 2001;68:211.
186. Brame LA, White KE, Econs MJ. Renal phosphate wasting disorders: clinical features and pathogenesis. *Semin Nephrol*. 2004;24:39.
187. Knochel JP. The pathophysiology and clinical characteristics of severe hypophosphatemia. *Arch Intern Med*. 1977;137:203.
188. Calvo MS, Uribarri J. The public health impact of dietary phosphorus excess on bone and cardiovascular health in the general population. *Am J Clin Nutr*. 2013;98:6.
189. Tonelli M, Pannu N, Manns B. Oral phosphate binders in patients with kidney failure. *N Eng J Med*. 2010;362:1312.
190. Allen DG, Trajenovska S. The multiple roles of phosphate in muscle fatigue. *Front Physiol*. 2012;3:463.

191. Palmer SC, Hayen A, Macaskill P, et al. Serum levels of phosphorus, parathyroid hormone, and calcium and risks of death and cardiovascular disease in individuals with chronic kidney disease. *JAMA*. 2011;305:1119.
192. Howard SC, Jones DP, Pui CH. The tumor lysis syndrome. *N Eng J Med*. 2011;364:1844.
193. Glassman K. Low serum phosphorus got you down? *Pract Gastroenterol*. 2013;37:26.
194. van der Veere CN, Jansen PLM, Sinaasappel M, et al. Oral calcium phosphate: a new therapy for Crigler-Najjar disease? *Gastroenterology*. 1997;112:455.
195. Brown KA, Dickerson RN, Morgan LM, et al. A new graduated dosing regimen for phosphorus replacement in patients receiving nutrition support. *JPEN J Parenter Enteral Nutr*. 2006;30:209.
196. Marinella MA. The refeeding syndrome and hypophosphatemia. *Nutr Rev*. 2003;61:320.
197. Brown AR, DiPalma JA. Bowel preparations for gastrointestinal procedures. *Curr Gastroenterol Rep*. 2004;6:395.
198. Schwetz BA. Review: oral sodium phosphate. *JAMA*. 2001;286:2660.
199. Carbonero F, Benefiel AC, Alizadeh-Ghamsari AH, et al. Microbial pathways in colonic sulfur metabolism and links with health and disease. *Front Physiol*. 2012;3:article 448.
200. Markovich D. Slc13a1 and Slc26a1 KO models reveal physiological roles of anion transporters. *Physiology*. 2012;27:7.
201. Jahoor F. Effects of decreased availability of sulfur amino acids in severe childhood undernutrition. *Nutr Rev*. 2012;70:176.
202. Iron therapy. The importance of iron. http://www.irontherapy.org/iron-essentials/importance-iron#
203. Hurrell R, Egli I. Iron bioavailability and dietary reference values. *Am J Clin Nutr*. 2010;91(Suppl):1461S.
204. Standing Committee on the Scientific Evaluation of Dietary Reference Intakes, Food and Nutrition Board, Institute of Medicine. *Dietary Reference Intakes for Vitamin A, Vitamin K, Arsenic, Boron, Chromium, Copper, Iodine, Iron, Manganese, Molybdenum, Nickel, Silicon, Vanadium, and Zinc*. Washington, DC: National Academies Press, 2002.
205. Sandberg AS, Brune M, Carlsson G, et al. Inositol phosphates with different numbers of phosphate groups influence iron absorption in humans. *Am J Clin Nutr*. 1999;70:240
206. Abizari AR, Moretti D, Schuth S, et al. Phytic acid-to-iron molar ratio rather than polyphenol concentration determines iron bioavailability in whole-cowpea meat among young women. *J Nutr*. 2012;142:1950.
207. Afify AE, El-Beltagi HS, El-Salam SM, et al Bioavailability of iron, zinc, phytate, and phytase activity during soaking and germination of white sorghum varieties. *PLoS One*. 2011;6:e25512.
208. Hurrell RF. Phytic acid degradation as a means of improving iron absorption. *Int J Vitam Nutr Res*, 2004;74:445.
209. Olivares M, Pizarro F, Ruz M. Zinc inhibits nonheme iron bioavailability in humans. *Biol Trace Elem Res*. 2007;117:7.
210. Hunt JR. Bioavailability of iron, zinc, and other trace minerals from vegetarian diets. *Am J Clin Nutr*. 2003;78(Suppl 3):633S.
211. Correnti C, Strong RK. Mammalian siderophores, siderophore-binding lipocalins, and the labile iron pool. *J Biol Chem*. 2012;287:13524.
212. Blanck HM, Cogswell ME, Gillespie C,et al. Iron supplement use and iron status among US adults: results from the third National Health and Nutrition Examination Survey. *Am J Clin Nutr*. 2005;82:1024.
213. Hoppe M, Hulthen L, Hallberg L. The importance of bioavailability of dietary iron in relation to the expected effect from iron fortification. *Eur J Clin Nutr*. 2008;62:761.
214. Lopez MA, Martos FC. Iron availability: an updated review. *Int J Food Sci Nutr*. 2004;55:597.
215. Whittaker P, Tufaro PR, Rader JI. Iron and folate in fortified cereals. *J Am Coll Nutr*. 2001;20:247.
216. Joosten E, Vanderelst B, Kerkhofs P, et al. Does dietary iron intake influence the iron status in hospitalized elderly patients? *J Nutr Health Aging*. 1999;3:8.
217. Hastka J, Lasserre JJ, Schwarzbeck A, et al. Laboratory tests of iron status: correlation or common sense? *Clin Chem*. 1996;42:5.
218. Wormwood M. The laboratory assessment of iron status—an update. *Clin Chim Acta*. 1997;259:3.
219. Weiss G, Goodnough LT. Anemia of chronic disease. *N Engl J Med*. 2005;352:1011.
220. Northrop-Clewes CA. Interpreting indicators of iron status during an acute phase response—lessons from malaria and human immunodeficiency virus. *Ann Clin Biochem*. 2008;45:18.
221. Finch CA, Cook JD. Iron deficiency. *Am J Clin Nutr*. 1984;39:471.
222. Sackett DL, Richardson WS, Rosenberg W, et al. *Evidence-based Medicine*. New York: Churchill Livingstone, 1997:124.

223. Thurnham DI, McCabe LD, Haldar S, et al. Adjusting plasma ferritin concentrations to remove the effects of subclinical inflammation in the assessment of iron deficiency: a meta-analysis. *Am J Clin Nutr*. 2010;92:546.
224. Aguilar-Martinez P, Schved JF, Brissot P. The evaluation of hyperferritinemia: an updated strategy based on advances in detecting genetic abnormalities. *Am J Gastroenterol*. 2005;100:1185.
225. Beguin Y. Soluble transferring receptor for the evaluation of erythropoiesis and iron status. *Clin Chim Acta*. 2003;329:9.
226. Eschbach JW. Iron requirements in erythropoietin therapy. *Best Pract Res Clin Haematol*. 2005;18:347.
227. Kroot JJ, Kemna EH, Bansal SS, et al. Results of the first international round robin for the quantification of urinary and plasma hepcidin assays: need for standardization. *Haematologica*. 2009;94:1748.
228. Vermeulen E, Vermeersch P. Hepcidin as a biomarker for the diagnosis of iron metabolism disorders: a review. *Acta Clin Belg*. 2012;67:190.
229. Bergamaschi G, Di Sabatino A, Albertini R, et al. Serum hepcidin in inflammatory bowel diseases: biological and clinical significance. *Inflamm Bowel Dis*. 2013;19:2166.
230. Tussing-Humphreys L, Nemeth E, Fantuzzi G, et al. Elevated systemic hepcidin and iron depletion in obese premenopausal females. *Obesity*. 2010;18:1449.
231. Guyatt GH, Oxman AD, Ali M, et al. Laboratory diagnosis of iron-deficiency anemia: an overview. *J Gen Intern Med*. 1992;7:145.
232. Psaty BM, Tierney WM, Martin DK, et al. The value of serum iron studies as a test for iron-deficiency anemia in a county hospital. *J Gen Intern Med*. 1989;2:160.
233. Thompson WG, Meola T, Lipkin M Jr, et al. Red cell distribution width, mean corpuscular volume, and transferrin saturation in the diagnosis of iron deficiency. *Arch Intern Med*. 1988;148:2128.
234. Adams PC. Population screening for hemochromatosis. *Hepatology*. 1999;29:1324.
235. Whitlock EP, Garlitz BA, Harris EL, et al. Screening for hereditary hemochromatosis: a systematic review for the U.S. Preventive Services Task Force. *Ann Intern Med*. 2006;145:209.
236. Beaumont C, Delaby C. Recycling iron in normal and pathological states. *Semin Hematol*. 2009;46:328.
237. Finch CA, Huebers W. Perspectives in iron metabolism. *N Engl J Med*. 1982;306:1520.
238. Cook JD. Adaptation in iron metabolism. *Am J Clin Nutr*. 1990;51:301.
239. Andrews NC, Fleming MD, Gunshin H. Iron transport across biologic membranes. *Nutr Rev*. 1999;57:114.
240. Anderson GJ, Frazer DM. Recent advances in intestinal iron transport. *Curr Gastroenterol Rep*. 2005;7:365.
241. van Dokkum W. Significance of iron bioavailability for iron recommendations. *Biol Trace Elem Res*. 1992;35:1.
242. Andrews NC, Schmidt PJ. Iron homeostasis. *Annu Rev Physiol*. 2007;69:1.
243. Latunda-Dada GO, Simpson RJ, McKie AT. Recent advances in mammalian haem transport. *Trends Biochem Sci*. 2006;31:182.
244. Theil EC. Iron homeostasis and nutritional iron deficiency. *J Nutr*. 2011;141:7245.
245. Zoller H, Pietrangelo A, Vogel W, et al. Duodenal metal-transporter (DMT-1, NRAMP-2) expression in patients with hereditary hemochromatosis. *Lancet*. 1999;353:2120.
246. West AR, Oates PS. Mechanisms of heme iron absorption: current questions and controversies. *World J Gastroenterol*. 2008;14:4101.
247. Collings R, Harvey LJ, Hooper L, et al. The absorption of iron from whole diets: a systematic review. *Am J Clin Nutr*. 2013;98:65.
248. Sargent PJ, Farnaud S, Evan RW. Structure/function overview of proteins involved in iron storage and transport. *Curr Medl Chem*. 2005;12:2683.
249. Theil EC. The iron responsive element (IRE) family of mRNA regulators: regulation of iron transport and uptake compared in animals, plants, and microorganisms. *Met Ions Biol Syst*. 1998;35:403.
250. Ganz T. Hepcidin and iron regulation, 10 years later. *Blood*. 2011;117:4425.
251. Evstatiev R, Gasche C. Iron sensing and signaling. *Gut*. 2012;61:933.
252. Franchini M, Montagnana M, Lippi G. Hepcidin and iron metabolism: from laboratory to clinical implications. *Clin Chim Acta*. 2010;411:1565.
253. Zhang AS, Enns CA. Iron homeostasis: recently identified proteins provide insight into novel control mechanisms. *J Biol Chem*. 2009;284:711.

254. Knutson MD. Iron-sensing proteins that regulate hepcidin and enteric iron absorption. *Annu Rev Nutr*. 2010;30:149.
255. Pantopoulos K, Prwal AK, Tratakoff A, et al. Mechanisms of mammalian iron homeostasis. *Biochemistry*. 2012;51:5705.
256. Philpott CC. Coming into view: eukaryotic iron chaperones and intracellular iron delivery. *J Biol Chem*. 2012;287:13518.
257. Mole DR. Iron homeostasis and its interaction with prolyl hydroxylases. *Antiox Redox Signal*. 2010;12:445.
258. Smith TG, Robbins PA, Ratcliffe PJ. The human side of hypoxia-inducible factor. *Br J Haematol*. 2008;141:325.
259. Lozoff B, Jimenez E, Hagen J, et al. Poorer behavioral and developmental outcome more than 10 years after treatment for iron deficiency in infancy. *Pediatrics*. 2000;105:E51.
260. Gordon N. Iron deficiency and intellect. *Brain Dev*. 2003;25:3.
261. Andrews NC. Disorders of iron metabolism. *N Engl J Med*. 1999;341:1986.
262. Khaodhiar L, Keane-Ellison M, Tawa NE, et al. Iron deficiency anemia in patients receiving home total parenteral nutrition. *JPEN J Parenter Enteral Nutr*. 2002;26:114.
263. Bayraktar UD, Bayraktar S. Treatment of iron deficiency anemia associated with gastrointestinal tract diseases. *World J Gastroenterol*. 2010;16:2720.
264. Weiss G, Gasche C. Pathogenesis and treatment of anemia in inflammatory bowel disease. *Haematologica*. 2010;95:175.
265. Sarzynski E, Puttarajappa C, Xie V, et al. Association between proton pump inhibitor use and anemia: a retrospective cohort study. *Dig Dis Sci*. 2011;56:2349.
266. Gomollon F, Gisbert JP. Intravenous iron in inflammatory bowel diseases. *Curr Opin Gastroenterol*. 2013;29:201.
267. Dec GW. Anemia and iron deficiency—new therapeutic targets in heart failure? *N Eng J Med*. 2009;361:2474.
268. Steinmetz HT, Tsamaloukas A, Schmitz S, et al. A new concept for the differential diagnosis and therapy of anaemia in cancer patients. *Support Care Cancer*. 2011;19:261.
269. Fretham SJ, Carlson ES, Georgieff MK. The role of iron in learning and memory. *Adv Nutr*. 2011;2:112.
270. Krayenbuieh PA, Battagay E, Breymann C, et al. Intravenous iron for the treatment of fatigue in non-anemic, premenopausal women with low serum ferritin concentration. *Blood*. 2011;118:3222.
271. O'Keefe ST. Secondary causes of restless leg syndrome in older people. *Age Aging*. 2005;34:349.
272. Connor JR, Boyer PJ, Menzies SL, et al. Neuropathological examination suggests impaired brain iron acquisition in restless leg syndrome. *Neurology*. 2003;61:304.
273. Dauvilliers Y, Winkelmann J. Restless legs syndrome: update on pathogenesis. *Curr Opin Pulm Med*. 2013;19:594.
274. Aorora RN, Kristo DA, Bista SR, et al. The treatment of restless legs syndrome and periodic limb movement disorder in adults—an update for 2012: practice parameters with an evidence-based systematic review and meta-analysis. *Sleep*. 2012;35:1039.
275. Finberg KE. Iron-refractory iron deficiency anemia. *Sem Hematol*. 2009;46:378.
276. De Silva AD, Mylanoki M, Rampton DS. Oral iron therapy in inflammatory bowel disease: usage, tolerance, and efficacy. *Inflamm Bowel Dis*. 2003;9:316.
277. Seligman PA, Caskey JH, Frazier JL, et al. Measurements of iron absorption from prenatal vitamin–mineral supplements. *Obstet Gynecol*. 1983;61:356.
278. Van Iperen CE, Kraaijenhagen RJ, Biesma DH, et al. In early period after surgery, iron cannot be utilized due to the inflammatory process. *Br J Surg*. 1998;85:41.
279. Ganz T. Molecular pathogenesis of anemia of chronic disease. *Pediatr Blood Cancer*. 2006;46:554.
280. Verdon F, Burnard B, Stubi CL, et al. Iron supplementation for unexplained fatigue in non-anemic women: double-blind randomized placebo controlled trial. *BMJ*. 2003;326:1124.
281. Gozzard D. When is high-dose intravenous iron repletion needed? Assessing new treatment options. *Drug Des Devel Ther*. 2011;5:51.
282. Burns DL, Mascioli EA, Bistrian BR. Effect of iron-supplemented total parenteral nutrition in patients with iron deficiency anemia. *Nutrition*. 1996;12:411.
283. Kumpf VJ. Update on parenteral iron therapy. *Nutr Clin Pract*. 2003;18:318.
284. Koutroubakis IE, Karmiris K, Makreas S, et al. Effectiveness of darbepoetin-alfa in combination with intravenous iron sucrose in patients with inflammatory bowel disease and refractory anemia: a pilot study. *Eur J Gastroenterol Hepatol*. 2006;18:421.

285. Dignass AU, Stein J. Management of iron deficiency anaemia in inflammatory bowel disease with special emphasis on intravenous iron. *Pract Gastroenterol.* 2011;35:17.
286. Auerbach M, Witt D, Toler W, et al. Clinical use of the total dose intravenous infusion of iron dextran. *J Lab Clin Med.* 1988;111:566.
287. Auerbach M, Winchester J, Wahab A, et al. A randomized trial of three iron dextran infusion methods for anemia in EPO-treated dialysis patients. *Am J Kidney Dis.* 1998;31:81.
288. National Kidney Foundation. Clinical practice guidelines for nutrition in chronic renal failure. *Am J Kidney Dis.* 2000;35(6 Suppl 2):S1.
289. Silverstein SB, Rodgers GM. Parenteral iron therapy options. *Am J Hematol.* 2004;76:74.
290. Bailie GR, Clark JA, Lane CE, et al. Hypersensitivity reactions and deaths associated with intravenous iron preparations. *Nephrol Dial Transplant.* 2005;20:1443.
291. Lyseng-Williamson KA, Keating GM. Ferric Carboxymaltose: a review of its use in iron–deficiency anemia. *Drugs.* 2009;69:739.
292. Anonymous, Ferumoxytol Feraheme—a new parenteral iron formulation. *Med Lett..* 2010;52:23.
293. Jahn MR, Andreasen HB, Futterer S, et al. A comparative study of the physicochemical properties of iron isomaltoside 1000 (Monofer), a new intravenous iron preparation and its clinical implications. *Eur J Pharm Biopharm.* 2011;78:480.
294. Fleming RE, Ponka P. Iron overload in human disease. *N Eng J Med.* 2012;366:348.
295. Brittenham GM. Iron-chelatinog therapy for transfusional iron overload. *N Engl J Med.* 2011;364:146.
296. Donangelo CM, Zapata CL, Woodhouse LR, et al. Zinc absorption and kinetics during pregnancy and lactation in Brazilian women. *Am J Clin Nutr.* 2005;82:118.
297. Hunt JR, Matthys LA, Johnson LK. Zinc absorption, mineral balance, and blood lipids in women consuming lactoovovegetarian and omnivorous diets for 8 weeks. *Am J Clin Nutr.* 1998;67:421.
298. Brown KH, Peerson JM, Allen LH. Effect of zinc supplementation on children's growth: a meta-analysis of intervention trials. In: Sandstrom B, Walter P, eds. *Role of Trace Elements for Health Promotion and Disease Prevention.* Davis, CA: University of California, 1998:76.
299. Briefel RR, Bialostosky K, Kennedy-Stephenson J, et al. Zinc intake of the U.S. population: findings from the Third National Health and Nutrition Examination Survey, 1988–1994. *J Nutr.* 2000;130:1367S.
300. Freeland-Graves J. Mineral adequacy of vegetarian diets. *Am J Clin Nutr.* 1988;48:859.
301. King JE. Assessment of zinc status. *J Nutr.* 1990;120(Suppl 11):1474.
302. Lowe NM, Feket K, Decsi T. Methods of assessment of zinc status in humans: a systematic review. *Am J Clin Nutr.* 2009(Suppl):2040S.
303. Lu J, Stewart AJ, Sadler PJ, et al. Albumin as a zinc carrier: properties of its high-affinity zinc-binding site. *Biochem Soc Trans.* 2008;36:1317.
304. Wiesman K, Hoyer H. Serum alkaline phosphatase and serum zinc levels in the diagnosis and exclusion of zinc deficiency in man. *Am J Clin Nutr.* 1985;41:1214.
305. Rookani N, Hurrell R, Kilighedi R, et al. Zinc and its importance in human health: an interpretive review. *J Res Med Sci.* 2013;18:144.
306. Hess SY, Lonnerdal B, Hotz C, et al. Recent advances in knowledge of zinc nutrition and human health. *Food Nutr Bull.* 2009;10:55.
307. Gibson RS, Hess SY, Hotz C, et al. Indicators of zinc status at the population level: a review of the evidence. *Br J Nutr.* 2008;99(Suppl 3):S14.
308. Blanchard RK, Cousins RJ. Regulation of intestinal gene expression by dietary zinc: induction of uroguanylin mRNA by zinc deficiency. *J Nutr.* 2000;130:1393S.
309. Eide DJ. Zinc transporters and the cellular trafficking of zinc. *Biochim Biophys Acta.* 2006;1763:711.
310. Schlemmer U, Frolich W, Prieto RM, et al. Phytate in foods and significance for humans: food sources, intake, processing, bioavailability, protective role and analysis. *Mol Nutr Food Res.* 2009;53:S330.
311. Alpers DH. Intraluminal bioavailability of divalent cations. *Curr Opin Gastroenterol.* 2013;29:164.
312. Sandstrom B, Cederblad A, Kivisto B, et al. Retention of zinc and calcium from the human colon *Am J Clin Nutr.* 1986;44:501.
313. Lichten LA, Cousins RJ. Mammalian zinc transporters: nutritional and physiologic regulation. *Annu Rev Nutr.* 2009;29:153.
314. Hambidge KM, Miller LV, Westcott JE, et al. Zinc bioavailability and homeostasis. *Am J Clin Nutr.* 2010;91(Suppl):1478S.
315. King JC, Shames DM, Woodhouse LR. Zinc homeostasis in humans. *J Nutr.* 2000;130:1360S.
316. Manary MJ, Abrams SA, Griffin IJ, et al. Perturbed zinc homeostasis in rural 3–5-y-old Malawian children is associated with abnormalities in intestinal permeability attributed to tropical enteropathy. *Pediatr Res.* 2010;67:671.

317. Palacios O, Atrian S, Capdevilla M. Zn- and Cu-thioneins: a functional classification for metallothnioneins? *J Biol Inorg Chem.* 2011;16:991.
318. Cousins RJ. Zinc. In: Ziegler EK, Filer LJ, eds. *Present Knowledge in Nutrition,* 7th ed. Washington DC: ILSI, 1996:293.
319. Wang K, Zhou B, Kuo YM, et al. A novel member of a zinc transporter family is defective in acrodermatitis enteropathica. *Am J Hum Genet.* 2002;71:66.
320. Kim RE, Wang F, Dufner-Beattie J, et al. Zn^{2+}-stimulated endocytosis of the mZIP4 zinc transporter regulates its location at the plasma membrane. *J Biol Chem.* 2004;279:4523.
321. Krebs NF. Overview of zinc absorption and excretion in the human gastrointestinal tract. *J Nutr.* 2000;130:1374S.
322. Mills CF. Dietary interactions involving the trace elements. *Annu Rev Nutr.* 1985;5:173.
323. Whittaker P. Iron and zinc interactions in humans. *Am J Clin Nutr.* 1998;68:442S.
324. Lonnerdal B. Dietary factors influencing zinc absorption. *J Nutr.* 2000;130:1378S.
325. Stewart AJ, Blindauer CA, Berezenko S, et al. Interdomain zinc site on human albumin. *Proc Natl Acad Sci U S A.* 2003;100:3701.
326. Gaither LA, Eide DJ. Eurkaryotic zinc transporters and their regulation. *BioMetals.* 2001;14:251.
327. Fraker PJ, King LE, Laakko T, et al. The dynamic link between the integrity of the immune system and zinc status. *J Nutr.* 2000;130:1399S.
328. Rink L, Kirchner H. Zinc-altered immune function and cytokine production. *J Nutr.* 2000;130:1407S.
329. Haase H, Mocchegiani E, Rink L. Correlation between zinc status and immune function in the elderly. *Biogerontology.* 2006;7:421.
330. Prasad AS. Zinc deficiency in women, infants, and children. *J Am Coll Nutr.* 1996;15:113.
331. Wapnir RA. Zinc deficiency: malnutrition and the gastrointestinal tract. *J Nutr.* 2000;130:1388S.
332. Ruz M, Carrasco F, Rojas P, et al. Zinc absorption and zinc status are reduced after Roux-en-Y gastric bypass: a randomized study using 2 supplements. *Am J Clin Nutr.* 2011;94:1004.
333. Haider BA, Bhutta ZA. The effect of therapeutic zinc supplementation among young children with selected infections: a review of the evidence. *Food Nutr Bull.* 2009;30:541.
334. Hoque KM, Binder HJ. Zinc in the treatment of acute diarrhea: current status and assessment. *Gastroenterology.* 2008;130:2201.
335. Yakoob MY, Theodoratou E, Jabeen A, et al. Preventive zinc supplementation in developing countries: impact on mortality and morbidity due to diarrhea, pneumonia and malaria. *BMC Public Health.* 2011;11(Suppl 3):523.
336. Terrin G, Canani RB, Passariello A, et al. Zinc supplementation reduces morbidity and mortality in very low birth weight preterm neonates: a hospital based randomized, placebo-controlled trial in an industrialized country. *Am J Clin Nutr.* 2013;98:1468.
337. Takuma Y, Nours K, Makino Y, et al. Clinical trial: oral zinc in hepatic encephalopathy. *Aliment Pharmacol Ther.* 2010;32:1080.
338. Anonymous. Infertility, zinc and other metals. *Arbor Clin Nutr Uptdates.* 2010;323:1.
339. Brocard A, Dreno B. Innate immunity: a crucial target for zinc in the treatment of inflammatory dermatosis. *J Eur Acad Dermatol Venerol.* 2011;25:1146.
340. Osaki T, Ohshima M, Tomita Y, et al. Clinical and physiological investigations in patients with taste abnormality. *J Oral Pathol Med.* 1996;25:38.
341. Henkin RI, Schecter PJ, Friedewald WT, et al. A double blind study of the effects of zinc sulfate on taste and smell dysfunction. *Am J Med Sci.* 1976;272:285.
342. Hodkinson CF, Kelly M, Alexander HD, et al. Effect of zinc supplementation on the immune status of healthy older individuals aged 55–70: the ZENITH study. *J Gerontol A Biol Sci Med Sci.* 2007;62:598.
343. Brewer GJ, Kanzer SH, Zimmerman EA, et al. Subclinical zinc deficiency in Alzheimer's disease and Parkinson's disease. *Am J Alzheimers Dis Other Demen.* 2010;25:572.
344. Brewer GJ. Copper excess, zinc deficiency, and cognitive loss in Alzheimer's disease. *Biofactors.* 2012;38:107.
345. Belbraouet S, Biaudet H, Tebi A, et al. Serum zinc and copper status in hospitalized vs healthy elderly subjects. *J Am Coll Nutr.* 2007;26:650.
346. Aslam T, Delcourt C, Skilva R, et al. Micronutrients in age-related macular degeneration. *Ophthalmologica.* 2013;239:75.
347. Walker CF, Kordas K, Stoltzfus RJ, et al. Interactive effects of iron and zinc on biochemical and functional outcomes in supplementation trials. *Am J Clin Nutr.* 2005;82:5.
348. Marshall I. Zinc for the common cold. *Cochrane Database Syst Rev.* 2000;(2):CD001364.
349. Marshall S. Zinc gluconate and the common cold. Review of randomized controlled trials. *Can Fam Physician.* 1998;44:1037.

350. Prasad AS, Fitzgerald JT, Bao B, et al. Duration of symptoms and plasma cytokine levels in patients with the common cold treated with zinc acetate: a randomized, double-blind, placebo-controlled trial. *Ann Intern Med*. 2000;13:245.
351. Hulisz D. Efficacy of zinc against common cold viruses: an overview. *J Am Pharm Assoc*. 2004;24:255.
352. Patel AB, Mamtani M, Badhoniya N, et al. What zinc supplementation does and does not achieve in diarrhea prevention: a systematic review and meta-analysis. *BMC Infect Dis*. 2011;11:122.
353. Brooks WA, Santosham M, Naheed A, et al. Effect of weekly zinc supplements on incidence of pneumonia and diarrhea in children younger than 2 years in an urban, low-income population in Bangladesh: randomized controlled trial. *Lancet*. 2005;366:999.
354. Hambridge M. Human zinc deficiency. *J Nutr*. 2000;130:1344S.
355. Gletsu-Miller N, Wright BN. Mineral malnutrition following bariatric surgery. *Adv Nutr*. 2013;4:506.
356. Fosmire GJ. Zinc toxicity. *Am J Clin Nutr* 1990;51:225.
357. Smith JC, Zeller JA, Brown ED, et al. Elevated zinc: a heritable anomaly. *Science*. 1976;193:496.
358. Hedera P, Fink JK, Bockenstedt PL, et al. Myelopolyneuropathy and pancytopenia due to copper deficiency and high zinc levels of unknown origin: further support for existence of a new zinc overload syndrome. *Arch Neurol*. 2003;60:1303.
359. Sampson B, Fagerhol MK, Sunderkotter C, et al. Hyperzincaemia and hypercalprotectinaemia: a new disorder of zinc metabolism. *Lancet*. 2002;360:1742.
360. Fessatou S, Fagerhol MK, Roth J, et al. Severe anemia and neutropenia associated with hyperzincemia and hypercalprotectinemia. *J Pediatr Hematol Oncol*. 2005;27:477.
361. Sugiura T, Goto K, Ito K, et al. Effects of cyclosporine A in hyperzincaemia and hypercalprotectinaemia. *Acta Paediatr*. 2006;95:857.
362. Klevay LM, Medeiros DM. Deliberations and evaluations of the approaches, endpoints and paradigms for dietary recommendations about copper. *J Nutr*. 1996; 126:2419S.
363. Hughes J, Buttriss J. An update on copper: contributions of MAFF-funded research. *Nutr Bull*. 2000;25:271.
364. Pennington JT, Calloway DH. Copper content of foods. *J Am Diet Assoc*. 1973;63:143.
365. Linder MC, Hazegh-Azam M. Copper biochemistry and molecular biology. *Am J Clin Nutr*. 1996;63:797S.
366. Harvery LJ, McArdle HJ. Biomarkers of copper status: a brief update. *Br J Nutr*. 2008;99 (Suppl 3):S10.
367. Brewer GJ, Yuzbasiyan-Gurkan V. Wilson disease. *Medicine*. 1992;71:139.
368. Stremmel W, Meyerrose KW, Niederau C, et al. Wilson disease: clinical presentation, treatment, and survival. *Ann Intern Med*. 1991;115:720.
369. Wang Y, Hodgkinson V, Zhu S, et al. Advances in the understanding of mammalian copper transporters. *Adv Nutr*. 2011;2:129.
370. Roberts EA, Sarkar B. Liver as a key organ in the supply, storage, and excretion of copper. *Am J Clin Nutr*. 2008;88(Suppl):851S.
371. Gunshin H, Mackenzie B, Berger UV, et al. Cloning and characterization of a mammalian proton-coupled metal-ion transporter. *Nature*. 1997;388:482.
372. Prohaska JR, Gybina AA. Intracellular copper transport in mammals. *J Nutr*. 2004;134:1003.
373. Schilsky ML. Wilson disease: new insights into pathogenesis, diagnosis, and future therapy. *Curr Gastroenterol Rep*. 2005;7:26.
374. Kaler SG. ATO7A-related copper transport diseases—emerging concepts and future trends. *Nat Rev Neurol*. 2011;7:15.
375. Robinson NJ. A platform for copper pumps. *Nature*. 2011;475:41.
376. Eisenstein RS. Discovery of the ceruloplasmin homologue hephaestin: new insight into the copper/iron connection. *Nutr Rev*. 2000;58:22.
377. Triplett WS. Clinical aspects of zinc, copper, manganese, chromium, and selenium. *Nutr Int*. 1985;1:60.
378. Blackman AE, Bailey E. Management of copper deficiency in cholestatic infants: review of the literature and a case series. *Nutr Clin Pract*. 2013;28:75.
379. Danks DM. Copper deficiency in humans. *Annu Rev Nutr*. 1988;8:235.
380. Kodama H, Fujisawa C, Bhadhprasit W. Inherited copper transport disorders: biochemical mechanisms, diagnosis, and treatment. *Curr Drug Metab*. 2012;13:327.
381. Turner Z, Horn N, Tonnesen T, et al. Early copper-histidine treatment for Menkes disease. *Nat Genet*. 1996;12:11.

382. Klevay LM. Cardiovascular disease from copper deficiency—a history. *J Nutr.* 2000;130:489S.
383. Kumar N, Low PA. Myeloneuropathy and anemia due to copper malabsorption. *J Neurol.* 2004;251:747.
384. Kumar N. Metabolic and toxic myelopathies. *Semin Neurol.* 2012;32:173.
385. Tan JC, Burns DL, Jones HR. Severe ataxia, myelopathy, and peripheral neuropathy due to acquired copper deficiency in a patient with history of gastrectomy. *JPEN J Parenter Enteral Nutr.* 2006;30:446.
386. Gabreyes AA, Abbasi HN, Forbes KS, et al. Hypocupremia associated cytopenia and myelopathy: a national retrospective review. *Eur J Haematol.* 2013;90:1.
387. Stern BR. Essentiality and toxicity in copper health risk assessment: overview, update and regulatory considerations. *J Toxicol Environ Health A.* 2010;73:114.
388. Hodgkinson V, Petris MJ. Copper homeostasis at the host-pathogen interface. *J Biol Chem.* 2012;287:13549.
389. Bremner I. Manifestations of copper excess. *Am J Clin Nutr.* 1998;67 (Suppl 5):S1069.
390. Fontana L, Klein S, Holloszy JO, et al. Effect of long-term calorie restriction with adequate protein and micronutrients on thyroid hormones. *J Clin Endocrinol Metab.* 2006;91:3232.
391. Rohner F, Zimmermann M, Jooste P, et al. Biomarkers of nutrition for development-Iodine review. *J Nutr* 2014;144:1322S.
392. Stanbury JB, Dunn JT. Iodine and iodine deficiency disorders.. In: Bowman BA, Russell RM, eds. *Present Knowledge in Nutrition*, 8th ed. Washington, DC. ILSI Press 2001:344.
393. Wright EM. Glucose transport families SLC5 and SLC50. *Mol Aspects Med.* 2013;34:183.
394. Daniels GH, Haber DA. Will radioiodine be useful in treatment of breast cancer? *Nat Med.* 2000;6:859.
395. Kavishe F. Iodine deficiency disorders. In: Sadler MJ, Strain JJ, Caballero B, eds. *Encyclopedia of Human Nutrition.* London: Academic Press, 1998:1136.
396. Hetzel BS. Iodine and neuropsychological development. *J Nutr.* 2000;130:493S.
397. Zimmermann M, Delange F. Iodine supplementation of pregnant women in Europe: a review and recommendations. *Eur J Clin Nutr.* 2004;58:979.
398. Costeira MJ, Oliveira P, Ares S, et al. Parameters of thyroid function throughout and after pregnancy in an iodine-deficient population. *Thyroid.* 2010;20:995.
399. Anonymous. Iodine and the brain. *Arbor Clin Nutr Updates.* 2010;325:1.
400. Lee K, Bradley R, Dwyer J, et al. Too much versus too little: the implications of current iodine intake in the United States. *Nutr Rev.* 1999;57:177.
401. Angermayr L, Clar C. Iodine supplementation for preventing iodine deficiency disorders in children. *Cochrane Database Syst Rev.* 2004;(2):CD003819.
402. Yeng W, Shan Z, Teng X, et al. Effect of iodine intake on thyroid diseases in China. *N Engl J Med.* 2006;354:2783.
403. Nielsen FH. Micronutrients in parenteral nutrition: boron, silicon, and fluoride. *Gastroenterology.* 2009;137:555.
404. Rao GS. Dietary intake and bioavailability of fluoride. *Annu Rev Nutr.* 1984;9:115.
405. Dhar V, Bhatnager M. Physiology and toxicity of fluoride. *Indian J Dent Res.* 2009;20:350.
406. Anonymous. Position of the American Dietetic Association: the impact of fluoride on health. *J Am Diet Assoc.* 2000;100:1208.
407. Sanders TAB. Diet and general health: dietary counselling. *Caries Res.* 2004;38 (Suppl 1):3.
408. Freeland-Graves JH, Turnlund JR. Deliberations and evaluations of the approaches, endpoints and paradigms for manganese and molybdenum dietary recommendations. *J Nutr.* 1996;126:2435S.
409. Aschner JL, Aschner M. Nutritional aspects of manganese homeostasis. *Mol Aspects Med.* 2005;26:353.
410. Burch RE, Sullivan JR. Diagnosis of zinc, copper, and manganese abnormalities in man. *Med Clin North Am.* 1976;60:655.
411. Friedman BJ, Freeland-Graves JH, Bales CW, et al. Manganese balance and clinical observations in young men fed a manganese-deficient diet. *J Nutr.* 1987;117:113.
412. Hardy G. Manganese in parenteral nutrition: who, when, and why should we supplement? *Gastroenterology.* 2009;137:529.
413. Fitzgerald K, Mikalunas V, Rubin H, et al. Hypermanganesemia in patients receiving total parenteral nutrition. *JPEN J Parenter Enteral Nutr.* 1999;23:333.
414. Wardle CA, Forbes A, Roberts NB, et al. Hypermanganesemia in long-term intravenous nutrition and chronic liver disease. *JPEN J Parenter Enteral Nutr.* 1999;23:350.

415. Anderson RA. Nutritional factors influencing the glucose/insulin system: chromium. *J Am Coll Nutr*. 1997;16:404.
416. Jeejeebhoy KN. The role of chromium in nutrition and therapeutics and as a potential toxin. *Nutr Rev*. 1999;57:329.
417. Zhitkovich A. Chromium in drinking water: sources, metabolism, and cancer risks. *Chem Res Toxicol*. 2011;24:1617.
418. Ducros V. Chromium metabolism. A literature review. *Biol Trace Elem Res*. 1992;32:68.
419. Wang ZQ, Cefalu WT. Current concepts about chromium supplementation in type 2 diabetes and insulin resistance. *Curr Diab Rep*. 2010;10:145.
420. Vincent JB. Quest for the molecular mechanism of chromium action and its relationship to diabetes. *Nutr Rev*. 2000;58:67.
421. Shenkin A. Micronutrients in health and disease. *Postgrad Med J*. 2006;82:559.
422. Anderson RA. Chromium metabolism and its role in disease processes in man. *Clin Physiol Biochem*. 1986;4:31.
423. Vincent JB. Recent advances in the nutritional biochemistry of trivalent chromium. *Proc Nutr Soc*. 2004;63:41.
424. Jomova K, Valko M. Advances in metal-induced oxidative stress and human disease. *Toxicology*. 2011;283:65.
425. Standing Committee on the Scientific Evaluation of Dietary Reference Intakes, Food and Nutrition Board, Institute of Medicine. *Dietary Reference Intakes for Vitamin C, Vitamin E, Selenium, and Beta-carotene and Other Carotenoids*. Washington, DC: National Academies Press, 2000.
426. Rayman MP. The importance of selenium to human health. *Lancet*. 2000;356:233.
427. Hardy G, Hardy I. Selenium: the Se-XY nutraceutical. *Nutrition*. 2004;20:590.
428. Fairweather-Tait SJ, Collings R, Hurst R. Seleium bioavailability: current knowledge and future research requirements. *Am J Clin Nutr*. 2010;91(Suppl):1484S.
429. Diplock AT. Indexes of selenium status in human populations. *Am J Clin Nutr*. 1993;57:256S.
430. Beckett GJ, Arthur JR. Selenium and endocrine systems. *J Endocrinol*. 2005;184:455.
431. Epidemiologic studies on the etiologic relationship of selenium and Keshan disease. *China Med J*. 1979;92:477.
432. Jacobson S, Plantin LO. Concentration of selenium in plasma and erythrocytes during total parenteral nutrition in Crohn's disease. *Gut*. 1985;26:50.
433. Al-Matary A, Hussain M, Ali J. Selenium: a brief review and a case report of selenium responsive cardiomyopathy. *BMC Pediatr*. 2013;13:39.
434. Moreno-Reyes R, Suetens C, Mathieu F, et al. Kashin-Beck osteoarthropathy in rural Tibet in relation to selenium and iodine status. *N Engl J Med*. 1998;339:1112.
435. Andrews PJD. Selenium and glutamine supplements: where are we heading? A critical care perspective. *Curr Opin Clin Nutr Metab Care*. 2010;13:192.
436. Jacobs ET, Jiang R, Alberts DS, et al. Selenium and colorectal adenoma: results of a pooled analysis. *J Natl Cancer Inst*. 2004;96:1669.
437. Anonymous. Selenium and cancer treatment. *Arbor Clin Nutr Updates*. 2010;317:1.
438. Rannem T, Ladefoged K, Hylander E, et al. Selenium depletion in patients with gastrointestinal diseases: are there any predictive factors? *Scand J Gastroenterol*. 1998;33:1057.
439. Reyes H, Baez ME, Gonzalez MC, et al. Selenium, zinc and copper plasma levels in intrahepatic cholestasis of pregnancy, in normal pregnancies and in healthy individuals in Chile. *J Hepatol*. 2000;32:542.
440. Combs GF Jr. Current evidence and research needs to support a health claim for selenium and cancer prevention. *J Nutr*. 2005;135:343.
441. Moyad MA. Selenium and vitamin E supplements for prostate cancer: evidence or embellishment? *Urology*. 2002;59(Suppl 4A):9.
442. Clark LC, Combs GF Jr, Turnbull BW, et al. Effects of selenium supplementation for cancer prevention in patients with carcinoma of the skin. A randomized controlled trial. *JAMA*. 1996;276:1957.
443. Lippman SM, Kean EA, Goodman PJ, et al. Effect of selenium and vitamin E on risk of prostate cancer and other cancers: the Selenium and Vitamin E Cancer Prevention Trial (SELECT). *JAMA*. 2009;301:39.
444. Yang GQ, Wang SZ, Zhou RH, et al. Endemic selenium intoxication of humans in China. *Am J Clin Nutr*. 1983;37:872.

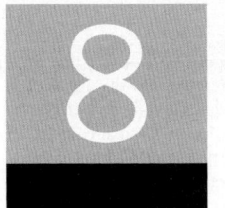

Dietary Supplements

A dietary supplement is a product or compound that is taken orally and meant to supplement the diet. A wide variety of dietary supplements include herbal products, vitamins, minerals, amino acids, and biochemical intermediates such as carnitine and creatine (1). In some countries, supplements are defined as foods, and in others as drugs or natural health products. No such distinction is made in the United States of America by the Food and Drug Administration (FDA). Dietary supplements are consumed widely in the United States and elsewhere; in the United States alone, many billions of dollars are spent on dietary supplements each year. A large percentage of the US population use supplements, accounting for a major proportion of the estimated average requirement (EAR) for many micronutrients (2).

For some dietary supplements, good scientific data are available to support safety and efficacy, whereas for others, no such data exist. Few large, controlled clinical trials have assessed the safety and efficacy of dietary supplements. In contrast, large, controlled trials are required by law for the approval of prescription drugs. For this reason, far less information is available to assess the safety and efficacy of dietary supplements than to assess prescription drugs. To address this lack of data, the National Institutes of Health (NIH) Office of Dietary Supplements (ODS) has developed a website that serves as a clearing house for peer-reviewed information on dietary supplements, http://ods.od.nih.gov/publications/publications.html.

REGULATION OF DIETARY SUPPLEMENTS

The FDA requires that prescription drugs have been proved safe and effective for their labeled use before they are marketed; however, no such requirement applies to dietary supplements provided they are not marketed as a treatment for a specific disease. Dietary supplements are regulated under the Dietary Supplement Health and Education Act (DSHEA) of 1994. These regulations, which are largely favorable to the manufacturers of dietary supplements, were enacted by Congress in response to an effort by the FDA to remove some herbal products from the market. The negative public response to this effort caused the government to relax the regulations on dietary supplements.

Subsequent to the passage of the DSHEA, the FDA in 2007 implemented a policy to ensure that dietary supplements "are produced in a quality manner, do not contain contaminants or impurities, and are accurately labeled," using current good manufacturing practices (GMPs) (3). Audits in 2011 and 2012, however, showed that approximately 70% of supplement manufacturers were currently not compliant with GMP, and also were under-reporting adverse events (4). To remove a product from the market, the FDA must prove that the product is unsafe, but the FDA is underfunded to test most of the products. The FDA's final rule on GMPs means that the products must meet the conditions to prevent adulteration under the Federal Food, Drug, and Cosmetic Act (3). It is not surprising that contamination and false labeling are not uncommon (5). An attempt was made in 2010 to require enforcement of the DSHEA (Dietary Supplement Full Implementation and Enforcement Act, S3414), but it did not become law (6).

The FDA does require that the labels of dietary supplements include an "information panel," similar to the "nutrition facts" panel required on food labels. The information panel must describe the part of the plant used, the suggested serving size, and the amount of specific nutrients included (e.g., vitamins and minerals). For herbal products in particular, such labeling is not informative because herbs contain many different compounds, the levels of which vary according to the soil and climate conditions where the herbs are grown. Moreover, for many herbs, the specific active ingredient is unknown, and therefore the amount present in a product cannot be stated.

The manufacture of prescription pharmaceuticals is carefully regulated to ensure that standards of purity and dosing are maintained. Herbal remedies are exempt from this regulation, and there is considerable variation in the composition of herbal products among manufacturers and among lots. There are also discrepancies between label information and actual content. In addition to problems with inconsistency of composition, there are problems with contamination. Herbal remedies have been contaminated with drugs, toxic metals, pesticides, fumigating agents, microbial toxins, microorganisms, and other botanicals (7). More than 400 recalls of dietary supplements "spiked" with pharmaceutical compounds have occurred since 2008 (8).

In addition to issues with safety, there are problems with claims for dietary supplements. All ingredients in a product are required by law to be declared on the label. The manufacturer does not have to provide evidence to back up whatever claims are made, but it is not legal to market a dietary supplement product as a treatment or cure for a specific disease (9). Under the DSHEA, the labels of dietary supplements can include "statements of nutritional support," but not claims of their efficacy in the treatment of specific diseases. Statements of nutritional support may describe the ability of a supplement to affect the function or structure of an organ, or promote general well-being. Thus, the label of a dietary supplement can claim that the supplement "improves memory," "supports cardiovascular health," or "enhances mental well-being," but it cannot claim that the supplement is effective in the treatment of Alzheimer disease, coronary artery disease, or depression. The standards for the evidence required as a basis for the statements of nutritional support are quite lax. When a product claims to affect a structure or function of the body, a disclaimer is required that states, "This statement has not been evaluated by the FDA. This product is not intended to diagnose, treat, cure, or prevent any disease" (9). It is not surprising that many qualified health claims have been submitted to the FDA regarding a wide variety of dietary supplements (10). These can be followed online by the savvy consumer and health-care worker, as the FDA tries to provide a summary of the validity of the claim. In addition, the FDA maintains a website on Tips for the Savvy Supplement User: Making Informed Decision and Evaluating Information (11).

Exact frequencies of adverse events from dietary supplements are difficult to find, as such events are surely under reported (12). In the United States of America, the problems involve both inadequate as well as poor-quality reporting (13).

In Germany, where herbal products are widely used, a government agency, the German Federal Institute for Drugs and Medicinal Devices, formed a commission to evaluate the safety and efficacy of a large number of herbal remedies. The report of that commission was translated into English and published as *The Complete German Commission E Monographs: Therapeutic Guide to Herbal Medicines* (Blumenthal M, ed. Austin, TX: American Botanical Council, 1998). This publication is a comprehensive and objective guide to the efficacy and safety of herbal medicines.

"FUNCTIONAL" FOODS AND SUPPLEMENTS

The definition of food in the Food, Drug, and Cosmetic Act of 1938 is very general, and includes anything that is eaten or drunk by humans (foods, beverages, chewing gum). "Functional" foods were defined in this Act as "articles intended for the diagnosis, cure, mitigation, treatment, or prevention of disease." Subsequently, they have been defined as "any food or food ingredient that may provide a health benefit beyond that conferred by the nutrients the food contains" (14). The European definition is by consensus the following: "A food can be regarded as functional if it is satisfactorily demonstrated to affect beneficially one or more target functions in the body, beyond adequate nutritional effects, in a way which is relevant to either the state of well-being and health or the reduction of the risk of a disease" (15). "Functional food" is used to describe physiologically active foods and is often used synonymously with the terms *nutraceutical, designer food*, and *medical food*. The older term for these foods was "foods for special dietary use." The orphan drugs amendment to the Food, Drug, and Cosmetic Act (1988) defines *medical food* as "a food which is formulated to be consumed or administered enterally under the supervision of a physician and which is intended for the specific management of a disease or condition for which distinctive nutritional requirements, based on recognized scientific principles, are established by medical evaluation." Examples of medical foods include oral rehydration solutions and enteral formulas. However, medical foods are not subject to regulation by the FDA, and in 1990, the National Labeling Education Act exempted medical foods from its labeling requirements (16).

Infant formulas are another category of food, and the Infant Formula Act (1980) gives the FDA authority to create standards for these foods. Dietary supplements are defined by the DSHEA as products other than tobacco that contain one or more dietary ingredients, including "a vitamin, mineral, herb or other botanical, or amino acid," and are provided to increase dietary intake. It can be provided as "a concentrate, metabolite, constituent, extract, or combination of any of the aforementioned ingredients." Products are marketed as supplements, functional foods, "dietetic" foods, nutraceuticals, and phytochemicals. Their purpose is to improve function not only in healthy people but also in patients with restricted diets. Such use has been spurred by the passage of the DSHEA of 1994, which formally defined dietary supplements. Because these supplements were regulated as foods and not as drugs, manufacturers did not have to prove efficacy. As of March 1999, all vitamin, mineral, herbal, and supplement products must include "nutrition facts" in their label. Nutrients are listed as percentage of daily value, although the dose is called a "serving." Nutrients labeled "high potency" must supply at least 100% of the daily value, and multivitamins must supply 100% of the daily value of two-thirds of the contents. "Antioxidants" must prevent chemical damage in vitro. However, neither label means that the product is effective. For any health claims, the label must carry the following disclaimer: "This statement has not been evaluated by the Food and Drug Administration." The NIH ODS views a supplement as any substance consumed in addition to the regular diet—that is, in addition to meals, snacks, and beverages (14). The American Dietetic Association has published a useful guide to many of these supplements (17).

Table 8-1 lists many of the supplements that are specific nutrients. Those that are micronutrients (vitamins and minerals) are discussed in Chapters 6 and 7. The NIH ODS and the Consumer Healthcare Products Association have initiated a bibliography to highlight scientifically sound research on dietary supplements and their role in health maintenance. Copies of the document are posted on the Internet (*http://ods.od.nih.gov/publications/publications.html*) and are available from the ODS at *ods@nih.gov* or by ordering from 301-435-2920.

Currently, the FDA has approved health claims for some foods in the prevention of chronic disease, and other claims are pending (Table 8-2). These claims include fiber-containing products for cancer and cardiovascular disease (CVD), fruits and vegetables for cancer, and calcium for osteoporosis (18). It also recognizes the relationship between saturated fat and cholesterol and the risk for CVD, dietary fat and cancer, sodium and hypertension, and sugar alcohols and dental caries (14,16). The DSHEA of 1994, which exempts dietary supplements from regulation as drugs and food additives, also allows structure/function claims to be made and literature about functional foods to be distributed. Claims can be made that functional foods are modifiers of oxidative damage, anticarcinogens, enhancers of gastrointestinal (GI) function (including probiotics and prebiotics), and agents of immunomodulation, neuroregulation, cholesterol metabolism, blood pressure control, and allergic responses. Prebiotics and probiotics are considered "functional" foods by some because they contain or produce components similar to those in some functional foods (19). Table 8-3 lists some of the compounds included in functional foods and the claims that may be made for them (17).

In this chapter, we review some of the supplement groups and a few of the hundreds of alternative nutritional products that are available commercially (Table 8-4). The nutritional products presented in this chapter were chosen because of wide use (e.g., *Ginkgo biloba*, *Echinacea*), some evidence of efficacy (e.g., fish oil, phytosterols), or significant safety issues (e.g., ma huang). A larger range of dietary supplements is reviewed in *The Health Professional's Guide to Popular Dietary Supplements* (20). The "evidence" supporting the value of most supplements in human health comes largely from in vitro studies using cell lines or ex vivo tissues, or in some cases in vivo animal preparations that are not models for the human disease of interest. When human studies are available, in general, the results are derived from inadequately designed or powered studies, and these results are conflicting or positive only for unvalidated surrogate markers of disease. When randomized controlled trials (RCTs) are examined, most involve vitamin supplements, but have included selenium, calcium, glucosamine, lipids, and some herbal preparations (gingko, St. John's wort, saw palmetto, milk thistle, garlic, *Echinacea*). Only those using vitamin D and omega-3 (ω-3) fatty acids have sufficient support for specific clinical end points in specific

TABLE 8-1 Selected Nutritional Dietary Supplements

Supplement	Marketing Claims	Efficacy	Adverse Effects
Alanine	Spares muscle	Not proven	None
	Stabilizes blood glucose	Equivocal	
Arginine	Helps prevent CV disease	Possibly	None
	Helps immune Fx	Equivocal	
	Builds muscle mass	Not proven	
Boron	Prevents osteoporosis	Not proven	Toxic >50 mg/day
	Improves memory, libido		
BCAA	↑ Muscle mass, exercising	Not proven	↑ NH_3 if >20 g/day
Calcium	Prevents osteoporosis	Proven	UL 2,500 mg/day
	↓ Blood pressure	Possibly	↑ Absorption of Fe, other drugs
	↓ Colon cancer risk	Equivocal	
L-Carnitine	Helps heart, immune function	Not proven	Diarrhea >6 g/day
β-Carotene	↑ Cancer prevalence	Probably not	May ↑ lung cancer in male smokers
	↓ Immunity, helps prevent CV disease	No	
Chromium	Helps control diabetes	Possibly	Safe daily intake 50–200 µg
	Lowers cholesterol	Equivocal	
	↓ Body fat	No	
Creatine	↑ Muscle strength	Equivocal	Water retention
	↑ Muscle mass	Not proven	
Folate	Prevents birth defects	Yes	Masks B_{12} deficiency at >400 µg/day, Anticonvulsants >5 mg/day
	Prevents colon cancer	Not proven	
	Prevents depression	Not proven	
Fructo-oligosaccharides	Supports GI tract health	Equivocal	Bloating, cramps, diarrhea at >50 g/day
	Controls blood glucose, cholesterol	Not proven	
Glucosamine	Relieves arthritis pain	Possibly	None
Glutamine	Enhances immune system	Equivocal	None
Lecithin	Helps prevent Alzheimer's, memory loss	No	Diarrhea >20 g/day
Lysine	↓ Herpes virus effect	Equivocal	↓ Arginine absorption
	↓ Angina	Not proven	
Magnesium	↓ CV disease, BP	Equivocal	UL 350 mg/day
	↓ Migraine, PMS	Equivocal	
Pantothenate	Blocks stress, ↑ cholesterol	Not proven	None
Phosphatidylserine (source, bovine brain extract)	Improves memory in elderly	Equivocal	Contains B_{12}
	Raises IQ	Not proven	
Potassium	↓ Blood pressure	Possibly	GI ulcer, bleeding >6 g/day ↑ [K], inhibits ACE
Pyruvate	↓ Cholesterol, weight	Not proven	Flatus, diarrhea

TABLE 8-1 Selected Nutritional Dietary Supplements *(continued)*

Supplement	Marketing Claims	Efficacy	Adverse Effects
Selenium	↓ Cancer risk	Possibly	Toxic >750 µg/day
	Helps heart, immune function	Not proven	
Vitamin A	Improves immunity	Possibly	Toxic >50,000 IU/day
	Improves skin disease	Yes	Teratogenic
	Reverses skin aging	Not proven	>3,000 IU/day
Vitamin B_1	↑ Energy	No	None
B_2	↑ Energy, helps migraine	No	None
B_3	↓ Cholesterol	Yes	Flushing, diarrhea
B_6	Improves PMS, autism	Equivocal	Nerve damage
	Improves heart Fx	Possibly	>500 mg/day
B_{12}	Improves dementia, energy	No	None
	↑ Function in elderly deficient	Yes	
Vitamin C	Improve cold Sx, ↓ heart disease	Equivocal	Diarrhea >3 g/day
	Protects vs. cancer, cataracts	Possibly	↑ Fe absorption in hemochromatosis, ↑ oxalate excretion
Vitamin D	↑ Ca^{++} absorption, bone health	Yes	UL 1,000 IU (50 µg)
	↓ Cancer risk	Equivocal	↑ Increased if on anticoagulants
Vitamin E	Improves diabetes, immunity	Possibly	
	↓ Heart attack, cataracts	Possibly	
	Improves lung Fx, psychiatric illness	Possibly	
Zinc	Improves cold Sx, taste	Not proven	↑ Cu absorption >100 mg/day
	↑ Immunity, fertility, skin	No	↑ Cholesterol, nausea at high dose

Explanation of efficacy: Yes, several controlled trials in humans; possibly, preliminary data from controlled trials; equivocal, conflicting controlled data in humans; not proven, not enough data in humans or data are poor; no, human data not supportive. A detailed listing of many supplements is available in the *PDR for Nutritional Supplements*, 1st ed., Hendlor SS, Rorvak D, eds., Medical Economics, Montvale NJ, 2001.
UL, upper limit recommended by Food and Nutrition Board, National Academy of Science;
PMS, premenstrual syndrome; ACE, angiotensin-converting enzyme; BCAA, branched-chain amino acid.

populations (21). There is not much evidence to support the use of dietary supplements in a general Western population. However, before addressing individual supplements, it is worth considering groups of supplements designed to attract certain disease markets, as that is how consumers are attracted to an individual supplement.

Supplement Groups

Nutritional supplements are only one component of products offered in the field of complementary and alternative medicine (CAM) (22). "Products" are offered in fields known as "energy medicine" (e.g., vibrational or touch techniques), "herbal medicine" (including products

TABLE 8-2   FDA-Approved and Qualified Health Claims for Nutrients

Dietary Substance	Approved Claim	Permitted Qualified Claim
Calcium	Osteoporosis	Bone fractures, cancer, menstrual disorders, hypertension, renal stones
Chromium picolinate		Insulin resistance, diabetes
Dietary lipids (fat)	Cancer	
Dietary saturated fat and cholesterol	Coronary heart disease	
Omega-3 fatty acids (supplements/food)		Coronary heart disease
Monounsaturated fatty acids (olive oil)		Coronary heart disease
Dietary noncariogenic sweeteners	Dental caries	
Fiber-containing grain products, fruits, and vegetables	Cancer	
Fruits and vegetables	Cancer	
Soluble fiber from certain foods	Coronary heart disease	
Whole-grain foods	Heart disease and certain cancers	
Soy protein	Coronary heart disease	
Plant sterol/stanol esters	Coronary heart disease	
Folic acid	Neural tube defects	
0.8 mg folic acid (supplement)		Neural tube defects
Sodium	Hypertension	
Selenium (dietary supplement)		Cancer
Vitamin C or E (supplement)		Cancer
Green tea		Cancer (prostate)
Tomatoes, lycopene containing tomato-based products		Cancer (prostate, ovarian, gastric, pancreatic)
Nuts (almonds, hazelnuts, peanuts, pistachio nuts, walnuts)		Heart disease
Vitamin B_6, B_{12} and/or folic acid		Vascular disease
Phosphatidylserine (supplement)		Cognitive dysfunction, dementia

Source: US FDA. Health claims that meet significant scientific agreement are approved by the FDA Center for Food Safety & Applied Nutrition, website available at: www.cfsan.fda.gov/~dms/lab-ssa.html. In 2002, the FDA began allowing qualified health claims that did not meet the standard of "significant scientific agreement" and that would be misleading without such qualification. These are available on the qualified health claims website at: www.fda.gov/Food/UbgreduebtsPackaging Labeling/Labeling/Nutrition/ucm073992.html. Details of the criteria for each of these claims are reviewed by Turner et al. (18).

that contain pharmaceutical agents), "homeopathic products" (based on the theory that compounds causing symptoms in large doses will minimize symptoms when given in markedly diluted doses), "mind–body medicine" (techniques focused on the stress response), and "physical medicine" (including chiropracty, massage therapy, and osteopathy) (22). Only nutritional and herbal supplements will be considered further here, as the other topics are unrelated to the focus of this manual. Some diets based on nutritional or herbal "principles" (defined by elimination of certain foods) are prescribed by alternative practitioners, but their value is undocumented (23). Such diets include the alkaline diet, Ayurvedic diet, macrobiotic diet, and paleo diet. The use of the gluten-free diet for patients without evidence of celiac disease and diets for irritable bowel syndrome (IBS) will not be discussed in this chapter, but the evidence-supported uses of these diets are included in Chapter 12.

TABLE 8-3 Physiologically Active Compounds in Functional Foods

Compound	Food Source	Potential Health Benefit
Isothiocyanates	Cruciferous vegetables	Chemoprevention of cancer by altering drug-metabolizing enzymes
Epigallocatechin	Green tea	↓ Cancer/heart disease by antioxidation
Carotenoids	Tomatoes, carrots, citrus fruits, yams	↓ Cancer/heart disease by antioxidation
Lactoferrin	Milk	Stimulate immune system, antimicrobial
Conjugated linoleic acid	Dairy products	Prevention of cancer/atherosclerosis
Genestein and other isoflavones	Soybeans, soy foods	↓ Menopausal symptoms, osteoporosis, cancer, heart disease
Diallyl disulfide	Garlic, onions	Prevention of cancer, ↑ immune function, ↓ serum cholesterol, triglyceride
Limonene	Citrus fruits	Prevention of cancer
Nondigestible oligosaccharides	Garlic, asparagus, chicory	↓ Immune function, ↓ serum cholesterol
Omega-3 fatty acids	Algae, fish	↓ Serum cholesterol/heart disease, suppress immune function
Coumarins	Vegetables, citrus fruits	↓ Blood clotting, anticarcinogenic

Table 8-4 Examples of Probiotic Food Products Commercially Available in The United States of America

Product	Food Type	Claims	Probiotic Strains	Dose/Serving
Activia	Yogurt	Helps regulate the digestive system	Bifidobacterium animalis	10 billion
Align	Capsule	Clinically proven to protect against GI symptoms	B. infantis	1 billion
Attune	Nutrition bar	Supports digestive health	Lactobacillus acidophilus, L. casei, B. lactis	6.1 billion
Culturelle	Capsule	Promotes digestion	L. rhamnosus GG	10 billion
DanActive/Actimel	Yogurt	Regulates intestinal function	L. bulgaris, L. casei, S. thermophilus	10 billion
Danimals	Cultured milk	Keeps kids healthy	L. rhamnosus GG	Billions
Florajen	Capsules	Maintains balance of intestinal flora	L. acidophilus	Billions
Florastor	Capsule	Maintains balance of intestinal flora	Saccharomyces boulardii	5 billion
Good Belly	Fruit drink	Supports digestive and immune health	L. plantarum	20 billion
Naked Juice	Fruit drink	Promotes healthy digestive and immune system	B. lactis	Billions

(Continued)

Table 8-4 Examples of Probiotic Food Products Commercially Available in The United States of America (*Continued*)

Product	Food Type	Claims	Probiotic Strains	Dose/Serving
Nestle Good Start Protect Plus	Powdered infant formula	Supports baby's healthy immune system	B. lactis	10 million
Original kefir	Cultured milk	Balances digestive health	L. lactis, L. rhamnosus, S. diacetylactis, L. plantarum, L. casei, S. florentinus, B. longum, B. breve, B. lactis, L. acidophilus, L. reuteri	7–10 billion
Phillips' Colon Health	Capsules	Defends against gas, diarrhea, constipation	L. gasseri, B. bifidum, B. longum	
Stonyfield Farm	Yogurt	Enhances digestive and immune health	L. rhamnosus, B. lactis, L. acidophilus, L. casei	1 billion
VSL#3	Packet	Aids in dietary management of UC, IBS, and ileal pouch	B. breve, B. infantis, L. casei, B. longum, L. acidophilus, L. bulgaricus, L. plantarum, Streptococcus thermophiles	450 billion

Data from Salminen SJ, Guiemonde M, Isolauri E. Probiotics that modify disease risk. *J Nutr.* 2005;13:1294.

Supplements for Weight Loss

Various supplements have been offered as aids to weight loss, including Ayurvedic preparations, chitosan (a cationic polysaccharide derived from crustaceans), chromium picolinate, *Ephedra sinica*, *Garcinia cambogia*, glucomannan, guar gum, hydroxymethylbutyrate, *Plantago psyllium*, pyruvate, yerba mate in combination with other herbs, and yohimbe. While the rationale for each differs, none of the evidence from double-blind, randomized controlled trials (DBRCT) with these over-the-counter (OTC) agents (or meta-analyses using these trials) has produced convincing evidence of efficacy (24).

Antioxidants for Cancer and Chronic Diseases

The "standard" antioxidant supplement components include β-carotene, vitamin A, vitamin C, vitamin E (see Table 6-42), and selenium. These components do not include all of the possible antioxidant compounds in the body, but have been the most widely used. A review of RCTs with these components found no evidence to support their use to prevent mortality in healthy persons and in those with various stable diseases (25). However, there have been individual studies that have suggested a benefit for certain groups of patients taking certain antioxidant compounds. At this time, there is no consistent pattern of benefit, nor have many of these studies been replicated, a difficult standard, since the studies are complex. Although selected studies will be discussed below, it is important to realize that these are examples of potential benefit, but cannot constitute an endorsement of the use of antioxidants to prevent any specific disease.

One DBRCT on male physicians showed that daily multivitamin supplementation produced a significant but modest decrease in the risk for total cancer (26). Although antioxidants do not prevent GI cancers in the general population, some studies suggest an effect on prevention of gastric and esophageal cancer, especially in populations at high risk (27). One must keep in mind that some studies on cancer prevention show that high doses of some supplements (β-carotene, vitamin E) were shown to increase cancer risk (28). The reproducibility of these findings is just as subject to critical evaluation as are the results suggesting benefit.

A consensus statement from the American Cancer Society concludes that dietary supplements do not lower cancer risk (29). Other consensus statements from the World Cancer Research Fund (2007), the Agency for Healthcare Research and Quality (2006), an NIH State of the Science Conference (2006), and a US Preventive Services Task Force (2003) agree with this overall conclusion for prevention of chronic disease as well as cancer (28). These guidelines are based on studies of vitamin and antioxidant supplements that have been tested for prevention of chronic degenerative disease other than cancer. A review of 50 DBRCT for prevention of CVDs showed no benefit (30).

The use of antioxidant in improving cognitive function has been suggested by epidemiologic studies, but when total ferric-reducing antioxidant power of the diet was tested in the Nurses' Health Study, no effect of diet on cognition was found (31). However, the most compliant subgroup of subjects in the Supplementation with Antioxidant Vitamins and Minerals Trial (SU.VI.MAZ) was found to have improved verbal memory, but not other tasks (32). More suggestive is the demonstration of slowing of the accelerated rate of brain atrophy in elderly patients with mild cognitive impairment by addition of homocysteine-lowering B vitamins (33). Moreover, in an elderly community-dwelling population, the addition of folic acid and vitamin B_{12} led to improvement in immediate and delayed memory performance (34). These data suggest that with prolonged use in the correct population, some prevention in the decline of specific aspects of cognition (primarily memory) may occur with vitamin treatment, but the best current data are with the use of vitamins that are not considered as antioxidants (B vitamins).

There are some data suggesting a benefit of antioxidant micronutrients in other special populations. A systematic review of 21 DBRCTs in critically ill patients showed a significant reduction in mortality and in the duration of mechanical ventilation (35). The results seemed more evident in patients with higher risk of death. Antioxidant mixtures in small studies with various study designs have shown a decrease in pain (intensity or days with pain) in patients with chronic pancreatitis (36). A review of DBRCTs of antioxidant vitamin or mineral supplements on the progression of age-related macular degeneration found one large trial in a well-nourished USA population that showed a reduction in progression of disease (37). Cross-sectional data from results in the NHANES 2001–2004 database showed that higher intakes of β-carotene, vitamin C, and magnesium were associated with lower risks of hearing loss (38). For each of these indications, what is needed are more and larger intervention trials. These are difficult trials to perform and harder to duplicate, and they take years of follow-up. No definitive recommendations on the use of antioxidant mixtures can be made at this time.

Polyphenols and Other Food Components and Risk of Metabolic Disorders

Polyphenols, products of plant metabolism, range from phenols to highly polymerized compounds, such as tannins and lignins. Distinctions are made according to the number of phenol rings they contain, leading to classification as phenolic acids (one ring), stilbenes and lignans (two rings), and flavonoids (three rings) (39). These chemicals include isothiocyanates and indoles in cruciferous vegetables, genistein in soybeans and tofu, saponins in many legumes, and lycopene in tomatoes.

Fruits and beverages (e.g., tea, red wine) provide the main sources of dietary polyphenols, but in most cases, the mix of polyphenols is complex and poorly characterized. The food content is greatly affected by climate, soil type, rainfall, and other environmental factors. Polyphenols are easily oxidized, so food content is affected by storage and food preparation. For example, onions and tomatoes lose about three-quarters of their initial quercetin content after boiling for 15 minutes. Most of them are not currently included in the determination of dietary fiber, but lignin is the exception. Lignin is not a carbohydrate and constitutes about 12% of plant organic compounds. It comprises a group of phenyl propane polymers of varying sizes because polymerization continues as the plant ages. It reinforces the cellulose support structure and inhibits microbial cell wall digestion. Thus, lignin is variably degraded by anaerobic digestion systems and is only partially metabolized in the colon, as are the cell wall polysaccharides. It represents only a small part of the human diet by weight (~0.2%).

Phenolic acids and aldehydes, such as vanillin, are common, but the most common of the plant phenolics are the flavonoids, which consist of two aromatic rings linked through three carbons that form an oxygenated heterocyclic ring (39). Flavonoids and other polyphenols are ubiquitous in plants and beverages. Comprising over 4,000 compounds, flavonoids are the most abundant polyphenols in plant foods (40). They are found in tea and contribute to the bitterness of that and other beverages (41). Flavonoid intake in human diets is estimated to range from 20 to 200 mg per day, depending upon how much tea is ingested. No dietary reference intake (DRI) or upper intake level (UL) has been established for flavonoids (40). Polyphenols usually account for less than 1% of the dry matter of plants, but they can reach concentrations of 4,000 to 7,000 mg per mL in red wines and fruit juices (39). The dietary intake of polyphenols in the United States is 1 to 1.1 g per day, with flavonoids accounting for about 4% of the total. Polyphenols can quench free radicals in vitro, and so are considered potential antioxidants.

Resveratrol, a component of grapes and red wine, is one of the most widely investigated polyphenolic compounds. Multiple mechanisms have been identified in cell culture systems and in preclinical animal studies. Many trials in animals have been performed to show efficacy, but they have used high doses, short exposures, and physiological end points that may or may not be related to human physiology (42). Resveratrol has a low bioavailability (<1%), and very high doses would be needed in humans to match the biological activity reported in animals (43). Although the major sites of metabolism of resveratrol are the intestine and liver, colonic bacterial metabolism may be more important than is currently appreciated. Most of the studies performed in humans have measured only physiological end points, with uncertain relevance to disease states or clinically relevant outcomes (44). Whether any clinical benefit is provided by resveratrol or related compounds is not completely settled, and there seems no evidence currently to support the use of this supplement.

In the past, there have been no extensive food composition tables to allow observational epidemiologic studies of polyphenol intake, and the claims for these compounds have been limited to small interventional studies. There are now two food composition databases for flavonoids, from the USDA and from the UK Food Standards Agency (45,46). These data have been used in the large European Prospective Investigation into Cancer and Nutrition Study (EPIC) to show an association between flavonoid intake and gastric adenocarcinoma (47). Total flavonoid intake in the 90th percentile was estimated at more than 900 mg per day. More studies using these new databases are needed.

There are not enough data to make recommendations for general use for total flavonoids or for specific foods, but the diet should contain a wide variety of flavonoid-rich foods (fruits, vegetables, and beverages like tea) as part of a balanced healthy diet. Recommendations for intake of specific compounds vary according to the companies selling the supplements. Some recommend 50 mg per day of isoflavones or 100 to 300 mg per day of grape seed extracts rich in proanthocyanidins in order to approximate the intake derived from ingestion of soy products in Japan, or in grapes or wine in European nations (39). Other available tablets or capsules contain much more of this type of compound, amounting to approximately 100 times the polyphenol intake in a Western diet (48). Examples would include one to six doses per day of quercetin 300 mg, citrus flavonoids 1 g, or resveratrol 20 mg. Ingestion of excess polyphenols may not be without risk, as potential hazards identified from the oxidative products of these compounds include carcinogenicity or teratogenicity, thyroid toxicity, estrogenic activity of isoflavones, inhibition of nonheme iron, and interactions with pharmaceuticals (48). The dosing suggestions from commercial products, however, are not based on clinical data, and, like the products they represent, should not be recommended.

Green Tea

Like other components of fiber, polyphenols are degraded and absorbed in the colon, but the effect of these compounds on short-chain fatty acid production and microflora depends on the type of compound and the microorganisms present. Polyphenols bind proteins and precipitate in the intestinal lumen, and they can increase the fecal excretion of nitrogen and fat. They also inhibit iron absorption. The antioxidant effects of polyphenols have been of interest, particularly as they relate to carcinogens and low-density lipoproteins (LDLs), but under some circumstances, they can act as pro-oxidants (49). Their antioxidant effects depend on solubility and chelating potential, among other properties. The blacker the tea, the greater the degree of oxidation of the polyphenols and the weaker the possible effects of these compounds. Herbal teas are not true teas (*Camellia sinensis*), and their flavonoid content is much lower. Tea contributes more than 60% of dietary flavonoids and onions about 13%; grapes, apples, red wine, and dairy products provide most of the rest. The consumption of one to two cups of tea per day has been associated with health benefits in epidemiologic studies (41,50).

Catechins in green tea (esp. epigallocatechin gallate) and theaflavins and thearubigins derived from black tea are the major substances responsible for the physiological effects of tea in vitro on cells (51). These compounds have been shown to have pro-oxidant as well as antioxidant effects (as well as other effects), and high concentrations have been used to demonstrate effects in many cell cultures. Thus, the biological relevance in vivo of these effects is still very much in doubt. The overall antioxidant potency of polyphenol-rich beverages in the United States has been measured (pomegranate juice and red wine head the list), but this does not prove in vivo biological activity (52). Urinary metabolites of polyphenols have been measured, but at best they document intake, not biological activity (53). Even then, only some of the metabolites (a few isoflavones) correlate well with intake, whereas catechins and flavonones correlate less well with intake. Green tea contains polyphenolic flavonoids that account for up to 40% of the dry weight of green tea, as well as caffeine and other methyl xanthines (54). Many health benefits (cancer and atherosclerosis prevention among them) are claimed for heavy ingestion of green tea (up to 20 cups per day) (50). However, current evidence does not support or refute a definitive effect of green tea intake on cancer prevention, even for breast and prostate cancer (55). Some studies show a positive effect of green tea extract on fat metabolism at rest and during exercise, and this effect has been proposed to be useful in weight loss by increasing fat oxidation, but the data are inconclusive (56). There are many confounding factors in evaluating the effect of tea, such as patient compliance, habitual caffeine intake, polyphenol content of the beverages ingested, and genetic predisposition to obesity (57). A meta-analysis of studies on the effect of green tea on glycemic control suggests a favorable effect on fasting glucose, but no effect on insulin sensitivity (58). These studies do not provide overall definitive support for an effect on chronic metabolic disease and/or atherosclerosis.

The other major component of green tea that enhances metabolism and is thermogenic is caffeine. However, the effects of caffeine by itself on energy expenditure are evident only at rest or with mild exercise, and effects on fat metabolism are small at best (59). Most of the suggestions about the value of caffeine in disease prevention come from epidemiological studies, such as the lower risk of type 2 diabetes mellitus with coffee intake in the Nurses' Health Study (60). As with other suggestions from epidemiology, this hypothesis needs to be confirmed by prospective intervention trials. The data described above show only associations, not causation. Thus, it is not possible to recommend the consumption of large amounts of phenolics as foods or supplements until more data are available.

Ox-LDL may play a significant role in atherogenesis, and has been identified as a risk factor for CVD. However, flavonoid-rich foods (e.g., olive oil, tea, red wine, soy) have not been shown to have a consistent effect on this risk factor (61). The combination of these products with fruits, vegetables, and ω-3 polyunsaturated fatty acids (PUFAs) does appear to decrease the rate of oxidation of LDL. It is possible that the lack of consistent effect of flavonoid supplements might be due to the variety and quantity used of the supplements or compounds. Nonetheless, the data do not currently justify use of these products for prevention of heart disease.

Olive Oil

Polyphenols are components of many foods, including olive oil. Olive oil contains greater than 30 of these compounds (e.g., tyrosol and hydroxytyrosol containing oleocanthol), along with other components such as vitamin E, to which are attributed antioxidant and anti-inflammatory properties. A large study using a Mediterranean diet supplemented with one of two polyphenol-rich sources, olive oil and nuts reported prevention of CVD with such supplements (62). The amount of olive oil used in this study was very large (1 L per week for 16 weeks), providing 14 g per day as polyphenols, if polyphenols account for 10% of olive oil by weight. This intake was as large as the highest olive oil intake for any population, that of the island of Crete (63). By way of contrast, the estimated intake of olive oil in the United States of America is 0.9 L per year. However, the diets similar to those used in the intervention study lower blood pressure (not necessarily an effect of polyphenols alone) and the only cardiovascular end point that was statistically affected was stroke, an expected result from lower blood pressure. Thus, the results of this widely publicized trial are still not very conclusive for an effect of polyphenols, especially at the commonly achieved intake of dietary polyphenols.

The health benefits of olive oil were first suggested by Ancel Keys, who noted a low rate of CVD in people on the island of Crete (63). The benefits were also related to the content of monosaturated fatty acids, as olive oil has a ratio of mono-/polyunsaturated fatty acids of approximately 5:1. In vegetable oils, this ratio is reversed. One difficulty in recommending olive oil for health benefits is that the qualities and content of "extra virgin olive oil," while seemingly regulated by the European Union and the International Olive Council established in 1959 by the United Nations, are difficult to ascertain owing to lack of application of the regulations that outline a series of chemical requirements, including free fatty acid content of 0.8% or less, and peroxides of <20 mEq per kg. True extra virgin olive oil is thus expensive to produce and does not have a long shelf life. These issues have led to the widespread use of adulteration of olive oils by other vegetable oils (64). The detection of such adulteration is very difficult, however, and not widely used by the industry overall (65). The most reliable source of extra virgin olive oil is from single producers, but high cost does not always equate with high quality (64). Thus, when recommending olive oil as part of a diet, it is difficult to know whether the product will contain the level of antioxidant and anti-inflammatory components that have been thought to exert health benefits. Evidence for specific effects of olive oil has been suggested to be sufficient to advance labeling claims. For example, olive oil has been shown in some studies to decrease the amount of circulating oxidized LDL. Thus, the claim that "olive oil polyphenols contribute to the protection of blood lipids from oxidative stress" has been allowed on olive oils containing at least 5 mg of hydroxytyrosol and its derivatives per 20 g of oil (66).

Chocolate

Chocolate and cocoa powder contain flavanols (e.g., epicatechins) and procyanidins that can be metabolized to strong antioxidants, as well as other active ingredients such as theobromine and magnesium (67). Dark chocolate contains about three times the amount of polyphenols as milk chocolate (185 mg versus 64 mg per 40 g serving), and white chocolate contains none, as it has no cocoa powder. In vitro and animal testing of individual components highlight possible mechanisms as increased nitric oxide (NO) production (epicatechins), and dilation of blood vessels. Of the greater than 70 clinical studies performed in recent years, study design and end points varied greatly, but no clinical end points were shown to improve (67). On the basis of observational studies, chocolate consumption was associated with a reduction of risk for cardiovascular disorders, but no randomized trials have been carried out (68). Effects on endothelial function, and lowering of blood pressure and serum cholesterol, have been noted, but these effects may have been modified by the high calorie and sugar content of the cocoa used for such studies. No recommendations about the use of chocolate for prevention of heart disease can be made at this time.

Other Nutritional Supplements for Prevention and Treatment of Chronic Disease

Only about one-third of people in the United States engage in regular physical exercise—mostly walking, swimming, bicycling, running, and step aerobics. A deficiency of certain vitamins (including all B vitamins) adversely affects physical performance (e.g., by causing anemia, muscle weakness, fatigue, or peripheral neuropathy). Exercise can increase the need for some nutrients, as in the GI blood loss seen during prolonged exercise (69). In addition, some vitamins are considered to be important in reducing the risk for CVD. These include vitamin E and the vitamins that lower serum homocysteine levels (vitamin B_6, folate, and vitamin B_{12}). The role of each of these vitamins is discussed in Chapter 6.

The new DRIs include separate recommendations for persons over the age of 70 (70) (see also Chapter 2). In the Survey in Europe on Nutrition and the Elderly, a Concerned Action (SENECA) Study, evidence of low vitamin intake/deficiency based on serum levels was found in 47% of European elderly persons for vitamin D, 23% for vitamin B_6, 2.7% for vitamin B_{12}, and 1% for vitamin E (71). Neurocognitive function can be decreased in deficiency states of vitamins B_6 and B_{12} and folate (72), the same vitamins that help to regulate homocysteine levels. The intake of these vitamins is often inadequate in the elderly. Because on average the elderly ingest only about 50% of the recommended dietary allowance (RDA) for any vitamin, special care must be taken to ensure that the full RDA (or DRI) is taken.

Not only may micronutrient deficiency play a role, but energy intake is often insufficient in elderly populations, and may be associated with cognitive impairment (73). At the other end of life, poor early weight gain appears to be associated with chronic disease. Stunting in children and adults from regions with chronic enteric infection is associated with central obesity, insulin resistance, hypertension, and low LDL cholesterol in adults (74). However, even when malnutrition is recognized as part of a chronic disease, as in cirrhosis, there is no evidence that oral or enteral supplements alter clinical outcomes (75). Some supplements that can improve cholesterol lowering to a modest degree include niacin, ω-3 fatty acids, tocotrienols, plant sterols, soluble fibers, probiotics, soy, and mixed nuts (76). Substances that are ineffective include garlic, ginseng, coenzyme Q, and chromium. It is instructive that the supplements with some efficacy have associated mechanisms to explain the effect.

Vitamins and Minerals

The use of multivitamin and mineral supplements has increased greatly, with some populations reporting a use that approaches 50%. These preparations contain many potentially active nutrients such as so-called antioxidant vitamins, magnesium, and selenium, all of which have been postulated to have an effect on CVD. Many observational studies and one RCT provided mixed results for an effect on myocardial infarction (MI). One RCT in Swedish women showed that multivitamins alone or with minerals was associated with a 27% decrease in the rate of MI after 10 years in women without a history of CVD, but not in those with such a history. The decline in MI rates was even greater in those patients who had used multivitamins for greater than 5 years (77). However, no preventive effect was noted in those women using other supplements. This result will need to be replicated before it can be accepted as definitive. However, the effect does have a possible mechanism in the proposed relationship of degenerative diseases to mitochondrial decay (78).

In addition to their potential role in preventing CVD, vitamins and other supplements have been suggested to have a role in cancer chemoprevention (see Chapter 15) and in preventing cataracts, particularly the vitamins with antioxidant properties (vitamin A, β-carotene, and vitamin E) (79). Some studies have suggested a preventive role for B vitamins, but other data suggest no effect, or even an increased risk of colorectal cancer with folate supplementation under the conditions of the trials (80,81). The data are not yet sufficient to suggest that regular use of these vitamins prevents cancer or nuclear cataracts or CVD (79,82). In addition, the use of vitamin supplements (e.g., vitamin E, B_{12}, folic acid) has not prevented cognitive impairment or Alzheimer disease in patients at risk for such clinical outcomes (83). If vitamins and minerals are effective in these settings, however, the guidelines from professional societies and the US government recommend obtaining adequate amounts of these micronutrients from food (84). Small amounts of regular and enriched foods improve vitamin concentrations in frail, elderly patients, so deficiency is not a problem of malabsorption (85). In physically active people without deficiency, there is no well-documented effect of supplemented vitamins and minerals if they are ingesting a balanced diet (86).

However, despite the absence of evidence supporting the widespread use of multivitamin supplementation in the general population, evidence continues to accrue suggesting that some supplements may benefit some groups in terms of prevention of chronic disease. The challenge is to identify the populations at risk, to select the specific appropriate nutrient(s), and to provide consistent data demonstrating efficacy.

The question of a role for supplements in patients with chronic disease is even more complex, and positive effects have not been reproducibly documented. As with antioxidant supplements, much of the data to support a role in disease prevention comes largely from in vitro studies. However, more studies in humans are being performed with valid clinical end points, and these continue to suggest a role for vitamins and/or minerals in chronic conditions. Some of these will be highlighted below, and others included in discussions of the individual vitamins and minerals in Chapters 6 and 7.

Coenzyme Q10 (CoQ10) supplements have been studied for years in patients with chronic congestive heart failure. A meta-analysis of 12 RCTs found that CoQ10 may improve ejection fraction, although the effect size was small (3.6%) (87). Studies reported before 1993 tend to be positive, while later ones were negative (88). Results from the Q-SYMBIO trial on CoQ10 supplementation (2 mg/kg/day) were reported at a conference in 2012, and all-cause mortality was said to be lower (88). The published results will be awaited with great interest. The proposed mechanism would be to improve mitochondrial function, by either correcting deficiency, bypassing a block in electron transport, or acting as an antioxidant (89). However, CoQ10 supplementation has yet to be found effective in genetic mitochondrial diseases in which abnormal mitochondrial function is the known culprit (89).

Suggestive reports for other vitamins and minerals continue to emerge, although none have reached the point at which clinical recommendations can be made. An observational study showed a significant association of cobalamin and folate status with cognitive function in North Indian children (90). These data are consistent with the effect of B vitamin supplement on brain atrophy in adults (33). B_{12} status can be followed, as there is a dose–response relation between B_{12} intake and methylmalonic acid concentrations in serum (91). Vitamin D supplementation (1,000 and 4,000 IU per day) to African Americans showed a fall in systolic (but not diastolic) blood pressure of 3.4 and 4.0 mm Hg, respectively, calculating a fall of 0.2 mm Hg for each 1 ng per mL elevation in 25-hydroxy vitamin D (92).

Mineral supplementation has been used to control various manifestations of CVD. Calcium supplements have been studied in patients with CVD, because calcium has been shown to lower blood pressure by 3 to 4 mm Hg. However, no efficacy has been found, and even a possible increase in CVD mortality has been reported in men (93). Selenium is a component of the oxidative machinery, and observational studies suggested an inverse relationship between selenium intake and CVD risk. However, the limited trials of selenium supplementation do not support such an association (94). Chromium has an effect on insulin sensitivity, and supplementation was proposed as a weight control mechanism. However, the effect on weight in obese patients, if real, is very small (0.5 kg) (95).

Each of these proposed roles for micronutrients assume that nothing else in the diet is changing. However, unknown "supplements" may be present and influence results. As one example, the role of drinking-water nitrate has been examined, and concerns about a link to cancer and neural tube defects have been voiced (96). Such complex interactions with other nutrients are the reason why only consistent effects of supplements in well-defined populations should lead eventually to clinical recommendations.

Immune-Modulating Polysaccharides

As immune function declines with age and in certain chronic diseases, natural health products have been advocated as preventive measures. However, the data supporting their use is inconsistent (97). Certain polysaccharides have been suggested to affect immune function, including glucans, pectins, and heteroglycans. A total of 62 studies, including 15 in humans, have shown some sort of positive result (98). The most positive results were in animal studies, and several human studies reported improved "biomarkers" of disease. Several studies using glucans from the *Coriolus versicolor* mushroom have been reported to increase survival in patients with colorectal or gastric cancer (98). This mushroom has been used in Chinese medicine (yun zhi). The American Cancer Society did not find that the available evidence supported a role for extracts of this mushroom in cancer therapy (99). Currently, no medicine from this mushroom is approved in Western countries, and the mechanism of any effect is not known.

Chondroitin Sulfate and Glucosamine

These compounds are among the most commonly used "natural" agents in chronic disease, and are sold separately but are more commonly ingested in combination. Both of these compounds are produced endogenously in joints. Chondroitin sulfate, a glycosaminoglycan that is formed from repeating disaccharides of galactosamine sulfate and glucuronic acid, is found in articular cartilage, where it is secreted by chondrocytes. It inhibits the enzymes that degrade cartilage and holds water in cartilage, thereby increasing its elasticity. Glucosamine is an aminosugar found in cartilage, tendons, and synovial fluid; it stimulates the synthesis of proteoglycans and glycosaminoglycans. However, there is no evidence that these compounds are absorbed intact in humans, and thus they are very unlikely to reach the target organ, the joint (100). If they have any effect, it would have to be related to some local effect on the intestine, either by altering microflora or the permeability barrier.

A meta-analysis of 17 studies of chondroitin sulfate and glucosamine in osteoarthritis concluded that they are effective in improving outcomes, but the magnitude of their effect is unclear because of inconsistencies in the study methods and dependence on industry support for execution of the studies (101). A meta-analysis of placebo-controlled trials of chondroitin alone for osteoarthritis indicated that the symptomatic benefit of chondroitin alone was minimal or nonexistent (102). A meta-analysis of placebo-controlled studies of glucosamine alone for osteoarthritis indicated that the glucosamine product made by Rotta was superior to placebo in the treatment of pain and functional impairment, whereas non-Rotta products were not superior to placebo (103). A further review of four meta-analyses showed a high degree of heterogeneity and concluded that the minimal symptomatic benefit was based on 3/20 studies (104). Finally, a review of 10 large-scale randomized trials found no effect of the supplements alone or in combination on joint pain or on radiological progression of the disease (105). Despite the popularity of these supplements, there is no evidence to support their use. Typical dosing for chondroitin sulfate is 1,200 mg per day; for glucosamine, it is 1,500 mg per day. There are no safety issues with these compounds, but that is consistent with the lack of evidence of significant bioavailability.

Herbal Products (Including Phytoestrogens) and Hepatic Toxicity

Many claims are made for mixtures of herbal compounds, with traditional Indian (Ayurvedic), Chinese, and Japanese (Kampo) medicine providing the most common examples (22). These herbal mixtures are part of a system and philosophy that includes a proper lifestyle, but in Western nations, the herbal compounds are often used alone. Other mixtures or combinations of other herbs have been proposed to enhance, for example, brain function (106) and to treat benign prostatic hyperplasia (107). Claims for health benefits abound, with limited data to support these claims. For example, Japanese herbal medications have been studied in functional GI disorders, but there are few well-designed RCTs using standardized medications (108). Although 406 RCTs of herbal medicine interventions were found up to 2011, the quality of these studies was rather poor with inadequate reporting of important characteristics of the studies (109). Findings from such trials do not usually allow firm conclusions to be made regarding efficacy (e.g., for glycemic control in diabetes), although the herbs are generally found to be safe (110). However, hepatotoxicity has been reported for a number of herbal compounds (see below). A number of databases exist that provide information on herbal preparations, including camLine (http://www.camline.ca), HerbMed (http://www.herbmed.org), U Texas MD Anderson Cancer Center, Complementary/Alternative Medicine (www.medanderson.org/departments/CIMER/index.cfm), NIH ODS (http://www.ods.od.nih.gov), Natural Medicines Comprehensive Database (www.naturaldatabase.com), and Natural Standard (www.naturalstandard.com). Several of the more commonly available herbal compounds will be discussed below, but this selection is not meant either to be comprehensive or to imply a recommendation.

Curcumin

Turmeric is an approved food additive, containing approximately 2% to 5% curcumin as its most active ingredient. Curcumin is a polyphenol with known structure that has been shown to have antisolubility and poor bioavailability (111). It has shown efficacy in many cell systems and in some animal models (112). Phase-I studies in humans have demonstrated that doses up to 15 g per day are safe. Because of the limited bioavailability, potential effects on the GI tract have been considered as this mucosa is exposed to very high doses, and some suggestive results have been reported in small trials (113). However, only two RCTs involving 99 patients with inflammatory bowel disease (IBD) have been reported, and the results are insufficient for any conclusion (114). Curcumin has been tried as a chemo- and radiosensitizer for tumors (115), and for cancer chemoprevention (116). Although a number of small phase-I and phase-II studies have been completed, evidence for efficacy is generally lacking. Well-designed studies in large numbers of patients are needed to know whether any efficacy is present and reproducible, given the very poor bioavailability of the compound, along with the observation that only low nanomolar (nM) concentrations have been found in plasma, and picomolar (pM) concentrations in tissues, in contrast to the millimolar (mM) concentrations used to demonstrate effects in cells in culture (111). Curcumin is available in tablets of 400 to 500 mg, but quality control data are lacking for these preparations.

Echinacea

Three of the nine species of the genus *Echinacea* are commonly found in herbal preparations. The most commonly used is *Echinacea purpurea*, the purple coneflower. Both the above-ground parts and the root have been used as herbal medicines. Extracts of the plant show antiviral, antimicrobial, and immune–modulatory activities in vitro, which appear to be due to multiple components (117). *Echinacea* has been used to treat or prevent the common cold and influenza and as a stimulant to the immune system. The efficacy of *Echinacea* in reducing the viral load was tested in 437 healthy adults exposed to rhinovirus. No differences were seen in the rate of infection, the severity of symptoms, or viral titers (118). There are some suggestions that *Echinacea* preparations might be effective for the early treatment of colds in adults, but the results are not consistent (119). Three studies of induced rhinovirus colds show some effect on symptoms (120). The effects on immune modulation in vitro have led to interest in supplementing trained athletes, but studies showing efficacy are lacking (121). *Echinacea* is available as the root or the herb; some formulations contain both. Commercial products include tinctures, tablets, capsules, lozenges, and teas. Typical daily dosing is 300 to 900 mg of dried extract, but dosing is difficult to analyze because of the wide range of formulations available. Allergic reactions and asthma have been reported with *Echinacea*. Hepatotoxicity has been seen after prolonged use. Thus, *Echinacea* should be used cautiously. One anaphylactic reaction to an *Echinacea* extract has been reported.

G. biloba

An extract of the leaves of the ginkgo tree is used to improve memory and increase peripheral blood flow. It is one of the top-selling herbs in the United States. Ginkgo leaves contain flavonoids, sesquiterpenes, and terpenes called *ginkgolides*. Biological activities demonstrated in vitro include scavenging free radicals, lowering oxidative stress, reducing neural damage, reducing platelet aggregation, and anti-inflammatory, antitumor, and antiaging activities (122). A meta-analysis of nine trials in dementia detected only a moderate effect on cognition without an effect on activities of daily living (123). A 5-year trial of ginkgo extract for prevention of Alzheimer disease showed no reduction in the risk of progression from mild cognitive impairment to Alzheimer's (124). However, a direct comparison among placebo, a German *G. biloba* product (eGb761), and a second-generation cholinesterase inhibitor (donepezil) in patients with Alzheimer disease demonstrated that both ginkgo and donepezil were better than placebo but there was no difference between ginkgo and donepezil (125). Single trials in other degenerative diseases have reported positive results, but these remain to be confirmed. In a 24-week, double-blinded, placebo-controlled trial of 111 patients with peripheral vascular disease, superior, pain-free walking and maximal walking distance were noted in those who received *G. biloba* extract (120 mg per day) (126). Two separate small trials showed modest effects on vision in age-related macular degeneration (127). However, trials in many other areas have shown no efficacy, despite multiple studies, for example, in tinnitus (128). *G. biloba* extract is available as tincture, tablets, and capsules. Typical dosing is 40 to 80 mg three times a day. Ginkgo is thought to be a platelet-activating factor antagonist and may potentiate the effects of antiplatelet drugs and anticoagulants.

Ginseng

The term ginseng includes American ginseng (*Panax quinquefolius*) and Asian ginseng (*P. ginseng* and *P. japonicus*). Siberian ginseng (*Eleutherococcus senticosus*) is not a true ginseng, but is promoted and sold as ginseng. *P. ginseng* is the species most widely available in the United States and also the most widely studied. The plant part used is the root. There are three types, depending on how it is processed: fresh ginseng (<4 years old), white ginseng (4 to 6 years old and air-dried), and red ginseng (harvested at 6 years, not peeled, and steam-treated root). Saponins (ginsenosides) are thought to be the active ingredients, although their mechanism of action is unknown. Twenty randomized trials in Korea using either Asian or American ginseng showed no results that could be interpreted as positive, but methodological problems made interpretation very difficult (129). In addition, 65 randomized studies were reviewed using *P. ginseng* without documenting a single clearly efficacious result (130). Clinical end points tested ranged from psychomotor performance to cancer. The Asian, American, and Siberian forms of ginseng are available as tablets, capsules, powders, teas, and tinctures. Most commercial products contain 100 to 400 mg of extract (equivalent to 0.5 to 2.0 g of root). The levels of ginsenosides vary widely among different commercial products. High doses of ginseng are associated with central nervous system (CNS) excitation, hypertension, sleeplessness, and nervousness. Drug interactions may occur with corticosteroids, estrogens, and digitalis preparations. *P. ginseng* produces hypoglycemic effects, perhaps by accelerating hepatic lipogenesis, and should be used cautiously in patients with diabetes.

Hoodia Gordonii

The genus *Hoodia* is one of a group of succulent plants grown in South Africa and Namibia. The National Food Research Institute, CSIR in Pretoria, S. Africa, in 1963 investigated indigenous plants used as food and observed an appetite-suppressing activity in mice. Although no efficacy has yet been demonstrated in humans, research has resulted in an active compound, and licensing of the patent to international companies, along with a license to a Khoisan community to make and sell the product (131). The importance of this product, therefore, is not in the demonstration of its efficacy in humans, but in its acceptance by and support from a government agency. It is not clear whether its availability for Western communities will increase with time.

Ma Huang (E. sinica)

The dried root of the herb *E. sinica* has been used in Chinese medicine for centuries. It contains the alkaloids ephedrine and pseudoephedrine and is used as a bronchodilator in asthma, a nasal decongestant, and an aid to weight loss. Ephedrine, which is used to treat asthma, is a sympathomimetic agent that can induce tachycardia, raise blood pressure, and cause urinary retention and restlessness. Pseudoephedrine is found in many OTC cold medicines.

Ephedrine is an effective bronchodilator, and pseudoephedrine is an effective nasal decongestant. The ephedrine and pseudoephedrine in ma huang provide no advantage over the same substances in prescription drugs and OTC medications. Because of the inability to quantify the alkaloid content of ma huang, both underdosing and overdosing (with toxicity) are possible; the use of prescription drugs or OTC medications containing ephedrine poses no such risks when used at recommended doses. Ephedrine, frequently in combination with caffeine, has been used in a number of weight loss programs. When ephedrine and caffeine are combined with a low-calorie diet, a marginally greater weight loss is achieved than with a low-calorie diet alone, but at the expense of a high incidence of insomnia, tremors, and dizziness (132). In addition, ma huang is one of the herbal products (along with Siberian ginseng, bitter orange, and licorice) that has been consistently associated with increased blood pressure (133). Ma huang is available as teas, tinctures, capsules, and tablets. The alkaloid content of commercial ma huang products varies from 0.3 to 56 mg. In comparison, prescription asthma medications contain 24 mg of ephedrine, and OTC cold preparations contain 60 to 120 mg of pseudoephedrine. Ma huang has been associated with stroke, MI, and death (134). More common side effects include tremors, insomnia, and urinary retention. The risk for adverse events associated with ma huang is increased when it is given to patients with preexisting hypertension, coronary artery disease, thyroid disease, and benign prostatic hypertrophy (BPH). The FDA recommends that everyone avoid ma huang.

Phytosterols (γ-Oryzanol)

Plants contain sterols that are structurally similar to cholesterol but are poorly absorbed from the GI tract. These plant sterols (which include sitosterol/stigmasterol, sitostanol, and campesterol) are collectively called *phytosterols*. Vegetable oils contain significant levels of phytosterols. In general, vegetable oils containing large amounts of PUFAs (e.g., corn oil) have more phytosterols than oils containing smaller amounts of PUFAs (e.g., palm oil, coconut oil). Purification and processing can remove phytosterols from vegetable oils.

The clinical evidence that phytosterols lower serum cholesterol levels is excellent (135,136). The mechanism of this effect is not definitely known, but it may be that phytosterols diminish cholesterol absorption from the intestine. The poor absorption of phytosterols from the intestine supports the suggestion that they act in the intestinal lumen to impair cholesterol absorption. No blinded studies of the effects of γ-oryzanol on serum cholesterol levels have been performed in humans.

The FDA currently allows no claims for supplements containing free phytosterols, although it allows conventional foods containing free and/or esterified phytosterols to make claims for reducing the risk of coronary heart disease (CHD), and broadens the range of foods allowed to make such claims (http://www.gpo.gov/fdsys/phg/FR-2010-12-08/pdf/2010-30386.pdf). Other companies claim that combination of free phytosterols and phytostanols can decrease LDL cholesterol, but only very modestly (4.9%) in patients with primary hypercholesterolemia, and when taken in addition to using the National Cholesterol Education Program (NCEP) Therapeutic Lifestyle Change (TLC) diet (137). Other studies confirm a cholesterol-lowering effect, but no DBRCT is available that shows an effect of plant sterols on hard cardiovascular end points (138).

γ-Oryzanol, which is prepared commercially from rice bran oil, is a mixture of ferulic acid esters of phytosterols. Sitosterol esters are available as an additive to margarine (Benacol™). γ-Oryzanol is available in tablets and capsules in doses of 100 to 500 mg per day. There are no safety issues for this product. However, stigmasterol as a component of soy oil–based lipid emulsions used for parenteral nutrition has been implicated in the cholestatic liver damage (parenteral-associated liver disease) seen mostly in infants and young children (http://www.nature.com/nrgastro/journal/v10/n12/full/nrgastro.2013.206.html). This damage does not occur to the same degree using fish oil–based emulsion.

Phytoestrogens (Soy Protein)

Soy protein preparations also contain phytoestrogens-like activity. Isoflavones, which are found primarily in soy products, are weak estrogens. The major isoflavones in soy protein preparations are genestein, daidzein, and glycetein. Isoflavone-containing soy products appear to improve endothelial function, which might provide a rationale for influencing the health of vessels (139). They also bind to estrogen receptors, providing support for use of these products in menopause. As a result, the claims for phytoestrogens are wide-ranging, including improvement in heart disease, menopausal symptoms, and prevention of osteoporosis and breast cancer (140). Soy protein also lowers serum cholesterol; whether or not the effects of soy proteins on serum cholesterol are mediated through isoflavones is not known. A meta-analysis evaluated the results of 38 controlled trials of the effects of soy protein (average intake of 47 g per day) on serum cholesterol. Soy protein was associated with decreases in total cholesterol (9.3%), LDL cholesterol (12.9%), and triglycerides (10.5%) (141). In all of these trials, large amounts of soy protein were consumed, amounts so large that major reductions of other dietary components would be needed to accommodate the increase in soy protein. The FDA allows commercial products containing at least 6.25 g of soy protein to carry a label claiming a role for soy protein in reducing the risk for coronary artery disease when combined with a diet low in cholesterol and saturated fat.

Because of their estrogenic effects, soy products containing isoflavones have been used to relieve hot flashes and other menopausal symptoms. It has been suggested that phytoestrogens relieve menopausal symptoms without causing the adverse effects seen with hormone replacement therapy, particularly the increased risk for breast cancer. Botanical compounds and dietary supplements (e.g., black cohosh, red clover, soy products) are often used by patients to control symptoms of menopause. Phytoestrogen extracts, including soy foods and red clover, do not seem to have much effect, although they appear to have positive effects on plasma lipid concentrations (142). Black cohosh does seem to be safe and to alleviate hot flashes. In a 12-week trial, postmenopausal women received placebo or 40 g of soy protein isolate containing 76 mg of isoflavones. In the women who received soy, hot flashes were reduced by 45%, whereas in those receiving placebo, they were reduced by 30% (143). This is clearly a large amount of soy protein, and the consumption of this amount of soy protein would require a major change in dietary habits. Despite this positive report, a review of 21 trials of soy proteins on hot flashes and night sweats failed to demonstrate any benefit (144).

Soy proteins are available as soy flour, soy milk, soy protein isolates, natto (fermented soy beans), tofu, and textured soy protein. These preparations contain 1 to 10 mg of isoflavones per gram of protein. The dosage of isoflavones used to treat menopausal symptoms is 76 mg per day or more. Genestein supplements are also available. There are no safety issues. However, because of the binding of phytoestrogens to the estrogen receptor, and a large amount of preclinical data suggesting that endocrine function and development may be disrupted, the question of the long-term safety of these products is still debated (140).

Saw Palmetto

Saw palmetto berry is the ripe dried fruit of *Serenoa repens*, a dwarf palm tree that grows in the southern United States. Commercial preparations are extracts containing phytosterols and polysaccharides from these berries. Saw palmetto has been used to treat BPH. Some evidence indicates that it inhibits 5-α-reductase, the enzyme that converts testosterone to dihydrotestosterone, a steroid that promotes prostate growth. Saw palmetto is promoted as an agent that reduces symptoms associated with BPH. A series of double-blinded, randomized, placebo-controlled trials have demonstrated decreases in nocturia, increases in peak urine flow, and decreases in residual volume in patients with BPH who receive saw palmetto (145). Although the evidence that saw palmetto relieves the symptoms of BPH is suggestive, no evidence has been found that it reduces an enlarged prostate or prevents prostatic cancer. Saw palmetto, prepared as whole berries or as a lipophilic extract, is available as capsules, tablets, and tinctures. Typical dosing is 1 to 2 g of berries or 160 to 320 mg of lipophilic extract per day. A number of commercially available formulations provide subtherapeutic doses. A single case of hepatic toxicity has been ascribed to saw palmetto.

St. John's Wort

The dried, above-ground parts of *Hypericum perforatum* have been used extensively to treat depression and as a mood elevator. Several mechanisms of action have been proposed, including increases of serotonin levels and monoamine oxidase activity, but little evidence is available to support any specific mechanism. St. John's wort appears to be better than placebo in the short-term management of mild to moderate depression (146–148). However, 8-week studies in major depression did not reveal any advantage over placebo (149,150). In one of these studies, a conventional antidepressant, sertraline, was used as an active comparator and was found to be superior to both placebo and St. John's wort (150). St. John's wort is available as tablets, capsules, tinctures, powders, and teas. Typical daily dosing is 900 mg of standardized extract. St. John's wort may induce photosensitivity; allergic reactions with hives and skin rash have occurred. Common side effects include fatigue, dyspepsia, and sleep disturbances. Pretreatment with St. John's wort reduces the area under the curve for a number of drugs, including digoxin, amitriptyline, midazolam, and the active metabolite of simvastatin (1).

Adverse Effects of Herbal Medicines

Herbal medicines have been reported to be responsible for a variety of adverse effects, most commonly liver damage, but also kidney damage, colon perforation, carcinoma, coma, and death. The single herbals associated with most severe effects were *Herbae pulvis standardisatus*, *Larrea tridentata*, *Piper methysticum*, and *Cassia senna* (151). Herbals also produce drug interactions, about 40% due to altered pharmacokinetics (152). The most common herbals leading to contraindications for use with other drugs include flaxseed, *Echinacea*, and yohimbe.

Liver injury has been reported as well with the use of complex herbal mixtures, including Herbalife and Hydroxycut products, and products containing usnic acid (153), Ayurvedic and Chinese herbs, black cohosh, and germander (154), and *Ephedra* compounds (155). The list of herbal preparations that cause hepatotoxicity grows each year, and will continue to do so. Recent additions to the list include White Flood, a muscle-building supplement containing the Chinese herbal agents *Evodia ruaecarpa* and *Huperzia serrata*, vinpocetine from the *Vinca* plant, along with other ingredients (156), Limbrel, or flavocoxid, a proprietary blend of plant-derived bioflavonoids (157), and the Chinese herbal *Fructus Psoraleae* (Bol-gol-zhee) (158).

Food supplements increasingly have contained cyanobacteria (most often the genera *Spirulina/Arthrospira* and *Aphanizomenon*). These bacteria produce anatoxin-α, microcystin, and nodularin (159), which carry risks of hepatotoxicity, neurotoxicity, and allergy (160). With global warming, the risk of increased blooms of blue-green algae and contamination of the herbal and food supplies is a real possibility (161). Although renal toxicity is less common than hepatotoxicity with herbal preparations, renal damage has been a well-documented risk for decades, most commonly involving the *Aritolochia* genus of plants, with most exposure still occurring in Asia (162).

Amino Acids (Glutamine, Arginine, Taurine) and Products (L-Carnitine, Creatine, and 5-Hydroxytryptophan)

The concept of conditionally essential amino acids has been proposed, because of the importance of certain amino acids in the stress response to acute illness (e.g., glutamine [Gln], arginine). In addition, other amino acids (e.g., arginine, leucine, citrulline) may alter the balance between muscle protein synthesis and breakdown, leading to muscle protein anabolism in chronic and acute disease states (163). The most commonly used compounds available as supplements will be reviewed below.

Glutamine

Gln, along with aspartate, is an important energy source for the small intestine, but it has not been classified as an essential amino acid (164). A special role for Gln has been suggested for critically ill patients, as it is the most abundant extracellular amino acid, is utilized at high rates by intestine, CNS, and immune cells, and its serum levels fall during critical illness. However, the data do not clearly support such a claim (165–167). Clinical efficacy of supplemental Gln (either p.o. or parenteral in doses from 10 to 60 g per day) led in some studies to some improvement in immunologic measures, reduction in costs, in rates of infectious complications (166), and in treatment of mucositis from chemo- or radiotherapy (168), although not all reports confirm these conclusions. One study with surgical ICU patients showed an increase in mortality (6.2% in controls to 17.7% in those supplemented with Gln 0.25 to 0.5 g/kg/day) (169). The problems with assessing the considerable literature on Gln are many, and include the greatly different patient populations, the variety of end points tested, the relatively short follow-up, the lack of adequately powered studies, and the lack of reproducible improvement of significant end points (167). Studies examining the effect of Gln on clinically relevant outcomes have suggested that in a well-defined group of critically ill patients, Gln can have its greatest chance to improve mortality and morbidity if it is given in doses greater than 035 g/kg/day and for longer than 5 days (170). However, when 30 g per day of a Gln-containing dipeptide delivering 0.35 g/kg/day was given orally within 24 hours of admission to critically ill patients for up to 28 days, no beneficial effect on clinical outcomes was seen, but mortality was increased in those patients with multiorgan failure (171). In neonates with GI disease (172) or those with very low birth weight (173), no reduction in infectious complications was found. Thus, despite the attractive characteristics of Gln to modify cell function during stress, further studies are needed before Gln supplementation can be recommended for use in critically ill (or any other) patients.

The other use for Gln that has been recommended is to stimulate small intestinal growth in patients with short bowel syndrome. All of the studies have combined oral Gln with parenteral recombinant human growth hormone (GH), providing both substrate and hormonal stimulation to enterocyte growth, although neither stimulus is specific for the intestine. Most of the early studies were open label and not controlled. One randomized double-blind controlled trial of 41 patients has shown some efficacy for the combination (174). Patients receiving GH + Gln + diet had a larger reduction in parenteral nutrition volume per week than either Gln + diet or diet alone. There was no effect of Gln alone, nor was there any added effect of Gln to GH when compared to GH alone. GH alone may be indicated in patients with less than 150 cm of small bowel remaining or with 60 to 90 cm of small bowel with a portion of functioning colon, if a specialized diet is included, one rich in protein (~20% of calories), low–moderate fat content (~30%), and high in complex carbohydrates (~50%). However, it is not clear how many patients are able to be weaned from parenteral nutrition completely. Current data do not support the addition of Gln to this program. Direct comparison with another agent that has a modest effect on weaning from parenteral nutrition, parenteral GLP-2 (teduglutide/Gattex), has not been reported to date.

Arginine

Arginine is not considered an essential amino acid according to the current Institute of Medicine recommendations (171). However, as in the case of Gln, it is suggested that critical illness, in this case sepsis, produces a state of conditional deficiency (175). Arginine is a precursor for NO, and its potential benefits are related to replacing NO in severe illness (176). Consistent with its effect as a precursor for NO, 11 trials of oral arginine at doses from 4 to 24 g per day in patients with hypertension demonstrated a lowering of systolic pressure by 5.4 mm Hg, and of diastolic pressure by 2.7 mm Hg (177). Arginine can be provided safely at doses of 12 to 14 g per L parenterally (2 L per day) or 30 g orally per day, and can improve certain laboratory end points in some studies, but evidence for clinical efficacy is still uncertain in critical illness (178). Most studies providing arginine do so when combined with n-3 fatty acids, branched-chain amino acids, and nucleotides in commercial products that are marketed to modulate immunity. The benefits reported include reductions in infectious complications, increased immune function, and length of hospital stay, similar to the range of benefits suggested for Gln supplementation (179). The same problems with study design that are found with Gln recur in studies with arginine supplementation. Reviews of the data either do (180–182) or do not support the recommendation of providing arginine or other immunomodulatory substances to critically ill patients (183–185). If there is a role for such intervention, it is not clear at what degree of severity the benefit would begin, or which component(s) of the commercial immunonutrition products are important. Currently, it is not possible to make a recommendation for routine addition of arginine or the commercial immunonutrition products that contain it. Further studies are needed to see whether there is indeed an effect on infectious complications, the situation in which the data are the most suggestive of a benefit.

Gln contributes to the synthesis of arginine via citrulline released from the small intestine, and preclinical data suggest that the combination of the amino acids might be of greater benefit than each one alone (186). However, there are almost no clinical data to support this combination in humans, even in IBDs in which intestinal mucosal metabolism is altered (187).

Taurine

Taurine is a semi-essential amino acid that is not incorporated into proteins. The major route for biosynthesis of taurine is from cysteine (derived from methionine) via the enzyme cysteine sulfinate decarboxylase (CSD), requiring oxidation of hypotaurine to form taurine (188). It is the most abundant free amino acid in the heart, retina, skeletal muscle, and leukocytes, reaching 20 to 50 mM in the latter tissue (189). Taurine is present as the most abundant amino acid in all ocular tissues. The intracellular concentration is largely controlled by the synthetic enzymes cysteine dioxygenase (CDO) and CSD, and the taurine transporter, TauT (190). Taurine scavenges perchlorate (HOCl) formed by myeloperoxidase activity to form the less toxic Tau-Cl. It is this action, it is thought to contribute to its anti-inflammatory action in animal models. Taurine shows antihypertensive effects in animal models, but it is unclear these effects are due to its anti-inflammatory actions (191). Taurine is an essential amino acid for preterm neonates to prevent retinal damage, and is provided in breast milk. Individuals at risk for deficiency who may benefit from supplementation include premature and newborn infants on parenteral nutrition, and those with chronic hepatic, heart, or renal failure (192).

The diet is the usual source of taurine, although it can be synthesized from methionine and cysteine in the presence of vitamin B_6. Taurine is included in commercially produced mixtures of amino acids. Trophamine was designed for term and premature infants up to age 3 months, and replicates the serum amino acid concentrations of a breast-fed infant. A 1.6% solution contains 4 mM taurine. Taurolidine (Geistlich Pharma, AG, Wolhusen, Switzerland) is a derivative of taurine that is used in Europe, the United Kingdom, and the United States as adjunctive treatment for infections. This use is related to the finding of low plasma taurine in the setting of sepsis in trauma patients, suggesting a relative deficiency state (193). Taurolidine is composed of two taurolidine rings derived from taurine and three molecules of formaldehyde to form a two-ringed structure. It has a short half-life, and its activity may be due to more than just the taurine components. When impregnated into catheters, taurolidine has been effective in preventing bloodstream infections in a few studies (194). However, it does not appear to be antibacterial enough to be useful in a serious infection, such as bacteremia (195). Further studies will be needed to determine the benefits of replenishing taurine pools or adding taurine routinely to parenteral nutrition regimens.

L-Carnitine

Carnitine is essential for neonates (196). L-Carnitine is a short-chain carboxylic acid formed from lysine and methionine. It serves as a carrier molecule for the transport of fatty acids across the mitochondrial membrane into the mitochondria, where they undergo oxidation (59). Carnitine is found primarily in skeletal and cardiac muscle, which contains large numbers of mitochondria. Humans can synthesize carnitine from lysine and methionine. The major dietary source of carnitine is meat.

Carnitine functions to transfer long-chain fatty acids into mitochondria, improves glucose disposal, and may reduce insulin resistance (197). Carnitine is made in the liver and kidney, and is available in the diet in milk and meat products. Various disease states can alter carnitine status (198). Increasing loss from the body is a common cause, including renal tubular dysfunction, chronic renal failure, and dialysis. Inborn errors of fatty acid oxidation or branched-chain amino acid metabolism or liver cirrhosis can decrease synthesis, and certain drugs (e.g., valproic acid, zidovudine) can cause deficiency. Decreased intake from malnutrition, malabsorption, or total parenteral nutrition (TPN) can lower carnitine levels, and increased requirements for carnitine can occur following trauma, sepsis, or burns. Mitochondrial function (e.g., in HIV infection) may also cause conditional deficiency. Levocarnitine (Carnitor) is approved for such deficiencies, but data for improved clinical outcomes are not available for all the conditions listed above. Levocarnitine produces modest effects when given at 2 g per day to patients with anemia of renal failure (199).

Use L-carnitine has been approved for reimbursement by the Centers for Medicare and Medical Services for anemia and intradialytic hypotension, despite the absence of adequate data. The supplement has an attractive rationale and appears safe, so the definitive trials needed to prove efficacy likely will not be performed (200). Another promising use is in dialysis patients with resistance to human recombinant erythropoietin (201). The Medicare criteria for levocarnitine use are in patients who have been on hemodialysis for at least 3 months, and who have documented carnitine deficiency (plasma-free carnitine level <40 μmol per L) along with signs and symptoms of resistance to erythropoietin.

L-carnitine and propionyl-L-carnitine have been used in a variety of disorders, including cardiac and muscle ischemia (202). Theoretically, L-carnitine prevents loss of high energy phosphate stores by increasing fatty acid transport into mitochondria, and in deficient states might improve heart recovery. The use of 9 g per day after coronary artery bypass surgery for 5 days and 6 g per day orally for 12 months attenuated left ventricular dilatation. Propionyl-L-carnitine has higher affinity for muscle carnitine transferase, creating potentially better efficiency of the Krebs cycle during hypoxia by providing propionate, and may be the preferred form to use for prevention of ischemic heart disease (203). However, it is possible that exogenous carnitine promotes atherosclerosis, through metabolism by intestinal bacteria to a proatherogenic species, trimethylamine-*N*-oxide (TMAO) (204).

Long-term treatment has been shown to improve exercise duration and oxygen consumption when taken at 1.5 g per day for 1 to 6 months (202). This study is difficult to interpret because of the high dropout rate. It has been suggested that carnitine may improve exercise performance by enhancing fatty acid oxidation and decreasing lactic acid production. When carnitine was given to athletes immediately before exercise, serum carnitine levels increased, but no improvements in respiratory exchange ratios, muscle lactate accumulation, plasma lactate levels, or exercise performance were noted (205).

Acetyl-L-carnitine (Alcar) has been used to improve symptoms in early Alzheimer disease (206). In this meta-analysis, doses of 1.5 to 3.0 g per day taken for 3 to 12 months showed improvement in Clinical Global Impression, but another meta-analysis using mostly the same studies found no difference (207). Acetyl-L-carnitine has also been found to be deficient in diabetes, and analysis of two randomized, placebo-controlled trials suggests that 1 g t.i.d. improves pain and vibratory sensation in patients with chronic diabetic neuropathy (208). Carnitine deficiency can impair fatty acid oxidation, and rarely can lead to hyperammonemia and hepatic encephalopathy, which is resistant to standard therapy (209).

Carnitine is available in capsules or tablets as L-carnitine, propionyl-L-carnitine, and L-acetylcarnitine. Dosing is 2 to 4 g per day in two or three divided doses. Very high doses can cause diarrhea and nausea.

Creatine and Other "Ergogenic" Compounds for Muscle Maintenance

Creatine is a nitrogenous organic acid synthesized endogenously from arginine, glycine, and methionine in a two-step process in skeletal muscle and other organs, and dietary creatine is not required. Exogenous creatine is taken up into muscle and increases muscle levels of creatine. Creatine and phosphocreatine are involved in the storage and transmission of phosphate bond energy; phosphocreatine is an important reservoir of chemical energy in muscle. It has been suggested that increased amounts of phosphocreatine can shorten the recovery time of muscle adenosine triphosphate levels after exercise.

A large number of blinded, placebo-controlled studies of the effect of creatine on athletic performance has been performed (210,211). In a typical study, 32 swimmers were timed in sprints and then received placebo or creatine (20 g per day) for a week. No difference in performance was observed between the placebo- and creatine-treated groups after a week of therapy (212). A review of creatine supplementation and exercise performance concluded that creatine supplementation has not consistently proved to enhance exercise performance (213). There is some evidence from randomized trials that creatine supplementation of at least 0.03 g per kg body weight improved muscle strength in patients with muscular dystrophies and was well tolerated, although no effect in similar trials was seen in patients with metabolic myopathies (214).

Creatine is available in pills and powders as creatine monohydrate. Many formulations combine creatine with carnitine and amino acids. Typical dosing is a loading dose of 20 g per day for

5 or 6 days followed by a maintenance dose of 2 g per day. Creatine holds water in muscle; increases in intramuscular water may contribute to muscle cramping and dehydration. Creatine should not be given to patients with renal disease. Some athletes consume doses of creatine that are higher than recommended; whether excessive doses lead to additional adverse events is unclear (215).

Many substances other than creatine have been suggested for muscle maintenance and recovery in patients with loss of muscle mass. These substances include branched-chain amino acids and leucine, β-hydroxy-β-methylbutyrate, fish oil, ornithine α-ketoglutarate, and protein (216). Although some of these compounds increase nitrogen retention in animal models and improve some parameters of human muscle metabolism, there is as yet no evidence of improvement in clinically relevant end points. Similarly, many compounds have been used to improve performance in team-sport athletes. Caffeine has been shown to improve single- and multiple-sprint performance modestly, but evidence is not convincing for β-alanine, and no evidence is available to support the use of branched-chain amino acids or β-hydroxy-β-methylbutyrate, or ribose, especially in well-trained athletes (217). There is even less information available from any sort of controlled studies for the use of these so-called ergogenic compounds in untrained persons participating in sports.

β-Alanine has been used to improve exercise performance, with the presumed mechanism being to increase intracellular muscle carnosine (β-alanyl-L-histidine). Despite a large literature, most studies involve a small number of subjects. Supplementation with greater than 150 g per day provides only modest benefit, with improvement of 2.85% in an exercise test (CI, 0.37% to 10.49%), and the benefit was seen only between 60 and 240 seconds into the test (218). A review of 19 RCTs (mostly of moderate quality) examined the role of β-alanine in increasing exercise tolerance or improving athletic performance. The authors suggested that the supplement might increase power output, working capacity, and tissue carnosine levels (219). Side effects, however, have been under reported. Another review felt that more studies were needed to measure more relevant outcomes of exercise (220). In addition, optimal dosing has not been established, in part because no standard objective measures of efficacy have been agreed. Doses used are high (up to 6.4 g per day) for as long as 10 weeks, with paresthesias as the only reported side effect (221). Many fewer studies have been made using carnosine itself as the supplement (222). β-Alanine is included in many preworkout supplements along with caffeine, creatine, arginine, taurine, and other compounds, but data on efficacy and safety of such combinations are scant (223). This does not seem to be a supplement that can be recommended currently.

5-Hydroxytryptophan

5-Hydroxytryptophan (5-HTP) is a supplement marketed for the treatment of depression and mood enhancement, and for promotion of normal sleep (224). It is an intermediate step in the biosynthesis of serotonin from tryptophan. However, the data available from 108 studies in patients with depression or dysthymia, and treated with 5-HTP or L-tryptophan, were not sufficiently supportive of efficacy (225). There is no indication for taking 5-HTP or L-tryptophan, although side effects are usually mild (especially nausea), but it is possible that at high doses, 5-HTP supplements could cause serotonin syndrome (226).

Supplements and Foods to Improve the Lipid Profile (v-3 and v-6 Essential Fatty Acids and Fish Oil)

Many clinical trials have shown that lowering LDL cholesterol levels reduces the risk for CHD. Moreover, higher circulating ω-3 PUFA levels are associated with lower total mortality, especially from CHD (227). Statins are effective and usually well tolerated, but there are a significant number of patients who require additional or alternate therapy. Among the supplements that show an LDL-cholesterol lowering effect after RCTs are a Mediterranean diet, fiber, phytosterols, soy protein, whole-grain foods, low-fat diet, nuts, and ω-3 fatty acid supplements (228,229). There is no difference in the effects of plant sterols or plant stanols (230).

The metabolic ω-3 products, eicosapentaenoic acid (EPA) and docosahexaenoic acid (DHA), are synthesized by oceanic microorganisms and are thus abundant in fish and fish oils. Fish oil contains large amounts of highly unsaturated fatty acids, including DHA, which has six double bonds, and EPA, which has five. In these fatty acids, the last double bond is located three carbons from the end (ω-3), whereas in the PUFAs from plants, the last double bond is typically located six carbons from the end (ω-6). EPA and DHA can serve as substrates for cyclooxygenase, the rate-limiting step in prostaglandin production, and for lipoxygenase, the rate-limiting step in leukotriene production. The metabolic products of EPA and DHA derived through these pathways are less biologically active than the metabolites of arachidonic acid, the more typical substrate for these enzymes. Thus, one effect of fish oil is to diminish the production of conventional eicosanoids, including thromboxane A_2, prostaglandin E_2, and leukotriene B_4. By blocking the synthesis of thromboxane A_2, fish oil inhibits platelet aggregation and so acts as an antithrombotic agent. By blocking the synthesis of prostaglandin E_2, fish oil reduces the increased blood flow and edema associated with inflammation. Finally, by reducing the synthesis of leukotriene B_4, fish oil reduces the neutrophil infiltration associated with inflammation.

It has been proposed that ω-3 fatty acids play a role in preventing or treating many diseases, including coronary artery disease, Crohn disease, autoimmune disorders, and various cancers, but it is premature to recommend their routine use (231,232). The best data on prevention of sudden death from MI are those from the large Italian trial (233). Using 1 g per day of ω-3 PUFAs and vitamin E (300 mg per day) on top of other drug therapy and optimal life-style, reduction in cardiovascular and total mortality was approximately one-third in the first year of treatment. Other studies testing only ω-3 supplementation have not been so positive (234). A daily dose of 1,800 mg of EPA in addition to statins in patients with elevated cholesterol levels showed a 0.7% decrease (3.5% to 2.8%) in major coronary events (235). Patients with chronic heart failure given 1 g per day of ω-PUFA showed a 2% absolute decrease in cardiovascular and all-cause mortality compared with placebo over nearly 4 years (236). The mechanism of the effect of moderate amounts of ω-3 PUFAs is not known, but the effect on mortality from sudden death is greater in patients with systolic dysfunction (237). Replacing saturated fatty acids with ω-6 PUFAs has no effect on all-cause or cardiovascular mortality (238). While moderate amounts of ω-3 PUFAs as supplements or food additives may afford some benefit, saturated fatty acids and trans fats may not in themselves be harmful (239). The adverse effects of fats may be related to oxidative products of PUFAs as well as other fats. Thus, preingestion processing of fats may be more important than appreciated.

The FDA has approved a limited health claim for ω-3 fatty acids regarding CHD (240). The American Heart Association endorses the benefits of fish oil in heart disease and recommends 1 g per day of ω-3 supplements in those with CHD and 2 to 4 g per day in those with hypertriglyceridemia (241). Despite this recommendation, there is no uniformity on what the evidence shows. Several different meta-analyses have selected RCTs that differ by over 40%, and it is not surprising that these analyses have reached diverse conclusions (242–245). One of these (a systematic review as well) examined not only ω-3 and ω-6 supplementation but also the role of saturated fatty acid (245). Its findings did not support current cardiovascular guidelines that promote high consumption of ω-3, ω-6, and PUFAs with reduction of total saturated fatty acids. Some of the conflicting evidence will be discussed below.

Most studies have looked at the ability of ingested EFA supplements to lower mortality. A large (12,513 patients) study compared daily supplements of 1 g of ω-3 fatty acids (both EPA and DHA) with placebo over 5 years of follow-up, given to patients with multiple cardiovascular risk factors or demonstrated atherosclerotic vascular disease, but no MIs (246). No effect was seen on cardiovascular mortality or morbidity. The difficulty in making conclusions from these extensive data is that the type of pathology in the trials has varied, and the populations have varied in terms of baseline EFA blood levels. There is also a question as to whether results apply only to fish oils that are rich in EPAs or also to plant-derived α-lipoic acid, and the extent to which this is converted to EPA.

Fish oil supplementation might beneficially affect persons with CVD by at least three mechanisms. It reduces plasma triglycerides (3 to 12 g per day) by about 30% (247) and reduces blood pressure by a small but statistically significant amount (248). Fish oil also has antithrombotic properties; it reduces platelet aggregation by decreasing thromboxane production. A meta-analysis of 10 large (a total of 14,727 subjects) randomized trials of fish oil versus placebo revealed decreases of both total mortality and MI-related mortality in patients with CVD disease receiving fish oil (mean exposure 37 months) (249). But prospective studies provide no evidence that fish oil supplements prevent CVD (either primary or secondary prevention), either in diabetics or in the general population, or improve recurrences of atrial fibrillation, although they can lower serum triglycerides (250). A meta-analysis of 20 trials showed no reduction by ω-3 PUFA supplements in all-cause or cardiac mortality, sudden death, MI, or stroke, when compared with control (251). Thus, the recommendation on use of ω-3 PUFA supplementation is limited to lowering serum triglyceride levels, and that effect is modest.

Other dietary PUFAs may play a role in cardiovascular health, but they are not as available as EPA and DHA in the form of supplements. α-Linolenic acid, an ω-6 fatty acid with two double bonds is the primary ω-6 fatty acid in the diet. It is not synthesized by humans, and is found primarily in plant oils (corn, sunflower, safflower, soy), but the conversion to EPA and DHA is very low. Replacement of dietary saturated fats from animal sources with ω-6 PUFAs from safflower oil and margarine did not reduce all-cause mortality or mortality from CHD (238). On the other hand, the 2009 advisory from the American Heart Association concluded that ω-6 PUFAs at 5% to 10% of energy intake were beneficial for CHD prevention (252). Conjugated linoleic acids (CLAs) are synthesized in the rumen of cattle, deer, sheep, and goats by biotransformation of PUFAs (e.g., oleic and linoleic acid), and can be made endogenously (253). Most CLAs are formed as ω-6 FAs. No consistent clinical outcomes have been identified with the intake of such fatty acid conjugates.

Eicosanoids have been identified as mediators of the inflammatory response in chronic inflammatory diseases, so it is not surprising that an agent that reduces eicosanoid production may be of therapeutic value in these diseases. After prolonged treatment (>3 months) with fish oil, joint tenderness and morning stiffness were decreased in patients with rheumatoid arthritis (254). Fish oil has also proved useful in the therapy of acute disease and in maintaining remission in IBD (255). The use of fish oil as a component of parenteral nutrition has been tested in critically ill hospitalized patients, but the results of secondary benefits, such as days of ICU or hospital stay or complication rate, are not conclusive (256). However, because vegetarians have low blood levels of ω-3 PUFAs, supplementation of these fatty acids has been suggested for this specific population (257).

The main source of ω-3 PUFAs is fatty fish, for example, salmon, tuna, although small amounts are present in nuts, seeds, and plant oils. Foods that contain high levels of ω-3 PUFAs include flaxseed oil (7.3 g per tbsp), walnut and canola oil (~1.4 g per tbsp), tofu (0.7g per half cup), salmon (1.5 g per 3 oz), sardines (2 g per 2 oz), and trout (0.8 g per 3 oz). ω-3 PUFA content of vegetable oils is approximately 7% for soy oil, up to 10% for walnut and canola oil, but less than 1% for corn, safflower, and sunflower oils (239). A proposed intake of 0.65 g per day has been suggested for EPA and DHA. One gram of fish oil contains about 300 g of these substances, and commercially available sources (e.g., EPA, Max EPA, Promega, SuperEPA, Sea-Omega, Marine Lipid Concentrate) contain from 300 to 800 mg of n-3 fatty acids per capsule. Other brands of fish oil are available OTC, some of them now validated for content by the US Pharmacopeia (www.usp.org). Fish oil is available in gelatin capsules and as liquid oil. Supplements typically contain 180 to 300 mg of EPA and 120 to 200 mg of DHA. Dosing in either cardiovascular or chronic inflammatory disease studies is 4 to 5.4 g per day (total of EPA and DHA). However, the commercial products are not the same mixture as fish oil, and the optimal dose has not been established. Moreover, while addition of DHA increases DHA in blood and breast milk, the same is not true for ALA or EPA (258). Doses of 10 to 20 g per day may be needed to produce a biochemical effect on LDL and HDL cholesterol. It is still uncertain whether these nutrients should be added to commercial supplements, such as infant formulas. Food enrichment with n-3 fatty acids has not been successful thus far because it causes a fishy taste, and oxidation occurs during processing. These fatty acids are not required for patients on a low-fat diet who are ingesting vegetable oils or fish.

Two prescription forms of ω-3 PUFA supplements are available in the United States of America. *Lovaza* contains DHA and EPA (1,000 mg per capsule), and is FDA-approved for treatment of hypertriglyceridemia greater than 500 g per dL, but *Vescapa*, containing only EPA (1,000 mg per capsule), is also approved for the same indication (259). The FDA has declared fish oil to be generally recognized as safe (GRAS) at doses up to 3 g per day. The major toxic effect is a prolonged bleeding time secondary to inhibition of platelet aggregation. Fish oil should be used cautiously by patients who have bleeding disorders or are taking anticoagulants. Patients taking large amounts of fish oil complain that they acquire a fishy odor. As with any nutrient taken in excess, some data suggest that ω-3 fatty acids from fish or supplements, when taken in excess, may act as tumor promoter, via overproduction of lipid peroxides (http://perfecthealthdiet.com/category/nutrients/omega-3-and-omega-6-fats/). This concern does not alter the recommendations for cardiovascular health, but suggests a caution regarding excessive use.

γ-Linolenic Acid (Evening Primrose Oil, Borage Oil, Black Currant Oil)

γ-Linolenic acid (GLA) is an ω-6 conditionally essential fatty acid that is endogenously synthesized in humans (260,261). Linolenic acid is converted to GLA by δ-6-desaturase. GLA is also available from the diet. Evening primrose oil (8% GLA), borage oil (23% GLA), and black currant oil (15% GLA) are especially rich dietary sources. GLA can be metabolized to a biologically inactive prostaglandin (prostaglandin E_1) and to a lipoxygenase product, 15-S-hydroxy-8,11, 13-eicosatrienoic acid, which blocks the synthesis of biologically active arachidonic acid metabolites (262). In certain disease states, including diabetes and hypercholesterolemia, the conversion of linoleic acid to GLA by δ-6-desaturase may be impaired. In addition, impaired synthesis of GLA has been associated with advanced age, alcoholism, and a variety of vitamin and mineral deficiencies. It has been suggested that supplying dietary GLA may compensate for impaired endogenous conversion of linoleic acid to GLA.

In a 24-week, double-blinded study, 37 patients with rheumatoid arthritis received placebo or GLA (1,400 mg per day) in borage oil. In the patients who received GLA, disease activity decreased during the 24 weeks, whereas in those who received placebo, it did not change or increased (263). It is possible that serum levels of certain fatty acids are altered in premenstrual syndrome (PMS). Levels of arachidonic acid and dihomo-γ-linolenic acid (DGLA), a metabolite of GLA, are decreased in PMS. However, a series of trials in which evening primrose oil was given to patients with PMS failed to reveal compelling evidence of a clinical benefit (264). GLA has been recommended for treatment of eczema, rheumatoid arthritis, menopause, and cancer, but no convincing evidence is available for its efficacy (265).

Evening primrose oil, borage oil, and black currant oil are all available in capsules or as liquid oil. The rate of endogenous synthesis of GLA in normal humans is 250 to 1,000 mg per day. Typical dosing of GLA is 500 to 3,000 mg per day. Drug interactions with anticonvulsants and tricyclic antidepressants may occur. GLA supplements appear to be safe, but patients taking potentially hepatotoxic drugs should not use GLA.

Probiotics for General Health and Specific Conditions (e.g., Diarrhea)

Probiotics have been defined as "a preparation of or a product containing viable, defined microorganisms in sufficient numbers, which alter the microflora (by implantation or colonization) in a compartment of the host and by that exert beneficial health effects in this host" (266). Major differences in diet type (e.g., Western, Japanese, Indian) can affect intestinal microflora, so it is possible that probiotics might reflect a downstream result of dietary alterations. To understand the role of probiotics, one must define the normal gut microflora. Less than 30% of gut microflora have been cultured, but most organisms are identified by sequencing the well-conserved 16S rRNA genes (267). Understanding the place of probiotics will require defining the collective genomes in the gut, using metagenomic methods. Using such methods, 647 new gene families were identified to be exclusively present in human gut microbiomes (268). Most of the organisms expressing these genes are in the colonic flora, which is present at concentrations of 10^{11} to 10^{12} cells per g of luminal content (269). These organisms are responsible for producing short-chain fatty acids that control proliferation and differentiation of colonic mucosal cells, but the bacteria can also produce toxins (e.g., hydrogen sulfide) that can damage the cells (270). Moreover, the microbiota of the human small intestine are being described, with changes evident in disease states, such as celiac disease and IBD (271,272).

The human intestinal tract is sterile at birth, but develops during infancy to the stable pattern seen in adults. Factors that lead to population of the neonatal gut include vaginal flora from the mother, flora from the hospital environment (for caesarean delivery), breast milk flora (esp. bifidobacteria), or prebiotic/probiotic supplementation from formula (273). It is not surprising that the correlation between microbiota of mother and child is not very strong. In the adult, the majority of gut microbiota are members of the phyla *Bacteroidetes* and *Firmicutes*. But the "minor" phylum *Proteobacteria* includes many of the intestinal pathogens and other organisms important for nitrogen fixation. And the most common probiotic organisms (e.g., bifidobacteria) belong to the phylum *Actinobacteria* (274). On the one hand, the endogenous bacteria make butyrate, acetate, propionic acid, and metabolize polyphenols, all of which may enhance growth, influence immune responses, and induce antioxidant and anti-inflammatory responses in the host (275). On the other hand, some bacteria can initiate inflammation and promote cancer formation in animals, and perhaps in humans. Nutrient loads can influence the overall gut microbial community in the short term (276). The core microbiome can regulate energy balance in the host, and lead to obesity. Obesity in mice and humans is associated with an increased proportion of *Firmicutes*, with reduced *Bacteriodetes*, or both (277). Despite the widespread use of probiotics, little is known about their impact on the autochthonous gut microbiota or on the host, in either the short- or long term. Despite these uncertainties, work is progressing to develop probiotics that are felt to be health-associated (278).

Probiotics have been proposed to modulate the existing microbial community and thereby improve gut integrity, inhibit the growth of pathogens, and regulate the immune system. The most common organisms used are lactobacilli (phylum *Firmicutes*) and bifidobacteria (phylum *Actinobacteria*) (279). These have been isolated from traditional fermented products and from the gut, feces, or breast milk of human subjects. The largest category of diseases that have been targets for probiotic therapy are infections, including infectious diarrhea and antibiotic-associated diarrhea in infants and children, traveler's diarrhea, necrotizing enterocolitis in infants, *Helicobacter pylori*, respiratory tract infections (RTIs), ENT infections, and infections in critically ill patients (280). Such studies usually lack power, do not identify pathogens, and report immune biomarkers thought to be related to underlying mechanisms.

Digestive diseases are another group of diseases that have been targeted for probiotic treatment, because of the close association between the gut lumen and the diseased organ (281). Twenty RCTs using probiotics to treat *Clostridium difficile* diarrhea have shown that probiotics reduced the diarrhea in patients receiving antibiotic treatment, although the effect was modest with a NNT (number needed to treat) ranging from 23 to 34 (282). Further analysis of 31 RCTs also showed the efficacy of probiotics for prevention of *C. difficile*– associated diarrhea, but not for *C. difficile* infection or length of hospital stay (283).

It is not clear whether there is a difference between specific probiotic agents. Probiotics appear to reduce mortality in necrotizing enterocolitis, to prevent diarrhea in antibiotic-associated diarrhea, and to decrease the severity and duration of diarrhea in children (281). Data in IBS and IBD are less convincing or conflicting, not surprising for such heterogeneous disorders. Although some data suggest that small bowel overgrowth is responsible for symptoms in IBS, the effect of probiotics in this disorder, if any, is probably due to the effect on colonic bacteria (284). The response to probiotics in IBS is complicated by the response of some patients to low carbohydrate intake, and to the lack of a consistently observed abnormal microbial community. Probiotics have a reasonable rationale for use in IBS, but it is unclear which organisms might be best, or even whether the same organism should be used for all patients. Probiotics seem to alleviate abdominal pain in IBS patients, but other symptoms are not always improved (285). The available studies are of very different design, and are complicated by a very high placebo response rate (286). The European Society for Primary Care Gastroenterology supported some evidence that certain probiotics help to reduce overall symptom burden in some IBS patients (287). Thus, conclusions about the use of probiotics in IBS must be very limited at this time.

Reports on probiotic use in IBD have been rather sparse. There is abundant evidence to support their use from animal studies, but none of these studies involve true IBD models (288). Probiotics (VSL#3) have improved pouchitis, and *Escherichia coli* Nissle 1917 and VSL#3 have shown activity in maintaining remission of ulcerative colitis, but response in Crohn disease has not yet been documented (288).

There is some rationale for the use of probiotics in allergic diseases, but the choice of strains and the timing of treatment are variables that have not been studied adequately (289). Moreover, a Cochrane meta-analysis of five studies found not significant difference in eczema severity (290). Based on existing studies, probiotics cannot be recommended for treating eczema in children. Rationale similar to that for allergy (anti-inflammatory, immune regulation) has been proposed for RTIs. Prophylactic use of probiotics by healthy volunteers or patients with a RTI did not reduce the incidence or the duration of RTI, although the severity of the symptoms was lessened (291).

Probiotics have been used for metabolic conditions, again presuming that alteration in immune function might be beneficial. A review of 13 studies adding probiotics to patients with high, borderline, and normal serum cholesterol levels found a modest effect on reducing serum cholesterol (mean 6.4 mg per dL) and LDL cholesterol (mean 4.9 mg per dL), but no significant effect on HDL cholesterol or on triglyceride (292). Critical illness is a risk factor for altering the gut microbiota and allowing the appearance of pathogenic bacteria. In 11 RCTs, the rate of infectious complications in critically ill patients was reduced by 18%, but hospital mortality and length of stay were not improved (293). However, most of the trials had a high risk of bias, so firm conclusions cannot be made (294).

Many probiotic food products are commercially available in the United States of America, including those that use a single lactobacillus (L) or bifidobacterium (B) species and those that use multiple organisms. The concentration of organisms differs, as do the claims for each product (Table 8-4) (295).

There is no agreement on the most appropriate organism (or combination of organisms) to use for efficacy, nor which are the most appropriate symptom or disease targets, nor the dose required for efficacy. In the United States of America, most probiotics claim to have GRAS status (generally regarded as safe), although because a probiotic has GRAS status as a food does not necessarily mean that it keeps the same status in a capsule or sachet. Probiotics are usually included as a dietary supplement, and can thus be widely sold (296).

Probiotics can produce gas, diarrhea, bloating, and other GI symptoms, but these are usually mild. Infections have occurred in very immunosuppressed or critically ill patients (297). Intestinal microflora can metabolize dietary components (e.g., phospholipids) to harmful products (in this case, the atherogenic TMAO) (298). The potential for probiotic strains to alter the balance between good and bad effects in the gut lumen is unknown, either acutely or chronically. However, probiotics appear to be fairly safe in the short term in otherwise healthy individuals.

Probiotics can affect T-helper cell balance and responsiveness (299). Thus, gut organisms may be able to modify disease risk by modulating cytokine production (300), although only about 10% of all species tested have strong immunomodulatory effects (301). If indeed probiotics are able to modulate overall inflammatory response of the body, there may be great potential for the use of such agents. On the other hand, without more specificity of organism or dose, or without more sensitivity of a general effect in the face of local tissue inflammatory responses, there are no current recommendations that can be made for the use of these supplements.

REFERENCES

1. De Smet PAGM. Herbal remedies. *N Engl J Med*. 2002;347:2046.
2. Fulgoni VL III, Keast DR, Bailey RL, et al. Foods, fortificants, and supplements: where do Americans get their nutrients? *J Nutr*. 2011;141:1847.
3. Wikipedia. Dietary supplement. http://en.wikipedia.org/wiki/Dietary_supplement.
4. Watson E. *Dan Fabricant: FDA "Somewhat Aghast" at Degree of cGMP Non-compliance*. 2012. http://www.nutraingredients-usa.com/Regulation/Dan-Fabricant-FDA-somewhat-aghast-at-degree-of-cGMP-non-compliance.
5. Larimore WL, O'Mathuna DP. Quality assessment programs for dietary supplements. *Ann Pharmacother*. 2003;37:893.
6. Denham BE. Dietary supplements-regulatory issues and implications for public health. *JAMA*. 2011;306:428.
7. De Smet PAGM. Toxicological outlook on the quality assurance of herbal remedies. In: De Smet PAGM, Keller K, Hansel R, et al, eds. *Adverse Effects of Herbal Drugs*. Berlin, Germany: Springer-Verlag, 1992:1–72.
8. Thompson CA. Some dietary supplements resemble drugs more than food. *Am J Health Syst Pharm*. 2012;69:736.
9. U.S. Food and Drug Administration. http://www.fda.gov/food/dietarysupplements/qadietary supplements
10. U.S. Food and Drug Administration. reference 10: http://www.fda.gov/food/ingredientspackaging labeling/labelingnutrition/ucm073992.htm
11. U.S. Food and Drug Administration. http://www.fda.gov/food/dietarysupplements/usingdietary supplements/ucm10567.htm.

12. Reichenbach S, Juni P. Medical food and food supplements: not always as safe as generally assumed. *Ann Intern Med.* 2012;156:894.
13. Gardiner P, Sarma DN, Dog TL, et al. The state of dietary supplement adverse event reporting in the United States. *Pharmacoepidemiol Drug Saf.* 2008;17:962.
14. Marriott BM. Functional foods: an ecologic perspective. *Am J Clin Nutr.* 2000;71(suppl):1728S.
15. Bidlack WR, Wang W. Designing functional foods. In: Shils ME, Olson JA, Shike M, et al, eds. *Modern Nutrition in Health and Disease*, 9th ed. Baltimore, MD: Williams & Wilkins, 1999:1823.
16. Ross S. Functional foods: the Food and Drug Administration perspective. *Am J Clin Nutr.* 2000;71(suppl):1735S.
17. DHHS/FDA. Food labeling: general requirements for health claims for food. *Fed Reg.* 1993;58:2478.
18. Turner RE, Degnan FH, Archer DL. Label claims for foods and supplements: a review of the regulations. *Nutr Clin Pract.* 2005;20:21.
19. Diplock AT, Aggott PJ, Ashwell M, et al. Scientific concepts of functional foods in Europe: consensus document. *Br J Nutr.* 1999;8(suppl):S1.
20. Fragakis AS, Thomson S. *The Health Professional's Guide to Popular Dietary Supplements.* 3rd ed. Chicago, IL: American Dietetic Association, 2006.
21. Marik PE, Flemmer M. Do dietary supplements have beneficial health effects in industrialized nations: what is the evidence? *JPEN J Parenter Enteral Nutr.* 2012;36:159.
22. Kiefer D, Pitluk J, Klunk K. An overview of CAM: components and clinical uses. *Nutr Clin Pract.* 2009;24:549.
23. Mullin GE. Popular diets prescribed by alternative practitioners—parts 1 and II. *Nutr Clin Pract.* 2010;25:212, 308.
24. Pittler MH, Ernst E. Complementary therapies for reducing body weight: a systematic review. *Int J Obes (Lond).* 2005;29:1030.
25. Bjelakovic G, Nikolova D, Gluud LL, et al. Antioxidant supplements for prevention of mortality in healthy participants and patients with various diseases. *Cochrane Database Syst Rev.* 2012;(3):CD007176.
26. Gaziano JM, Sesso HD, Chisten WG, et al. Multivitamins in the prevention of cancer in men: the Physicians' Health Study II randomized controlled trial. *JAMA.* 2012;308:1871.
27. Williams CD. Antioxidants and prevention of gastrointestinal cancers. *Curr Opin Gastroenterol.* 2013;29:195.
28. Martinez ME, Jacobs ET, Baron JA, et al. Dietary supplements and cancer prevention: balancing potential benefits against proven harms. *J Natl Cancer Inst.* 2012;104:732.
29. Kushi LH, Doyle C, McCullough M, et al. American Cancer Society Guidelines on nutrition and physical activity for cancer prevention: reducing the risk of cancer with healthy food choices and physical activity. *CA Cancer J Clin.* 2012;62:30.
30. Myung SK, Ju W, Cho B, et al. Efficacy of vitamin and antioxidant supplements in prevention of cardiovascular disease: systematic review and meta-analysis of randomized controlled trials. *BMJ.* 2013;346:f10. doi:1138/bmj.f10.
31. Devore EE, Kang JH, Stampfer MJ, et al. Total antioxidant capacity of diet in relation to cognitive function and decline. *Am J Clin Nutr.* 2010;92:1157.
32. Kesse-Guyot E, Amieva H, Castethon K, et al. Adherence to nutritional recommendations and subsequent cognitive performance: findings from the prospective Supplementation with Antioxidant Vitamins and Minerals 2 (SU.VI.MAX 2) study. *Am J Clin Nutr.* 2011;93:200.
33. Smith AD, Smith SM, de Jager CA, et al. Homocysteine-lowering by B vitamins slows the rate of accelerated brain atrophy in mild cognitive impairment: a randomized controlled trial. *PLoS One.* 2010;5:e12244.
34. Walker JG, Batterham PJ, Mackinnon AJ, et al. Oral folic acid and vitamin B-12 supplementation to prevent cognitive decline in community-dwelling older adults with depressive symptoms—the Beyond Aging project: a randomized controlled trial. *Am J Clin Nutr.* 2012;95:194.
35. Manzanares W, Dhaliwal R, Jiang X, et al. Antioxidant micronutrients in the critically ill: a systematic review and meta-analysis. *Crit Care.* 2012;16:R66. doi:10.1186/cc11316.
36. Hernandez N, Perez N, Patel S, et al. Antioxidant supplementation in chronic pancreatitis: current evidence and overview. *Pract Gastroenterol.* 2011;35:47.
37. Evans JR, Lawrenson JG. Antioxidant vitamin and mineral supplements for slowing the progression of age-related macular degeneration. *Cochrane Database Syst Rev.* 2012;(11):CD000254.
38. Choi YH, Miller JM, Tucker KI, et al. Antioxidant vitamins and magnesium and the risk of hearing loss in the U.S. general population. *Am J Clin Nutr.* 2014;99:148.

39. Manach C, Scalbert A, Morand C, et al. Polyphenols: food sources and bioavailability. *Am J Clin Nutr*. 2004;79:727.
40. Birt DF, Jeffery E. Flavonoids. *Adv Nutr*. 2013;4:576.
41. Trevisanato SI, Kim Y-I. Tea and health. *Nutr Rev*. 2000;58:1.
42. Tome-Carneiro J, Larrosa M, Gonzalez-Sarrias A, et al. Resveratrol and clinical trials: the crossroad from in vitro studies to human evidence. *Curr Pharm Des*. 2013;19:6064.
43. Walle T. Bioavailability of resveratrol. *Ann N Y Acad Sci*. 2011;1215:9.
44. Smoliga JM, Baur JA, Hausenblas HA. Resveratrol and health—a comprehensive review of human clinical trials. *Mol Nutr Food Res*. 2011;55:1179.
45. Neveu V, Perez-Jimenez J, Vos F, et al. Phenol-Explorer: an online comprehensive database on polyphenol contents in foods. *Database (Oxford)*. 2010;2010:bap024.
46. USDA. *USDA Database for the Flavonoid Content of Selected Foods*. Beltsville, MD: USDA, 2007.
47. Zamora-Ros R, Agudo A, Lajan-Barroso L, et al. Dietary flavonoid and lignan intake and gastric adenocarcinoma risk in the European Prospective Investigation into Cancer and Nutrition (EPIC) study. *Am J Clin Nutr*. 2012;96:1398.
48. Mennen LI, Walker R, Bennetau-Pelissero C, et al. Risks and safety of polyphenol consumption. *Am J Clin Nutr*. 2005;81(suppl):326S.
49. Decker EA. Phenolics: prooxidants or antioxidants. *Nutr Rev*. 1997;55:396.
50. Clement Y. Can green tea do that? A literature review of the clinical evidence. *Prev Med*. 2009;49:83.
51. Lorenz M. Cellular targets for the beneficial actions of tea polyphenols. *Am J Clin Nutr*. 2013;98(6 suppl):1642S.
52. Seeram NP, Aviram M, Zhang Y, et al. Comparison of antioxidant potency of commonly consumed polyphenol-rich beverages in the United States. *J Agric Food Chem*. 2008;56:1415.
53. Perez-Jiminez J, Hubert J, Hooper L, et al. Urinary metabolites as biomarkers of polyphenol intake in humans: a systematic review. *Am J Clin Nutr*. 2010;92:801.
54. Sander LC, Befdner M, Tims MC, et al. Development and certification of green tea-containing standard reference materials. *Anal Bioanal Chem*. 2012;402:473.
55. Yuan JM. Cancer prevention by green tea: evidence from epidemiological studies. *Am J Clin Nutr*. 2013;98(suppl 6):1676S.
56. Hodgson AB, Randell RK, Jeukendrup AE. The effect of green tea extract on fat oxidation: evidence of efficacy and proposed mechanisms. *Adv Nutr*. 2013;4:129.
57. Hursel R, Westerterp-Plantenga MS. Catechin- and caffeine-rich teas for control of body weight in humans. *Am J Clin Nutr*. 2013;98(6 suppl):1682S.
58. Liu K, Zhou R, Wang B, et al. Effect of green tea on glucose control and insulin sensitivity: a meta-analysis of 17 randomized controlled trials. *Am J Clin Nutr*. 2013;98:340.
59. Jeukendrup AE, Randall R. Fat burners: nutrition supplements that increase fat metabolism. *Obes Rev*. 2011;12:841.
60. Bhupathiraju SN, Pan A, Malik VS, et al. Caffeinated and caffeine-free beverages and risk of type 2 diabetes. *Am J Clin Nutr*. 2013;97:155.
61. Lapointe A, Couillard C, Lemieux S. Effects of dietary factors on oxidation of low-density lipoprotein particles. *J Nutr Biochem*. 2006;17:645.
62. Estruch R, Ros E, Salas-Salvado J, et al. Primary prevention of cardiovascular disease with a Mediterranean diet. *N Engl J Med*. 2013;368:1279.
63. Olive oil. http://en.wikipedia.org/wiki/olive_oil.
64. Mueller T. *Extra Virginity: The Sublime and Scandalous World of Olive Oil*. London, England: Atlantic Books, 2012.
65. Frankel EN. Chemistry of extra virgin olive oil: adulteration, oxidative stability, and antioxidants. *J Agric Food Chem*. 2010;58:5991.
66. Martin-Pelaez S, Covas MI, Filo M, et al. Health effects of olive oil polyphenols: recent advances and possibilities for the use of health claims. *Mol Nutr Food Res*. 2013;57:760.
67. Ellam S, Williamson G. Cocoa and human health. *Annu Rev Nutr*. 2013;33:105.
68. Buitrago-Lopez A, Sanderson J, Johnson L, et al. Chocolate consumption and cardiometabolic disorders: systematic review and meta-analysis. *BMJ*. 2011;343:d4488. doi:10.1136/bmj.d4488.
69. Haymes EM. Trace minerals and exercise. In: Wolinsky I, Hickson JF Jr, eds. *Nutrition in Exercise and Sport*. 2nd ed. Boca Raton, FL: CRC Press, 1994:224.
70. Russell RM. New views on the RDAs for older adults. *J Am Diet Assoc*. 1997;97:515.
71. Haller J. The vitamin status and its adequacy in the elderly: an international overview. *Int J Vitam Nutr Res*. 1999;69:160.

72. Selhub J, Bagley LC, Miller C, et al. B vitamins, homocysteine, and neurocognitive function in the elderly. *Am J Clin Nutr.* 2000;71:614S.
73. Jesus P, Desport JC, Massoulard A, et al. Nutritional assessment and follow-up of residents with and without dementia in nursing homes in the Limousin region of France: a health network initiative. *J Nutr Health Aging.* 2012;16:504.
74. Guerrant RL, DeBoer MD, Moore SR, et al. The impoverished gut-a triple burden of diarrhea, stunting and chronic disease. *Nat Rev Gastroenterol Hepatol.* 2013;10:220.
75. Ney M, Vandermeer B, van Zanten SJ, et al. Meta-analysis: oral or enteral nutritional supplementation in cirrhosis. *Aliment Pharmacol Ther.* 2013;37:672.
76. Houston MC, Fazio S, Chilton FH, et al. Nonpharmacologic treatment of dyslipidemia. *Prog Cardiovasc Dis.* 2009;52:61.
77. Rautianinen S, Akesson A, Levitan EB, et al. Multivitamin use and the risk of myocardial infarction: a population-based cohort of Swedish women. *Am J Clin Nutr.* 2010;92:1251.
78. Ames BN. Low micronutrient intake may accelerate the degenerative diseases of aging through allocation of scarce micronutrients by triage. *Proc Natl Acad Sci U S A.* 2006;47:17589.
79. Lyle BJ, Mares-Perlman JA, Klein BEK, et al. Serum carotenoids and tocopherols and incidence of age-related nuclear cataracts. *Am J Clin Nutr.* 1999;69:272.
80. Zschabitz S, Cheng TY, Neuhauser ML, et al. B vitamin intakes and incidence of colorectal cancer: results from the Women's Health Initiative Observational Study cohort. *Am J Clin Nutr.* 2013;97:332.
81. Wien TN, Pike E, Wisloff T, et al. Cancer risk with folic acid supplements: a systematic review and meta-analysis. *BMJ Open.* 2012;2:e000653. doi:10.1136/bmjopen-2011-000653.
82. US Preventive Services Task Force. Routine vitamin supplementation to prevent cancer and cardiovascular disease: recommendations and rationale. *Ann Intern Med.* 2003;139:51.
83. Dwyer J, Donoghue MD. Is risk of Alzheimer disease a reason to use dietary supplements? *Am J Clin Nutr.* 2010;91:1155.
84. Fairfield KM, Fletcher RH. Vitamins for chronic disease prevention in adults: scientific review. *JAMA.* 2002;287:3116.
85. de Jong N, Chin AP, de Groot LC, et al. Nutrient-dense foods and exercise in frail elderly: effects on B vitamins, homocysteine, methylmalonic acid, and neuropsychological functioning. *Am J Clin Nutr.* 2001;73:338.
86. Lukaski HC. Vitamin and mineral status: effects on physical performance. *Nutrition.* 2004;20:632.
87. Fotino AD, Thompson-Paul AM, Bazzano LA. Effect of coenzyme Q10 supplementation on heart failure: a meta-analysis. *Am J Clin Nutr.* 2013;97:268.
88. Stocker R, Macdonald P. The benefit of coenzyme Q10 supplements in the management of chronic heart failure: a long tale of promise in the continued absence of clear evidence. *Am J Clin Nutr.* 2013;97:233.
89. Stackpoole PW. Why are there no proven therapies for genetic mitochondrial diseases? *Mitochondrion.* 2011;11:679.
90. Strand TA, Taneja S, Ueland PM, et al. Cobalamin and folate status predicts mental development scores in North Indian children 12-18 mo of age. *Am J Clin Nutr.* 2013;97:310.
91. Dullemeijer C, Souverein OW, Doets EL, et al. Systematic review with dose-response meta-analyses between vitamin B-12 intake and European Micronutrient Recommendations Aligned's prioritized biomarkers of vitamin B-12 including randomized controlled trials and observational studies in adults and elderly persons. *Am J Clin Nutr.* 2013;97:390.
92. Forman JP, Scott JB, Ng K, et al. Effect of vitamin D supplementation on blood pressure in blacks. *Hypertension.* 2013;61:779.
93. Hulisz D. Do calcium supplements increase cardiovascular mortality? http://www.medscape.com/viewarticle/779420.
94. Rees K, Hartley L, Day C, et al. Selenium supplementation for the primary prevention of cardiovascular disease. *Cochrane Database Syst Rev.* 2013;(1):CD009671.
95. Onakpoya I, Posadzki P, Ernst E. Chromium supplementation in overweight and obesity: a systematic review and meta-analysis of randomized clinical trials. *Obes Rev.* 2013;14:496–507. doi:10.1111/obr.12026.
96. Ward MH, deKok TM, Levallois P, et al. Workshop report: drinking-water nitrate and health—recent findings and research needs. *Environ Health Perspect.* 2005;113:1607.
97. Haddad PA, Azar GA, Groom S, et al. Natural health products, modulation of immune function and prevention of chronic diseases. *Evid Based Complement Alternat Med.* 2005;1:513.
98. Ramberg JE, Nelson ED, Sinnott RA. Immunomodulatory dietary polysaccharides: a systematic review of the literature. *Nutr J.* 2010;9:54.

99. Coriolus versicolor. http://www.cancer.org/treatment/treatmentsandsideeffects/complementary andalternativemedicine/dietandnutrition/coriolus_versicolor.
100. Jackson CG, Plaas AH, Sandy JD, et al. The human pharmacokinetics of oral ingestion of glucosamine and chondroitin sulfate taken separately or in combination. *Osteoarthritis Cartilage*. 2010;8:297.
101. McAlindon TE, LaValley MP, Gulin JP, et al. Glucosamine and chondroitin for treatment of osteoarthritis: a systematic quality assessment and meta-analysis. *JAMA*. 2000;283:1469.
102. Reichenbach S, Sterchi R, Scherer M, et al. Meta-analysis: chondroitin for osteoarthritis of the knee or hip. *Ann Intern Med*. 2007;146:580.
103. Towheed TE, Maxwell L, Anastassiades TP, et al. Glucosamine therapy for treating osteoarthritis. *Cochrane Database Syst Rev*. 2005;(2):CD002946.
104. Monfort J, Martei-Pelletier J, Pelletier JP. Chondroitin sulphate for symptomatic osteoarthritis: critical appraisal of meta-analyses. *Curr Med Res Opin*. 2008;24:1303.
105. Wandel S, Juni P, Tendal B, et al. Effects of glucosamine, chondroitin, or placebo in patients with osteoarthritis of hip or knee: network meta-analysis. *BMJ*. 2010;341:c4675.
106. Kennedy DO, Wightman EL. Herbal extracts and phytochemicals: plant secondary metabolites and the enhancement of human brain function. *Adv Nutr*. 2011;2:12.
107. Espinosa G. Nutrition and benign prostatic hyperplasia. *Curr Opin Urol*. 2013;23:38.
108. Suzuki H, Inadomi IM, Hibi T. Japanese herbal medicine in functional gastrointestinal disorders. *Neurogastroenterol Motil*. 2009;21:688.
109. Gagnier JJ, Moher D, Roon H, et al. Randomized controlled trials of herbal interventions underreport important details of the intervention. *J Clin Epidemiol*. 2011;64:760.
110. Yeh GY, Kaptchuk TJ, Eisenberg DM, et al. Systematic review of herbs and dietary supplements for glycemic control in diabetes. *Diabetes Care*. 2003;26:1277.
111. Alpers DH. The potential use of curcumin in management of chronic disease: too good to be true? *Curr Opin Gastroenterol*. 2008;24:173.
112. Aggarwal BB, Sung B. Pharmacological basis for the role of curcumin in chronic diseases: an age-old spice with modern targets. *Trends Pharm Sci*. 2009;30:85.
113. Rajasekaran SA. Therapeutic potential of curcumin in gastrointestinal practices. *World J Gastrointest Pathophysiol*. 2011;2:1.
114. Taylor RA, Leonard MC. Curcumin for inflammatory bowel disease: a review of human studies. *Altern Med Rev*. 2011;16:152.
115. Goel A, Aggarwal BB. Curcumin, the golden spice from Indian saffron, is a chemosensitizer and radiosensitizer for tumors and chemoprotector and radioprotector for normal organs. *Nutr Cancer*. 2010;62:919.
116. Shehzad A, Wahid F, Lee YS. Curcumin in cancer chemoprevention: molecular targets, pharmacokinetics, bioavailability, and clinical trials. *Arch Pharm (Weinheim)*. 2010;9:489.
117. Hudson JB. Applications of the phytomedicine Echinacea purpurea (purple coneflower) in infectious diseases. *J Biomed Biotechnol*. 2012;2012:769896. doi:10.1155/2012/769896.
118. Turner RB, Bayer R, Woelkart K, et al. An evaluation of *Echinacea angustifolia* in experimental rhinovirus infections. *N Engl J Med*. 2005;353:341.
119. Linde K, Barrett B, Wokart K, et al. Echinacea for preventing and treating the common cold. *Cochrane Database Syst Rev*. 2006;(1):CD000530.
120. Schoop R, Klein P, Suter A, et al. Echinacea in the prevention of induced rhinovirus colds: a meta-analysis. *Clin Ther*. 2006;28:174.
121. Senchina DS, Shah NB, Doty DM, et al. Herbal supplements and athlete immune function— what's proven, disproven, and unproven? *Exerc Immunol Rev*. 2009;15:66.
122. Chan PC, Xia Q, Fu PP. Ginkgo biloba leave extract: biological, medicinal, and toxicological effects. *J Environ Sci Health C Environ Carcinog Ecotoxicol Rev*. 2007;25:211.
123. Weinmann S, Roll S, Schwarzbach C, et al. Effects of *Ginkgo biloba* in dementia: systematic review and meta-analysis. *BMC Geriatr*. 2010;10:14.
124. Vellas B, Coley N, Ousset PJ, et al. Long-term use of standardized *Ginkgo biloba* extract for the prevention of Alzheimer's disease (GuidAge): a randomized placebo-controlled-trial. *Lancet Neurol*. 2012;11:853.
125. Mazza M, Capuano A, Bria P, et al. *Ginkgo biloba* and donepezil: a comparison in the treatment of Alzheimer's dementia in a randomized placebo-controlled double-blind study. *Eur J Neurol*. 2006;13:981–985.
126. Peters H, Kieser M, Holscher U. Demonstration of the efficacy of *Ginkgo biloba* special extract EGb 761 on intermittent claudication—a placebo-controlled, double-blinded multicenter trial. *Vasa*. 1998;27:106.

127. Evans JR. *Ginkgo biloba* extract for age-related macular degeneration. *Cochrane Database Syst Rev.* 2013;(1):CD001775.
128. Hilton M, Stuart E. *Ginkgo biloba* for tinnitus. *Cochrane Database Syst Rev.* 2004;(2):CD003852.
129. Choi J, Kim TH, Choi TY, et al. Ginseng for health care: a systematic review of randomized controlled trials in Korean literature. *PLoS One.* 2013;8:e59978.
130. Shergis JL, Zhang AL, Zhou W, et al. Panax ginseng in randomized controlled trials: a systematic review. *Phytother Res.* 2013;27:949–965. doi:10.1002/ptr.4832.
131. van Heerden FR. *Hoodia gordonii*: a natural appetite suppressant. *J Ethnopharmacol.* 2008;119:434.
132. Astrup A, Breum L, Toubro S, et al. The effect and safety of an ephedrine/caffeine compound compared to ephedrine, caffeine, and placebo in obese subjects on an energy-restricted diet: a double-blinded trial. *Int J Obes Relat Metab Disord.* 1992;16:269.
133. Rasmussen CB, Glisson JK, Minor DS. Dietary supplements and hypertension: potential benefits and precautions. *J Clin Hypertens.* 2012;14:467.
134. Haller CA, Benowitz NL. Adverse cardiovascular and central nervous system events associated with dietary supplements containing ephedra alkaloids. *N Engl J Med.* 2000;343:1833.
135. Lin X, Racette SB, Lefevre M, et al. The effects of phytosterols present in natural food matrices on cholesterol metabolism and LDL-cholesterol: a controlled feeding trial. *Eur J Clin Nutr.* 2010;64:1481.
136. Lin X, Racette SB, Lefevre M, et al. Combined effect of ezetimibe and phytosterols on cholesterol metabolism: a randomized, controlled feeding study in humans. *Circulation.* 2011;124:596.
137. Maki KC, Lawless AL, Reeves MS, et al. Lipid-altering effects of a dieting supplement tablet containing free plant sterols and stanols in men and women with primary hypercholesterolemia: a randomized placebo controlled crossover trial. *Int J Food Sci Nutr.* 2012;63:476.
138. Silbernagel G, Benser B, Nestel P, et al. Plant sterols and atherogenesis. *Curr Opin Lipidol.* 2013;24:12.
139. Beavers DP, Beavers KM, Miller M, et al. Exposure to isoflavone-containing soy products and endothelial function: a Bayesian meta-analysis of randomized controlled trials. *Nutr Metab Cardiovasc Dis.* 2012;22:182.
140. Patisaul HB, Jefferson W. The pros and cons of phytoestrogens. *Front Neuroendocrinol.* 2010;31:400.
141. Anderson JW, Johnstone BM, Cook-Newell ME. Meta-analysis of the effects of soy protein intake on serum lipids. *N Engl J Med.* 1995;333:276.
142. Geller SE, Studee L. Botanical and dietary supplements for menopausal symptoms: what works, what does not. *J Womens Health.* 2005;14:634.
143. Albertazzi P, Pansini F, Bonaccorsi G, et al. The effect of dietary soy supplementation on hot flushes. *Obstet Gynecol.* 1998;91:6.
144. Balk E, Chung M, Chew P, et al. Effects of soy on health outcomes. *Evid Rep Technol Assess (Full Rep).* 2005;126:1.
145. Wilt TJ, Ishani A, Stark G, et al. Saw palmetto extracts for treatment of benign prostatic hyperplasia: a systematic review. *JAMA.* 1998;280:1604.
146. Williams JW Jr, Mulrow CD, Chiquette E, et al. A systematic review of newer pharmacotherapies for depression in adults: evidence report summary. *Ann Intern Med.* 2000;132:743.
147. Whiskey E, Werneke U, Taylor D. A systematic review and meta-analysis of *Hypericum perforatum* in depression: a comprehensive clinical review. *Int Clin Psychopharmacol.* 2001;16:239.
148. Mischoulon D. Update and critique of natural remedies as antidepressant treatments. *Psychiatr Clin North Am.* 2007;30:51.
149. Shelton RC, Keller MB, Gelenberg A, et al. Effectiveness of St. John's wort in major depression: a randomized controlled trial. *JAMA.* 2001;285:1976.
150. Hypericum Depression Trial Study Group. Effect of *Hypericum perforatum* (St. John's wort) in major depressive disorder; a randomized controlled trial. *JAMA.* 2002;287:1807.
151. Posadzki P, Watson LK, Erst E. Adverse effects of herbal medicines: an overview of systematic reviews. *Clin Med.* 2013;13:7.
152. Tsai HH, Lin HW, Pickard S, et al. Evaluation of documented drug interactions and contraindications associated with herbs and dietary supplements: a systematic literature review. *Int J Clin Pract.* 2012;66:1056.
153. Stickel F, Kessebohm K, Weimann R, et al. Review of liver injury associated with dietary supplements. *Liver Int.* 2011;31:595.
154. Bunchorntavakul C, Reddy KR. Review article: herbal and dietary supplement hepatotoxicity. *Aliment Pharmacol Ther.* 2013;37:3.
155. Chitturi S, Rarrell GC. Hepatotoxic slimming aids and other herbal hepatotoxins. *J Gastroenterol Hepatol.* 2008;23:366.

156. Cohen SM, Heywood E, Pillai A, et al. Hepatotoxicity associated with the use of White Flood, a nutritional supplement. *Pract Gastroenterol*. 2012;36:45.
157. Chalasani N, Vuppalanchi R, Vavarro V, et al. Acute liver injury due to Flavocoxid (Limbrel), a medical food for osteoarthritis. *Ann Intern Med*. 2012;156:857.
158. Cheung WI, Tse ML, Ngan T, et al. Liver injury associated with the use of *Fructus Psoaraleae* (Bol-gol-zhee or Bu-gu-zhi) and its related proprietary medicine. *Clin Toxicol*. 2009;47:683.
159. Rellan S, Osswald J, Saker M, et al. First detection of anatoxin-α in human and animal dietary supplements containing cyanobacteria. *Food Chem Toxicol*. 2009;47:2189.
160. Dittmann E, Wiegand C. Cyanobacterial toxins—occurrence, biosynthesis and impact on human affairs. *Mol Nutr Food Res*. 2006;50:7.
161. El-Shehawy R, Gorokhova E, Fernandez-Pinas F, et al. Global warming and hepatotoxin production by cyanobacteria: what can we learn from experiments? *Water Res*. 2012;46:1420.
162. Gokmen MR, Cosyns JP, Arlt VM, et al. The epidemiology, diagnosis, and management of aristolochic acid nephropathy. *Ann Intern Med*. 2013;158:469.
163. Jonker R, Englelen MP, Deutz NE. Role of specific amino acids in clinical conditions. *Br J Nutr*. 2012;108:S139.
164. Food and Nutrition Board, Institute of Medicine. *Dietary Reference Intakes for Energy, Carbohydrate, Fiber, Fat, Fatty Acids, Cholesterol, Protein, and Amino Acids (Macronutrients)*. Washington, DC: National Academies Press, 2005.
165. Buchman AL. Glutamine: commercially essential or conditionally essential? A critical appraisal of the human data. *Am J Clin Nutr*. 2001;74:25.
166. Novak F, Heyland DK, Avenell A, et al. Glutamine supplementation in serious illness: a systematic review of the evidence. *Crit Care Med*. 2002;30:2022.
167. Alpers DH. Glutamine: do the data support the cause for glutamine supplementation in humans? *Gastroenterology*. 2006;130:S106.
168. Savarese DMF, Savy G, Vahdat L, et al. Prevention of chemotherapy and radiation toxicity with glutamine. *Cancer Treat Rev*. 2003;29:501.
169. Schulman AS, Willcutts KF, Claridge JA, et al. Does the addition of glutamine to enteral feeds affect patient mortality? *Crit Care Med*. 2005;33:2501.
170. Kim M, Wischmeyer PE. Glutamine. *World Rev Nutr Diet*. 2013;105:90.
171. Heyland D, Muscedere J, Wischmeyer PE, et al. A randomized trial of glutamine and antioxidants in critically ill patients. *N Engl J Med*. 2013;368:1489.
172. Ong EG, Eaton S, Wade AM, et al. Randomized clinical trial of glutamine-supplemented versus standard parenteral nutrition in infants with surgical gastrointestinal disease. *Br J Surg*. 2012;99:929.
173. van den Berg A, von Zwol A, Moll HA, et al. Glutamine-enriched enteral nutrition in very low-birth-weight infants. *Arch Pediatr Adolesc Med*. 2007;161:1095.
174. Byrne TA, Wilmore DW, Iyer K, et al. Growth hormone, glutamine, and an optimal diet reduces parenteral nutrition in patients with short bowel syndrome. *Ann Surg*. 2005;242:655.
175. Luiking YC, Poeze M, Dejong CH, et al. Sepsis: an arginine deficiency state? *Crit Care Med*. 2004;32:2135.
176. Appleton J. Arginine: clinical potential of a semi-essential amino acid. *Altern Med Rev*. 2002;7:512.
177. Dong JY, Qun LQ, Zhang Z, et al. Effect of oral L-arginine supplementation on blood pressure: a meta-analysis of randomized, double-blind, placebo-controlled trials. *Am Heart J*. 2011;162:959.
178. Morris SM, Loscalzo J, Bier D, et al. Arginine metabolism: enzymology, nutrition, and clinical significance. *J Nutr*. 2004;134(suppl 10S):2741S.
179. Brijs N, Worner EA, Brinkmann SJ, et al. Novel nutritional substrates in surgery. *Proc Nutr Soc*. 2013;72:277.
180. Kudsk KA. Immunonutrition in surgery and critical care. *Annu Rev Nutr*. 2006;26:463.
181. O'Callaghan G, Beale RJ. The role of immune-enhancing diets in the management of perioperative patients. *Crit Care Resusc*. 2003;5:277.
182. Grimble RF. Immunonutrition. *Curr Opin Gastroenterol*. 2005;21:216.
183. Heyland DK, Dhaliwal R, Drover JW, et al. Canadian clinical practice guidelines for nutritional support in mechanically ventilated, critically ill patients. *JPEN J Parenter Enteral Nutr*. 2003;27:355.
184. Bistrian BR, McCowen KC. Nutritional and metabolic support in the adult intensive care unit: key controversies. *Crit Care Med*. 2006;34:1525.
185. Singer P, Berner MM, van den Berghe G, et al. ESPEN guidelines on parenteral nutrition: intensive care. *Clin Nutr*. 2009;28:387.
186. Coeffier M, Dechelotte P. Combined infusion of glutamine and arginine: does it make sense? *Curr Opin Clin Nutr Metab Care*. 2010;13:70.

187. Coeffier M, Marion-Letellier R, Dechelotte P. Potential for amino acids supplementation during inflammatory bowel diseases. *Inflamm Bowel Dis*. 2010;16:518.
188. Ripps H, Shen W. Review: taurine: a "very essential" amino acid. *Mol Vis*. 2012;18:2673.
189. Schuller-Levis GB, Park E. Taurine: new implications for an old amino acid. *FEMS Microbiol Lett*. 2003;226:195.
190. Tappaz ML. Taurine biosynthetic enzymes and taurine transporter: molecular identification and regulations. *Neurochem Res*. 2004;29:83.
191. Abebe W, Mozaffari MS. Role of taurine in the vasculature: an overview of experimental and human studies. *Am J Cardiovasc Dis*. 2011;1:293.
192. Lourenco R, Camilo ME. Taurine: a conditionally essential amino acid in humans? An overview in health and disease. *Nutr Hosp*. 2002;17:262.
193. Chiara C, Giovannini I, Siegel JH, et al. The relationship between plasma taurine and other amino acid levels in human sepsis. *J Nutr*. 2000;130:2222.
194. Koldehoff M, Zakrzewski JL. Taurolidine is effective in the treatment of central venous catheter-related bloodstream infections in cancer patients. *Int J Antimicrob Agents*. 2004;24:491.
195. Solomon LR, Cheesbrough JS, Ebah L, et al. A randomized double-blind controlled trial of taurolidine-citrate catheter locks for the prevention of bacteremia in patients treated with hemodialysis. *Am J Kidney Dis*. 2010;55:1060.
196. Carnitine: the science behind a conditionally essential nutrient (Proceedings of a conference, Bethesda, Maryland, March 25–26, 2004). *Ann N Y Acad Sci*. 2004;1033:1
197. Tein I. Carnitine transport: pathophysiology and treatment of known molecular defects. *J Inherit Metab Dis*. 2003;26:147.
198. Famularo G. Carnitine and its congeners: a metabolic pathway to the regulation of immune response and inflammation. *Ann N Y Acad Sci*. 2004;1033:132.
199. Golper TA, Goral S, Becker BN, et al. L-carnitine treatment of anemia. *Am J Kidney Dis*. 2003;41(4)(suppl 4):S27.
200. Wasserstein AG. L-carnitine supplementation in dialysis: treatment in quest of disease. *Semin Dial*. 2013;26:11.
201. Schreiber B. Levocarnitine and dialysis: a review. *Nutr Clin Pract*. 2005;20:218.
202. Ferrari R, Cicchitelli MG, Dele D, et al. Therapeutic uses of L-carnitine and propionyl-L-carnitine on cardiovascular diseases: a review. *Ann N Y Acad Sci*. 2004;1033:79.
203. Malaguarnera M. Carnitine derivatives: clinical usefulness. *Curr Opin Gastroenterol*. 2012;28:166.
204. Koeth RA, Wang Z, Levison BS, et al. Intestinal microbiota metabolism of L-carnitine, a nutrient in red meat, promotes atherosclerosis. *Nat Med*. 2013;19:576.
205. Brass EP, Hoppel CL, Hiatt WR. Effect of intravenous L-carnitine on carnitine homeostasis and fuel metabolism during exercise in humans. *Clin Pharmacol Ther*. 1994;55:681.
206. Montgomery SA, Thal LJ, Amrein R. Meta-analysis of double blind randomized controlled clinical trials of acetyl-L-carnitine versus placebo in the treatment of mild cognitive impairment and mild Alzheimer's disease. *Int Clin Psychopharmacol*. 2003;18:61.
207. Hudson S, Tabet N. Acetyl-L-carnitine for dementia. *Cochrane Database Syst Rev*. 2003; (2):CD003158.
208. Sima AAF, Calvani M, Merhra M, et al. Acetyl-L-carnitine improves pain, nerve regeneration, and vibratory perception in patients with chronic diabetic neuropathy: an analysis of two randomized placebo-controlled trials. *Diabetes Care*. 2005;28:89.
209. Ling P, Lee DJ, Yoshida EM, et al. Carnitine deficiency presenting with encephalopathy and hyperammonemia in a patient receiving chronic enteral tube feeding: a case report. *J Med Case Rep*. 2012;6:227.
210. Volek JS, Rawson ES. Scientific basis and practical aspects of creatine supplementation for athletes. *Nutrition*. 2004;20:609.
211. Kreider RB. Effects of creatine supplementation on performance and training adaptations. *Mol Cell Biochem*. 2003;244:89.
212. Burke LM, Pyne DB, Telford RD. Effect of oral creatine supplementation on single-effort sprint performance in elite swimmers. *Int J Sport Nutr*. 1996;6:222.
213. Williams MH, Branch JD. Creatine supplementation and exercise performance: an update. *J Am Coll Nutr*. 1998;17:216.
214. Kley RA, Vorgerd M, Tarnopolsky MA. Creatine for treating muscle disorders. *Cochrane Database Syst Rev*. 2007;24(1):CD004760.
215. Francaux M, Poortmans JR. Side effects of creatine supplementation in athletes. *Int J Sports Physiol Perform*. 2006;1:311.

216. Krenitsky J. Nutrition and nutraceuticals for muscle maintenance and recovery: hero or hokum? *Pract Gastroenterol.* 2012;36:27.
217. Bishop D. Dietary supplements and team-sport performance. *Sports Med.* 2010;40:995.
218. Hoffmann JR, Emerson NS, Stout JR. β-Alanine supplementation. *Curr Sports Med Rep.* 2012;11:189.
219. Quesnele JJ, Laframboise MA, Wong JJ, et al. The effects of beta-alanine supplementation on performance: a systematic review of the literature. *Int J Sport Nutr Exerc Metab.* 2014;24:14.
220. Caruso J, Charles J, Unruh K, et al. Ergogenic effects of β-alanine and carnosine: proposed future research to quantify their efficacy. *Nutrients.* 2012;4:585.
221. Hobson RM, Saunders B, Ball G, et al. Effects of β-alanine supplementation on exercise performance: a review by meta-analysis. *Amino Acids.* 2012;43:25.
222. Sale G, Artioli GG, Gualano B, et al. Carnosine: from exercise performance to health. *Amino Acids.* 2013;44:1477.
223. Eudy AE, Gordon LL, Hockaday BC, et al. Efficacy and safety of ingredients found in preworkout supplements. *Am J Health Syst Pharm.* 2013;70:577.
224. Iovieno N, Dalton ED. Fava M, et al. Second-tier natural antidepressants: review and critique. *J Affect Disord.* 2010;130:343.
225. Shaw K, Turner J, De Mar C. Tryptophan and 5-hydroxytryptophan for depression. *Cochrane Database Syst Rev.* 2002;(1):CD003198.
226. In brief: 5-HTP for depression. *Med Lett Drugs Ther.* 2012;54:16.
227. Mozaffarian D, Lemaitre RN, King IB, et al. Plasma phospholipid long-chain ω-3 fatty acids and total cause-specific mortality in older adults. *Ann Intern Med.* 2013;158:515.
228. Nijjar PS, Burke FM, Bloesch A, et al. Role of dietary supplements in lowering low-density lipoprotein cholesterol: a review. *J Clin Lipidol.* 2010;4:248.
229. Huang J, Frohlich J, Ignaszewski AP. The impact of dietary changes and dietary supplements on lipid profile. *Can J Cardiol.* 2011;27:488.
230. Talati R, Sobieraj DM, Makanji SS, et al. The comparative efficacy of plant sterols and stanols on serum lipids: a systematic review and meta-analysis. *J Am Diet Assoc.* 2010;110:719.
231. Hooper L, Summerbell CD, Higgins JP, et al. Dietary fat intake and prevention of cardiovascular disease: a systematic review. *BMJ.* 2001;322:757.
232. Swanson D, Block K, Mousa SA. Omega-3 fatty acids EPA and DHA: health benefits throughout life. *Adv Nutr.* 2012;3:1.
233. Marchioli R, Barzi F, Bomba E, et al. Early protection against sudden death by n-3 polyunsaturated fatty acids after myocardial infarction: time-course analysis of the results of the Gruppo Italiano per lo Studio della Sopravvivenza nell-Infarto Miocardico (GISSI)-Prevenzione. *Circulation.* 2002;105:1897.
234. McCowen KC, Bistrian BR. Essential fatty acids and their derivatives. *Curr Opin Gastroenterol.* 2005;21:207.
235. Yokoyama M, Origasa H, Matsuzaki M, et al. Effects of eicosapentaenoic acid on major coronary events in hypercholesterolaemic patients (JELIS): a randomized open-label, blinded end point analysis. *Lancet.* 2007;369:1090.
236. GISSI-HF investigators. Effect of n-3 polyunsaturated fatty acids in patients with chronic heart failure (the GISSI-HF trial): a randomized, double-blind, placebo-controlled trial. *Lancet.* 2008;372:1223.
237. Macchia A, Levantesi G, Franzosi MG, et al. Left ventricular systolic dysfunction: total mortality, and sudden death in patients with myocardial infarction treated with n-3 polyunsaturated fatty acids. *Eur J Heart Fail.* 2005;7:904.
238. Ramsden CE, Zamora D, Leelarthaepin B, et al. Use of dietary linoleic acid for secondary prevention of coronary heart disease and death: evaluation of recovered data from the Sydney Diet Heart Study and updated meta-analysis. *BMJ.* 2013;346:e8707.
239. Lawrence GD. Dietary fats and health: dietary recommendations in the context of scientific evidence. *Adv Nutr.* 2013;4:294.
240. Food and Drug Administration, Center for Food Safety and Applied Nutrition, Office of Premarket Approval. *EAFUS: A Food Additive Database*. Available at: http://www.accessdata.fda.gov/scripts/fcn/fcnnavigation.cfm?rpt=eafuslisting. Accessed October 20, 2007.
241. Kris-Etherton PM, Harris WS, Appel LJ; for the Nutrition Committee. AHA scientific statement: fish consumption, fish oil, omega-3 fatty acids, and cardiovascular disease. *Circulation.* 2002;106:2747.
242. Hooper L, Thompson RL, Harrison RA, et al. Risks and benefits of omega 3 fats for mortality, cardiovascular disease, and cancer: systematic review. *BMJ.* 2006;332:752.
243. Harper CR, Jacobson TA. Usefulness of omega-3 fatty acids and the prevention of coronary heart disease. *Am J Cardiol.* 2005;96:1521.

244. Wang C, Chung M, Lichtenstein A, et al. *Effects of Omega-3 Fatty Acids on Cardiovascular Disease.* Evidence Report/Technology Assessment Number 94, AHRQ Publication Number 04-E009-1. Rockville, MD: Agency for Healthcare Research and Quality, 2004.
245. Chowdhury R, Warnakula S, Kunutsor S, et al. Association of dietary, circulating, and supplement fatty acids with coronary risk: a systematic review and meta-analysis. *Ann Intern Med.* 2014;160:398.
246. The Risk and Prevention Study Collaborative Group. N-3 fatty acids in patients with multiple cardiovascular risk factors. *N Engl J Med.* 2013;368:19.
247. Harris WS, Ginsberg HN, Arunakul N, et al. Safety and efficacy of Omacor in severe hypertriglyceridemia. *J Cardiovasc Risk.* 1997;4:385.
248. Morris MC, Sacks F, Rosner B. Does fish oil lower blood pressure? A meta-analysis of controlled trials. *Circulation.* 1993;88:523.
249. Yzebe D, Lievre M. Fish oils in the care of coronary heart disease patients: a meta-analysis of randomized controlled trials. *Fundam Clin Pharmacol.* 2004;18:581.
250. Kwak SM, Myung SK, Lee YJ, et al. Efficacy of omega-3 fatty acid supplements (eicosapentaenoic acid and docosahexaenoic acid) in the secondary prevention of cardiovascular disease: a meta-analysis of randomized, double-blind, placebo-controlled trials. *Arch Intern Med.* 2012;172:686.
251. Rizos EC, Ntzani EE, Bika E, et al. Association between omega-3 fatty acid supplementation and risk of major cardiovascular events: a systematic review and meta-analysis. *JAMA.* 2012;308:1024.
252. Harris WS, Mozaffarian D, Rimm E, et al. Omega-6 fatty acids and risk for cardiovascular disease: a science advisory from the American Heart Association Nutrition Subcommittee of the Council on Nutrition, Physical Activity, and Metabolism; Council on Cardiovascular Nursing; and Council on Epidemiology and Prevention. *Circulation.* 2009;119:902.
253. Benjamin S, Spener F. Conjugated linoleic acid as functional food: an insight into their health benefits. *Nutr Metab (Lond).* 2009;6:36.
254. Fortin PR, Lew RA, Liang MH, et al. Validation of a meta-analysis: the effects of fish oil in rheumatoid arthritis. *J Clin Epidemiol.* 1995;48:1379.
255. Belluzzi A, Brignola C, Campieri M, et al. Effect of an enteric-coated fish-oil preparation on relapse in Crohn's disease. *N Engl J Med.* 1996;334:1557.
256. Calder PC, Deckelbaum RJ. Intravenous fish oil in hospitalized adult patients: reviewing the reviews. *Clin Nutr.* 2013;16:119.
257. Harris WS. Achieving optimal n-3 fatty acid status—the vegetarian's challenge—or not? *Am J Clin Nutr.* 2013;100(suppl 1):449S.
258. Brenna JT, Salem N Jr, Sinclair AJ, et al. Alpha-linolenic acid supplementation and conversion to n-3 long-chain polyunsaturated fatty acids in humans. *Prostaglandins Leukot Essent Fatty Acids.* 2009;80:85.
259. Fish oil supplements. *Med Lett Drugs Ther.* 2012;54:83.
260. Fan YY, Chapkin RS. Importance of dietary gamma-linolenic acid in human health and nutrition. *J Nutr.* 1998;128:1411.
261. Horrobin DF. Nutritional and medical importance of gamma-linolenic acid. *Prog Lipid Res.* 1992;31:163.
262. Kapoor R, Huang YS. Gamma linolenic acid: an inflammatory omega-6 fatty acid. *Curr Pharm Biotechnol.* 2006;7:531.
263. Leventhal LJ, Boyce EG, Surier RB. Treatment of rheumatoid arthritis with gamma-linolenic acid. *Ann Intern Med.* 1993;119:867.
264. Budeiri D, Li Wan Po A, Dornan JC. Is evening primrose oil of value in the treatment of premenstrual syndrome? *Control Clin Trials.* 1996;17:60.
265. Wong C. Health benefits of gamma-linoleic acid. http://www.altmedicine.about.com/od/efa/a/Gamma-Linolenic-Acid.htm.
266. Kappelman M, Bousvaros A. Probiotic therapies: the crossroads of traditional and alternative medicine. *Pract Gastroenterol.* 2005;29:20.
267. Fraher MH, O'Toole PW, Quigley EMM. Techniques used to characterize the gut microbiota: a guide for the clinician. *Nat Rev Gastroenterol Hepatol.* 2012;9:312.
268. Kubokawa K, Itoh T, Kuwahara T, et al. Comparative metagenomics revealed commonly enriched gene sets in human gut microbiomes. *DNA Res.* 2007;14:169.
269. Mai V, Morris JG Jr. Colonic bacterial flora: changing understandings in the molecular age. *J Nutr.* 2004;134:459.
270. O'Keefe SJD. Nutrition and colonic health: the critical role of the microbiota. *Curr Opin Gastroenterol.* 2008;24:51.

271. Cotter PD. Small intestine and microbiota. *Curr Opin Gastroenterol.* 2011;27:99.
272. Wu GD, Lewis JD. Analysis of human gut microbiome and associations with disease. *Clin Gastroenterol Hepatol.* 2013;11:774.
273. Marques TM, Wall R, Ross RP, et al. Programming infant gut microbiota: influence of dietary and environmental factors. *Curr Opin Biotechnol.* 2010;21:149.
274. Turroni F, Ribbera A, Foroni E, et al. Human gut microbiota and bifidobacteria: from composition to functionality. *Antonie Van Leeuwenhoek.* 2008;94:35.
275. Rooks MG, Garrett WS. Bacteria, food, and cancer. *F1000 Biol Rep.* 2011;3:12. doi:10.3410/B3-12.
276. Jumpertz R, Le DS, Turnbaugh PJ, et al. Energy-balance studies reveal associations between gut microbes, caloric load, and nutrient absorption in humans. *Am J Clin Nutr.* 2011;94:58.
277. Turnbaugh PJ, Gordon JI. The core gut microbiome, energy balance and obesity. *J Physiol.* 2009;587:4153.
278. Relman DA. Restoration of the gut microbial habitat as a disease therapy. *Nat Biotechnol.* 2011;21:25.
279. Fontana L, Bermudez-Brito M, Plaza-Diaz J, et al. Sources, isolation, characterisation and evaluation of probiotics. *Br J Nutr.* 2013;109:S35.
280. Wolvers D, Antoine JM, Myllyluoma E, et al. Guidance for substantiating the evidence for beneficial effects of probiotics: prevention and management of infections by probiotics. *J Nutr.* 2010;140:698S.
281. Gareau MG, Sherman PM, Walker WA. Probiotics and the gut microbiota in intestinal health and disease. *Nat Rev Gastroenterol Hepatol.* 2010;7:503.
282. Johnston BC, Ma SS, Goldenberg JZ, et al. Probiotics for the prevention of *Clostridium difficile*-associated diarrhea: a systematic review and meta-analysis. *Ann Intern Med.* 2012;157:878.
283. Goldenberg JZ, Ma SS, Saxton JD, et al. Probiotics for the prevention of *Clostridium difficile*-associated diarrhea in adults and children. *Cochrane Database Syst Rev.* 2013;5:CD006095.
284. Simren M, Barbara G, Flint HJ, et al. Intestinal microbiota in functional bowel disorders: a Rome foundation report. *Gut.* 2013;62:159.
285. McFarland LV, Dublin S. Meta-analysis of probiotics for the treatment of irritable bowel syndrome. *World J Gastroenterol.* 2008;14:2650.
286. Rogers NJ, Mousa SA. The shortcomings of clinical trials assessing the efficacy of probiotics in irritable bowel syndrome. *J Altern Complement Med.* 2012;18:112.
287. Hungin APS, Mulligan C, Pot B, et al. Systematic review: probiotics in the management of lower gastrointestinal symptoms in clinical practice—an evidence-based international guide. *Aliment Pharmacol Ther.* 2013;38:864.
288. Round JL, Mazmanian SK. The gut microbiota shapes intestinal immune responses during health and disease. *Nat Rev Immunol.* 2009;9:313.
289. Kalliomaki M, Antoine JM, Herz U, et al. Guidance for substantiating the evidence for beneficial effects of probiotics: prevention and management of allergic diseases by probiotics. *J Nutr.* 2010;140:713S.
290. Boyle RJ, Hextall FJ, Leonardi-Bee J, et al. Probiotics for the treatment of eczema: a systematic review. *Clin Exp Allergy.* 2009;39:1117.
291. Vouloumanou EK, Makris GC, Karageorgopoulos DE, et al. Probiotics for the prevention of respiratory tract infections: a systematic review. *Int J Antimicrob Agents.* 2009;34:197.
292. Guo Z, Liu XM, Zhang QX, et al. Influence of consumption of probiotics on the plasma lipid profile: a meta-analysis of randomized controlled trials. *Nutr Metab Cardiovasc Dis.* 2011;21:844.
293. Petrof EO, Dhallwal R, Manzanares W, et al. Probiotics in the critically ill: a systematic review of the randomized trial evidence. *Crit Care Med.* 2012;40:3290.
294. Koretz RL. Probiotics, critical illness, and methodologic bias. *Nutr Clin Pract.* 2009;24:45.
295. Quigley EMM, Sanders ME. Probiotic foods for gastrointestinal health. *Gastroenterol & Endoscopy News Special Edition.* September 2009:1. www.gastroendonews.com/download/ProbioticFood_GENSE09_WM.pdf.
296. Vanderhoof JA, Young R. Probiotics in the United States. *Clin Infect Dis.* 2008;46(suppl 2):S67.
297. Probiotics revisited. *Med Lett Drugs Ther.* 2013;55:3.
298. Tang WH, Wang Z, Levison BS, et al. Intestinal microbial metabolism of phosphatidylcholine and cardiovascular risk. *N Engl J Med.* 2013;368:1575.
299. Kalliomaki MA, Isolauri E. Probiotics and down-regulation of the allergic response. *Immunol Allergy Clin North Am.* 2004;24:739.
300. Salminen SJ, Guiemonde M, Isolauri E. Probiotics that modify disease risk. *J Nutr.* 2005;13:1294.
301. Bengmark S, Martindale R. Prebiotics and synbiotics in clinical medicine. *Nutr Clin Pract.* 2005;20:244.

SECTION III
Therapeutic Nutrition

9 Nutritional Support Decision Making

DEFINITION OF NUTRITIONAL SUPPORT

Feeding is not considered medical therapy under ordinary circumstances. When patients are unable to meet their daily requirements by consuming a normal diet or when assessment documents deficiencies, then nutritional planning becomes a part of medical therapeutics. Nutritional support is the planning of patient-specific nutritional therapy. The Nutrition Care Process as outlined by the Academy of Nutrition and Dietetics (Academy) is one way to approach nutritional therapy (1). In hospitalized patients, the goals of the Nutrition Care Process are to provide the appropriate macro- and micronutrients to replete existing deficiencies, minimize the patient's metabolic response to stress, aid in the prevention of oxidative cellular injury, support wound healing, and maximize the patient's immune function. This process consists of four parts, including nutrition screening, assessment, intervention, and monitoring (1).

SUCCESSFUL NUTRITION SCREENING (SEE ALSO CHAPTER 5)

A successful nutrition screening tool should be easy to use by nonnutritional professionals and adequately identify malnourished patients or those at nutritional risk who require further assessment (2). A comparison of 10 different tools found the Malnutrition Screening Tool (MST) to have the greatest validity and reliability in a variety of patients (3). This tool is simple to use, relying on unintentional weight loss and reduced appetite to screen for malnutrition. Other tools may be more beneficial in specific subsets of patients. Defining malnutrition has changed to an etiology-based approach, based on the presence or not of inflammation and whether the inflammatory response is acute or chronic (4,5). This classification system divides malnutrition into three types: starvation-related malnutrition (e.g., anorexia nervosa), chronic disease-related malnutrition (e.g., cancer, congestive heart failure), and acute disease-related malnutrition (e.g., sepsis, burn trauma) (6). Patients at nutritional risk have been shown to have worse clinical outcomes, including increased length of stay and mortality, than those at low risk (7–9).

Presence of specific nutrient deficiencies or protein–energy deficit may be identified in patients at risk for malnutrition. While vitamins and minerals are more easily replaced (see Chapters 6 and 7), these may not cure the underlying problem. For example, intravenous (IV) potassium supplementation may correct low serum potassium levels, but does not address the causative factor (e.g., hyperemesis gravidarum). Primary protein–energy deficit caused by inadequate intake is often reversible with nutritional therapy. The Joint Commission on Accreditation of Hospitals Organization requires hospitals to complete nutrition screening on all patients within 48 hours of admission. The advancement of the electronic patient medical record has enabled many institutions to surpass this requirement. Admission questionnaires, including nutritional questions completed by admitting or nursing personnel who generate nutrition consults based on the patient's responses, are frequently utilized to meet this requirement (Table 9-1).

TABLE 9-1 Example of Nutrition Screening Questions to Include in Admission Survey

1. How is your appetite?
2. Current home diet?
3. Do you take diet or nutritional supplements? If yes, what are they?
4. Do you understand your diet?
5. Do you follow your diet?
6. Have you had any recent weight loss or gain over the past 3 months? If yes, how much? Was it intentional?
7. Do you have any food intolerances?
8. Are you pregnant or lactating?

When screening a patient for nutritional risk, the above information may be combined with other data pulled from the admission survey, such as admission weight, usual weight, admission height, reason for admission, normal elimination, last bowel movement, and ability to prepare own meals to aid in the determination of the patient's present nutritional status.

NUTRITION ASSESSMENT

Nutrition assessment is the vital next step once a patient is identified to be at risk for malnutrition. The prevalence of hospital malnutrition has been documented at 20% to 50% (10,11). The economic, morbidity, and mortality impacts increase as the severity of the malnutrition increases (12,13). In October 2012, the Centers for Medicare and Medicaid Services approved severe malnutrition as a secondary diagnosis at discharge, recognizing the impact of this diagnosis on patient outcome and length of stay. One group classified the degree of malnutrition and determined the association with 1-year mortality in hospitalized patients (Figure 9-1) (14).

There is no "gold standard" for nutrition assessment, and the validity of surrogate markers depends heavily on the clinical situation. However, since micro- and macronutrient intake is an important component of body composition and physiologic function, the ultimate goal is to assess past and current intake. Nutrition assessment cannot be completed in a vacuum. The patient's clinical condition and medical treatments may also affect nutrient requirements. In general, patients who have lost greater than 10% of their body weight over the past 6 months

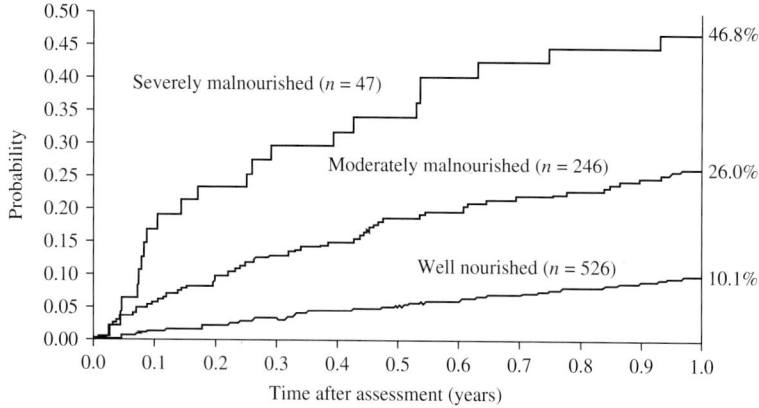

Figure 9-1 Incidence of malnutrition-associated mortality up to 1 year. P-value is <0.0005 between the three categories (2). (Adapted from Middleton MH, Nazarento G, Nivison-Smith I. Prevalence of malnutrition and 12-month incidence of mortality in two Sydney teaching hospitals. *Intern Med J*. 2001;31:455.)

or have a decreased body mass index (BMI), especially in combination with chronic disease or increased metabolic requirements, are at increased nutritional risk. A complete nutrition assessment should be completed to identify which patients will benefit from nutritional therapy. Optimally, the nutrition assessment should include medical and nutritional histories, a nutrition-focused physical examination, and a review of the appropriate laboratory studies (see Tables 9-2 and 9-3; also Table 4-12 for a mechanism-based approach to nutritional screening).

In the past, hepatic proteins were thought to be associated with a patient's nutritional status. Although a low serum albumin level is correlated with an increased incidence of morbidity and mortality, it is illness or injury, not malnutrition, which is responsible for the decreased albumin levels in sick patients (15,16). Even during chronic malnutrition, such as in the anorexic patient, little change is seen in the plasma albumin concentration (17,18). Further information regarding nutritional protein assessment tools is presented in Table 5-19.

NUTRITION INTERVENTION OR SUPPORT

Nutrition intervention or nutrition support may be achieved through several avenues (Figure 9-2). Prior to beginning nutritional support, the following questions should be addressed.

TABLE 9-2   Medical and Nutritional History Components

Diet/medication history	• Recent intake/intolerances/appetite changes • Swallowing/chewing difficulties • Diet restrictions • Supplement usage—herbal, dietary, vitamins, minerals • Present home medications • Over-the-counter medications
Medical/surgical history	• Preexisting conditions • Past surgeries • Present anatomy (bowel resections/ostomies)
Social/functional/family history	• Use of alcohol, tobacco, IV drugs • Present employment, living arrangements, social support • Functional status—ability to perform ADLs, exercise patterns • Family medical history • Religion, education, cultural factors
Gastrointestinal history	• Recent nausea/vomiting • Normal bowel habits • Changes/increase in diarrhea, constipation, steatorrhea, bloating, flatus
Anthropometrics	• Height • Usual body weight • Ideal body weight • Calculated BMI • Recent weight changes
Laboratory assessment	• Comprehensive metabolic profile • Serum magnesium • Serum phosphorus • Serum triglyceride • CBC • Hemoglobin A1C, routine blood glucose levels • Other laboratory tests as indicated: TSH, PTH, CRP, vitamin/mineral studies

ADL, activities of daily living; BMI, body mass index; CBC, complete blood count; CRP, C-reactive protein; IV, intravenous; PTH, parathyroid hormone; TSH, thyroid-stimulating hormone.

TABLE 9-3	Nutrition-Focused Physical Assessment
Vital signs	• Temperature • Blood pressure • Pulse • Respiration—work of breathing, abnormal breath sounds
Oral cavity	• Dry or inflamed mucosa • Cracked lips • Magenta tongue • Smooth, slick tongue • Excess caries, missing teeth • Bleeding gums • White patches/sores • Purple sores • Tumors
Skin	• Color • Turgor • Sores/pressure ulcers • Rashes • Moisture/dryness • Temperature
Face/hair/eyes	• Night blindness • Bitot spots (eyes) • Temporal wasting • Asymmetry • Drooling • Easily pluckable hair • Thinning hair • Moon face • Neck vein distention
Nails	• Spoon shaped • Pale, mottled
Abdomen	• Presence of distention • Percuss for tympany • Presence of scars, wounds, ostomies, feeding access
Other	• Inspect temporalis, deltoid, and quadriceps for muscle wasting • Presence of edema in extremities, sacral area • Swollen joints • Bow legs

Is the Patient Malnourished, and If So, What Type?

Many of the decisions regarding the urgency of instituting nutritional support, especially the intensive forms of support (i.e., tube feeding and total parenteral nutrition), revolve around the answer to this question. Clinical, anthropometric, and laboratory data are used to formulate a general opinion regarding the degree of depletion and type of malnutrition; the difficulties of arriving at a meaningful nutritional assessment are described in Chapter 5. By using current techniques, the physician can determine whether patients are malnourished and then divide these patients into three main clinical groups: (a) starvation-related malnutrition, (b) chronic disease-related malnutrition, and (c) acute disease-related malnutrition (6). Patients in all three of these categories may have mild, moderate, or severe micronutrient deficiencies. Micronutrient deficiencies should be repleted as outlined in Chapters 6 and 7. Malnourished patients should have nutrition support initiated as soon as possible. New data suggest that there may be some

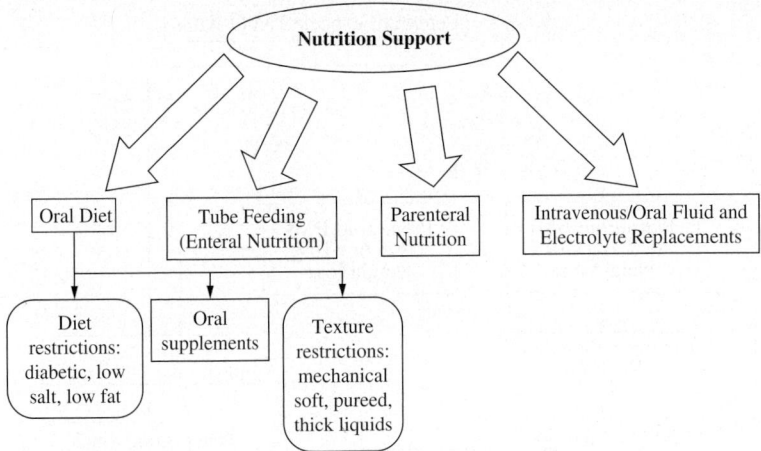

Figure 9-2 Avenues of nutrition support.

benefit in supplementing healthy patients, as well as malnourished patients, preoperatively to metabolically prepare for the "stress" of surgery (19–21). A review of prospective randomized controlled trials of perioperative parenteral or enteral nutrition found a significant reduction in postoperative complications and economic benefit in patients diagnosed with severe malnutrition who received preoperative nutrition support (22,23).

What Is the Anticipated Length of Time That Nutritional Support Will Be Required?

This will help to address both need and timing for nutrition support (see Figure 9-3). See Chapters 10 and 11 for more information on enteral and parenteral nutrition support and access. A review of several large trials demonstrates that the avoidance of underfeeding may improve clinical outcomes (24). Anticipating the length of time that energy and protein requirements will not be satisfied by normal diets (i.e., the cumulative result of negative balance) helps determine the urgency of instituting protein–calorie support. Estimation of the cumulative result of negative balance for the anticipated length of illness puts into perspective the end result of persistent negative energy balance. Representative estimates of weight losses incurred—depending on the degree of negative balance and the length of illness—are given in Table 9-4. This estimate is based on the assumption that a negative balance of 3,400 kcal represents a loss of 1 lb of body weight. In situations of metabolic stress, such a relationship is not as accurate as it is in situations of slow weight gain or loss, and this relationship does not remain constant as weight loss progresses. Also, the relationship does not take into account the adaptive processes that occur during starvation. However, it does help the clinician make a crude estimate of expected losses. A cumulative caloric deficit of 10,000 cal or more has been associated with a survival disadvantage in intensive care patients (25–28) See Ch 5 Energy Balance section for further discussion of estimated weight loss.

How Should the Nutrition Support Be Provided: Enteral versus Parenteral?

The usual guideline for choosing between enteral and parenteral nutritional support is to use enteral support whenever possible. Parenteral nutrition should be reserved for patients in whom enteral feeding is not an option and for those who are severely malnourished (Figure 9-4) (29). Enteral nutrition is preferred to parenteral nutrition for several reasons: enteral nutrition provides nutrients to the gastrointestinal mucosa that are not provided by parenteral nutrition (i.e., short-chain fatty acids) (30); nutrients in the intestinal lumen have been shown to protect the integrity of the gastrointestinal tract in animals and may be beneficial in humans (31); enteral

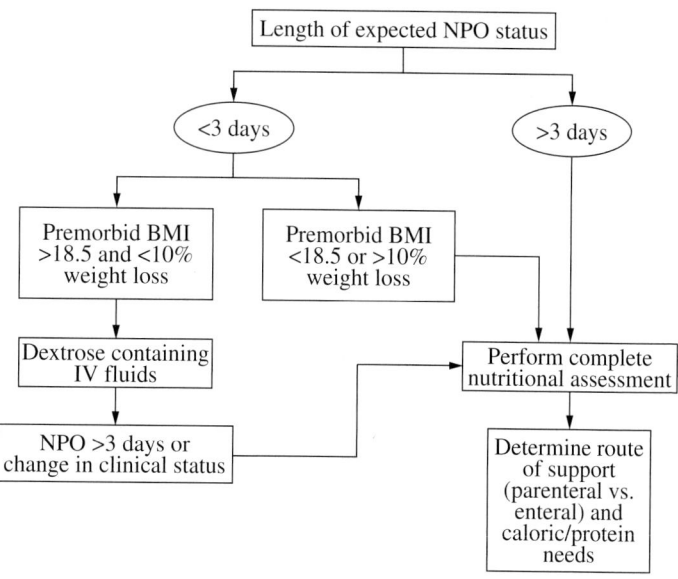

Figure 9-3 Timing of nutrition support.

nutrition is associated with fewer septic complications (29) than parenteral nutrition; and enteral nutrition is safer, more convenient, and less expensive (31,32). Even if full nutrition support by the enteral route is not feasible, it is unclear whether there is any benefit to instituting complementary parenteral nutrition (33).

What Are the Patient's Caloric and Protein Needs?

This question is covered in great detail in Chapter 5 for free-living and hospitalized patients. While malnutrition and hypocaloric feeding may decrease a patient's resting energy expenditure (REE) by 15% to 20%, metabolic stress will increase the REE by as much as 40% in patients with severe burns (34). Several equations exist to estimate the REE requirements; the most common of these (including Harris–Benedict, WHO, and BMI-based) are reviewed in Chapter 5. A task force convened by the Academy of Nutrition and Dietetics recently reviewed the use and reliability of

TABLE 9-4 Estimated Cumulative Effect of Negative Balance

Estimated Balance (kcal/d)	Cumulative Weight Loss During Illness (illness length in days)										
	2	4	6	8	10	12	14	16	18	20	22	24
	−5%[a]							−10%[a]				
−4,000	2.4[b]	4.7	7.1	9.4	11.8	14.1	16.5	18.8	21.2	23.2	25.9	28.2
−3,500	2.1	4.1	6.2	8.2	10.3	12.4	14.4	16.5	18.5	20.5	22.6	24.7
−3,000	1.8	3.5	5.3	7.1	8.8	10.6	12.4	14.1	15.9	17.6	19.4	21.2
−2,500	1.5	2.9	4.4	5.9	7.4	8.8	10.3	11.8	13.2	14.7	16.2	17.6
−2,000	1.2	2.4	3.5	4.7	5.9	7.1	8.2	9.4	10.6	11.8	12.9	14.1

[a]Percentage weight change for a 154-lb (70-kg) patient.
[b]Estimated weight loss in pounds.

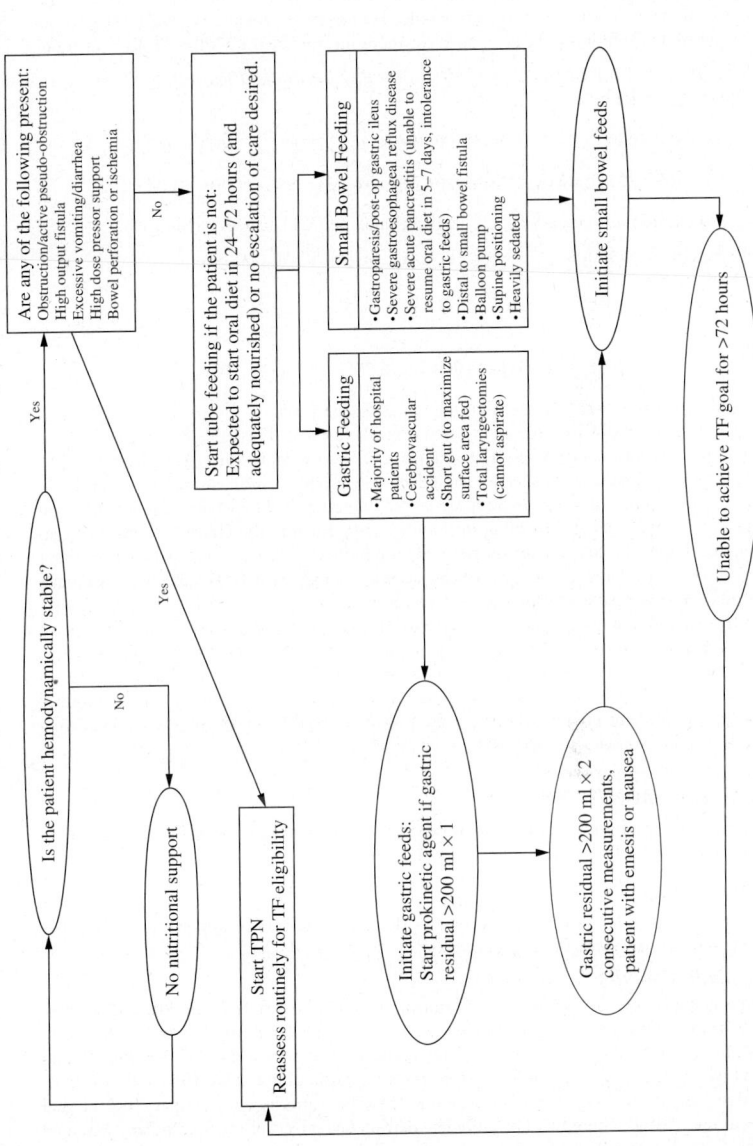

Figure 9-4 Determining the route of intensive nutrition support. TF, tube feeds; TPN, total parenteral nutrition.

these equations in the intensive care unit and in obese patients (35). In the absence of indirect calorimetry, the Penn State University ([PSU] 2003b) equation is recommended to determine RMR in critically ill, mechanically ventilated obese adults who are younger than 60 years and the PSU (2010) equation for obese patients 60 years or older. For nonobese patients, the PSU (2003b) equation is suggested (35). Both of the Penn State equations incorporate the Mifflin–St. Jeor equation.

REE Estimations for Critically Ill, Mechanically Ventilated Patients
Penn State Equations

$$\text{PSU (2003b): RMR} = \text{Mifflin} (0.96) + V_E (31) + T_{max} (167) - 6{,}212$$

$$\text{PSU (2010): RMR} = \text{Mifflin} (0.71) + V_E (64) + T_{max} (85) - 3{,}085$$

V_E, expired minute ventilation; T_{max}, highest temperature in degrees Celsius.

Mifflin–St. Jeor Equations
Men:

$$\text{REE (kcal/day)} = 10(W) + 6.25(H) - 5(A) + 5$$

Women:

$$\text{REE (kcal/day)} = 10(W) + 6.25(H) - 5(A) - 161$$

W, weight in kilograms; H, height in centimeters; A, age in years.

A simple method of REE prediction based on BMI (presented in Table 5-4) is based on the premise that, in general, energy given per kilogram of body weight is inversely related to BMI. The lower range within each category should be considered in insulin-resistant, critically ill patients, unless they are depleted in body fat, to decrease the risk of hyperglycemia and infection associated with overfeeding. Providing total daily energy equal to the Harris–Benedict calculation plus an additional 20% is a reasonable goal for nonobese, noncritically ill patients who have increased metabolic demands. It may be more accurate to utilize the BMI approach to estimate daily total energy for patients who are either very lean or obese.

Individual protein requirements are affected by several factors, such as the amount of nonprotein calories provided, overall energy requirements, protein quality, and the patient's nutritional status (see Chapter 5). In general, approximately 15% to 20% of total protein requirements should be in the form of essential amino acids in normal adults. Protein requirements during different clinical conditions are presented in Table 5-13. Illness, by increasing catabolism and metabolic rate, also increases requirements for protein.

NUTRITION MONITORING

Nutrition monitoring should address not only the tolerance of the nutritional support provided but also the continued adequacy and effectiveness.

Monitoring Plan

The monitoring plan for patients at nutritional risk receiving nutrition support should include a determination of daily actual nutrition intake.

Critically Ill Patients

In critically ill patients, provision of enteral nutrition within the first 48 hours with at least 60% to 70% of total estimated energy requirements received is associated with a decreased length of stay, time on mechanical ventilation, and infectious complications (36–38). Caution should be used when feeding critically ill patients as evidence exists of potential harm with overfeeding. Some researchers suggest that "overfeeding" may be achieving greater than 70% of goal intake in the critically ill population (39). The detrimental effects of overfeeding are presented in Table 5-25. The concept of short-term feeding of 50% to 60% of a patient's estimated caloric needs while providing nearly 100% of their protein needs during periods of severe metabolic stress has been termed "permissive underfeeding" (39). Although preliminary research suggested that there may be a benefit to underfeeding critically ill patients, a randomized trial in patients with acute lung injury demonstrated no additional benefit (40); another multicenter randomized trial in mixed ICU patients is underway to confirm these results (41,42).

Noncritically Ill Patients

Noncritically ill patients should be advanced to their caloric goal within 24 to 48 hours. However, there is some evidence to suggest that both critical and noncritical obese patients may benefit from the practice of permissive underfeeding, combining low calories with high protein provision (43). Other techniques to monitor intake in hospitalized patients are reviewed in Chapter 5.

Electrolytes

Electrolytes should be monitored during the administration of nutrition support. Patients at risk of refeeding (critically ill, >10% body weight loss, prolonged decreased oral intake) should be followed up closely as the consequences are potentially serious (see Table 5-26). Changes in clinical status (i.e., decreasing renal function) may lead to electrolyte abnormalities and a need for alteration of the nutrition prescription. Specific recommendations for monitoring patients receiving enteral and parenteral nutrition are presented in Chapters 10 and 11.

FORMULATING A FINAL PROTEIN AND CALORIE SUPPORT PLAN

The final plan is designed according to the previously mentioned considerations. The key questions lead to decisions regarding the urgency of support and methods of protein and calorie delivery. More than one suitable method of support is usually available. An appropriate plan does not interfere with usual medical care but rather is an effective adjuvant to medical and surgical therapeutics. Of importance to the clinician is the appropriate selection of patients for intensive nutritional support (tube feeding and total parenteral nutrition). The key questions can help select these patients. Figures 9-3 and 9-4 present algorithms that are useful in the selection of patients and determination of timing and route for intensive nutrition support. The following examples illustrate possible approaches to nutrition support.

Example 1

History

A 26-year-old man with a 7-year history of Crohn disease and two prior small-bowel resections enters the hospital because of an exacerbation of symptoms. Despite outpatient therapy with immunosuppressive medications, he has continued to experience fatigue, a poor appetite, crampy postprandial abdominal pain, diarrhea, and low-grade fevers, but he does not appear dehydrated. His weight has dropped from 142 (usual) to 130 lb (an 8.5% decrease) in the past 3 months. Physical examination reveals a thin man with a tender abdominal mass in the right lower quadrant. Laboratory data include the following values: hemoglobin, 12.2 g per dL; white blood cell count, 16,000 per mm^3 (he is receiving corticosteroids); 9% lymphocytes (total lymphocyte count, 1,440 per mm^3); serum albumin, 3.2 g per dL; and total iron-binding capacity, 270 mg per dL. A small-bowel radiographic study shows multiple skip lesions typical of Crohn disease in the remaining ileum, along with a very narrowed distal segment proximal to the prior anastomosis.

Impression and Plan

The patient meets the criteria for chronic disease-related malnutrition; however, the screening laboratory tests indicate that the degree of depletion is probably not severe. Despite the favorable assessment, total parenteral nutrition may be indicated in this situation because of the patient's poor appetite and to lessen his discomfort during the management of refractory extensive Crohn disease of the small bowel. The planned course of therapy will probably exceed 3 to 4 weeks.

Example 2

History

Fever and a productive cough have developed in a 72-year-old woman in previously good health. Because her appetite is poor and her fluid intake inadequate, she is admitted for therapy. She appears acutely ill and mildly dehydrated. Radiographic examination of the chest confirms the diagnosis of lobar pneumonia. Laboratory studies reveal normal hemoglobin and albumin levels and a normal lymphocyte count. Nutritional history estimates a recent daily intake of 650 kcal and 20 g of protein.

Impression and Plan
No historical features suggest malnutrition in this patient, and the laboratory data support the impression. Remember, however, that albumin levels are affected by hydration. Current intake does not match calculated requirements, but the illness is expected to be short. Oral liquid supplements are offered to improve fluid, protein, and calorie balance until the pneumonia resolves and a regular diet is tolerated.

Example 3
History
Progressive respiratory failure has developed in a 58-year-old man with chronic obstructive lung disease and several recent acute respiratory infections. He is admitted and requires mechanical ventilation. His weight has fallen from 166 to 156 lb (a 6% decrease) in the past 6 months. Current treatment includes 150 g of IV dextrose per day as the only calorie source.

Impression and Plan
Clinical and anthropometric data suggest severe chronic disease-related malnutrition. In this case, the anticipated duration of nutritional support is unclear. Because of the existing deficiencies, it is reasonable to proceed with intensive support. Tube feeding with a small-caliber nasoduodenal tube is initiated.

Example 4
History
A 52-year-old woman is transferred from another hospital after a complicated postoperative course. Within the past 8 weeks, she has undergone a vagotomy and pyloroplasty for peptic ulcer disease and then a reoperation for gastric outlet obstruction with creation of a gastrojejunostomy. The stoma is functioning poorly. She continues to require nasogastric suction because of vomiting, and a revision of the anastomosis will be necessary. She appears to be overweight (height of 65 inches), but her weight has fallen from 220 to 192 lb (a 13% decrease) in the past 2 months. She states that she is very weak. Laboratory values include a white blood cell count of 5,200 per mm^3, 12% lymphocytes (total lymphocyte count of 620 per mm^3), serum albumin level of 2.13 g per dL, and total iron-binding capacity of 180 mg per dL (estimated transferrin level, 100 mg per dL).

Impression and Plan
The history of recent operations and weight loss suggests that severe acute disease-related malnutrition may be present. In this case, initially excessive fat stores have prevented the appearance of wasting despite persistent negative balances and concomitant protein losses. On the basis of the current degree of negative balance (her only intake is IV 5% dextrose) and the fact that another laparotomy is necessary, it is felt that the anticipated duration of support may be long. The patient is appropriately selected for intensive nutritional support; because the intestinal tract is not readily available for use, total parenteral nutrition is instituted. It is decided to give the patient 3 weeks of total parenteral nutrition before her third laparotomy.

Example 5
History
A 66-year-old woman is admitted because of diarrhea, a poor appetite, and a 5% weight loss in the past 23 months. Twelve months ago, she completed a course of radiation therapy for carcinoma of the cervix. Small-bowel series reveals several long areas of fold thickening and speculation in the distal ileum, consistent with radiation enteritis. Laboratory values include a serum albumin level of 3.0 g per dL, serum transferrin level (estimated from the total iron-binding capacity) of 190 mg per dL, and total lymphocyte count of 1,200 per mm^3. A creatinine height index of 68% is calculated from a 24-hour urinary creatinine collection, originally ordered for determining creatinine clearance. Inpatient calorie counts reveal a daily intake of 800 to 900 kcal and 20 to 30 g of protein.

Impression and Plan
Chronic disease-related malnutrition is suggested by the history and screening laboratory tests. Protein losses may be occurring from the intestinal tract, and these losses would accelerate the rate of protein depletion. The nearly normal serum transferrin level may be a result of concomitant iron deficiency secondary to persistent gastrointestinal blood loss. The anticipated length of negative balance is uncertain, and attempts are made to increase oral intake with low-fat, high-protein commercial supplements. Antidiarrheal medications are also used. Although the diarrhea abates, repeated calorie counts suggest that the negative balance of about 500 kcal per day is persisting because of poor appetite. Tube feeding with similar formulas via a nasoduodenal tube is offered to the patient, but she chooses to continue to try oral supplements; she wishes to be discharged and be reevaluated in several weeks.

REFERENCES
1. Lacey K, Pritchett E. Nutrition Care Process and Model: ADA adopts road map to quality care and outcomes management. *J Am Diet Assoc.* 2003;103(8):1061–1072.
2. Jensen GL, Compher C, Sullivan DH, et al. Recognizing malnutrition in adults: definitions and characteristics, screening, assessment, and team approach. *JPEN J Parenter Enteral Nutr.* 2013;37(6):802–807.
3. Skipper A, Ferguson M, Thompson K, et al. Nutrition screening tools: an analysis of the evidence. *JPEN J Parenter Enteral Nutr.* 2012;36(3):292–298.
4. Jensen GL, Mirtallo J, Compher C, et al. Adult starvation and disease-related malnutrition: a proposal for etiology-based diagnosis in the clinical practice setting from the International Consensus Guideline Committee. *JPEN J Parenter Enteral Nutr.* 2010;34(2):156–159.
5. Jensen GL, Mirtallo J, Compher C, et al. Adult starvation and disease-related malnutrition: a proposal for etiology-based diagnosis in the clinical practice setting from the International Consensus Guideline Committee. *Clin Nutr.* 2010;29(2):151–153.
6. White JV, Guenter P, Jensen G, et al. Consensus statement of the Academy of Nutrition and Dietetics/American Society for Parenteral and Enteral Nutrition: characteristics recommended for the identification and documentation of adult malnutrition (undernutrition). *J Acad Nutr Diet.* 2012;112(5):730–738.
7. Lim SL, Ong KC, Chan YH, et al. Malnutrition and its impact on cost of hospitalization, length of stay, readmission and 3-year mortality. *Clin Nutr.* 2012;31(3):345–350.
8. Martins CP, Correia JR, do Amaral TF. Undernutrition risk screening and length of stay of hospitalized elderly. *J Nutr Elder.* 2005;25(2):5–21.
9. Koren-Hakim T, Weiss A, Hershkovitz A, et al. The relationship between nutritional status of hip fracture operated elderly patients and their functioning, comorbidity and outcome. *Clin Nutr.* 2012;31(6):917–921.
10. Ray S, Laur C, Golubic R. Malnutrition in healthcare institutions: a review of the prevalence of under-nutrition in hospitals and care homes since 1994 in England. *Clin Nutr.* 2013;doi:10.1016.
11. Ulltang M, Vivanti AP, Murray E. Malnutrition prevalence in a medical assessment and planning unit and its association with hospital readmission. *Aust Health Rev.* 2013;37(5):636–641.
12. Barker LA, Gout BS, Crowe TC. Hospital malnutrition: prevalence, identification and impact on patients and the healthcare system. *Int J Environ Res Public Health.* 2011;8(2):514–527.
13. Correia MI, Waitzberg DL. The impact of malnutrition on morbidity, mortality, length of hospital stay and costs evaluated through a multivariate model analysis. *Clin Nutr.* 2003;22(3):235–239.
14. Middleton MH, Nazarenko G, Nivison-Smith I, et al. Prevalence of malnutrition and 12-month incidence of mortality in two Sydney teaching hospitals. *Intern Med J.* 2001;31(8):455–461.
15. Myron Johnson A, Merlini G, Sheldon J, et al. Clinical indications for plasma protein assays: transthyretin (prealbumin) in inflammation and malnutrition. *Clin Chem Lab Med.* 2007;45(3):419–426.
16. Neel DR, McClave S, Martindale R. Hypoalbuminaemia in the perioperative period: clinical significance and management options. *Best Pract Res Clin Anaesthesiol.* 2011;25(3):395–400.
17. Winston AP. The clinical biochemistry of anorexia nervosa. *Ann Clin Biochem.* 2012;49(pt 2):132–143.
18. Krantz MJ, Lee D, Donahoo WT, et al. The paradox of normal serum albumin in anorexia nervosa: a case report. *Int J Eat Disord.* 2005;37(3):278–280.

19. Braga M, Gianotti L, Nespoli L, et al. Nutritional approach in malnourished surgical patients: a prospective randomized study. *Arch Surg.* 2002;137(2):174–180.
20. Luttikhold J, Oosting A, van den Braak CC, et al. Preservation of the gut by preoperative carbohydrate loading improves postoperative food intake. *Clin Nutr.* 2013;32(4):556–561.
21. Awad S, Varadhan KK, Ljungqvist O, et al. A meta-analysis of randomised controlled trials on preoperative oral carbohydrate treatment in elective surgery. *Clin Nutr.* 2013;32(1):34–44.
22. Jean-Claude M, Emmanuelle P, Juliette H, et al. Clinical and economic impact of malnutrition per se on the postoperative course of colorectal cancer patients. *Clin Nutr.* 2012;31(6):896–902.
23. Howard L, Ashley C. Nutrition in the perioperative patient. *Annu Rev Nutr.* 2003;23:263–282.
24. Singer P, Pichard C. Reconciling divergent results of the latest parenteral nutrition studies in the ICU. *Curr Opin Clin Nutr Metab Care.* 2013;16(2):187–193.
25. Nguyen NQ, Fraser RJ, Bryant LK, et al. The impact of delaying enteral feeding on gastric emptying, plasma cholecystokinin, and peptide YY concentrations in critically ill patients. *Crit Care Med.* 2008;36(5):1469–1474.
26. Doig GS, Heighes PT, Simpson F, et al. Early enteral nutrition reduces mortality in trauma patients requiring intensive care: a meta-analysis of randomised controlled trials. *Injury.* 2011;42(1):50–56.
27. Nguyen NQ, Besanko LK, Burgstad C, et al. Delayed enteral feeding impairs intestinal carbohydrate absorption in critically ill patients. *Crit Care Med.* 2012;40(1):50–54.
28. Alberda C, Gramlich L, Jones N, et al. The relationship between nutritional intake and clinical outcomes in critically ill patients: results of an international multicenter observational study. *Intensive Care Med.* 2009;35(10):1728–1737.
29. Gramlich L, Kichian K, Pinilla J, et al. Does enteral nutrition compared to parenteral nutrition result in better outcomes in critically ill adult patients? A systematic review of the literature. *Nutrition.* 2004;20(10):843–848.
30. Klein S. Short-chain fatty acids and the colon. *Gastroenterology.* 1992;102(1):364–365.
31. McClave SA, Heyland DK. The physiologic response and associated clinical benefits from provision of early enteral nutrition. *Nutr Clin Pract.* 2009;24(3):305–315.
32. Doig GS, Chevrou-Severac H, Simpson F. Early enteral nutrition in critical illness: a full economic analysis using US costs. *Clinicoecon Outcomes Res.* 2013;23:429–436.
33. Doig GS, Simpson F, Sweetman EA, et al. Early parenteral nutrition in critically ill patients with short-term relative contraindications to early enteral nutrition: a randomized controlled trial. *JAMA.* 2013;309:2130–2138.
34. Rousseau AF, Losser MR, Ichai C, et al. ESPEN endorsed recommendations: nutritional therapy in major burns. *Clin Nutr.* 2013;32(4):497–502.
35. Critical Care Workgroup CIGW. Determination of Resting Metabolic Rate. Academy of Nutrition and Dietetics Evidence Analysis Library, 2012. http://www.andeal.org/topic.cfm?menu=5302. Accessed November 15, 2013.
36. Huang HH, Hsu CW, Kang SP, et al. Association between illness severity and timing of initial enteral feeding in critically ill patients: a retrospective observational study. *Nutr J.* 2012; 11(1):30.
37. Dhandapani S, Dhandapani M, Agarwal M, et al. The prognostic significance of the timing of total enteral feeding in traumatic brain injury. *Surg Neurol Int.* 2012;3:31.
38. Heyland DK, Stephens KE, Day AG, et al. The success of enteral nutrition and ICU-acquired infections: a multicenter observational study. *Clin Nutr.* 2011;30(2):148–155.
39. Reid C. Frequency of under- and overfeeding in mechanically ventilated ICU patients: causes and possible consequences. *J Hum Nutr Diet.* 2006;19:13–22.
40. Needham DM, Dinglas VD, Bienvenu OJ, et al. One year outcomes in patients with acute lung injury randomised to initial trophic or full enteral feeding: prospective follow-up of EDEN randomised trial. *BMJ.* 2013;346:f1532.
41. Arabi YM, Haddad SH, Aldawood AS, et al. Permissive underfeeding versus target enteral feeding in adult critically ill patients (PermiT Trial): a study protocol of a multicenter randomized controlled trial. *Trials.* 2012;13:191.
42. Boitano M. Hypocaloric feeding of the critically ill. *Nutr Clin Pract.* 2006;21(6):617–622.
43. Choban P, Dickerson R, Malone A, et al. A.S.P.E.N. clinical guidelines: nutrition support of hospitalized adult patients with obesity. *JPEN J Parenter Enteral Nutr.* 2013;37(6):714–744.

10 Enteral Nutritional Therapy

GENERAL PRINCIPLES

This chapter outlines methods of providing macronutrients to individuals with inadequate intake or ineffective absorption of their usual diet. Enteral nutritional therapy may be accomplished by diet modifications of texture and content or provision of commercially available oral and forced enteral feeding products (Figure 10-1).

Modification of the Basic Diet

Modification of the basic diet may include texture or liquid consistency modifications. In addition, protein and caloric intake may also be supplemented or restricted by manipulating a patient's intake of certain whole foods.

Oral Supplements

Commercially available oral supplements are often used to improve a patient's daily intake of protein and calories. Many are now available in multiple flavors and forms to avoid taste monotony in long-term use.

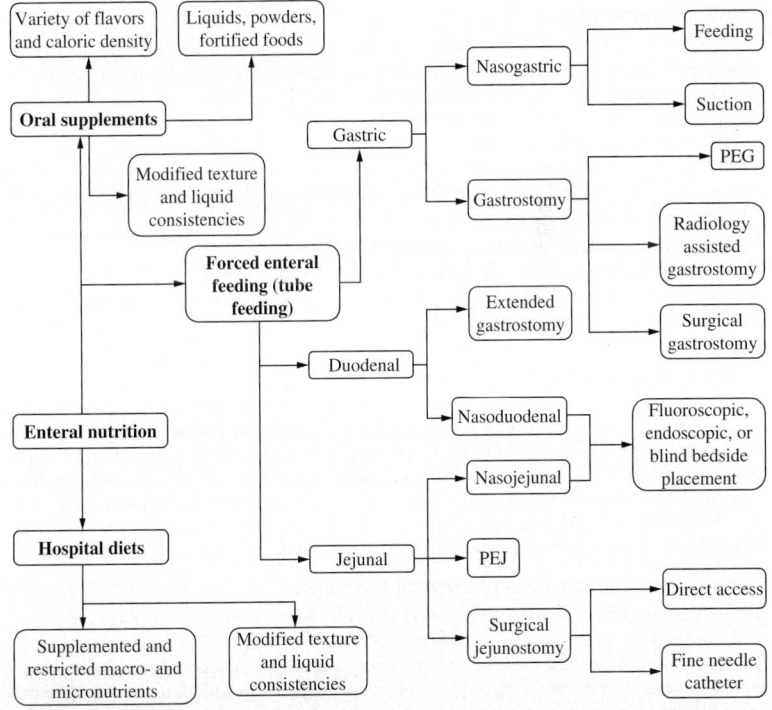

Figure 10-1. Overview of enteral nutrition therapy.

Forced Enteral Feeding

Forced enteral feeding, generally referred to as tube feeding (TF), is preferred to total parenteral nutrition (TPN) if the intestinal tract can be used to aid in maintaining the structural and functional integrity of the gastrointestinal (GI) tract as outlined in Chapter 9. According to the published guidelines of the American Society of Parenteral and Enteral Nutrition (1), TF is contraindicated in diffuse peritonitis, intestinal obstruction, intractable vomiting and diarrhea, paralytic ileus, and GI ischemia. Advances in the composition of TF products allow its use in conditions previously thought to be contraindicated, such as pancreatitis, short-bowel syndrome (SBS), and enterocutaneous fistulae.

INDICATIONS FOR ENTERAL THERAPY

Modification of Diet Texture and Content

Changes in diet texture and liquid consistency are often necessary in the nutritional management of certain diseases and neurologic conditions. In general, texture modifications are required in individuals with a neurologic deficit or head and neck abnormalities. Information on modified-texture diets can be found in Chapters 12 and 13. A change in diet content to supplement or restrict protein and calories is often required in patients with an increased metabolic rate (e.g., burns or sepsis), specific disease state (e.g., renal or liver failure), or varied oral intake. Improved nutritional intake and quality of life have been linked to patient modification of whole food texture and use of supplements to increase protein and calories (2). Macro- and micronutrient content may also need to be adjusted in patients with malabsorptive or inflammatory bowel disease. Techniques used in managing two special problems of protein and calorie absorption (pancreatic insufficiency and SBS) are discussed later in this chapter.

Oral Supplementation

Hospitalized patients are often plagued with inadequate protein or calorie intake to meet their daily requirements. Commercially available oral supplements (Table 10-1) are now available in a variety of forms (e.g., cereal, pudding, soups, and liquid supplements), consistencies (e.g., nectar-thick liquids, honey-thick liquids), and flavors (e.g., strawberry, butter pecan, cappuccino). It is often as easy, if not easier, to instruct a patient to take one or two oral supplement servings per day with a defined nutritional content as it is to suggest a selection of foods that may be unfamiliar or unappealing to the patient. Certain groups of people are particularly good candidates for oral dietary supplements.

Patients Chronically Ill with Associated Anorexia

Patients who are chronically ill with associated anorexia, as seen in cancer and HIV+ patients, may be unable to meet their caloric needs for weight maintenance with table foods alone. Dietary counseling and use of oral supplements or TF has been shown to improve quality of life and in some cases improved clinical outcomes (3).

Patients Requiring Liquid or Soft Diets

Patients requiring liquid or soft diets because of an inability to chew foods, painful oral lesions, strictures of the esophagus, or poor gastric antral motor activity may prefer commercially prepared supplements to the usual dietary liquids (e.g., milk, juice) or blenderized and puréed foods. Usual dietary liquids alone are deficient in daily requirements of vitamins and minerals. Commercial supplements can guarantee satisfactory vitamin and mineral allowances along with protein and calorie supplementation. The recent FOOD trial demonstrated the benefits of oral supplementation on weight maintenance or gain in this population (4).

Patients Preparing for Tests or Surgical Procedures

Radiographic studies may subject the patient to a negative caloric balance day after day in the hospital. Nutritional supplements, particularly in combination with a clear liquid diet, can minimize nutritional losses. Many low-residue commercially available supplements can be used in conjunction with the clear liquid diet. In most cases, low-residue supplements added to the diet while the colon is being prepared do not compromise the quality of a barium enema or colonoscopy. The Enhanced Recovery After Surgery (ERAS) Society recommends supplementation, specifically

TABLE 10-1 Examples of Commercially Available Products

Product Type	Nestlé Nutrition	Abbott Nutrition	Hormel Health Labs
Ready to feed	BOOST (high protein plus glucose control) Impact Carnation (Instant Breakfast, Instant Breakfast no sugar added) Nutren (1.0–2.0 with/without fiber, and pulmonary) Resource (2.0, Diabetishield, health shakes)	Ensure (high protein plus immune health, muscle health) Glucerna (1.0–1.5, advance shake, shake, hunger smart shake) Nepro with carb steady	Great shakes, Mighty shakes
Powdered	Carnation Instant Breakfast, Sugar-Free Instant Breakfast Modulen	Ensure powder	Instant mixes for shakes
Clear liquid	Boost Breeze (broth plus mix, Arginaid extra, fruit flavored beverage)	Ensure Clear Juven	
Fortified Foods	BOOST pudding Resource (cereal, cookie, custard, ice cream, pudding)	Ensure Pudding	Magic Cup

of carbohydrates, the night before and two hours prior to surgery as part of their protocols for various surgical procedures, all of which have led to improved outcomes (5,6). Provision of oral supplements preoperatively has been proven to decrease postoperative weight loss and complications, especially in patients with premorbid malnutrition (7). In addition, pre- and perioperative oral supplements have also been shown to decrease overall postoperative hospital costs (6).

Specific Dietary Needs
Patients with specific dietary needs may benefit from the special characteristics of many commercially available supplements.

Commercial Supplements
Most commercial supplements are low in residue because they contain no vegetable or meat fiber. Supplements containing no fiber and no fat probably add the least to the volume entering the colon. Soy polysaccharide has been added to several supplements to increase their fiber content. High-fiber products may be beneficial to selected patients with altered bowel habits resulting from functional motor disorders.

Many Lactose-Free Supplements Are Available
Corn syrup solids, sucrose, glucose, and other sugars serve as a source of carbohydrate; casein, soy protein, egg whites, or amino acids (or a combination of these) serve as a source of protein, so the need for milk additives or lactose is avoided.

Oral Supplements
Oral supplements with modified amino acid profiles have been developed for patients with renal failure and chronic liver disease.

Patients with Renal Failure. For patients with renal failure, essential amino acids added to a diet low in total protein content help to promote a positive nitrogen balance without causing unacceptable increases in blood urea nitrogen (BUN). The amino acid profiles in these supplements are designed to meet and exceed by several times the normal essential amino acid requirements. A review of available guidelines demonstrates a lack of consensus regarding the need for protein restriction in early chronic kidney disease (CKD); recommendations range from no restriction to 1.0 g/kg/ day (8), given the lack of benefit of a very low protein diet in halting the progression of renal failure (9). A diet providing less than 40 g of protein per day is not recommended for nondialysis patients, and 1.2 to 1.4 g//kg/day should be provided to patients undergoing dialysis (10). Undernutrition is common in patients with chronic renal failure with uremic syndrome. Common causes of undernutrition in these patients include reduced oral intake, restrictive dietary regimen, uremic toxicity, metabolic alterations, endocrine issues, and GI issues (11). Studies show that more than 50% of hemodialysis patients reported an intake of less than 1 g//kg/day of protein (12), suggesting the use of high-protein supplements may be beneficial in this patient population.

Patients with Chronic Liver Disease and Hepatic Encephalopathy. Patients with chronic liver disease and hepatic encephalopathy also have consistently abnormal plasma amino acid profiles, with an increase in aromatic amino acids (phenylalanine, tyrosine, tryptophan) and decreased proportions of branched-chain amino acids (BCAAs; isoleucine, leucine, valine). Protein supplements rich in BCAAs can be added to the protein-restricted diet to assist in establishing a positive nitrogen balance without precipitating encephalopathy (13,14). Disease-specific protein supplements are covered later in this chapter.

Indications for Tube Feeding

1. Patients with existing severe malnutrition or who are at nutritional risk due to poor intake or unintentional weight loss
2. Anorexia
3. Fractures of the head and neck or neurologic disorders preventing satisfactory oral feeding
4. Coma or depressed mental state
5. Need for prolonged assisted ventilation
6. Serious medical or surgical illnesses (e.g., burns) in which metabolic requirements are very high
7. Specific indications for the use of enteral feeding

Enterocutaneous Fistulae

Patients with enterocutaneous fistulae have been successfully delivered nutrition with goal enteral feeds infused via a feeding tube into the intestine distal to the fistula (fistuloclysis) (15,16). However, a series of studies reporting the use of enteral feeding for the primary treatment of enterocutaneous fistulae are small and uncontrolled. Complete bowel rest with the use of TPN has been employed more commonly as a nonsurgical attempt to close fistulae before definitive surgery.

Small-bowel Adaptation

Small-bowel adaptation occurs when intraluminal nutrients are again presented to the remaining small-bowel mucosa following massive intestinal resection. TPN may not be needed in these patients when vitamin and mineral supplements and large amounts of calories and protein are provided enterally (17,18). In addition, patients able to consume oral nutrition report a higher quality of life than those supported only with TPN (18).

Crohn Disease of the Small Bowel

Crohn disease of the small bowel can be managed with enteral nutrition (19). In children, exclusive enteral feeds are just as effective as corticosteroids in newly diagnosed patients (20). Enteral nutrition is well established as a first-line therapy in children; however, the same results do not hold true for adults. This may be related to poor compliance with enteral nutrition (19). Controlled trials have found elemental and intact-protein TF diets in adult patients to be equally effective; there is still debate in children, however, that is beyond the scope of this chapter (19).

Severe Acute Pancreatitis

Severe acute pancreatitis was for years considered an indication for TPN. Enteral nutrition was considered contraindicated because it was thought that it would worsen pancreatic damage. Now guidelines recommend the use of enteral nutrition in severe acute pancreatitis to prevent infectious complications and avoid TPN (21–25). Nasojejunal enteral feeds are well tolerated and are recommended as the first line of nutrition support in severe acute pancreatitis on the basis of theoretical considerations, but data showing a clear benefit over nasogastric feeding are not available (22).

METHODS OF PROVIDING ORAL ENTERAL NUTRITION THERAPY

Supplementation with Whole Foods

Supplementation with whole foods should be utilized for patients with normal appetites who are not meeting their daily protein and caloric requirements.

Protein Supplementation with Whole Foods

The quality of a protein supplement as a source of amino acids for growth is referred to as the biologic value of the protein. The protein content of various foods is listed in Table 10-2. Certain characteristics of these foods may limit their use, depending on coexisting intestinal disorders.

Milk Products

The lactose content is high; hard cheeses contain the least lactose per serving. The fat content is at least 4 g per serving (serving sizes are listed in Table 10-2) except for skim and nonfat dry milk, both of which have less than 1 g per cup. Most cheeses are high in fat, but a selection made with skim milk is available.

Eggs

Egg whites contain protein without lipid. The cholesterol is in the yolk.

Peanut Butter

Peanut butter contains 8 g of fat per tablespoon (50% of its weight is fat).

Beef, Poultry, and Fish

Flat fish are lowest in triglyceride, whereas steaklike fish have a fat content quantitatively similar to that of beef.

Calorie Supplementation with Whole Foods

Calorie supplementation with whole foods is conceptually attractive but often practically unfeasible. A normal diet with adequate calorie content restores glycogen and fat stores in the patient who has voluntarily or involuntarily starved. However, a lack of available calorie sources is not

TABLE 10-2 Common Foods That Should Be Included in a High-Protein Diet

Protein Source	Biologic Value	Food	Serving Size	Protein Content (g Per Serving)
Milk	85	Whole milk	1 cup	8.5
		Skim milk	1 cup	9
		Nonfat dry milk	1 tbsp	2.7
		Ice cream	1 cup	6
		Ice milk	1 cup	6
		Cottage cheese	1 cup	30
		Yogurt (low fat)	1 cup	8
		Cheese slice	1 oz	6–8
Egg	85	Egg	1 large	7
		Eggnog	1 cup	12
Nuts	70–75	Peanut butter	1 tbsp	4
Meat	75–90	Lean beef	1 oz	7
		Fresh fish	1 oz	7
		Tuna	1 oz	7
		Chicken/turkey (without skin)	1 oz	7
		Pork loin	1 oz	7

usually the reason for negative calorie balance and fat store depletion in the United States. If increasing the usual diet with good calorie sources satisfies the daily requirements, then this is the ideal way of managing calorie deficiency. In 2013, United States Department of Agriculture published an updated version of *Nutritive Value of Foods,* which is available online at http://www.ars.usda.gov/sp2UserFiles/Place/12354500/Data/SR26/sr26_doc.pdf. They also provide an online search engine of an extensive listing of foods available in the United States at http://ndb.nal.usda.gov/ndb/search/list. Nongovernment references are also available, including the newest edition of *Bowes and Church's Food Values of Portions Commonly Used* (26).

Supplementation with Commercially Available Modular Products

Almost all the familiar commercial products for oral supplementation or TF are "complete" formulas that provide a mixture of macronutrients and micronutrients. These products supply a person's nutritional needs completely if taken in sufficient quantity. In addition to the "complete" formulations, commercial sources produce feeding modules that provide a single macronutrient. These macronutrient modulars can be used to alter commercial formulas or as an oral supplement, to tailor both TFs and oral diets to a patient's unique nutritional requirements. The modulars are generally more expensive than "complete" formulations.

Protein Modulars
Protein modulars are generally a concentrated source of whey protein isolate that are designed to mix instantly into a wide variety of foods without affecting their taste or texture.

Carbohydrate Modulars
Carbohydrate modulars are usually composed of glucose polymers formed by the partial hydrolysis of starch. Modules with smaller polymers are sweeter and have a higher osmolality than those with large polymers.

Fat Modular
The only fat modular on the market at present consists of medium-chain triglycerides (MCTs) in an oil form. MCTs are fatty acids with chains that have 6 to 12 carbon atoms, whereas long-chain triglycerides (LCTs), the predominant lipid in both vegetable and animal fats, contain fatty acids with chains that have 14 or more carbon atoms. The advantages and disadvantages of MCT versus LCT are presented in Table 10-3. The theoretical caloric value is 8.3 kcal per g. The caloric value per serving is estimated at about 115 kcal per tbsp (15 mL). MCT oil can be used as a caloric supplement in patients with fat malabsorption of any cause.

FORMULAS FOR FORCED ENTERAL FEEDING OR TF

Formulas for forced enteral feeding or TF are available with many variations in specific characteristics and nutritional content. These formulas can be divided into four general categories: standard, elemental/semi-elemental, disease-specific, and immune-modulating products

TABLE 10-3 Medium-Chain Triglycerides—Advantages and Disadvantages

Advantages	Disadvantages
• Hydrolyzed more rapidly	• Lack linoleic and linolenic acids, so small amounts of LCTs[a] are needed to prevent EFAD[b]
• Bile acids not required for absorption	
• Absorbed as an intact triglyceride molecule	
• Highly water soluble	• More ketogenic and should be avoided in patients with diabetes, ketosis, or acidosis
• Transported to the liver directly via the portal vein	
• Does not require reesterification within chylomicrons	• Contraindicated in patients with cirrhosis (particularly those with portal systemic shunts)
• Crosses the mitochondrial membrane rapidly in the liver without carnitine	• May cause gastrointestinal symptoms of nausea, vomiting, and diarrhea if daily amount exceeds 500 calories per day
• Readily oxidized	

[a]Long-chain triglycerides.
[b]Essential fatty acid deficiency.

TABLE 10-4 Classification of Commercially Available Complete Enteral Nutrition Products

Standard 1.0–1.2 Calorie/ml
- IsoCal/IsoCal HN
- Nutren 1.0
- Osmolite/Osmolite 1 cal
- Osmolite 1.2 cal

1.5–2.0 Calories/ml
- IsoSource
- Nutren 1.5/Nutren 2.0
- Osmolite 1.5
- TwoCal HN

High Protein >18% of Calories
- IMPACT
- Promote

Fiber-Containing
- Fibersource/HN
- IsoSource 1.5
- Jevity 1.0–1.5
- Nutren Fiber

Disease-Specific
Pulmonary
- Nutren Pulmonary
- Pulmocare

Diabetic
- Diabetisource AC
- Glucerna

Renal
- Nepro Carb Select
- Novasource Renal
- Suplena Carb Select

Liver
- NutriHep

Elemental/Semi-Elemental Peptide-Based
- Oxepa
- Peptamen
- Peptamen AF
- Vital AF
- Pivot 1.5

Free Amino Acid–Based
- F.A.A.
- Vivonex TEN/RTF
- Vital RTF

(Table 10-4). A very large number of commercial enteral formulations are available, and new formulations are introduced frequently. The most suitable diet for an individual patient is one that provides the planned, desired allowances of macronutrients and micronutrients and also is appropriately restricted and varied according to any intestinal or metabolic disorders that are present. Table 10-5 groups commercial diets by the major categories and provides detailed nutritional information and the special characteristics of these formulas. For clarity, table definitions are provided.

Definitions

The following are definitions of some terms used in the tables:

Low Residue
This term is applied to diets that contain no meat or vegetable fiber.

Caloric Density
The caloric densities of commercial enteral products range from 1.0 to 2.0 kcal per mL.

Osmolality
Whole proteins and complex polysaccharides contribute a large number of calories to a formulation but relatively few milliosmoles. In contrast, free amino acids and monosaccharides contribute many more milliosmoles for the same number of calories. As a result, the osmolalities of elemental/semi-elemental and chemically defined diets tend to be higher than those of standard formulations with intact proteins and complex carbohydrates. The electrolyte content of the formulation also contributes to the osmolality without affecting caloric density. Isotonic formulations have an osmolality of about 300 mOsmol, which is similar to that of blood. Hypertonic solutions (>400 mOsmol) can cause delayed gastric emptying with nausea, vomiting, and distention. Hypertonic solutions entering the small bowel cause intestinal fluid secretion; if this fluid is not reabsorbed in the intestine, diarrhea and dehydration develop.

Ratio of Nonprotein Calories to Nitrogen
For most patients receiving forced enteral feeding, the quantity of amino acids provided in standard enteral formulas is large enough to provide for protein synthesis so long as enough formula is given to provide for caloric needs. In a few patients (e.g., those who have sustained severe

TABLE 10-5 Nutrient Analysis of Various Commercially Available Protein and/or Calorie Supplements and Diets

Product	Manufacturer	Oral (O)/Tube (T)	Macronutrient Major Sources Protein	CHO	Fat	Caloric Distribution (%) Protein	CHO	Fat	Caloric Density (kcal/mL)	Osmolality[a] (mOsmol/kg)	Fiber (g/1,000 kcal)
Boost	Nestle	O	M	CS, S	CA, C, SU	17	68	15	1	625	0
Boost HP	Nestle	O	C	CS, S	S	25	53	22	1	650	0
Boost Plus	Nestle	O	M, C	CS, S	C	15	50	35	1.5	670	8.4
Boost Very High Calorie	Nestle	O	C, S	CS, S	C, CA	16	34	50	2.25	950	0
Boost Glucose Control	Nestle	O	C	CS, F, FOS	CA	23	33	44	1.06	400	14.8
Carnation Breakfast Essential (CBE) (powder)	Nestlé	O	M	MD, S, L	MF	25	73	2	0.8	NA	0
CBE no sugar powder	Nestlé	O	M	MD, L	MF	33	63	4	0.56	NA	0
Diabeti-Source AC	Nestle	T	S, AR	CS, F, M	CA, FI	20	36	44	1.2	450	15.2
Ensure	Abbott	O, T	M, S	CS, S	CA, S, C	14	64	22	1.06	620	0
Ensure Plus	Abbott	O, T	M	CS, FOS	CA, C	15	57	28	1.5	680	12
Enlive	Abbott	O	W	CS		14	86	0	1.01	796	0
Fibersource HN	Nestle	O, T	S	CS	CA, MCT	18	53	29	1.2	490	12
Glucerna	Abbott	O, T	C	CS, F	SA, S, CA, F	16.7	34.3	49	1	355	14.4
Glucerna Shake	Abbott	O	C, S	CS, F, FOS	CA, SA	18	47	35	.93	530	10.8
Impact	Nestle	T	C, AR	CS	FI, SA	22	53	25	1	375	0
Impact with fiber	Nestle	T	C, AR	CS, SP	FI, SA	22	53	25	1	375	10
Impact Advanced Recover	Nestle	O	C, AR	S, CS	F, FI, MCT	22	53	25	1.4	930	10.4
Isosource 1.5	Nestle	T	C	CS, S	CA, MCT, S	18	44	38	1.5	650	5.4
Isosource HN	Nestle	T	S	CS	CA, MCT	18	52	30	1.2	490	0
Jevity 1 cal	Abbott	T	C	CS, FOS	MCT, C, S	16.7	54.3	29	1.06	300	14.4
Jevity 1.2	Abbott	T	CS, C, C	CS, FOS, MD	MCT, C, CA	18.5	52.5	29	1.2	450	18
Jevity 1.5	Abbott	T	CS, C, S	CS, FOS, MD	MCT, C, CA	17	53.6	29.4	1.5	525	22
Nepro w/carb steady	Abbott	O, T	C	FOS, CS, S	SA, C	18	34	48	1.8	745	7.2
Novasource Renal	Nestle	O, T	C, S	CS, S	CA	18	37	45	2	800	0
Nutren 1.0	Nestlé	O, T	C	MD, CS	MCT, CA	16	51	33	1	370	0
Nutren 1.0 with Fiber	Nestlé	O, T	C	MD, CS	MCT, CA, C	16	51	33	1	410	14
Nutren 1.5	Nestlé	O, T	C	MD, CS	MCT, CA, C	16	45	39	1.5	510	0
NutriHep	Nestlé	T	AA, HP	MD, CS	MCT, CA, C	11	77	12	1.5	650	0
Nutren Pulmonary	Nestlé	O	C	MD, S	CA, MCT	18	27	55	1.5	450	0
Optimental	Abbott	O, T	S, C	FOS, MD, S	F, MCT, CA	20.5	55	24.5	1	585	0
Osmolite 1 cal	Abbott	T	C, S	G	C, S, MCT	16.7	54.3	29	1.06	300	0
Osmolite 1.5	Abbott	T	C, S	MD	MCT, Ca, S	16.7	54.3	29	1.5	525	0
Oxepa	Abbott	O, T	C	MD, S	CA, MCT, FI	16.7	28.1	55.2	1.5	535	0
Peptamen	Nestlé	O, T	M	MD, ST	MCT, SU	16	51	33	1	270–380	0
Peptamen 1.5 w/ Prebio	Nestlé	O, T	HP	MD, CS, FOS	MCT, S	18	49	33	1.5	550	4.4

Per 1,000 kcal

Non Protein Calorie/ Nitrogen Ratio	Protein (g/ 1,000 kcal)	CHO (g/ 1,000 kcal)	Fat (g/ 1,000 kcal)	Na (mg)	K (mg)	Cl (mg)	Ca (mg)	P (mg)	Mg (mg)	Fe (mg)	I (mg)	Cu (mg)	Zn (mg)	Mn (mg)	Nutritionally Complete[a]
128:1	43	170	18	630	1932	1,440	1,270	1,060	420	15.2	161	1.7	19	3	Yes
80:1	57.5	132.5	24.4	833	1680	1142	1470	1260	420	18.9	159	2.1	18.9	2.9	Yes
139:1	39.2	126	39.2	559	974	836	559	559	224	10	84	1.1	11.1	1.6	Yes
131:1	41.8	87.4	57	532	798	517	475	475	152	11.9	114	1.33	28.5	1.9	Yes
89:1	57.5	82.5	48.9	1040	1,040	880	1104	880	320	14.4	120	1.6	12	1.6	Yes
NA	62.5	182	2.2	1018	2,400	NA	1,600	1,200	400	18	180	2	15	NA	NA
NA	82.5	157.5	4.4	1,105	3,158	NA	2,105	1,579	632	23.7	237	2.63	19.7	NA	NA
95:1	50	82.5	49	874	1320	528	660	660	264	11.9	99	1.32	15.8	3	Yes
146:1	36	160	24	800	1480	1120	1200	1000	400	18	152	2	15.2	4.8	Yes
144:1	37	142.5	31.3	638	1218	756	840	840	280	11.3	106	1.4	10.6	3.4	Yes
154:1	35	215	0	175	175	0	200	1000	40	9	187.5	1	15	3.5	No
115:1	44.5	132	32.3	990	1567	742	825	825	280	14.8	122	1.5	14.8	1.4	Yes
150:1	41.8	93.7	55.7	928	1,561	1,435	704	704	282	12.7	106	1.5	1.5	15.9	Yes
138:1	44.5	131.8	38.7	945	1665	1597	1125	1125	450	20.2	171	2.25	17.1	4.5	Yes
71:1	56	132	28	110	1,300	1,300	800	800	270	12	100	1.7	1.7	15	Yes
71:1	56	140	28	1,100	1,300	1,300	800	800	270	12	100	1.7	1.7	15	Yes
73:1	61.2	153	31.3	1190	1530	1360	918	816	262	13.6	170	2	17	2.38	No
116:1	45.3	113.3	43.3	867	1,400	1,067	733	733	287	12.7	107	1.4	21.3	1.4	Yes
116:1	44	130	34	924	1567	957	990	990	288	12.8	124	1.4	15.9	1.4	Yes
125:1	42	154	35	880	1,480	1,240	860	716	286	12.9	107	1.44	16.1	3.56	Yes
110:1	55.5	169	39	1125	1,541	1,250	1000	1000	333	15	125	1.6	19	4.1	Yes
122:1	42.5	144	33	933	1,433	906	800	800	266	12	100	1.3	15.3	3	Yes
121:1	45	85	53	588	588	470	589	389	117	10.5	89	1.1	14.4	1.1	Yes
113:1	45	91.3	50	472	472	399	420	410	98.7	9	75.6	1	10.9	2.1	Yes
133:1	40	127	38	880	1,248	1,200	668	668	268	12	100	1.4	14	2.7	Yes
133:1	40	127	38	876	1,248	1,200	668	668	268	12	100	1.4	14	2.7	Yes
131:1	40	113	45	500	1,253	1,000	693	693	333	12	100	1.3	13.3	2.7	Yes
209:1	26	193	14	213	880	1,000	667	667	267	12	101	1.3	10.1	2.7	Yes
116:1	45	67	63	415	528	505	686	343	105	9.5	78.9	NA	1.1	11.8	Yes
97:1	51.3	138.5	28.4	1113	1,701	1,340	1,050	1,050	425	13	160	1.9	16	3.6	Yes
125:1	42	135.6	32.8	880	1,480	1,360	715	715	286	13	107.2	1.43	16.08	3.57	Yes
125:1	42	135	32	924	1187	1133	555	555	267	12	100	1.3	15	3	Yes
125:1	45	100	47.5	872	1,308	1,125	703	703	287	12.7	107	1.4	16	3.7	Yes
131:1	40	127	39	500	1,252	1,000	800	700	400	12	100	1.4	14	2.7	Yes
116:1	45.9	124	37.8	688	1255	1174	675	675	270	18.2	151	2	24	2.7	Yes

(continued)

TABLE 10-5 Nutrient Analysis of Various Commercially Available Protein and/or Calorie Supplements and Diets (*Continued*)

Product	Manu-facturer	Oral (O)/Tube (T)	Protein	CHO	Fat	Protein	CHO	Fat	Caloric Density (kcal/mL)	Osmolality[a] (mOsmol/kg)	Fiber (g/1,000 kcal)
Peptamen AF	Nestlé	T	HP	MD, CS	MCT, FI, S	25	36	39	1.2	390	0
Peptamen Bariatric	Nestle	T	HP	CS, FOS, MD	FI, MCT, SA	37	31	32	1	345	4.4
Perative	Abbott	T	C, L, AR	CS	CA, MCT	20.5	55	25	1.3	460	5.12
Pivot 1.5	Abbott	T	C	CS, FOS	MCT, S, FI	25	45	30	1.5	595	5
Promote	Abbott	O, T	C, S	CS, S	CA, MCT	25	52	23	1	340	0
Promote with fiber	Abbott	O, T	C, S	CS, S	CA, MCT	25	50	25	1	380	14.4
Pulmocare	Abbott	O, T	C	S, CS	C, MCT, SA	16.7	28.1	55.2	1.5	475	0
Renalcal	Nestlé	T	AA, HP	MD, CS	MCT, C, FI	7	58	35	2	600	0
Resource 2.0	Nestle	O	M, C	CS, MD	C	17	43	40	2.0	790	0
Suplena	Abbott	O, T	C	CS, S, FOS	SA, S	10	42	48	1.8	780	7.2
Two Cal HN	Abbott	O, T	C	CS, S	C, MCT	16.7	43.2	40.1	2	725	2.5
Vital 1.0	Abbott	O, T	P, AA	MD, FOS	MCT, SA	16	51	33	1	390	4.2
Vital AF	Abbott	O, T	P, AA	MD, FOS	MCT, F	25	36	39	1.2	425	4.2
Vivonex RTF	Nestle	T	AA, AR	MD, CS	MCT	20	70	10	1	630	0

Formulations may have changed since the preparation of this table; consult the manufacturers' literature.
Protein sources: AA, amino acids; AR, arginine; C, casein salts; CH, casein hydrolysate; DL, delactosed lactalbumin; E, egg white solids; HP, hydrolyzed proteins other than casein; L, lactalbumin; M, milk proteins; P, mixed protein sources; S, soy protein. **Carbohydrate sources:** CS, cornstarch or corn syrup solids; F, fructose; FOS, fructose oligosaccharides; G, glucose; GO, glucon oligosaccharides; L, lactose; M, mixed carbohydrate sources; MD, malt dextrin; MS, monosaccharides; S, sucrose; SP, soy polysaccharides;

trauma), the requirements for protein synthesis are so great that a lower ratio of calories to protein may be optimal. This ratio is expressed as nonprotein calories to nitrogen (kilocalories per gram of nitrogen). The conversion of nitrogen to protein and vice versa is as follows:

$$\text{Grams of Nitrogen} = (\text{Grams of Protein})/6.25$$

Standard Formulas

Standard formulas contain intact proteins, lipid in the form of LCT, and possibly fiber. Most standard formulas are gluten- and lactose-free. The composition of these formulas will supply the reference values for macro- and micronutrients for a healthy population within a caloric value ($\sim$ 1,500 calories) that will meet the majority of patients' needs. In Table 10-5, the column labeled "Nutritionally Complete" indicates whether 1,500 calories of the enteral formula meets the RDA for the average adult. For many patients, the normal RDA will not be sufficient because of impaired absorptive function and intestinal losses.

Fiber-containing Enteral Formulas

Fiber-containing enteral formulas may be beneficial for patients with diarrhea or constipation. In most cases, soy polysaccharide is the fiber added to enteral formulas to increase stool bulk and regulate transit time. Fiber is fermented by colonic bacteria to short-chain (butyric, acetic, and propionic) fatty acids that serve as energy sources for colonocytes. Fiber also decreases the rate of gastric emptying and delays the absorption of dietary glucose. Theoretically, a reduction of the levels of short-chain fatty acids in the colonic lumen may be associated with adverse effects on the function of the colonic epithelium. Some manufacturers have added fructo-oligosaccharides to enteral nutrition formulations. Fructo-oligosaccharides are mixtures of oligomers composed

Non Protein Calorie/ Nitrogen Ratio	Protein (g/ 1,000 kcal)	CHO (g/ 1,000 kcal)	Fat (g/ 1,000 kcal)	Per 1,000 kcal											Nutritionally Complete[a]
				Na (mg)	K (mg)	Cl (mg)	Ca (mg)	P (mg)	Mg (mg)	Fe (mg)	I (mg)	Cu (mg)	Zn (mg)	Mn (mg)	
76:1	62.5	90	43	666	1,333	1,133	667	667	267	12	110	2	24	2.6	Yes
43:1	93.2	78	38	668	1332	1132	668	668	268	12	120	2	24	2.7	Yes
97:1	51	136	29	800	1,330	1,269	667	667	267	12	100	1.3	14	1.5	Yes
75:1	62.5	112	33	933	1,333	1,067	667	667	267	12	100	1.3	16	3.3	Yes
75:1	62.5	130	26	928	1,980	1,263	960	960	320	14.4	120	1.6	18	4	Yes
75:1	62.5	139	28	928	1,980	1,263	960	960	320	14.4	120	1.6	18	4	Yes
125:1	41.7	70.4	61.4	868	1302	1,126	704	704	282	12.7	106	1.4	1.4	15.9	Yes
300:1	17	145	41	30	40	14.6	30	50	10	0	0	0	7	0	No
116:1	42	109	44.1	399	756	596	525	525	210	9.5	78.7	1.1	7.9	1.1	No
251:1	25.4	111.3	54.4	456	648	528	600	425	120	11	89	1.1	14	1.1	Yes
125:1	41.7	108.2	45.3	653	1218	821	526	526	211	9.5	78.9	1.05	11.85	2.63	Yes
131:1	39.9	129	37.8	1050	1386	1050	697	693	277	12.6	105	1.4	21	3.5	Yes
75:1	62.3	91.7	44.8	1050	1400	1050	700	700	280	12.6	105	1.4	21	3.5	Yes
111:1	50	176	11.6	700	1200	800	668	668	268	12	106	1.32	12	1.32	No

T, tapioca starch. **Fat sources:** C, corn; CA, canola oil; F, mixed fat sources; FFA, free fatty acids; FI, fish oil; MCT, medium-chain triglycerides; MF, milk fat; S, soy oil; SA, safflower oil; SU, sunflower.
Other abbreviations: CHO, carbohydrates; NA, not available.

[a]When served full strength prepared in the usual way or diluted to suggested caloric density. The supplement or diet is said to be nutritionally complete if 2,000 mL or less meets the recommended dietary allowance (RDA) of all vitamins and minerals for the average adult.

primarily of β-D-fructose monomers linked by β2-1 glycosidic bonds. Fructo-oligosaccharides are fermented by bacteria in the colon to form short-chain fatty acids (see Chapter 12). Long-term ingestion of an elemental diet in rats results in diminished production of short-chain fatty acids in the colonic lumen and atrophy of the colonic mucosa (27,28). A significant reduction in inflammation was noted in the defunctionalized colon when short-chain fatty acids were instilled in the affected portion of the colon of patients with diversion colitis (27). In view of the important role of short-chain fatty acids in the maintenance of colonic structural and functional integrity, the use of fiber-containing formulations should be seriously considered in any patient for whom TFs are expected to be the sole source of nutrition for an extended period of time, especially patients with intestinal disease or injury.

Calorically Dense Formulas

Calorie-dense formulas may be beneficial in patients with fluid overload (e.g., renal failure, congestive heart failure, and ascites). Adults require 1 mL of water per kilocalorie or 30 to 35 mL per kg of their usual body weight. Tube-fed patients may not get enough free water, especially when nutrient-dense formulas are used. Denser formulas are frequently hypertonic; the added osmolar load may cause diarrhea (although hypertonicity is not a common cause of the diarrhea seen with enteral feeding).

Elemental/Semi-elemental Formulas

Elemental formulas contain free amino acids and glucose polymers. They are low in fat with only about 2% to 3% of calories derived from LCTs. In general, elemental products are used in patients with severe fat malabsorption or a chyle leak. However, these costly products are often not palatable, requiring administration via a feeding tube. Semi-elemental formulas contain proteins that have been hydrolyzed (oligopeptides), containing some free amino acids, dipeptides, and tripeptides, but larger peptides predominate. These formulas also include carbohydrate in the form of simple sugars, glucose polymers, or starch along with fat generally with a higher MCT:LCT ratio than a standard product. Often, semi-elemental formulas are labeled "elemental," since these products contain some free amino acids, but the terms are not regulated by any governing body. Theoretically, dipeptides and tripeptides are more easily absorbed than free amino acids or intact proteins because of the specific transport mechanisms for their intact uptake (29–32). These formulas may be beneficial in patients with some degree of malabsorption; generally, they can be used as a bridge to standard formulas as tolerance improves. At present, only small studies support the suggestion that oligopeptides are advantageous in patients with small-bowel disease (33,34). However, these results have not been reproduced in large prospective randomized control trials (32,35–37).

Disease-Specific Formulas

Disease-specific formulas include formulas that have been altered in their macro- or micronutrient content to address the needs of a specific disease and/or digestive or metabolic disorder, including pulmonary failure, hepatic insufficiency, renal failure, diabetes, and critical illness. In general, the clinical advantage of the majority of these disease-specific formulas over less expensive, standard intact-protein formulas remains controversial (38,39).

Pulmonary Disease

When a calorie of carbohydrate is metabolized, more carbon dioxide is produced than when a calorie of fat is metabolized. The rapid administration of a large carbohydrate load to a patient with severe pulmonary disease may increase the carbon dioxide tension. Several companies make calorically dense enteral formulas that have a higher fat-to-carbohydrate ratio for patients with severe pulmonary disease. However, the usefulness of these formulas when compared with standard products has not been proven in randomized trials (40). It is important to remember that the amount of carbon dioxide produced is more a function of the number of calories consumed than of the macronutrient source of the calories. Overfeeding should be avoided in patients with pulmonary disease. Early evidence suggested that products with a higher ratio of omega-3 fatty acids to omega-6 fatty acids are beneficial in patients with an acute lung inflammatory process such as acute respiratory distress syndrome (ARDS) (41–44). However, a large randomized double-blind, placebo-controlled multicenter trial did not demonstrate any benefit in clinical outcomes when a twice-daily enteral supplement of omega-3 fatty acids, linolenic acid, and antioxidants was provided (45).

Hepatic Disease

Chronic liver disease is associated with an abnormal pattern of circulating amino acids; the concentrations of aromatic amino acids (phenylalanine, tyrosine, and tryptophan) are increased, and the concentrations of BCAAs (leucine, isoleucine, and valine) are decreased. It has been postulated that this imbalance contributes to encephalopathy because it leads to the production of false neurotransmitters. A double-blind randomized trial compared 1 year of nutritional supplementation with BCAAs, leucine, isoleucine, and valine, containing formula with two standard formulas in 174 patients with advanced cirrhosis (14). The BCAA arm experienced a significantly lower average hospital admission rate, stable or improved nutritional parameters and liver function tests, as well as improved health-related quality of life (14). Other studies have reported only small differences. The special hepatic formulations are very expensive, and their use can be justified only in patients who are encephalopathic (see Chapter 12). Alcoholism, the most frequent cause of chronic liver disease, is associated with other nutritional problems, including deficiencies of thiamine, folate, vitamin C, zinc, and magnesium. According to a meta-analysis, abstinence and nutrition support remain the cornerstones of management of alcoholic liver disease (46). Chronic liver disease is frequently associated with ascites and edema. Control of salt and water balance is an important component of the management of chronic liver disease. The sodium content of enteral formulas rarely exceeds 2 g per day when meeting a patient's caloric requirements. A calorically dense (1.5 to 2.0 kcal per ml) formula aids in the restriction of fluids in these patients.

Renal Disease

In chronic renal failure, the ability of the kidney to excrete urea and electrolytes is limited. An important part of the management of chronic renal disease is the adjustment of dietary and fluid intake to accommodate for the diminished functional capacity of the kidneys. One estimate of the demands placed by a nutritional product on the kidneys is the renal solute load, which is determined primarily by the protein and electrolyte content of the formula. The major contributors to the renal solute load are urea, the end product of protein digestion, and the electrolytes (sodium, potassium, and chloride). The greater the renal solute load, the greater the obligatory water loss through the kidneys. As renal function decreases, the ability of the kidney to concentrate solutes is diminished. Thus, the greater the impairment of renal function, the greater the obligatory water loss for a given solute load. Commercial enteral formulas developed specifically for patients with chronic renal disease not receiving dialysis are calorically dense and electrolyte- and protein-restricted with a high percentage of essential amino acids. The diminished protein content combined with a high percentage of essential amino acids allows for adequate protein synthesis with minimal urea production. These formulas also have an altered vitamin and mineral content. Supplementation with vitamin and mineral formulation developed for patients in renal failure may be necessary. Patients with renal disease on enteral nutrition should be monitored frequently. Particular attention should be given to serum electrolytes, daily weights, and inputs and outputs. Patients who have milder degrees of renal impairment or on dialysis can be managed with standard calorically dense formulas (see discussion of the dietary management of renal disease in Chapter 13).

Diabetes

In diabetes, use of complex carbohydrates, such as fructose, cornstarch, and fiber, improves glycemic control by delaying gastric emptying and reducing intestinal transit time. With regard to macronutrients, the American Diabetes Association recommends counseling by a dietitian so the mix of carbohydrate, protein, and fat may be adjusted to meet the metabolic goals and individual preferences. Individuals should monitor carbohydrate intake either by carbohydrate counting choices or by experience-based estimation. Saturated fat intake should be limited to less than 7% of total calories; in addition, trans fat should be minimized (46). Commercially available diabetic formulas are based on the recommendations by the Academy of Nutrition and Dietetics (Academy) and the European Dietetic Association (47,48). Few long-term studies of diabetic formulas in a hospital population exist, making it impossible to draw firm conclusions about the benefit of these formulas. One study reported better glycemic control with the use of a diabetic formula compared with a standard formula, and several others have reported lower mean, fasting, and/or postprandial glucose levels, glycemic variability, and lower short-acting insulin requirements (49–54). However, although a trend toward reduced infections and hospital length of stay (LOS) has been mentioned, no significant differences in clinical outcome (LOS, ventilator support, infection rate, or mortality) have been reported. Hence, while the use of a diabetic formula can affect blood glucose levels, the effect has yet to be shown to be clinically important. Now that there is greater attention to glycemic control in the hospitalized setting, the utility of these products is further diminished.

Immune-Modulating Formulas

Over the last 10 years, more than 500 articles have been published addressing the benefits and risks of immunonutrition. Immunonutrition formulas are supplemented with any single or combination of immune stimulants, such as arginine, glutamine, omega-3 fatty acids, and nucleotides. Patients shown to have favorable outcomes with the use of immune-modulating formulations include patients post trauma and burn injury and those undergoing major elective GI surgery or surgery for head and neck cancer (54,55). A meta-analysis of randomized clinical trials comparing immunonutrition with standard products in surgical patients concluded there were significant effects on risk of acquired infections wound complications and LOS. No difference was found for mortality (56). A higher mortality rate has been observed in septic patients receiving immunonutrition when compared with similar patients receiving parenteral nutrition (57). However, in the same study, a significant reduction in infectious complications and LOS was observed in elective surgery patients. Interpreting the data on immunonutrition is hampered by differing study populations, inconsistent use of blinding, the use of different control feeds, and small sample sizes. Similarly, studies reviewing the effect of a single nutrient or class of nutrients demonstrate minimal benefit. Keep in mind that any recommendations regarding components of immunonutrition products are based on current data, most of which involves safety. The evidence that these products or individual components are efficacious is rather sparse and/or conflicting (see Chapter 15, specifically Table 15-9).

Glutamine

Glutamine is a nonessential amino acid that accounts for about 8% of the amino acids in dietary protein and can be synthesized by virtually all tissues in the body. Glutamine is involved in acid–base balance, protein synthesis, nitrogen transport, energy generation, and provision of nitrogen for nucleic acid synthesis. In catabolic states, glutamine is released from skeletal muscle and is taken up by the intestine, where it is burned for fuel. Depletion of plasma glutamine is associated with loss of intestinal integrity, villous atrophy, ulcerations, and necrosis. In rats, mucosal atrophy predisposes to bacterial translocation and the development of sepsis. This would be especially undesirable in severely ill patients; however, evidence is scarce that this occurs in humans (58). All standard enteral formulas contain glutamine ($\sim$ 2.9 g per 1,000 calories); however, several commercial companies offer immunonutrition products that contain especially high levels (>10 g per 1,000 calories). Supplementation with high levels of glutamine is used because some investigators believe that glutamine is a "conditionally essential" amino acid in catabolic states (59). In a double-blind, randomized trial of 48 severe burn patients, enteral glutamine treatment of 0.5 g/kg/day compared with a control group receiving 0.5 g per kg of glycine led to a shorter hospital stay (p <0.05) (60). This study did not report on infectious morbidity or mortality. In a large multicenter trial of both enteral and parenteral glutamine in critically ill patients, there was an increased 28-day mortality (32.4% vs. 27.2%; adjusted odds ratio, 1.28; confidence interval [CI], 1.00 to 1.64; p = 0.05); furthermore in-hospital (37.2% vs. 31%; p = 0.02) and 6-month mortality (43.7% vs. 37.2%; p = 0.02) was associated with the supplementation (see Chapter 8) (61). At present, practitioners should consider using enteral glutamine products for burn patients. Future research may help determine which subsets of critically ill patients may benefit from glutamine supplementation.

Circulating Levels of Antioxidants

Circulating levels of antioxidants (β-carotene, vitamin A, vitamin C, vitamin E, zinc, and selenium) are known to decrease rapidly in sepsis, trauma, or surgery and possibly remain low for a prolonged period of time (62–63). A prospective randomized control trial of enteral micronutrient/antioxidant supplementation in critically ill patients found an increase in circulating levels of vitamin E and selenium; however, no difference in clinical outcomes, including mortality, infectious complications, and LOS, were noted (64). A large meta-analysis that aggregated the results of 14 randomized controlled trials (n = 1,468) demonstrated micronutrient supplementation was associated with a significant reduction (RR 0.78, 95% CI 0.67 to 0.90, p = 0.0009) in overall mortality in patients suffering from burns, trauma, or critical illness (65). However, supplementation was not associated with a decrease in infectious complication or LOS in the ICU or hospital (see Chapter 6) (65). A trial of vitamin C and E supplementation in 170 patients with type 2 diabetes mellitus reported significant increases (p <0.001) in enzyme activity of superoxide dismutase and glutathione peroxidase, as well as significant improvements in fasting blood sugar (p <0.05) and HbA1c (p <0.001) (66). A more extensive review of trials with vitamins and minerals is provided in Chapter 6.

Arginine

Arginine is also considered "conditionally essential" in injury or stress situations (67). Plasma arginine levels are affected by surgery (decrease of 30% to 50% seen in abdominal surgery patients), burn (decrease of 57% in severely burned children), and sepsis (70% drop in septic patients when compared with healthy controls) (68). The interaction of arginine with growth hormone is thought to be involved in tissue repair and immune cell function (69). Arginine has been associated with maintaining T-cell immune function (70) after trauma, reducing the cellular immune suppression associated with injury, and enhancing collagen synthesis at the wound site (such as during tissue repair and wound healing) (71,72). An observational study of spinal patients with pressure ulcers supplemented with arginine demonstrated significantly shorter healing time when compared with historical controls (73).

Omega-3 Fatty Acids

Marine oil (Menhaden oil) is a rich source of omega-3 fatty acids and contains EPA (eicosapentaenoic acid) and DHA (docosahexaenoic acid). Increasing the omega-3 fatty acid content of the diet may displace the omega-6 fatty acids within the cell membrane, thereby favoring production of the less inflammatory eicosanoids. The literature suggests omega-3 fatty acids are less inflammatory and more immunostimulatory than omega-6 fatty acids (74). A ratio of 4:1 (omega-6:omega-3) has been suggested for healthy adults; a lower ratio may be appropriate for short periods of time when excessive inflammation is a factor and modified immune support is desired. Three small prospective randomized controlled trials compared a high omega-3 fatty acid containing formula with a high omega-6 fatty acid formula on patients with ARDS (42,44,75). Patients receiving the omega-3 fatty acid formula had significant improvement in gas exchange, required significantly fewer days on the vent, and had decreased LOS in the ICU (42,44,75). However, a large randomized double-blind placebo-controlled trial in 272 adults with acute lung injury (ALI) requiring mechanical ventilation comparing twice-daily enteral supplementation of omega-3 fatty acids, linolenic acid, and antioxidants with an isocaloric control was stopped early for futility. Patients receiving the omega-3–based supplementation did not have increased ventilator-free days, yet did have a trend toward increased mortality (45). Some authors suggest the different findings in this large trial were due in part to the delivery method of the supplements (bolus versus continuous) and the fact that the control group received a higher protein load (76). Future research may clarify if enteral formulas with fish oils, borage oils, and antioxidants should be considered for use in patients with ALI and ARDS.

CHOOSING AN ENTERAL PRODUCT FOR TF

There is generally more than one product that would be acceptable for any given patient (Figure 10-2). Therefore, the algorithm suggests product types based on patient assessment as according to a combination of the 2002 ASPEN guidelines for use of parenteral and enteral nutrition in adult patients (77), the Canadian Critical Care Nutrition Guidelines (78), and the 2009 Society of Critical Care Medicine and ASPEN guidelines for critically ill patients (55).

Enteral Feeding Access Devices

Physical characteristics are presented in Table 10-6. These devices vary in the type of construction material, length and diameter, presence of a stylet or guidewire, weighting of the tube, number of lumens, number of exit ports, and the presence of a Y-port.

Material

Most enteral feeding tubes are constructed with polyurethane, silicone, or a combination of these materials. Silicone tubes are the softest; however, they may collapse when checking for gastric residuals. Occasionally, Foley catheters will be used for long-term feeding access; however, the practitioner should remember these are made of latex, which can be irritating to the skin of some patients and dangerous to those who have latex allergies. In addition, Foley catheters have been shown to migrate, with the balloon often obstructing the pylorus or duodenum (79,80). In general, all tubes designed for enteral feeding delivery are completely radiopaque or have a radiopaque strip to facilitate radiographic confirmation of placement.

Tube Length and Diameter

The length of the enteral feeding tube is determined both by the site of insertion and desired site of feeding. The shortest surgically implanted tubes are called "button" or "skin-level" tubes. Surgically placed gastrojejunostomy tubes are available with a shorter gastric lumen for decompression and a longer jejunal limb for feeding. Some percutaneous endoscopically gastrostomy tubes can accommodate placement of a jejunal tube through the gastric part, allowing for simultaneous feeding and decompression. In addition to differing lengths, the diameters of tubes can also vary. The tube diameter is measured in French units (one French unit = 0.33 mm). Smaller diameter tubes are more comfortable for the patient and less likely to produce sinusitis, but they are also more likely to clog following infusion of medications or viscous TF product, especially if flushing is inadequate.

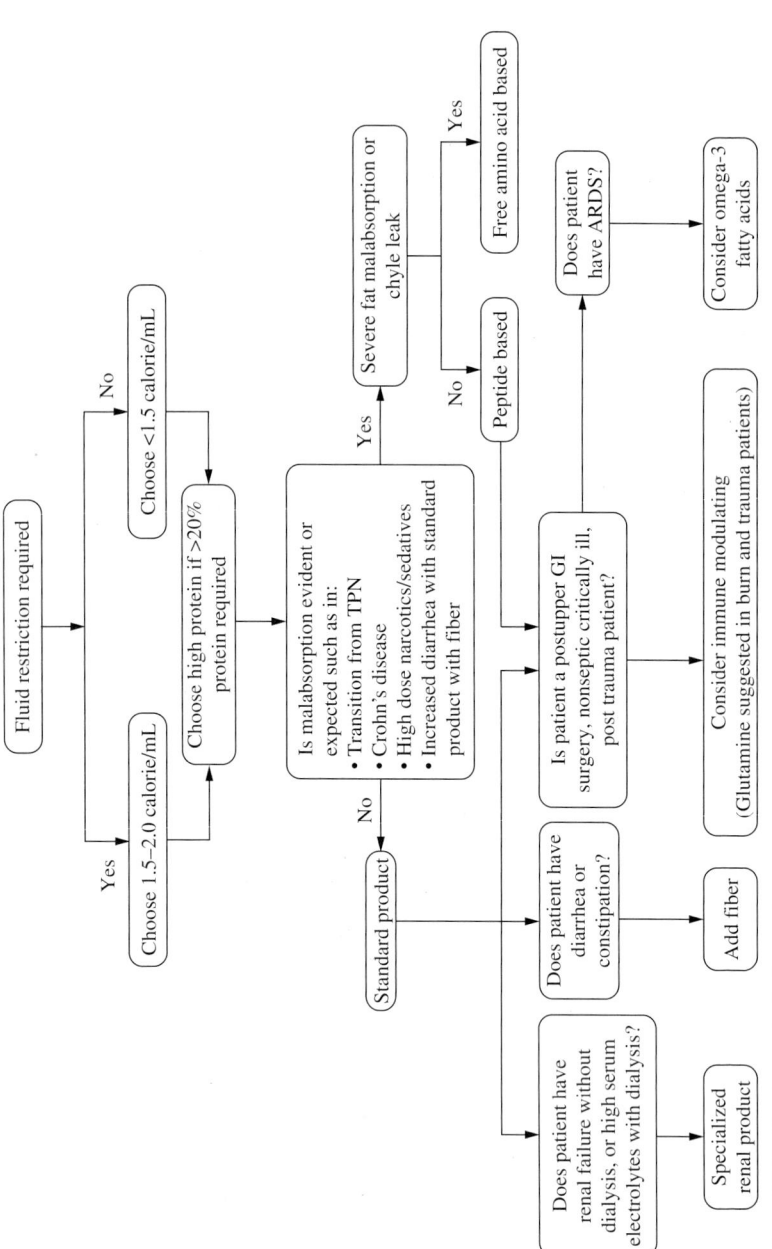

Figure 10-2. Choosing a tube-feeding product.

TABLE 10-6 Characteristics of Adult Enteral Access Devices

Tube Type	Material	Length	French (Fr) Size	Stylet or Guidewire	Manufacturers
Nasogastric Salem sump	Polyvinyl chloride or silicone	36–48 inches	12–20 Fr	No	Covidien
Nasoenteric feeding tube	Polyurethane, silicone, or mixture	36–60 inches	8–14 Fr	Yes/no	Corpak, Cook, Covidien
PEG	Silicone or polyurethane	Cut to fit	14–24 Fr	Yes/no	Wilson-Cook, BARD, Corpak, Kimberly-Clark, Covidien
Gastrostomy	Silicone or polyurethane	4–6 inches	12–28 Fr	No	Wilson-Cook, BARD, Corpak, Covidien, Kimberly-Clark
Jejunostomy	Silicone or polyurethane	6–10 inches	8–14 Fr	No	Wilson-Cook, BARD, Corpak, Kimberly-Clark
Jejunostomy via PEG	Silicone or polyurethane	35–45 inches	8–10 Fr	Yes	Wilson-Cook
Gastrojejunostomy	Silicone or polyurethane	Jejunal length: 35–45 inches	G port: 22–24 Fr J port: 8–12 Fr	Yes	Kimberly-Clark

PEG, percutaneous endoscopic gastrostomy.

Stylets
Stylets are frequently used to stiffen polyurethane or silicone feeding tubes to facilitate placement. Stylets generally have a flow-through design that allows flushing of air or water through the tube ports while the stylet is in place. The stylets do not extend the entire length of the tube, and they end in a blunt loop or a spring tip to decrease the risk of tube puncture during placement.

Y-ports
Y-ports on the end of nasoenteric feeding tubes allow for tube flushing and medication administration without disconnection of the feeding administration set. This can minimize contamination of the nutrition formulation. If only a single port is present on the end of the feeding tube, generally a Y extension set can be added. The ports should be labeled clearly to avoid confusion with respect to the purpose (e.g., "gastrostomy port," "feed," "for flushing only").

Tungsten Tips
Tungsten weighted or nonweighted tips are available on nasoenteric feeding tubes. Initially, it was believed the weighted tip would facilitate tube placement into the small bowel; however, some studies suggest increased ease of placement with nonweighted tubes (81,82). Presently, the preference of the person placing the tube determines the use of weighted versus nonweighted tips.

Feeding Methods
Enteral feedings can be infused either continuously or intermittently. Continuous feedings require a feeding pump to regulate the infusion rate. Intermittent feedings may be administered by gravity (over 20 to 40 minutes), by using a gravity drip bag or pump assisted, or via a syringe to provide a bolus feeding (over 5 to 15 minutes).

Feeding Equipment

Administration Sets

Administration sets are designed for either gravity or pump feedings, or to provide simultaneous continuous or intermittent bolus water flushing. Administration sets are preattached to hydration, gravity, or pump-feeding bags, which prevent separation. The gravity-feeding delivery sets have a roller clamp to help control the flow rate. Generally, the sets designed for continuous feeding are pump-specific. For safety purposes, many pump sets have an anti–free-flow device to avoid inadvertent delivery of a large feeding bolus. In addition, the connectors on a feeding set cannot attach to an intravenous (IV) needle or a Luer connector, making it virtually impossible to inadvertently administer enteral feeding into an IV line.

Enteral Feeding Containers

Enteral feeding containers vary in size and hold different volumes. Bag sets are used with cans of formula and typically hold a maximum of 1 L. The bag and administration set should be discarded after 24 hours. However, if formula remains in the bag for longer than 8 hours, both the formula and the bag should be discarded. Closed-system containers are available in bag or hard plastic form and are prefilled with a specific volume, generally 1 to 1.5 L. A spike set is necessary to access the enteral product in a closed-system container. In general, for safety purposes the closed containers and spike sets are clearly marked "not for IV use." In the near future, feeding ports will be "non-IV" compatible. Per most manufacturers, a closed system may hang for 48 hours after initial spiking when clean techniques are followed and only one new feeding set are used; otherwise, the hang time reverts to 24 hours. Theoretically, the closed system should decrease the risk of contamination. However, to avoid wasting enteral product, it may be prudent to use cans during initial patient testing or in the intensive care setting where the patient's clinical status may change quickly.

Enteral Feeding Pumps

Enteral feeding pumps should be accompanied by clear instructions and should be simple to use. Feeding pumps should be quiet, provide accurate volumetric delivery, and have both audio and visual alarms to protect against overinfusion. Pumps provided with an 8- to 24-hour battery backup and built-in IV pole clamp are highly desirable.

Feeding Tube Tip Location

The optimal feeding tube tip location for the patient continues to be debated (83–85). Some common indications, advantages, and disadvantages of various tubes are listed in Table 10-7. In a meta-analysis, small-bowel feeding was found to reduce the risk of pneumonia in critically ill patients without affecting mortality, LOS, or duration of mechanical ventilation. A subset analysis demonstrated this association was strongest for trauma patients.

Gastric (Prepyloric)

Gastric (prepyloric) feeding advantages include preservation of the reservoir function of the stomach, which allows for a large volume of hyperosmolar feeding without cramping, distention,

TABLE 10-7 Gastric Versus Small-Bowel Feeding

Gastric Feeding	Small-Bowel Feeding
• Majority of ICU patients	• Gastroparesis/post-op gastric ileus
• Cerebrovascular accident	• Severe gastroesophageal reflux disease
• Short gut (to maximize surface area fed)	• Severe acute pancreatitis (unable to resume diet in 5–7 days)
	• Intolerance to gastric feeds (despite prokinetic use)—high residuals, emesis
	• Patient status does not allow for elevated head of bed
	• Heavy sedation

ICU, intensive care unit.

or vomiting; easy tube placement for short-term access; and decreased cost because a pump is not required. The disadvantages are related to prolonged retention of formula in the stomach (high residuals) with delayed gastric emptying. This could lead to delay in the achievement of caloric goals, reflux, and possible tracheobronchial aspiration. However, a meta-analysis of six randomized controlled trials and six prospective observation studies suggests that, in general, monitoring of gastric residual volume (GRV) to guide nutrition appears unnecessary in the ICU (86). One observational study suggested surgical patients with a GRV greater than 200 ml more than once was associated with an increased frequency of aspiration (87).

Small Bowel (Postpyloric)
Small-bowel (postpyloric) feeding advantages include bypassing the pylorus if gastric emptying is a problem and a theoretical decreased risk of aspiration (88). The decreased risk of aspiration pneumonia associated with small-bowel feeding as opposed to gastric feeding continues to be debated. A study of almost 6,000 tracheal secretions was assayed for pepsin; 31.3% were found to be positive. In the study, patients with pneumonia on day 4 had a significantly higher percentage of pepsin-positive tracheal secretions than did those without pneumonia ($P < 0.001$) (89). The disadvantages of small-bowel feeding relate to the increased costs associated with the additional use of equipment (feeding pump) and availability of trained personnel for placement (bedside, endoscopy, or fluoroscopy) (90,91). There also may be a safety risk associated with intrahospital transport (92).

Insertion of Feeding Tubes
The selection of a specific device and placement technique to install enteral feeding is based, in part, on whether the patient will be fed into the stomach (prepyloric feeding) or the small bowel (postpyloric feeding) and whether the patient is likely to need short-term (<4 weeks) or long-term (≥4 weeks) enteral access. An overview of various tube types and their associated access duration, placement techniques, advantages and disadvantages, and potential patients in whom placement would be appropriate is presented in Table 10-8.

Short-Term Access
Short-term access feeding devices are utilized when enteral feeding is required for less than 4 weeks. These tubes are nasally or orally placed (in the event a patient has facial or sinus fractures) and may terminate in the stomach or small bowel. Many hospitalized patients will have a large-bore tube inserted for gastric decompression. Frequently, these tubes will be used for medication and feedings when decompression is no longer needed. Unfortunately, these tubes are uncomfortable, may harden over time, and are more likely to cause sinusitis or nasal necrosis than a smaller-bore, more flexible nasoenteric feeding tube (93,94). The bedside nurse can place a nasogastric flexible enteric feeding tube. If the patient's condition precludes gastric feeding, a nasoduodenal or nasojejunal enteric feeding tube can be placed. Trained personnel are required for the placement by any method of a nasoduodenal or nasojejunal tube. Success rates of blind bedside placement of small-bowel feeding tubes by a placement team are approaching those of endoscopic- or fluoroscopic-assisted placement (90,91,95). Several techniques for blind placement of small-bowel feeding tubes have been described in the literature (82,96–98). An example of one technique is presented in Table 10-9. Given the increasing popularity of bedside placement secondary to reduced costs and decreased risk to the patient by avoiding intrahospital transport, several devices to assist with placement have been developed. Devices include an external handheld magnet combined with a feeding tube fitted with a small magnet at the tube's distal end (99), an electrocardiographically (ECG) guided verification technique (97), and, most recently, a technique involving a styleted feeding tube with an electromagnetic transmitter on the tip of the stylet in combination with a receiver unit placed at the patient's xiphoid process with the signal of the tube's path displayed on a computer monitor (100). Regardless of the technique used, abdominal radiographs were still used to confirm placement prior to use.

Long-Term Feeding Access
Long-term feeding access, or surgical placement of a feeding tube, should be considered if feeding is expected for longer than 4 weeks. These tubes are generally less disturbing to the patient and will eliminate the risk of sinusitis and nasal necrosis. Because implanted feeding tubes

TABLE 10-8 Tube Types and Associated Characteristics

Tube Type	Access Duration	Placement Technique and Expertise Level	Advantages	Disadvantages and Risks	Patient Types
Nasogastric Salem sump	Short term	Bedside/RN	Large bore; less clogging; nasal or oral route; staff RN can replace if needed; used for decompression	Aspiration risk; patient discomfort; sinusitis; nasal necrosis	Normal gastric emptying; low risk of aspiration
Nasoenteric feeding tube—gastric or small-bowel placement	Short term	Bedside gastric placement/RN; Bedside small-bowel placement/trained RN, RD, MD endoscopy, fluoroscopy/MD	Softer, more flexible material for improved patient comfort; nasal or oral placement; patient can swallow "around" tube; if larger than 8 French unlikely to clog with good flushing techniques; available for immediate use after placement verification	Cannot be used for decompression, sinusitis; if placed in stomach, may migrate easily into the small bowel; aspiration risk; if placed in small bowel, tube may "flip" back to stomach; may not be able to be placed in patients with altered anatomy	Gastric—low risk of aspiration; Small bowel—delayed gastric emptying, increased risk of aspiration secondary to condition or positioning
PEG or fluoroscopically placed gastrostomy	Long term	Endoscopy, fluoroscopy/MD	Large bore; low risk of clogging; may feed via intermittent or syringe method; may accommodate a small-bowel feeding tube, if necessary	Hemorrhage; infection at insertion site; risk of peritonitis; may have to wait 24 hours to use; persistent gastrocutaneous fistula if tract does not close when removed; cannot be placed if endoscopy unable to be done	Normal gastric emptying; low risk of aspiration; need for long-term enteral feeding
Surgical gastrostomy	Long term	Surgical/MD	Large bore; low risk of clogging; may feed via intermittent or syringe method	Requires surgical placement; hemorrhage; infection at incision or insertion site; anesthetic complications; may have to wait 24 hours to use; persistent gastrocutaneous fistula if tract does not close when removed	Normal gastric emptying; low risk of aspiration; need for long-term enteral feeding; unable to place gastrostomy via endoscopic or fluoroscopic techniques

Type	Duration	Placement	Advantages	Disadvantages	Contraindications/Risks
PEG	Long term	Endoscopy/MD	Decreased risk of aspiration; can provide supplemental feeds at night; may use immediately postplacement; bypasses the stomach if decreased gastric motility a problem	Hemorrhage; infection at insertion site; risk of peritonitis; may "flip" back into stomach; difficult to replace; cannot check residuals; requires continuous infusion; smaller bore; may occlude easily; persistent gastrocutaneous fistula if tract does not close when removed. Cannot be placed if endoscopy unable to be done	Increased risk of aspiration; gastric motility disorders
Jejunostomy via PEG	Long term	Endoscopy, fluoroscopy/MD	Decreased risk of aspiration; can provide supplemental feeds at night; may use immediately postplacement; simultaneous gastric decompression and small-bowel feeding possible	May be difficult to get tube in position, jejunal extension may "flip" back into stomach; requires continuous infusion; smaller bore; may occlude easily	Increased risk of aspiration, gastric motility disorders
Double lumen gastrojejunostomy	Long term	Surgical/MD	Decreased risk of aspiration; can provide supplemental feeds at night; may use immediately postplacement; simultaneous gastric decompression and small-bowel feeding possible	Requires surgical placement; hemorrhage; infection at incision or insertion site; anesthetic complications; jejunal extension may "flip" back into stomach; small-bore tube; may clog easily; unable to be replaced if inadvertently pulled; persistent gastrocutaneous fistula if tract does not close when removed	Increased risk of aspiration; motility disorders; endoscopic placement not feasible
Surgical jejunostomy	Long term	Surgical/MD	Decreased risk of aspiration; can provide supplemental feeds at night; may use immediately postplacement; bypasses the stomach if decreased gastric motility a problem	Requires surgical placement; hemorrhage; infection at incision or insertion site; anesthetic complications; small-bore tube may clog easily; unable to easily replace if inadvertently pulled	Increased risk of aspiration, motility disorders, gastric-outlet obstruction or other anatomy precluding gastric placement

PEG, percutaneous endoscopic gastrostomy; PEJ, percutaneous endoscopic jejunostomy; RD, registered dietitian; RN, registered nurse.

TABLE 10-9 Sample Bedside Small-Bowel Feeding Tube Placement Policy and Procedure

Bedside Small-Bowel Feeding Tube Placement
A variation of the "10-10-10" protocol

Policy Statement: A Nutrition Support Service member or APN who has shown clinical competency with insertion will place a small-bowel feeding tube (SBFT) at the bedside with verification of placement by KUB prior to initiation of feeding.

Description: A protocol involving the insertion of all but **10** cm of a nonweighted 43" or 55" Corpak feeding tube with a stylet. If first attempt unsuccessful, give 10 mg IV metoclopramide, wait **10** minutes, then reattempt advancement of SBFT.

Procedure:

1. Administer 10 mg IV metoclopramide (5 mg if patient in renal failure) over 1–2 minutes ∼ 10 minutes prior to tube insertion.
2. Put on gloves.
3. If NGT or OGT in place obtain aspirate, noting color and pH, clamp NGT/OGT for SBFT insertion.
4. Set the hub of the stylet firmly into main port of feeding tube, close the medication port with cap.
5. Flush tube with ∼ 10 cc tap water to check for patency or leaks; activate lubricant.
6. Elevate patient's HOB as tolerated.
7. Insert SBFT into nostril and advance to nasopharynx and into esophagus. Flexion of patient's neck or having patient swallow will facilitate passage of tube into esophagus.
8. Advance tube to 55–60 cm and auscultate over the epigastric area and attempt to aspirate gastric contents comparing aspirate with previous NGT aspirate if available. Gastric aspirate is bilious in appearance. The pH may range from 1–7 depending on the use of gastric prophylaxis medication.
9. Continue to advance SBFT slowly with a gentle touch. Infuse ∼ 60 cc air slowly starting at 70–75 cm to help open the pylorus. Never force the tube; if resistance is met, pull back and attempt to readvance. Continue to advance to the 100-cm mark. There should be a vacuum present on the syringe when the tube is in the small bowel.
10. Aspirate and check pH and color of output when tube at 100-cm mark. Color of small-bowel aspirate is generally yellow in appearance with a pH of 7+.
11. Remove stylet and check for kinks or loops, then attempt to reinsert. The stylet should be easy to insert. Upon reinsertion of stylet, if any resistance is met, pull tube back until stylet is easily inserted. After stylet is in place, readvance tube.
12. When tube is in position, remove stylet and secure tube with tape to nose. Place stylet in plastic bag to use in future if SBFT needs to be repositioned.
13. Return NGT to suction, if on prior to procedure.
14. Order KUB to verify placement.
15. If SBFT pulled back from original insertion cm marking, reinsert stylet and advance SBFT per above procedure. Obtain KUB to verify position.

APN, advanced practice nurse; HOB, head of bed; IV, intravenous; NGT, nasogastric tube; OGT, orogastric tube.

transverse two epithelial barriers—the skin and mucosa of the GI tract—risk of infection at the insertion site is increased (101,102). In addition, if the tube is inadvertently removed before the tube tract has matured (generally 2 to 3 weeks postplacement when significant adhesions form between the stomach and the abdominal wall), an operative procedure may be needed to prevent spillage of GI contents into the peritoneum (103). Several options are available for the placement of gastrostomy tubes; currently, the most common technique is the percutaneous endoscopic gastrostomy or PEG (104,105). Percutaneous techniques have advantages over surgical techniques in that they are less expensive and do not require general anesthesia. Placement of a PEG requires passage of an endoscope into the stomach to see and manipulate the insertion site. The PEG procedure can be accomplished with either a push or pull technique, in that the gastrostomy tube may either be pulled through the stomach and out the anterior abdominal wall or pushed over a guidewire into the stomach and out the hole in the abdominal wall (106). After placement, an external bolster holds the tube in position and keeps the stomach up against the abdominal wall to prevent leakage of feedings or gastric contents. At present, good documentation regarding the benefit of a PEG versus feeding via a nasogastric tube (NGT) does not exist. In FOOD trial, 3 of 321 dysphagic stroke patients allocated to either a PEG or NGT, PEG was associated with an increase in absolute risk of death of 1.0% (95% CI 10.0 to 11.9; $p = 0.9$) and an increased risk of death or poor outcome of 7.8% (95% CI 0.0 to 15.5; $p = 0.05$) (107).

Basic Requirements for Use of the PEG Technique
The basic requirements for use of the PEG technique include ability to pass the endoscope (not possible in some patients with severe neurologic disease), ability of the patient to tolerate sedation, an unobstructed esophagus if the pull-through technique is used, absence of excessive obesity, and no history of a complicated surgical procedure in the upper abdomen that may have caused bowel loops to adhere between the stomach and the abdominal wall.

The general practice is to wait 24 hours postinsertion to initiate feedings, although there is evidence that feeding can begin as early as 4 to 6 hours postplacement (108). Major complications (peritonitis, necrotizing fasciitis, severe hemorrhage) and lesser complications (tube extrusion or migration, gastrocolic fistula) occur less often in patients receiving a PEG as compared with a surgical gastrostomy (109,110). However, for patients who have conditions that preclude endoscopic placement as stated above, or who are undergoing laparotomy for other reasons, a surgical gastrostomy is a viable alternative. Although a higher complication rate is associated with a surgical approach, because the stomach is secured to the abdominal wall directly, the risk of leakage of gastric contents is usually lower than with other techniques (111).

Short Silicone Post Low-Profile Tube
A short silicone post low-profile tube (e.g., "the button tube") may be used to replace a standard gastrostomy tube. The intragastric component of the post is a mushroom tip, and the external part is a small, tablike crosspiece. An attached flap closure provides a flush surface. During feeding, a tube is inserted into the open post. This device, which can be placed 4 to 6 weeks or more after the gastrostomy procedure, allows a better cosmetic effect and the regression of granulation tissue from the original tube in some patients, and it reduces skin irritation. The button is designed as a one-way antireflux valve. A special adapter is needed to cannulate the valve and check the residual volume (RV) or detect decompression.

Long-Term Small-Bowel Access
If long-term small-bowel access is desired, some PEGs will accommodate the passage of a jejunal extension through the gastrostomy and into the duodenum or jejunum. Alternatively, a percutaneous endoscopic jejunostomy (PEJ) can be placed using a technique similar to that for a PEG, with the tube positioned endoscopically beyond the pylorus into the jejunum (108,112). Some authors believe a direct PEJ placement is preferable to a PEG tube with jejunal extension because of the ability to place a larger-bore tube that can be anchored in the jejunum, preventing proximal migration into the stomach (113). One group reports a single-incision laparoscopic surgery technique where access was obtained through the umbilicus with the selected loop of jejunum exteriorized through this incision, feeding tube placed and loop returned into the abdomen. Under laparoscopic guidance, the tube is brought externally through the abdomen (114). The same benefit is obtained by placing a feeding jejunostomy at the time of laparotomy via a surgically constructed serosal tunnel. Smaller-bore needle catheter jejunostomy tubes are a viable alternative when enteral feeding is only required for a short period of time because patency may be difficult to maintain, and the tube cannot be replaced if inadvertently removed (115).

Care of the Insertion Site
Care of the insertion site for both short- and long-term tubes should begin as soon as the tube is placed and continue until the tube is removed and the exit site is healed (Table 10-10). As previously mentioned, a tube inadvertently removed before the tract has matured leaves the

TABLE 10-10 Care of The Tube Insertion Site

Type of Placement	Evaluate	Assess	Care	Precautions
Nasal or oral	Daily	Redness, dryness, or fissures noted around nose or mouth	Lubricate nares with water-soluble lubricant. Change anchoring method	If condition worsens, may need to change site of insertion
Nasal or oral	Twice daily	Decreased oral hygiene	Mouth care	
Nasal	Daily	Sores or increased nasal drainage	Replace via the oral route, may require antibiotics	May indicate sinusitis, report to physician
Gastrostomy or jejunostomy	Daily—start 24 hours postplacement	Check exit site	Clean tube site twice daily with soap and water and the area immediately around the skin opening. If covered by a bolster, use cotton swab for cleaning	
	Immediately postplacement, then daily	Increased bleeding or drainage at exit site	Place additional gauze dressing around the site and the tube	Do not place dressings directly under the external bolster—may dislodge tube, report to physician
	Daily	Increased tenderness, swelling, or redness	More frequent cleaning, cap feeding ports when not in use, possibly antibiotics or tube removal	Report immediately to physician; may be signs of an infection
	Daily	Inadvertent tube removal	Contact physician—may be able to reinsert through established tract if done quickly	If tract not mature, this should be considered a medical emergency

patient at risk of leakage of gastric contents into the peritoneal cavity and should be considered a medical emergency. A mature tract should be recannulated within a few hours to avoid permanent closure.

Maintenance of Tube Patency

Small-bore, more flexible enteric feeding tubes are more prone to clogging than the larger-bore stiffer decompression tubes. The best method to prevent clogging continues to be regular flushing with water or normal saline. The tube should be flushed with a minimum of 30 ml of water or saline before and after each intermittent feeding and medication administration. If the patient is fed continuously, a 30-ml flush is recommended every 4 hours. Medications should never be mixed with the enteral formula because either coagulation of the formula and clogging of the tube or precipitation of the medication and loss of its effectiveness could occur. If enteral feedings are held for any reason, the tube should continue to be flushed every 4 hours to maintain patency. If the enteral feeding tube does become clogged, several maneuvers can be attempted to clear the tube (Table 10-11) (116).

TABLE 10-11 Steps to Unclog Enteral Access

1. Irrigate the tube with warm water and alternate with aspiration of the tube[a].
2. If unsuccessful with step 1, infuse crushed pancrelipase dissolved in a bicarbonate solution, and allow to sit for 30 minutes.
3. Repeat step 1.
4. If tube remains clogged, it must be replaced.

[a]To prevent rupture of the tube, avoid applying excessive pressure by using a 60-mL syringe.

Initiation of Enteral Feedings

Regardless of the route and feeding-tube type, enteral feeds are generally started at a low rate and gradually increased over a 24-hour period to a final infusion rate calculated from the desired daily provision of calories and protein (Figure 10-3). Authors have shown that enteral feeds can be initiated at full feeding without significant differences in tolerance (117).

Maintaining a 45-degree Elevation

Maintaining a 45-degree elevation of the head of the bed during TF infusion is still one of the best defenses against tracheobronchial aspiration (89). It is good practice to keep the head elevated even when feeding ports are near or distal to the ligament of Treitz. Patients receiving

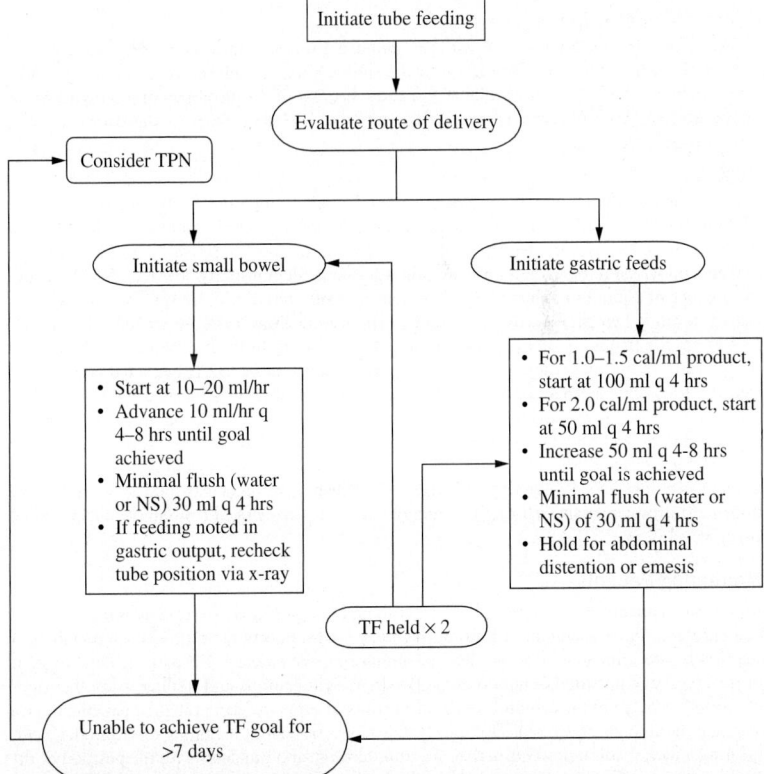

Figure 10-3. Initiation of tube feeding.

gastric TFs should not recline for at least 2 hours after instillation of a feeding, even one as small as 100 mL. Regurgitation is possible with a NGT because it interferes with the function of the upper and lower esophageal sphincters, which normally prevent tracheobronchial aspiration during recumbency.

Feeding Formulas in Cans or Closed Systems
These systems do not need to be refrigerated. If they are refrigerated, they should be brought to room temperature before infusion. Formula in cans should be allowed to hang no more than 8 hours in a feeding solution administration set. The longer the formula hangs in the bag at room temperature, the higher the level of bacterial contamination (118). Ready-to-hang or closed systems hang times range from 24 to 48 hours. Absence of microbial growth in enteral feeding samples from a closed system was demonstrated at the completion of a 48-hour hang time with strict adherence to label instructions for clean technique (118,119). Optimally, the feeding bag and administration set should be discarded after 24 hours. However, in home settings this may not be feasible secondary to cost; therefore, the feeding bag should be washed thoroughly every 24 hours to prevent bacterial contamination. Theoretical complications related to bacterial growth in the feeding formula rarely develop into true clinical problems.

Intermittent or Bolus Feeding
Intermittent or bolus feeding directly into the small bowel through nasoduodenal or jejunostomy tubes is not recommended because the secretory osmotic response of the small bowel to hypertonic bolus feedings will generally lead to dumping syndrome.

Constant-infusion Techniques
Constant-infusion techniques used with nasoduodenal tubes also can be used for gastrostomy and NGT feeding. Constant infusion into the stomach may be advantageous in a few conditions, including SBS (17). However, in most cases, because of the possibility of gastric retention of the infusate, intermittent feeding through tubes with feeding ports in the stomach is the recommended technique.

Aspirate
Aspirate through the nasogastric or gastrostomy tube before initiating the feeding to determine whether retained gastric secretions are present. Although almost all centers use the RV as a guide to managing TFs, the recommended cutoff volume varies considerably, and few data are available on which to base a recommendation. One study demonstrated low RVs did not assure the absence of aspiration events (120). The frequency of aspiration was 23% when RV was less than 150 ml. When the RV trigger to hold gastric feedings was increased to 200 ml and then to 400 ml, the frequency of aspiration did not change significantly, 21.6% and 22.6%, respectively (120). In another study focusing on aspiration, a subset of 182 patients fed consistently into the stomach was analyzed to determine the risk of aspiration associated with RV. While the overall mean RV was greater in the patients experiencing aspiration than those not aspirating, the finding had no clinical or statistical significance ($p = 0.058$) (89). However, if there is concern for aspiration, the use of prokinetic agents and caloric dense formula can be used in an attempt to reduce RVs. Persistent gastric retention of feeding formula may indicate gastric-outlet obstruction, proximal small-bowel obstruction, or ileus involving the stomach and proximal small bowel.

Monitoring Patients
Monitoring patients receiving enteral nutrition should be completed in a regular fashion to detect complications and evaluate the efficacy of the nutritional support (Table 10-12). All members of the health-care team should be involved in monitoring the enterally fed patient. Positive signs of the efficacy of nutritional support come slowly. Weight gain, wound healing, and other signs of anabolism may not be seen until weeks of nutritional support. Many tube-fed patients receive less than the amount prescribed. This may be due to several factors, including tube dislodgement, GI intolerance, medical procedures that interrupt feeding, and problems with the position of the feeding tube. In a large observational cohort study of over 1,200 patients from 167 ICUs, patients overall received only 59.2% of the energy and 56% of the protein prescribed (121).

TABLE 10-12 Monitoring The Patient Receiving Tube Feedings

Assessment	Frequency/Rationale
Gastric residuals (gastric feedings alone)	Before each feeding. Amounts >250 mL twice in succession should be evaluated for appearance. If TF product is noted in residual, this may indicate delayed gastric emptying. Consider prokinetic agent. If residuals continue, consider small-bowel access.
Emesis	May indicate delay of gastric emptying, follow recommendations for high residuals
Auscultate bowel sounds and abdominal exam, patient complaints	Every 8 hours. Absent bowel sounds and abdominal distention and patient complaints of fullness may indicate ileus
Bowel movements	Every 8 hours. Change in consistency may indicate malabsorption (diarrhea) or decreased bowel motility (constipation), requiring addition of fiber or change in product
Head of bed	Should be kept at 45° during gastric feeding and for 2 hours postfeeding
Vital signs—temp, respiratory rate, effort, and breath sounds	Daily. Increased temperature, respiratory rate, and effort may be associated with pneumonia. Breath sounds should be clear
Weight	Daily. Weight gain of 1 to 1½ pounds per week may indicate actual weight gain; daily increases are more indicative of fluid status
I/O	Daily at first, then as needed. To aid in monitoring fluid status and potential need to adjust caloric density of enteral product
Laboratory Data	
Serum sodium, potassium, chloride, bicarbonate, BUN, creatinine	Daily until stable, then biweekly. To evaluate for changing metabolic status and renal function
Potassium, magnesium, and phosphorus	Daily until stable. To evaluate for refeeding syndrome
Liver function tests, albumin, calcium, hematocrit, prothrombin time	Baseline, then once a week
Triglycerides, cholesterol	Follow in patients at risk of pancreatitis, history of hyperlipidemia
Glucose	Nondiabetics: check every 6 hours; diabetics: check every 4 hours until within normal limits, then every 8–12 hours to determine glycemic control. Cover with sliding-scale insulin as needed. For diabetics, begin basal and scheduled insulin as indicated

BUN, blood urea nitrogen; I/O, inputs/outputs; TF, tube feeding.

COMPLICATIONS OF TFS
Metabolic Complications

Fluid and electrolyte problems are common in patients receiving TFs, and in many cases, the formula must be modified to solve these problems. Hypokalemia, hyponatremia, hypophosphatemia, and hyperglycemia are among the most frequent metabolic complications. Some of the complications result from the use of commercial products, all of which have fixed electrolyte content. This disadvantage is easily outweighed by their convenience of use and modest expense.

Electrolyte Disturbances

The mineral contents of the formulas are given in Table 10-4 and are based on the usual requirements (see Chapter 7). Some patients may require additional supplements or may not tolerate the preestablished amounts of individual minerals. Problems are especially likely to develop in patients with renal, hepatic, or cardiac disease. Periodic monitoring of serum levels of sodium, potassium, chloride, calcium, phosphorus, and magnesium detects the most frequent electrolyte abnormalities.

Deficiencies of Trace Minerals

Deficiencies of trace minerals may appear in patients on long-term TF. Clinically relevant zinc deficiency has been noted. Zinc deficiency is especially likely in patients with zinc loss from the GI tract, as in active Crohn disease. Patients receiving defined formulas as their only source of nutrition for prolonged periods must be observed for micronutrient deficiencies.

Hyperosmolarity Syndrome

Hyperosmolarity syndrome is an uncommon complication resulting from inadequate intake of free water despite continuous ingestion of a high osmotic load. The clinical syndrome includes lethargy, obtundation, appearance of dehydration, and at times fever. Serum electrolytes reveal hypernatremia and hyperosmolarity. The treatment includes increasing daily free water by supplementing the usual routine with water. IV 5% dextrose in water or 0.45% sodium chloride solution may be necessary, as in the management of hypernatremia, if changes in mental status are significant.

Refeeding Syndrome

Refeeding syndrome may develop when patients who are severely malnourished are begun on enteral (or parenteral) nutrition. With refeeding, potassium, phosphate, and magnesium move from the extracellular to the intracellular space, causing hypokalemia, hypophosphatemia, and hypomagnesemia. Patients with decreased levels should be repleted before the start of feeding. Serum magnesium, potassium, and phosphate levels should be monitored carefully in all patients who are being refed (see Table 5-27).

Warfarin Resistance

Warfarin resistance may result from the unsuspected delivery of vitamin K in enteral supplements or feeding formulas. The estimated safe and adequate daily intake of vitamin K is 70 to 140 µg, yet the average diet in the United States contains 300 to 500 µg of this vitamin. Warfarin resistance is an uncommon development with the vitamin K content of currently available products.

Nonmetabolic Complications

Diarrhea and Constipation

Diarrhea and constipation are common complications of enteral feeding, occurring in as many as 20% of patients. Steps to take with troubleshooting diarrhea and constipation are outlined in Table 10-13. The incidence of diarrhea in TF depends on the definition of diarrhea. If diarrhea is defined broadly (one or more liquid stools per day), the incidence in tube-fed patients is more than 70%; if a more stringent definition is used (four or more liquid stools per day or five or more stools per day), the incidence falls to 21% (122).

Esophagitis or Esophageal Ulcer

Nasally placed tubes can cause esophagitis by directly irritating the esophageal mucosa and by interfering with normal protective mechanisms against esophageal damage by gastric acid. Competence of the lower esophageal sphincter, normal esophageal stripping by primary and secondary peristalsis, and swallowing of saliva all appear to help prevent reflux esophagitis in normal persons; and all these mechanisms may be impaired in patients with feeding tubes.

Complications

Very rare complications include small-bowel perforation, pneumatosis intestinalis, rupture and division of the feeding tube, and inadvertent IV administration of the formula. Bronchopulmonary complications, including perforation of the lung, can occur if a stylet is used and the tube inadvertently enters the trachea during placement. This complication can occur even in the presence of an inflated tracheostomy tube cuff.

ADMINISTERING MEDICATIONS THROUGH FEEDING TUBES

For many patients with feeding tubes, especially those at home or in extended-care facilities, the tube is the only practical avenue for administering medications. However, not all medications can be administered successfully by feeding tube. Some general guidelines have been developed, but the guidelines may not be applicable to certain combinations of drugs, enteral formula, and feeding tube.

TABLE 10-13 Troubleshooting Tube-Feeding Complications of Diarrhea or Constipation

Diarrhea

First quantify the diarrhea; a tube-fed patient may experience 4–5, moderate amount, loose- to soft-formed stools per day normally. If the patient is experiencing diarrhea or an increase in their normal stooling, try the following:

1. Review all medications: Often when enteral access is obtained, medicines are changed to the enteral route. If the diarrhea is severe, change medicines to IV form at least as a trial. Medications that may contribute to diarrhea include antibiotics, antineoplastics, magnesium-containing antacids, potassium and phosphate supplements, laxatives, medications with sorbitol base (i.e., theophylline), and colchicine.
2. Check for *Clostridium difficile*.
3. Try adding fiber (i.e., Benefiber^R 1 tbsp t.i.d.).
4. If infusing a hypertonic formula, change to an isotonic product.
5. Once infectious causes are ruled out (and bowel surgery patients are at least 10–14 days post-op) and if diarrhea persists, try an antidiarrheal agent on a routine dose: loperamide 2 mg q 6 hours, increase to 4 mg q 6 hours if diarrhea persists.
6. KEEP FEEDING!!!

Constipation

Constipation is defined as no bowel movement for >3 days after tube feedings are at goal or difficulty passing stools.

1. Check for signs of dehydration—increased Na, Cl, BUN; dark and/or decreased amount of urine—if present, increase amount of water flush.
2. Try adding fiber.
3. Start patient on docusate 100 mg/day.
4. Rectal examination.
5. Bisacodyl suppository prn.

BUN, blood urea nitrogen; IV, intravenous; prn, as needed; t.i.d., three times per day; tbsp, table-spoon.

The Tube

The location of the tube must be considered. Drugs administered beyond the pylorus are absorbed more rapidly. Antacids and Carafate should not be delivered beyond the pylorus. The diameter of the tube must be considered. The smaller the diameter, the more likely it is to become clogged. Thick liquids such as antacids should not be administered through a tube with a diameter smaller than 10 F.

The Drug

1. Slow-release drugs (e.g., Calan SR, Cardizem, Isordil Tembid) and enteric-coated drugs (e.g., MI-Cebrin, Azulfidine EN-tabs) should not be crushed because crushing may increase the rate of absorption (for slow-release formulations), expose the drug to degradation in the stomach, or cause gastric upset.
2. Pancreatic enzymes (e.g., pancreas) are usually enteric-coated. If they are crushed and administered by NGT, they can be inactivated by gastric acid. However, powdered Viokace may be mixed in 30 mL of water and administered via the feeding tube.
3. The use of liquid preparations is generally preferable to crushing and dissolving tablets. A liquid formulation of a drug should be used if it is available.

Administration

1. Crushed tablets should be reconstituted in at least 10 to 15 mL of water.
2. Hard gelatin capsules should be opened and the powder dissolved in at least 10 to 15 mL of water.
3. Drugs that are hypertonic or that irritate the GI mucosa should be dissolved in larger volumes of water before administration.

4. Drugs should not be added to the enteral formula.
5. The enteral formula should be stopped before medication is administered.
6. The feeding tube should be flushed with water to remove residual formula before medication is administered.
7. The feeding tube should be flushed with water (10 to 30 mL) after the drug is administered.
8. For patients on intermittent gastric feeding schedules, the timing of administration of medications that should be taken on a full or empty stomach should be adjusted according to the patient's feeding schedule.

Drugs with Specific Requirements

The absorption of several medications may be impaired when given via the enteral feeding access (Table 10-14) (123–128). To decrease this effect, the TF should be held for 1 hour before and after the time of medication dosing if possible (126). In addition, when applicable, blood levels of medication should be monitored. Many medications may form a precipitate when combined with enteral formula and clog the feeding tube (Table 10-14) (127). If at all possible, these medications should be given via a separate enteral access or with adequate tube flushing before and after administration to prevent clogging. In the event the feeding tube becomes occluded, a review of the literature suggests warm sterile water should be used first in an attempt to unclog the tube due to proven efficacy, low cost, and lack of adverse effects (128,129). Powdered Viokace (pancreatic enzyme) mixed with bicarbonate has also been shown to be efficacious (128). Carbonated beverages or cranberry juice have not been proven to be beneficial (128). The use of commercial products containing papain along with digestive enzymes has been successful; however, these are costly (129). Mechanical products designed to remove a clog whether caused by enteral formula or medications are also available. A flexible catheter of some type is inserted into the tube to dislodge the obstruction. These products are designed for single use and may also be costly (128).

Patients receiving medications with a high sorbitol content (Table 10-14) should be monitored closely for diarrhea, abdominal cramping, and bloating. Any medications given directly into the small bowel should be diluted with water prior to administration, given the lack of a reservoir and the potential for ulceration (127,128). Given the increased usage of enteral feeding in the hospital setting and the potential for errors, a quality improvement effort may lead to decreased morbidity as well and should be considered for implementation.

PANCREATIC DISEASE
Chronic Pancreatitis

Chronic pancreatitis is a chronic irreversible inflammatory process of the pancreas that may lead to fibrosis with calcification (129). Eventually, the patient will experience impairment of endocrine and exocrine function of the pancreas. The patient with chronic pancreatitis generally presents with chronic abdominal pain and normal or mildly elevated pancreatic enzyme levels. Diabetes mellitus and steatorrhea will present as the pancreas loses its endocrine and exocrine function (129). Fat malabsorption does not become significant until lipase output is less than 10% of normal, and consequently, a considerable portion of the gland must be destroyed before fat malabsorption is clinically recognized (130,131). Steatorrhea usually occurs prior to protein deficiencies since lipolytic activity decreases faster than proteolytic activity. The Toxic-Metabolic, Idiopathic, Genetic, Autoimmune, Recurrent and Severe Acute Pancreatitis, Obstructive (TIGAR-O) classification system is used to categorize causes and associated factors of chronic pancreatitis (130). In the United States, one of the most common etiologies of exocrine pancreatic insufficiency in adults is alcoholism (129). Abstinence from alcohol, dietary modifications, and pancreatic enzyme supplementation are sufficient in over 80% of patients with chronic pancreatitis (132).

Diet

A diet low in fat (50 to 70 g per day) and high in protein (1.0 to 1.5 g per kg) and complex carbohydrates provided over six small meals should be tried initially in patients with steatorrhea (132). Adequate nutritional therapy combined with pain management may have a positive effect on nutritional status by allowing for increased caloric intake after an attenuation of postprandial pain. If steatorrhea persists, fat intake should be reduced to 0.5 g//kg/day and pancreatic enzymes initiated (Table 10-15). The largest groups of patients in need of these enzymes are

TABLE 10-14 Potential Medication and Enteral Feeding Interactions

Medications That Cause Precipitates and May Clog Feeding Tubes (≤10 French)
Brompheniramine/phenylephrine (Dimetane)
Brompheniramine/phenylpropanolamine (Dimetapp)
Calcium glubionate (Neo-calglucon)
Chlorpromazine (Thorazine Concentrate)
Clarithromycin (Biaxin)
Ferrous sulfate (Feosol)
Guaifenisin (Robitussion products)
Lithium citrate (Cibalith-S)
Lansoprazole (Prevacid)
MCT oil—separates and clogs tube
Metoclopramide (Reglan)
Monobasic sodium phosphate (Fleet Phospho-Soda)
Opium tincture (Paragoric)
Potassium chloride
Pseudoephedrine (Sudafed)
Sodium biphosphate (Fleets Phospho-Soda)
Thioridazine (Mellaril Concentrate)
Zinc sulfate capsules

Medications That Have Increased or Decreased Bioavailability When Given with Enteral Feeding
Alendronate—decreases absorption
Carbamazepine (Tegretol)—May bind with tube and have 10% to 20% loss of medication. Flushing with NS decreases this interaction
Ciprofloxin (Cipro) (Possibly other quinolones such as levofloxacin, etc.)—inactivates medication
Ketoconazole—inactivates medication
Itraconazole (Sporonax)—inactivates medication
Levodopa (Sinemet)
Phenytoin (Dilantin)—inactivates medication
Quinolones—reduce serum levels
Theophylline (Theolair)—inactivates medication
Tetracycline

Medications Containing High Levels of Sorbitol
Acetaminophen elixir
Aluminum hydroxide gel
Aluminum hydroxide/magnesium carbonate (Gaviscon)
Aluminum hydroxide/magnesium hydroxide (Maalox)
Amantadine H Cl (Amantadine)
Aminocaproic acid (Amicar)
Carbamazepine (Tegretrol)
Charcoal, activated (Actidose with sorbitol)
Guaifenesin/dextromethorphan syrup (Mucinex DM)
Lithium citrate syrup
Phenylephrine hydrochloride/brompheniramine maleate elixir
Pseudoephedrine syrup (Sudafed)
Sodium polystyrene sulfonate suspension (kayexalate)
Tetracycline hydrochloride suspension
Theophylline oral solution

TABLE 10-15 Pancreatic Enzyme Preparations[a]

	Lipase (Units)	Amylase (Units)	Protease (Units)	Distributor
Pancrelipase Products				
Delayed-release capsules				
Enteric-Coated Minimicrospheres				
Creon 6000	6,000	30,000	19,000	Abbott
Creon 12000	12,000	60,000	38,000	Abbott
Creon 24000	24,000	1,20,000	76,000	Abbott
Enteric-Coatedminitablets				
Ultresa 13800	13,800	27,600	27,600	Aptalis
Ultresa 20700	20,700	46,000	41,400	Aptalis
Ultresa 23000	23,000	46,000	41,400	Aptalis
Enteric-Coated Beads				
Zenpep 3000	3,000	16,000	10,000	Eurand
Zenpep 5000	5,000	27,000	17,000	Eurand
Zenpep 10000	10,000	55,000	34,000	Eurand
Zenpep 15000	15,000	82,000	51,000	Eurand
Zenpep 20000	20,000	1,09,000	68,000	Eurand
Zenpep 25000	25,000	1,36,000	85,000	Eurand
Pancrealipase	5,000	17,000	27,000	X-Gen
Enteric-Coatedmicrotablets				
Pancreaze 4200	4,200	17,500	10,000	McNeil Peds
Pancreaze 16800	16,800	70,000	40,000	McNeil Peds
Pancreaze 21000	21,000	61,000	37,000	McNeil Peds
Pertzye 8000	8,000	28,750	30,250	Digestive Care
Pertzye 16000	16,000	57,500	60,500	Digestive Care
Non-Enteric-Coated Tablets				
Viokace	10,440	39,150	39,150	Aptalis
Viokace	20,880	78,300	78,300	Aptalis

[a]This is not meant to be a complete listing. Products may have changed since this list was compiled.

those with the diagnosis of cystic fibrosis. The intake of fat can be liberalized (to 30% of calories) as control of diarrhea with supplemental enzymes is achieved. If steatorrhea is persistent, then MCTs can be administered to provide approximately 400 calories per day (~4 tbsp per day). However, MCTs are not very palatable and may induce abdominal pain and diarrhea at higher doses, making it difficult to determine when the chronic pancreatitis symptoms are subsiding. Protein supplementation via oral supplements is generally recommended because the intake of dietary protein is restricted along with the intake of fat. TF is indicated only if the patient cannot ingest enough calories for weight maintenance.

Enzyme Replacement

Enzyme replacement is used to aid digestion in patients with pancreatic enzyme deficiency. Several commercial preparations exist (Table 10-15). Pancrelipase is a lipase-enriched extract. Tablets, capsules, and enteric-coated preparations may all be effective in reducing or abolishing steatorrhea if adequate amounts of enzymes are supplied. Approximately 30,000 IU of lipase must be taken with each meal to eliminate steatorrhea completely, and even then enzyme is inactivated by gastric acid. Taking all the tablets at once with a meal is as effective as taking them intermittently with and after a meal. The usual doses of products with in vitro enzyme activity that can be given to reduce steatorrhea are given in Table 10-15.

Vitamin Supplementation

Fat-soluble vitamin supplementation is rarely needed once the previously mentioned measures are taken to reduce steatorrhea because the concentrations of bile acids required to solubilize the fat-soluble vitamins are usually normal. Moreover, the fat-soluble vitamins do not depend on pancreatic hydrolysis for absorption. Vitamin B_{12} deficiency can result from pancreatic insufficiency. Pancreatic proteolytic enzymes are needed to digest haptocorrin and so liberate ingested cobalamin and bind to intrinsic factor. Enzyme supplementation partially corrects this error, but vitamin B_{12} supplements should still be given to ensure that chronic neural damage does not develop.

Acute Pancreatitis

Acute pancreatitis is an earlier pathological stage than chronic pancreatitis. In acute pancreatitis, inflammation exists even between clinical episodes, but acinar and endocrine cell function is preserved. In acute pancreatitis, the patient presents with acute and severe abdominal pain, nausea, and vomiting. The pancreas is acutely inflamed (neutrophils and edema), and the serum levels of pancreatic enzymes (amylase and lipase) are elevated. The severity of acute pancreatitis is classified by the Atlanta criteria (133). Approximately 80% of the patients have mild disease associated with minimal or no organ dysfunction or necrosis (134). These patients are usually managed with analgesics, IV fluids, and NPO status for 5 to 7 days, after which they are generally able to resume an oral low-fat (<30% of calories) diet. Typically, nutritional management is not required in this patient subset. In the most severe cases, mortality can rise to 25% to 50% with infected necrosis (134,21). Historically, it was believed enteral nutrition was harmful secondary to stimulation of the exocrine pancreatic secretion. This was considered a risk for exacerbating the autodigestive process. In animals, enteral nutrition was found to be superior to parenteral nutrition in maintaining the gut barrier by helping to modify the lactulose/mannitol ration, lower the plasma endotoxin level, maintain the normal gut microbiota, and decrease the risk of bacterial translocation (135). Theoretically, by maintaining the gut barrier and, consequently, the immune function, the patient is at a decreased risk for infectious complications. A recent meta-analysis found that enteral nutrition started within 48 hours of admission for severe acute pancreatitis leads to a significant reduction in infections, hyperglycemia, length of hospital stay, and mortality (136).

Diet

In severe necrotizing pancreatitis, 80% of the patients are catabolic with high energy expenditure (137). In all likelihood, these patients will be unable to consume an oral low-fat diet without pain within 5 to 7 days. In one study, previously healthy men who developed severe pancreatitis who were not fed for at least 5 days developed decreased muscle function proportional to decreased protein stores (138). This, combined with the SCCM/ASPEN recommendations to provide nutrition support to patients expected to have a prolonged NPO status of greater than 7 days, suggests nutrition support should be instituted when the patient is hemodynamically stable. Two landmark trials and a recent observation study comparing enteral with parenteral nutrition in patients with severe acute pancreatitis found enteral nutrition significantly attenuated the acute phase response in these patients when compared with parenteral nutrition, and led to a decrease in infectious complications (138–140). Several other authors have demonstrated the benefit of enteral nutrition (delivered in the jejunum) over parenteral nutrition or NPO status in these patients (141–144) as well. Caloric provision, combined with a higher infection rate in TPN-treated patients, may be the reason for the improved results. The preferred site to deliver enteral feeds, the jejunum, is based on the theoretical benefit that decreasing pancreatic enzyme and bicarbonate secretion stimulation will be associated with jejunal feeding and that such a decrease will have clinical benefit. However, in a recent study, tolerance was demonstrated in patients fed into the stomach (22). Most of the trials mentioned previously provided peptide-based enteral formulations, although one of the more recent trials demonstrated tolerance with a polymeric formula (143). At present, the following recommendations can be made based on the evidence:

1. Small-bowel feeding is as safe as gastric feeding, and is well tolerated, but clinical outcomes may not be improved.
2. Obtain small-bowel feeding access, if easily done. Do not persist in attempting small-bowel access, as gastric feeding is an equally valid alternative.
3. Begin enteral feeds utilizing a peptide-based product at a slow rate of 10 to 20 mL per hour as soon as the patient is hemodynamically stable.
4. Advance the enteral feeds slowly over 48 hours to the patient's goal rate.
5. Most patients' needs can be met by providing 25 to 30 calories per kg and 1.0 to 1.5 g per kg protein.

SHORT-BOWEL SYNDROME

SBS, which usually results from extensive small-bowel resection, is not strictly defined. Several potential nutritional consequences exist in SBS, including malabsorption of fluid, electrolytes, minerals, and other essential nutrients, which may lead to malnutrition and dehydration. The degree to which nutrition support will be required depends on the extent and site of the surgical resection, the underlying disease, and level of intestinal adaptation in the remaining bowel (145,18). Massive surgical resection of diseased, ischemic small bowel (arterial or venous occlusion, strangulation in hernia, volvulus) is the leading cause of the most severe form of the syndrome. Gradual "whittling away" of the small intestine with multiple resections for Crohn disease (146,147), on the other hand, is a common cause of the less-severe clinical picture. Parenteral nutrition is the mainstay of treatment in SBS with severe malabsorption. Patients who require long-term parenteral nutrition experience complications, which contribute to morbidity and mortality (18). Therefore, any therapies that decrease reliance on parenteral nutrition are of benefit to the patient. In less severe cases, maintenance of adequate protein and calorie balance is the only major problem, which can generally be overcome by oral supplementation.

Intestinal Adaptation after Massive Resection

Intestinal adaptation after massive resection is highly individualized, and maximal adaptation may take up to 2 years (145,18). Enteral nutrition is essential to aid in maximal adaptation. However, most patients with SBS will require at least short-term TPN during the initial postoperative period, the initial adaptation phase. The ability of the bowel to adapt will depend on a number of things.

1. The length of remaining bowel: greater than 50% usually requires no significant intervention; 25% to 50% often requires dietary modifications, antimotility agents, and vitamin and mineral supplementation; less than 25% will most likely require long-term parenteral nutrition or intestinal transplantation (145,18,147–149).
2. The presence of the colon: while malabsorption of energy can be an issue in patients with or without a colon, those without do not derive energy from anaerobic bacterial fermentation of carbohydrate to the short-chain fatty acids, which has been shown to provide 5% to 10% of energy in healthy subjects (150). In addition, the colon aids with fluid and electrolyte reabsorption.
3. The presence of the ileocecal valve, which acts as the "ileal brake," slowing transit time (148). Patients lacking this valve may have a higher requirement for antimotility medications.

Initiate TPN

To prevent nutritional deterioration during the restoration of electrolyte and water balance, TPN should be initiated. Gradual attempts at enteral feeding can be made while the functional capacity of the remaining bowel is assessed. The major objective of nutrition support in SBS is to reduce or eliminate the need for parenteral nutrition. Recently, a recombinant human GLP-2 analog (teduglutide) was approved in the United States for the treatment of adults with SBS who are dependent on parenteral nutrition (18). In clinical studies, teduglutide was shown to increase villus height and crypt depth, improving intestinal absorption (151).

Monitor

Monitor serum electrolytes, calcium, phosphorus, and magnesium regularly. Calcium supplementation in Crohn disease patients with SBS who have been on steroids for long periods of time is essential, given their increased risk for bone fractures, osteopenia, and osteoporosis at baseline (146). Patients with SBS may have significant losses of zinc and selenium, requiring additional supplementation (18,149). In addition, these patients may develop magnesium deficiencies while maintaining a normal serum concentration; therefore, measurement of 24-hour urine magnesium levels may be beneficial (152).

Following Adaptation after Massive Resection, or for Long-Term Management of Less Severe SBS

Diet Therapy

In general, food should be provided over 5 to 6 small meals per day. Depending on the amount of malabsorption, 130% to 150% of estimated caloric and protein needs may be necessary. Fluid intake should exceed stool losses to maintain hydration. Complex carbohydrates are preferred to simple carbohydrates, since simple carbohydrates will increase the hyperosmolar load in the intestine and therefore decrease the fluid absorption.

High-Carbohydrate, Low-fat Diet

A high-carbohydrate (60%), low-fat (20%) diet in patients with SBS and a normally functioning colon leads to a significant (P <0.001) increase in energy absorption compared with patients fed an isocaloric low-carbohydrate (20%), high-fat (60%) diet (153). No difference in caloric absorption was noted between the two diets when given to SBS patients without a colon. Patients with a colon have a higher risk of developing calcium oxalate renal stones and may benefit from a low-oxalate diet.

Patients with an Ileostomy or a Jejunostomy

Patients with an ileostomy or jejunostomy are more likely to experience deficiencies in fluid, electrolyte, vitamin, and mineral status. These should be monitored frequently and supplementation adjusted as needed. Vitamin and mineral supplementation is important, especially in patients not receiving parenteral nutrition. Specific supplementation will depend on the remaining bowel; potential requirements are presented in Table 10-16. If ≥60 cm of terminal ileum is resected, a vitamin B_{12} deficiency, is likely and supplementation should be started.

Lactose

Lactose is restricted initially until the symptoms are under best control. Liberalization with monitoring of the clinical response is then appropriate.

Enteral Feeding

Enteral feeding during both the adaptation and postadaptation periods is feasible. It has been suggested that a peptide-based product may be more readily absorbed than one with intact protein in patients with SBS. While a few small studies support this conclusion, none found a significantly increased absorption of energy, fat, electrolytes, fluid, or minerals (35,154,155). Enteral TFs should be provided continuously in the stomach to increase the contact time between the luminal nutrients and the intestinal mucosa allowing for maximal absorption.

TABLE 10-16 Vitamin and Mineral Supplementation in Short-Bowel Syndrome (152,168)

Supplement (Representative Product)	Dose	Route
Prenatal multivitamin with minerals[a]	1 tab q day	PO
Vitamin D[a]	1,600 U DHT daily	PO
Calcium[a]	300–800 mg elemental daily	PO
Vitamin B_{12}[b]	1 mg q day	PO/nasally
	100–500 µg q 1–2 mo	SC
Vitamin A[b]	5,000–20,000 U q day	PO
Vitamin K[b]	5 mg/day	PO
(Mephyton; AquaMEPHYTON)	5–10 mg/wk	SC
Vitamin E[b] (Aquasol E(®))	30–400 IU/day	PO
Magnesium gluconate[b] (Magonate(®) or magnesium oxide capsules (URO-MAG)	50–500 mg elemental daily	PO
Magnesium sulfate[b]	290 mg elemental 1–3 times/week	IM/IV
Zinc sulfate[b]	220–440 mg/day	PO
Selenium[b]	60–100 µg/day	PO
Ferrous sulfate[b,c]	60 mg elemental iron t.i.d.	PO
Iron dextran[b,c]	≤100 mg elemental iron per day based on formula or table	IV

[a]Recommended routinely for all patients.
[b]Recommended for patients with documented nutrient deficiency or malabsorption.
[c]For a more complete list of iron supplements, see Table 7-39 (Oral) and Table 7-41 (Parenteral)
DHT, dihydrotachysterol; IM, instramuscular; IV, intravenous; PO, oral; SC, subcutaneous.

TABLE 10-17 Oral Rehydration Solutions

Product	Na meq/L	K meq/L	Cl meq/L	Citrate meq/L	kcal/L	CHO g/L	mOsm
CeraLyte 70(®)[a]	70	20	98	30	165	40	235
CeraLyte 90(®)[a]	90	20	98	30	165	40	260
Gatorade(®)[b]	20	3	N/A	N/A	210	45	330
WHO	90	20	80	30	80	20	200
Washington University	102	3	75	10	75	18	260

[a]Cumberland Pharmaceuticals, Nashville, TN.
[b]Not to be used as an oral rehydration solution—included for comparison purposes alone.

Home Recipes
WHO (World Health Organization) formula: Mix 3/4 tsp sodium chloride, 1/2 tsp sodium citrate, 1/4 tsp potassium chloride, and 4 tsp glucose (dextrose) in 1 L (4 1/4 cups) of distilled water.
Washington University formula: Mix 3/4 tsp sodium chloride + 2 tsp sodium citrate + 32 oz bottle of G2 Gatorade. Mix formulas with sugar-free flavorings as needed for palatability.

Oral Rehydration Solutions

Oral rehydration solutions (ORSs) (Table 10-17) may aid with sodium and fluid absorption by taking advantage of both the passive and the active transport of sodium in the jejunum (in Chapter 7, see Table 7-10 for a list of products) (156). Maximal absorption is achieved with a solution containing 120 mmol per L of sodium; however, if the patient finds this unpalatable, a 90 mmol per L solution can be tried. ORSs are encouraged over restricted sugar-containing beverages (hyperosmotic) and hypoosmotic solutions, such as water. Hypo- and hyperosmotic solutions in large amounts will lead to increased diarrhea, and thus increased fluid and electrolyte losses. For best results, fluids should be taken in small amounts between meals throughout the day to avoid dumping syndrome (increased bowel movements shortly after eating) (157).

Adjunctive Medications

These can prove useful in the management of patients with SBS.

Antimotility Agents

Antimotility agents will be useful in helping to reduce food-induced diarrhea. An example approach is as follows:

Begin with 2 mg of loperamide every 6 hours, gradually increasing the dosage up to 10 mg every 6 hours if needed. If this approach is unsuccessful, discontinue the loperamide and start 3 drops (0.15 ml) of deodorized tincture of opium 4 times per day, increasing to 15 drops (0.75 ml) per dose as needed. If the deodorized tincture of opium alone is unsuccessful, clonidine may be tried, starting at 0.05 mg b.i.d., increasing to a maximum of 0.15 mg b.i.d. Case reports have demonstrated the successful use of clonidine in patients with SBS (158).

Control Gastric Hypersecretion

About 50% of patients who have undergone massive resection have transient gastric hypersecretion that can result in severe peptic ulcer disease. The mechanism is unclear but is felt to be hormonal (loss of an inhibitory control mechanism). Proton-pump inhibitors or histamine$_2$-receptor antagonists may be required for 6 months after surgery (148).

If the fluid losses exceed 3 L per day, the use of long-acting somatostatin analog octreotide may be useful to decrease secretory diarrhea. However, studies in animals suggest that octreotide may impair intestinal adaptation (159,160).

REFERENCES

1. Druyan ME, Compher C, Boullata JI, et al; American Society of Parenteral and Enteral Nutrition. Clinical guidelines for the use of parenteral and enteral nutrition in adult and pediatric patients: applying the GRADE system to development of A.S.P.E.N. clinical guidelines. *JPEN J Parenter Enteral Nutr.* 2012;36:77.

2. van den Berg MG, Rutten H, Rasmussen-Conrad EL, et al. Nutritional status, food intake, and dysphagia in long-term survivors with head and neck cancer treated with chemoradiotherapy: a cross-sectional study. *Head Neck*. 2014;36:60.
3. Langlus JA, Zandbergen MC, Eerenstein SE, et al. Effect of nutritional interventions on nutritional status, quality of life and mortality in patients with head and neck cancer receiving (chemo) radiotherapy: a systematic review. *Clin Nutr*. 2013;32:671.
4. Dennis MS, Lewis SC, Warlow C; The Food TrialCollaboration. Routine oral nutritional supplementation for stroke patients in hospital (FOOD): a multicentre randomised controlled trial. *Lancet*. 2005; 365(9461):755.
5. Lassen K, Coolsen MM, Slim K, et al; ERAS⁻ Society; European Society for Clinical Nutrition and Metabolism; Interanational Association for Surgical Metabolism and Nutrition. Guidelines for perioperative care for pancreaticoduodenectomy: Enhanced Recovery After Surgery (ERAS⁻) Society recommendations. *Clin Nutr*. 2012;31:817.
6. Gustafsson UO, Scott MJ, Schwenk W, et al. ERAS® Society. Guidelines for perioperative care in elective colonic surgery: Enhanced Recovery After Surgery (ERAS®) Society recommendations. *Clin Nutr*. 2012;31:783.
7. Norman K, Pirlich M, Smoliner C, et al. Cost-effectiveness of a 3- month intervention with oral nutritional supplements in disease-related malnutrition: a randomized controlled pilot study. *Eur J Clin Nutr*. 2011;65:735.
8. Lope-Vargas P, Tong A, Sureshkumar P, et al. Prevention, detection and management of early chronic kidney disease: a systematic review of clinical practice guidelines. *Nephrology*. 2013;18:592.
9. Menon V, Kopple JD, Wang X, et al. Effect of a very low-protein diet on outcomes: long-term follow-up of the Modification of Diet in Renal Disease (MDRD) study. *Am J Kidney Dis*. 2009;53:208.
10. Kopple JD. National kidney foundation Kidney Disease Outcomes Quality Initiative clinical practice guidelines for nutrition in chronic renal failure. *Am J Kidney Dis*. 2001;37(Suppl 2):S66.
11. Cano N, Fiaccadori E, Tesinsky P, et al. ESPEN Guidelines on enteral nutrition: adult renal failure. *Clin Nutr*. 2006;25:295.
12. Dowell SA, Welch JL. Use of electronic self-monitoring for food and fluid intake: a pilot study. *Nephrol Nurs J*. 2006;33:271.
13. Kawaguchi T, Shiraishi K, Suzuki K, et al. Branched-chain amino acids prevent hepatocarcinogenesis and prolong survival of patients with cirrhosis. *Clin Gastroenterol Hepatol*. 2014;12:1012.
14. Marchesini G, Bianchi G, Merli M, et al. Nutritional supplementation with branched-chain amino acids in advanced cirrhosis: a double-blind, randomized trial. *Gastroenterology*. 2003;124:1792.
15. Wright SJ, Daniells S, Keogh GW. Fistuloclysis: a high-calorie, polymeric formula can be successful. *JPEN J Parenter Enteral Nutr*. 2013;37:550.
16. Teubner A, Morrison HR, Ravishankar ID, et al. Fistuloclysis can successfully replace parenteral feeding in the nutritional support of patients with enterocutaneous fistula. *Br J Surg*. 2004;91:625.
17. Jeejeebhoy KN. Management of short bowel syndrome: avoidance of total parenteral nutrition. *Gastroenterology*. 2006;130(2 Suppl 1):S60.
18. Kelly DG, Tappenden KA, Winkler MF. Short bowel syndrome: highlights of patient management, quality of life and survival. *JPEN J Parenter Enteral Nutr*. 2014;38:427.
19. Guo Z, Wu R, Shu W, et al. Effect of exclusive enteral nutrition on health-related quality of life for adults with active Crohn's disease. *Nutr Clin Pract*. 2013;28:499.
20. Soo J, Malik BA, Turner JM, et al. Use of exclusive enteral nutrition is just as effective as corticosteroids in newly diagnosed pediatric Crohn's disease. *Dig Dis Sci*. 2013;58:3584.
21. Tenner S, Baillie J, DeWitt J, et al; American College of Gastroenterology. American College of Gastroenterology guideline: management of acute pancreatitis. *Am J Gastroenterol*. 2013;108:1400.
22. Chang YS, Fu HQ, Xiao YM, et al. Nasogastric or nasojejunal feeding in predicted severe acute pancreatitis: a meta-analysis. *Crit Care*. 2013;17(3):R118.
23. Wereszczynska-Siemiatkowska U, Swidnicka-Siergiejko A, Siemiatkowski A, et al. Early enteral nutrition is superior to delayed enteral nutrition for the prevention of infected necrosis and mortality in acute pancreatitis. *Pancreas*. 2013;42:640.
24. Nathens AB, Curtis JR, Beale RJ, et al. Management of the critically ill patient with severe acute pancreatitis. *Crit Care Med*. 2004;32:2524.
25. Meier R, Ockenga J, Pertkiewicz M, et al. ESPEN guidelines on enteral nutrition: pancreas. *Clin Nutr*. 2006;25:275.
26. Pennington JA, Spungen JS. *Bowes & Church's Food Values of Portions Commonly Used*. 19th ed. New York: Lippincott Williams and Wilkins, 2010.

27. Harig JM, Soergel KH, Komorowski RA, et al. Treatment of diversion colitis with short-chain fatty acid irrigation. *N Engl J Med.* 1989;320:23.
28. Koecher KJ, Thomas W, Slavin JL. Healthy subjects experience bowel changes on enteral diets; addition of a fiber blend attenuates stool weight and gut bacteria decreases without changes in gas. *JPEN J Parenter Enteral Nutr.* 2013 (Nov. 14).
29. Hua Z, Turner JM, Mager DR, et al. Effects of polymeric formula vs elemental formula in neonatal piglets with short bowel syndrome. *JPEN J Parenter Enteral Nutr.* 2014;38:498.
30. Silk DB, Fairclough PD, Clark ML, et al. Use of a peptide rather than free amino acid nitrogen source in chemically defined "elemental" diets. *JPEN J Parenter Enteral Nutr.* 1980;4:548.
31. Silk DB. Digestion and absorption of dietary protein in man. *Proc Nutr Soc.* 1980;39:61.
32. Ksiazyk J, Piena M, Kierkus J, et al. Hydrolyzed versus nonhydrolyzed protein diet in short bowel syndrome in children. *J Pediatr Gastroenterol Nutr.* 2002;35:615.
33. Rees RG, Hare WR, Grimble GK, et al. Do patients with moderately impaired gastrointestinal function requiring enteral nutrition need a predigested nitrogen source? A prospective crossover controlled clinical trial. *Gut.* 1992;33:877.
34. Brinson RR, Hanumanthu SK, Pitts WM. A reappraisal of the peptide-based enteral formulas: clinical applications. *Nutr Clin Pract.* 1989;4:211.
35. Cosnes J, Evard D, Beaugerie L, et al. Improvement in protein absorption with a small-peptide-based diet in patients with high jejunostomy. *Nutrition.* 1992;8:406.
36. Tiengou LE, Gloro R, Pouzoulet J, et al. Semi-elemental formula or polymeric formula: is there a better choice for enteral nutrition in acute pancreatitis? Randomized comparative study. *JPEN J Parenter Enteral Nutr.* 2006;30:1.
37. Lochs H, Dejong C, Hammarqvist F, et al. ESPEN Guidelines on Enteral Nutrition: Gastroenterology. *Clin Nutr.* 2006;25:260.
38. Russell MK, Andrews MR, Brewer CK, et al. Standards for specialized nutrition support: adult hospitalized patients. *Nutr Clin Pract.* 2002;17:384.
39. Russell MK, Charney P. Is there a role for specialized enteral nutrition in the intensive care unit? *Nutr Clin Pract.* 2002;17:156.
40. Malone AM. The clinical benefits and efficacy of using specialized enteral feeding formulas. *Support Line.* 2002;24:3.
41. Pontes-Arruda A, Aragao AM, Albuquerque JD. Effects of enteral feeding with eicosapentaenoic acid, gamma-linolenic acid, and antioxidants in mechanically ventilated patients with severe sepsis and septic shock. *Crit Care Med.* 2006;34:2325.
42. Gadek JE, DeMichele SJ, Karlstad MD, et al; Enteral Nutrition in ARDS Study Group. Effect of enteral feeding with eicosapentaenoic acid, gamma-linolenic acid, and antioxidants in patients with acute respiratory distress syndrome. *Crit Care Med.* 1999;27:1409.
43. Pacht ER, DeMichele SJ, Nelson JL, et al. Enteral nutrition with eicosapentaenoic acid, gamma-linolenic acid, and antioxidants reduces alveolar inflammatory mediators and protein influx in patients with acute respiratory distress syndrome. *Crit Care Med.* 2003;31:491.
44. Singer P, Theilla M, Fisher H, et al. Benefit of an enteral diet enriched with eicosapentaenoic acid and gamma-linolenic acid in ventilated patients with acute lung injury. *Crit Care Med.* 2006;34:1033.
45. Rice TW, Wheeler AP, Thompson BT, et al. Enteral omega-3 fatty acid, gamma-linolenic acid, and antioxidant supplementation in acute lung injury. *JAMA.* 2011;306:1574.
46. Zhang FK, Zhang JY, Jia JD. Treatment of patients with alcoholic liver disease. *Hepatobiliary Pancreat Dis Int.* 2005;4:12.
47. American Diabetes Association. Standards of Medical Care in Diabetes 2012. *Diabetes Care.* 2012; 35(Suppl 1):S11.
48. Inzucchi SE, Bergenstal RM, Buse JB, et al. Management of hyperglycemia in type 2 diabetes: a patient-centered approach: position statement of the American Diabetes Association and the European Association for the Study of Diabetes. *Diabetes Care.* 2012;35:1364.
49. Ceriello A, Lansink M, Rouws CH, et al. Administration of a new diabetes-specific enteral formula results in an improved 24h glucose profile in type 2 diabetic patients. *Diabetes Res Clin Pract.* 2009;84:259.
50. Garg A, Grundy SM, Koffler M. Effect of high carbohydrate intake on hyperglycemia, islet function, and plasma lipoproteins in NIDDM. *Diabetes Care.* 1992;15:1572.
51. Alish CJ, Garvey WT, Maki KC, et al. A diabetes-specific enteral formula improves glycemic variability in patients with type 2 diabetes. *Diabetes Technol Ther.* 2010;12:419.
52. Leon-Sanz M, Garcia-Luna PP, Sanz-Paris A, et al. Glycemic and lipid control in hospitalized type 2 diabetic patients: evaluation of 2 enteral nutrition formulas (low carbohydrate-high monounsaturated fat vs high carbohydrate). *JPEN J Parenter Enteral Nutr.* 2005;29:21.

53. McCargar LJ, Innis SM, Bowron E, et al. Effect of enteral nutritional products differing in carbohydrate and fat on indices of carbohydrate and lipid metabolism in patients with NIDDM. *Mol Cell Biochem*. 1998;188:81.
54. Falewee MN, Schiif A, Boufflers E, et al. Reduced infections with perioperative immunonutrition in head and neck cancer—exploratory results of a multicenter, prospective, randomized, double-blind study. *Clin Nutr*. 2013; S0261–5614(13)00265.
55. McClave SA, Martindale RG, Vanek VW, et al. Guidelines for the provision and assessment of nutrition support therapy in the adult critically ill patient: Society of Critical Care Medicine (SCCM) and American Society for Parenteral and Enteral Nutrition (A.S.P.E.N.). *JPEN J Parenter Enteral Nutr*. 2009;33:277.
56. Marik PE, Zaloga GP. Immunonutrition in high-risk surgical patients: a systemic review and analysis of the literature. *JPEN J Parenter Enteral Nutr*. 2010;34:378.
57. Bertolini G, Iapichino G, Radrizzani D, et al. Early enteral immunonutrition in patients with severe sepsis: results of an interim analysis of a randomized multicentre clinical trial. *Intensive Care Med*. 2003;29:834.
58. Alpers D. Is glutamine a unique fuel for small intestinal cells? *Curr Opin Gastroenterol*. 2000;16:155.
59. Lacey JM, Wilmore DW. Is glutamine a conditionally essential amino acid? *Nutr Rev*. 1990;24:297.
60. Peng X, Yan H, You Z, et al. Clinical and protein metabolic efficacy of glutamine granules-supplemented enteral nutrition in severely burned patients. *Burns*. 2005;21:342.
61. Heyland D, Muscedere J, Wischmeyer PE, et al. A randomized trial of glutamine and antioxidants in critically ill patients. *N Engl J Med*. 2013;368(16):1489–97.
62. Alonso de Vega JM, Diaz J, Serrano E, et al. Oxidative stress in critically ill patients with systemic inflammatory response syndrome. *Crit Care Med*. 2002;30:1782.
63. Motoyama T, Okamoto K, Kukita I, et al. Possible role of increased oxidant stress in multiple organ failure after systemic inflammatory response syndrome. *Crit Care Med*. 2003;31:1048.
64. Schneider A, Markowski A, Momma M, et al. Tolerability and efficacy of a low-volume enteral supplement containing key nutrients in the critically ill. *Clin Nutr*. 2011;30:599–603.
65. Visser J, Labadarios D, Blaauw R. Micronutrient supplementation for critically ill adults: a systematic review and meta-analysis. *Nutrition*. 2011;27:745–758.
66. Rafighi Z, Shiva A, Arab S, et al. Association of dietary vitamin C and E intake and antioxidant enzymes in type 2 diabetes mellitus patients. *Glob J Health Sci*. 2013;20:183–187.
67. Bansal V, Syres KM, Makarenkova V, et al. Interactions between fatty acids and arginine metabolism: implications for the design of immune-enhancing diets. *JPEN J Parenter Enteral Nutr*. 2005;29 (1 Suppl):S75.
68. Popovic PJ, Zeh HJ, Ochoa JB. Arginine and immunity. *J Nutr*. 2007;137:1681S.
69. Collier SR, Casey DP, Kanaley JA. Growth hormone responses to varying doses of oral arginine. *Growth Horm IGF Res*. 2005;15:136.
70. Zhu X, Pribix JP, Rodriguez PC, et al. The central role of arginine catabolism in T-cell dysfunction and increased susceptibility to infection after physical injury. *Ann Surg*. 2014;259:171.
71. Wittmann F, Prix N, Mayr S, et al. L-arginine improves wound healing after trauma-hemorrhage by increasing collagen synthesis. *J Trauma*. 2005;59:162.
72. Stechmiller JK, Childress B, Cowan L. Arginine supplementation and wound healing. *Nutr Clin Pract*. 2005;20:52.
73. Brewer S, Desneves K, Pearce L, et al. Effect of an arginine-containing nutritional supplement on pressure ulcer healing in community spinal patients. *J Wound Care*. 2010;19:311.
74. Mizock BA, DeMichele SJ. The acute respiratory distress syndrome: role of nutritional modulation of inflammation through dietary lipids. *Nutr Clin Pract*. 2004;19:536.
75. Pontes-Arruda A, Aragao AM, Albuquerque JD. Effects of enteral feeding with eicosapentaenoic acid, gamma-linolenic acid and antioxidants in mechanically ventilated patients with severe sepsis and septic shock. *Crit Care Med*. 2006;34:2325.
76. Cook DJ, Heyland DK. Pharmaconutrition in acute lung injury. *JAMA*. 2011;12:1599.
77. ASPEN Board of Directors and the Clinical Guidelines Task Force. Guidelines for the use of parenteral and enteral nutrition in adult and pediatric patients. *JPEN J Parenter Enteral Nutr*. 2002;26(1 Suppl):1SA.
78. Dhaliwal R, Cahill N, Lemieux M, et al. The Canadian Critical Care Nutrition Guidelines in 2013: an update on current recommendations and implementation strategies. *Nutr Clin Pract*. 2013;29:29.
79. Date RS, Das N, Bateson PG. Unusual complications of ballooned feeding tubes. *Indian Med J*. 2002;95:181.

80. O'Keefe KP, Dula DJ, Varano V. Duodenal obstruction by a nondeflating Foley catheter gastrostomy tube. *Ann Emerg Med*. 1990;19:1454.
81. Lord LM, Weiser-Maimone A, Pulhamus M, et al. Comparison of weighted vs unweighted enteral feeding tubes for efficacy of transpyloric intubation. *JPEN J Parenter Enteral Nutr*. 1993;17:271.
82. Levenson RTW, Dyson A, Zike L, et al. Do weighted nasoenteric feeding tubes facilitate duodenal intubations? *JPEN J Parenter Enteral Nutr*. 1988;12:135.
83. Adam MD, Rupinder D, Andrew GD, et al. Comparisons between intragastric and small intestinal delivery of enteral nutrition in the critically ill: a systematic review and meta-analysis. *Crit Care*. 2013;17:R125.
84. Alhazzani W, Almasoud A, Jaeschke R, et al. Small bowel feeding and risk of pneumonia in adult critically ill patients: a systematic review and meta-analysis of randomized trials. *Crit Care*. 2013;17:R127.
85. Jabbar A, McClave SA. Pre-pyloric versus post-pyloric feeding. *Clin Nutr*. 2005;24:719.
86. Kuppinger DD, Rittler P, Hartl WH, et al. Use of gastric residual volume to guide enteral nutrition in critically ill patients: a brief systematic review of clinical studies. *Nutrition*. 2013;29:1075.
87. Metheny NA, Schallom L, Oliver DA, et al. Gastric residual volume and aspiration in critically ill patients receiving gastric feedings. *Am J Crit Care*. 2008;17:512.
88. Heyland DK, Drover JW, MacDonald S, et al. Effect of postpyloric feeding on gastroesophageal regurgitation and pulmonary microaspiration: results of a randomized controlled trial. *Crit Care Med*. 2001;29:1495.
89. Metheny NA, Clouse RE, Chang YH, et al. Tracheobronchial aspiration of gastric contents in critically ill tube-fed patients: frequency, outcomes, and risk factors. *Crit Care Med*. 2006;34:1007.
90. Ott DJ, Mattox HE, Gelfand DW, et al. Enteral feeding tubes: placement by using fluoroscopy and endoscopy. *AJR Am J Roentgenol*. 1991;157:769.
91. Stone SJ, Pickett JD, Jesurum JT. Bedside placement of postpyloric feeding tubes. *AACN Clin Issues*. 2000;11:517.
92. Shirley PJ, Bion JF. Intra-hospital transport of critically ill patients: minimizing risk. *Intensive Care Med*. 2004;30:1508.
93. Caplan ES, Hoyt NJ. Nosocomial sinusitis. *JAMA*. 1982;247:639.
94. Montgomery RC, Bar-Natan MF, Thomas SE, et al. Postoperative nasogastric decompression: a prospective randomized trial. *South Med J*. 1996;89:1063.
95. Taylor B, Schallom L. Bedside small bowel feeding tube placement in critically ill patients using a dietitian/nurse team approach. *Nutr Clin Pract*. 2001;16:258.
96. Zaloga GP. Bedside method for placing small bowel feeding tubes in critically ill patients. A prospective study. *Chest*. 1991;100:1643.
97. Slagt C, Innes R, Bihari D, et al. A novel method for insertion of post-pyloric feeding tubes at the bedside without endoscopic or fluoroscopic assistance: a prospective study. *Intensive Care Med*. 2004;30:103.
98. Taylor B, Schallom M, Muckova N. Bedside small bowel placement in over 1200 critically ill patients—a success story. *Crit Care Med*. 2003;31(Suppl):A85.
99. Gabriel SA, Ackermann RJ. Placement of nasoenteral feeding tubes using external magnetic guidance. *JPEN J Parenter Enteral Nutr*. 2004;28:119.
100. Mathus-Vliegen EM, Duflou A, Spanier MB, et al. Nasoenteral feeding tube placement by nurses using an electromagnetic guidance system. *Gastrointest Endosc*. 2010;71:728.
101. Shellito PC, Malt RA. Tube gastrostomy: techiniques and complications. Ann Surg. 1985;201:180.
102. Ephgrave KS, Buchmiller C, Jones MP, et al. The cup is half full. *Am J Surg*. 1999;178:406.
103. Steed H, Barrett D, Emm C, et al. Unsedated percutaneous endoscopic gastrostomy insertion: a safe, effective and well-tolerated method. *JPEN J Parenter Nutr*. 2012;36:231.
104. Gauderer MW, Ponsky JL, Izant RJ. Gastrostomy without laparotomy: a percutaneous endoscopic technique. *J Pediatr Surg*. 1980;15:872.
105. Gauderer MW. Percutaneous endoscopic gastrostomy—20 years later: a historical perspective. *J Pediatr Surg*. 2001;36:217.
106. Hogan RB, DeMarco DC, Hamilton JK, et al. Percutaneous endoscopic gastrostomy—to push or pull: a prospecitve randomized trial. *Gastrointest Endosc*. 1986;32:253.
107. Dennis M, Lewis S, Cranswick G, et al. FOOD Trial Collaboration. FOOD: a multicentre randomised trial evaluating feeding policies in patients admitted to hospital with a recent stroke. *Health Technol Assess*. 2006;10:1.

108. Stayner JL, Bhatnagar A, McGin AN, et al. Feeding tube placement: errors and complications. *Nutr Clin Pract*. 2012;27:738.
109. Rustom IK, Jebreel A, Tayyab M, et al. Percutaneous endoscopic, radiological and surgical gastrostomy tubes: a comparison study in head and neck cancer patients. *J Laryngol Otol*. 2006;120:463.
110. Ljungdahl M, Sundbom M. Complication rate lower after percutaneous endoscopic gastrostomy than after surgical gastrostomy: a prospective randomized trial. *Surg Endosc*. 2006;20:1248.
111. DeLegge RL, DeLegge MH. Percutaneous endoscopic gastrostomy evaluation of device materials: are we "failsafe?" *Nutr Clin Pract*. 2005;20:613.
112. Duh QY, Senokozlieff-Englehart AL, Siperstein AE, et al. Prospective evaluation of the safety and efficacy of laparoscopic jejunostomy. *West J Med*. 1995;162:117.
113. Baron TH. Direct percutaneous endoscopic jejunostomy. *Am J Gastroenterol*. 2006;101:1407.
114. Mohiuddin SS, Anderson CE. A novel application for single-incision laparoscopic surgery (SILS): SIL jejunostomy feeding tube placement. *Surg Endosc*. 2011;25:323.
115. Chin KF, Townsend S, Wong W, et al. A prospective cohort study of feeding needle catheter jejunostomy in an upper gastrointestinal surgical unit. *Clin Nutr*. 2004;23:691.
116. Taylor B, Mazuski J. Enteral access devices and placement techniques. *Support Line*. 2005;27:3.
117. Needham DM, Dinglas VD, Bienvenu OJ, et al. One year outcomes in patients with acute lung injury randomized to initial trophic or full enteral feeding: prospective follow-up of EDEN randomized trial. *BMJ*. 2013;19:346.
118. Kohn CL. The relationship between enteral formula contamination and length of enteral delivery set usage. *JPEN J Parenter Enteral Nutr*. 1991;15:567.
119. Chan L. Evaluation of the bacteriological contamination of a closed feeding system for enteral nutrition. *Med J Malaysia*. 1994;49:62.
120. McClave SA, Lukan JK, Stefater JA, et al. Poor validity of residual volumes as a marker for risk of aspiration in critically ill patients. *Crit Care Med*. 2005;33:324.
121. Alberda C, Gramlich L, Jones N, et al. The relationship between nutritional intake and clinical outcomes in critically ill patients: results of an international multicenter observational study. *Intensive Care Med*. 2009;35:1728.
122. Chang SJ, Huang HH. Diarrhea in enterally fed patients: blame the diet? *Curr Opin Clin Nutr Metab Care*. 2013;16:588.
123. Kotake T, Takada M, Goto T, et al. Serum amiodarone and desethylamiodarone concentrations following nasogastric versus oral administration. *J Clin Pharm Ther*. 2006;31:237.
124. Beringer P, Nguyen M, Hoem N, et al. Absolute bioavailability and pharmacokinetics of linezolid in hospitalized patients given enteral feedings. *Antimicrob Agents Chemother*. 2005;49:3676.
125. Heldt T, Loss SH. Drug-nutrient interactions in the intensive care unit: literature review and current recommendations. *Rev Bras Ter Intensiva*. 2013;25:162–167
126. Klang M, McLymont V, Ng N. Osmolality, pH, and compatibility of selected oral liquid medications with an enteral nutrition product. *JPEN J Parenter Enter Nutr*. 2013;37:689.
127. Dandeles L, Lodolce A. Efficacy of agents to prevent and treat enteral feeding tube clogs. *Ann Pharmacother*. 2011;45:676–680.
128. Williams NT. Medication administration through enteral feeding tubes. *Am J HealthSyst Pharm*. 2008;65:2347–2357.
129. Forsmark, CE. Management of chronic pancreatitis. *Gastroenterology*. 2013;144:1282.
130. Etemad B, Whitcomb DC. Chronic pancreatitis: diagnosis, classification and new genetic developments. *Gastroenterology*. 2011;120:682.
131. Fieker A, Philpott J, Armand M. Enzyme replacement therapy for pancreatic insufficiency: present and future. *Clin Exp Gastroenterol*. 2011;4:55.
132. Kadiyala V, Suleiman SL, Conwell DL. Pancreatic insufficiency: part 2 of 2: treatment and therapeutic considerations. *Gastroenterology & Endoscopy News*. June 2012. www.gastroendonews.com/download/PancreaCaPart2_WM.pdf. Accessed on March 11, 2014.
133. Acevedo-Piedra NG, Moya-Hoyo N, Rey-Riveiro M, et al. Validation of the determinant-based classification and revision of the Atlanta classification systems for acute pancreatitis. *Clin Gastroenterol Hepatol*. 2014;12:311.
134. Khanna AK, Meher S, Prakash, et al. Comparison of Ranson, Glasgow MOSS, SIRS, BISAP, APACHE II, CTSI Scores, IL-6, CRP and procalcitonin in predicting severity, organ failure, pancreatic necrosis and mortality in acute pancreatitis. *HPB Surg*. 2013;2013:367581
135. Qin HI, Su ZD, Gao Q, et al. Early intrajejunal nutrition: bacterial translocation and gut barrier function of severe acute pancreatitis in dogs. *Hepatobiliary Pancreat Dis Int*. 2002;1:150.

136. Li JY, Yu T, Chen GC, et al. Enteral nutrition within 48 hours of admission improves clinical outcomes of acute pancreatitis by reducing complications: a meta-analysis. *PLoS ONE.* 2013;8:e64926.
137. Dickerson RN, Vehe KL, Mullen JL, et al. Resting energy expenditure in patients with pancreatitis. *Crit Care Med.* 1991;19:484.
138. Windsor ACJ, Kanwar S, Li AGK, et al. Compared with parenteral nutrition, enteral feeding attenuates the acute phase response and improves disease severity in acute pancreatitis. *Gut.* 1998;42:431.
139. Davies AR, Morrison SS, Ridley EJ, et al. Nutritional therapy in patients with acute pancreatitis requiring critical care unit management: a prospective observational study in Australia and New Zealand. *Crit Care Med.* 2011;39:462.
140. Kalfarentzos F, Kehagias J, Mead N, et al. Enteral nutrition is superior to parenteral nutrition in severe acute pancreatitis: results of a randomized prospective trial. *Br J Surg.* 1997;84:1665.
141. Abou-Assi S, Craig K, O'Keefe SJD. Hypocaloric jejunal feeding is better than total parenteral nutrition in acute pancreatitis: results of a randomized comparative study. *Am J Gastroenterol.* 2002;97:2255.
142. O'Keefe SJ, Lee RB, Anderson FP. Physiological effects of enteral and parenteral feeding on pancreaticobiliary secretion in humans. *Am J Physiol Gastrointest Liver Physiol.* 2003;284:G27.
143. Gupta R, Patel K, Calder PC. A randomised clinical trial to assess the effect of total enteral and total parenteral nutritional support on metabolic, inflammatory and oxidative markers in patients with predicted severe acute pancreatitis. *Pancreatology.* 2003;3:406.
144. Austrums E, Pupels G, Snippe K. Postoperative enteral stimulation by gut feeding improves outcomes in severe acute pancreatitis. *Nutrition.* 2003;19:487.
145. Matarese LE, Steiger E. Dietary and medical management of short bowel syndrome in adult patients. *J Clin Gastroenterol.* 2006;40(suppl):S85.
146. Thompson JS, Iyer KR, DiBaise JK, et al. Short bowel syndrome and Crohn's disease. *J Gastrointest Surg.* 2003;7:1069.
147. Uchino M, Ikeuchi H, Bando T, et al. Risk factors for short bowel syndrome in patients with Crohn's disease. *Surg Today.* 2012;42:447.
148. Buchman AL, Scolapio J, Fryer J. AGA technical review on short bowel syndrome and intestinal transplantation. *Gastroenterology.* 2003;124:1111.
149. Jeejeebhoy KN. Short bowel syndrome: a nutritional and medical approach. *CMAJ.* 2002;166:1297.
150. McNeil NI. The contribution of the large intestine to energy supplies in man. *Am J Clin Nutr.* 1984;39:338.
151. Jeppesen PB, Sanguinetti EL, Buchman A, et al. Teduglutide (ALX-0600), a dipeptidyl peptidase IV resistant glucagon-like peptide 2 analogue, improves intestinal function in short bowel syndrome patients. *Gut.* 2005;54:1224.
152. Fleming CR, George L, Stoner GL, et al. The importance of urinary magnesium values in patients with gut failure. *Mayo Clin Proc.* 1996;71:21.
153. Nordgaard I, Hansen BS, Mortensen PB. Colon as a digestive organ in patients with short bowel. *Lancet.* 1994;343:373.
154. Levy E, Frileux P, Sandrucci S, et al. Continuous enteral nutrition during the early adaptive stage of the short bowel syndrome. *Br J Surg.* 1988;75:549.
155. McIntyre PB, Fitchew M, Lennard-Jones JE. Patients with a high jejunostomy do not need a special diet. *Gastroenterology.* 1986;91:25.
156. Fordtran JS. Stimulation of active and passive sodium absorption by sugars in the human jejunum. *J Clin Invest.* 1975;55:728.
157. Matarese LE. Nutrition and fluid optimization for patients with short bowel syndrome. *JPEN J Parenter Enteral Nutr.* 2013;37:161.
158. McDoniel K, Taylor B, Huey W, et al. Use of Clonidine to decrease intestinal fluid losses in patients with high-output short-bowel syndrome. *JPEN J Parenter Enteral Nutr.* 2004;28:265.
159. Bass BL, Fischer BA, Richardson C, et al. Somatostatin analogue treatment inhibits postresectional adaptation of the small bowel in rats. *Am J Surg.* 1991;172:107.
160. Peeters M, Van den Brande J, Francque S. Diarrhea and the rationale to use Sandostatin. *Acta Gastroenterol Belg.* 2010;73:25.

Parenteral Nutritional Therapy

GENERAL PRINCIPLES

Parenteral nutrition (PN) can be used to supply all the essential nutrients without the use of the intestinal tract. In most cases, PN is reserved for patients who are unable to meet their nutritional requirements through enteral routes, as infusing nutrients directly into the bloodstream is the least preferred method of providing nutritional therapy (1). However, for patients with no other option for nutrition support, PN is a lifesaving therapy. While recognizing that there are issues specific to needs during childhood, this chapter will discuss issues pertinent only to adults.

Background

The successful establishment of a positive nitrogen balance and growth by means of PN was demonstrated successfully more than 30 years ago (2). Since then patients have been maintained on PN at home and have survived for many years. According to the American Society of Parenteral and Enteral Nutrition (ASPEN), in the hospital setting PN should be reserved for those patients without a functioning gastrointestinal (GI) tract, who cannot, should not, or will not eat adequately for a "prolonged" period of time and in whom the benefits outweigh the risks (3). In general, "prolonged" is defined as 14 days for well-nourished patients and 7 to 10 days in those with preexisting medical illnesses or high levels of metabolic stress. The recommendation for use only after a period of time is based on the lack of clear efficacy for "early" use of PN. Two large trials have demonstrated conflicting results; one reinforced the potential adverse impact on patient outcome from early use of PN in postelective surgery patients (4), and the other suggested no difference in mortality in critically ill patients started on early PN when enteral nutrition (EN) was contraindicated (5). In regard to preoperative use, only in severely malnourished patients has PN been shown to be beneficial when EN was not an option (6,7). A review of four meta-analyses involving more than 5,000 patients showed that total parenteral nutrition (TPN) given 7 to 10 days before surgery in "severely malnourished patients" (defined as >20% body weight loss or serum albumin <2.5 g per dL) had fewer noninfectious complications than their better nourished counterparts (5% vs. 43%, respectively) (7). In a meta-analysis, intravenous (IV) fluids alone were associated with a significantly higher risk for mortality ($P < 0.05$) and a trend toward higher rate of infection when compared with use of PN (8). A prospective controlled multicenter trial randomized 2,312 patients to receive PN 48 hours after ICU admission (early) and 2,328 patients to receive PN 8 days after ICU admission (late). Both groups were started on EN per protocol, and PN was discontinued when EN met 80% of caloric goals. The late PN group had fewer ICU infections ($P = 0.008$), fewer days of renal replacement therapy ($P = 0.008$), less time on mechanical ventilation ($P = 0.006$), but no difference in mortality (9).

Indications for Parenteral Nutrition

Indications for PN can be divided into three subcategories: those patients in whom PN is *indicated*, *possibly indicated*, and *contraindicated* (Table 11-1) (3,10).

Complete Bowel Rest

Complete bowel rest combined with PN has often been used to treat patients with certain GI disorders. The premise is that excluding all oral intake minimizes trauma to and contractile activity in the diseased bowel. The GI tract maintains a cyclic motility pattern even during fasting. Periodic surges of pancreatic and gastric secretion also occur in relation to the migrating motor complex, which in humans cycles at approximately 2-hour intervals. PN does not alter this periodic activity in laboratory animals. Despite continued motor and secretory activity

TABLE 11-1 Indications, Possible Indications, and Contraindications for PN

PN Indicated in:
- Documented severe malabsorption of nutrients from the GI tract as in:
  Massive small-bowel resection (at least initially)
  Intractable diarrhea
  Radiation enteritis
  Scleroderma of the bowel
- Complete bowel obstruction
- Inability to obtain enteral access for feeding for at least 7 to 10 days
- Persistent GI bleeding
- High output fistula (>500 mL) and inability to gain enteral access distal to fistula
- Diffuse peritonitis
- GI ischemia
- Catabolic state with or without malnutrition when GI tract not usable for 7 to 10 days
- Preoperatively in severely malnourished patients without functioning GI tract
- Severe acute pancreatitis with documented abdominal pain with jejunal enteral feeds

PN Possibly Indicated in:
- Enterocutaneous fistula if poor tolerance of distally infused enteral nutrition
- Inflammatory bowel disease not responding to medical therapy
- Chylous ascites or chylothorax if increased output continues with low fat enteral nutrition
- Intractable vomiting (such as in hyperemesis gravidarum) and jejunal feeding is not an option
- Prolonged small-bowel ileus expected for at least 7 to 10 days
- Severe acute pancreatitis in ventilated patient with signs of malabsorption of jejunal feeding

PN Contraindicated in:
- Functional GI tract
- Inability to access GI tract anticipated to be <7 days
- Venous access not available
- When the associated risks of PN determined to outweigh the potential benefit

---

between periods of digestion, most experience supports the idea that limiting oral intake reduces symptoms of abdominal pain and diarrhea in patients with GI disorders, at least for the duration of the therapy. However, satisfactory data to support the careful use of bowel rest and PN as primary therapy does not presently exist either for acute pancreatitis (1), closure of fistula, or for inflammatory bowel disease (11,12).

Nutritional deficiencies are frequently seen in the two most common forms of inflammatory bowel disease, Crohn disease and ulcerative colitis. Often, decreased oral intake, malabsorption, accelerated nutrient losses, increased requirements, and drug–nutrient interactions are the culprits of these deficiencies. In many cases, EN is effective in inducing clinical remission in adults. Use of EN in these patients is reviewed in Chapter 10.

Crohn disease of the small bowel remits with complete bowel rest, so that most patients experience symptomatic improvement, but the effect is not specific. Four early studies compared short-term remission rates in patients treated with either PN combined with bowel rest or EN. All of these studies found similar remission rates in the two groups (Table 11-2).

Ulcerative colitis involving the entire colon, often referred to as pan-colitis, usually prohibits enteral feeding, making PN the nutritional therapy of choice. However, in less severe cases, enteral feeding is often an option.

Enterocutaneous fistulas are often a consequence of active inflammatory bowel disease. In cases of high fistula output, PN combined with bowel rest is generally used to correct and

TABLE 11-2 Incidence of Short-term Remission in Patients Receiving Parenteral Nutrition Plus Bowel Rest Versus Enteral Nutrition in Crohn Disease

Study	PN + Bowel Rest	EN
Lochs et al. (82)	7/10 (70%)	8/10 (80%)
Jones (83)	14/19 (88%)	11/17 (85%)
Greenberg et al. (84)	12/17 (71%)	11/19 (58%)
Wright and Adler (85)	4/5 (80%)	3/6 (50%)
Total	38/51 (75%)	32/52 (62%)

PN, parenteral nutrition; EN, enteral nutrition.

prevent nutritional disturbances. A review of the literature regarding nutrition and management of enterocutaneous fistulas found malnutrition to be a common problem; the administration of nutrition support initially PN transitioning to EN, including provision of EN via the fistula itself (known as fistuloclysis), appeared to reduce the mortality rate and allow for spontaneous fistula closure in some of the patients (12).

The adaptation period after intestinal resection in short-bowel syndrome may need to be managed with PN if attempts of EN are plagued with continued nutrient and electrolyte deficiencies secondary to malabsorption. EN management of short-bowel syndrome is reviewed in Chapter 10. Patients who have undergone resection of more than 75% of the small bowel usually require long-term PN, whereas those with less than 75% resection may not require permanent PN support (13)

Severe acute pancreatitis may be an indication for PN in patients experiencing pain with enteral feeding or those with complications such as necrosis, abscess, pseudocyst, fistula, and ascites. However, even in the presence of these complications, enteral feeding should be considered. Although most investigators recommend feeding beyond the ligament of Treitz, this has not been proven to be significantly superior to gastric feeding in this patient population (14). Pancreatitis is sometimes accompanied by hypertriglyceridemia. Lipid emulsions should not be given to any patient with a serum triglyceride level above 400 mg per dL (1).

Types of Parenteral Nutrition

Types of PN are not defined by the initial point of entry into the vascular system, but by the position of the distal catheter tip. Access information will be covered in more depth in the next section (Venous Access).

Central parenteral nutrition (CPN) is delivered via a central venous access with the catheter tip located in the superior vena cava. In cases where intravascular access is limited, the inferior vena cava may be used. CPN is the most commonly utilized form of PN. This route is chosen when a central catheter is already in position for other reasons, or the expected length of therapy is long term (>7 days).

Peripheral parenteral nutrition (PPN) is delivered via a peripheral venous access with the catheter tip located outside of the inferior or superior vena cava. This route is chosen when the expected length of therapy is short term (≤7 days).

VENOUS ACCESS

The various types of venous access for PN and the general disadvantages and advantages are presented in Table 11-3.

Central Venous Catheter

The central venous catheter (CVC) is most commonly used in patients receiving PN, as this allows for the infusion of solutions with an osmolarity greater than 900 mOsm per L. Central PN solutions range from approximately 1,400 to 2,600 mOsm per L. A central venous access may be tunneled (i.e., Hickman, Broviac, Groshong), nontunneled (Hohn, general multilumen

TABLE 11-3 Venous Access Devices: Advantages and Disadvantages (6,13)

Line Type	Advantages	Disadvantages	Dwell Time
Peripheral Lines			
Short peripheral catheter	• Easily inserted by nurse or other trained personnel • Least expensive • Minimal care and maintenance • Low risk of catheter-related sepsis • Easy to remove	• Lasts for only 48 to 72 h; need to change frequently • Risk of phlebitis high • Patient may not have adequate peripheral veins • Limited to osmolality 600 to 900 mOsm/L, so can use only peripheral PN • Cannot instill acidic solutions (pH < 5) or medications that cause severe phlebitis	48 to 72 h
Midline peripheral catheter	• Same as short • May last 3 to 5 days longer (not proven if used for PPN) • Allows access to larger vessel (still not a central line)	• Same as short • Higher cost than short • Higher level of training required for placement	48 to 72 h
Central lines	Able to give solutions >900 mOsm/L		
Peripheral inserted central catheter (PICC)	• No risk of pneumothorax or puncture of internal carotid or subclavian arteries • Bedside insertion • Inserted by specially trained nurses • Available in single, double, and triple lumens • External portion can be repaired if damaged • Lower risk of catheter-related sepsis than CVC • Less costly than CVC • Can be used for short- or long-term PN	• Smaller diameter and greater length than CVC, increasing risk of occlusion • Insertion site on arm may increase risk of dislodgement and hinder self-care of catheter • Placement unsuccessful in 25% of attempts • More likely to coil than CVC • More difficult to draw blood than CVC	Up to 1 year
Nontunneled CVC	• Low cost • Can be removed by trained RN • May be placed at bedside or radiology by MD • Multiple lumens	• Increased infection rate compared with single lumen and tunneled catheters • Only for use in acute care	2 weeks

TABLE 11-3	Venous Access Devices: Advantages and Disadvantages (6,13) *(continued)*		
Line Type	Advantages	Disadvantages	Dwell Time
Tunneled CVC (Hickman, Broviac)	• Long-term catheter • May have multiple lumens	• Requires surgical procedure for placement and removal • Higher cost • Removal by MD	Several years
Port	• Lowest infection risk of all options • Site care needed only when accessed • Useful for intermittent access • Access underneath the skin	• Requires surgical procedure for placement and removal • Requires "stick" to access with Huber needle	Several years

catheters), peripherally inserted (PICC), or provided as an implanted IV port device. The three most common sites for CVC insertions are the subclavian vein, and internal jugular and femoral veins. If a CVC has multiple lumens, the most distal lumen should be designated for PN to decrease the risk of contaminated blood draws and mixing of PN with other medications (15). A chest x-ray should always be obtained postplacement to confirm position prior to catheter use. Complications of CVC can be divided into early and late complications.

Potential early complications of CVC placement include the following:
1. Pneumothorax
2. Brachial plexus injury
3. Subclavian and carotid artery puncture
4. Hemothorax
5. Thoracic duct injury
6. Chylothorax

Mechanical complications are less likely to occur if the CVC is inserted by a more experienced physician, not placed in the femoral vein, and placed with the use of ultrasound guidance during internal jugular placements (15).

To avoid the possibility of an **air embolus**, never disconnect the tubing from an unclamped catheter with the patient in an upright position. Air embolism can also occur during insertion or afterward if the connection between the catheter and the IV tubing is not well secured.

Late complications associated with CVC include the following:
1. Catheter dislodgement
2. **Catheter occlusions** are commonly related to the formation of a thrombus within the lumen, the formation of a fibrin sheath around the catheter end, the malpositioning of a catheter tip against the vessel wall or within a small branch vessel, or the presence of thrombosis or stenosis in the native vein.
3. **Catheter thrombosis** may be treated with thrombolytic agents, such as tissue-type plasminogen activator (tPA), e.g., alteplase (Activase; Genentech, Inc., South San Francisco, CA) or reteplase (Retavase; Centocor Inc., Malvern, PA). This technique should be completed by a physician or nurse with special training (15). However, there is inadequate evidence to draw strong conclusions on the efficacy or safety of these drugs. At present, their use is based on low quality evidence, and therefore cautions should be used when prescribing these medications (16). If this technique is used, the entire lumen of the catheter is filled with approximately 2 mg of tPA diluted in the appropriate volume to fill the catheter.

TABLE 11-4   Common Types of Catheter-related Infections

Type	Description
Catheter colonization	Present if the catheter is removed or exchanged over a guidewire and >15 CFU of microorganisms grow from a culture from a catheter segment and the patient has no signs of systemic sepsis
Catheter-related blood stream infection	The most severe catheter infection, diagnosed when line tip culture and a peripheral blood culture grow the same microorganism and the patient has systemic sepsis with no other identifiable source: fever, leukocytosis, or tachycardia
Exit-site infection	Erythema, tenderness, induration, or purulence within 2 cm of the CVC skin exit site

This is left in place for 15 to 30 minutes. Care must be taken to infuse just enough solution so that it fills only the lumen of the catheter and to prevent systemic administration of the thrombolytic agent. After the appropriate time, the thrombolytic agent is aspirated.

4. Catheter-related infections (Table 11-4). Blood stream infections are most commonly caused by *Staphylococcus epidermidis* and *S. aureus*. In long-term PN patients, *Enterococcus*, *Candida* species, *Escherichia coli*, *Pseudomonas*, *Klebsiella*, *Enterobacter*, *Acinetobacter*, *Proteus*, and *Xanthomonas* should also be considered. Table 11-5 reviews one suggested management approach for suspected catheter-related infection (17).

Techniques to decrease infectious risk associated with CVC (17,18) are as follows:
1. **Femoral access should be avoided if at all possible.** The lowest infectious risk exists with subclavian catheterization, the highest with femoral sites.
2. **Use of maximal** sterile-barrier precautions **during catheter insertion:** mask, cap, sterile gown, sterile gloves, and large sterile drape have been shown to reduce the rate of infection.

TABLE 11-5   Management of Suspected Catheter-related Infection

1. Initial evaluation:
    a. Evaluate catheter insertion site and culture any drainage
    b. Obtain blood cultures from both peripheral and central veins
    c. Look for other causes of infection (e.g., urinalysis, chest X-ray, sputum, wounds)
2. Stop TPN for 48 to 72 h
3. Indications for central venous catheter removal:
    a. Immediate removal
        (1) Purulent discharge or abscess at insertion site
        (2) Septic shock without another etiology for the source of infection
    b. Positive culture from both sites or persistent signs of infection without other cause for infection identified
4. Antibiotic therapy
    c. Empiric antibiotic therapy administered through central venous catheter until culture results are back:
        (1) Vancomycin 1 g q 12 h (adjust dose for creatinine/GFR)
        (2) Cefepime 1 g q 12 h (if gram negative infection suspected)
    d. Specific antibiotic therapy administered through central venous catheter once culture results are available
    e. If a catheter is "irreplaceable," consider trial of antibiotic therapy with line in place
    f. Duration of antibiotic therapy usually ranges from 2 to 6 weeks depending on patient, organism, and whether central line has been left in place
5. Repeat blood cultures in 48 and 72 h to ensure clearance of bacteremia
6. Fever should resolve within 72 to 96 h if given appropriate antibiotics; remove catheter if fever persists

3. **Avoid the use of antibiotic ointments**, which may increase the rate of fungi colonization and promote the development of antibiotic-resistant bacteria.
4. **Do not change catheter routinely** (i.e., every 7 days) as this does not reduce the risk of infection. In fact, routine exchange over a guidewire is associated with a trend toward a higher infection rate.
5. **Antimicrobial CVCs**, silver-platinum-carbon–impregnated catheters and rifampicin-minocycline–coated catheters should be considered in patients whose catheter is expected to remain more than 5 days in facilities with above-average central line-associated bloodstream infection (CLABSI) rates even after implementing safe practices.
6. Antibiotic lock prophylaxis in patients with long-term catheters should be used only in patients with a history of multiple CLABSI despite optimal adherence to aseptic technique.

Peripheral Venous Catheters

Peripheral venous catheters are the quickest, simplest, least expensive, and most common method of venous access. However, peripheral veins are prone to phlebitis and subcutaneous (SC) infiltration, and the catheter should not remain in one site for longer than 48 to 72 hours (19). Peripheral catheters should be used to infuse only PPN in patients with adequate peripheral veins. They are contraindicated in patients with poor peripheral veins, requiring PN for longer than 7 days, or with intolerance to fluid load. Given the need to restrict the osmolality of solutions infused to less than 900 mOsm per L, PPN requires a relatively large fluid volume to administer significant amounts of protein and calories.

Catheter Maintenance

Tubing and Filters

Tubing should be changed every 24 hours. Use of unnecessary tubing and extension sets is discouraged. A stopcock should not be part of the tubing assembly because it is easily contaminated. In addition, the catheter–tubing junction should be wiped with alcohol before being disconnected to avoid inadvertent contamination of the catheter hub.

In-line filters are recommended by the Food and Drug Administration (FDA) for use when PN is being infused. This recommendation was prompted by two deaths caused by calcium phosphate precipitates in three-in-one PN admixtures, referred to as total nutrient admixtures (TNAs) (see discussion of TNAs under Designing the Solution for Parenteral Nutrition). A 0.22-μm filter is used for base solutions (dextrose and amino acids only); however, this is too small to allow for lipid emulsions to be administered. Filters with larger pores (≥ 1.2 μm) are used with TNA. Insertion of the filter creates an additional opportunity for contamination in the tubing assembly. Despite their filtering capabilities, in-line filters do not appear to significantly reduce catheter infection rates. However, filters do reduce the infusion of particulate matter in the solution.

Occlusive Dressing

An occlusive dressing is an important part of CVC maintenance. The dressing must be occlusive on all sides to prevent catheter contamination. Gauze dressings are often initially used at the time of CVC placement and should be changed within 24 hours to a transparent dressing of a porous synthetic material (Op-Site). This dressing allows for visualization of the catheter entry site and can be left in place for 7 days as long as it remains dry and occlusive.

Aseptic Maintenance

Aseptic maintenance of the catheter and tubing system cannot be emphasized enough for the safe administration of long-term PN through a CVC. The following precautions should be followed in addition to the techniques mentioned above.

1. Avoid a bulky dressing. A single folded 4×4-inch pad should be adequate.
2. Make sure the dressing is occlusive on all sides.
3. Tape all connections to avoid accidental disconnection or contamination.
4. Clean all connections, including the catheter–tubing connection, with alcohol or povidone-iodine before any tubing changes are made.
5. Change the catheter dressing if it is wet. If the replaced dressing also becomes damp, then the catheter–tubing junction and exposed catheter should be examined carefully. Under no

TABLE 11-6 Energy and Substrate Guidelines for Adult Patients on Parenteral Nutrition

	Critical Care	Acute Care
Energy		
Obese (BMI ≥ 30)	15–20 kcal/kg/day	15–20 kcal/kg/day
Nonobese (BMI 15–29)	20–35 kcal/kg/day	25–35 kcal/kg/day
Undernourished (BMI < 15)[a]	35–40 kcal/kg/day	30–40 kcal/kg/day
Protein	1.2–2.0 g/kg/day	0.8–1.0 g/kg/day[b]
Carbohydrate (dextrose)	<4 g/kg/day	<7 g/kg/day
Lipid	<1 g/kg/day	<1–2 g/kg/day
Fluid	Minimum needed to deliver prescribed formula	30–35 mL/kg/day + losses

[a]If refeeding risk starts at 15 kcal/kg.
[b]If patient catabolic increases to 1.2 to 2.0 g/kg/day.

circumstances should this examination be performed in a casual way without adhering to the usual aseptic technique. If the catheter dressing must be removed, sterile precautions should be taken to avoid accidental contamination of the catheter insertion site.

6. Once infusion from a solution bag is started, the bag should not hang for more than 24 hours so that bacterial growth is minimized.

NUTRIENT REQUIREMENTS DURING PARENTERAL NUTRITION

The calculation of calorie and protein requirements is covered in Chapter 5. Dietary vitamin and mineral requirements are discussed in Chapters 6 and 7. The usual goals for protein, carbohydrate, fat, and fluid intake for adult patients on PN are similar for like patient types not on PN and are presented in Table 11-6 (1,10,20).

Nonprotein Calories Versus Total Calories

Total calories are used to determine intake for patients receiving all forms of enteral feeding. However, when administering PN, some clinicians do not count amino acids as a calorie source. This is based on the expectation that some of the amino acids will be incorporated into new protein rather than metabolized. However, this implies that one can direct protein utilization. It may make more physiologic sense to include amino acids as a calorie source in the expectation that more will be metabolized than incorporated into new protein (21,22). This assumption helps prevent overfeeding and hyperglycemia.

Fluid Requirements

Fluid requirements will vary depending on the capacity of the patient to excrete an osmotic load and the estimate of fluid losses. Increased losses may occur in patients with fever, open abdomen, high drain or ostomy outputs, frequent emesis, and diarrhea. Electrolyte concentrations in various GI fluids are presented in Table 7-6 in Chapter 7. Understanding of a patient's electrolyte losses will aid in their repletion. In general, the euvolemic patient will require 30 to 40 mL/kg/day. The PN should not be used as the primary source for fluid and electrolyte repletion, especially in critically ill patients whose status may change from the time PN is ordered to completion (~36 h). However, in circumstances where fluid restriction is desired, it may be beneficial to make changes to the PN solution. For example, increase the base component of the PN (i.e., acetate) as opposed to starting a separate sodium bicarbonate infusion in a patient with renal failure and a metabolic acidosis.

Vitamin Requirements

Vitamin requirements during parenteral therapy are uncertain because they are not based on balance studies. Refer to Chapter 6 for a discussion of specific vitamin requirements and monitoring for vitamin deficiencies. The requirements for an adult parenteral multivitamin drug product were last amended by the FDA in 2003 (23). At that time, it recommended an increase in vitamins B_1, B_6, C, and folic acid to better meet estimated needs and to include 150 µg of vitamin K. The present

TABLE 11-7 Adult Parenteral MVI Products

Vitamin	MVI Adult (Hospira) (per 10 mL)	MVI-12 (Hospira) (per 10 mL)	Infuvite Adult (Baxter) (per 10 mL)
A[a] (retinol)	1 mg[a]	1 mg[a]	3,300 units
D[a]	5 µg[a] (ergocalciferol)	5 µg[a] (ergocalciferol)	200 units (cholecalciferol)
E[a] (d-alpha tocopheryl acetate)	10 mg[a]	10 mg[a]	10 units
K (phytonadione)	150 µg	None	150 µg
C (ascorbic acid)	200 mg	200 mg	200 mg
B-1 (thiamine)	6 mg	6 mg	6 mg
B-2 (riboflavin)	3.6 mg	3.6 mg	3.6 mg
Niacinamide	40 mg	40 mg	40 mg
Dexpanthenol	15 mg	15 mg	15 mg
B-6 (pyridoxine)	6 mg	6 mg	6 mg
B-12 (cyanocobalamin)	5 µg	5 µg	5 µg
Biotin	60 µg	60 µg	60 µg
Folic Acid	600 µg	600 µg	600 µg
Others:			
Aluminum	43–183 µg/L[b]	43–78 µg/L[b]	70 µg/L[bc]
Polysorbate 80	160 mg	160 mg	140 mg
Polysorbate 20	2.8 mg	2.8 mg	None
Propylene Glycol	3 g	3 g	3 g

[a]1 mg vitamin A = 3,300 USP units, 5 µg vitamin D = 200 USP units, 10 mg vitamin E = 10 USP units.
[b]Maximum, labeled concentration at product expiration date; Hospira products vary depending on whether it is a unit vial, single-dose or multi-dose packaging.
[c]Product label revised, 9/2007.

adult parenteral Multivitamin (MVI) formulations are presented in Table 11-7. In 2012, an ASPEN advisory board convened and published their recommendations to adjust the current IV MVI formulations on the market (24). There is some debate regarding the correct dosing of vitamin D. Patients receiving home PN have been shown to have insufficient vitamin D status that is not corrected by oral dosing, leaving some researchers to suggest an alternate route of supplementation or an increase in the current formulation (25). Patients with increased oxidative stress may benefit from the antioxidant properties of vitamin A, C, and E. The intake of antioxidant vitamins below 66% of RDA leads to worsening in oxidative stress parameters, compared with intake of at least 66% of the RDA (26). A small group of patients provided an IV infusion of 500 mg per day of vitamin C post GI surgery, demonstrated a decrease in a marker of oxidative stress when compared with patients receiving only 100 mg per day (27). However, a large trial of over 1,200 critically ill patients demonstrated no benefit in clinical outcomes from the addition of parenteral and enteral antioxidants and glutamine (28). Critically ill patients and those at risk of refeeding syndrome (see Clinical Applications of Nutritional Status Assessment in Chapter 5) may also be at risk for thiamine deficiency and may benefit from the addition of 100 mg thiamine to the PN solution for 3 to 4 days (29,30). Risk factors for folate deficiency in the hospital patient include extensive tissue damage due to sepsis, trauma or surgery, acute renal failure requiring renal replacement therapy, or recent alcohol abuse (31). In a study of the erythropoietin response in critical illness, 13% of patients were found to have iron, B$_{12}$, folate, or a combination deficiency on admission to the ICU (32). Although information was not provided on the admitting nutritional status of the deficient patients, it may be beneficial to provide an additional 1 mg folate for 3 to 4 days to critically ill patients.

Shortages of parenteral vitamin and mineral mixtures on the US market over the past several years have led to signs and symptoms of deficiencies in long-term PN patients. A recent ASPEN survey indicates the shortages are having a profound effect on clinical practice, leading many practitioners to ration existing supplies for those patients with the most severe deficiencies (33). The shortages and subsequent rationing have led to adverse outcomes including lactic acidosis, Wernicke encephalopathy, altered skeletal development, and rashes and skin conditions. The effects are most profound in infants (34). Public and professional concern led to the approval by the FDA for the importation of trace elements from Europe in 2012 (http://www.nutritioncare.org/News/Industry_and_Product_News/FDA_Announces_Importation_of_Trace_Elements/ Accessed March 12, 2014).

Mineral Requirements

Mineral requirements may vary considerably from patient to patient and for an individual patient during a course of PN therapy. Ranges of major minerals and reasons for adjustments in CPN are listed in Table 11-8. For optimal nitrogen repletion, adequate supplementation of these minerals is required.

Potassium requirements may fluctuate based on the presence of a catabolic state. As a patient's metabolic stress decreases, potassium requirements decrease as well. In addition, potassium requirements may also be affected by certain medications (i.e., diuretics) or changes in renal function of hospitalized patients. If the patient is at risk for refeeding, potassium should be adequately supplemented prior to starting PN.

Phosphate should also be repleted prior to initiating PN. The phosphate required varies with the number of calories provided. In general, the PN solution should be supplemented with

TABLE 11-8 Electrolytes Administered via the PN Solution

Suggested Electrolytes (per L)	Conditions That May Require Alteration of Amount Provided	Electrolyte Carriers
Sodium 60–150 mEq	• Renal function • Fluid status • GI losses • Traumatic brain injury	Sodium chloride Sodium acetate Sodium phosphate
Potassium 40–120 mEq	• Renal function • GI losses • Metabolic acidosis • Refeeding	Potassium chloride Potassium acetate Potassium phosphate
Phosphate 10–30 mM	• Renal function • Refeeding • Bone disease • Hypercalcemia • Rapid healing[a] • Hepatic function	Sodium phosphate Potassium phosphate
Chloride 60–120 mEq	• Renal function • GI losses (gastric) • Acid–base status	Sodium chloride Potassium chloride
Acetate 10–40 mEq	• Renal function • GI losses (small bowel) • Acid–base status • Hepatic function	Sodium acetate Potassium acetate
Calcium 4.5–9.2 mEq	• Hyperparathyroidism • Malignancy • Bone disease • Immobilization • Acute pancreatitis • Renal function	Calcium gluconate Calcium chloride
Magnesium 8.1–24.3 mEq	• Renal function • Refeeding • Hypokalemia	Magnesium sulfate

[a]Rapid healing examples being burn, and young trauma patients who have rapid tissue generation.

TABLE 11-9 Recommended Daily IV Delivery of Essential Trace Minerals to Adults

Element	Stable Adult	Comments
Zinc	2.5–4.0 mg	Increase dose with catabolic state; increase dose with intestinal fluid losses: 12.2 mg/L small-bowel fluid loss 17.1 mg/kg stool/ileostomy
Copper	0.3–0.5 mg	Reduce or hold dose with biliary disease
Chromium	10–15 µg	Increase dose to 20 µg with intestinal losses, reduce in renal disease
Manganese	60–100 µg	Reduce dose with biliary disease
Selenium	20–40 µg	
Molybdenum[a]	20–130 µg	Reduce dose with renal disease

[a]Molybdenum is not presently included in the combination commercial trace element product.

7 to 9 mmol per 1,000 kcal. However, this amount may need to be reduced in patients with renal failure. At present, there is a nationwide shortage of phosphate solutions compatible with PN.

Other trace minerals may not need to be supplemented daily in short-term PN. However, syndromes have been caused by the omission of zinc, chromium, and copper from long-term PN. Recommendations for parenteral supplementation of these minerals were established by the ASPEN Advisory Group and are listed in Table 11-9 (24). The amounts of trace minerals in previously available commercial products are listed in Table 11-10. Owing to decreased productivity by the companies producing MVI formulations, there is currently a nationwide shortage. The FDA has approved importation of a European product (Table 11-10) for use during times of shortage.

The acid–base balance of the patient is influenced by the chloride and acetate content of the PN formula. Acetate can be converted to bicarbonate, which raises the pH. In cases of metabolic acidosis, the acetate content of the formula should be increased and the chloride content decreased. Increasing the acetate content of the PN solution is also useful in cases of large bicarbonate loss, as in pancreatic fistula. In contrast, the chloride content should be increased in metabolic alkalosis. The chloride content should also be increased when nasogastric tube drainage results in a significant loss of stomach acid.

Essential Fatty Acids

Essential fatty acids (EFA) must be supplied for all patients receiving PN. This is done with the addition of linoleic and linolenic acid, 18-carbon EFA. Although a large amount of adipose storage fat

TABLE 11-10 Commercially Available Intravenous Trace Mineral Products for Adults

Product	Chromium (µg)	Copper (mg)	Manganese (mg)	Zinc (mg)	Selenium (µg)
Multitrace-4	4	0.4	100	1	0
Multitrace-5	4	0.4	100	1	20
Multitrace-4 concentrate	10	1	500	5	0
Mutitrace-5 concentrate	10	1	500	5	60
Addamel N[a]	1	0.13	0.027	0.65	3.2

[a]Addamel N also contains (per 1 mL): Iron 0.11 mg, Molybdenum 1.9 µg, Iodine 0.013 mg, Fluorine 0.095 mg. Normal dosing 5–10 mL.
Amounts of trace elements are for a 1mL dose in a previously manufactured product, amounts may change in future products.
Single trace element products are also available for chromium, copper, manganese, zinc, selenium, molybdenum, and iodine.

is linoleic acid (8%–10%), fatty stores are largely inaccessible during the infusion of concentrated carbohydrate solutions. High plasma levels of insulin, resulting from the infusion of concentrated glucose, prevent the breakdown of stored triglycerides and release of the EFAs into the circulation. Linoleic acid deficiency has been reported in patients on glucose-based PN without lipids for as little as 2 weeks. Currently available IV fat emulsions (IVFE) contain approximately one-half to two-thirds of their fatty acids as linoleic acid and approximately 5% to 10% as linolenic acid.

Manifestations of EFA deficiency, which often appears 3 to 4 weeks after the initiation of lipid-free PN, include the following:
1. Dry, cracked, scaling skin with impetigo and oozing in intertriginous folds
2. Coarsened hair
3. Hair loss
4. Impaired wound healing
5. Alterations in platelet function

Tests for deficiency include measuring the triene:tetraene ratio. Deficiency is present when the ratio exceeds 0.2 and is combined with the before-mentioned clinical manifestations. The ratio of linoleic acid to arachidonic acid also can be measured. Normal values average 1.67 ± 0.62. Ratios of approximately 1.2 are seen in EFA deficiency.

In patients who do not tolerate parenteral lipids, either **cutaneous application of safflower oil** (~3 mg/kg/day) or oral supplementation of 15 mL corn oil or medium-chain triglyceride oil may be used to prevent EFA deficiency (35).

DESIGNING THE SOLUTION FOR PARENTERAL NUTRITION

The base solution is the amino acid and dextrose combination to which electrolytes, vitamins, and minerals are added. The dextrose–amino acid combination is often prepared in the hospital pharmacy or centralized pharmacy with sterile technique by combining concentrated dextrose solutions with commercially available amino acid preparations. Two-in-one (dextrose–amino acid) or three-in-one (dextrose–amino acid–lipids) parenteral solutions are also commercially available. Characteristics of various commercially available amino acid solutions are given in Tables 11-11 to 11-13.

Commercial Amino Acid Solutions

Commercial amino acid solutions may contain various amounts of electrolytes, as noted in Table 11-11. This becomes important when the final electrolyte content of combined solutions is calculated. Many of the 3% to 5% solutions are used in PPN. Higher concentrations of electrolytes have been added to these solutions so that they can be ordered without additional electrolyte supplementation. Most of the more concentrated amino acid solutions have a low concentration of electrolytes so that individualized combinations of total daily electrolytes can be prepared. The standard solutions profiles presented in Table 11-12 are based on amino acid concentrations in normal serum with modifications to stimulate anabolism. Disease-specific solutions are also available (Table 11-13). In general, these solutions should not be used for longer than 2 weeks since they do not provide a complete amino acid profile (35).

Amino acid solutions designed for **patients with renal failure not receiving dialysis** have an increased concentration of essential amino acids (Table 11-13). The benefit of these solutions has not been proven in controlled trials. In addition, they are more expensive and are available only in low concentrations, which may lead to problems with fluid overload.

Solutions with **increased** branched-chain amino acids (BCAAs) were developed to be used in patients with increased metabolic stress or hepatic failure with encephalopathy (Table 11-13). Standard amino acid solutions have total BCAA concentrations of 20% to 25%. Again, the high cost of these formulas combined with lack of evidence regarding their benefit outside of patients with encephalopathy limits their usefulness.

During catabolism, intracellular levels of glutamine fall, and, it has been theorized, supplementation would be beneficial. However, a randomized trial of parenteral and enteral glutamine supplementation in critically ill patients with shock and multiorgan failure demonstrated a trend toward increased mortality when compared with patients who did not receive glutamine (32.4% vs. 27.2%, $P = 0.05$) (26). No difference in mortality was noted in a trial of patients

TABLE 11-11 Electrolyte and Nitrogen Content of Crystalline Amino Acid Solutions for Parenteral Nutrition

	Sodium (mEq/L)	Potassium (mEq/L)	Magnesium (mEq/L)	Acetate (mEq/L)	Chloride (mEq/L)	Phosphorus (mmol of P per L)	Nitrogen (g/L)	Osmolarity (mEq/L)	pH
Standard									
Aminosyn 10%	0	5.4	0	148	0	0	15.7	1,000	5.3
Aminosyn 8.5% w/o lytes	0	5.4	0	90	35	0	13.4	850	5.3
Aminosyn 8.5% with lytes	65	66	10	142	98	30	13.4	1,160	5.3
Aminosyn II 10%	45	0	0	72	0	0	15.3	873	5.0–6.3
Aminosyn II 8.5%	33	0	0	61	0	0	13	742	5.0–6.5
FreAmine III	10	0	0	72	2	10	13.0	810	6.6
Procalamine 3%	35	24	5	47	41	3.5	4.6	735	6.8
Travasol 10%	0	0	0	87	40	0	16.5	1,000	6.0
Travasol 8.5% w/o lytes	3	0	0	73	34	0	9.3	520	6.0
Travasol 8.5% with lytes	70	60	10	141	70	30	14.3	1,160	6.0
Travasol 3.5% M	25	15	5	54	25	7.5	5.9	525	6.0
Catabolic State									
Aminosyn-HBC 7%	7	0	0	70	42	0	NA	665	5.2
BranchAmin 4%	0	0	0	0	0	0	4.43	316	6.0
FreAmine HBC 6.9%	10	0	0	57	<3	0	9.7	620	6.5
Hepatic Failure									
HepatAmine 8%	10	0	0	62	<3	10	12.0	785	6.5
Renal Failure									
Aminess 5.2%	0	0		50	0	0	6.6	416	6.4
Aminosyn-RF 5.2%	0	0	0	105	0	0	7.7	475	5.2
NephrAmine 5.4%	5	0	0	44	<3	0	6.5	435	6.5
RenAmin 6.5%	0	0	0	60	31	0	10	600	5.0–7.0
Pediatric									
Aminosyn-PF 10%	3.4	0	0	46	0	0	15.2	834	5.0–6.5
Trophamine 10%	5	0	0	97	<3	0	15.5	875	5.0–6.0

Formulations may have changed since the preparation of this table. Consult prescription information.

TABLE 11-12 Amino Acid Profiles of Standard Crystalline Amino Acid Solutions for Parenteral Use[a]

Amino Acid	Aminosyn 10%	Aminosyn II 10%	FreAmine III 10%	Novamine 15%	ProcalAmine 3%	Travasol 10%
Essential Amino Acids (g/dL)						
Lysine	0.72	1.05	0.75	1.18	0.31	0.58
Tryptophan	0.16	0.20	0.15	0.25	0.05	0.18
Phenylalanine	0.44	0.30	0.56	1.04	0.17	0.56
Methionine	0.40	0.17	0.53	0.75	0.16	0.40
Threonine	0.52	0.40	0.40	0.75	0.12	0.42
Leucine	0.94	1.00	0.91	1.04	0.27	0.73
Isoleucine	0.72	0.66	0.69	0.75	0.21	0.60
Valine	0.80	0.50	0.66	0.96	0.20	0.58
Nonessential Amino Acids (g/dL)						
Histidine	0.30	0.30	0.28	0.89	0.08	0.48
Glutamate	—	0.74	—	0.75	—	—
Proline	0.86	0.72	0.63	0.89	0.34	0.68
Aspartate	—	0.70	—	0.43	—	—
Serine	0.42	0.53	0.59	0.59	0.18	0.50
Arginine	0.98	1.02	0.95	1.47	0.29	1.15
Alanine	1.28	0.99	0.71	2.17	0.21	2.07
Glycine	1.28	0.50	1.40	1.04	0.42	1.03
Tyrosine	0.04	0.27	—	0.04	—	0.04
Cysteine	—	—	<0.02	—	<0.02	—

[a]Values are given for a single concentrated solution available in each product line.
Formulations may have changed since the preparation of this table. Consult prescribing information.

with inflammatory bowel disease (36). A review of prospective randomized clinical trials of glutamine supplementation in patients with short-bowel syndrome, during cancer chemotherapy and in bone marrow transplantation, and in surgical, burn, and intensive care unit patients, was completed, and it was concluded, based on present evidence, that no firm recommendation regarding the use of supplemental parenteral glutamine can be made at this time (37,38) (see Chapter 11 for further discussion of glutamine).

Dextrose

Dextrose is the primary energy source for the human body. The **dextrose monohydrate** used in IV solutions provides 3.4 kcal per gram. The brain, erythrocytes, leukocytes, lens of the eye, and renal medulla exclusively require or preferentially use glucose to meet their needs. Dextrose is available in concentrations of 5% to 70%. The percent concentration is grams of solute per 100 mL of solution. For example, 10% dextrose (D10) contains 10 g dextrose per 100 mL of solution or 100 g per L. The most common concentrations used to compound CPN are 50% and 70% dextrose.

> Minimum requirement: 1 mg/kg/min
> Maximum tolerated: 4 mg/kg/min in critically ill patients
> 7 mg/kg/min in stable hospitalized patients

Higher rates are associated with hyperglycemia and fatty liver (3).

Intravenous Fat Emulsions

Currently, soybean oil–based lipids are primarily used for adults in the United States. In Canada and Europe, medium-chain triglyceride, olive oil– and fish oil–based alternatives are also available.

IVFE of soybean or safflower oil in combination with glycerol and emulsifiers are available in 10%, 20%, and 30% concentrations. The emulsified particles are about the same size as

TABLE 11-13 Amino Acid Profiles of Modified Crystalline Amino Acid Solutions for Specialized Parenteral Use

	Catabolic State			Renal Failure			Hepatic Failure	Pediatric Growth Formulas	
Amino Acid	Aminosyn-HBC 7%	BranchAmin 4%	FreAmine HBC 6.9%	Aminess 5.2%	Aminosyn-RF 5.2%	Nephr-Amine II 5.4%	Ren-Amin 6.5%	HepatAmine 8%	Aminosyn-PF 10%	Trophamine 10%
Essential Amino Acids (g/dL)										
Lysine	0.25	—	0.41	0.60	0.54	0.64	0.45	0.61	0.47	0.49
Tryptophan	0.09	—	0.09	0.19	0.16	0.20	0.16	0.07	0.12	0.12
Phenylalanine	0.23	—	0.32	0.82	0.73	0.88	0.49	0.10	0.30	0.29
Methionine	0.21	—	0.25	0.82	0.73	0.88	0.50	0.10	0.12	0.20
Threonine	0.27	—	0.20	0.38	0.33	0.40	0.38	0.45	0.36	0.25
Leucine	1.58	1.38	1.37	0.82	0.73	0.88	0.60	1.10	0.83	0.84
Isoleucine	0.79	1.38	0.76	0.52	0.46	0.56	0.50	0.90	0.53	0.49
Valine	0.79	1.24	0.88	0.60	0.53	0.64	0.82	0.84	0.45	0.47
Nonessential Amino Acids (g/dL)										
Histidine	0.15	—	0.16	0.41	0.43	0.25	0.42	0.24	0.22	0.29
Glutamate	—	—	—	—	—	—	—	—	0.58	0.30
Proline	0.45	—	0.63	—	—	—	0.35	0.80	0.57	0.41
Aspartate	—	—	—	—	—	—	—	—	0.37	0.19
Serine	0.22	—	0.33	—	—	—	0.30	0.50	0.35	0.23
Arginine	0.51	—	0.58	—	0.60	—	0.63	—	0.86	0.73
Alanine	0.66	—	0.40	—	—	—	0.56	0.77	0.49	0.32
Glycine	0.66	—	0.33	—	—	—	0.30	0.90	0.27	0.22
Tyrosine	0.03	—	—	—	—	—	0.04	—	0.04	0.14
Cysteine	—	—	<0.02	—	—	<0.02	<0.02	—	—	<0.02
Taurine	—	—	—	—	—	—	—	—	0.05	0.02

Formulations may have changed since the preparation of this table. Consult prescribing information.

chylomicrons. The most commonly used in PN solutions are 10% and 20% emulsions that provide 1.1 kcal per mL and 2.0 kcal per mL, respectively. The additional nonfat calories come largely from glycerol. Egg phospholipids are used as an emulsifier. Patients with an egg allergy should not be given lipids. The IVFE should not be given to patients who have triglyceride concentrations of greater than 400 mg per dL. Moreover, patients at risk for hypertriglyceridemia should have serum triglyceride concentrations checked at least once during IVFE infusion to ensure adequate clearance. Characteristics of several commercially available lipid emulsions are given in Table 11-14. Because the emulsions are isotonic, administration together with the base solution reduces the overall osmolarity of the infused fluids, an advantage in PPN. The optimal percentage of calories from fat is not known; however, 20% to 60% of calories from fat have been administered without detrimental effects. Problems (decreased reticuloendothelial system function, impaired immune response, fat overload syndrome) have been associated with very high rates of lipid administration (>1 kcal/kg/h). *Limiting the rate of lipid administration to 0.03 to 0.05 g/kg/hour has been recommended* (3,38).

Vitamin K is included in most commercial lipid emulsions (Table 11-14). The vitamin K content is affected by the proportion of safflower oil to soybean oil (higher concentration of vitamin K) as well as the lipid concentration, doubling with an increase from 10% to 20% lipid (39).

Lipid emulsions containing **fish oil as a source of** omega-3 fatty acids (**n-3 lipids**) in addition to a fixed combination of long-chain triglycerides (LCT), LCT/medium-chain triglyceride mixture, with or without olive oil-based lipid emulsion, are primarily available in the European market. Omegaven, an omega-3 fatty acid–based emulsion manufactured in Germany, is available for research purposes and single patient use with FDA approval (http://www.fda.gov/Drugs/DevelopmentApprovalProcess/HowDrugsareDevelopedandApproved/ApprovalApplications/InvestigationalNewDrugINDApplication/ucm368740.htm.). A recently approved product, ClinOleic (20% lipid emulsion, a mixture of olive and soybean oil), by Baxter, will soon be approved for distribution in the United States. A secondary analysis of a prospective multicenter study in adult ICU patients found that compared with soybean oil, patients receiving olive or fish oil–based lipids had improved clinical outcomes including shorter length of ICU stay and time on ventilator (40). Concern regarding the use of n-6 lipids in critically ill patients has prompted guidelines recommending holding soy-based lipids the first week in these patients (41). Soybean-based emulsions were found to be potentially harmful in patients with severe pulmonary failure and sepsis (42). However, a retrospective review of surgical/trauma ICU patients before/after a change in standard of practice to withholding lipids for 7 to 10 days

TABLE 11-14 Characteristics of Lipid Emulsions for Parenteral Use

Product	Parent Oil	Average Droplet Size (µg)	Osmolarity (mOsmol/L)	Caloric Content (kcal/mL)	Linoleic Acid (% total fat)	Linolenic Acid (% total fat)
Intralipid 10%	Soybean oil	0.5	260	1.1	50	9
Intralipid 20%	Soybean oil	0.5	268	2.0	50	9
Intralipid 30%	Soybean oil	0.5	200	3.0	50	9
Liposyn II 10%	Soybean and safflower oils	0.4	320	1.1	66	4
Liposyn II 20%	Soybean and safflower oils	0.4	340	2.0	66	4
Liposyn III 10%	Soybean oil	0.4	284	1.1	54	8
Liposyn III 20%	Soybean oil	0.4	292	2.0	54	8
ClinOleic 20%	Olive Oil (80%) + Soybean oil (20%)	0.45	270	2.0	15	65
Omegaven	Fish Oil (10%) + glycerol (2.5%)		308–376	1.1		

post admission demonstrated no differences in infectious complication or mortality (43). It is known that n-6 lipids serve as a precursor of the cyclooxygenase and lipoxygenase pathway for the production of highly inflammatory mediators (prostaglandin E2 and leukotriene B4). Emulsions with n-3 lipids change the synthesis to mediators with less inflammatory potential (prostaglandin E3 and leukotriene B5). The shift in lipid mediator generation and the incorporation of n-3 lipids into cell membrane phospholipids has been confirmed in several studies (44–47).

Several prospective randomized controlled studies have been completed comparing n-6 sparing lipids to n-6 lipids, primarily in ICU and trauma patient populations (41,48–52). A meta-analysis of these studies demonstrates a trend toward a reduction in mortality, ICU length of stay, and duration of ventilation. The 2013 Canadian critical care nutrition guidelines suggest that if parenteral lipids are used, options to reduce the load of n-6 fatty acids/soybean oil emulsions should be considered if available; otherwise, n-6 lipids should be held for patients in whom PN is required for less than 10 days (38).

Lipid emulsions can be given at different times from the base solution, at the same time as the base solution in a single bag (refer to earlier section on Nutrient Requirements during Parenteral Nutrition) or at the same time as the base solution in a separate bag. In the latter case a Y-tube arrangement of the two bags is used to mix the base solution and lipid emulsion just before they enter the patient. Issues of stability have become more important as home PN has become more common and delays between the preparation and use of PN formulas are longer. In general, admixtures are less stable than base solution and lipids in separate bags. Homecare patients now have the option of a product that has the base solution and lipid in separate compartments of one bag. The compartments are separated by a zipper, which is opened just before use.

Total Nutrient Admixture

TNA, also known as a three-in-one PN, provides the lipid emulsion and base solution combined in a single bag. This approach allows a hospital pharmacy to combine all the components of a patient's PN formula for a whole day in a single 3-L bag. Physical manipulation of the central line is reduced, as is the risk for infection. Reduced requirements for nursing time and equipment (bags, tubes) lead to cost savings. However, certain disadvantages and advantages are associated with TNAs as presented in Table 11-15. The emulsion may break down, with fat droplets combining to form larger fat droplets, and if deterioration progresses, the fat and water components separate. The safe use of TNAs requires visual inspection for signs of deterioration before administration. Deterioration takes place in stages:

1. **Aggregation**—larger fat droplets form and are distributed throughout the solution; reversible with gentle shaking.

TABLE 11-15 Advantages and Disadvantages Associated with Total Nutrient Admixture

Disadvantages
- Lipid droplets (0.33 to 0.5 μm) can clog filters; thus a larger filter is needed that may not trap all organisms, increasing risk of contamination
- Some medications that are compatible with base solutions are incompatible with TNA (55)
- Lipid emulsions are a good medium for growth of bacteria and fungi
- It is more difficult to see particulates, such as precipitated salts
- The emulsion may break down with the fat and water components separating

Advantages
- Only one bag of solution to compound and administer
- Less manipulation during administration
- Less risk of contamination
- Possible benefit in fluid-restricted patients
- May be more cost-effective overall

2. **Creaming**—the formation of a thin (1- to 2-cm) layer of aggregated fat droplets on the surface of the solution; reversible with gentle shaking.
3. **Coalescence**—the further fusion of fat droplets to create a thicker (10-cm), dense layer at the surface; if coalescence develops, the infusion must be discontinued.
4. **Oiling out**—occurs when fat droplets separate from the solution and appear as a clear layer on the surface; if oiling out is observed, the infusion should be discontinued. The likelihood that a lipid emulsion will deteriorate increases with time and temperature. TNAs should not hang at room temperature for more than 24 hours.

Electrolyte and Trace Mineral Preparations for Parenteral Use

These should be added to base solutions for PN in pharmacy IV additive rooms under controlled, aseptic conditions. The use of laminar flow hoods has reduced the incidence of contaminated fluids.

Electrolyte Additives

Electrolyte additives can be added by specifying the actual additive (e.g., sodium chloride) or, ideally, by specifying the final content of the individual cations and anions. Electrolyte salts often used in PN solutions, the normal ranges of requirements for the patient receiving PN, and conditions that may require an alteration of the amount provided are listed in Table 11-8. Additional electrolytes may also be needed to compensate for increased losses from wounds, gastric suction, fever, surgical drains, emesis, and diarrhea. Although the approximate electrolyte content of GI losses is known (Table 7-6, Chapter 7), if there is any question, an aliquot of the output can be sent for analysis.

Vitamins

Vitamins are ordered daily or every other day from the outset of PN therapy based on availability of product. The formulation for the MVI Adult is presented in Table 11-7. As previously mentioned, the present standard MVI preparations contain vitamin K.

Vitamin K was included in the new formulation with the intention of providing the patient with a consistent daily supply. This addition raised concerns regarding the potential impact on patient management. Prior to this change, physicians were prescribing vitamin K separately either as a SC or as an intramuscular (IM) injection. Theoretically, the consistent and modest amount of vitamin K added to the new formulation should increase the ease of maintaining a desired level of hypoprothrombinemia in patients on anticoagulant therapy with warfarin (53).

Trace Mineral Supplements

US Commercial Trace Metal Solutions provide *chromium, copper, zinc, manganese, selenium, iodide,* and *molybdenum* in various combinations to provide the recommended daily adult dose in 0.8 to 3 mL of solution, depending on the manufacturer. The components of commonly used trace elements supplementation for CPN are presented in Table 11-10. Current drug shortages have led to FDA clearance for temporary importation of a product from Europe (Addamel N) that has a few additional components (see Table 11-10)

Zinc

Additional zinc may be added as zinc sulfate; however, it should not exceed 10 mg in TNAs. The addition of 5 mg of elemental zinc (commonly found in combination supplements) meets the average daily requirements of most patients who do not have additional intestinal losses.

Iron

Iron deficiency can be corrected with the administration of parenteral iron (e.g., iron dextran) IM or IV (see Chapter 7, under Trace Minerals). The IM administration of iron dextran rarely has been associated with pain, the formation of sterile abscesses, and tissue atrophy. As a result, IV administration is the preferred route. The usual daily requirements are met by the monthly administration of 1 mL of iron dextran (50 mg of elemental iron), which may be added directly to a base solution but not to a TNA. Two other preparations commonly used are sodium ferric gluconate (1 mL = 12.5 mg of elemental iron) and iron sucrose (1 mL = 20 mg elemental iron). For a complete list of preparations, see Table 7-4 in Chapter 7. If abnormal amounts of iron are being lost from the GI tract or other sites of bleeding, larger replacement doses are necessary.

Iron replacement should be titrated to laboratory indices of iron status. The parenteral administration of iron dextran is associated with anaphylaxis. The precautions to be taken in administering parenteral iron are outlined in Chapter 7, and these must be carefully observed. Because of the large stores of iron and the low rate of turnover in iron-repleted patients, the problems associated with iron administration can be avoided in many cases by not giving parenteral iron at all. Patients with normal iron stores prior to starting PN who require less than 2 months of therapy will most likely not need supplementation.

Additional Points

Iodine deficiencies have been described in infants (53) and adult patients on long-term PN. Iodine must be ordered individually as sodium or potassium iodide; the suggested daily dose is 1.0 μg of iodine per kg. There is some concern that the amount of **manganese** added to the standard trace element formulations may lead to toxicity in patients receiving long-term PN. Whole blood manganese levels should be monitored periodically (54). **Molybdenum** (20 μg) also may be provided within the PN for patients on long-term support (55).

Other Additives

Other additives may be included directly in the PN formula or administered safely in piggyback fashion with the base solution or TNA. Compatibility is a complex issue that is influenced by the exact components of the nutrient solution (including electrolytes, vitamins, and minerals), pH, concentration of the additive, and mixing sequence.

Medications

Medications that will come in direct contact with the PN (admixture in container or co-infusion through the same IV tubing), compatibility, and stability of the various components should be known. Otherwise, the medications should be administered separate from the PN. Incompatible medication and PN formulations can lead to precipitates that can obstruct blood flow through the pulmonary capillaries, leading to pulmonary embolism. Most pharmacies have a short list of medications that are commonly added directly to PN formulations (histamine2-receptor antagonists, insulin, vitamins). Other additives are better given in piggyback fashion. Table 11-16 lists common additives reported to be compatible with base solutions or three-in-one admixtures (56,57). References for the compatibility of specific additives appear in Rombeau and Rolandelli (58) and in Trissel (59).

Insulin

Regular insulin reduces hyperglycemia when added directly to the PN solution. Hypoglycemia is less apt to result from a decrease in the fluid rate or inadvertent interruption of the PN fluid if the insulin is added directly to the fluid rather than given by SC injection. Insulin is not routinely added to all TPN solutions; however, when added, only regular human insulin should be used.

- Insulin-requiring diabetics: Add 0.1 unit of insulin for each g of dextrose. For example, if the PN solution contains 250 g dextrose, 25 units of insulin should be added. Supplement with additional SC insulin as dictated by the blood glucose (BG) level.
- On day 2 of PN for insulin-requiring diabetics: Increase the added insulin by two-thirds of the additional SC insulin given in the previous 24 hours.
- All patients started on PN should have their BG levels monitored q 4 hours while the PN is infusing, covering with SC insulin as needed. Oral hypoglycemics should be discontinued when TPN is initiated.

Heparin

Heparin has been advocated by some as an additive to prevent fibrin plugging of the CVC. Sodium heparin is compatible at all concentrations with the PN solution, but probably is of little benefit and is not currently recommended for routine TPN use (60,61).

METABOLIC COMPLICATIONS ASSOCIATED WITH PARENTERAL NUTRITION

The morbidity associated with PN is the greatest deterrent to its use in many institutions. Complication rates are effectively reduced when teams that include physicians, dietitians, nurses, and pharmacists are organized to administer PN (60–62). Serious complications develop in

TABLE 11-16 Medication Compatibilities with PN

Additive	2-in-1	TNA	Additive	2-in-1	TNA
Acetazolamide	I	X	Hydrocortisone	C	X
Acyclovir	I	I	Ifosfamide	C	C
Albumin	C	I	Imipenem-Cilastatin sodium	C	C
Amikacin	C	I	Indomethacin sodium trihydrate	I	X
Aminophylline	C	C	Insulin	C	C
Amoxicillin	I	I	Iron dextran	C	I
Amphotericin B	I	I	Isoproterenol	C	C
Ampicillin sodium	C	C	Kanamycin	C	C
Ascorbic acid	C	C	Lidocaine	C	C
Aztreonam	C	C	Linezolid	C	X
Carbenicillin	C	X	Lorazepam	C	I
Cefazolin	C	C	Mannitol	C	C
Cefepime[a]	C	I	Meropenem[a]	C	C
Cefoxitin	C	C	Meperidine	C	X
Ceftazidme	C	C	Methotrexate	I	C
Ceftriazone sodium	C	C	Methylprednisolone	C	C
Cephalothin	C	X	Methicillin	C	X
Cephapirin	C	C	Metoclopramide[a]	C	C
Chloramphenicol	C	X	Metronidazole	I	I
Ciprofloxacin lactate	I	C[b]	Methyldopate	C	I
Cisplatin	I	C[b]	Mezlocillin	C	X
Clindamycin	C	C	Midazolam	I	I
Cyanocobalamin	C	X	Morphine sulfate	C	X
Cyclosporine	C	C	Multivitamins	C	C
Cytarabine	C	X	Nafcillin sodium	C	C
Dexamethasone	C	C	Norepinephrine bitartrate	C	C
Digoxin	C	C	Octreotide	I	I
Dipehnhydramine HCl	C	C	Ondansetron HCl	C	I
Dobutamine HCl	C	C	Oxacillin	C	C
Dopamine	C	C	Pantoprazole	I	I
Doxycycline	C	X	PenicillinG potassium	C	C
Enalaprilat	C	C	Pentobarbitol sodium	C	I
Epinephrine HCl	C	X	Phenobarbitol sodium	C	I
Erythromycin	C	C	Phenytoin sodium	I	I
Esomeprazole[a]	I	I	Phytonadione	C	C
Famotidine	C	C	Piperacillin sodium	C	C
Fentanyl[a]	C	C	Promethazine HCl	C	C
Fluconazole	C	C	Ranitidine	C	C
Foscarnet	C	X	Tacrolimus	C	C
Furosemide	C	C	Ticarcillin disodium	C	C
Gentamicin	C	C	Tobramycin	C	C
Haloperidol lactate	C	I	Urokinase	C	X
Heparin sodium	C	I	Vancomycin	C	C

[a]Compatibility only studied for 4 hours.
[b]Discoloration at 4 hours.
C, compatible; I, incompatible; X, no information.

fewer than 5% of patients treated with TPN at institutions where a team approach has been implemented. The complications of PN can be categorized as metabolic or nonmetabolic depending on whether they are related to the nutritional formula or the mechanical technique of delivery. Mechanical or nonmetabolic complications were addressed earlier in this chapter.

Hyperglycemia and Hyperosmolarity

A common complication resulting from the delivery of concentrated dextrose, hyperglycemia is more likely to develop during periods of intense catabolic stress. Hyperglycemia can adversely affect fluid balance, immune function, inflammation, and outcome; glucose control has been shown to lessen these effects (63). Because this appears to be true for patients with and without a known diagnosis of diabetes, hyperglycemia should be aggressively treated in all patients (64). The ability to handle the glucose load may improve as PN continues. Hyperosmolarity results from the insufficient administration of free water or from persistent glycosuria and free water diuresis. The insidious development of hyperglycemia and glycosuria during an apparently stable course of PN can indicate the onset of a new catabolic stress, such as catheter sepsis or other infectious source. Hyperglycemia secondary to insulin resistance is often seen in the stressed hospital patient as well. Overfeeding (receiving more calories than needed) will cause hyperglycemia as well. Short-term overfeeding causes hyperglycemia; long-term overfeeding causes fatty liver and can result in impaired immune function. Overfeeding with resultant hyperglycemia is one of the most common and most serious problems associated with PN (65). The concern for the metabolic complications of overfeeding has led to growing support for hypocaloric feeding (66); however prolonged hypocaloric feeding is associated with its own deleterious effects and should be avoided (67). Many protocols now exist to aid with glycemic control of the hospitalized patient (64). There remains debate regarding the desired target BG range for different patient populations; however, the majority agree BG levels should be maintained less than 150 to 160 mg per dL (64).

Abnormalities of Serum Electrolyte Concentration

Abnormalities of any serum electrolyte concentration can develop during PN; requirements vary considerably from patient to patient and during an individual patient's course of therapy. Potassium requirements may be high initially because of fluxes from the extracellular to the intracellular space (secondary to insulin and glucose administration) and because of reversal of the catabolic state. This initially high requirement is likely to decrease during the course of PN. Hyperchloremic acidosis was once a frequent complication of PN because of the high chloride content of early amino acid solutions. Currently available solutions are low in chloride, and this complication is now less frequent. Still, one should *keep the chloride content equal to or below the sodium content in the daily prescription to prevent hyperchloremia* unless unusual chloride losses are occurring. Phosphorus requirements increase with the initiation of protein and may result in hypophosphatemia shortly after PN is initiated. If feasible, oral or per tube phosphate formulations should be initiated at the same time as PN in times of shortages of parenteral forms. The PN formula should not be used as the "repletion" route for low electrolyte levels due to the rate of infusion. For example, a PN formulation containing 80 mEq of potassium given over a 24-hour period would only provide 3.3 mEq per hour. This may be too long to delay repletion. In general, patients should be given an IV piggyback supplementation, with the amount in the PN adjusted to reflect what has been given with the goal of maintenance as opposed to repletion.

Bone Disease/Liver Dysfunction

Complications of long-term PN include metabolic bone disease and liver dysfunction. These are discussed in detail later in this chapter.

ORDERING AND INITIATING PARENTERAL NUTRITION FOR CENTRAL VENOUS CATHETER

The decision to begin PN need never be made in haste. PN should be initiated under controlled conditions and according to a defined protocol (Table 11-17). Orders must be carefully written because of the multiple additives needed on a daily basis. A special order form is recommended to avoid transcription errors and accidental omission of important nutrients. Figure 11-1 is an example of a CVC PN order form that offers four different TNAs based on amino acid content, and the option to provide only a base solution of amino acid/dextrose with separate or no lipid emulsion. The TNAs provide percent calories for all macronutrients within recommended ranges. According to this order form, PN bags are sequentially numbered throughout a patient's

TABLE 11-17 Calculation of Macronutrient Additives for TPN

1. Calculate patient's caloric and protein needs:
   70 kg × 25 kcal/kg = 1,750 calories
   70 kg × 1.2 g pro/kg = 84 g protein
2. Determine amino acids first:
   84 g = 336 calories
   10% amino acid solution = 10 g/100 mL of solution
   12.5% = 12.5 g/100 mL
   8% = 8 g/100 mL
   Example: 10 g/100 mL = 84 g/? mL
   $$\frac{84 \text{ g} \times 100 \text{ ml}}{10 \text{ g}} = ? \text{ mL of 10\% amino acid solution}$$
   = **840 mL of 10% amino acid solution**
3. Determine dextrose requirements next:
   Assume patient is a nondiabetic = 55% calories from carbohydrate
   1,750 × .55 = 962 calories
   962 calories ÷ 3.4 (kcal/kg dextrose) = 283 g dextrose
   Based on 70% dextrose base: 70 g/100 mL = 283 g/? mL
   $$\frac{283 \text{ g} \times 100 \text{ ml}}{70 \text{ g}} = ? \text{ mL of D70}$$
   = **404 ml of D70 (70% dextrose) solution**
4. Leftover calories as lipid (or withhold these calories if lipids to be held)
   1,750 calories − (336 protein calories + 962 dextrose calories) = 452 calories
   10% lipid emulsion = 1.1 kcal/mL   452 ÷ 1.1 = **411 mL 10% lipid solution**
   20% lipid emulsion = 2.0 kcal/mL   452 ÷ 2.0 = **226 mL 20% lipid solution**

course of therapy. Note that all the additives are ordered on the same order form so that the daily prescription of nutrients can easily be seen.

1. **Review patient assessment and baseline labs** (Table 11-18).
2. **Determine patient's caloric and protein requirements as previously outlined** (Table 11-6).
3. **Determine which standard formula would come closest to meeting the patient's estimated needs.** On the example form, the grams of each macronutrient per 1,000 calories are provided. For example, if it is determined that the patient requires 1,500 calories (1.5 × 1,000 calories): 1,500 calories of the Intermediate Nitrogen solution will provide 60 g protein (40 g × 1.5 = 60), whereas 1,500 calories of the High Nitrogen solution will provide 75 g protein. Therefore, the practitioner would decide whether the patient would benefit more from 60 or from 75 g protein per day.
4. **Whether or not to start at full calories is based on patient tolerance.** Patients who have poor glycemic control, are critically ill, or are at risk of refeeding syndrome should be started with 100 to 200 g or 10% to 15% dextrose. If BG levels remain less than 180 mg per dL and electrolytes are within normal limits, the dextrose concentration should be advanced to goal over 1 to 2 days. If the patient is critically ill or septic, consideration should be given to withholding the lipids for the first 7 to 10 days. Although it is unproven that withholding n-6 lipids in these patients will improve outcomes, it will allow for increased medication compatibility with Y-site administration in patients often plagued with limited IV access. In this case, the base solution formula would be used. The example presented in Table 11-17 demonstrates how to determine the milliliters needed from each macronutrient solution.
5. **Begin electrolytes, MVI, and trace elements based on the patient's lab values and general requirements as outlined in Tables 11-7 to 11-9.** The breakdown of the electrolyte salts used and MVI and trace element formulations, in addition to the intrinsic electrolytes included in the amino acid solution as they appear on the back of the sample order form, are presented in Figure 11-2.

PARENTERAL NUTRITION ORDERS

TPN cut-off time for ordering is **1400**

DATE DUE: _____ BAG #: _____ Calories to the nearest 100 Kcal per 24 hours: _____. Hang time is **2000**.

Check One	STANDARD SOLUTIONS	% Total Kcals Provided As			GM / 1000 Kcal			Approx. Volume Per 1000 Kcal
		Amino Acid	Dextrose	Fat	Amino Acid	Dextrose	Fat	
	a) Intermediate Nitrogen	16%	60%	24%	40	176	27	761 ml
	b) High Nitrogen	20%	55%	25%	50	162	28	843 ml
	c) Very High Nitrogen	24%	56%	20%	60	165	22	920 ml
	d) Low Nitrogen	12%	65%	23%	30	191	26	680 ml
	e) Modified (Approval Required)	__%	__%	__%	---	---	---	----------
	f) Peripheral	16%	32%	52%	40	94	58	1429 ml
	g) Amino Acid / Dextrose	10% Amino Acid _____ ml			70% Dextrose _____ ml			
	Lipids (as separate infusion)	☐ 100 ml ☐ 250 ml ☐ 500 ml ☐ 20% Intralipid rate _____ ml/hour						

ELECTROLYTES	Suggested Daily Amount	Quantity Ordered
Sodium	60-120 mEq	mEq
Potassium	30-80 mEq	mEq
Chloride	80-140 mEq	mEq
Acetate*	*	BALANCE
Calcium	4.6-9.2 mEq	mEq
Magnesium	8.1-24.3 mEq	mEq
Phosphorus	12-24 mMol	mmol
MICRONUTRIENTS		
MVI-Adult	10 ml/day	ml
Trace Elements - 5	1 ml/day	ml
MEDICATIONS		
Insulin for glycemic control	Regular Humulin only	units

WEIGHT: _____ HEIGHT: _____
BMI: _____
(Used for nutritional calculation)

Plasma BMP

Na^+ | Cl^- | BUN \
                                      glu
K^+ | HCO_3 | Cr

Mg^{++} _____
PO_4 _____
Ca^{++} _____

Comments: _____

☐ Order transcribed then read back and verified with prescriber. (REQUIRED)
☐ Telephone/Verbal order taken by: _____ Dietitian from: _____ M.D.
Date: _____ Physician Signature: _____ Printed Name: _____ Pager: _____

Page Nutrition Support Service at 790-4677 for assessment prior to initiating TPN

DO NOT WRITE BELOW THIS LINE

Figure 11-1. Sample parenteral nutrition ordering form, page 1.

6. Recommendations for monitoring patients on PN are presented in Table 11-18. Metabolic complications occur frequently, and the results of routine monitoring should be used not only to adjust the PN formula but also to regulate the frequency of monitoring. Thus, if a patient is found to be hypokalemic on routine monitoring, the appropriate response is not only to increase the potassium content of the PN formulation but also to monitor the serum potassium level more frequently.

7. **The appropriate protocol for discontinuing PN** has been controversial, and practice patterns vary from hospital to hospital. Some investigators have recommended infusing 10% dextrose to avoid hypoglycemia if PN is interrupted, and slow tapering of PN solutions to avoid hypoglycemia when PN is discontinued. In these circumstances, the potential for hypoglycemia is thought to be related to the continued secretion of insulin when the

TABLE 11-18 Monitoring the Acute Care Patient on PN

Parameter	Baseline	Initiation Period	Critically ill	Stable Patient
Vitals, temp	Yes	q 6 h	q 8 h	q 12 h
Weight	Yes	3 times/day	Daily	3 times/week
Intake/Output	Yes	Daily	Daily	As indicated
Blood glucose	Yes	q 4 h	q 1–4 h based on control	q 4–72 h based on control
CBC	Yes	Daily	2 times/week	Weekly
Basic metabolic profile (Na, K, Cl, CO_2, BUN, Creat, Glu, Ca)	Yes	Daily	Daily	2–3 times/week
Mg, PO_4	Yes	Daily	3–4 times/week	Weekly
Triglyceride	Yes	Day 1–2	As needed	As needed
LFTs—ALT, AST, ALP, total bilirubin	Yes	Day 1–2	Weekly	Monthly
Line site	Yes	Daily	Daily	Daily
Dressing change		Day 1–2 post-line placed, replace gauze with transparent dressing	Transparent dressing q week or if nonocclusive	Transparent dressing q week or if nonocclusive

Salts Used
Sodium chloride, Sodium acetate, Sodium phosphate
Potassium chloride, Potassium acetate, Potassium phosphate
Calcium gluconate
Magnesium sulfate

Trace Elements-5	Amount per 1 ml
Zinc	5 mg
Copper	1 mg
Manganese	0.5 mg
Chromium	10 mcg
Selenium	60 mcg

MVI-Adult	Amount per 10 ml
Ascorbic acid (Vitamin C)	200 mg
Retinol (Vitamin A)	1 mg
Ergocalciferol (Vitamin D)	5 mcg
Thiamine (Vitamin B_1)	6 mg
Riboflavin (Vitamin B_2)	3.6 mg
Pyridoxine (Vitamin B_6)	6 mg
Niacinamide	40 mg
d-Panthenol	15 mg
Vitamin E	10 mg
Biotin	60 mcg
Folic acid	0.6 mcg
Cyanocobalamin (Vitamin B_{12})	5 mcg
Phylloquinine (Vitamin K_1)	150 mcg

Travasol 10%- Intrinsio Electrolytes	Amount per 1 liter
Acetate	87 mEq
Chloride	40 mEq

Figure 11-2. Sample parenteral nutrition ordering form, page 2.

infusion of high-glucose solutions is stopped. Others have noted there was no symptomatic hypoglycemia, and glucose profiles returned to a similar baseline level in those whose PN was abruptly stopped when compared with those in the tapered group (68).
8. **Cycling PN** is a method of PN in which the base solution or TNA is infused over a 12- to 16-hour period, usually at night. One guideline for deciding the duration of the infusion during cycling is that the patient should not receive more than 0.5 g of glucose per kg of body weight per hour. Cycling has no physiologic disadvantage over continuous infusion and may actually be better. The fluids are discontinued in the morning so that the patient is free to perform his or her usual daily activities. This method of PN delivery is used for patients who will ultimately be sent home on PN and is also suitable for selected patients expected to undergo long courses of PN in the hospital (e.g., patients receiving bone marrow transplantation). Cyclic PN may not be suitable for patients with diabetes, especially those requiring insulin, because of the risks for hypoglycemia. Cyclic PN may also be unsuitable for patients with heart failure, who cannot tolerate the higher rates of fluid administration.

- **A period of stability (>24 h)** on conventional PN therapy (24-h infusions) should be demonstrated prior to initiating cyclic PN.
- **The use of a volumetric infusion pump** is required. Cyclic PN is facilitated by using a single 2- or 3-L bag for the entire night's infusion. The TNA system is ideal for cyclic infusion if lipid emulsions are required.
- **BG levels should be checked while the infusion is running and 1 to 2 hours post completion.** Given the half-life of regular insulin, the effects of any insulin in the PN may be seen for 1 to 2 hours post completion. The goal should be to keep BG levels greater than 70 mg per dL when the patient is off the PN. Cycling is not advisable for patients who are persistently hyper- or hypoglycemic or who have erratic insulin requirements.
- **Use sterile technique each time the catheter is handled** to connect or disconnect the tubing. A sterile cap should be placed over the catheter tip when it is not in use. Be certain to clamp the catheter before disconnecting it from the solution tubing.
- **Flush the catheter port with heparinized saline solution** immediately before beginning an infusion and when discontinuing the infusion. We use 1:100 heparinized saline solution for permanent catheters and 1:10 for temporary catheters. The volume of the flush varies from 1 to 5 mL and is determined by the length and internal diameter of the catheter.

ORDERING AND INITIATING PERIPHERAL PARENTERAL NUTRITION
General Principles
Providing PN through a peripheral vein is more difficult than through a central vein because peripheral veins tolerate concentrated hypertonic solutions poorly. Daily volume limitations in combination with the requirement for less concentrated solutions may prevent delivery of the desired number of calories. However, protein, vitamin, and mineral requirements can usually be met. In most institutions, CPN is viewed as the procedure of choice for almost all patients requiring PN; however, some investigators advocate supplemental PPN in elderly patients with poor intake and intolerance to short-term feeding tubes (69,70). Need to change access site and phlebitis were noted as downsides to this approach. Premade PPN formulations (e.g., ProcalAmine) are available on the market, lessening the labor cost and concerns for incompatibilities.

Basic Rules for Planning Peripheral Parenteral Nutrition
1. Keep the osmolarity of the final infusate below 800 to 900 mOsmol per L and the dextrose concentration at 10% or less (Table 11-19).
2. Utilize lipid emulsions to increase the nonprotein calories delivered per day, and decrease the osmolarity of the final infusate. An example of a standard PPN formula is a TNA with a caloric distribution of 32% dextrose, 16% protein, and 52% fat and a caloric density of 0.7 cal per mL. Three liters of this TNA contain 2,100 calories and 84 g of protein. Possible immunosuppressive effects have been associated with formulations in which lipids provide such a high portion of the calories.
3. Do not allow fats to provide more than 60% to 70% of the total daily nonprotein calories (>2.5 g per kg of body weight per day).

TABLE 11-19 Osmolarity and Caloric Content of Concentrated Dextrose Solutions

Dextrose Concentration (wt/vol)	Osmolarity (mOsmol/L)	Caloric Content[a] (kcal/dL)
5%	250	17
10%	500	34
20%	1,000	68
50%	2,500	170
70%	3,500	237

[a]Based on the caloric value of dextrose monohydrate used in commercial preparations (3.4 kcal/g).

4. Make sure that both the physician and the pharmacist understand the electrolyte content of the ordered solution. Many of the 3.0% to 3.5% amino acid solutions for peripheral venous administration contain significant amounts of electrolytes. The ordering physician should be aware of the electrolyte content before adding additional electrolytes to the daily PN prescription (Table 11-11).
5. Change the IV infusion site regularly and at the first sign of thrombophlebitis.
6. The osmolarity of PPN solutions may be calculated as follows:

$$\text{Osmolarity (mOsm/L)} = (\text{grams dextrose/L}) \times 5 + (\text{grams amino acid/L}) \times 10 + (\text{grams lipids/L}) \times 0.67 + (\text{mEq cations/L}) \times 2$$

Home Parenteral Nutrition

Home parenteral nutrition (HPN) allows for the increased survival of patients with diseases prohibiting adequate intake and absorption of nutrients via the oral or enteral route. Primarily includes patients with short-bowel syndrome, cancer (causing obstruction or malabsorption), or severe inflammatory bowel disease. ASPEN has recently established a national patient registry (Sustain) for HPN patients to get a better understanding of the number of home patients and to collect data in order to improve patient outcomes. According to the Sustain website in 2002, approximately 39,000 people worldwide received HPN at a cost of $125,000 to $250,000 per year (http://www.nutritioncare.org/ASPEN_Sustain/About_Sustain/). According to the Oley Foundation, a nonprofit organization supporting HPN and EN patients (http://oley.org/index.html), in 2003 approximately 7,000 people in the United States were receiving HPN (71). The first patient discharged home on PN was in the late 1960s (72). While many patients have been on HPN over 10 years, a few are nearing 30 years. The underlying diagnosis is the single most important factor with regard to outcome. For example, a cancer patient has a greater than 70% mortality rate per year, while a Crohn patient has a 4% mortality rate per year. While some factors are absolute, such as diagnosis, length of remaining bowel, and patient's age, others are not, such as use of narcotics and sedatives, treatment by multidisciplinary professionals with experience in HPN, adequate patient/caregiver training, and participation in a HPN support group (73). Regardless, a long-term patient accrues a 10% to 15% chance of dying from a complication of the HPN.

COMPLICATIONS ASSOCIATED WITH LONG-TERM HOME PARENTERAL NUTRITION

Line Sepsis

Line sepsis is the most common cause of fever in a HPN patient. In general, line or catheter sepsis occurs in 1.3% to 26.2% of patients using the catheter to administer HPN. An outcome analysis in 50,470 patients with central venous access found that the most common catheter complications, in descending order, were catheter dysfunction (primarily thrombotic occlusion), catheter site infections, and bloodstream infections. The fewest complications were associated with a chest port followed by tunneled catheter. Midline and nontunneled catheters were associated with increased complications (74).

Metabolic Bone Disease

In some patients receiving long-term CPN (>2 to 3 months), severe pain develops in the periarticular regions, lower extremities, and back despite apparent improvement in the overall nutritional status. Bone biopsies reveal patchy osteomalacia and decreased mineralization, although serum levels of calcium, phosphorus, parathyroid hormone, and total 25-hydroxyvitamin D are normal. Low serum levels of 1,25-dihydroxyvitamin D have been reported in patients on long-term CPN; thus, an altered vitamin D metabolism may be involved in the pathogenesis of the syndrome. Symptoms resolve and 1,25-dihydroxyvitamin D levels normalize after CPN is discontinued. Abnormalities have also been found in the bone biopsy specimens of asymptomatic patients. A study that evaluated 943 bone mass scans (spinal, hip, and forearm) in 75 patients on HPN found a statistically significant decline over time ($P < 0.005$) (75). However, the decline was not significantly different than that of healthy well-matched controls for age and sex. Other factors contributing to bone disease include hypercalciuria during the CPN infusion (likely related to glucose loading or an increased burden of organic sulfate) and possibly improper administration of trace minerals.

Detection
The pathogenesis is not well understood; no good serum marker is available at this time. Symptoms usually include pain in the periarticular regions, lower extremities, and back. Bone mineral density is required for diagnosis.

Treatment
Temporary or permanent discontinuance of CPN and, potentially the removal of vitamin D from the solution are the only currently known therapies.

Liver Dysfunction

Liver dysfunction in patients receiving CPN ranges from mild complications such as elevated transaminases (aspartate aminotransferase, alanine aminotransferase) to steatosis, cholestasis, cirrhosis, liver failure, and even death (76). The mild complications seen in short-term CPN generally resolve with the discontinuation of CPN and rarely lead to severe abnormalities (77). Delayed elevations or persistent elevations (>20 days) of enzymes may represent toxic hepatitis, thought to be related to the amino acid infusion (possibly from products of tryptophan degradation). A reduction in liver enzyme levels has been reported with the use of antibiotics (78). A retrospective review also suggested that liver enzymes are less likely to be elevated in patients receiving metronidazole (78). This effect is possibly related to a reduction in the anaerobic bacterial overgrowth in the small bowel that occurs during CPN. Such organisms may produce hepatotoxic substances, for example, endotoxins, or lithocholic acid. In some patients, elevated liver enzymes and painful hepatomegaly result from acute fat accumulation during carbohydrate feeding. The administration of glucose at rates above 7 mg/kg/min is associated with the development of fatty liver. A recent study of liver disease in patients on HPN found high rates of liver disease (79). Chronic cholestasis developed in 65% of patients after an average of 6 months of HPN. The prevalence of complicated liver disease was 26% after 2 years of HPN and 50% after 6 years.

Detection
Liver disease is detected by regular monitoring of common liver function tests (78) (Table 11-18).

Treatment
Focus should be on prevention of CPN-associated liver disease by avoiding overfeeding (specifically glucose and lipids). Steatosis, fatty liver, often resolves with a reduction of the total calories provided. In addition, lipid intake of greater than 1 g/kg/day has been associated with CPN-induced liver disease (80). Elevated liver enzymes per se are not an indication for discontinuation of CPN. Cycling of the CPN formula over 12 to 14 hours is associated with a decreased metabolic load to the liver. In a study of 107 patients with impaired liver function, 36 were prophylactically cycled, and there were 71 control patients. Time to hyperbilirubinemia was longer in the prophylactically cycled group ($P = .005$). This difference held true after 25 and 50 days of PN. At any time patients in the continuous group were 4.76 times more likely to develop hyperbilirubinemia (95% CI, 1.62 to 14.00) (81). The onset of hepatic encephalopathy requires a reduction in protein delivery and possibly discontinuance of amino acid infusion if significant hepatic toxicity is suspected.

REFERENCES

1. Lipman TO. The chicken soup paradigm. *JPEN J Parenter Enteral Nutr*. 2003;27:93–99.
2. Dudrick SJ, Wilmore DW, Vars HM, et al. Long-term total parenteral nutrition with growth, development, and positive nitrogen balance. *Surgery*. 1968 64(1):134–142.
3. American Society of Parenteral and Enteral Nutrition. Guidelines for the use of parenteral and enteral nutrition in adult and pediatric patients. *JPEN J Parenter Enteral Nutr*. 2002;26(1 suppl):1SA.
4. Casaer MP, Mesotten D, Hermans G, et al. Early versus late parenteral nutrition in critically ill adults. *N Engl J Med*. 2011;365:506–517.
5. Doig GS, Simpson F, Sweetman EA, et al. Early parenteral nutrition in critically ill patients with short-term relative contraindication to enteral nutrition: a randomized controlled trial. *JAMA*. 2013;22:2130–2138.
6. Detsky AS; Veterans Affairs TPN Cooperative Study Group. Parenteral nutrition—is it helpful? *N Engl J Med*. 1991;325:573.
7. Howard L, Ashley C. Nutrition in the perioperative patient. *Annu Rev Nutr*. 2003;23:263–282.
8. Braunschweig CL, Levy P, Sheean PM, et al. Enteral compared with parenteral nutrition: a meta-analysis. *Am J Clin Nutr*. 2001;74:534–542.
9. Cove ME, Pinsky MR. Early or late parenteral nutrition: ASPEN vs ESPEN. *Crit Care*. 2011;15:317.
10. Madsen H, Frankel EH. The hitchhiker's guide to parenteral nutrition management for adult patients. *Pract Gastroenterol*. July 2006:46–68.
11. Triantafillidis JK, Papalois AE. The role of total parenteral nutrition in inflammatory bowel disease: current aspects. *Scand J Gastroenterol*. 2014;49:314.
12. Polk TM, Schwab CW. Metabolic and nutritional support of the enterocutaneous fistula patient: a three-phase approach. *World J Surg*. 2012;36:524–533.
13. Matarese LE. Nutrition and fluid optimization for patients with short bowel syndrome. *JPEN J Parenter Enteral Nutr*. 2013;37:161–170.
14. Chang YS, Fu HQ, Xiao YM, et al. Nasogastric or nasojejunal feeding in predicted severe acute pancreatitis: a meta-analysis. *Crit Care*. 2013;17:R118.
15. Boullata JI, Gilbert K, Sacks G, et al. ASPEN Clinical guidelines: parenteral nutrition ordering, order review, compounding, labeling and dispensing. *JPEN J Parenter Enteral Nutr*. 2014;38:334–377.
16. van Miert C, Hill R, Jones L. Interventions for restoring patency of occluded central venous catheter lumens. *Cochrane Database Syst Rev*. 2012;4:CD007119. doi:10.1002/14651858.CD007119.pub2
17. O'Grady NP, Alexander M, Burns LA, et al; The Healthcare Infection Control Practices Advisory Committee (HICPAC). CDC guidelines for the prevention of intravascular catheter-related infections, 2011. http://www.cdc.gov/hicpac/pdf/guidelines/bsi-guidelines-2011.pdf. Accessed December 26, 2013.
18. Weber DJ, Rutala WA. Central line-associated bloodstream infections: prevention and management. *Infect Dis Clin North Am*. 2011;25:77–102.
19. Malach T, Jerassy Z, Rudensky B, et al. Prospective surveillance of phlebitis associated with peripheral intravenous catheters. *Am J Infect Control*. 2006;34:308–312.
20. Frankenfield DC, Ashcraft CM. Estimating energy needs in nutrition support patients. *JPEN J Parenter Enteral Nutr*. 2011;35:563–570.
21. Van Way CA. Total calories vs nonprotein calories. *Nutr Clin Pract*. 2001;16:271–272.
22. Miles JM, Klein J. Should protein calories be included in caloric calculations for a TPN prescription? Point-counterpoint. *Nutr Clin Pract*. 1996;11:204–206.
23. Food and Drug Administration (FDA). Parenteral multivitamin products; drugs for human use; drug efficacy study implementation; amended (21 CFR5.70). *Fed Reg*. 2000;65:21200–21201.
24. Vanek VW, Borum P, Buchman A, et al. ASPEN position paper: recommendations for changes in commercially available parenteral multivitamin and multi-trace element products. *Nutr Clin Pract*. 2012;27:440–491.
25. Kumar PR, Fenton TR, Shaheen AA, et al. Prevalence of vitamin D deficiency and response to oral vitamin D supplementation in patients receiving home parenteral nutrition. *JPEN J Parenter Enteral Nutr*. 2012;36:463–469.
26. Abiles J, de la Cruz AP, Castano J, et al. Oxidative stress is increased in critically ill patients according to antioxidant vitamins intake, independent of severity: a cohort study. *Crit Care*. 2006;10:R146.
27. Yamazaki E, Horikawa M, Fukushima R. Vitamin C supplementation in patients receiving peripheral parenteral nutrition after gastrointestinal surgery. *Nutrition*. 2011;27:435–439.
28. Heyland D, Muscedere J, Wischmeyer PE, et al. A randomized trial of glutamine and antioxidants in critically ill patients. *N Engl J Med*. 2013;368:1489–1497.
29. Crook MA, Hally V, Panteli JV. The importance of the refeeding syndrome. *Nutrition*. 2001;17:632–637.

30. Manzanares W, Hardy G. Thiamine supplementation in the critically ill. *Curr Opin Clin Nutr Metab Care.* 2011;14:610–617.
31. Geerlings SE, Rommes JH, van Toorn DW, et al. Acute folate deficiency in a critically ill patient. *Neth J Med.* 1997;51:36–38.
32. Rodriguez RM, Corwin HL, Gettinger A, et al. Nutritional deficiencies and blunted erythropoietin response as causes of the anemia of critical illness. *J Crit Care.* 2001;16:36–41.
33. Mirtallo JM, Holcombe B, Kochevar M, et al. Parenteral nutrition product shortages: the ASPEN strategy. *Nutr Clin Pract.* 2012;27:382–391.
34. Hanson C, Thoene M, Wagner J, et al. Parenteral nutrition additive shortages: the short-term, long-term and potential epigenetic implications in premature and hospitalized infants. *Nutrients.* 2012;4:1977–1988.
35. Gasser E, Parekh N. Parenteral nutrition: macronutrient composition and requirements. *Support Line.* 2005;27:6–22.
36. Ockenga J, Borchert K, Stuber E, et al. Glutamine-enriched total parenteral nutrition in patients with inflammatory bowel disease. *Eur J Clin Nutr.* 2005;59:1302–1309.
37. Murray SM, Pindoria S. Nutrition support for bone marrow transplant patients. *Cochrane Database Syst Rev.* 2009;1:CD002920.
38. Dhaliwal R, Cahill N, Lemieux M, et al. The Canadian critical care nutrition guidelines in 2013: an update on current recommendations and implementation strategies. *Nutr Clin Pract.* 2014;29:29–43.
39. Fogle P. Vitamin K and lipid emulsions. *Support Line.* 2001;23:3–8.
40. Edmunds CE, Brody RA, Parrott JS, et al. The effects of different IV fat emulsions on clinical outcomes in critically ill patients. *Crit Care Med.* 2014;42:1168–1177.
41. McClave SA, Martindale RG, Vanek VW, et al. Guidelines for the Provision and Assessment of Nutrition Support Therapy in the Adult Critically ill Patients: Society of Critical Care Medicine (SCCM) and American Society for Parenteral and Enteral Nutrition (ASPEN). *JPEN J parenteral Enteral Nutr.* 2009;33:277–316
42. Suchner U, Katz DP, Furst P, et al. Impact of sepsis, lung injury, and the role of lipid infusion on circulating prostacyclin and thromboxane A(2). *Intensive Care Med.* 2002;28:122–129.
43. Gerlach AT, Thomas S, Murphy CV, et al. Does delaying early intravenous fat emulsion during parenteral nutrition reduce infections during critical illness? *Surg Infect (Larchmt).* 2011;12:43–47.
44. Morlion BJ, Torwesten E, Lessire H, et al. The effect of parenteral fish oil on leukocyte membrane fatty acid composition and leukotriene synthesizing capacity in patients with postoperative trauma. *Metabolism.* 1996;45:1208–1213.
45. Koller M, Senkal M, Kemen M, et al. Impact of omega-3-fatty acid enriched TPN on leukotriene synthesis by leukocytes after major surgery. *Clin Nutr.* 2003;22:59–64.
46. Senkal M, Haaker R, Linseisen J, et al. Preoperative oral supplementation with long-chain omega-3-fatty acids beneficially alters phospholipid fatty acid patterns in liver, gut mucosa and tumor tissue. *JPEN J Parent Enteral Nutr.* 2005;29:236–240.
47. Grimm H, Mertes N, Goeters C, et al. Improved fatty acid and leukotriene pattern with a novel lipid emulsion in surgical patients. *Eur J Clin Nutr.* 2006;45:55–60.
48. Friesecke S, Lotze C, Kohler J, et al. Fish oil supplementation in the parenteral nutrition of critically ill medical patients: a randomized controlled trial. *Intensive Care Med.* 2008;34:1411–1420.
49. Wang X, Li W, Zhang F, et al. Fish oil-supplemented parenteral nutrition in severe acute pancreatitis patients and effects on immune function and infectious risk: a randomized controlled trial. *Inflammation.* 2009;32:304–309.
50. Barbosa VM, Miles EA, Calhau C, et al. Effects of a fish oil containing lipid emulsion on plasma phospholipid fatty acids, inflammatory markers, and clinical outcomes in septic patients: a randomized control clinical trial. *Crit Care.* 2010; 14(1):R5.
51. Umpierrez GE, Spiegelman R, Zhao V, et al. A double-blind, randomized clinical trial comparing soybean oil-based versus olive oil-based lipid emulsions in adult medical-surgical intensive care unit patients requiring parenteral nutrition. *Crit Care Med.* 2012;40:1792–1798.
52. Helphingstine CJ, Bistrian BR. New food and drug administration requirements for inclusion of vitamin K in adult parenteral multivitamins. *JPEN J Parenter Enteral Nutr.* 2003;27:220–224.
53. Ibrahim M, de Escobar GM, Visser TJ, et al. Iodine deficiency associated with parenteral nutrition in extreme preterm infants. *Arch Dis Child Fetal Neonatal Ed.* 2003;88:56–57.
54. Abdalian R, Saqui O, Fernandes G, et al. Effects of manganese from a commercial multi-trace element supplement in a population sample of Canadian patients on long-term parenteral nutrition. *JPEN J Parenter Enteral Nutr.* 2013;37:538–543.
55. Sardesai VM. Molybdenum: an essential trace element. *Nutr Clin Pract.* 1993;8:277–281.

56. Bouchoud L, Fonzo-Chirste C, Klinguller M, et al. Compatibility of intravenous medications with parenteral nutrition: in vitro evaluation. *JPEN J Parenter Enteral Nutr.* 2013;37:416–424.
57. Robinson CA, Lee JE. Y-site compatibility of medications with Parenteral Nutrition. *J Pediatr Pharmacol Ther.* 2007;12:53–59.
58. Rombeau JL, Rolandelli RH, eds. *Clinical Nutrition: Parenteral Nutrition.* Philadelphia: Saunders; 2000.
59. Trissel LA. *Handbook on Injectable Drugs*, 17th ed. Bethesda, MD: American Society of Hospital Pharmacists; 2013.
60. Schiffer CA, Mangu PB, Wade JC, et al. Central venous catheter care for the patient with cancer: American Society of Clinical Oncology clinical practice guideline. *J Clin Oncol.* 2013;31:1357–1370.
61. Haqiwara S, Mori T, Tuchiya H, et al. Multidisciplinary nutritional support for autologous hematopoietic stem cell transplantation: a cost-benefit analysis. *Nutrition.* 2011;27:1112–1117.
62. Martinez MJ, Martinez MA, Montero M, et al. Hypophosphatemia in postoperative patients with total parenteral nutrition: influence of nutritional support teams. *Nutr Hosp.* 2006;31:657–660.
63. Van den Berghe G, Wouters P, Weekers F, et al. Intensive insulin therapy in critically ill patients. *N Engl J Med.* 2001;345:1359–1367.
64. Jacobi J, Bircher N, Krinsley J, et al. Guidelines for the use of an insulin infusion for the management of hyperglycemic in critically ill patients. *Crit Care Med.* 2012;40:3251–3276.
65. McMahon MM. ASPEN clinical guidelines: nutrition support of adult patients with hyperglycemia. *JPEN J Parenter Enteral Nutr.* 2013;37:23–36.
66. Boitano M. Hypocaloric feeding of the critically ill. *Nutr Clin Pract.* 2006;21:617–622.
67. Berger MM, Chiolero RL. Hypocaloric feeding: pros and cons. *Curr Opin Crit Care.* 2007;13:180–186.
68. Nirula R, Yamada K, Waxman K. The effect of abrupt cessation of total parenteral nutrition on serum glucose: a randomized trial. *Am Surg.* 2000;66:866–869.
69. Thomas DR, Zdrodowski CD, Wilson MM, et al. A prospective randomized clinical study of adjunctive peripheral parenteral nutrition in adult subacute care patients. *J Nutr Health Aging.* 2005;9:321–325.
70. Schoevaerdts D, Gazzotti C, Cornette P, et al. Peripheral parenteral nutrition in geriatric wards. *Acta Clin Belg.* 2006;61:170–175.
71. Wilson E. The Oley Foundation celebrates 20 years. *Support Line.* 2003;25:6–10.
72. Shils ME, Wright WL, Turnbull A, et al. Long term parenteral nutrition through external arteriovenous shunt. *N Engl J Med.* 1970;283:341–344.
73. Opilla M. Epidemiology of bloodstream infection associated with parenteral nutrition. *Am J Infect Control.* 2008;36:S173.
74. Moureau N, Poole S, Murdock MA, et al. Central venous catheters in home infusion care: outcomes analysis in 50,470 patients. *J Vasc Interv Radiol.* 2002;13:1009–1016.
75. Haderslev KV, Tjellesen L, Haderslev PH, et al. Assessment of the longitudinal changes in bone mineral density in patients receiving home parenteral nutrition. *JPEN J Parenter Enteral Nutr.* 2004;28:289–294.
76. Buchman AL. Complications of long-term home total parenteral nutrition: their identification, prevention and treatment. *Dig Dis Sci.* 2001;46:1–18.
77. Gunsar C, Vatansever S, Var A, et al. Antibiotic treatment is superior to ursodeoxycholic acid on total parenteral nutrition associated hepatic dysfunction. *Pediatr Surg Int.* 2010;26:479–486.
78. Lambert JR, Thomas SM. Metronidazole prevention of serum liver enzyme abnormalities during total parenteral nutrition. *JPEN J Parenter Enteral Nutr.* 1985;9:501.
79. Cavicchi M, Beau P, Crenn P, et al. Prevalence of liver disease and contributing factors in patients receiving home parenteral nutrition for permanent intestinal failure. *Ann Intern Med.* 2000;132:525.
80. Tillman EM. Review and clinical update on parenteral nutrition-associated liver disease. *Nutr Clin Pract.* 2013;28:30–39.
81. Jensen AR, Goldin AB, Koopmeiners JS, et al. The association of cyclic parenteral nutrition and decreased incidence of cholestatic liver disease in patients with gastroschisis. *J Pediatr Surg.* 2009; 44:183–189.
82. Lochs H, Meryn S, Marosi L, et al. Has total bowel rest been a beneficial effect in the treatment of Crohn's disease? *Clin Nutr.* 1983;2:61.
83. Jones VA. Comparison of total parenteral nutrition and elemental diet in induction of remission of Crohn's disease. *Dig Dis Sci.* 1987;32(suppl 12):100S.
84. Greenberg GR, Fleming CR, Jeejeebhoy KN, et al. Control trial of bowel rest and nutritional support in the management of Crohn's disease. *Gut.* 1988;29:1309.
85. Wright RA, Adler EC. Peripheral parenteral nutrition is no better than enteral nutrition in acute exacerbation of Crohn's disease: a retrospective trial. *J Clin Gastroenterol.* 1990;12:396.

12 Use of Diets and Dietary Components in Clinical Practice

GENERAL PRINCIPLES

In many diets useful in managing disease, a particular element (e.g., fat or lactose) is *restricted*. In such cases, care must be taken to ensure that a balanced diet, providing all the major required macronutrients and micronutrients, is offered. Sometimes, supplements must be added to a restrictive diet (e.g., calcium to a low-lactose diet). In other diets, a nutrient that may be required in larger amounts than can be obtained from a usual, well-balanced diet (e.g., protein or calcium) is *added*. Finally, in some cases, either the *consistency* of a diet or the content of indigestible residue or fiber is *altered*. The availability of required nutrients is not changed in a major way, but such diets are useful in the treatment of certain intestinal disorders. This chapter begins with a review of the components of a usual, well-balanced diet because many patients do not maintain such diets, either through ignorance or a wish to avoid certain foods that seem to cause symptoms. Useful source books for information on diets are available (1,2).

Normal Diet

To obtain all the essential nutrients, foods from each of the five major groups—dairy products, meat (including nuts), cereals and grains, fruits, and vegetables—should be included in the diet. Macronutrients are required for different reasons. Protein is needed to supply essential amino acids (see Chapter 5 for a discussion of requirements). The essential amino acid content of plant proteins is lower than that of animal proteins. To obtain a mix of essential amino acids comparable with that in animal proteins, protein from various sources must be consumed (Table 12-1). Fats are needed to supply essential fatty acids (see Chapter 11) and vary the flavor of food. When fat is cooked, chemical changes occur that markedly affect food palatability.

Carbohydrates are needed to provide texture and blandness, which offset the stronger flavors of protein and fats to make food pleasant-tasting. However, no carbohydrate is essential for the maintenance or growth of tissue. The distribution of macronutrients in some common foods is listed in Table 12-2. The values in the table refer to unprepared foods. Cooking can modify the components of food greatly (e.g., fried foods) or not at all (e.g., milk).

Micronutrients are distributed widely among the major food classes, but the distributions differ for the individual vitamins and minerals. The food sources for each micronutrient are

TABLE 12-1 Use of Vegetarian Sources to Provide Adequate Essential Amino Acids

Group	Major Components	Limiting Amino Acids	Other Group Needed for Complete Proteins
A[a]	Whole grains, cereals	Lysine, threonine, tryptophan (sometimes)	B or D ± C
B	Legumes, including peanuts	Methionine, tryptophan	A
C	Nuts and seeds, except peanuts	Lysine	A + B or D
D	Vegetables, especially potato	Methionine	A

[a]Also provides iron and riboflavin.
Data from *Mayo Clinic Diet Manual.* 6th ed. Toronto: BC Decker, 1988.

TABLE 12-2 Food Sources of Macronutrients

Food Group	Serving	Protein (g)	Carbohydrate (g)	Fat (g)	kcal
Dairy					
Milk					
Whole	1 cup	8.5	12	8.5	160
2% with nonfat milk solids	1 cup	10	15	5	145
Skim	1 cup	9	12	0.2	88
Ice cream	1 cup	6	27	14	287
Butter	1 tsp	—	—	5	45
Cream, coffee	2 tbsp	1	1.0	6	64
Cheese, slice	1 oz	8	0.5	8	105
Meat, Fish, Peanut Butter					
Chicken, turkey	3 oz	21	—	15	220
Fresh fish	3 oz	21	—	15	220
Lean meats	3 oz	21	—	15	220
Egg	1	7	—	5	75
Shrimp, medium	3 oz	21	—	—	124
Tuna	3 oz	21	—	15	220
Peanut butter	1 oz	7	—	5	75
Cereals and Grains					
Bread	1 slice	2	15	—	70
English muffin	1	2	15	—	70
Bagel	½	2	15	—	70
Unsweetened cereals	3/4 cup	2	15	—	70
Pasta, cooked	1/2 cup	2	15	—	70
Rice, cooked	1/2 cup	2	15	—	70
Cooked hot cereal	1/2 cup	2	15	—	70
Fruits and Vegetables					
Potato chips	1 oz	2	15	12	170
Corn	1/2 cup	2	15	—	70
Peas, beans, lentils (dried and cooked)	1/2 cup	2	15	—	70
Potatoes, baked	1	2	15	—	70
Squash, baked	1/2 cup	2	15	—	70
Other vegetables	1/2 cup	2	15	—	70
Fruit juices					
Apple, grapefruit, orange	1/2 cup	—	10	—	40
Apricot, cranberry, grape	1/4 cup	—	10	—	40
Hi-C, prune juice					
Berries, melon	1 cup	—	10	—	40
Orange, peach, pear, apple	1 (medium)	—	10	—	40
Grapefruit, banana	½	—	10	—	40

covered in Chapters 6 and 7, and the information is summarized in Tables 12-3 and 12-4. The content of vitamins and minerals is often higher in more brightly colored fruits and vegetables. For example, vitamin A and carotenoids are more abundant in bright-orange vegetables and fruits and in dark-green leafy vegetables. Fortified foods are enriched with some micronutrients.

Occasionally, certain foods that are sources of nutrients have special features that must be considered when the foods are used to maintain a balanced diet. For example, avocados provide fiber,

TABLE 12-3 Food Source of Vitamins

Vitamin	Meat/Fish/Eggs	Grains	Vegetables/Fruits	Dairy	Nuts/Beans	Comments
B_1	+	++	+	++	+	Grain products enriched
B_2	++	+	+	+	+	Especially organ meats
Niacin	++	+	+	—	—	Grain products enriched
B_6	+	++	+	+	—	Produced by bacteria
Folate	+	+	++	+	++	Especially green leafy vegetables, organ meats, eggs, whole grains, dried beans
B_{12}	++	—	—	++	—	Foods of animal origin only
C	—	—	++	—	—	Especially citrus fruits, green vegetables
A	++	—	++	+	—	Especially liver, pigmented vegetables, fruits
D	++	—	—	++	—	Milk enriched; made in skin; high levels in liver, fish, and eggs
E	++	—	++	+	+	Only in animal or vegetable fat
K	+	—	++	—	—	Especially green leafy vegetables; made by enteric bacteria

Estimates of content refer to raw food. Water-soluble vitamins are extracted into the cooking water.
+, present in appreciable amounts; ++, daily portion contains about 25% of RDA.

folate, potassium, vitamin C, and vitamin B_6 in good amounts, but each ounce contains about 50 kcal and 5 g of fat (3). Both of these foods are excellent components of a balanced diet, but the special features of each should be noted. The common macronutrients, vitamins, and minerals contained in foods are listed in Table 12-5, which provides guidelines for maintaining a balanced diet.

US Department of Agriculture Food Guides

Methods for educating consumers about a balanced diet have been devised by the US Department of Agriculture (USDA) since the 1940s (4). The first guide divided foods into seven groups (leafy yellow vegetables, citrus fruits and tomatoes, potatoes and other vegetables, dairy products, meat and nuts, bread and cereals, and butter and margarine), but the recommendations lacked serving sizes. In 1956, the Basic Four Food Guide was introduced (dairy products, vegetables and fruits, meat and nuts, and bread and cereal). This specified amounts from each of these groups, but did not give guidance on calorie intake, fats, or sugars. This guide was expanded in 1979 by adding a fifth group to provide guidance on intake of fats, sweets, and alcohol. The Food Wheel was introduced in 1984 using the five food groups but giving daily amounts of food at three calorie levels. The Food Pyramid guide was launched in 1992 with goals for nutrient adequacy and moderation. Added fats and sugars were visualized throughout the five food groups and at the tip of the pyramid. The pyramid was expanded in 2005 to MyPyramid, including daily amounts of food at 12 calorie levels, and added a band for oils and the concept of physical activity. The latest version is MyPlate, introduced in 2011 at the same time as the 2010 Dietary Guidelines for Americans (DGA). The shape of the icon has been modified to a plate, as

TABLE 12-4 Food Source of Minerals

Mineral	Meat/Fish/Eggs	Grains	Vegetables/Fruits	Dairy	Nuts/Beans	Comments
Na	+	+	—	++	+	Especially processed food
K	++	+	++	+	+	Especially meat, milk, fruits
Ca	+	—	+	++	++	Especially dairy, meat, fish
P	+	+	+	+	+	Widely distributed
Mg	+	+	+	+	+	Widely distributed
Fe	++	—	+	—	++	Heme iron best
Zn	++	+	—	—	—	Complexes in grain less bioavailable
I	++	—	—	+	—	Seafood best, salt enriched
Cu	++	—	+	—	++	Shellfish, organ meats best
Mn	+	++	+	—	++	Organ, not muscle meats
F	+	+	+	+	+	Drinking water enriched
Cr	+	+	+	+	+	Widely distributed
Se	++	+	—	—	—	Especially organ meats, fish

+, present in appreciable amounts; ++, daily portion contains about 25% of RDA.

the pyramid proved confusing, with the most restricted foods at the top of the pyramid. However, MyPlate continues the personalized approach started with MyPyramid. This brief summary of the USDA Food Guides is meant to underline the continued use of food groups and serving sizes, and the continuous development of the concept for consumer use. In fact, MyPlate and MyPyramid are just different ways of illustrating the same principles.

Dietary Guidelines for Americans 2010

Many guidelines have been developed to provide a diet to minimize the risks for major chronic conditions, such as heart disease, cancer (see Chapter 15), stroke, diabetes, hypertension, dental caries, alcoholism, and obesity. The DGA are evidence-based federal recommendations developed every 5 years, and "designed to prevent and reduce diet-related chronic diseases, while promoting good health and healthy weight among Americans ages two and older" (5). In response to focus groups and the current marketing of foods, the 2010 Dietary Guidelines focused on two concepts: to maintain calorie balance over time that achieves and sustains a healthy weight and to focus on consumption of nutrient-dense foods and beverages. The key recommendations of the 2010 Guidelines are listed in Table 12-6. These recommendations have been used to create the advice presented in MyPlate, so each program reinforces the other. In addition, MyPlate notes the importance of physical activity to accompany any dietary program. MyPlate offers the following tips (3):

- Build a healthy plate.
  - Make half your plate fruits and vegetables.
  - Switch to skim or 1% milk.
  - Make at least half your grains whole.
  - Vary your protein food choices, using fish, beans, and lean meats.
- Cut back on foods high in solid fats, added sugars, and salt.
  - Choose foods and drinks with little or no added sugars.
  - Look out for salt (sodium) in foods you buy.
  - Eat fewer foods that are high in solid fats.

TABLE 12-5 Distribution of Nutrients among Food Groups for Balanced Meals

Minimum Recommended Number of Servings[a]

Food Group	Major Nutrients	Child	Teenager	Adult	Pregnant Woman	No meat	No Milk
Dairy products	Calcium, vitamin D[b], protein, vitamins B_1 and B_2, vitamin A[b]	3	4	2	4	4	0
Meat and meat alternates (beans, nuts, peas)	Protein, Zn, Fe, vitamins B_1, B_2, B_6, and B_{12}, folate, niacin	1–1 1/2	2	4	3	3 (legumes)	6 (2 legumes)
Fruits and Vegetables[c]							
Vitamin A–rich	Vitamin A, Mg, vitamins C and B_6, folate	1/2	1	1	1	1 1/2	3
Vitamin C–rich	Vitamins C and A, niacin, folate, carbohydrate	1/2	1	1	1	3	3
Others	Vitamin B_6, folate, niacin, K, carbohydrate	2	2	2	2	0	0
Enriched or whole-grain cereals and breads	Vitamins B_1[b] and B_2[b], niacin, [b] protein, carbohydrate, Fe[b], Mg	4	4	4	4	6	3
Oils and fats	Essential fatty acids, vitamins E and A[b]	Depends on caloric need					

[a]A serving equals 1 cup milk or milk products; 3 oz meat, poultry, or fish; 3/4 cup cooked legumes; 1 oz nuts; 3/4 cup cooked or 1 cup raw vegetables or fruit; 1 oz dry cereal; 1/4 cup cooked cereal or pasta; 1 slice bread; 1 tbsp oil.
[b]Often fortified in the food.
[c]Representative fruits and vegetables: vitamin A—broccoli, green peppers, collards, carrots, spinach, sweet potato, cantaloupe, plums, squash; vitamin C—citrus fruits and juices, tomatoes, strawberries, green pepper, watermelon, brussels sprouts; other—banana, apple, pear, grapes, potatoes, corn, peas, green beans.

- Eat the right amount of calories for you.
  - Enjoy your food, but eat less.
  - Cook more often at home.
  - When eating out, choose lower-calorie menu options.
- Be physically active your way.
  - Pick activities that you like and do as much as you can regularly.
- Use food labels to help you make better choices.

MyPlate offers, as did MyPyramid, a daily food plan that provides specific recommendations at 12 different calorie-intake levels. Table 12-7 presents such a plan for a 2,000-calorie pattern.

TABLE 12-6 Key Recommendations of the Dietary Guidelines for Americans 2010

Balancing Calories to Manage Weight	Building Healthy-Eating Patterns
Prevents and/or reduce overweight through improved eating and physical activity behavior	Select an eating pattern that meets nutrient needs over time
Control total calorie intake to manage body weight	Account for all foods and beverages consumed
Increase physical activity and reduce sedentary behavior	Follow food safety recommendations to reduce risk of foodborne illness
Foods and Food Components to Reduce	**Foods and Nutrients to Increase**
Sodium intake to <2.3 gm, and further to 1.5 gm for persons >51 years old and with high BP, diabetes, or chronic renal disease	Vegetable and fruit intake
<10% of calories from saturated fat	Dark-green, red, and orange vegetables
<300 mg of dietary cholesterol	>Half of all grains as whole grains
Limit trans fatty acids (e.g., hydrogenated oils)	Fat-free or low-fat milk and milk products
Reduce intake of solid fats and added sugars	Seafood, lean meat and poultry, eggs, beans and peas, soy products, nuts, and seeds as protein sources
Limit refined grain foods, esp. with added sugar	Use oils to replace solid fats when possible
Alcohol in moderation (1 drink/d for women, 2 for men)	Foods that provide potassium, dietary fiber, calcium, and vitamin D

Modified from Development of 2010 Dietary Guidelines for Americans. http://www.health.gov/dietaryguidelines/dga2010/dietaryguidelines2010.pdf.

The DGA aims to reduce diet-related chronic diseases. Vegetarian diets achieve many of these objectives because they reduce the risks for hypertension, coronary artery disease, diabetes (type 2), and gallstones (6,7). Diets designed to prevent cancer or heart disease are based on similar recommendations (see also Chapter 15). The dietary recommendations outlined above and discussed in Chapters 2 and 3 are intended for general populations in the United States. However, some special considerations should be emphasized for African Americans and other minority groups. The diets of middle-aged African Americans may be lower in calcium, magnesium,

TABLE 12-7 Daily Food Plan on a 2,000-Calorie Pattern

Food Group	Amount	Comments
Grains	6 oz	Aim for at least 3 oz of whole grains
Vegetables	2.5 cups	Vary types, aim for each week: dark-green veggies 1.5 cups, red/orange veggies 5.5 cups, beans/peas 1.5 cups, starchy veggies 5 cups, other veggies 4 cups
Fruits	2 cups	Eat a variety of fruit, whole or cut-up rather than juices
Dairy	3 cups	Low-fat (1%) or fat-free milk, yogurt, and cheese
Protein foods	5.5 oz	Use seafood 2x/week; vary protein to choose beans, peas, nuts, and seeds more; keep meat/poultry portions small and lean
Fats, sugars, salt	Limit	Oils to 6 tsp/d, calories from solid fats and added sugars to 260 kcal/d, sodium to <2300 mg/d
Physical activity	150 min/wk	

Adapted from www.chooseMyPlate.gov.

iron (for women), folacin, and zinc. Obesity is more prevalent in African American women than in White women, and it may be more difficult for them to achieve a desirable weight. Hispanic-Americans tend to consume a diet higher in fiber and with less animal fat. Overweight has been a greater problem in Hispanic-Americans than in Anglo-Americans. The diet of Asian/Pacific-Americans is generally higher in fish, shellfish, and fruits and vegetables but lower in dairy products and calcium. As these populations become more assimilated into Anglo-American societies, group differences may diminish.

The American Heart Association has issued its comments on the DGA 2010, which largely confirm its own 2006 Guidelines, designed to reduce the risk of cardiovascular disease (CVD) (8). These recommendations are very similar to their 2006 document, and to all other evidence-based healthy diets. Recommendations include the suggestions to

- Achieve and maintain a healthy body weight (body mass index [BMI] 18.5 to 24.9).
- Consume a diet rich in vegetables and fruits (especially those that are deeply colored).
- Select whole-grain, high-fiber foods (half of grain intake should be whole grain).
- Consume fish at least twice a week (especially oily fish rich in ω-3 fatty acids).
- Limit intake of saturated fat to less than 7% of calories, *trans* fat to less than 1% of calories, and cholesterol to less than 300 mg per day by selecting lean meats, skim and low-fat dairy products, and minimizing intake of partially hydrogenated fats by substituting solid margarines with liquid vegetable oils.
- Minimize intake of beverages and foods with added sugars (especially sucrose and corn syrup).
- Choose and prepare foods with little or no salt (limit to 2.3 g of sodium per day).
- Consume alcohol in moderation (less than two drinks per day for men, one drink per day for women).

Other Important Factors in Maintaining a Healthy Diet

Practical Advice

Food should be consumed as three daily meals. This practice avoids periods of great hunger with subsequent overeating and provides energy for tasks to be performed throughout the day. Snacks can certainly be a part of the diet and can include foods from any of the major groups. *Junk* or *fast foods* also can be included in a balanced diet. It is only when most of the daily calories are derived from these foods that they pose a problem. Fast foods often contain many calories in the form of fat and carbohydrates, with lesser amounts of protein. Moreover, they usually do not include fruits and vegetables and so do not provide all the micronutrients needed. The term *empty calories*, which has been used to describe the nutritive value of these foods, is a poor one. The caloric value of fast foods is as real as that of any other foods because all calories are equal. The foods lack many of the other nutrients, but the caloric value is the same.

The best way to entice a patient to follow a *balanced diet* is to review food lists, identify the perceived problems in the intake of all foods, and provide specific recommendations for foods in each major group. In addition, the health-care provider must discover what behavioral patterns accompany the abnormal or irregular intake of food if an attempt to correct the diet is to be made.

The average *hospital house diet* is balanced as far as nutrients are concerned, although the palatability is not always good because the flavors are usually quite bland. The hospital diet provides each day between 2,000 and 2,500 kcal, 60 to 80 g of protein, 2.5 to 3.5 g of sodium, 3.5 to 4.5 g of potassium, 1.0 to 1.3 g of calcium, 1.1 to 1.5 g of phosphorus, 300 to 400 mg of magnesium, 7 to 9 mg of iron, and 13 to 14 mg of zinc. However, many teaching hospitals do not design house diets to meet nationally recognized dietary recommendations (9). Moreover, they do not always provide enough information for the patients to select appropriate and healthful choices.

Alcohol

Alcohol is a component of many diets, and the carbohydrate and caloric load should be appreciated, as these can be considerable (Table 12-8).

Taste and Smell

One major factor in maintaining an adequate oral intake is the presence of normal taste and smell. It is now clear that the gustatory system, unlike other sensory systems, is comprised of

TABLE 12-8 Nutritional Composition of Alcoholic Beverages

Beverage	Serving Size (oz)	Alcohol (% vol)	Calories (kcal)	Carbohydrate (g)
Beer	12	4–5	140–150	10–11
Light beer	12	~4.3	~110	6–7
Wine, red	5	11.7	105	2.5
Wine, dry white	5	11.7	94	1.3
Gin and tonic	7	13.8	190	15.5
Martini	2	40.7	119	0.1
Bloody Mary	4.6	15.7	120	4.5
Frozen daiquiri	4.7	19.3	190	15.5
Manhattan	2.3	38.2	137	3.4
Margarita	3.5	41.4	221	11.3
Pina colada	6	24.1	644	91.8
Screwdriver	7	13.8	208	16.1

Mixed drink source: www.drinkmixer.com; wine data source: USDA Nutritional Database SR17, 2004; calorie and carbohydrate source: Borushek A. *The Doctor's Calorie Fat and Carbohydrate Counter*, Family Health Publications, 2004.

many (~50) different receptors concentrated in only a few cell types, providing clues to perceive thousands of different taste sensations by a combination of receptor activation (10). Thus, sensing sweet, salt, bitter, and amino acids is probably coordinated within the brain. Moreover, genetic variations in bitter taste perception can cause great variability in the acceptance and use of certain foods, particularly vegetables (11). Central representation of taste discrimination may be the reason why people lose smell and taste acuity as they age, and this change is associated with poorer appetite and food intake (12). In addition, many elderly people are unaware of this impairment in smelling acuity. The basal forebrain cholinergic system sends projections to the olfactory bulb and to other brain regions involved in the perception of memory and cognition (13). Thus, it is not surprising that olfactory loss also occurs early in Alzheimer and Parkinson diseases and other degenerative brain disorders. Other important causes of altered taste and smell include depression, the postmenopausal state, and many medications, particularly halide salts that are concentrated in salivary secretions.

Sweet-tasting products also can produce satiety, and may be important in the reward mechanism in response to food (14). While taste receptors in the mouth may mediate much of this feedback, it is clear that luminal contents in the intestine are recognized by specialized enteroendocrine cells in the intestinal epithelium that can act on nerve endings to transmit signals (15). Molecular signals are best described for sugars (transporters and G protein–coupled receptors), but fatty acid receptors and transporters (including CD36) have been implicated in nutrient sensing, as have peptide and amino acid G protein–coupled receptors.

"Health-promoting" Diets Other Than DGA 2010

Vegetarian Diets

The vegetarian diets include strict vegan (without milk or eggs), lacto–vegetarian, ovo–vegetarian, and lacto–ovo–vegetarian. The strict vegan diet compared with an omnivore diet contains lower fat, less saturated fat, a high polyunsaturated/saturated fat ratio, no cholesterol, about 50% to 100% more fiber, and somewhat less protein (6). A lacto–ovo–vegetarian diet contains intermediate ranges of these components. The more milk and cheese is ingested, the higher the animal fat and cholesterol content. But all vegetarian diets contain more plant foods, bringing with them higher intake of fiber, folate, antioxidants, and phytochemicals. These components are thought to account for many of the lower risks that have been observed for developing cancer (especially colon and lung), obesity, heart disease, type 2 diabetes, hypertension, constipation, and gallstones (7). The risks of vegetarian diets are mostly seen with strict vegan diets, and include osteopenia from low calcium intake, vitamin B_{12} deficiency, and impaired growth from low energy intake. Vegetarian diets are now considered to offer more health benefits than risks (16). However, the value of a vegetarian diet may not be universal in all cultures. A review of eight Asian nation cohort studies in Bangladesh, China, Japan, Korea, and Taiwan did not show a higher rate of mortality for total meat intake (17). In fact, meat intake was inversely associated with CVD mortality among men in these Asian countries.

Vegetarian diets are also good sources of most vitamins and minerals, but not vitamin B_{12} or iron. Plant foods that contain as much calcium as one cup of cow's milk include 1 cup of calcium-fortified juice or soy milk, or calcium-set tofu (18). Natural sources (e.g., 2 cups of broccoli or kale) may contain as much calcium, but the bioavailability will not equal that of milk. Vegetarian diets can also provide vitamin D_3, either from fortified plant milk (40 to 120 IU per cup) or from commercial mushrooms (~380 IU per cup) (18).

Nitrates and Nitrites

Another concern about diets that contain a large amount of fruits and vegetables (vegetarian, DASH [dietary approaches to stop hypertension], Mediterranean, Nordic, etc.) is that these foods contain about 80% of dietary nitrates, and these diets probably exceed the World Health Organization's (WHO) Acceptable Daily Intake for nitrate by five- to sixfold (19). Nitrates are present in up to 50 mg per L in drinking water, the permissible concentration recommended by the WHO. Estimated average nitrate intakes from food are 31 to 185 mg per day in Europe and approximately 40 to 100 mg per day in the United States of America, with a bioavailability of 100% (19). Nitrite content of foods is approximately 10% or less that for nitrates. The WHO Acceptable Daily Intake for nitrate ions is 3.7 mg per kg body weight, and for nitrites 0.06 mg per kg (20). The Environmental Protection Agency recommendations are approximately 7.0 mg per kg of nitrate. Exogenous nitrate is converted to nitrite on the tongue by bacterial nitrate reductases, and in the tissues by mammalian reductases. Nitrite ions are converted to nitric oxide (NO), which has beneficial effects on blood pressure and blood vessels (15,21). Endogenous NO is produced from L-arginine.

Vegetable sources rich in nitrate include broccoli, carrots, cauliflower, and cucumber (20 to 50 mg per 100 g fresh weight), cabbage, turnip (50 to 100 mg per 100 g), celeriac, Chinese cabbage, endive, fennel, kohlrabi, leek, parsley (100 to 250 mg per 100 g), and celery, cress, lettuce, red beetroot, spinach, and arugula (>250 mg per 100 g) (22). Current regulatory limits for exogenous intake of nitrates are easily exceeded by normal daily intakes of individual foods, especially spinach and soya milk. There are data suggesting that dietary nitrate and/or nitrite might improve cardiovascular (CV) health (e.g., by lowering blood pressure), but the current regulatory limits are based on concerns of carcinogenicity and methemoglobinemia, generated by data largely from animal experiments. Although in vitro and animal data suggest that nitrates are converted to carcinogenic N-nitrosamines, there are few data in humans that nitrates are carcinogenic (19). This view is supported by the review by the WHO Committee on Food Additives (23), and epidemiological studies suggesting that abundant intake of vegetables decreases the risk for cancer. Current data are not sufficient to generate an accurate benefit/risk assessment for nitrate intake, in part because of the lack of inclusion of nitrate/nitrite concentrations in standard food databases.

Mediterranean Diet

The Mediterranean diet reinforces the plant-based core of the dietary pattern of MyPlate, but also emphasizes cultural and lifestyle activities, including conviviality, culinary activities, physical activity, and adequate rest (24). The key components of the diet itself include eating largely plant-based foods (fruits, vegetables, whole grains, legumes, and nuts), replacing butter with olive or canola oil, using herbs and spices for seasoning instead of salt, limiting red meat to only a few times a month, eating fish and poultry at least twice a week, and drinking red wine in moderation. The health benefits of this diet have included lower overall mortality, lower CVD and cancer incidence or mortality, and lower risk for neurodegenerative disease (25). This diet has been well accepted in Southern Europe, where it fits the needs and lifestyle of that cultural region.

Nordic Diet

The Nordic diet was developed as a regional diet stressing locally available foods, as the Mediterranean diet was not easily reproduced in Northern Europe. This diet emphasizes the use of native berries, cabbage and related cruciferous vegetables, native fish and other seafood, wild and pasture-fed animals (e.g., moose, deer, reindeer, hare, goose, duck, grouse), rapeseed/canola oil as the source of monounsaturated fat, and oat/barley/rye grains in preference to wheat (26). Such a diet has been shown to lower mortality and to improve insulin resistance (27). The importance of the Nordic diet has been the emphasis on diets and food that can be delivered regionally. Part of this delivery system has been the concept of "shop centers" at which families receive dietary instruction and collect most of their foods (28). While purchasing of foods has been high at these centers during study trials, it needs to be confirmed that the concept could be expanded on a larger scale.

DIETS OF ALTERED CONSISTENCY
Clear Liquid Diet

A clear liquid diet consists of liquids that can be seen through (e.g., water, broth, plain gelatin) that are easily digested and leave no undigested residue. It is often used before tests, procedures (e.g., colonoscopy), or surgeries. A clear liquid diet meets the daily requirement for water but minimally stimulates the gastrointestinal tract. This effect is achieved at the cost of minimal ingestion of protein and fat—macronutrients that are potent stimuli of gastric and pancreatic secretions and gastrointestinal motility. In addition, the diet is low in fiber. Because few unabsorbed components are provided, fecal weight and bacterial mass are decreased.

A clear liquid diet is used in the following cases: to treat dehydration resulting from excessive diarrhea or vomiting (if the vomiting has ceased), in mild or moderate pancreatitis as a prelude to introducing full feeding, to decrease output from enterocutaneous fistulae, to manage diarrhea resulting from inflammatory bowel disease (IBD), to maintain nutrient intake during chemotherapy or radiation therapy for cancer, and to prepare a patient for bowel surgery or for colonoscopic examination (29). In the surgical setting, a clear liquid diet is useful in the recovery phase of abdominal or other surgery when partial ileus is present. This restriction may not be applicable to patients after gastrointestinal surgery once bowel sounds have been heard. Early refeeding by tube or per os of either liquid or solid food has been used successfully after gastrointestinal surgery and may be beneficial for reducing hospital stay and complications (30). There seems to be no clear advantage to withholding feeding from patients following lower-bowel surgery, and perhaps even after upper-abdominal surgery. A clear liquid diet may be useful preoperatively as well, as some data suggest that preoperative fasting has adverse consequences for the patient, especially insulin resistance (31). No studies are available demonstrating an effect of preoperative fasting on differences in morbidity and mortality.

The identification of foods that are easily digested may be more culturally than scientifically derived (32). Thus, the use of limited diets, such as clear liquid, has persisted for a long time. Following gastrointestinal or gynecological surgery, the small bowel recovers normal motility first (6 to12 h), followed by the stomach (12 to 24 h) and colon (48 to 72 h). Thus, early feeding (fluids or food within the first 24 h postoperatively) has been shown to be safe and to shorten hospital stay, although such a schedule is limited in some patients by nausea (33). While the timing of feeding has been studied, the initial choice of diet has been much less studied. Clear liquids are usually offered, but a regular or soft bland diet has been equally well tolerated (34). The Enhanced Recovery After Surgery (ERAS) Group recommendations suggest solids allowed up to 6 hours before colorectal surgery, and early feeding and oral supplements from the day of surgery until "normal" food intake is achieved (35). Thus, the time-honored progression from clear liquid to full liquid to soft solid no longer seems necessary for most patients with colorectal or gynecological surgery (or with other nonabdominal surgeries). The same thinking applies to mild acute pancreatitis, for which nonliquid soft or solid diets are as well tolerated as liquid ones, and lead to earlier discharge from hospital (36).

Increased intake of calorie-containing beverages (150 to 300 kcal per day) has been associated with an increase in weight in the United States. A Beverage Guidance Panel was organized and has issued a report (37). This panel concluded that drinking water should be the preferred beverage to fulfill daily water needs, followed by tea and coffee, low-fat and skim milk, noncalorically sweetened beverages, beverages with some nutrients (juices, whole milk, alcohol, and sport drinks), and least of all calorically sweetened but otherwise nutrient-poor beverages. Beverages sweetened with sugar or high-fructose corn syrup (HFCS) pose a risk for fatty liver (fructose increases hepatic lipogenesis), obesity (as intake of beverages does not replace other calories), and hypertriglyceridemia (due to fructose) (38). The clear liquid diet designed for medical purposes needs to use caloric beverages, but it is worth remembering that in other circumstances, it is better to drink calorie-poor beverages, mainly water.

The clear liquid diet is largely water and sugar and provides few other nutrients unless supplements are added. Without supplements, the diet provides about 1,200 kcal per day (300 g of carbohydrates) along with 1.0 g of sodium, 50 to 60 mg of calcium and magnesium, 2,000 to 2,500 mg of potassium, less than 100 mg of phosphorus, 1.2 mg of iron, and only 0.33 mg of zinc. To obtain even this supply of nutrients, one must ingest about 1,500 mL of strained fruit juice, 600 mL of gelatin or fruit ice, and 30 g of sugar added to coffee or tea. Intake of these volumes can be achieved by healthy or younger patients. The diet of an elderly or ill patient may be even more restricted because intake is smaller.

Multiple vitamin and iron supplementation is suggested if the patient is to be on the diet for more than 3 weeks, or sooner if deficiency is present when the diet is initiated. If the diet is to be continued beyond 3 days or if fluid intake is limited, it can be supplemented with carbohydrate and a small amount of protein in addition to some micronutrients. Table 12-9 lists these modifications. The supplemented clear liquid diet provides about half the daily adult protein allowance, and it meets or exceeds allowances for vitamins E and C, folic acid, thiamine, riboflavin, niacin, vitamins B_6 and B_{12}, and iron. Vitamin A, calcium, and phosphorus are provided at about 60% of the daily allowance. Carbonated beverages can be substituted for Polycose™ as a source of carbohydrate, but they have many fewer calories. The use of supplements depends on the acceptability of fruit juices and gelatins as the major caloric source for the patient. Foods allowed include coffee, tea, carbonated beverages, broth, bouillon, strained fruit juices, gelatin, sugar, and sugar candies. Side effects do not develop if supplements are provided. Calories, protein, vitamins, and minerals are needed in the usual circumstances during long-term use.

Caffeine

It is generally agreed that the caffeine content of various beverages alters certain aspects of gastrointestinal function (e.g., transit time is shortened), and causes (unwanted) alertness and a jittery feeling. For this reason, the inclusion of caffeinated beverages may not be desirable in other diets. However, these drinks are usually included in a clear liquid diet. Table 12-10 lists the caffeine content of some foods and drugs.

TABLE 12-9   Nutritive Value of Clear Liquid Diets

Diet	Protein (g/d)	Fat (g/d)	Carbohydrate (g/d)	Total Calories Per Day
No supplements (~2.5 L intake)	12	0	300	1,200
No supplements (<1 L intake)	6	0	74	320
+ Ensure Clear (Institutional) (five 6.8-oz servings) (Abbott Nutrition)	35	0	215	1,000
+ Polycose (two cups) (Abbott Nutrition)	0	0	186	760
+ Citrotein Punch Clear Liquid (four 10-oz servings) (Novartis Nutrition)	42	0	128	680
Vivonex Plus (with flavor pack, four 300 mL servings) (Nestle Nutrition)	54	8	228	1,200
	40	0	260	1,200
RESOURCE fruit beverage (five 177 mL servings) (Nestle Nutrition)	30	0	270	1,050
NuBasics Juice Drink (four 163 mL servings) (Nestle Clinical Nutrition)	37.2	0.6	204	932

Vivonex Plus, RESOURCE, and NuBasics Juice Drink are commercially available clear liquid supplements that are intended to serve as the total daily nutritional provision. They contain varying amounts of sodium (183, 100, and 50 mg per serving, respectively) and potassium (294, 50, and 50 mg per serving, respectively), and all are hyperosmolar (650, 750, and 430 mOsm per kg of water, respectively).

TABLE 12-10 Caffeine Content of Foods and Drugs

Food	Unit	Caffeine Content[a] (mg/unit)
Prepared Coffee	6-oz cup	
Instant, freeze-dried		61–72
Percolated		97–125
Drip		137–174
Starbuck's Coffee Grande[b]	16-oz cup	330
Dunkin Donuts Coffee with Turbo Shot[c]	20-oz cup	436
Decaffeinated Coffee	6-oz cup	
Ground		2–4
Instant		0.5–1.5
Tea, Bagged or Loose	**6-oz cup**	**15–75**
Black, 5-min brew		40–60
Green, Japan, 5-min brew		20
Iced	12-oz cup	67–76
Starbuck's Teas	16-oz cup	80–135
Cocoa Beverages	**6-oz cup**	**10–17**
Chocolate		
Chocolate milk	8 oz	2–7
Milk chocolate	1 oz	1–15
Semi-sweet	1 oz	5–35
Baker's	1 oz	26
Syrup	1 oz	4
Bar	One	60–70
Carbonated Drinks	**12-oz can**	
Colas[c]		45–55
Mountain Dew		54
Diet colas		35–47
Root beer, citrus		0
Ginger ale, tonic, other nondiet		0–22
Drugs	**Tablet**	
Cold tablets		30–32
Alertness tablets		100–200
Weight control tablets		140–200
Pain relief OTC		32–65
Prescription pain tablets		30–100
Sport/Energy Drinks[c]		
AMP energy	8.5 oz	75
AMP Energy Boost Original	16 oz	142
Five Hour Energy	1.9 oz	208
Full Throttle	16 oz	200
Monster Energy	16 oz	180
Red Bull	8.5 oz	80
SoBe No Fear	16 oz	174
V8 V-Fusion + Energy	8 oz	80

[a]The ranges represent the range of figures from the literature because the method of preparation affects caffeine content of some beverages.
[b]Data from *Mayo Clinic Diet Manual* (www.mayoclinic.com/health/caffeine); Adapted from Nagy M. Caffeine content of beverages and chocolate. *JAMA*. 1974;29:337; Bunker ML, McWilliams M. Caffeine content of common beverages. *J Am Diet Assoc*. 1979;74:28.
[c]Data from Center for Science in the Public Interest. http://www.cspinet.org/new/cafchart.htm, updated Dec 2012.

The caffeine content of beverages depends on the amount of water used, method of brewing, and type of coffee or tea. Because caffeine is water-soluble, the longer the exposure to hot water, the greater the extraction of caffeine. Coffee is a complex mixture of chemicals and provides more than caffeine alone, including those with biological effects, such as phenolic compounds, magnesium, and quinides that can alter insulin sensitivity. Many of these compounds are not found in the coffee bean itself, but result from coffee metabolism in the small intestine and colon (39). Unfiltered coffee contains the diterpenes cafestol and kahweol that have been implicated in elevating cholesterol (40).

Low doses (<50 mg per day) probably have little effect on gastrointestinal function. The actual caffeine content of cocoa is not certain because of the wide variation in reported figures and the fact that most hospitals and homes now use instant cocoa mix, a prepared product. Theobromine, not caffeine, is the major methylxanthine stimulant in cocoa (~250 mg per cup) and chocolate. Caffeine is also a component of some over-the-counter analgesics and of many dietary supplements. These sources should be considered when caffeine intake seems important.

The health consequences of caffeine ingestion are not severe (41). For those patients with hypertension or hyperhomocysteinuria, or for groups that might be more vulnerable to the effects of caffeine (elderly, children, adolescents), limiting intake may be helpful. A subset of patients with restless leg syndrome may have attacks triggered by caffeine (42). No consistent epidemiologic evidence has been found of an effect on birth-related outcomes, including low birth weight, prematurity, spontaneous abortion, and congenital anomalies. However, many studies have not been controlled for smoking, alcohol, or medication. In one case-control study, more spontaneous abortions occurred in nonsmoking women who ingested more than 100 mg of caffeine a day when the fetus had a normal karyotype (43). The risk was proportional to the dose of caffeine ingested. Moreover, high caffeine intake is associated with the risk for late miscarriages, stillbirths, and infants who are small for their gestational age (44). One might cautiously allow reduced caffeine intake during early pregnancy, limiting coffee consumption to 3 cups per day (40). The hypercalciuric effect of 300 mg of caffeine has been well established in women with a diet low in calcium (<600 mg per day), but the mechanism is not clear. However, no effects have been noted on bone health, and caffeine is not considered an important risk factor for osteoporosis, except possibly when used on a long-term basis by persons with a dietary calcium deficiency. The pharmacologic effects on the CV, renal, respiratory, gastrointestinal, and central nervous systems have been studied extensively (41). Consumption of up to 500 mg of caffeine does not cause arrhythmias, but some patients may be especially sensitive to caffeine and should limit their intake. Although data have been reported on both sides of the issue, it does not appear that caffeine causes hypertension or coronary artery disease, nor are the data convincing that caffeine causes hyperlipidemia or fibrocystic breast disease, nor does it appear to increase the risk of chronic disease (45).

Studies are limited on coffee ingestion in relationship to all-cause mortality. Several studies have shown a positive association between higher levels of coffee consumption and CV mortality (46), but other studies have shown an inverse association, and other studies have suggested a U-shaped or J-shaped relationship between coffee ingestion and health outcomes (46). A large US-based study (Aerobics Center Longitudinal Study) confirmed a positive association between high coffee consumption (>4 cups per day) and all-cause mortality in men and women under 55 years of age (46). Although the NIH-AARP study found that coffee consumption was inversely associated with total and cause-specific mortality, there are many confounding issues and alternative explanations for the results arising from this large database that also apply to other large databases (47). Thus, the role of coffee ingestion in any effect on life span is still uncertain.

Because coffee contains many more chemicals than caffeine, studies of coffee intake have shown some interesting differences from that of caffeine alone. Coffee ingestion is associated with a lower risk of type 2 diabetes, but prospective studies are needed to confirm the relationship (48). In fact, irrespective of the caffeine content, sugar-sweetened beverages are associated with a higher risk for type 2 diabetes mellitus (T2DM), while coffee intake (not necessarily caffeine) was again associated with a lower risk (49). Coffee intake does not seem to increase the risk of heart disease or cancer, and 3 to 4 cups per day (300 to 400 mg caffeine) appear not to carry any long-term health risk (40). Although no increased risk of colon and rectal cancer was seen with ingestion of caffeinated coffee or tea, ingestion of more than 2 cups of decaffeinated coffee was associated with a decreased risk of rectal cancer (50). Tea ingestion may improve endothelium-dependent vasodilation. A meta-analysis of prospective cohort studies concluded that an increase in tea consumption of 24 oz per day was associated with a 11% decrease in myocardial infarction (51). But the results of subsequent studies have been inconsistent, and firm conclusions cannot be made (37).

Yet another association has been made regarding the benefits of coffee ingestion, which is on the risk of hepatocellular cancer. A meta-analysis of 16 studies showed a relative risk reduction of approximately one-third in both case-control and cohort studies, and over 50% reduction for high consumption (3 cups or more per day), regardless of a history of alcohol or liver disease (52). Although coffee contains multiple bioactive compounds other than caffeine (e.g., phenols, diterpenes), decaffeinated coffee does not seem to be protective. However, as with other associations, prospective studies are needed to show causation.

Although habituation to caffeine is common, it is not considered a drug of abuse, and it does not fulfill the Diagnostic and Statistical Manual-IV criteria for psychoactive substance dependence. Headache is a frequent withdrawal symptom. However, "energy drinks" are taken by persons with higher levels of risk-taking. It is possible that the neuropharmacologic effects of caffeine might play a role in enhancing alcohol addiction, although there is no evidence that taking energy drinks with alcohol increases alcohol consumption or increases alcohol dependence (53). Caffeine reverses alcohol-related slower reaction time, but did not alter the impairment of performance caused by alcohol (54). Thus, because no benefit of adding caffeine to alcoholic beverages could be demonstrated, a settlement was reached with two national breweries who agreed to remove caffeine and other stimulants from their products. In November 2011, the Food and Drug Administration (FDA) announced that caffeine is an unsafe food additive to alcoholic beverages, citing that caffeine obscured "some of the sensory cues individuals might normally rely on to determine their level of intoxication" (55). However, "energy drinks" may also pose a risk to health. These drinks contain high levels of caffeine per drink (ranging from 80 to 208 mg), while other drinks contain more than 400 mg of caffeine per serving (Table 12-10). Currently, the FDA sets the maximal allowable caffeine for cola-like drinks at 71 mg per 12-oz serving, but this limit does not apply to energy drinks (56). There are many other components in energy drinks (e.g., taurine, ginseng, glucuronolactone, B vitamins), but there is no evidence that any of these components alter physical or cognitive performance (57).

Full Liquid Diet

The full liquid diet is designed to provide adequate nourishment in a form that requires no chewing. Such a diet can also be useful when the esophagus is narrowed and solid food cannot pass. The full liquid diet (or mechanical soft diet) is indicated for patients who cannot chew properly or who have esophageal or stomach disorders interfering with the normal digestion of solid foods. Liquid supplements (500 kcal) given to patients postoperatively after major abdominal surgery led to improved weight (58). This diet can be used in conjunction with dilation in the management of esophageal stricture. Available methods for dilation include bougienage with mercury-weighted rubber catheters or with metal (olive) dilators.

The diets in which table foods are used can be maintained for long periods only when appropriate supplementation is provided or when all allowed food groups are included. Otherwise, this diet can be nutritionally incomplete. Alternatively, commercially available liquid diets can be used alone (see Chapter 10). However, long-term acceptability is greater when table foods are used as the major source of nutrition.

Full liquid diets can be given through a gastrostomy tube to bypass esophageal obstruction. In such cases, enteral supplements that supply all nutritional needs may be preferred (see Chapter 10) because taste is no longer a factor. Full liquid diets can be helpful temporarily after many types of surgery for debilitated patients who may not have recovered sufficient strength to chew food. Usually, this phase of recovery lasts no more than a few days, except after laryngectomy, when soreness and swelling are present and a new swallowing technique must be learned. In such instances, the use of creamier foods and thicker liquids makes it easier for patients to relearn how to swallow.

Practical Aspects
Certain characteristics of this diet should be kept in mind, especially for successful long-term use:

1. Foods need not be bland.
2. Milk-based foods form an important part of the diet. Lactose intolerance presents a problem when this diet is used, but many milk substitutes are now available, based on either corn syrup or soy.
3. Flavoring is helpful for some milk-based liquids, but natural or vanilla flavor is best tolerated for long-term use.
4. Caloric intake should be maintained near the estimated requirement.
5. Medications should be given in liquid form if possible.
6. Table foods allowed on a full liquid diet include all beverages, broth, bouillon, strained cream soups, poached or scrambled eggs, cereal (e.g., cream of wheat, farina, strained oatmeal), strained fruit juices, ice cream, sherbet, gelatin, custards, puddings, tapioca, yogurt without fruit, margarine, butter, cream, and all spices.
7. The full liquid diet easily provides adequate calories, protein, and essential fatty acids but not certain vitamins, notably ascorbic acid and thiamine, unless fruit juices and cereals are routinely included. The average hospital full liquid diet provides 1,900 to 2,000 kcal per day, along with 40 to 50 g of protein, 3 to 4 g of sodium, 3 to 4 g of potassium, 1.8 g of calcium, 1.3 g of phosphorus, 200 to 300 mg of magnesium, 3 mg of iron, and 8 to 9 mg of zinc.

Side Effects
The diet can be boring, and it is wise to include some items from the mechanical soft diet. If lactose intolerance is present, diarrhea may result, and milk substitutes can be used. If meat soups or brewer's yeast are not used, the diet will be deficient in folic acid, iron, and vitamin B_6.

Supplements Required
No supplements are required if all food groups are used. However, a multiple vitamin and mineral preparation, preferably liquid, is not unreasonable if this diet is to be used for a long time.

Mechanical Soft Diet
The mechanical soft diet is designed to provide a greater variety of foods than the full liquid diet for patients who find it difficult to chew or have an anatomic stricture. Patients with dysphagia may require a liquid or soft solid diet. A history of coughing or choking during meals, prolonged eating time, hoarseness after eating, regurgitation of liquid or food into the nose, frequent drooling, recurrent respiratory infections, and weight loss should lead to an evaluation of oral or pharyngeal swallowing problems. The diet must be planned individually depending on the reason for the restriction. The entire range of solid and liquid foods is used so that the diet is nutritionally balanced. One attempts to provide easily masticated foods. Because texture is an important part of taste, patients must choose the foods that they tolerate best and are most acceptable to them.

A mechanical soft diet is indicated for patients who have difficulty chewing because of advanced age or infirmity, postoperative weakness, or dental problems. It is also indicated for patients with anatomic strictures of the esophagus, especially those caused by carcinoma. For patients with strictures in other parts of the intestinal tract, such as the duodenum in active Crohn disease, only certain restrictions may be necessary because gastric grinding/mixing softens food, and allows only food particles of approximately 5 mm in diameter to enter the duodenum.

Practical Aspects
Spices (except hot peppers) are allowed and are in fact desirable to make food more palatable. Food thickeners, largely gums and modified starches, are available as an aid in swallowing to avoid aspiration. Patients with oral or pharyngeal dysphagia should eat slowly, sit up as straight as possible, keep their head in an optimal position for swallowing (as determined by swallowing studies), and ingest small amounts at any one time.

1. **Foods allowed on a mechanical soft diet.** All beverages and soups are allowed. Whole tender meat is permissible, as is ground or puréed meat, but not fibrous meat. Eggs and

cheese are permissible. Melted cheese or nonfat dry milk can be used to increase protein content. All potatoes and starches are allowed. Breads and cereals are acceptable, except for high-fiber cereals and hard, crusty breads. Cooked or refined ready-to-eat cereals are often better. Vegetables can be included if they are well cooked or puréed, but raw vegetables must be shredded or chopped. Foods that are hard to chew must be chopped, ground, or blended. Canned or fresh fruits without skin or seeds are acceptable, but not other fresh or dried fruits. Nuts are not allowed. Desserts are acceptable if they do not contain nuts.

2. The bland diet is often combined with a mechanical soft diet and has been used for years in the treatment of ulcer disease. However, no evidence has been found of the value of a bland diet that restricts spices or coarse foods.

3. Some dietary maneuvers have been helpful in the past in the management of acid peptic disease, such as the use of small, frequent feedings to minimize acid secretion after a meal and the avoidance of snacks before bedtime to prevent acid stimulation during sleep. Other dietary modifications in peptic disease have included the elimination of alcoholic and caffeine-containing beverages and smoking. However, with the current availability of potent acid-suppressing medications, these restrictions are now usually unnecessary.

4. Certain dietary restrictions also may benefit patients with gastroesophageal reflux disease (GERD). Foods that increase lower esophageal sphincter pressure include tomatoes and tomato juice, citrus fruits, chocolate, peppermint, and very fatty foods. However, the value of restricting fatty foods in the treatment of GERD has been questioned (59).

Side Effects
No side effects have been associated with this diet.

Supplements Required
Supplements are not required.

Modified-fiber Diets

Dietary fiber is not one chemical substance, nor is it completely indigestible. It is a component of the diet that either by itself or through its metabolites produces certain physiologic effects in humans, although the nature and importance of these effects are as yet poorly delineated. *Fiber* is not the same as *residue*. The latter term refers to all stool solids that result from the ingestion of any given diet. In addition to fiber, residue includes bacteria, exfoliated cells, and mucus. A full or clear liquid diet is best for minimizing fecal residue. Bacteria comprise the largest component of stool solids on a Western diet (~50%), with fiber comprising only approximately 17% (60). Fiber alters the bacterial environment by providing a diluent of luminal contents, and by adding mass to promote colonic movement, but fiber does not promote a large bacterial mass in healthy subjects (61). However, in patients with short-bowel syndrome (SBS) who deliver more fat and calories to the colon, the amount of bacteria excreted in the stools and their fat content is increased, leading to an underestimate of the digestibility of ingested energy and fat (62).

Definition
The definition of dietary fiber has changed over time, developing by consensus. Trowell in 1972 first defined fiber as the proportion of food that is derived from the cellular walls of plants and is poorly digested by humans. The accepted definition of dietary fiber by the American Association of Cereal Chemists (2000) is "the edible parts of plants or analogous carbohydrates that are resistant to digestion and absorption in the human small intestine with complete or partial fermentation in the large intestine. Dietary fiber includes polysaccharides, oligosaccharides, lignin, and associated plant substances. Dietary fibers promote beneficial physiological effects including laxation, and/or blood cholesterol attenuation, and/or blood glucose attenuation" (63). About the same time as the AACC document was prepared, the Institute of Medicine (IOM) prepared a volume on dietary reference intakes (DRIs) that included fiber, recognizing that nondigestible carbohydrates could be isolated and when added to products might produce a health benefit (64). The IOM definitions are as follows: "Dietary fiber consists of nondigestible carbohydrates and lignin that are intrinsic and intact in plants. Functional fiber consists of isolated, nondigestible carbohydrates that have beneficial physiological effects in humans. Total fiber is the

sum of dietary fiber and functional fiber." The European Commission defined fiber as carbohydrate polymers with three or more monomeric units that are neither digested nor absorbed in the human small intestine (Statement of the Scientific Panel on Dietetic Products, Nutrition, and Allergies, July 6, 2007, at the 17th plenary session, www.efsa.europa.eu/en/efsajournal/pub/1060.htm). This definition included edible carbohydrate polymers occurring naturally in foods and those that have been obtained from food raw materials.

Fiber Content

The fiber content of foods is most commonly based on the rather indirect and imprecise measurement of *crude fiber*—the residue of food that remains after sequential acid and alkali treatment. The relationship between the measurement (of the residue that escapes digestion) and the physiologic role of the residue is confusing. A proposal for a definition of methods of analysis has been made by the Codex Committee on Nutrition and Foods for Special Dietary Uses. This group has stated that nondigestible material is composed of carbohydrate polymers with a degree of polymerization greater than 3, and that these polymers can be present in food when raw or prepared, or added back as synthetic polymers. This opinion has been confirmed by a consensus reached at the Ninth Vahouny Fiber Symposium, which agreed also on the functions of dietary fiber that is not digested or absorbed in the small intestine as increased stool bulk, decreased transit time, increased colonic fermentation and short-chain fatty acid production, positive modulation of colonic microflora, reduced blood total or LDL cholesterol (LDL-C), reduced postprandial blood glucose or insulin levels, weight loss in adiposity, and increased satiety. All these definitions and inclusions have caused a major issue with regulators and consumers (66). The division of fiber into dietary and functional (i.e., added) fiber has created much of this confusion. Although US labeling does not distinguish dietary from functional fiber, many products called functional fiber are on the market. Canadian regulators have concluded that a synthetic or "novel" fiber, when produced and added back to food, can be included in the total for dietary fiber if it meets the accepted definitions (is not digested and is polymerized enough) and has a proven physiological function (67). However, this is a difficult hurdle, as only a small number of novel fibers have been approved since 1985 (ground bleached oat hulls, soy cotyledon, sugar beet fiber, and psyllium seed husk) (66), and wheat bran soluble fiber, rich in arabinoxylan oligosaccharides (Bran Vita™). For an understanding of the uses of altered-fiber diets, the definition, measurement, metabolism, and possible functions of dietary fiber and functional fibers should be considered.

Classes of Fiber

The major chemical classes of dietary and functional fiber are cellulose, noncellulose polysaccharides, and lignin (Table 12-11). These classes can also be arranged based on those that are water insoluble/less fermented (cellulose, hemicellulose, and lignin), and water soluble/well fermented (pectin, gums, and mucilages) (68). All of these classes are all included in the category of nonstarch polysaccharides (NSPs), referring to the naturally occurring cell-wall material in plant foods. Although the NSP content of cereals is high, the ratio of NSP to dry matter (DM) is much greater in fruits and vegetables than in cereals (69). The total fiber content of plants, as exemplified by their content of NSP, is what has been considered the factor leading to health benefits, rather than individual components of NSP. Cereals and grains are rich in arabinoxylans (xylose polymers), cellulose (β-glucans/glucose polymers), and polymers of arabinose, mannose, and galactose. Fruits and vegetables are rich in pectins (uronic acid polymers), cellulose (glucose only), and polymers of rhamnose and fucose in addition to the other polymers found in cereals. The fiber components that are not found in the cell wall (gums, fructo-oligosaccharides, resistant starch) are the major sources of fiber that are added to foods and called "functional" fiber. Because of this label, it is often assumed that they are more beneficial than plant wall–derived fiber, but this is not the case. Most health benefits have been shown to be due to the use of whole plants in the diet, and it is not possible to make independent claims for most of the components of dietary fiber (69).

Cellulose

Cellulose is a straight-chain polymer of glucose with a β-1,4 linkage. It is not digested by pancreatic or small-bowel enzymes. Cellulose is a major structural component of cell walls but rarely accounts for more than 20% of total polysaccharides. It is highly represented in wheat

TABLE 12-11 Properties of Components of Dietary Fiber

Component	Plant Function	Major Food Sources	Effects
Cellulose	Cell wall structure	Bran, whole wheat/other flours, legumes, root vegetables, apples	↑ Fecal bulk, ↓ transit time, ↓ micronutrient absorption (impact), binds bile salts
Noncellulose polysaccharides (hemicellulose)	Cell wall stability	Bran, cereals, whole grains	Same as cellulose
Pectins[a]	Cell wall stability	Citrus fruits, berries, apples, bananas, carrots, potatoes	Alters food consistency, ↓ cholesterol absorption, ↑ fecal water, ↓ gastric emptying
Gums and mucilages[a] (psyllium, guar gum)	Secretions	Oatmeal, dried legumes, used in food industry (baking, dressings, juice stabilizers)	↓ Cholesterol absorption, ↑ fecal water, ↓ vitamin/mineral absorption
Lignins	Cell wall strength	Old/tough vegetables, wheat	↑Fecal bulk, ↓transit time
Fructo-oligosaccharides, polydextrose[a]	Cell structure, secretions	Onions, bananas, tomatoes, honey, barley, garlic, wheat	Prebiotic, alters fecal flora, ↑ SCFAs, prevents colon cancer
Resistant starch	Storage form	Processed grains, flours	↓Glycemic index, ↓ colon cancer

[a]Included in the category of functional fiber.
SCFA, short-chain fatty acid.

bran, apple and pear skin, and strawberries. Related to celluloses are the β-glucans, composed of straight polymers of β-1,4 glucose and β-1,3 glucose (70).

Hemicelluloses

Hemicelluloses are linear and highly branched polysaccharides of xylose, arabinose, mannose, glucomannans, galactomannans, galactoglucomannans, and glucuronic acid. They act as plasticizers and intertwine with lignin between the cellulose fibers of the cell wall. *Nonstructural polysaccharides*, including pectins, gums, and mucilages, are branched polymers containing many uronic acids that hold water and form gels. They are highly branched in growing plants and become less branched as the support structure becomes more developed. They act as adhesives and are insoluble in unripe fruit, becoming soluble only as the fruit matures. Thus, the amount extracted may vary with the age of the fruit.

Resistant Short-Chain Carbohydrates

These include those nonglycemic carbohydrates that are soluble in 80% ethanol, other than highly polymerized sugar alcohols. The resistant short-chain carbohydrate (RSCC) fraction includes carbohydrates otherwise referred to as nondigestible oligosaccharides, and includes inulin, fructo-oligosaccharides, polydextrose, methylcellulose, and resistant maltodextrins.

Resistant Starches

Resistant starches are defined as starches that enter the colon. RS1 is physically inaccessible because of its particle size or entrapment in food. RS2 and RS3 resist amylase action because of their compact (unbranched) structure; RS2 is unbranched, and RS3 is retrograded (i.e., altered during processing) (71). Some starches are relatively resistant because they become available slowly in the intestinal lumen. Most resistant starches are produced during food preparation, a process that can either increase or decrease the amount of RS. The food properties that determine whether or not carbohydrate is digestible are determined in vitro by measuring the release of rapidly and slowly available glucose (RAG/SAG); what is left is RS (69). Cereals and bakery products have lower SAG values than do pasta and whole grains. The intake of such starches in a Western diet is estimated at 5 to 10 g per day.

Common Commercial Ingredients High in Dietary Fiber

Acacia gum (gum Arabic) is produced from two species of tree. The gum is a large and complex polysaccharide consisting mainly of arabinogalactans, contributing to soluble fiber. β-Glucan is a component of cell walls from fungi, algae, and grains, although the location of the glucan within the cereal grain varies. This variability leads to large differences in yield when various cereals are processed (72). Chitin and chitosan are β- 1→4 linked insoluble polysaccharides found in arthropods, some fungi, and yeasts. These compounds are the second most abundant (after cellulose) fiber polymer in nature, and are widely produced and consumed in supplements. Algal polysaccharides include alginates, agars, carrageenans, ulvanes, and fucoidans, and are widely used in foods and pharmaceutical products (73). Because these products are largely water soluble, they are easily added to products for thickening and texture, and have been touted as having many health benefits.

Corn bran contains nearly 90% of weight as insoluble fiber, two-third hemicelluloses with some cellulose, is widely available, and has high water-binding capacity (72). Inulin is a soluble fiber composed of a linear chain of fructose molecules that is present in thousands of plants and vegetables. Plants with the highest inulin content include onion, leek, garlic, Jerusalem artichoke, artichoke, and chicory. This fiber is added to provide viscosity and to stabilize emulsions, but is available as a prebiotic as well, promoting the growth of bifidobacteria (72). Oat bran contains from approximately 30% to 90% dietary fiber, much of which is β-glucan. Pectins are linear chains of galaturonic acid with some rhamnose component. Pectin does not contribute much to fecal bulk or transit time.

Polydextrose is a synthetic soluble fiber made from glucose molecules with mainly 1,6 linkages that consequently delivers only approximately 1 kcal per g of energy. It also contains approximately 10% sorbitol and 1% citric acid. Polydextrose is often used as a replacement for sugar, starch, and fat, and as a bulking agent and dietary fiber source in food products, in part because it is stable and very water soluble. It has also been shown to promote the growth of beneficial bacteria, and is used as a prebiotic (72). If a serving contains more than 15 g of polydextrose per serving, the label must contain a statement about laxation. Thus, commercial products tend to limit the content of polydextrose. Like many other dietary fiber components, polydextrose is not specifically identified by usual food analysis for dietary fiber (see below).

Psyllium/ispaghula is the common name used for members of the plant genus *Plantago*, whose seeds are harvested for production of mucilage. The husk of the seeds provides approximately 70% soluble fiber as a polymer of arabinose, galactose, rhamnose, and galacturonic acid (72). Psyllium increases stool weight and water content, and the number of bowel movements, and is a common component in many commercial fiber products (e.g., Metamucil™, Correctol™, Effersyllium™, Fiberall™, Hydrocil™, Konsyl™, Perdiem™, and Syllact™). Psyllium is also used as a thickener and is used in frozen desserts, as its viscosity property is little affected by changes in temperature.

Rice bran is a by-product of white rice production, containing approximately 20% to 33% insoluble fiber, mostly cellulose and lignin. Thus, it is used mostly in rice flours and breakfast cereals. Soy bran is made from the hull of the bean, and contains 65% to 95% insoluble fiber. Soy fiber contains approximately 75% dietary fiber as a mixture of insoluble and soluble fiber, with much less cellulose than soy bran. Soy bran and fiber are used in multigrain breads, muffins, noodles, breakfast cereals, snack foods, and other baked products (72). Wheat bran contains approximately 45% dietary fiber (cellulose and hemicellulose) with protein and starch making up the rest of the product. Wheat bran is often marketed by itself as a fiber source. Wheat fiber is a further-refined product, almost completely composed of dietary fiber. This product is used for baking because of its high water-holding capacity and storage stability.

Measurement

Four methods for measuring dietary fiber have provided enough data to be useful in assessing the fiber content of foods.

Crude Fiber

Crude fiber is the residue of plant food left after sequential extraction with solvent, dilute acid, and dilute alkali. Early chemists thought that residue-resisting alkali and acid treatment was indigestible. The crude fiber procedure was developed in the 19th century and was favored because of the purity of the residue, which was low in ash and nitrogen content. Extraction and loss of hemicelluloses (>80%) and lignin (50% to 90%) are a consequence of solubility at acid and alkaline pH. All components of dietary fiber are at least partially soluble in these solutions. However, the degree of extraction varies with food preparation, particle size, and presence of other fiber components. Crude fiber is still the measure of fiber reported in some food tables and was the original basis for all altered-fiber diets, but it provides an incomplete and inaccurate assessment of fiber because hemicellulose and lignin are extracted more than cellulose. Crude fiber is slowly being replaced by other methods. The relation of crude fiber to plant cell wall polysaccharide content depends on the proportions of pectins, cellulose, and hemicelluloses, which vary among vegetables and fruits. Monocotyledons in general are high in hemicelluloses and lignin and low in crude fiber. Legumes are higher in lignin but low in hemicelluloses and are intermediate for crude fiber. Dicotyledonous nonlegume vegetables have the highest proportion of cellulose and crude fiber.

Neutral Detergent Residues

These were developed by Van Soest and McQueen (74) and refined further by Englyst et al. (75), and Anderson and Bridges (76). Neutral detergent fiber or residue results from extraction with boiling sodium lauryl sulfate and ethylenediaminetetraacetate (EDTA) and is nonhydrolytic. Pectins and mucilages are removed completely, and the residue contains cellulose, lignin, and hemicelluloses (i.e., the cell wall components of fiber). This residue contains other nonlignin components that are not polysaccharides. Because neutral detergent residue includes all the major plant cell wall components, it continues to be used to assess the dietary fiber content of foods.

The Method of Southgate (77)

This method is the most complex but probably the most accurate because it measures both soluble polysaccharides (mucilages, gums, and pectins) and cell wall components. A series of extractions with organic solvents and acids is followed by enzymatic treatment and hydrolysis. Data derived by this method or a modification of the method are recorded as "total dietary fiber," which includes noncellulose polysaccharides (hemicelluloses, gums, mucilages, and pectins) and lignins.

Association of Official Analytical Chemists Method

In the Association of Official Analytical Chemists (AOAC) method, enzymes and gravimetry are used. After fat is extracted from food, dried samples are gelatinized and then digested with protease and amyloglucosidase to remove protein and starch. The soluble dietary fiber is precipitated with ethanol, dried, and ashed. Total dietary fiber equals ethanol-precipitated-residue weight minus ashed-residue weight. This is the method now used by the USDA for its tables of food fiber content (see www.usda.gov).

The "correct" assessment of fiber content cannot be made from these data because the physiologic importance of each component is not known. In addition, the preparation of food may alter the measurements by removing soluble and loosely bound components. Thus, fiber supplements should be offered with an understanding of the nonequivalent nature of the product sources.

Fermentation of Fiber

Variations in Degradation

The proportion of cellulose digested in the colon varies widely, from 47% to 80%. Purified cellulose is handled differently from dietary cellulose and is less degraded, about 25% (78). Bran cellulose is less degraded, perhaps because of its high lignin content. Cellulose metabolism is increased by slow transit, as in the elderly. Noncellulose polysaccharides are in general more completely degraded. Wheat bran is among the most poorly digested sources of dietary fiber, for reasons not related solely to its chemical composition. The digestion of NSPs is variable and unpredictable. Most freshly cooked foods and uncooked cereals contain a high percentage of readily digested starch. However, a cooled, cooked potato is less digestible than a freshly cooked one. Thus, it is not true that starch is completely digested and absorbed in the small intestine. Moreover, the fermentation products of starch and NSPs differ in the large intestine. Factors that affect starch digestibility in humans include (besides the physical form) transit time, food processing, and the presence of amylase inhibitors, lectins, or phytates (79). In a Western-type diet, the amount of fermentable carbohydrate entering the colon includes, on average, 12 g of NSPs and a variable amount of starch.

Volatile Fatty Acids

Volatile fatty acids are probably the main product of fiber polysaccharides and are well absorbed by the human colon. Thus, some of the nutritive value of dietary fiber is recovered by the absorption of fermentation products. It has been estimated that from 20 g of dietary fiber, 100 mEq of volatile fatty acids is produced, of which about 20% is excreted and the rest absorbed or used by bacteria.

Fermentation

The overall fermentation process as it is now understood can be defined quantitatively. Fermentation of resultant soluble hexoses is about 60%. Hydrogen produced in large amounts is converted to methane in the ruminating animal. Of humans, only 30% to 40% produce methane, so hydrogen gas is excreted in large amounts. The gas by-products of carbohydrate fermentation are odorless but carry with them the more noticeable by-products of protein breakdown (putrefaction). The volatile fatty acids (acetate, propionate, and butyrate) are available in part as energy sources. Some of the available energy supports bacterial growth. It has been estimated that fermentation of 100 g of carbohydrate supports the growth of 30 g of bacteria. The effect of bacterial growth on other colonic functions has not been determined.

Functions of Dietary Fiber

A high-fiber diet increases stool bulk, produces more frequent stools, and decreases transit time through the intestine. Fecal bile acids appear to be increased when fiber is included in the diet. Table 12-11 reviews the properties of fiber components that may be responsible for the (known and postulated) effects of dietary fiber. However, the intake of fiber must be adequate if the potential benefits are to be realized. Intake in the United States remains lower than the recommended 25 g per day, averaging 17 g per day in the third National Health and Nutrition Examination (NHANES III) (80).

Factors Related to Increased Stool Weight

Even when a function of dietary fiber has been established (water-holding capacity), that function does not necessarily correlate with the crude fiber or total dietary fiber content of foods (Table 12-12). Moreover, the increment in stool weight is not linearly related to either the in vitro water-holding capacity or the water content of the food. It is possible that more than one factor (e.g., volatile fatty acid production in addition to water-holding capacity) is responsible for the observed result—an increase in stool weight. The practical aspect of this information is that not all fiber sources are alike, and the effect of a high-fiber diet may depend on the exact mixture of foods used.

Decreased Intake of Food. Obesity is rare in populations that consume a high-fiber diet, possibly because of a lower caloric intake or increased satiety (81). Dietary fiber intake is lower for obese subjects and BMI is lower in subjects who have higher fiber ingestion (82). Supplementing 14 g per day of fiber is associated with modest weight loss (1.9 kg over 3.8 months), but decreased intake was found mostly in obese subjects (83). The mechanism for this weight loss is unclear but might include satiation, altered glycemic responses, decreased energy absorption, altered gastric emptying, or decreased food intake at a later meal (82). Convincing evidence for most of these mechanisms is lacking. Supplements proposed to work by increasing satiety have shown some effect (glucomannan, guar gum) or no effect (psyllium), but the positive trials showed only modest results in small numbers of subjects (84). Intervention studies show that a very large amount of fiber (~30 g per meal) is needed to decrease energy intake taken after the fiber-containing meal, but this is much beyond what most subjects could tolerate (64). The data are rather better to support a role for dietary fiber in limiting weight gain, especially when compared with high meat intake (85).

TABLE 12-12 Water-Holding Capacity of Various Foods

Food	Crude Fiber Content (g/100 g of raw food)[a]	Aoac Fiber Content (g/100 g of raw food)[a]	Capacity of Fiber in 100 g of Raw Vegetables to Absorb Water (g)[b]	Moisture (g/100-g edible portion)[a]
Potato, fresh	0.5	1.5	41	75.4
Tomato	0.5	1.3	71	94
Cucumber	0.4	1.0	77	96
Celery	0.6	1.6	97	94.7
Lettuce	0.6	1.0	99	95.7
Pear	1.4	2.6	113	83.8
Orange	0.5	2.4	122	86.8
Corn	0.7	3.7	129	69.6
Apple	0.6	2.2	177	83.9
Carrot	1.0	3.2	208	87.8
Wheat bran	9.4	35.3	447	2.9

[a]McConnell AA, Eastwood MA, Mitchell WD. A comparison of methods of measuring "fiber" in vegetable material. *J Sci Food Agric.* 1974;25:1457.
[b]Human Nutrition Information Service, U.S. Department of Agriculture. *Provisional table on dietary fiber content of selected foods,* HNIS/PT-106, 1988, and updated *Appendix* Tables 8-19, 1991; and 8-20, 1989.
AOAC, Association of Official Analytical Chemists.

Coronary Heart Disease. Coronary heart disease has been inversely related to fiber intake, for example, in the Nurses' Health Study, in which each increase of total daily dietary fiber of 10 g was associated with a relative risk reduction of 0.81 (86). Of the various sources of dietary fiber, only cereal fiber was strongly associated with a reduced risk for coronary heart disease (relative risk reduction of 0.63 per 5 g daily). Soluble fiber decreases serum total and LDL-C, risk factors for CVD, but there are no epidemiologic studies that link functional fiber (mostly soluble fibers) with the risk of coronary artery disease (64). Moreover, most epidemiological studies link high fiber intake from cereal products with lower rates of CVD. Higher fiber intake, mostly from cereals and vegetables, is associated with lower mortality, particularly from circulatory, digestive, and inflammatory diseases (87). The association was similar for men and women and after correcting for confounding lifestyle and dietary factors.

Diabetes. Fiber ingestion by diabetic patients leads to some delay in gastric emptying, improvement in glucose tolerance, and reduction of hyperinsulinemia and hyperlipidemia (88). The diet used for this study contained 25 g each of soluble and insoluble fiber, and the effect was greater than that seen when the American, British, and Canadian Diabetes Association recommendations were used (8 g of soluble and 16 g of insoluble fiber per day). Total fiber intake may decrease the risk of diabetes and improve postprandial glucose responses, although it may be difficult to separate any positive effect from an improvement in weight (89).

Mineral Availability. Binding by fiber of minerals and trace elements has been shown consistently in vitro, but has not been consistently reported in clinical studies. When a wide variety of food is available and ingested, it is not known whether fiber intake affects mineral availability, and micronutrient supplements are not needed when fiber intake is increased. In fact, oligofructans have been reported to improve calcium absorption and calcium balance in experimental models (90).

Colonic Disorders. The evidence for the inverse association of dietary fiber with diverticular disease, cancer of the colon, and irritable bowel syndrome (IBS) is incomplete, and much of it is based on epidemiologic data (64). In one prospective study, a low intake of fiber (13 g per day) was associated with an increase in the relative risk for the development of symptomatic diverticular disease of 2.35 (91). Some data suggest that a fiber intake of 30 to 35 g per day is inversely related to the risk for colon cancer (see references 92 and 93 for reviews of case-control studies), but the data do not unequivocally support a protective role for fiber. Nine large epidemiological studies examining the relationship between fiber and colorectal cancer (CRC) have been analyzed; four studies showed a statistically significant lower risk for CRC associated with higher fiber intake, but five did not (94). It is possible that the highest levels of fiber intake might show a preventive effect against colon tumors, but the data are not available for very high fiber intakes. Studies have suggested a protective role for fiber against colorectal adenomas (95–97). When other dietary risk factors (smoking, alcohol, folate, red meat, total milk, and total energy) are accounted for in prospective cohort studies, the significance of the association disappeared (98). Because it is difficult to single out one dietary component in relation to cancer prevention (see also Chapter 15), it is not possible to make a recommendation for altering fiber content at this time, except to suggest that the DRI of fiber be followed (Table 12-13).

Although dietary fiber is known to improve the number and bulk of bowel movements in normal subjects, the evidence for its value in IBS is not evident. Some randomized controlled trials (RCTs) show benefit, but most do not (99). It is not clear whether the effect, if and when it occurs, does so in patients with diarrhea compared with constipation or with the mixed bowel pattern, but it is unlikely that fiber is effective against the entire symptom complex (pain, bloating, etc). Any use of fiber in IBS patients should be individualized, especially if a trial of use appears to be helpful.

Lowering Cholesterol Levels. Soluble gel-forming fiber (β-glucans, pectins, guar gum) decreases serum total and LDL-C concentrations and improves insulin resistance (100). The effect may be mediated by cholesterol binding, altered gastric emptying, or both. Sources of insoluble fiber (wheat bran, cellulose) have no effect. Rice bran lowers cholesterol, but the effects appear to be produced by nonfiber components. The cholesterol-lowering effect is small but within the practical range of intake. For example, 3 g of soluble fiber from oatmeal (84 g) decreases total and LDL-C by about 0.13 mmol per L (101). The addition of psyllium supplements (10.2 g per day) to a prudent American Heart Association diet can lower total cholesterol by about 5% and LDL-C by 8.6% (102). Although a decreased intake of saturated fat is the most important dietary factor in lowering serum cholesterol, the effect of soluble fiber is comparable with decreasing dietary cholesterol to below 200 mg per day and with a weight loss of 5 kg (103).

Treatment of Inflammatory Colitis. Some products of the fermentation of fiber (especially short-chain fatty acids, primarily butyrate) are an important energy source for colonic mucosal cells. Infusions of sodium butyrate (100 mmol per L) in the form of enemas may relieve ulcerative colitis (UC) and diversion colitis, but the data are not consistent, and a strong recommendation cannot be made with current information (104). Based on data mostly in rodents, it is possible that dietary fiber plays a role in immunomodulation, as evidenced by changes in inflammatory markers, but data in humans are virtually absent (105).

Indications for Modified-fiber Diets
Current Consumption Levels

Total dietary fiber intake has been only about half of the recommended intake in recent decades in the United States, estimated as 11 to 13 g per day in NHANES II (1976–1980) (92) and as

TABLE 12-13 Adequate Intake Values (g/day) for Total Fiber

Life Stage (year)	Male	Female
1–3	19	19
4–8	25	25
9–13	31	26
14–18	38	26
19–50	38	25
51–>70	30	21
Pregnancy/lactation		28/29

Source: Food and Nutrition Board, Institute of Medicine, Dietary Reference Intakes for Energy, Carbohydrate, Fiber, Fat, Fatty Acids, Cholesterol, Protein, and Amino Acids (Macronutrients). Washington DC: National Academies Press, 2005.

10 to 14 g per day in NHANES III (1988–1991) (80,106). Fewer grain products are consumed on average than in the 1930s and 1940s, but more fresh fruits and vegetables are now consumed throughout the year than previously.

Recommended Intake

The recommendations of the IOM committee on macronutrients considered the availability of food fiber and added (or functional) fiber, as well as the amount of fiber needed to deliver possible health benefits when estimating the dietary recommended intake for fiber. Not enough data were available to provide an estimate average requirement (EAR), so an adequate intake (AI) was used to meet the average needs of a healthy population (Table 12-13).

Low-Fiber Diet

This diet is indicated whenever decreased fecal bulk is desired, as during preparation for barium studies or intestinal surgery, although a clear liquid diet is often preferred in such cases. A low-fiber diet may be used in *acute diarrheal illnesses*, such as gastroenteritis and UC, and in SBS when the colon is still present. This diet is not indicated for the long-term treatment of diverticular disease or IBS. In patients with diverticulitis presenting with a chronic partial obstruction of the colon, a low-fiber diet may be used temporarily. *Partial obstruction of any part of the intestinal tract* (e.g., pylorus, colon) may be managed either by mechanical softening of foods (more useful for upper intestinal obstructions) or by a low intake of fiber (more useful for lower-intestinal obstructions).

Partial Low-Fiber Diet

Sometimes, a diet with only a moderate restriction of fiber is indicated. When an ileal segment is very narrow in a patient with *Crohn disease*, only the most indigestible of the fiber sources need be eliminated (bran buds, corn, nuts); the other fiber-rich foods often can be consumed in moderation. *Gastric phytobezoars* can be treated initially with a full low-fiber diet; however, to prevent recurrences, the elimination of pulpy fruits (citrus fruits, pears) and persimmons from the diet is sometimes sufficient. Alternatively, a modified low-fiber diet can be used, in which only the foods highest in fiber (Table 12-13) are avoided. Examples include fruits (oranges, grapefruits, prunes, raisins, figs, cherries, persimmons, apples, grapes, berries), vegetables (celery, pumpkin, sauerkraut, lettuce, broccoli, brussels sprouts, potato skins), and others (bran, coconut, peanut, popcorn, kidney beans). An unusual food therapy for gastric phytobezoars is the use of Coca-Cola, based on no known mechanism. Forty-six patients have been reported in 24 publications, using 0.5 to 3 L per day for 1 day to 6 weeks, and demonstrating efficacy in most cases (107). However, none of the reports is controlled, and there is every reason to think that high-volume washing of the stomach might be effective.

High-Fiber Diet. A high-fiber diet is used in the long-term treatment of recurrent diverticulitis (not simple diverticulosis) and irritable bowel disease when altered bowel habit is a major symptom. A high-fiber diet is not essential for every healthy adult who is ingesting the recommended amount of dietary fiber per day (Table 12-13). It is sometimes used nonspecifically in the treatment of chronic diarrhea to produce semiformed, less liquid stools, especially as a fiber-supplemented enteral formula (108). However, the effect is often produced at the expense of an increase in the number or volume of stools. Moreover, if a high-fiber supplement is administered to a patient through a small-bore tube, the tube may become obstructed. For these reasons, a high intake of fiber must be used cautiously in most cases of diarrhea.

Practical Aspects

A clear liquid diet may be substituted for a low-fiber diet, but only for a short time because caloric intake is insufficient. Alternatively, commercially prepared liquid diets can be used (see Chapter 10). Table 12-14 lists total dietary fiber per average serving. Both high-fiber and low-fiber diets can be derived from such tables. Low-fiber diets are adequate in protein and fat. If dairy products are eliminated from the diet because of lactose intolerance, protein and calcium intake from other sources should be increased.

Commercial Psyllium Powders

These powders contain about 3.4 g of psyllium mucilloid per teaspoon. Because preparations are produced and packaged differently, the instructions for use of each product should be carefully followed and not transferred to other products. Some plants (e.g., *Plantago*) are very rich in psyllium, which comprises 10% to 12% of soluble fiber. The exact conversion of grams of psyllium

TABLE 12-14 Fiber Content/Serving of Commonly Used Foods

Total Dietary Fiber 5 g
Baked beans (1/4 cup)
Split peas (1/2 cup)
Chick peas, kidney beans, lentils (1/2 cup)
Butter beans, cooled (1/2 cup)
Blackberries (1/4 cup)
Grapes, white (12)
Raspberries (1/2 cup)
Bran wheat (1/4 cup)
All-Bran, raisin bran (1/3 cup)
Shredded Wheat (2 biscuits)
Almonds (15)
Grapenuts (1 cup)
Prunes, stewed (1/2 cup)

Total Dietary Fiber ~4 g
Peas, fresh or canned (1/2 cup)
Turnip greens (1/2 cup)
Broccoli (1 cup)
Cranberries (1 cup)
Prunes, dried (3)
Pear with skin (1 medium)
Apricots (5)
Apple (1 large)
Figs, dried (2)

Total Dietary Fiber ~3 g
Beets, boiled (1/2 cup)
Potato with skin, baked (one 2 1/2-in diameter)
Rye crackers (4)
Fruit pie (9-in diameter, 1/6 of pie)
Corn flakes (1 cup)

Total Dietary Fiber ~2 g
Banana (1 small)
Peach (1 medium)
Potato (1 medium with skin)
Corn on cob (small ear)
Carrot (1 medium)
Cabbage, boiled (1/2 cup)
Tomato (1 medium)
Turnips (2/3 cup)
Cauliflower, raw (1 cup)
Rhubarb (1/4 cup)
Strawberries (10 large)
Plums (2 medium)
Orange (flesh) (1 small)
Tangerine (1 large)
Cherries (15)
Puffed wheat (1 cup)
Corn flakes (1 cup)
Flour, wholemeal (3 tbsp)
Peanut butter (2 tbsp)
Bran, powdered (1 tbsp)

(continued)

TABLE 12-14 Fiber Content/Serving of Commonly Used Foods *(continued)*

Rye bread (1 slice)
Whole wheat bread (2 slices)
Total Dietary Fiber ~1 g
Onion (1 small)
Cauliflower, boiled (1/2 cup)
Celery, raw (1/2 cup)
Potato, boiled, no skin (1 medium)
Asparagus, boiled (4 spears)
Cucumber, raw (2 cups)
Rice Krispies (3/4 cup)
Special K (3/4 cup)
White bread (1 slice)
Popcorn (1 cup)
Raisins (1 tbsp)
Nectarines (1 medium)
Melon, all types (1/4 melon)
Pineapple, fresh (1/2 cup)
Grapefruit (1/2)
Rice, boiled white (1/2 cup)
Flour, white (3 tbsp)
Peanuts (12)
Total Dietary Fiber <0.2 g
Fruit juices, strained (1 cup)
Sugar, white (1 tbsp)
Mayonnaise (1 tbsp)
Fruit jellies (1 tbsp)
Fats (2 tbsp)
Milk (1 cup)
Egg (1 medium)
Meat, fish, poultry (3 oz)
Coffee, tea, soda (1 cup)

to total dietary fiber is uncertain, but a 1:1 equivalence is probably nearly correct, and a suitable estimate for practical application.

Sources of Fiber

High-fiber diets can be based on foods with moderate or high amounts of fiber. Commercial psyllium seed may be used instead of, or in addition to, a high-fiber diet or a bran preparation, but this is not recommended for increasing fiber intake in healthy populations. The type of fiber is different in each source, and the effects are occasionally additive. Most often, however, a patient responds to one or another source of fiber. The psyllium seed preparations are easy to take, their effects are reproducible, and they eliminate the need to use a special diet. However, in some instances, they are ineffective, whereas other types of fiber relieve symptoms. Most dietary fiber in a Western-type diet comes from fresh fruits, vegetables, and cereals. Usual servings of fruits, vegetables, and cereals contain 2 to 4 g of dietary fiber (Table 12-14).

High-Fiber Diet

High-fiber diets should aim to add the equivalent of at least 10 g of total dietary fiber to the diet. This increment may be accomplished by adding a normal distribution of fiber-containing foods to the previous diet, or the use of a single, concentrated source of fiber may be required. The importance of obtaining a dietary history is obvious. Psyllium seed provides 6 to 7 g of fiber in a dosage of 2 tsp per day; All-Bran cereal contains 11.2 g of dietary fiber in each cup; wheat bran contains about 5 g of dietary fiber in each tablespoon. In general, ingestion of two to three doses per day provides 10 g of additional dietary fiber. Keep in mind that not all sources of fiber produce the same effect (Table 12-11). Thus, it is best to increase foods containing dietary fiber. If added (or functional) fiber is used, it may be necessary to try different types of fiber supplement before finding one that improves symptoms or is well tolerated.

Prebiotics are an increasingly common source of fiber that are available over the counter. The major sources of prebiotics available in Europe and the United States are inulin (derived from chicory roots), fructo-oligosaccharides or oligofructose (derived from the hydrolysis of chicory inulin or synthesized from sucrose), galacto-oligosaccharides (synthesized from lactose), and soybean oligosaccharides (extracted from soybeans). The average chain lengths of most of these are quite short, with only three to four residues, except for inulin, which has an average of 10 residues, and they comprise the classification of RSCCs (68). They are used as fat or sugar replacements and to add body to a variety of products, including dairy products, breakfast cereals, baked goods and breads, chocolate and confections, dietetic products, table spreads and salad dressings, and meat products. These supplements should be included on the label of the food products to which they are added, although the amount added may not be specified.

Fiber is being included in enteral feeding formulas for use both in hospital and in the community. Forty-three RCTs have been analyzed, demonstrating a decrease in the diarrhea caused by enteral feedings (109). Bowel frequency was reduced when baseline frequency was high, and increased when it was low. Xanthan gum, a polysaccharide secreted by the bacterium *Xanthomonas campestris*, is a common food additive used as a thickening agent. It has been provided as a powder to thicken food and beverages for patients with oropharyngeal dysphagia (Resource Thicken Up Clear™), and provides 7 g of fiber per tbsp.

Low-Fiber Diet
Allowed foods are mainly animal foods (eggs, meats, milk), fats, white bread or rice, strained juices, and low-fiber fruits and vegetables, such as peaches without skin and peeled cucumber.

Side Effects
An excess of fiber can increase the frequency of stools in the absence of constipation or worsen the symptoms of chronic constipation. Thus, fiber should be used cautiously to treat constipation as an isolated symptom. Excess fiber may obstruct a structural narrowing of the intestinal tract. When a low-fiber diet is used inappropriately to treat diverticulitis or irritable bowel disease, symptoms may worsen.

Supplements Required
A strict low-fiber diet containing 3 cups of milk per day and some meat servings is adequate for all nutrients except vitamin A (unless liver is eaten) and iron (for female patients). The caloric intake also may be inadequate, depending on the patient. In most cases, the diet is used only for a short time, and nutritional deficiency is not a problem for the nutrient-replete patient.

DIETS THAT RESTRICT OR SUPPLEMENT INDIVIDUAL COMPONENTS
Low-available-carbohydrate Diet
Principles
When gastric emptying is rapid or when food enters the small intestine at an unregulated rate, the presence of small-molecular-weight foodstuffs is to be avoided. Because it is permeable in both directions, the upper small bowel rapidly corrects hypertonic or hypotonic luminal contents to isotonicity. Most meals are hypertonic, so a net loss of fluid into the lumen of the intestine leads to a decreased plasma volume and distention of the upper intestine. The decrease in plasma volume and corresponding increase in intestinal distention accounts for many of the symptoms associated with the dumping syndrome.

Small-molecular-weight soluble substances exert a greater osmotic pressure than do macromolecules. The low-molecular-weight dietary components present in high concentrations are monosaccharides and disaccharides (e.g., dextrose, lactose, sucrose). Free amino acids or dipeptides are rarely encountered in the stomach. Therefore, a diet designed to decrease the osmolarity of ingested food is one low in the type of carbohydrate that is readily available for absorption. Of course, starch can be digested rapidly to maltose and glucose, and so starch also contributes to luminal osmolarity. Because milk sugar is a disaccharide, a low-available-carbohydrate diet is also a low-lactose diet. However, within a given range of osmolarity for liquid solutions such as oral rehydration solutions, it is the carbohydrate content rather than the osmolarity that determines the rate of gastric emptying (110). In people with normal stomachs, high-carbohydrate content decreases gastric emptying, but when the stomach delivers food more rapidly after gastric resection, the mechanism by which carbohydrate regulates gastric emptying is lost, and increased carbohydrate is delivered to the duodenum where it generates increased osmotic pressure.

Different starchy foods are digested at different rates. Moreover, simple sugars vary in their effect on blood glucose levels. Glucose produces a greater effect than sucrose or fructose. Some starches produce a greater effect on blood glucose than do some simple sugars. Factors that affect starch digestibility include particle size, nature of the starch, processing of the starch, presence and type of fiber, and starch–protein–fat interactions (111,112). Because of the difficulty in predicting the effects of starchy or sugar-containing foods on blood glucose levels, the glycemic index (GI) was developed. The GI is defined as follows:

$$[\text{Area under the 2-h glucose curve for food} \div \text{area under the 2-h glucose curve for an equivalent weight of reference sugar}] \times 100$$

The original reference sugar was glucose, but bread baked from flour of known composition has proved a better standard. A lower mean glycemic load (GL) in the diet (GI of food times total daily carbohydrate intake) was associated with a twofold lower risk for the development of diabetes and CVD in the large Nurses' Health Study (86). Review of 11 RCTs found that a low GI or low GL decreased glycated hemoglobin, HbA1c, with no increase in hypoglycemic episodes (113). Review of 24 RCTs found that a low GI lowered serum cholesterol and LDL-C modestly, but no effect was found on HDL cholesterol and triglycerides (114).

Despite this apparent effect on some CV risk factors, a meta-analysis of 15 RCTs using low–GI diets showed only a weak effect on reducing coronary heart disease, but these studies also showed none on LDL or HDL cholesterol (115). A low-carbohydrate diet may not be enough to alter the natural history of CV disease. Follow-up of two large prospective studies involving more than 120,000 patients found that a low-carbohydrate diet, including animal fat and protein, was associated with a higher all-cause mortality, but a low-carbohydrate diet based on vegetable sources was associated with a lower all-cause and CV disease mortality rates (116). When a low-carbohydrate diet is coupled with behavioral treatment, leading to weight loss of approximately 8 kg, there are favorable changes in serum lipids at 1 year, although these improvements were no longer evident at 2 years (117). Thus, the data are not yet consistent enough for a clear recommendation. Moreover, it is not clear what role various factors play in modifying the glycemic potency of foods, and its use in routine clinical management is still controversial.

Indications

Dumping Syndrome

The low-available-carbohydrate diet is useful after vagotomy with or without a drainage procedure because many patients have vasomotor and abdominal symptoms of the dumping syndrome (postprandial nausea, vomiting, weakness, dizziness, cramping, diarrhea, flushing, palpitations) during the early postoperative period (118). The rate of gastric emptying of fluids is enhanced at this time. However, the rate eventually returns to normal and the symptoms subside. Only a few patients must maintain the full diet on a long-term basis, although a large number may remain on a somewhat restricted diet. Some of the symptoms associated with dumping occur 1 to 3 hours after a meal; these may be caused by reactive hypoglycemia (see below). The diet also diminishes such symptoms by decreasing the carbohydrate load. The anatomic configuration of patients who have undergone *gastric bypass* for obesity (not gastroplasties) is associated with the dumping syndrome because the fundus of the stomach is anastomosed to the jejunum, and such patients often must remain on a low-available-carbohydrate diet.

Reactive Hypoglycemia

This occurs rarely in the absence of gastric surgery, sufficient in degree to produce symptoms (dizziness, hunger, weakness, sweating, palpitations). However, these symptoms are nonspecific and often related to anxiety. The true incidence of reactive hypoglycemia is probably much lower than the frequency of the diagnosis suggests. The definitive diagnosis requires the production of typical symptoms during a 5-hour glucose tolerance test, accompanied by a low plasma glucose level (<50 mg per dL). When reactive hypoglycemia is present, the low-carbohydrate diet is helpful.

SBS Without a Colon

Although it is not widely accepted that an increased intake of fat may be indicated therapeutically, a few reports suggest the possible usefulness of such a maneuver. The rationale is that fat delays gastric emptying and prolongs small-bowel transit time via a humorally mediated mechanism termed the ileal brake (119). A high-fat diet has been used in some cases of SBS (120). The rationale is that in a person with a short bowel and no colon, the importance of unabsorbed fatty acid derivatives as colonic secretagogues is limited. Thus, water secretion is regulated by the osmolarity of the diet, which is lower with a low intake of complex carbohydrate and a high intake of fat. Gastric emptying may also be delayed by a high-fat meal, preventing too rapid presentation of calories to the remaining small intestine, but the same effect probably occurs with high-complex-carbohydrate diets (121).

Sucrase–Isomaltase Deficiency

Congenital sucrase–isomaltase deficiency is a rare autosomal recessive disorder, but the incidence of heterozygotes in the United States of America is estimated to be as high as 8.9% (122). For infants with sucrase–isomaltase deficiency, glucose or fructose may be added to formulas that contain no carbohydrate (see Chapter 10). Sucrose is added to many commercial baby foods, especially puréed fruits. Labels should be read carefully. Older children with this disorder become more tolerant to sucrose, and the diet is less necessary. An unsupplemented low-sucrose diet may be limited in ascorbic acid and folic acid, and perhaps also iron, thiamine, and niacin. An FDA-approved oral solution is available containing sucrase from *Saccharomyces cerevisiae* (baker's yeast), marketed as Sucraid (sacrosidase) (www.sucraid.net). The usual dose is 1 to 2 mL per meal. About three-fourths of treated patients can be reasonably asymptomatic while ingesting sucrose. The most common side effects are abdominal pain, vomiting, and allergic reactions.

Low-Carbohydrate Diet for Obesity and CVD

The basis for the low-carbohydrate diet for metabolic disorders remains unproven. It is clear that weight loss can occur, but the effect is not long-lasting (123), and it could be due to a decrease in food intake, secondary to limited food choices that achieves portion control in a manner that is not specific to meal content. In fact, a review of low-carbohydrate diets found that it is the duration of diet and restriction of energy intake, not restriction of carbohydrates, that leads to weight loss (124). With current information, a low-carbohydrate diet itself cannot be recommended to decrease weight long term or to decrease the risk of metabolic disorders.

Low-Carbohydrate Diet Postoperatively Following Bariatric Surgery That Includes Gastric Bypass

When a gastric bypass is created, food from the small fundic pouch moves directly into the jejunum, creating an anatomical situation that produces dumping syndrome. The diet is restricted in volume, but also avoids concentrated sugars and alcohol (125). Patients should eat and drink slowly, take small bites, and chew well to avoid distending the gastric pouch or producing staple dehiscence.

Functional Gastrointestinal Disorders and Low–FODMAP Diet

In the early 2000s, an elimination diet (FODMAP) was introduced to reduce symptoms in patients with functional gastrointestinal disorders (FGIDs), but has achieved its widest use in IBS. FODMAP is an acronym for fermentable oligosaccharides, disaccharides, monosaccharides, and polyols. These diet components are either osmotically active themselves or ferment rapidly in the colon and/or small bowel to become osmotically active. The theory is that by producing more intraluminal volume and altering intestinal microflora, these food components lead to GI symptoms (126). Indeed, such food components have been shown to increase stool volume and gas production. Evidence that diets restricted in FODMAP components improve symptoms in patients with FGIDs, however, is more controversial. Several studies show that 75% of FGID (127) or IBS (128) patients show improvement in bloating, abdominal pain, or gas. However, these results have been achieved in patients who complain of those symptoms and who tend to be ingesting FODMAP–containing foods. Thus, the diet may be most useful in patients who are exaggerating the symptoms from their underlying disorder because of ingestion of foods that induce luminal gas and fluid production. The best way to establish the validity of eliminating such foods is by a double-blind placebo-controlled food challenge, but this is not practical in practice (129). The best approach is to provide individual guidance regarding FODMAP–rich foods, often with the assistance of a trained dietitian (126,129,130). The long-term implications of such a diet are unclear in that the FODMAP elimination diet removes many fruits and vegetables felt to be otherwise foods that might prevent some chronic diseases, and reduces luminal Bifidobacteria, a so-called "good" bacterial genus (131). This uncertainty about microbial composition, along with uncertainty about efficacy, has led to caution about advocating this diet for all patients with FGID (132). One should instead ascertain whether foods likely to be rich in FODMAPs are being ingested and contributing to symptoms, prior to restricting them on a trial basis.

Fructose Intolerance

Fructose absorption is more limited than that of glucose, but is quite variable, ranging from 5 to 50 g in absorption studies with fructose administration alone (133). This is because the intestinal transport of fructose is mediated by the facilitative transporters GLUT5 and GLUT2 (134). GLUT7 is another facilitative hexose transporter that accepts fructose as a substrate (135). However, fructose malabsorption can be modulated by glucose, possibly by increasing solvent drag. Most dietary forms of fructose (sucrose, honey) contain fructose and glucose in a 1:1 ratio, thus limiting the clinical effect of fructose malabsorption (133). HFCS may contain more fructose relative to glucose, but many preparations of HFCS contain high-molecular-weight glucose polymers that provide variable available glucose. Fruits such as apples, pears, and watermelon contain more fructose than glucose, but the ratio in vegetables is close to 1:0. Thus, it is difficult to interpret the correlation of hydrogen breath tests (suggesting malabsorption) with symptoms, as this must be tested using usual dietary intake with glucose. Whether patients do demonstrate true fructose intolerance must be decided on an individual basis. The most common setting appears to occur in patients who ingest large volumes of beverages containing HFCS. In such cases, what is needed is restriction of HFCS ingestion, not a fructose-restricted diet.

There is a large literature suggesting that excessive fructose ingestion is a risk factor for metabolic diseases, including fatty liver (136). However, it is unclear whether the effect, if real, is due to fructose or to HFCS, or whether the metabolic changes simply reflect differences in caloric intake (137). The available evidence suggests that fructose in its natural form is not associated with adverse effects, but that fructose in the form of HFCS may overwhelm the ability of tissues to handle large amounts of fructose. Excessive intake of refined sugar may explain, in part, the high incidence of metabolic disease, but rapidly absorbed sources of sugar (present either free or as part of high GI starch) also contribute to cardiometabolic disease (138). It also seems unlikely that replacing fructose with glucose will suffice to reverse the metabolic changes seen with HFCS, as increased calories and high GI can produce similar results (138).

Practical Aspects

1. **Timing.** Food should be taken as six dry meals per day. Because liquids leave the stomach faster than solids, it is better to allow solid foods, with a potentially high osmotic load, to liquefy slowly and be diluted with endogenous secretions. Liquids should be taken 30 to 45 minutes after solids and limited to 1 cup per meal.
2. Milk in all forms, including ice cream and other frozen desserts, should be avoided. Even lactose substitutes contain high concentrations of monosaccharides, disaccharides, or both. Only calorie-free beverages should be consumed.
3. Sugar, sweets, candy, syrup, chocolate, and gravies should be avoided.
4. The stomach should not be overloaded.
5. Foods likely to be high in sugars have the following listed as the first or second ingredient: brown or invert or table sugar, corn sweetener, corn syrup, dextrose, fructose, fruit juice concentrate, glucose, HFCS, honey, lactose, maltose, malt syrup, molasses, sucrose, or syrup.

6. Patient education materials on a diet for dumping syndrome are also available on the Internet from the University of Pittsburgh Medical Center (http://www.upmc.com/patients-visitors;education/nutrition/pages/dumping-syndrome-diet.aspx) and from the University of Virginia (http://www.medicine.virginia.edu/clinical/departments/medicine/division/digestive-health/nutrition-support-team/patient-education/postgastrectomy%20-%20dumping?2011-2010.pdf).
7. **Osmolarity of foods.** Simple sugars and low-molecular-weight carbohydrates, in addition to electrolytes and amino acids, all contribute to the osmolarity of food, either as a preformed liquid or after liquefaction in the intestinal lumen. Dietary fats are relatively water-insoluble and do not increase osmolarity significantly.

    One major aim of a low-available-carbohydrate diet is to reduce the osmolarity of ingested foods. This diet eliminates foods with a sugar content likely to increase the osmolarity of the gastric contents. The osmolarity of the gastric contents is usually hypertonic after a meal, but iso-osmolar liquids are emptied most efficiently by the stomach. A diet low in available carbohydrate is used to lower the gastric and intestinal osmolarity as much as possible.

    In acute disorders such as gastroenteritis, in which gastric emptying is impaired, or in chronic disorders such as diabetic gastroparesis, the use of iso-osmolar foods is helpful. Unfortunately, such a diet may be low in calories because it is the calorie-containing components of food that contribute most to osmolarity. Moreover, fat decreases the rate of gastric emptying, so low-fat liquids are needed for rapid gastric emptying. During acute illnesses, however, iso-osmolar low-calorie liquids can be used for short periods alone.

    Nearly all liquid or semisolid foods are hyperosmolar (1) (Table 12-15). When nausea or vomiting is among the symptoms to be treated, the use of these fluids should be modified so that appropriate dilutions decrease the osmolarity to about 280 to 300 mOsmol per L.
8. Foods allowed include those containing protein, fat, or complex polysaccharides.

    Foods containing simple sugars should be avoided. Table 12-16 lists the fructose, glucose, sucrose, and starch contents of many foods. In this table, foods are ranked in decreasing order of simple sugar content—that is, monosaccharides and disaccharides. Foods high in simple sugars should be avoided or taken in small amounts. Fructose in excess of glucose is the main determinant of fructose malabsorption and diarrhea. This excess is seen especially in honey, apples, and pears. However, the largest source of dietary fructose is as a sweetener in dietetic foods and soft drinks and in corn syrups (~50% fructose) (139). The mean daily intake of free fructose in the United States is 20 g. Sorbitol is ingested in fruits along with fructose, and as a sweetener in candy, mints, "sugarless" chewing gum, and dietetic foods. As much as 2 g of sorbitol can be contained in one stick of gum. The decreased carbohydrate absorption of fruit juices in young children is related to the sorbitol content of the juice (140). The lactose contents of milk products are listed in Table 12-17, and these should also be limited. In congenital sucrase–isomaltase deficiency, a rare disorder, only foods containing little sucrose can be ingested. As seen in Table 12-16, this diet eliminates many fruits and vegetables and most sweets.

TABLE 12-15 Osmolarity of Commonly Used Beverages

Food	mOsmol/L	Food	mOsmol/L
Gatorade	330	Eggnog	695
Ginger ale	510	Apple juice	683
Gelatin dessert	735	Orange juice	614
Tomato juice	595	Malted milk	940
7-Up	640	Ice cream	1,150
Coca-Cola	680	Grape juice	863
Sherbet	1,225		

TABLE 12-16 Carbohydrate Content of Selected Foods

Food	Fructose[a]	Excess Free Fructose[b]	Glucose	Reducing Sorbitol	Sugars[c]	Maltose	Sucrose	Starch	Total Simple Sugars[d] (g/100-g portion)
			(g/100-g edible portion)						
Fruits									
Figs, dried	30.9	—	40	—	—	—	0.1	—	73
Dates, dried	—	—	—	—	16.2	—	45.4	—	61.6
Banana, ripe	2–4	0	4.5	—	—	—	11.9	—	19.9
Grapes, white	8.0	0	8.1	0.2	—	—	0.2	—	16.1
Cherries	5–7	0	4.7	1.4–2.1	12.5	—	0.1	—	12.6
Apple juice	6–8	2–7	1–4	0.3–1.0	8.0	—	4.2	—	12.2
Plums, sweet	1–4	0	4.5	0.3–2.8	7.4	—	4.4	—	11.8
Apple	6–8	2–7	1.7	0.2–1.0	8.3	—	3.1	0.6	11.4
Banana, green	—	—	—	—	5.0	—	5.1	—	10.1
Peaches	1.6	—	1.5	—	3.1	—	6.6	—	9.7
Orange	2.7	0	2.5	—	5.0	—	4.6	—	9.6
Pears	5–9	3–8	2.5	1.2–3.5	8.0	—	1.5	—	9.5
Watermelon	—	—	—	—	3.0	—	4.9	—	7.9
Apricots	0.4	—	1.9	—	—	—	5.5	—	7.8
Orange juice, frozen	2–6	0	—	—	4.6	—	3.2	—	7.8
Melon, cantaloupe	0.9	—	1.2	—	2.3	—	4.4	—	6.7
Strawberries	2.3	0	2.6	—	—	—	1.4	—	6.3
Grapefruit	1.2	0	2.0	—	—	—	2.9	—	6.1
Prunes	15	0	30	9.4–18.8	—	—	—	—	
Vegetables									
Beets, sugar	—	—	—	—	—	—	12.9	—	12.9
Onions	1	0	2	—	—	—	0.1	—	8.3
Carrots, raw	1	0	1	—	—	—	1.2	—	7.9
Peas, green	<0.1	0	<0.1	—	5.8	—	5.5	4.1	5.5
Potatoes, sweet	0.3	—	0.4	—	0.8	1.6	4.1	16.5	4.9
Cauliflower	—	—	2.8	—	—	—	0.3	—	3.1
Beans, green	1–1.5	0–1	0.5–1	—	1.7	—	0.5	2.0	2.2
Potatoes, white	0.1	—	0.1	—	0.8	—	0.1	17.0	0.9

514

Food							
Squash, summer	0.2	—	—	—	—	0.1	0.7
Cucumber	—	—	—	—	—	0.5	0.6
Dry legumes							
Beans, soy	—	—	1.6	—	—	7.2	1.9	8.8
Lentils	—	—	—	—	—	2.1	28.5	2.1
Beans, navy	—	—	—	—	—	—	35.2	—
Nuts							
Peanuts	—	—	0.2	—	—	4.3	4.0	4.5
Almonds	—	—	0.2	—	—	2.3	—	2.5
Peanut butter	—	—	0.9	—	—	—	5.9	0.9
Cereals							
Wheat flour	—	—	2.0	—	—	0.2	34.7	2.2
Rice, polished	—	—	—	—	—	0.4	72.9	0.4
Oats	—	—	—	—	—	—	56.4	—
Sweets							
Honey	40.5	7	34.2	—	—	—	1.9	88.6
Maple syrup	—	—	—	—	—	62.9	—	64.4
Molasses	6.8	—	6.8	26.9	—	36.9	—	63.8
Jellies	—	—	—	—	—	40–65	40–65	40–65
Chocolate, sweet, dry	—	—	—	—	—	56.4	56.4	56.4
Corn syrup	21.2	—	—	26.4	—	34.7	47.6

[a] Adapted from Rumessen JJ. Fructose and related food carbohydrates. Source, intake, absorption, and clinical implications. *Scand J Gastroenterol.* 1992;27:819. Mainly monosaccharides plus maltose and lactose.

[b] Free fructose as monosaccharides in excess of free glucose.

[c] Adapted from Hardinger MG, Swarner JB, Crooks H. Carbohydrates in food. *J Am Diet Assoc.* 1965;46:197.

[d] Total "simple" sugars equals reducing sugars plus sucrose; where total reducing sugar content is not available, the sum of the published figures for fructose, glucose, and/or maltose has been substituted.

Foods are listed with groups according to their monosaccharide and disaccharide content per 100-g edible portion. Thus, the total sugar added to the diet must take into account the size of the portion. See also *Sugar content of selected foods*, Report No. 48. Human Nutrition Information Service, U.S. Department of Agriculture.

TABLE 12-17 Lactose Content of Selected Milk Products

Product	Lactose Content (g/unit)
Whole milk (1 cup)	11
2% Milk (1 cup)	9–13
Skim milk (1 cup)	11–14
Chocolate milk (1 cup)	10–12
Sweetened condensed milk (1 cup)	35
Reconstituted dry whole milk (1 cup)	48
Buttermilk (1 cup)	9–11
Light cream (1 tbsp)	0.6
Half and half (1 tbsp)	0.6
Whipped cream topping (1 tbsp)	0.4
Low-fat yogurt (1 cup)	11–15
Cheeses	
Hard (Parmesan, blue, Gouda) (1 oz)	0.6–0.8
Semihard (American, Cheddar) (1 oz)	0.4–0.6
Soft (Camembert, Limburger) (1 oz)	0.1–0.2
Spread (added cream) (1 oz)	0.8–1.7
Cottage	
Regular (1 cup)	5–6
Low-fat (1 cup)	7–8
Ice creams	
Regular (1 cup)	9
Sherbet (1 cup)	4
Ice milk (1 cup)	10
Sorbets, ices (1 cup)	0
Butter (1 tbsp)	0.15
Oleomargarine	0

Data from Welsh JD. Diet therapy in adult lactose malabsorption: present practices. *Am J Clin Nutr.* 1978;31:592.

Most beverages contain available sugars and should be limited. These include beer, sodas, and iced tea or lemonade made with sugar. Canned fruits often contain extra sugar in the packing fluid; if these are used, the fluid should be drained away before the fruits are eaten.

9. **Fructose** has been singled out as an important component of available carbohydrate in the diet. Average consumption of fructose in the United States is approximately 30 g per year, half from sucrose and half from HFCS. Fructose enters the glycolytic pathway at the level of triose phosphates, thus bypassing the major control point at which glucose enters, that is, phosphofructokinase. Fructose can serve, therefore, as an unregulated source of acetyl CoA for hepatic lipogenesis. Fructose has been shown in short-term studies to increase energy intake and body weight, to decrease insulin sensitivity, and to increase postprandial plasma triglyceride levels (141). A low-carbohydrate diet should also be low in fructose.

10. **FODMAP elimination diet.** The major problem with the suggested FODMAP elimination diet is that there has been no standardization in foods or amounts allowed. Foods with high FODMAP content include those rich in oligosaccharides (e.g., artichokes, asparagus, broccoli, cabbage, onions, peas, wheat, watermelon), lactose (e.g., dairy products), fructose (e.g., apples, pears, peaches, honey, HFCS), and polyols, primarily sorbitol (e.g., cherries, plums, prunes, grapes, avocado, mushrooms, cauliflower) (90). Complex carbohydrates such as fructans are found in most wheat products. Acceptable foods include most vegetables and some fruits (e.g., banana, berries, citrus fruits), along with meat and fish. Many sites offer suggestions for a low–FODMAP diet; these diets also limit many high-fiber foods. Suggested sites include http://stanfordhospital.org/digestivehealth/

nutrition/DH-Low-FODMAP-Diet-Handout.pdf, and http://shepherdworks.com.au/disease-information/low-fodmap-diet.

11. Sweeteners. Sweeteners are often grouped as nutritive and nonnutritive. Nutritive sweeteners include mono- and disaccharides (4 kcal per g) and sugar alcohols or polyols (2 kcal per g). The former include glucose, fructose, galactose, sucrose, maltose, corn-based sweeteners (including HFCS), and agave nectar (containing fructans and oligosaccharides). These are reviewed in the position paper of the Academy of Nutrition and Dietetics on the Use of Nutritive and Nonnutritive Sweeteners (http://download.journals.elsevierhealth.com/pdfs/journals/2212-2672/PIIS2212267212003255.pdf). Polyols have been used to decrease the intake of carbohydrates that elevated blood glucose levels. These are used alone or more often in combination, and include the monosaccharides sorbitol, mannitol, xylitol, erythritol, and D-tagatose, and the disaccharide polyols isomalt, lactitol, maltitol, isomaltulose, and trehalose.

The US FDA has approved five nonnutritive sugar substitutes—*saccharin, aspartame, neotame, acesulfame-K*, and *sucralose*. Other sweeteners are under review (http://vm.cfsan.fda.gov/~dms/fdsugar.html). The American Dietetic Association Position Paper on Sweeteners concludes that these substances can be safely ingested as part of a diet, if general guidelines for individual health goals are followed, as exemplified in the DRIs (142).

Saccharin (*Sweet and Low, Sweet Twin*). Despite the concerns about saccharine as a carcinogen, it remains on the market; it is 300 times sweeter than sugar and has been used safely for decades, and the dose required to see tumors in laboratory animals is huge. Moreover, the physiology in the male rat bladder (high pH, calcium phosphate, and protein concentration) was considered sufficiently different from the human situation that the warning label concerning a health hazard was removed in 2000.

Aspartame (*NutraSweet, Equal*) is a dipeptide (phenylalanine–aspartic acid) that is 180 times sweeter than sugar. The FDA has reviewed more than 100 toxicologic and clinical studies that attest to its safety, although claims continue to arise regarding its possible role in causing various diseases. The very small number of patients who have phenylketonuria should not use this compound, but otherwise, it appears to be safe. Urticaria has been reported with aspartame and confirmed by rechallenge (143). It is postulated that the product of degradation may form amide bonds with proteins and act as an antigen. Based on animal toxicology, there has been a concern about carcinogenicity for aspartame, as with other artificial sweeteners, but the epidemiological data have not supported such a conclusion (144).

Aspartame is one of only a few food additives for which there are any substantial human trial data for safety. However, setting acceptable dietary intakes (ADIs) for food additives is a daunting job. The amounts of any one additive ingested are small, exposure may occur over a lifetime, synergism in toxic effects is not known between the hundreds of additives permitted, and postmarketing adverse reaction reporting is difficult because of the presence of additives like aspartame in many foods. Thus, most data on toxic effects of additives come from animals (mostly rodent). The statement that approved additives have been "proven to be safe" is superficially correct based on the available data, but the statement needs to be accepted with some qualification.

Neotame is a derivative of aspartame, with a 3,3-dimethylbutyl moiety attached to the aspartic acid residue. This addition blocks peptidase activity, thus prolonging stability of the sweetener. Neotame is 7,000 to 13,000 times sweeter than sucrose, and is added to many commercial products. However, it does not have to be listed as a separate ingredient, so its use is difficult to track. Like aspartame, it is degraded into potentially toxic substances (formaldehyde, formic acid, diketopiperazine), but evidence for human toxicity is not currently available.

Acesulfame potassium (*Sunett, Sweet and Safe, Sweet One*) is approved for use in baked goods, frozen desserts, candies, and beverages. It is 200 times sweeter than sugar and is often combined with other sweeteners. It is not degraded when cooked or baked. No evidence of toxicity has been reported.

Sucralose (*Splenda*) is 600 times sweeter than sugar and is approved for use as a table sweetener and in baked goods, nonalcoholic beverages, chewing gum, frozen dairy desserts, fruit juices, and gelatins. It is now approved as a general-purpose sweetener for all foods. It tastes like sugar because it is made from sucrose, but it cannot be digested. It is considered safe to use. Animal data suggest that nonnutritive sweeteners might modify postprandial hormonal responses, perhaps via action on "taste" receptors in the proximal intestine, but such changes have not been consistently reported in healthy humans (145). One report shows that sucralose increases plasma glucose and insulin levels after a glucose load in obese subjects (146). Thus, a role for sweeteners beyond simple taste is still possible.

Stevia rebaudiana (**Bertoni**) *(Truvia, PureVia, Sweet Leaf, Sun Crystals)* is a sweet herb native to South America. The sweetness is derived from glycosides, including rebaudioside A and C (147). In the United States of America, these glycosides are considered GRAS (generally recognized as safe). In 2008, the FDA issued a "no objection" letter in response to a request to include these glycosides as sweeteners in a variety of drinks, and as a tabletop sweetener. In contrast to the purified glycosides, whole-leaf *Stevia* or crude extracts of the plant cannot be used in foods as it has not been approved as a food additive. The European Food and Safety Authority has determined an acceptable daily intake of 4 mg per kg for the purified glycosides (147). Stevia is now a major tabletop sweetener and component of juices, dairy products, and bakery items.

Swingle (*S. prosverorii*) *(PureLo)* is a Chinese vine producing a sweet-tasting fruit (lo han kuo in Chinese, also called monk fruit). The sweetness is related to a group of aglycones. A clarified concentrate of the fruit received a "no question" letter from the FDA in 2010 in response to a request for GRAS status. The fruit extracts are found in soft drinks, nutritional and energy shakes, cereals, and granola products.

12. **Sugar alcohols** are not technically considered artificial sweeteners, but they do not promote tooth decay or raise blood sugar, as sugar does. They include sorbitol, xylitol, lactitol, mannitol, and maltitol. Sugar alcohols are used to sweeten "sugar-free" candies, cookies, and chewing gums. Fructose is also often added to foods because, like sugar alcohols, it is less sweet than dextrose. However, these sugars are absorbed less efficiently, and ingestion of more than 10 g (0.14 g per kg body weight) can produce diarrhea, gas, bloating, and cramps. Fructose is a major ingredient of soft drinks (about 40 g in a 16-oz cola). Sorbitol is added to diet gums (up to 2 g per stick) and processed apple juice (up to 0.7 g per 3 oz). Labels should be read carefully for the content of these sweeteners if symptoms occur regularly after ingestion of sweetened processed foods.

13. **The glycemic index (GI)** has been recommended as an alternative way to classify carbohydrate-containing food. The GI ranks sources of carbohydrate according to their ability to raise blood glucose. The area under the curve for blood glucose is calculated as a percent of the curve for glucose. Foods with a score of 70 are classified as having a high GI, those with a score of 50 or less as low, and those in between as medium. If this were practical, it would have a major effect on the development of a low-carbohydrate diet for any individual. Most grains and potatoes are rapidly hydrolyzed and have a high GI, but nonstarchy vegetables, fruits, legumes, and nuts have a low GI. GL has been defined as the arithmetic product of GI and carbohydrate content. Extensive articles and diet books have been published on this topic, and extensive lists of GI and GL values of common foods have been published (111). In general, the factors that affect the glycemic response include the amount of carbohydrate, the nature of the starch (amylase, amylopectin, resistant starch) or monosaccharide components (glucose, fructose, galactose), the food processing (particle size, chemical modification, resistant starch content), and other factors such as dietary fiber content (89). Examples of GI and GL include baked potato (GI 85, GL 20.3 g for 110-g serving), white bread (GI 70, GL 21 g for two slices), spaghetti (GI 41, GL 11.8 g for 110-g serving), lentil beans (GI 29, GL 5.7 g for 110 mL cooked serving), and skim milk (GI 32, GL 4.2 for 225 mL) (148).

Despite much controversy, the effects of low–GI diets on weight loss, insulin resistance, and risks of CVD are small (115,148). Moreover, the diets are complicated, and low energy diets probably accomplish as much. A major problem is that of consistency, and the experts disagree about the importance of the variability noted (www.asbmb.org/asbmbtoday/asbmbtoday_article.aspx?id=49410). The concept of GI fits with the food pyramid and healthy diet recommendations for the United States, but whether a low–GI diet has a role in improving insulin sensitivity or hyperlipidemia is not known. The clinical usefulness of GI and GL is still controversial, but has not yet been accepted as a standard recommendation for dietary management in the prevention of chronic disease. The US DGA, 2010, states that "Strong and consistent evidence shows that glycemic index and/or glycemic load are not associated with body weight and do not lead to greater weight loss or better weight maintenance. Abundant, strong epidemiological evidence demonstrates that there is no association between glycemic index or load and cancer. A moderate body of inconsistent evidence supports a relationship between glycemic load and type 2 diabetes. Strong, convincing evidence shows little association between glycemic load and type 2 diabetes. Due to limited evidence, no conclusion can be drawn to assess the relationship between either glycemic index or load and cardiovascular disease." (http://1.usa.gov/1gnFLVa).

Side Effects
A low-lactose diet may be low in calcium. If the diet is severely limited in fruits and vegetables, vitamin supplements, especially ascorbic acid and folic acid, may be necessary. Such severe restriction is only rarely, if ever, indicated with this diet. Because the diet is high in protein and fat, care should be taken to avoid increasing serum lipid levels in susceptible persons.

Supplement Required
If the diet is used on a long-term basis, 0.5 to 1.0 g of elemental calcium should be given daily.

Low-Lactose Diet

Principles
Most Caucasians are lactose-tolerant, but the other peoples of the world are largely lactose-intolerant. To avoid symptoms of flatulence, bloating, cramps, and diarrhea, a low-lactose diet is indicated. However, most people who have low levels of lactase are not lactose-intolerant (149). African Americans, a population thought to often be symptomatic from lactose intolerance, can usually tolerate ingesting 1 cup of milk without developing symptoms, even though they can be shown by specific testing to maldigest lactose (150). This situation arises because of differences in rates of gastric emptying and intestinal transit, composition of ingested food, capture of lactose fermentation products by colonic absorption, and perhaps individual tolerance. However, there are patient populations who develop lactose intolerance fairly consistently, including patients with active celiac sprue, those with SBS, and following acute gastroenteritis. The diagnosis is usually made either by a trial of lactose elimination or by administering a hydrogen breath test after lactose ingestion (151).

Lactose is commonly used as a sweetening agent in prepared foods because it is inexpensive to prepare and its taste is not excessively sweet. Thus, it is difficult to devise a diet completely free of lactose. In most cases, complete elimination of lactose is unnecessary because symptoms, when they occur, are dose-related. Each person has a threshold dose below which few symptoms occur.

Lactose, or milk sugar, is contained in human, cow, and goat's milk and in milk products. The whey contains all the lactose; any lactose in the curds represents contamination by whey. Whey is now added to more foods than before because large amounts of whey are available as a by-product of cheese production. Milk is a remarkable food that contains more than lactose. Many nutrients are lost from the diet when lactose is restricted; however, except for calcium, most of them are readily provided by the rest of a balanced diet.

Indications
Patients with symptoms of *lactose intolerance* are candidates for the diet. Because only 50% of lactose-intolerant persons have a history of intolerance, a useful first step is to place the patient suspected of being lactose-intolerant on a low-lactose diet for 3 to 4 days. If the response is uncertain, challenge tests can help to diagnose lactose intolerance.

A positive lactose-tolerance test result is defined as a rise in blood sugar of less than 20 mg per dL after a lactose load of 50 g per m^2 in children or 50 g in adults. The hydrogen breath test is a better means of diagnosis. It is more sensitive than the oral lactose-tolerance test and can detect malabsorption of as little as 2 g of lactose. Thus, a lower test dose (12.5 g) can be used, an amount equal to the lactose content of one glass of milk. A rise of less than 20 ppm is consistent with lactose intolerance. More recent criteria suggest a 6 ppm rise at 6 hours after the carbohydrate load, or more than 15 ppm over a 2-hour period from 5 to 7 hours after ingestion of carbohydrate (152). Certain pitfalls are encountered in interpreting the results of a hydrogen breath test. A small percentage of normal persons do not produce hydrogen gas, oral antibiotics can suppress hydrogen-producing bacteria, and smoking causes an increase in breath hydrogen concentration that is unrelated to carbohydrate intake.

The low-lactose diet is also appropriate for *patients requiring a low-available-carbohydrate diet* after gastric surgery or during the course of an intestinal disorder. A low-lactose diet is used during the acute phase of *diarrheal illnesses*, when intestinal transit is rapid and transient lactase deficiency can develop. These illnesses include acute gastroenteritis, UC, and Crohn disease. However, it is not necessary to restrict lactose from the diet in all such cases. In *sprue*, the enzyme lactase is decreased before treatment, and a low-lactose diet is helpful in the initial phase of therapy until the normal enzyme level is restored. However, restoration to normal levels may take many months.

Galactosemia is the only indication for very severe restriction of lactose. Virtually, all dietary galactose is derived from lactose, and in galactosemia, small amounts of galactose cause symptoms. Thus, adherence to the diet must be complete.

Supplemental milk is offered in schools in the United States, even when the racial mixture includes a large proportion of children who would be expected to have lactase deficiency. Tolerance to a small amount of milk, such as part or even all of the cup offered with school lunches, is quite good, and the Committee on Nutrition of the American Academy of Pediatrics supports the use of milk as a good food supplement even in areas of the world where the incidence of lactose intolerance is high (153).

Practical Aspects

Management of lactose intolerance need not include a generalized low-lactose diet, as many patients can tolerate small amounts of lactose (~4 g), such as contained in aged cheese or milk chocolate. When small amounts are ingested along with other foods or ingredients, the rate of gastric emptying is decreased and symptoms are less likely to occur. This is the rationale for the use of chocolate milk in small amounts.

1. **Milk and liquid milk products** should be avoided or used sparingly. Milk or cream should not be used in cooking. Small amounts of cheese and butter may be tolerated. Table 12-17 lists the major dietary sources of lactose in milk products.
2. **Labels** should be read carefully. Products containing milk, milk products, milk solids, whey, curd, casein, lactose, galactose, skim milk powder, skim milk solids, or milk sugar contain lactose. Foods that may contain "hidden" lactose include "nondairy" creamers, powdered sweeteners, breads and cakes, creamed soups, pancakes and waffles, puddings and custards, and candies. Many patients can tolerate small doses of lactose and need not be so cautious about restricting their intake of prepared foods containing small amounts of lactose. Often, however, the amount of lactose is not stated on the label. Practical information can be obtained from many Internet sites, listed on the No Milk page (www.panix.com/~nomilk) along with sites for milk allergy and casein intolerance.
3. **Commercially available fermented milk products** (buttermilk, yogurt) are sometimes sweetened by adding cream or milk and are not necessarily low in lactose. The lactose content of homemade yogurt and Greek-style yogurt will be lower, but some lactose will remain. Nearly complete fermentation produces an inedible product. Yogurt is better tolerated by lactose-intolerant persons because the fermentation of lactose continues in the intestinal lumen (154). However, tolerance must be individualized. Frozen yogurt does not contain active bacterial cultures and is less well tolerated than fresh yogurt.
4. The average lactose-intolerant patient becomes symptomatic after ingesting 12 g of lactose, the approximate content of an 8-oz glass of milk. More lactose may be tolerated when it is ingested with other foods that delay gastric emptying. Some patients become symptomatic

after ingesting as little as 3 g of lactose (155). These people must take great care to avoid foods that contain even small amounts of lactose. Patients with both lactase deficiency and IBS are often extremely sensitive to small amounts of lactose.

5. **Prepared foods** that contain lactose. Not all samples of the foods listed below contain lactose, but the labels of such food groups should be read with care.

    Foods with large amounts of lactose: cakes and sweet rolls, caramels, fudge, coated candies, cheese spreads, infant formulas, party dips, powdered soft drinks, puddings, sour cream, white sauces.

    Foods with small amounts of lactose (1 g per 100 g): canned or frozen fruits and vegetables, cookies and cookie sandwich fillings, cordials and liqueurs, dietetic and diabetic preparations, dried soups, French fries, corn cereals, instant coffee, instant potatoes, meat products prepared with fillings (e.g., frankfurters), pie crusts and fillings, salad dressings, liquid antibiotics, vitamin and mineral mixtures.

    Lactose-free foods: plain meat, fish, poultry, peanut butter, broth-based soups, cereals, fruits, vegetables (plain), tofu and tofu products, breads and desserts made without any milk products.

6. **Hospital diets** provide lactose-containing foods with most meals. Lactose-intolerant patients may become symptomatic in the hospital, especially if they are given a modified-consistency diet with many milk products but little selection. Many commercially available protein and calorie supplements are now lactose-free (see Chapter 10).

7. **Medications used for gastrointestinal conditions.** Many medications used to treat GI conditions can contain lactose (most in the range of 40 to 100 mg per tablet), in sufficient quantities to complicate symptoms in a sensitive individual (156). Such medications include loperamide, domperidone, metoclopramide, lactulose, Budenofalk, Asacol, Imuran, generic amitriptyline, and citalopram. A few medications contain considerable lactose. 16 mg per day of Imodium contains 1 g of lactose, 80 mg per day of domperidone contains 450 mg of lactose, 9 mg per day of budesonide as Budenofalk contains 1.8 g of lactose, and 150 mg per day of lactulose contains 10.2 g of lactose, equivalent to 216 mL of milk.

8. **Enzyme replacement.** Lactose-depleted milk can be prepared by hydrolyzing the lactose with a yeast enzyme preparation (e.g., LactAid, Dairy Ease, Lactrase). Mix five drops of LactAid liquid enzyme, which contains lactase from the yeast *Kluyveromyces lactis*, with 1 qt of milk or 12 oz of "liquid diet" or "instant breakfast" formulas at 4°C results in 70% hydrolysis of lactose in 1 day and 90% hydrolysis in 2 or 3 days. Patients with limited tolerance to lactose can use this milk, which is sweeter than regular milk but well accepted in cooking or on cereal. Dairy products other than milk cannot be treated in this way. Table 12-18 lists many of the sources of the enzyme lactase, along with milk substitutes. Lactase in tablets is not always from the same source. For example, Lactrase, derived from *Aspergillus oryzae*, is stable at both acid and alkaline pH, and this stability may be advantageous in some cases. One to three capsules are ingested with milk or food, depending on the amount of lactose ingested and on individual sensitivity. Alternatively, the capsule can be opened and sprinkled on the food or liquid containing lactose. Lactaid tablets come in three sizes—regular, extra, and ultra—containing 3,000, 4,500, and 9,000 lactase units per tablet. The corresponding recommended doses with food are three, two, and one tablet, respectively.

9. **Milk substitutes.** Chemically defined products are now available that simulate milk; corn solids are used as the carbohydrate source (Table 12-17). These products can be used as milk substitutes if the taste is acceptable, but the sugar content is 12 g per 8-oz glass and the vegetable fat content is 5%, as in whole milk. Some of these products are cholesterol-free, and some contain micronutrient supplements.

10. **Ice cream substitutes.** A wide variety of lactose-free frozen desserts are now available that provide 300 to 440 kcal per cup and contain little or no calcium. In most of the desserts, tofu is used as the base. Although they are cholesterol-free, they are high in polyunsaturated fat (10 to 26 g of fat per cup). Some widely marketed varieties are Tofutti and Tofu Lite. Frozen desserts that are both lactose-free and fat-free include fruit sorbets and ices. Low-lactose

TABLE 12-18	Selected Lactase Replacement Products and Milk Substitutes	
Lactase Products[a]	**Nondairy Creamers**	**Milk Substitutes**[b]
Lactaid	Cremora	Crowley
Lactrase	Coffee-mate	Bordens Plus
Say Yes to Dairy	Coffee Rich	Dairy Ease (70% ↓)
Prevail dairy enzyme	Hood	Lactaid (100%, 70% ↓)
Milk Digest-Aid	Taam Tov	NutriMil
Super Lactase	Cool Whip	Parmalat-Zymil
Swanson softgels	Rich Whip	Swiss Whey (70% ↓)
Dairy Relief LactoZYME		Soy milk (many)
Country Life		
Nature's Way		
Puritan's Pride Softgels		
Lacto-zyme Dairy Eze		
Solaray		
Solger		

[a] All products available as capsules or chewable tablets, and contain from 1,675–9,000 lactase/FCC units per dose. The suggested minimally effective dose is 1,500 units. List updated 2008.
[b] All products are lactose-free, except where listed. Lactaid is available as lactose-free and reduced lactose. Many supermarkets carry their own brand of lactose-free/reduced milk or lactose-free soy milk.
From: Steve Carper's Lactose Intolerance Clearing House/The Product Clearinghouse (http://www.stevecarper.com/li/The_Product_Clearinghouse.htm).

desserts can be tolerated by some patients. LactAid brand ice cream contains about 2 g of lactose per cup, compared with 9 g for regular ice cream. Frozen yogurt contains 5 g per cup but may not be tolerated because the action of the bacteria in yogurt is diminished by freezing.

11. **Lactose-free supplements** include Ensure drink and powder, Boost pudding, Slimfast powder with soy protein, and Slimfast fruit juice powder or cans with soy protein. Care must be taken to read labels, as products with similar trade names do contain lactose. These include Ensure bars (2 to 3 g per bar), Ensure pudding (5 g per 4 oz serving), Carnation Instant Breakfast (8 g per powder packet or 9 to 13 g per can), Slimfast powder (15 to 16 g per scoop with milk) or Slimfast cans (10 to 12 g per can).

Websites

National Library of Medicine/NIH http://www.nlm.nih.gov/medlineplus/lactoseintolerance.html

National Digestive Diseases Information Clearinghouse http://www.niddk.nih.gov/digest/pubs/lactose/lactose.htm

The Lactose Intolerance Nutrition Guide (American Dietetic Association) www.eatright.com/catalog/cat.php?CatNum=307x

Steve Carper's Lactose Intolerance Clearing House. http://www.stevecarper.com/li.com

Side Effects

A negative calcium balance may result if meat, nuts, and vegetables do not provide 0.8 to 1.0 g of calcium daily. Symptoms similar to those of lactose intolerance may develop when milk substitutes are used, which are also high in available carbohydrates.

Supplement Required

Calcium supplements (0.8 to 1.2 g of elemental calcium) should be given (see Chapter 7) if other sources are not ingested.

Low-fat Diet

Principles

Different Types of Fat

Fatty acids derived from triglycerides supply energy and essential fatty acids and help absorb lipid-soluble compounds, such as fat-soluble vitamins. Saturated fats are found in high-fat dairy products, fatty fresh and processed meats, skin and fat of poultry, and lard, palm, and coconut oils. They tend to raise serum cholesterol levels. Levels of *trans* fatty acids, which also tend to raise serum cholesterol, are high in partially hydrogenated vegetable oils (margarines, shortenings) and in some commercially fried foods and bakery goods. *Trans* fatty acids are not essential and have no known benefit to humans. Like saturated fatty acids (SFAs), there is a linear trend with intake and LDLs, so that it is recommended that intake be kept as low as possible. Dietary sources include dairy products, meats, and commercially prepared products (64). Unsaturated fats, which tend to keep blood cholesterol levels low, are found in vegetable oils, nuts, olives, avocados, and fatty fish. Conjugated linoleic acid occurs in foods derived from ruminants. There is a suggestion that one of its isomers may reduce body fat and enhance lean body mass (157). Nuts provide a dense source of polyunsaturated fatty acids (PUFAs) (Table 12-19).

The three types of fat (saturated, *trans*, and polyunsaturated) are equivalent calorically, all produce symptoms of malabsorption, and all must be decreased in a low-fat diet designed to reduce gastrointestinal symptoms. Dietary cholesterol, found in liver and other organ meats, egg yolks, and dairy fats, is not of concern in this diet. Diets designed to lower serum cholesterol are based on an altered ratio of intake of these fats (see Chapter 13).

Essential fatty acids (linolenic, linoleic) are found in high levels in vegetable oils (especially flaxseed, canola, and soy oils) and human milk, and dietary deficiency is rare in persons ingesting a balanced diet. Lack of linoleic acid leads to rough, scaly skin, and an increased plasma ratio of eicosatrienoic acid:arachidonic acid (triene:tetraene). The AI is 17 g per day for young men and 12 g per day for young women. α-Linolenic acid (ALA), the other essential dietary fat, has an AI of 1.6 g per day and 1.1 g per day for men and women, respectively (64). NHANES III mean data show that intake of total fat and saturated fat in the United States is 34% and 15% of total calories, respectively (158). Carnitine is a nonessential nutrient (synthesized from lysine and methionine) required for the entry of long-chain fatty acids into mitochondria. It is abundant in the diet, but some infant and other non–milk-based formulas are supplemented with carnitine. Sphingolipids occur widely in food (consumption ~0.3 to 0.4 g per day in the United States) and have some role in colon cancer prevention and lowering cholesterol in animals (159). Their role in human nutrition is not yet known.

The reduced-fat diets advocated to prevent chronic diseases stipulate a reduction in fat intake of no more than 30% (160) (see Chapter 2). These diets are not as restrictive as the low-fat diet required for patients with fat malabsorption, and the labeling terms "light" and "lite," which

TABLE 12-19 Lipid Content of Nut-Derived Oils

Nut	PUFA (%)	Fatty Acids Unsat/Sat (ratio)	Vitamin E α-Tocopherol (μg/100 g oil)	β-Tocopherol (μg/100 g oil)	Phytosterol and Sitosterol
Almonds	85	10.8	440	13	2071
Hazelnuts	87	9.9	310	61	991
Macadamia	58	5.6	122	trace	1507
Peanuts	45	5.45	88	60	1363
Walnuts	45	9.5	200	300	1130

Data from Maguire LS, O'Sullivan SM, Galvin K, et al. Fatty acid profile, tocopherol, squalene, and phytosterol content of walnuts, almonds, peanuts, hazelnuts, and the macadamia nut. *Int J Food Sci Nutr.* 2004;55:171.

mean fewer calories (see below), must be understood. However, many of the practical points relevant to a low-fat diet are also useful in a moderately reduced-fat diet. To achieve the recommended fat intake, the USDA recommends the following upper limit of fat intake at different levels of calorie consumption:

Total kcal/day	Saturated Fat (g/day)	Total Fat (g/day)
1,600	≤18	53
2,200	≤24	73
2,800	≤31	93

Indications

Patients with Malabsorption

Steatorrhea of any cause is relieved when the triglyceride intake is decreased. Fat malabsorption typically predominates in disorders in which the secretion or absorption of bile acids is limited; bile acids are needed for micelle formation and the absorption of fat, but not protein or carbohydrate. Both fat malabsorption and protein malabsorption occur in pancreatic insufficiency or diffuse small-bowel mucosal disorders. When protein malabsorption accompanies fat malabsorption, it produces few symptoms except perhaps that the putrid smell of feces is increased. Severe carbohydrate malabsorption causes some of the symptoms often associated with fat malabsorption (diarrhea, bloating, gas). The demonstration of steatorrhea or carbohydrate malabsorption by itself does not always determine which factor is most important in causing symptoms in an individual patient. Response to a trial of either a low-fat or a low-carbohydrate diet is often needed to resolve this issue in patients with "global" malabsorption.

As used for this indication, the term *fat* refers to triglycerides in food, not to other lipid components, such as cholesterol. Diarrhea is relieved by a low-fat diet because the diarrhea associated with steatorrhea is partly caused by the formation of hydroxyl fatty acids that act as secretagogues in the colon (162). If fewer fatty acids reach the colon, the diarrhea is diminished and the colonic absorption of other nutrients (especially short-chain fatty acids) improves. The low-fat diet is relatively rich in other sources of calories, especially carbohydrate, and is difficult to use when carbohydrate restriction is also desired. Low-fat diets are used to control symptoms of diarrhea, bloating, and gas—not to reverse abnormal physiology. Therefore, no single level of restriction is appropriate for all patients. A low-fat diet is also relatively low in protein because most sources of protein in a Western-type diet contain triglycerides. When malabsorption is severe and strict fat restriction is required, protein supplements must sometimes be given.

Many disorders of digestion or absorption are characterized by steatorrhea. In general, patients with disorders in which steatorrhea is significant require a low-fat diet. These include diseases in which bile acids are poorly absorbed in the entire small bowel (e.g., sprue) or terminal ileum (e.g., Crohn disease with or without resection, short-bowel syndromeSBS) or in which triglyceride absorption is limited (e.g., pancreatic insufficiency). When the coefficient of fat absorption is 85% to 95% (normal, ≥95%), fat restriction need not be stringent to achieve good results. For example, in a patient with a daily intake of 80 g of triglyceride and 90% efficient absorption (mildly abnormal), the fecal output would be only 8 g per day. However, if absorption is only 60% efficient, restriction must be more severe; with an intake of 50 g, 20 g of fat would still be excreted per day.

In some disorders, fat malabsorption is severe and is present at birth (e.g., chylomicron retention disease). In these disorders, a very low long-chain triglyceride intake is needed is needed to control symptoms, but the triglycerides in the diet need to be polyunsaturated, to supply essential fatty acids (163). In addition, vitamin E must be supplemented to allow normal development of the nervous system to progress.

Patients with Nonspecific Intestinal Symptoms

Many patients complain that fatty foods cause a variety of intestinal symptoms. For such patients, it is usually enough to avoid fried foods and very fatty meats (bacon, sausage). Because the ingestion of fat is usually not specifically related to the symptoms of cholecystitis, ulcer, IBS, and similar disorders, a low-fat diet is usually not indicated. Because protein is also a potent stimulus of intestinal and gastric motility, a selective restriction of fat intake serves no purpose.

Obesity
Adherence to low-calorie diets is one key factor for long-term success in losing weight. In addition, it is possible that maintaining a low-fat diet may be another, as a significant association has been shown between the amount of fat in the diet and the amount of food eaten (163).

SFA vs. PUFA for CVD Prevention (see also Chapter 8, Supplements and foods to improve the lipid profile)
Current recommendations suggest reducing SFA intake as a factor in reducing the risk of CVD. Replacement of 1% of energy from saturated fats with PUFAs lowers LDL-C and probably reduces CVD incidence by approximately 2% (164). However, ω-6 PUFAs can have detrimental effects on blood clotting and lipid peroxidation, and these can be modified by ω-3 PUFAs (165). Moreover, substituting carbohydrate for SFA has been a factor in increasing obesity. There is evidence that a diet high in SFAs could raise serum cholesterol, but it was not clear that SFAs themselves were a risk factor in diets in general, nor is it clear that replacing them would prevent CVD. It is clear that not all SFAs are the same physiologically; thus, the role of SFAs in the production of CVD is still controversial, although the existing recommendations have not been modified. The 2002 recommendations from the American Heart Association suggest eating two fish meals per week.

In the past few decades, the use of statins, antithrombotics, β-blockers, and angiotensin-converting enzyme inhibitors has increased greatly, perhaps leading to the lack of effect of the more recent large trials of PUFA addition for CVD prevention (166). However, these studies differed greatly in the type of ω-3 PUFA provided, the formulation, and the duration of dosing. Because the fate of PUFAs in the body is so complex, the original idea that the effect was related to eicosanoid-mediated effects is probably too simple (167). PUFAs are oxidized to other reactive compounds, such as peroxides and aldehydes, and these may be mediating the effects (good or bad) on the development of CVD. Ω-3 PUFAs also modify and reorganize lipid rafts, possibly leading to altered signaling in cells with improvement in immune and other functions (168). More information will be needed to determine whether PUFAs as a class are helpful in preventing CVD, or whether specific PUFAs will be useful.

Trans fats are another form of fat that can increase LDL-C and perhaps increase the risk of CVD (169). This association has led to an increasing movement to remove trans (hydrogenated) fats (the majority from soy oil) from the food chain (170). On the other hand, one of these trans fats, trans-palmitoleic acid, endogenously synthesized and found in whole-milk dairy products, has been associated with lower insulin resistance and incident diabetes (171). Thus, it is possible that only exogenous trans fats may carry a risk for CVD.

The use of low–SFA diets and replacement with PUFAs related to diabetes has also produced conflicting results. A diet that offered multiple components (plant sterols, fiber, and PUFAs in the form of soy oil and nuts) lowered LDL-C better than a low–SFA diet (172). However, other trials of PUFA supplementation at "standard" doses decreased serum triglycerides, but had varying effects on LDL-C (173). The risk of diabetes in the Singapore Chinese Health Study showed an inverse association between ω-3 PUFA intake and diabetes incidence, but the association was due to intake of ALA, and not of eicosapentaenoic acid (EPA)/docosahexaenoic acid (DHA) (174). ALA is the major vegetable oil ω-3 PUFA, raising the question whether vegetable oil might be preferable to fatty fish. This concept would be consistent with the possible effect of vegetable and fruit intake on disease prevention.

Other claims related to PUFA intake have even less to recommend them. There is no support for a role of ω-3 PUFA in preventing depression (175). The hypothesis that low-fat diets in patients grouped according to blood group type might be useful in lowering LDL-C has not received experimental support (176).

Non–Alcoholic Fatty Liver Disease

Non–alcoholic fatty liver disease (NAFLD) was once thought to be part of a spectrum from fatty liver to non–alcoholic steatohepatitis (NASH), but these two extremes are now felt to be two separate entities (177). The key to formation of NASH appears to be insulin resistance leading to increased uptake and synthesis of fatty acids. This leads to fatty liver. But subsequently, there is a problem with lipid disposal that triggers lipid peroxidation through reactive oxygen species and altered adipokine production, but other pathways are also important, including altered fatty acid transporters (178). This syndrome is comorbid with obesity, T2DM, and dyslipidemia. Diagnosis is usually made by abnormal liver enzymes and/or imaging with MRI or ultrasound. Because NAFLD is characterized by an imbalance between fatty acid input to the liver and fatty acid disposal, weight loss diets characterized by low-glycemic food, decreased SFA, and increased mono- and PUFA are usually recommended (179). If 7% to 10% of body weight is lost, improvement is seen in insulin resistance and hepatic histology. If this weight loss is maintained, it is possible that the natural history of NASH might be altered. The diet is probably indicated for hepatic steatosis, but mostly for weight loss, as the steatosis is not usually progressive. If diet alone is not sufficient, either treatment with insulin sensitizers and/or bariatric surgery may be indicated.

Hypertriglyceridemia to Prevent Pancreatitis

Severe hypertriglyceridemia ($\geq$5.65 mM per L or 500 to 2,000 mg per dL) is associated with acute pancreatitis, and can be a manifestation of absolute or relative deficiency of lipoprotein lipase (LPL), associated with either heterozygous or more rarely homozygous LPL deficiency. When this occurs with pancreatitis, treatment includes very-low-fat diet along with medications (fibrates, statins, ω-3 PUFAs, and insulin sensitizers) (180). When the hypertriglyceridemia is asymptomatic, the need for treatment for the purpose of preventing pancreatitis is much less clear. The progression of asymptomatic hypertriglyceridemia to the development of pancreatitis is rare (181). The prevalence of hypertriglyceridemia in patients with pancreatitis is nearly the same (2.1%) as that of the general population (1.7%). Despite this skepticism, the National Cholesterol Education Program Adult Treatment Panel III (ATPIII) still recommends that those rare cases with asymptomatic elevated triglycerides above 5.65 mmol per L should be treated with very-low-fat diets (<15% of caloric intake), weight reduction, increased exercise, and a triglyceride-lowering drug (182).

Practical Aspects

General Instructions

1. Broil, bake, or boil meats and fish.
2. Use chicken and turkey without skin as major sources of meat. The flat fish fillets usually served with sauces (flounder, sole) contain less fat than steaklike fish (salmon, halibut, tuna, trout, mackerel). Red meat trimmed of all fat or USDA select-grade meat (8% fat content) also can be used in smaller amounts.
3. Use skim milk.
4. Avoid most desserts (cakes, cookies, pies, pastry, candy).
5. Avoid cream sauces and gravies.
6. **Label information for fat content.** As of May 1994, all manufacturers of processed foods are required by the FDA to use uniform definitions of claims such as "light" or "low-fat." *Light* means only that the product has one-third fewer calories or one-half the fat of its original version. Under the new law, the "% fat-free" claim appears only on low-fat products. The total grams of fat is the most important item and it is found in the middle of the label, where it may not be seen at first glance. Also, the "% daily value for calories" refers to a 2,000-calorie diet needed by "the average person." This estimate may be excessive for many people (see Appendix B for further discussion of the new food labels).

Beef, pork, and lamb products also may appear with labels indicating approval by the Nutritional Effects Foundation (NEF), a new nonprofit organization. Most producers must apply for approval and comply with limits on fat content. "NEF-1" meat contains 3.5% fat or less by weight, and "NEF-2" contains 6% fat or less. This compares with the 15% to 20% fat content in the usual meat choices.

Nearly all hard cheeses are high in fat. Part-skim cheeses are lower in fat, but most (>50%) of the calories are still derived from fat.

Specific Recommendations

To suggest a given intake of fat, the content of table foods must be known. A list of some foods with their fat content appears in Table 12-20. Based on the values for fat in this table, a general scheme of low fat intake can be offered.

1. **When the fat intake must be 40 g per day,** foods allowed each day include most vegetables and fruits, breads, cereals with skim milk, two servings of lean meat (3 oz each), one egg, and 1 tsp of margarine.
2. **When fat intake must be 60 g per day,** in addition to the preceding foods, one can add 2 cups of 2% milk or one more ounces of meat or one egg with each serving or four more teaspoons of margarine or oil.
3. **When fat intake is 75 g per day,** in addition to foods allowed on the 60-g diet, the patient can ingest whole milk instead of 2% milk *or* two slices of bacon *or* 4 oz of ice cream *or* two larger servings of lean meat (6 oz each).
4. **Low-fat substitutes** are available for many foods, including whole milk (skim milk), cream (evaporated skim milk), butter/oils (apple or prune sauce, no-stick sprays), eggs (egg substitute), cheese, salad dressings, coffee cream, and ice cream (ice milk, sorbet).

Side Effects

The low-fat diet is a high-carbohydrate, high-osmolarity diet, and carbohydrate-induced diarrhea may occur. In such a case, the restriction of fat must be titrated to individual needs. When meats and fish must be severely restricted to control fat intake, low-fat dietary supplements may be needed to deliver adequate protein and calories (see Chapter 10). A low-fat diet is often quite bland because fat supplies much of the flavor in foods. Care must be taken to season foods so that adequate caloric intake is maintained.

Fat Supplements

When steatorrhea is present, fat-soluble vitamins often must be replaced. Bile acids are necessary for the absorption of fat-soluble vitamins; thus, the requirements are greatest in patients who have disorders associated with bile acid depletion (e.g., most cases of SBS). The large doses of vitamins needed to treat malabsorption are often available only as the individual vitamin, not as part of a multivitamin preparation. A discussion of vitamins A, D, E, and K is included in Chapter 6. If pancreatic insufficiency is the cause of steatorrhea, enzyme replacement is needed. When fat restriction is severe, medium-chain triglycerides (MCTs) or fat substitutes can be added to the diet.

Fat Substitutes

Because fat contains the highest energy (kcal per g) of any macronutrient, the food industry has tried many ways to replace fat. Traditional techniques involve removing fat by substituting water or air for fat, using lean meats or skim milk, and baking instead of frying. Fat may be replaced by formulating foods with lipid, protein, or carbohydrate-based ingredients. Such foods include baked goods, salad dressings, frozen desserts, margarine or shortening, confectionery, processed meat products, dairy products, soups or sauces, and snack products (183). Two types of fat replacers have been used. Fat substitutes are macromolecules that physically and chemically resemble triglycerides. Examples of fat substitutes include sucrose polyesters (Olestra™), emulsifiers such as lecithin or propylene glycol esters, and polyether polyols. Structured triglycerides have been used to include short- or medium-chain fatty acids in order to deliver fewer calories. The most common example is medium-chain triglycerides, but other structured lipids (e.g., Benefta™) are used in the baking industry.

TABLE 12-20 Fat Content of Selected Table Foods

Food	Fat (g/unit)
Milk Products	
Milk	
Whole (1 cup)	8.6
2% (1 cup)	4.9
1% (1 cup)	2.5
Skim (1 cup)	0.2
Buttermilk (1 cup)	2.4
Ice cream	
Regular (1 cup)	14.1
Rich grade (1 cup)	23.8
Ice milk (1 cup)	6.7
Yogurt	8.3
Cheese and Butter	
Butter	
Regular (tbsp)	11.5
Whipped (tbsp)	7.6
Margarine (tbsp)	11.5
Cheese	
Blue (1 oz)	8.6
Cheddar (1 oz)	9.1
Cottage (1 oz)	1.2
Cream (1 oz)	10.7
Parmesan (1 oz)	8.7
Swiss (1 oz)	7.9
American (1 oz)	8.5
Vegetables	
Eggplant (1/2 cup)	0.6
Peas, green (1/2 cup)	0.3
Spinach, cooked (1/.2 cup)	0.3
Sweet potato (1/2 cup)	2.8
Beans, dry (1/2 cup)	2.0
Avocado (1)	37
All others (1/2 cup)	<0.3
Grains and Cereals	
Bread (1 slice)	0.8
Cereal, dry (3/4 cup)	0.3
Rice, cooked (1/2 cup)	0.1
Roll (1)	0.6
Spaghetti, cooked (1/2 cup)	0.4
With tomato sauce and meatballs (1/2 cup)	5.8
Noodles (8 oz)	0.4
Meats (Yield from 3 oz Cooked)	
Beef	
Chuck with fat	13.5
Chuck, lean	5.6
Chuck steak	10.9
Trimmed	3.4
Flank steak	4.1
Porterhouse steak with bone	23.9
Trimmed	3.4
T-bone with bone	23.9
Trimmed	3.2

TABLE 12-20 Fat Content of Selected Table Foods *(continued)*

Food	Fat (g/unit)
Club steak with bone	21.2
Trimmed	3.9
Sirloin with bone	18.6
Trimmed	3
Rib roast with bone	22.6
Trimmed	4.9
Rump roast with bone	14.5
Trimmed	3.8
Ground beef	12.4
Lean	7.1
Corned beef	25.9
Chicken	
White, no skin	2.9
Dark, no skin	5.4
Chicken, fried	
White, no skin	5.2
Dark, no skin	7.9
Turkey	
Roasted with skin	14
White, no skin	3.3
Dark, no skin	7.1
Lamb	
Leg	9.4
Chops with bone	15.8
Shoulder	13.7
Liver, fried	9.8
Pork	
Chop with bone	13.2
Bacon (2 slices)	7–12
Sausages	
Liverwurst (1 slice)	2.7
Boiled ham (1 slice)	4.8
Pork sausage (1 link)	5.7
Salami (1 slice)	1.9
Frankfurters (1)	15.2
Bologna (1 slice)	1.0
Fruit	
Apple (1)	0.6
Pear (1)	0.3
Watermelon (1 cup)	0.4
All others (1)	0.3
Fats and oils	
Lard (1 tbsp)	13
Oils, corn, olive, peanut, soy, sesame (1 tbsp)	13.6
Salad dressing (1 tbsp)	6.2–9
Desserts	
Cake	
Chocolate (1 slice)	6.7
Devil's food (1 slice)	12.3
Pound (1 slice)	8.9
Sponge (1 slice)	1.9

(continued)

TABLE 12-20 Fat Content of Selected Table Foods *(continued)*

Food	Fat (g/unit)
White (1 slice)	9.7
Yellow (1 slice)	9.5
Candy	
Chocolate, milk (1 oz)	9.2
Fudge (1 piece)	5.3
Cookies	
Brownie (1 piece)	5
Chocolate chip (1)	3
Ginger snap (1)	0.6
Oatmeal (1)	2
Sugar (1)	1.3
Pies (1/8 of pie)	7–23
Fish (yield from 3 oz cooked)	
Flatfish fillets (sole, flounder)	4.8
Steaklike fish (swordfish, salmon)	6.5
Salmon, canned	11.9
Tuna, canned	
Canned in oil	17.5
Solids only	7
Canned in water	0.7
Shrimp	
Boiled	0.9
Fried	9.2
Lobster, boiled	1.3
Oysters, raw	0.5
Sardines, canned (1 fish)	1.3
Nuts	
Almonds, roasted (1 cup)	97
Peanuts, roasted (10 nuts)	4.5
Pecans (10 nuts)	10
Sesame seeds (1 tbsp)	4.3
Peanut butter (1 tbsp)	8.1
Miscellaneous and Snack Foods	
Egg	
Boiled (1)	5–6
Fried (1)	7–9
Popcorn (1 cup)	2
Potatoes	
French fried (3 oz)	11.3
Chips (1 oz)	11.3
Salad (1 cup)	7
Olives (10)	8.3

Medium-Chain Triglycerides

MCTs are composed of fatty acids with 6 to 12 carbon residues and are found in high concentration in kernel oils (e.g., palm oil) and coconut oil. The commercially available MCT oil is made from coconut oil; it contains mostly fatty acids with 8 to 10 carbon atoms (vs. 16 to 18 for dietary fats) and very rapidly undergoes β-oxidation. MCT oil provides 8.3 kcal per g; 1 tbsp weighs 14 g and provides 116 kcal. MCTs are relatively water-soluble and can be hydrolyzed in the absence of bile salts and with minimal concentrations of pancreatic enzymes, so they are ideal for use as a caloric supplement in fat malabsorption (184). Much interest has been shown in using MCTs as an aid to weight loss (185) and as a rapid source of energy, especially during prolonged endurance exercising, because they are metabolized more rapidly than other fats. However, little convincing evidence has been found that MCTs are useful in these roles. Human studies show that the addition of MCTs (10 g) to a mixed meal increases postprandial thermogenesis by 5% (186), but the role of MCTs in treatment of obesity is not clear.

Axona is a medical food with the major ingredient as caprylic acid triglyceride (fractionated coconut oil) that is marketed to improve cognition in Alzheimer disease. The proposed mechanism of action is to provide ketones as an alternate energy source for brain cells that no longer use glucose adequately. MCTs have been shown to have very modest effects on increasing energy expenditure and decreased weight, but no data are available on ketone production in humans (187). Axona is available by prescription, but the manufacturer decided not to perform phase 3 studies to achieve FDA approval as a drug. Thus, only fragmentary data are available regarding its possible efficacy.

Precautions

The rapid oxidation of MCTs leads to ketone formation. Thus, they are contraindicated in patients prone to ketosis. In cirrhosis, reduced hepatic clearance leads to increased serum MCT levels and hyperventilation, lactic acidemia, and symptoms compatible with hepatic encephalopathy (HE). Side effects of MCT oil include nausea, vomiting, diarrhea, and abdominal cramps when the dose is excessive, either at one feeding or daily. Symptoms may be a consequence of the hyperosmolarity that develops during rapid hydrolysis of MCTs.

Practical Aspects

1. Give divided doses of 1/2 tbsp up to six times a day.
2. For palatability, even though the oil is tasteless, add MCT oil (1 tbsp per 8 oz) to fruit juice or flavored beverages.
3. Use MCT oil in cooking or baking if the temperature does not exceed 300° to 325°F.
4. Use MCT oil as a salad or vegetable dressing.
5. Information on sources of MCT can be obtained from the Fatty Oxidation Disorders website (www.fodsupport.org/nutrition.htm). MCT oil formerly distributed by Mead Johnson is now available from Nestle Nutrition. However, other sources are said to be of equivalent quality and are less expensive (e.g., NOW and Premium MCT Gold, available through Health & Sport). Links to both sources are provided in the FOD website.

Fat mimetics are substances that have physical properties like triglycerides, but which do not replace fat. These are often protein- or carbohydrate-based. They provide limited calories (0 to 4 kcal per g) and absorb water. They cannot be used for frying because of their water content or because they caramelize at high temperatures, and they are less flavorful than fats. Table 12-21 includes a list of replacers that are classified as GRAS, and so can be added to foods and beverages. Two fat replacers are FDA-approved.

Simplesse is made from egg white and milk protein processed in such a way as to produce a creamy liquid with the texture of fat. It is marketed in an ice cream product (Simple Pleasures), and in other products, such as mayonnaise, salad dressings, dips, sour cream, yogurt, and cheese spreads. It cannot be used in cooking because the creamy texture is lost.

Olestra, a compound in which up to eight fatty acids from vegetable oil are linked to a sucrose core, is resistant to the action of pancreatic lipase. It can be used in cooking and has been approved for deep-fried snacks such as potato and corn chips. In a short-term (6-week) randomized, controlled trial of snack foods containing olestra or triglycerides, no clinically meaningful gastrointestinal symptoms were caused by the ingestion of snacks that contained olestra (188). Because olestra is a nonabsorbed lipid, it can cause a false-positive reaction in measurements of stool fat (189). Minor changes have been reported in serum fat-soluble vitamin concentrations, but the significance of these changes is not clear (190).

TABLE 12-21 Fat Replacers in Current Use

Classification	Product	Composition	Examples™
Fat substitutes	Emulsifiers	Vegetable mono- or diglycerides	Dur-Lo, ECt-25
	Sucrose fatty acid esters	Made from sucrose and edible fats	Olestra
	Salatrim	TG with long and short chain Fas	Benefat
	MCT oil	Medium-chain triglycerides from coconut oil	Many
Protein-based	Microparticulated proteins	Whey or egg protein	Simplesse
	Modified whey protein concentrate	Made by controlled thermal denaturation	Dairy-Lo
	Protein–carbohydrate blends	Egg white and milk proteins	K-Blazer, Ultra-Bake, Ultra-Freeze, Lita
Carbohydrate-based	Cellulose	Ground to microparticles	Avicel, Methocel, Solka-Floc
	Dextrins	Food sources such as tapioca, corn, potato, wheat, contains 4 kcal/g	Amylum, CrystLean, Lorelite, Lycadex, Maltrin, Paseille D-Lite, Star-Dri
	Fiber	Soluble or insoluble fiber, adds moisture and stability	Opta, Oat Fiber, Z-trim
	Gums/hydrophilic colloids	Guar gum, gum Arabic, locust bean gum, xanthan gum, carrageenan, pectin	Kelcogel, Keltrol, Slendid
	Inulin	Extract of chicory root	Faftiline, Fruitafit, Fibruline
	Oatrim	Enzyme-treated oat flours containing β-glucan fiber	Beta-Trim, TrimChoice
	Polydextrose	Dextrose polymer with bits of sorbitol and citric acid, contains 1 kcal/g	Litesse, Sta-Lite
	Polyols	Synthetic, contain 1.5–3.0 kcal/g	Many brands
	Modified food starch	From potato, corn, oat, rice, wheat, tapioca, 1–4 kcal/g	Amalean, FairnexVA, Instant Stellar, N-Lite, OptaGrade, AX-1, Pure-Gel, Sta-Slim

Modified from The Calorie Control Council, Glossary of Fat Replacers, http://www.caloriecontrol.org/articles-and-video/feature-articles/glossary-of-fat-replacers

Conditionally Essential Lipids

Choline

Choline is a precursor for acetylcholine, phospholipids, and the methyl donor betaine. Choline can be synthesized in sufficient amounts to support normal metabolism of normal animals and humans, so in the past has not been considered an essential nutrient. 5-Adenosylmethionine (AdoMet) is the major methyl donor in mammals. The methyl group in AdoMet is derived from the diet (methionine, choline, and betaine) and from *de novo* synthesis with the methyl group supplied by 5-methyltetrahydrofolate (191). The major consumer of these methyl groups had been thought to be creatine, but is more likely to be phosphatidylcholine synthesis via phosphatidylethanolamine methyltransferase (PEMT). Also, it had been thought that when intake of the labile methyl group (from choline and betaine) was decreased, methylneogenesis was enhanced by decreasing creatine synthesis.

However, in some pathological conditions and even in normal neonates, this nutrient is considered essential (192). A choline deficiency syndrome has never been described in humans, but the Food and Drug Nutrition Board of the IOM now classifies choline as an essential nutrient (192), based on the development of fatty liver or muscle damage when healthy humans were placed on a choline-deficient diet (193). Other evidence for the essential nature of choline includes the higher requirement for choline in postmenopausal compared with premenopausal women (194), and the development of more liver fibrosis in postmenopausal women with decreased choline plasma levels and non–alcoholic fatty liver (195). In addition, some data in patients on total parenteral nutrition suggest a partial reversal in hepatic abnormalities following choline supplementation (196). A population-based case-control study of birth defects in which subsequent dietary histories were taken found evidence for decreased risk of cleft lip with or without cleft palate in mothers ingesting the highest quartile of choline, methionine, and total protein (197).

Choline is absorbed from the intestine, but it is not clear if this process is related to the high-affinity choline transporter (CHT1) that mediates endocytosis in neural tissue. Foods with high choline content include liver, eggs, shrimp, collard greens, Swiss chard, cauliflower, spinach, beef, chicken/turkey, peanut butter, and milk, but lower amounts occur in all raw foods. The most common form of supplemental choline is lecithin, usually extracted from soybean, although choline bitartrate is widely available. Human intake is estimated at approximately 0.6 to 1.0 g per day. Gut flora degrades choline in part to betaine and methylamines. The AI for infants was set at 17 to 18 mg per kg, and for adults at 440 mg per day for men and 425 mg per day for women. A 20% lipid emulsion for TPN provides 11.6 to 13.2 mmol per L of phosphatidylcholine. The UL for choline is 3.5 g per day, the limiting factors being hypotension and a fishy body odor from a metabolite, trimethylamine (192).

Butyrate

Butyrate is a short-chain fatty acid produced by microbial fermentation in the colon from dietary fiber, and is an important energy source for colonic epithelial cells (198). It is absorbed via the monocarboxylate transporter 1, which is down-regulated in inflamed colonic mucosa, leading to intracellular butyrate deficiency as a possible explanation for decreased butyrate utilization in IBDs (199). Some studies with small numbers of patients show benefit of butyrate enemas in active distal UC, and possibly in other colitides, but much larger and better designed studies are needed to establish efficacy (200). Many other treatments are available for most causes of colitis and proctitis, so the new studies will need to be convincing (201). Butyrate has been used in colitides that have been difficult to treat with existing measures, for example, radiation colitis (202) and shigella colitis (203). It may be in these conditions that butyrate treatment may find a role.

High-Fat (Ketogenic) Diets

The major use for a high-fat very-low-carbohydrate diet has been to treat epilepsy in children (ketogenic diet). This diet uses 4 g of fat for every gram of protein and carbohydrate combined (204). For example, a 1,000 kcal diet of this type would contain 100 g fat, 18 g protein, and 7 g carbohydrate. Two modified versions of the diet have appeared. The first diet delivers approximately 1 g protein per kg, uses carbohydrates with a low GI, and provides more than 60% of calories from fat. The diet requires measuring or estimating foods in household measures, and is offered when the "classical" diet is too difficult to deliver (205). A second more liberal version is the modified Atkins diet that provides 65% of calories as fat (206). These diets can be used at any age. The usual indication is for patients who are poor candidates for epilepsy surgery, but is also the treatment of choice for inherited disorders where glucose metabolism is impaired, and ketones can be an alternate source of fuel for the cells, for example, glucose-1–deficiency syndrome and pyruvate dehydrogenase deficiency (204). The ketogenic diet has been suggested for diabetes and weight loss (207), but whether such severe carbohydrate restriction provides benefit over standard diets is not clear.

Low-Protein Diet

Principles

Pathophysiology

In chronic hepatic disease with cirrhosis and portal–systemic shunting, exogenous protein bypasses the liver, and the products of protein degradation induce HE. Protein restriction is most effective when liver disease is stable and the episodes of encephalopathy are related to exogenous sources. When encephalopathy is caused by active hepatic disease and an inability to utilize endogenous amino acids, the diet is less effective. The cause of encephalopathy is uncertain. The "false-neurotransmitter" theory suggests that biogenic amines derived from tyrosine and phenylalanine may be involved in the development of HE. In cirrhosis, the ratio of branched-chain amino acids (BCAAs) (leucine, valine, and isoleucine) to tyrosine and phenylalanine is decreased from between 3 and 3.5 to less than 1.0. Because BCAAs compete with aromatic and sulfur amino acids for transport into the brain, it is rational to use either a low intake of protein or a relative increase in BCAAs in the diet to prevent this effect (208).

However, it is not known whether BCAA mixtures are superior to standard amino acid mixtures. Protein-sparing nutritional support produces some improvement in liver function, but it is not clear that such support alters mortality or morbidity (209). Guidelines for nutritional management of alcoholic liver disease have been developed by the American College of Gastroenterology and by the European Society for Parenteral and Enteral Nutrition (210) (Table 12-22).

TABLE 12-22 Nutritional Support Guidelines for Management of Protein Intake in Patients with Alcoholic Liver Disease

Disease/ Complications	Aim of Support	Calories (g/kg)	Protein (g/kg)	CHO	Lipid	Other
Fatty liver	EtOH abstinence	Decreased	Nr	Nr	Nr	Nr
Alcoholic hepatitis	Prevent PEM	40	1.5–2.0	4–5	1.2	Vitamins
Cirrhosis, no malnutrition	Prevent PEM	35	1.3–1.5	4–5	1–1.5	
Cirrhosis + malnutrition	Prevent PEM	35–40	1.5–2.0	3–4	2–2.5	Vitamins
Protein intolerance	Prevent encephalopathy	~25	0.3–0.5	2.5–3.5	1–1.5	Fluid restrict
Ascites, edema		BCAA Recompensate				Fluid 1–1.5 L/day Na restrict

EtOH, ethanol; Nr, no recommendation; PEM, protein–energy malnutrition; BCAA, branched-chain amino acids; Na, sodium.
Data from Stickel F, Hoehn B, Schuppan D, Seitz HK. Review article: nutritional therapy in alcoholic liver disease. *Alimen Pharmacol Ther*. 2003;18:357.

BCAAs are recommended only for protein intolerance. A systematic review of 11 randomized studies comparing BCAA with isonitrogenous regimes showed that for a median intake of 28 g per day (range 11 to 57) and mean duration of 7 days (range 4 to 90 days), BCAA increased the percent of patients improving from encephalopathy (59% versus 41%), but without evidence of improved survival or adverse events (211,212). Some studies show a high frequency of noncompliance and side effects when BCAAs are used, factors that limit the practicality of using this form of supplement (213).

Chronic Renal Failure

In chronic renal failure, a low-protein diet is used to decrease the production of nitrogenous waste products that must be excreted (e.g., urea, uric acid). This diet stresses the essential amino acids because they tend to be used preferentially for protein synthesis and are not deaminated with subsequent production of urea. Restriction of dietary protein to about 0.6 g per kg of body weight reduces the relative risk for renal failure by about 33% (214). The details of this special use of the low-protein diet are discussed in Chapter 13.

Hospitalized Patients

Many elderly hospitalized patients meet less than 50% of their recommended protein and energy requirements, so the risk for a poor outcome is increased (215). This unintended low-protein diet is a consequence of many factors, including a decreased appetite and the administration of medications. Supplementing the hospital diet with 20 g of milk protein per day (up to about 1.0 g of total protein per kilogram per day) slowed the rate of bone loss, increased levels of insulin-like growth factor 1, and shortened hospital stay in patients after hip fracture (216). Whether supplementation with specific growth factors is needed or whether protein replacement alone is enough is still a matter of considerable debate (217).

Indications

In patients with **chronic liver disease** and HE, a low-protein diet can be useful. However, the diet must still supply protein at the required rate of 0.5 to 0.8 g/kg/day, and for most patients who show no evidence of protein intolerance, 1.0 to 1.5 g protein per kg is recommended (218). For this reason, restricted diets that provide less than 40 g per day for an adult or 1.0 to 2.5 g of protein per kg daily for a growing child may be associated with a negative nitrogen balance. However, identifying and correcting precipitating events, along with lactulose and nonabsorbable antibiotics comprise the standard of care for HE. Thus, diet alone is not usually acceptable. Moreover, current evidence does not support protein restriction in the management of HE (219).

In **hyperammonemia** of any cause, such as certain *inborn errors of metabolism* (e.g., isovaleric acidemia), this diet decreases available substrate.

Renal failure, whether acute or chronic, must be treated with a low-protein diet (see Chapter 13).

Practical Aspects

General Instructions

1. The caloric intake as carbohydrate should be sufficient to prevent the use of protein in muscle for energy (25 to 40 kcal per g of protein). For patients too ill to eat, parenteral administration is appropriate.
2. For patients with renal disease, 80% of the daily protein allotment should be protein of high biologic value—eggs, meat, fish, poultry, milk.
3. For patients with HE, the intestinal absorption of protein by-products should be reduced by concomitant treatment with lactulose (30 mL three or four times daily to produce loose stools) or neomycin (1 g two to four times daily).
4. An intake of 40 g of protein barely maintains nitrogen balance. Lesser amounts of protein can be used acutely but should not be prescribed on a long-term basis. Vegetable protein may be better tolerated than animal protein because it contains less tryptophan and sulfur amino acids, which are thought to contribute to HE.
5. The use of BCAA supplements is still not established, and no convincing data are available to indicate that such supplements are more effective in relieving acute or chronic encephalopathy than are standard amino acid mixtures (209). The guidelines for patient selection

and the endpoint of therapy are unclear, as is the demonstration of clear long-term benefit to the patient. Recommended doses of the oral products (e.g., Hepatic-Aid) are 15 to 60 g per day; for IV use (e.g., HepatAmine), they are 80 to 120 g per day (see Chapters 10 and 11 for the composition of these products). HepatAmine contains three amino acids (methionine, phenylalanine, and tryptophan) thought to contribute to HE. The doses mentioned above are recommended by the manufacturer and may be too high. Because efficacy is not proven, these products should be used with caution, especially at the recommended high doses.

6. For patients with renal disease, sodium and potassium must also be restricted.

Specific Instructions

Each ounce of meat, fish, poultry, or cheese contains about 7 g of protein, an egg contains 6 g, and 1 cup of milk contains 8 g. One-half cup of cereal, bread, pasta, or a vegetable contains 2 g of protein, whereas the same amount of dried beans, peas, or nuts contains 5 g or more. Table 12-23 lists the protein content of various foods. The National Kidney Foundation

TABLE 12-23 Protein Content of Selected Foods

Food	Protein (g/unit)	Food	Protein (g/unit)
Egg, 1 Large (100)[a]	6.5		
Milk Products (93)		**Breads and Cereals** (65)	
Milk		Bread (1 slice)	2.2
Whole (1 cup)	8.5	Cereal, dry (3/4 cup)	1.1–2.1
Skim (1 cup)	8.8	Rice, cooked (1/2 cup)	2.0
Buttermilk (1 cup)	8.1	Roll (1)	2.6
Ice cream (1 cup)	9.6	Spaghetti, cooked (1/2 cup)	3.4
Cheese (1 oz)	6.6–7.5		
Yogurt, low-fat, fruit (1 cup)	9.8	**Vegetables** (72)	
Meat, Fish, Poultry (75)		Asparagus, cooked (2/3 cup)	2.2
Hamburger (3 oz)	21.9	Broccoli, cooked (2/3 cup)	1.7
Sirloin steak (3 oz)	22.2	Cabbage, raw (1/2 cup)	1.3
Lamb chop (3 oz)	19.2	Cauliflower, cooked (2/3 cup)	2.3
Lamb leg (3 oz)	23.4	Cucumber, raw (1/2 cup)	0.3
Pork chop (3 oz)	22.2	Eggplant, cooked (1/2 cup)	2.0
Liver, beef (3 oz)	23.7	Lettuce (4 leaves)	1.7
Chicken, white meat (3 oz)	21.6	Green pepper, raw (1)	1.2
Chicken, dark meat (3 oz)	18.6	Spinach, cooked (1/2 cup)	3.0
Frankfurter (3 oz)	18.6	Green beans (1/2 cup)	0.8
Fish		Tomato (1)	1.1
Cod (3 oz)	25.5	Green peas, cooked (1/2 cup)	4.3
Halibut (3 oz)	22.8	Legumes, dried (1 oz)	6.7
Salmon, canned (3 oz)	17.7	**Fruits**	
Tuna, canned (3 oz)	26.1	Apple (1)	0.2
Shellfish		Apricots (1)	0.5
Crabmeat (3 oz)	12.9	Bananas (1)	1.2
Lobster (3 oz)	12.6	Cantaloupe (quarter)	1.0
Shrimp (3 oz)	14.4	Orange (1)	1.0
Bacon (2 slices)	6.0	Orange juice (1/2 cup)	0.7
Nuts (55)			
Peanuts (6 nuts)	2.6	Pear, peach (1)	0.6
Peanut butter (1 tbsp)	4.2	Watermelon (1 cup)	0.9

[a]Biologic value is based on the ability of the protein to produce positive nitrogen balance. The numbers in parentheses correspond to an average value for that food group versus 100% for egg.

(116 East 27th Street, New York, New York 10016) provides further information useful for patients. See Chapter 13 for details of the use of protein restriction in renal disease.

Side Effects
When protein restriction is too severe, catabolized muscle mass provides the amino acids needed for daily use (see Chapter 5). It is not wise to restrict protein to less than 0.4 g per kg of body weight (~30 g of protein for the average 70-kg patient). If the symptoms of HE or uremia do not respond to this degree of restriction, it is unlikely that more stringent restriction will help. When the intake of meat and milk is restricted, it is possible that calcium, iron, and B vitamins (thiamine, riboflavin, niacin) will be needed.

Supplements Required
In renal failure, calcium is often needed to compensate for hypocalcemia and a decreased calcium intake. Iron deficiency resulting from bleeding gastrointestinal lesions often complicates renal failure, but iron is sometimes needed even in the absence of overt gastrointestinal bleeding.

High-Protein Diet and Protein Supplements

High-Protein Diet
The traditional diet for reducing the risk of obesity, heart disease, and cancer has been a high-carbohydrate, low-fat diet (~15%, 15%, and 70% of calories as protein, fat, and carbohydrate, respectively), but results have been disappointing. The average diet in the United States contains approximately 14%, 34%, and 48% of calories as protein, fat, and carbohydrate, respectively (220). The success of the low-carbohydrate, high-protein (~30%, 30%, and 40% of calories as protein, fat, and carbohydrate, respectively) diet in causing initial weight loss (220, and Chapter 14) has led to a number of new observations on the relative effects of these two diets. Obesity is currently viewed as a problem equally as important as lowering lipoprotein levels, and the high-protein diet has become popular. There is little evidence that the high-protein diet can maintain weight loss for an extended period of time (123), nor that such diets can prevent heart disease (221). There is some evidence that some CV risk factors may be modified by ketogenic/high-protein diets, but no long-term clinical benefit has been documented (207). Although ketogenic diets can worsen glucose tolerance and stimulate the development of NAFLD in mice (222), some advantages have been noted in short-term human studies in terms of sparing of lean body mass, lowering of triglyceride levels, and improved glycemic control, when comparing high-protein with high-carbohydrate diets (223). The lack of long-term benefit may be due to compliance, as longer-term outcomes are similar, when comparing diets that differ in macronutrient content.

The DRI Committee of the IOM has allowed a higher amount of protein in the DRI than previously allowed, suggesting 10% to 35% of calories as an acceptable protein proportion (64). Although high protein intake can increase urinary calcium and nitrogenous waste products, the DRI Committee found no evidence that a high protein intake increases the risk of renal stones, cancer, osteoporosis, or CVD. However, the effect of consumption of large amounts of protein (30% to 35% of calories) on kidneys and bones is not known. Moreover, high-protein diets restrict other healthful foods, and are not recommended for weight loss by the American Heart Association (220). The updated AHA recommendations still take this position, because high-protein animal foods are also high in saturated fat, possibly increasing the risk of CVD (224).

Protein Supplements (see Chapter 8)

Gluten-Restricted Diet

Definitions
There is not complete agreement on the spectrum of celiac disease (CD), and as a result of that uncertainty, it is not always clear which patients should receive a gluten-free diet (GFD). The term "gluten" includes the related insoluble prolamins from wheat, rye, and barley, but probably not oats. However, contamination of foods thought to be "gluten-free" (GF) can complicate this definition. Four groups have published consensus statements regarding the

classification of gluten-related disorders, with recommendations for diagnosis and therapy (225–228). Terms used to describe patients with "gluten-related disorders" include typical/classical/overt/symptomatic CD, atypical/nonclassical/asymptomatic CD, silent/latent/potential CD, and gluten intolerance/gluten sensitivity/non–celiac gluten sensitivity (NCGS) (226). The entity of wheat allergy is separate from CD (227), and will be discussed below under "Elimination diets." The consensus between these groups is that CD is an autoimmune disease, consisting of three groups: symptomatic CD, silent CD, and potential CD (229). All three groups have abnormal serology (tissue transglutaminase [tTG], endomysial, and/or antigliadin antibodies), but only the first two groups have abnormal small-bowel mucosa. The separation of the groups is further confused by the wide range of symptoms associated with CD, ranging from infertility and osteopenia to psychiatric disorders, arthritis, and cardiomyopathy.

The fourth group, NCGS is characterized by negative CD serology and small-bowel biopsy, but symptoms that respond to a GFD. Occasionally, these patients will have antigliadin antibodies (230). NCGS was suggested by a study in IBS patients that demonstrated a symptomatic response to a GFD in a randomized double-blind placebo-controlled trial (231). However, a later trial studying similar patients with IBS and NCGS, a crossover design tested a diet containing low fermentable carbohydrate diet (FODMAP) against a diet containing gluten, and found that symptomatic worsening occurred equally with both diets (232). This result suggests that the response to a GFD in the absence of CD might be related to the high fructan content of wheat. These studies show the difficulty in establishing a diagnosis of NCGS based on symptomatic response alone. The American College of Gastroenterology guidelines suggest that a response to a GFD *not* be used to diagnose either CD or NCGS (228). The problem arises when patients present on a GFD stating that they improved on it. In such a situation, serology testing is not always definitive, as serology can become negative in a patient with CD on a GFD. HLA-DQ2/DQ8 testing can be used here, as a positive result will support a diagnosis of CD in a patient who has responded to a GFD, but such a patient could fall under the category of "potential CD." A challenge with gluten may be necessary to document the response, but even this must be distinguished from response to other carbohydrates that induce symptoms.

It is important to separate CD from NCGS for several reasons. First, the clinical validity of a definable and reproducible syndrome of NCGS has not been established, so one is always wondering if the patient will develop signs or symptoms of CD itself. Second, making a diagnosis of CD makes one look for associated autoimmune disorders, especially T2DM. In fact, many patients with CD are discovered by screening patients with highly associated autoimmune disorders (e.g., thyroid disease, dermatitis herpetiformis) and highly associated signs or symptoms (e.g., anemia, osteopenia, peripheral neuropathy, infertility, growth failure). Considering the significance of this diagnostic distinction is becoming more important, as patients are increasingly being started on a GFD as first-line therapy for disorders as diverse as attention-deficit hyperactivity disorder (ADHD), chronic fatigue syndrome, multiple sclerosis, IBD, and a variety of functional pain syndrome, including fibromyalgia (228).

Toxic Grain Products

Nontropical sprue (celiac sprue, gluten-sensitive enteropathy) is a disorder characterized by sensitivity to certain glutens. Glutens are a family of proteins found in many grains, including corn and rice, which are safe for patients with CD. The glutens that produce symptoms in this disorder are those in wheat, rye, and barley (233) (Table 12-24). Foods containing gluten include bread, pasta, cereals, gravies, sauces, pastries, cakes, cookies, crackers, soups, and any food with bread or grain additives from the list in Table 12-25. The data implicating oats have been shown to be misleading, because there is a high risk of gluten contamination in their preparation. Oats have been well tolerated in patients with dermatitis herpetiformis, a related disorder (234). No clinical or biopsy differences were seen in adults with CD ingesting oats over a 5-year period (235).

Substitutions. Glutens from corn and rice, in addition to those from wheat starch, potato flour, soybean flour, and tapioca, may be used as substitutes for the omitted cereal grains. Other

TABLE 12-24 Classification of Grains According to Gluten Content

Gluten-Containing	Gluten-Free
Barley	Amaranth
Bran	Buckwheat/kasha, whole or cracked grain
Bulgur	Corn, whole grain and flour
Couscous	Millet, whole grain
Durum wheat	Oats (some products may be contaminated with wheat)
Farro	Popcorn
Farina	Potato flour
Graham flour	Quinoa, whole grain
Kamut	Rice, brown/white/wild
Orzo	Sorghum, whole grain
Rye	Soybeans
Spelt	Teff, whole grain
Wheat, any type	Tapioca

Data from See J, Murray JA. Gluten-free diet: The medical and nutrition management of celiac disease. *Nutr Clin Pract.* 2006;21:1.

"grains" that do not contain disease-causing gluten include amaranth, millet, quinoa, sorghum, teff, wild rice, and buckwheat. The latter is not a true cereal grain, and when toasted is known as kasha. Its flour is used to produce the unique flavor of crepes from the region of Normandy in France. Approaches to approximate GF status for products, other than using gluten-free grains, include gluten removal by genetic modification, enzymatic pretreatment of wheat flour, oral enzyme gluten hydrolases, and polymeric gluten binders, but none of these have reached commercial availability (236).

Wheat Products are Used as Fillers in Many Processed Foods. It is helpful for the patient with sprue to develop an extensive list of acceptable products.

Duration of Diet

Although a GFD was formerly thought to be needed only until remission occurred in some patients, it is now clear that use of the diet should be lifelong (237). No convincing evidence indicates that the diet is useful for the nonspecific therapy of other diarrheal illness. However, acute intestinal damage resulting from conditions other than sprue may cause temporary gluten intolerance, especially in children. The long-term use of this diet should be limited to patients with gluten-induced enteropathy.

Relationship to Traditional Allergy

The abnormal response to wheat and other glutens in sprue differs from other food allergies in that the process is not mediated by immunoglobulin E (IgE). However, abnormalities of the intestinal immune system are involved in some way. In some cases, treatment with glucocorticosteroids can supplement dietary management of the disease (161).

Indications

A gluten-restricted diet is necessary for patients with biopsy-proven *nontropical sprue* or the related disorder *dermatitis herpetiformis*.

Practical Aspects

General Instructions

1. Eliminate foods containing wheat, rye, barley, and probably oats (Table 12-23 and Table 12-25). These glutens are the components that give form to dough. The flours allowed on a gluten-restricted diet produce flat or crumbly baked products. Any commercial product with a crown contains forbidden gluten. To meet the codex standard to be labeled "gluten-free" the product must contain less than 20 ppm of gluten, that is, if the total nitrogen content of the product gluten does not exceed 0.05 g per 100 g based on DM (WHO standard).

TABLE 12-25 Sources of Gluten[a]

Food Groups	Foods that Contain Gluten	Foods that may Contain Gluten	Foods that do *Not* Contain Gluten
Beverage	Cereal beverages (e.g., Postum), malt Ovaltine, beer, and ale	Commercial chocolate milk; cocoa mixes; other beverage mixes; dietary supplements; commercial rice and corn cereals[b]	Coffee; tea; decaffeinated coffee, carbonated beverages; chocolate drinks made with pure cocoa powder; wine; distilled liquor
Meat and meat substitutes		Meat loaf and patties; cold cuts and prepared meats; sausage; stuffing; breaded meats; cheese foods and spreads; commercial soufflés, omelets, and fondues; soy protein meat substitutes	Pure meat, fish, fowl, egg, cottage cheese, cheeses, and peanut butter
Fat and oil		Commercial salad dressing and mayonnaise, gravy, white and cream sauces, non-dairy creamer	Butter, margarine, vegetable oil
Milk	Milk beverages that contain malt	Commercial chocolate milk	Whole, low-fat, and skim milk; buttermilk
Grains and grain products	Bread, crackers, cereal, and pasta that contain wheat; oats; rye; malt and malt flavoring; graham flour, durum flour, pastry flour; bran or wheat germ; barley; millet; pretzels; communion wafers	Commercial seasoned rice and potato mixes, commercial corn, rice, and potato snacks	Specially prepared breads made with wheat starch[c], rice, potato, or soybean flour, or cornmeal; pure corn or rice cereals; hominy grits; white, brown, and wild rice; popcorn; low-protein pasta made from wheat starch
Vegetable		Commercial seasoned vegetable mixes; commercial vegetables with cream or cheese sauce; canned baked beans	All fresh vegetables; plain commercially frozen or canned vegetables
Fruit		Commercial pie fillings	All plain or sweetened fruits; fruit thickened with tapioca or cornstarch
Soup	Soup that contains wheat pasta; soup thickened with wheat flour or other gluten-containing grains	Commercial soup, broth, and soup mixes	Soup thickened with cornstarch, wheat starch, or potato, rice, or soybean flour; pure broth

TABLE 12-25 Sources of Gluten[a] (continued)

Food Groups	Foods that Contain Gluten	Foods that may Contain Gluten	Foods that do *Not* Contain Gluten
Desserts	Commercial cakes, cookies, and pastries; commercial dessert mixes	Commercial ice cream and sherbet	Gelatin; custard; fruit ice; specially prepared cakes, cookies, and pastries made with gluten-free flour or starch; pudding and fruit filling thickened with tapioca, cornstarch, or arrowroot flour; some commercial ice creams
Sweets		Commercial candies, especially chocolates	
Miscellaneous		Catsup; prepared mustard; soy sauce; commercially prepared meat sauces and pickles; vinegar; flavoring syrups (syrups for pancakes or ice cream)	Monosodium glutamate; salt; pepper; pure spices and herbs; yeast; pure baking chocolate or cocoa powder; flavoring extracts; artificial flavoring

[a]The terms *commercially prepared* and *commercial* are used to refer to partially prepared foods purchased from a grocery or food market and to prepared foods purchased from a restaurant.
[b]Check up-to-date lists of gluten-free commercial products.
[c]Wheat starch may contain trace amounts of gluten. Avoid if not tolerated.
Data from *Mayo Clinic Diet Manual*. 6th ed. Toronto: BC Decker, 1988.

Although many foods carry a "gluten-free" label, not all such foods when tested have been found to contain less than 20 ppm of gluten (238). The risk of ingesting such foods labeled as "gluten-free" is not high (18 per 10,000 patients), but it is finite (239). Moreover, not all methods to detect gliadin fragments also detect glutenin and its fragments.

The FDA in 2007 released a proposed rule for GF labeling of foods (240). In this proposed rule, a food labeled GF
- Will not contain an ingredient that is derived from a prohibited grain and has not been processed to remove gluten, for example, wheat germ, wheat bran, barley malt, malt vinegar
- Can contain an ingredient derived from a prohibited grain only if the final product contains less than 20 ppm of gluten
- This definition has been confirmed in the gluten-free label guidelines suggested by the FDA in 2013 (see Appendix B).

2. Read labels carefully. Avoid products that contain wheat, rye, barley, oats, unspecified flour or starch, emulsifiers, stabilizers, hydrolyzed plant/vegetable protein, vegetable monoacylglycerols or diacylglycerols, and natural flavorings. Other grains that might contain gluten include faro, spelt, kamut, farina, emmer, and triticate (wheat + rye). Some of these products may in fact be GF, but the absence of gluten should be verified with an up-to-date GF product list, or the company should be contacted. Wheat-free is not the same as GF. Any multi-ingredient product has the potential to be contaminated with gluten.

3. The foods most likely to contain glutens include cereal beverages (beer, Ovaltine), some commercial ice creams, commercial cakes and cookies, salad dressings, canned or processed meats, soups, candy bars, catsups, mustards, frozen foods with sauces, processed cheeses, chocolate milk, cream soups, most soy sauces, and breaded, creamed, or scalloped vegetables. Other foods that might contain gluten include thickeners, syrup, malt cereals or beverages, colorings, icings, and frostings (241). An additive that has created some confusion is "meat glue" or a microbial analog of tTG that binds proteins together and gives shape to processed meats. This product in pure form (e.g., Activa RM, Ajinomoto) contains no known gluten, and the enzyme is inactivated by cooking. The FDA does not require food companies to list this microbial tTG, because the product is considered a "processing aid." When it is listed, it is called "TGP enzyme," or "enzyme," or meats are called "formed" or "reformed." It is probable that the products are GF, but as with all multicomponent products, checking with the manufacturer is a useful precaution.
4. Products made from cornmeal, cornstarch, corn flour, rice, rice flour, tapioca, soybean, potato starch, or arrowroot may be used. For baking, 1 cup of wheat flour may be replaced by 1 cup of corn flour, 1 cup of fine cornmeal, 3/4 cup of coarse cornmeal, 10 tbsp of potato flour, or 14 tbsp of rice flour. For thickening, 1 tbsp of wheat flour can be substituted with 1/2 tbsp of cornstarch, potato flour, rice, or arrowroot starch or 2 tbsp of quick-cooking tapioca.
5. Fresh meats, milk, fish, eggs, fresh vegetables, and fruits are all acceptable.

A low-lactose diet may be needed in the early stages of treatment if lactose intolerance is present.

Over-the-counter and prescription medications and vitamin/mineral supplements may contain gluten (starch, dextrins, etc.) as an inert component in the capsule or coating, or mixed with the medication itself. Products made with generic ingredients should be avoided unless the manufacturer can confirm the source of the product components.

Specific Recommendations
Patient-Support Groups. Each of these groups can provide recipes, lists of GF commercial products, and information on gluten content in medications.

CSA/USA (Celiac Sprue Association)
PO Box 31700, Omaha, NE 68131-0700
Tel: 402-558-0600, url: www.csaceliacs.org.

The website contains useful information on grains and flours, GFDs, and lactose intolerance.

Gluten Intolerance Group of North America
15110 10th Ave SW, Suite A, Seattle, WA 98166
Tel: 206-246-6652, url: www.gluten.net.
Celiac Disease Foundation
13251 Ventura Blvd, Suite 1, Studio City, CA 91604-1838
Tel: 818-990-2354, url: www.celiac.org
Coeliac Society of the United Kingdom (www.coeliac.co.uk)
Canadian Celiac Association
5170 Dixie Road, Suite 204, Mississauga, ON L4W1E3, Canada
Tel: 905-507-6208, url: www.celiac.ca
North American Society for Pediatric Gastroenterology, Hepatology, and Nutrition
www.naspghan.org
www.glutenfreeliving.com
Recipe search site: www.totalrecipesearch.com

GF Cookbooks. Many large retail bookstores have such books. Several available online include
The Gluten-Free Cookbook. Heather Whinney, DK Books, 2012Good Food: Gluten Diet Recipes, S Cook, BBC Publications, 2012

Safe Commercial Products. The new Food Allergen and Consumer Protection Act of January 1, 2006, should be helpful to consumers. If any product contains one of the top eight allergens (milk, egg, soybean, tree nuts, peanuts, shell fish, fish, or wheat), the ingredient must be clearly identified on the label. However, the new law does not require foods with barley or rye to be identified. Among the many foods that often contain offending glutens, it is possible to select products that are safe. Therefore, another brand name should not be substituted for one known to be GF unless it, too, is known to be GF. The Celiac UPC database (www.brandbeach.com/celiac/upc/index.html) has been created to help patients with CD determine whether a product is GF according to the product's UPC code. The database can be used online or on a handheld personal computer. For a "complete" list of products, one of the patient-support groups can also be contacted. The chain health food store, Wild Oats, maintains a GF product guide (www.wildoats.com). An approach to providing effective education and resources for patients emphasizes the overlooked sources of gluten, and provides many book titles, magazines and newsletters, cookbooks, travel and dining resources, and other helpful items (242). Useful websites for obtaining grain substitutes include www.arrowheadmills.com, www.thebirkettmills.com, www.bobsredmill.com, www.quinoa.com, and www.wholegrainscouncil.org.

Gluten in Drug Products. Gluten is often added as an "inert" filler in tablets, capsules, and suspensions. Possible gluten sources in medications include unspecified starch (pregelatinized, starch glycolate, grain flour, dextrates and dextrins, dextrimaltose or caramel coloring, maltodextrins, and starch derivatives). Most major manufacturers do not use gluten. The CSA/USA has a listing of relevant pharmaceuticals.

Gluten When Eating Out. The physician/dietitian should be able to assist patients in eating out in restaurants. The factors to keep in mind are the gluten content of the foods, how they have been prepared, and whether they might have come into contact with any source of gluten. The patient should announce that they have an allergy to wheat, and then ask whether the food has been marinated in soy sauce, teriyaki sauce, or Worcestershire sauce, whether it has been dusted with flour before pan-frying, whether it was cooked in oil or a utensil that was also used to cook breaded products, whether there are croutons in the salad, and whether artificial products that might contain gluten are used, such as mashed potato mix, seitan (meat substitute), imitation crabmeat, or artificial bacon. Menu terms that include flour include au gratin, béchamel, a la meuniere, encrusted, dusted, fricassee, fritter, gnocchi, gravy, roux, scallopini, tempura, and veloute. Terms that include soy sauce (unlikely to be GF) include marinade and teriyaki sauce.

Side Effects
The gluten-restricted diet can be well balanced for all nutrients and so no side effects are associated. However, such diets can be low in thiamin, riboflavin, and niacin, and in fiber, because of the restriction in intake of grains, so attention should be paid to these aspects of the diet.

Supplements Required
No supplements are needed unless the malabsorption has caused specific deficiencies or unless the lactose intolerance is permanent and calcium supplements are required. CD is an important cause of osteoporosis, and adequate calcium (1,200 mg per day) and vitamin D (400 IU) must be provided to restore bone density in patients whose axial bone density is decreased.

Low-Oxalate Diet

Principles
Hyperoxaluria resulting from an increased absorption of dietary oxalate occurs in disorders in which bile acids are poorly absorbed, enter the colon, and increase its permeability (161). The degree of oxaluria in such cases is inversely correlated with the degree of fat absorption. The excessive free fatty acids in the lumen of the small bowel that result from fat malabsorption bind calcium, which is then not available to form the insoluble calcium oxalate salt. Consequently, the more soluble sodium oxalate forms and is absorbed in the colon. However, only about 10%

of the body oxalate is normally derived from the diet. Therefore, a low-oxalate diet is not always effective in reducing hyperoxaluria.

Indications

This diet is used in cases of *hyperoxaluria* (>40 mg per day). Hyperoxaluria develops in a subset of patients with renal stones (idiopathic hyperoxaluria) and in patients with *steatorrhea* resulting from *bile acid malabsorption* (e.g., SBS). The diet can begin before calcium oxalate stones have formed. After the diet has been started, urinary excretion should be remeasured to ascertain that the diet is effective.

Calcium supplements often must be added in cases of SBS because poor calcium absorption and a negative calcium balance can lead to osteopenia. When luminal calcium is increased, the calcium oxalate salt may reform and the hyperoxaluria decrease without use of the diet. In some instances, both treatments are given together.

Practical Aspects

The low-oxalate diet is often part of the regimen of patients requiring a *low-fat diet*. In evaluating the progress of a patient on a restrictive diet, one should determine the patient's compliance. General guidelines for reducing the risk of developing renal stones have been provided by the American Dietetic Association's *Nutrition Care Manual* (243). The oxalate content of foods varies according to soil conditions, ripeness of the food, and processing. There are differences in analytic methods as well that make it difficult to provide precise values for food. With these caveats, a full listing of oxalate content of selected foods is available from the General Clinical Research Center, University of California, San Diego Medical Center (Brzezinski E, Durning AM. Oxalate content of selected foods with recipes and menu suggestions. 2002). To order, call 800/520-7323.

Foods High in Oxalate

Certain snack foods are high in oxalates, such as cola beverages, nuts, potatoes, tea, and foods containing chocolate. Meats and dairy products are generally low in oxalate. Only recently has the oxalate content of flours been published, and it is clear that whole-grain wheat, especially durum wheat, has a high oxalate content (244). Foods with a very high content (>10 mg per serving) should be avoided completely. A detailed listing of the oxalate content of foods can be found in standard diet manuals and nutrition textbooks (1,2,245). The following paragraphs indicate the oxalate content of selected foods.

Foods very high in oxalate (>10 mg per serving): spinach, rhubarb, cocoa, chocolate, tea, Ovaltine, beer, peanut butter, green beans, beets, Swiss chard, collards, kale, eggplant, sweet potatoes, blueberries, Concord grapes, strawberries, raspberries, fruit cocktail, wheat germ, wheat bran, whole-grain wheat bread or other whole wheat grain products, pepper (>1 tsp per day), turmeric, tomato soup, nuts (especially peanuts, pecans, walnuts, almonds). Indian or Chinese teas made from *Camellia sinensis* are rich in oxalate; herbal teas, which are not true teas but derived from other plant sources, contain much less oxalate (175).

Foods moderately high in oxalate (2 to 20 mg per serving): parsley, turnip greens, brussels sprouts, tomatoes, lima beans, lettuce, corn, broccoli, figs, oranges, cola beverages, juices (orange, tomato, grape), apple, pear, pineapple, sardines.

Side Effects

None.

Supplements Required

None.

Elimination Diets for Allergy or Intolerance to Foods

Principles

Food Allergy and Intolerance

The Committee on Adverse Reactions to Foods of the American Academy of Immunology defines *food allergy* as a reaction to a specific food that is mediated by classic immune mechanisms (246,247). These definitions and guideline for diagnosis and management of food allergy have

TABLE 12-26　Classification of Food-Induced Reactions

IgE–Mediated	Not IgE–Mediated	Food Intolerance	Food Aversion
Urticaria/angioedema	Dermatitis herpetiformis	Lactose/sucrose	Chronic fatigue
Atopic dermatitis	Contact dermatitis	Fructose/sorbitol dermatitis	Irritable bowel
Rhinoconjunctivitis	Celiac disease	Histamine (scombroid)	Depression
Oral allergy syndrome	Eosinophilic enteritis	Bacterial enterotoxins	Phobias
Anaphylaxis	Heiner syndrome	Plant/phytotoxins syndrome[a]	ADHD
Food protein enteropathies	Migraine headaches	Food additives	IBD, flatus

[a]Heiner syndrome is milk-induced alveolitis and hemorrhagic gastroenteritis in infants.
ADHD, attention-deficit hyperactivity disorder; IBD, inflammatory bowel disease.

been summarized by a consensus panel of experts for the National Institute of Allergy and Infectious Diseases (NIAID) (248). Summaries of these guidelines are available on line for use by practitioners, dietitians, and nurses (http://www.niaid.nih.gov/topics/foodallergy/clinical/documents/faguidelinesexecsummary.pdf). In the absence of evidence of classic immune mechanisms, it is better to refer to such a reaction as *food intolerance* (Table 12-26). Even in the latter case, the food should provoke a clear reaction that recurs each time the food is eaten. This sequence is lacking in many cases of so-called food intolerance.

True Allergic Reactions to Food

Allergic reactions to food, which occur infrequently in adults, are most often caused by fruit juices, tree nuts, peanuts, chocolate, milk, eggs, soy, wheat, and shellfish (249). Onset of symptoms is rapid, and severe reactions can result. The organs usually affected are the skin (~45%), respiratory tract (~25%), and gastrointestinal tract (~20%). In the oral allergy syndrome, the most common form, early symptoms develop within minutes of ingestion and include swelling of the lips, tingling in the throat, and rhinorrhea. Later symptoms (developing within 2 hours of ingestion) may include asthma, urticaria, eczema, vomiting, diarrhea, abdominal pain, headache, and general malaise. Allergens can be inhaled as well as ingested (e.g., flour, spices, egg white, steam produced when legumes or crustaceans are cooked), and inhalation leads to respiratory symptoms.

Diagnostic Tests

The best diagnostic test for suspected food allergy is the controlled double-blind food challenge (250). Tests that identify immunoglobulin G (IgG) antibodies (e.g., radioallergosorbent test, enzyme-linked immunosorbent assay) do not prove the presence of an IgE immune complex. Allergies are more common in children because their IgE levels are much higher than those of adults. For this reason, most of the diagnostic procedures have been validated and used most extensively in children. Most reactions to fruits/juices disappear by age 3. Allergy to pollen-related food is the most common food allergy in adults in countries where tree pollen allergy is common. Primary pulmonary sensitization to pollen from trees, grasses, or herbs can give rise to food allergies when epitopes are shared. These cross-reactions lead most often to symptoms of the oral allergy syndrome and occur most often in patients with hay fever. Birch pollen proteins cross-react with proteins in apple, carrot, cherry, apricot, plum, and celery; ragweed pollen cross-reacts with melons; and grass pollen cross-reacts with peach, potato, tomato, and cherry (251). Because these proteins are labile, cooked fruits and vegetables do not produce symptoms. For example, natural latex dermatitis can be associated with food allergies to banana or avocado and birch pollen allergy can be associated with hazelnut or kiwi food allergy (246). The value of an elimination diet is that an offending food is identified by adding a single food at a time. This maneuver is necessary when the history does not provide the clue, and it can be used to identify allergies to both food additives and natural food components. The history remains the best means of identifying symptom complexes caused by true allergies.

Diagnosis

Foods

Foods most commonly implicated include milk, eggs, nuts, and shellfish. Less commonly involved are wheat, chocolate, cheese, soft fruits, and meat. Artificial coloring agents in addition to virtually all foods have been implicated in nonimmunologic adverse food reactions. One should remember the rules for food labeling when trying to determine the presence of a food allergen. The Food Allergen Labeling and Consumer Protection Act of 2004 (FALCPA) mandates that major food allergens be specifically declared on the label after January 1, 2006, for all FDA-regulated foods (252). Exemptions are raw agricultural commodities or ingredients specifically exempt from the definition of a major food allergen. A major food allergen is defined as an ingredient that contains protein derived from milk, egg, fish, crustacean shellfish, tree nuts, wheat, peanuts, or soybeans. To avoid confusion, the plain language name of the allergen must be used. Included in this labeling requirement are flavorings, colorings, or incidental additives.

Tests

If anaphylaxis occurs, no challenge should be given. If the response is mild, skin tests and food challenge may be used. Skin prick tests are recommended to assist in the identification of a food allergen, but should not be considered diagnostic (248). If the response is sporadic, a food diary may help. Double-blinded challenge may be needed because many patients are placebo reactors, and food intolerance is demonstrated in only a few of the adults in whom it is suspected (253). Both skin tests and radioallergosorbent tests give many false-positive results, and cross-reactions between allergens occur. The use of native food allergens seems to give better results than commercial extracts. Using native allergens, a large wheal diameter (e.g., 7 mm for egg, 8 mm for cow's milk) appears to be fairly specific (254). In most patients with IBS presenting with possible food allergy, symptom overreporting related to psychiatric disease may be a major cause of symptoms (255). Other tests have been suggested for diagnosis (249). These include radioallergosorbent tests for total serum IgE and allergen-specific IgE. Microdot arrays on chips can reliably identify antibodies against food allergens for those patients who have IgE–mediated allergy (256). Food allergen–specific IgE serum concentrations have been correlated with the outcome of food challenge tests to develop diagnostic decision-making cutoff values for a few allergens (e.g., peanut, egg, milk, and fish), but these values vary among authors and populations (257). Atopy patch tests (APTs) involve the application of intact protein allergens in a patch directly onto the skin. The test is quite reliable for some allergens, less so for others. The European Task Force on Atopic Dermatitis has developed a standardized APT technique (258), but the test is still not as well validated as the other tests. The NIAID consensus panel does not recommend the use of any of these tests for routine use, and it recommends against the use of skin prick, serum IgE, and APTs in combination to make a diagnosis of food allergy (248).

Double-Blinded Oral Control Challenge

This is the "gold standard" but is difficult to carry out in clinical practice and can be dangerous if anaphylaxis is suspected. It is usually more convenient to use an open or single-blinded food challenge. Both negative and positive results are highly predictive of the correct answer. When a positive allergic history is present or a food allergy is strongly suspected, an *elimination diet* can be tried. This diet is usually reserved for patients having daily or almost daily symptoms.

Non-IgE–Mediated Immunologic Adverse Reactions to Food

IgE–mediated reactions to food are usually immediate, whereas non–IgE and mixed reactions are chronic or at least delayed. The most common conditions are eosinophilic gastrointestinal diseases and allergic contact dermatitis. The most commonly encountered eosinophilic gastrointestinal (GI) disease is eosinophilic esophagitis (EoE), but this must be distinguished carefully from gastrointestinal reflux disease (GERD) by endoscopic appearance and degree of eosinophilia in blood and tissue (259). Both disorders can respond to proton-pump inhibition (PPI), so the response to PPIs cannot be diagnostic by itself (260). In most patients with EoE, an offending food can be identified by standard screening tests and elimination diets (261,262). Elimination of six common food proteins (cow's milk, soy, wheat, egg, peanut, and seafood) can relieve symptoms and improve esophageal histology (263).

Food elimination based on the presence of IgG antibodies in patients with IBS and migraine has been suggested by positive results from RCTs (264,265). However, subsequent trials in both disorders have not confirmed these results (266,267). Because other studies have not validated the use of IgG antibodies to foods as a diagnostic method for food allergy, it is better to rely on blinded elimination trials to diagnose food allergy in those non–IgE–mediated conditions that are not known to be associated with food allergies.

Practical Aspects
True Food Allergies (Adults)
The strictest diet, which is rarely needed, consists of lamb, rice, dry puffed rice, salt, and water for 5 to 7 days. One new food is then added each day, with relatively nonallergenic foods usually added first. Allergenic foods such as milk, eggs, wheat, and corn are finally added. No fat can be added to any prepared food. Salt or baking soda must be used to brush the teeth (246).

A less-strict initial diet (modified from Golbert TM. In: Patterson R, ed. *Allergic Diseases.* Philadelphia: JB Lippincott Co, 1972:362) allows the following foods and beverages (all fruits and vegetables *must be cooked*): lamb, poi, rice, rice cereals, water, pineapple, apricot, cherries, blueberries, lettuce, artichokes, beets, spinach, celery, sweet potatoes, salt, sugar, and tapioca. Any vegetable oil is allowed except oleomargarine and soy oil. Mazola margarine contains no milk and is acceptable. Specific foods to be avoided include pork, beef, fish and seafood, eggs, milk and milk products, and baked goods made with wheat, oats, corn, or rye flour. Also to be avoided are butter, margarine, tea, coffee, cola, soft drinks, chewing gum, alcohol, and chocolate. This diet may be more useful for outpatient use. Egg is often hidden in such foods as pastries, ice creams, marshmallows, sausages, salad dressings, instant coffee, and root beer.

Another version of the elimination diet avoids the top food allergens in the 6 most common groups: dairy, eggs, soy, gluten, nuts/tree nuts, and fish/shellfish for 6 weeks (http://gitract.mngastro.com/mngi.nsf/patient_education/51CF8EC239EE571186257815006A1691/$File/Elimination%20Diet%208%2011.pdf). This diet is commonly used to manage EoE.

Addition of Other Foods. The patient is instructed to continue the basic diet for 5 to 7 days. On each successive day, a single cooked food is added. The patient keeps a diet diary and records the time foods are ingested, with any untold reactions. For those unable to begin with such a strict diet, the same basic diet can be used, with the following foods added: chicken, turkey, beef, boiled ham, bacon, potatoes, potato chips, carrots, soybeans, asparagus, maple syrup, ginger ale, plums, prunes, lentils, navy beans, and kidney beans. These are poorly allergenic foods that can be added in the early stages of an elimination diet. When foods must be added in double-blinded fashion, dried foods can be placed into gelatin capsules. A dose of 8 g of each food is commonly used.

Foods should be cooked in the strictest diets because heating can denature proteins and render them less allergenic. Patients with a history of severe (anaphylactic) reactions to eggs or chicken should be tested with intradermal extracts before receiving egg-derived vaccines.

Milk Allergy (Infants)
In infants with suspected milk allergy, formulas containing casein hydrolysates (e.g., Pregestimil, Nutramigen, Alimentum) work well. Because 20% of milk-allergic patients react to soy protein, soy-based formulas are not suggested.

Oral Immunotherapy (Food Desensitization)
Evidence for the usefulness of this method in treating food allergy is generally lacking, particularly because reactions to low doses are not uncommon, and the nature of reactions are unpredictable (268). The NIAID consensus panel does not recommend immunotherapy to treat food allergy (248).

Elimination Diet for Intolerance to Foods
A low-lactose diet for lactose intolerance is discussed separately in this chapter. The other intolerance most commonly encountered is to gas-producing foods (primarily flatus). Although it is not clear that gas production or the perception of gas production is related to the intake of

TABLE 12-27 Foods to be Avoided in a Diet for Gassy Food Intolerance (Elimination on a Trial Basis)

Class	Examples
High-lactose foods	Dairy products
Vegetables	Legumes (beans, peas, lentils)
	Cruciferous vegetables (broccoli, cauliflower, brussels sprouts)
	Root vegetables (radishes, onion, rutabaga), cabbage, kohlrabi, cucumber, sweet peppers
Fruits	Prunes, apples, raisins, bananas
Grains	Whole wheat bread, bran cereals
Fatty foods	Fried foods, cream sauces, gravies
Artificial sweeteners	Fructose (soft drinks), sorbitol

specific foods, some foods undoubtedly contain oligosaccharides (e.g., stachyose, raffinose) or components of dietary fiber that escape digestion in the small bowel and are fermented in part in the colon. For the occasional patient with intolerance to gas-producing foods, an elimination diet can be suggested (269) (Table 12-27).

The enzyme **α-galactosidase (Beano)**, derived from a mold, is marketed with the claim that it prevents gas from occurring with a high fiber intake. The manufacturer recommends that three to eight drops of Beano be added to a food after it has cooled below 130°F. Some evidence indicates that the treatment may be effective (270).

Adverse Reactions to Food Additives

The same range of symptoms seen in food allergy can be caused by food additives. However, food allergies are much less common, and it may not be necessary to eliminate foods with troublesome additives from the diet completely. The mechanisms for many of the reactions are unknown but may be pharmacologic, toxic, or truly allergic. These reactions are most often to salicylates, tyramine, sulfites, food coloring, and monosodium glutamate (MSG).

- **Pharmacologic reactions:** caffeine (see earlier section in this chapter), MSG (headache, asthma), tyramine, phenylethylamine in chocolate (headache), nitrite and nitrates (headache), histamine-releasing foods such as egg white, strawberry, shellfish (anaphylactoid reaction), histamine poisoning from foods with high histamine content, such as tuna, mackerel, Swiss cheese, pickled cabbage, red wine (anaphylactoid reaction), sodium metabisulfite (asthma), and salicylates in candies. The reactions caused by histamine occur especially in subjects with a genetic defect in the metabolism of exogenous histamine (Maintz L, Novak N, Am J Clin Nutr 2007;85:1185).
- **Toxic reactions:** ethanol, acid juices (heartburn), toxins from infectious agents
- **Allergic reactions to common food chemicals:** tartrazine, menthol in breakfast cereals, candy, gum (urticaria), EDTA in mayonnaise and salad dressings (dermatitis), erythrosine in maraschino cherries and fruit cocktail, breakfast cereals (photosensitivity), sodium benzoate in catsup (purpura), quinine in tonic water, bitter lemon (purpura), sulfites

Side Effects
Care must be taken to provide a well-balanced diet, including foods from all basic groups.

Supplements Required
None.

Restricted Diets for Allergy or Intolerance to Food Additives

Salicylates/Tartrazine
The most common drug allergy for which an altered diet is important is salicylate hypersensitivity. Salicylates and tartrazine, a salicylate-related compound, can produce chronic urticaria in the sensitive patient. Most patients sensitive to aspirin also react to tartrazine.

Food Sources
Food sources of salicylates include many colas, Dr. Pepper, root beer, most carbonated soft drinks, many cereals and baked goods mixes, many fruits (apples, oranges, peaches, plums, cherries, grapefruit, berries), prepared meats, nondairy creamers, yogurt, ice cream, sherbet, most commercial dessert mixes, prepared pies and cakes, frostings, puddings, rolls, and candies. Methyl salicylate is commonly used as a flavoring agent under the name *wintergreen*. Candies containing wintergreen include gums, mints, and jelly beans. Cereals containing salicylate include breakfast squares and fruit turnover pastries. Tartrazine is included in many yellow and green candies, fruit crushes, and many antibiotic capsules and vitamin preparations.

Salicylate or Tartrazine-Free Foods
Included in this category are milk and milk products, most vegetables (except cucumbers, peppers, broccoli, asparagus, okra, spinach, squash, sweet potato, zucchini, and tomatoes), all fish, red meat, cheese, eggs, poultry, pasta, rice, white potatoes, most breads, all fats, sugar, syrup, and molasses. A more complete list of foods allowed has been published (271).

Supplements Required
A salicylate-free diet is adequate for all nutrients except vitamin C. Supplements (60 mg per day) can be provided for such patients.

Tyramine
Population at Risk
Patients taking monoamine oxidase inhibitors are at risk for the development of headache, palpitations, nausea, vomiting, and in some cases hypertensive crises if they ingest sympathomimetic drugs (methyl dopa, L-dopa, dopamine, epinephrine, ephedrine) or foods with a high concentration of tyramine. Tyramine is a biogenic amine derived from tyrosine metabolism. Inhibition of tyramine metabolism can cause hypertensive crises, which begin 30 to 60 minutes after the offending food is ingested, with headache, palpitations, nausea, and vomiting. At high doses (60 mg per kg of body weight), tyramine can cause cardiac arrhythmias, with a loss of P waves, atrial ectopies, ventricular and atrial premature beats, junctional rhythm, bigeminy, and Wenckebach phenomenon (272). It is not known whether the intake of tyramine-rich foods should be decreased in patients with arrhythmias.

Drugs That Inhibit Monoamine Oxidase
Included in this widely distributed complex enzyme system are furazolidone (Furoxone), isocarboxazid (Marplan), phenelzine sulfate (Nardil), procarbazine (Matulane), selegiline HCl (Eldepryl), transdermal selegiline (Emsam), linezolid (Zyvox) and tranylcypromine (Parnate). Patients taking these drugs should also refrain from taking medications containing sympathomimetic drugs, especially nose drops and cold capsules, and most antidepressant medications.

Restricted-Tyramine Diet
A restricted-tyramine diet should be followed by patients taking these drugs, as they may be intolerant of ingested tyramine. The details of this diet, which provides less than 2 mg of tyramine per day, are listed in Table 12-28. Usually, more than 6 mg of tyramine must be ingested to cause symptoms when it cannot be metabolized. Cheeses with the highest content of tyramine (>200 mg per g in some cheeses) are cheddar, Camembert, and Stilton. Most tyramine-rich foods are not components of hospital diets, so the restrictions are more appropriate for patients ingesting free-choice diets (273).

Sulfites
Uses and Abundance
Six sulfiting agents have been declared safe by the FDA. These chemicals are listed on labels as sulfur dioxide, sodium sulfite, sodium and potassium bisulfite, and sodium and potassium metabisulfite. Sulfites are widely used in the processing of wine and beer and in restaurants to maintain the crispness and freshness of salads, fruits, and potatoes. They are also used for bleaching food starches and in producing cellophane for food packaging. The FDA prohibits the use of sulfites in foods that are important sources of thiamine because they destroy the vitamin.

TABLE 12-28 Restricted-Tyramine Diet

Food Group	Unrestricted Foods (<5 µg/g)	Foods Allowed in Moderation (5–20 µg/g)	Foods to Avoid (>20 µg/g)
Cheese	Cottage cheese, ricotta, cream cheese	Processed American cheese, Gouda	Aged cheeses—brick, blue, cheddar, Camembert, Swiss, Romano, Roquefort, Stilton, mozzarella, Parmesan, provolone, Emmentaler, boursin, sour cream, Brie
Beverages	Milk	Coffee, hot chocolate, cola drinks (1–3 cups per day)	Ale, beer, sherry, red and white wines[a], yogurt, bouillon
Meats	Fresh or fresh-frozen meat, poultry		Canned meats, chicken liver, beef liver, fermented (hard) sausage or salami, pepperoni, summer sausage, bologna, Genoa salami
Fish	Fresh or fresh-frozen fish or shellfish		Salt herring, dried fish, caviar, pickled herring
Vegetables	Most		Italian flat beans, Chinese pea pods, broad (fava) beans, mixed Chinese vegetables, eggplant
Fruit	Most		Figs, avocados
Miscellaneous			Chocolate, soy sauce, protein extracts, yeast concentrates or products made with them

[a]Fermentation of wine and beer does not ordinarily involve processes that result in the production of tyramine. Despite this, levels in beer are variable. The production of appreciable amounts of tyramine in red wines results from contamination with other than the usual fermenting organisms and from the inclusion of grape pulp and seeds in the process. These potential sources of amino acids are not used in making white wines. Because of the unpredictable variability in tyramine levels, all the beverages listed are generally excluded (*Med Lett Drugs Ther.* 1976;18:32).

In 1986, the FDA also banned the use of sulfites in fruits and vegetables meant to be eaten raw. Sulfite sensitivity can develop even in persons without an allergic history, and it is not certain that all reactions are mediated by allergy. Symptoms include wheezing, hives, nausea, and diarrhea. Rarely, anaphylaxis may occur. With increased awareness and restricted use, adverse reactions to sulfites are now relatively uncommon. Updated information can be obtained from the FDA website (http://vm.cfsan.fda.gov/~dms).

Foods containing sulfites are so common that the average person ingests 2 to 3 mg per day, and when beer or wine is included in the diet, this figure can reach 5 to 10 mg per day. Foods frequently preserved with sulfites include instant tea, beer, wine, wine coolers and spirits, dried citrus fruit beverage mixes, condiments and relishes, confections and frostings, canned soups, dried mixes, seafood (especially shrimp), baked goods, processed and dried fruits, gelatin, puddings and fillings, jams and jellies, corn and maple syrup, molasses, breading, batters, noodle mixes, and processed vegetables (vegetable juices; canned, pickled, dried vegetables; potato chips).

Treatment is complicated by the widespread presence of the chemical, which makes the problem difficult to diagnose before the episode is complete. Moreover, several treatments for acute allergic response may contain potassium metabisulfite as a preservative, especially epinephrine and some IV solutions and medications. Terbutaline can be used safely in such a situation.

Monosodium Glutamate

Use in Foods

MSG is the sodium salt of glutamic acid. It is made by fermenting starch, sugar beets, sugar cane, or molasses and is used to enhance flavor, perhaps by stimulating glutamate receptors on the tongue. Foods labeled "no MSG" may in fact contain hydrolyzed protein, a source of free glutamate. Some products containing protein hydrolysates with substantial amounts of glutamate are labeled "contains glutamate."

Safety

MSG has been classified as GRAS, but because of its presumed role in "MSG syndrome" and asthma attacks, its use is subject to repeated review by the FDA, American Medical Association, European Communities, and WHO. All have found the additive to be safe. The most recent FDA/Federation of Associated Societies of Experimental Biology (FASEB) review (1995) concluded that a symptom complex may develop in an unknown percentage of people after the ingestion of 3 g or more of MSG without other food (http://vm.cfspan.fda.gov/~lrd). Most food servings contain no more than 0.5 g of MSG. The syndrome includes burning and numbness in the neck and arms, chest pain, facial pressure, headache, nausea, tachycardia, weakness, and bronchospasm in patients with asthma. However, no evidence for causation of other medical illnesses has been documented.

Benzoate–Cinnamon–Free Diet

Patients with orofacial granulomatosis (OFG) present with swelling of the lips primarily, but also of the gingivae, buccal mucosa, floor of the mouth, and other parts of the oral cavity. Unlike the usual orofacial presentation of food allergy, this condition also has chronic inflammatory changes in those sites. Common allergens on patch testing in this condition include cinnamon, cinnamaldehyde, chocolate, food additives, perfumes and flavorings, and benzoate. Benzoate is a common preservative, and occurs naturally in many foods, especially fruits. Cinnamic aldehyde, a constituent of cinnamon, is one of the compounds lending the typical odor and flavor to the spice, and is used as flavoring in mixed spices, soft drinks, chewing gum, ice cream, cakes, toothpaste, and mouthwashes. A diet free of these compounds provides benefit in 54% to 78% of patients, but gave complete relief in only about one-quarter of patients (274). The benzoate–cinnamon–free diet includes avoidance of dishes using products including benzoate or cinnamon, for example, dishes with a spicy sauce, many ready-to-eat meals, fruits (many of which are naturally high in benzoate), bleached-flour pasta, fats with hydrolyzed lecithin (requiring preservative), tea, some carbonated beverages, tartar-control toothpaste, some mouthwashes, mixed spice, allspice, curry powder, cinnamon, and chocolate. The mouth and oral cavity are exposed to many antigens aside from the diet, including those in drugs, cosmetics, toothpastes, microorganisms, and dental filling materials. It would not be surprising if other allergens are identified that contribute to symptoms in this condition. Cinammon and benzoate are phenolic acids, but the diet free of these components may still contain related polyphenols that are degraded to phenolic acids in the gut. Thus, a more restrictive diet low in phenolic acid (supplemented with micronutrients) has been tried in a small number of patients with a suggestion of better long-term response (275). This diet avoids yogurts, blue-veined cheeses, potatoes, wholemeal grain products, butter, margarine, vegetable oils, fruit juices, flavored waters, red wine, beer, dried fruit, most jams and foods with added flavorings. Thus, it will be difficult diet to follow.

Low-Sodium Diet

Principles

Disorders in which sodium retention or hypertension is a prominent feature are treated with a low-sodium diet. The usual intake of sodium in a Western-style diet is greatly in excess of daily needs. Moreover, many processed foods contain sodium (see Chapter 7). Therefore, the diet seems quite restrictive. When sodium is retained, the ability to excrete excess ingested sodium is limited. The less sodium ingested, the easier the task of removing excess sodium from the body. Potassium salts are often used to replace sodium. A high-sodium diet alone will not cause hypertension in an otherwise normotensive person. Thus, the diet is probably not needed to prevent hypertension.

Indications

A low-sodium diet is used in the management of *acute and chronic congestive heart failure, chronic hepatic failure with ascites, acute and chronic renal failure,* and *hypertension*. Less often, it may be indicated when the administration of exogenous corticosteroids causes salt retention in women with premenstrual edema. A low-sodium diet is often used together with diuretic agents. In certain cases, only one or the other of these therapies is necessary. In disorders associated with sodium retention and low levels of urinary sodium, the diet may be very important. In many cases of hypertension, drug therapy, perhaps in conjunction with mild sodium restriction, may be more useful, with better patient compliance. Convincing data support the effectiveness in controlling all-cause and CV mortality, and in lowering blood pressure and catecholamine levels and improving renal function (276,277).

The American Heart Association has developed guidelines for diet-related lifestyle modifications that are useful in lowering blood pressure (278). These include weight loss to achieve a normal BMI, reduced salt intake, DASH–type dietary patterns, increased potassium intake, and moderation of alcohol intake. Salt (sodium chloride) intake is to be lowered as much as possible, ideally to approximately 65 mmol per day of sodium (1.5 g per day of sodium or 3.8 g per day of sodium chloride). The DASH diet includes a rich supply of fruits and vegetables (8 to 10 servings per day) and low-fat dairy products (2 to 3 servings per day), while it is reduced in fat and cholesterol. Potassium intake should be increased to 120 mmol per day (4.7 g per day), the level provided in DASH–like diets. Alcohol intake is suggested at no more than two drinks per day for men, and one for women.

It is not a single dietary component that has the most influence on blood pressure, but the overall dietary pattern, as in the DASH diet. The DASH diet reduces systolic pressure by approximately 8 to 14 mm Hg, compared with a reduction of approximately 5 to 20 mm Hg for weight loss, and approximately 2 to 8 mm Hg for reduced sodium intake alone (279). The DASH diet shows the most efficacy in African Americans. Sympathetic tone increases with stimulation of the rennin–angiotensin–aldosterone system (RAAS), and is under the influence of salt intake. When the amount of urinary salt is accounted for (as a reflection of salt intake), polymorphisms of components of the RAAS show correlations with autonomic regulation of the CV system (280). These correlations are not yet far enough advanced to make genetic testing a practical addition to hypertension management, but that is the goal of the European Project on Genes in Hypertension (280).

Practical Aspects
General Instructions

1. The degree of sodium restriction required differs greatly among patients; a no-added-salt diet may suffice, or one that strictly limits salt-containing foods may be necessary.
2. Sodium is present in table salt, drinking water (depending on the source), medicines, and baked goods in which regular baking powder or soda is used. It is also present in foods seasoned with MSG; preserved with brine, sodium benzoate, or sodium sulfite; or processed with sodium hydroxide, sodium alginate, or sodium propionate.
3. Many products used in food preparation contain sodium. Products that should not be used in food preparation unless their sodium content is known include baking powder, baking soda, barbecue sauce, beverages (fruit-flavored mixes, many carbonated sodas), bouillon cubes, canned broth, catsup, celery salt, celery flakes, celery seed, chili sauce, consommé, garlic salt, horseradish (prepared), instant cocoa mixes, olives, onion salt, commercial gelatin (Jell-O), MSG, mustard (prepared), meat extract and sauces, meat tenderizers, molasses, parsley flakes, pickles, relishes, soy sauce, salad dressing, sodium saccharine, Worcestershire

sauce, rennet tablets, some salt substitutes, mayonnaise, bacon bits, maraschino cherries, and salted nuts.
4. The **sodium content** given for foods is approximate but much larger than usually appreciated. It is helpful to consider which foods are equivalent to a given amount of sodium. For example:

   50 mg of sodium: 1 tsp salted butter or margarine, 1/2 cup raw carrots, 1 1/2 tsp mayonnaise, one small egg, 1/2 cup ice cream or sherbet

   250 mg of sodium: 1 oz canned tuna, 2/3 cup buttermilk, 1/2 cup canned vegetables, five salted crackers, 1 1/2 tbsp salad dressing, one large strip of bacon, 1/2 cup cold cereal, 1/4 cup cottage cheese, one-eighth of a 9-in pie, two slices of bacon

   500 mg of sodium: 1/4 scant tsp salt, 3/4 tsp MSG, one-half bouillon cube, 2/3 cup canned tomato juice, one average-sized frankfurter, seven or eight green olives (small), 2 tsp regular soy sauce

   800 to 1,000 mg of sodium: one dill pickle, 1 cup canned vegetable soup (preparations vary)

5. **Sodium labeling.** The daily value for sodium is 2,400 mg in the United States.

   Sodium-free: <5 mg per serving

   Very low in sodium: ≤35 mg per serving

   Low in sodium: ≤140 mg per serving

   Light in sodium/lightly salted: ≤50% reduction in sodium per serving versus reference food

   Reduced in sodium or less sodium: ≤25% reduction in sodium per serving versus reference food

6. Cooking "from scratch" is usually the best way to prepare foods. Salt should not be added in cooking unless the patient can tolerate the added sodium. Patients should cook with oil or with unsalted butter or margarine.
7. Lemon juice, onion, red pepper, Tabasco sauce, and garlic are excellent substitute seasonings for meats and fish. See Table 7-10 for a list of other natural seasonings that can be substituted for salt to flavor foods.
8. Low-sodium baking powder is available in many stores that sell dietetic foods. If it is not available, the pharmacist can make it up with the following formula:

Potassium bicarbonate	39.8 g
Cornstarch	28.0 g
Tartaric acid	7.5 g
Potassium bitartrate	56.1 g

   If the patient is on a diet that limits potassium, excessive amounts of potassium-containing baking powder should not be ingested.
9. A large number of **cookbooks for low-sodium diets** are available in most retail bookstores. Two suggested titles are *American Heart Association Low-salt cookbook*, 4th edition, Clarkson Potter, 2013; and *No-salt, lowest-sodium cookbook*, Donald Gazzaniga, St Martin's Griffin, 2002. The recipes use small amounts of salt that can be replaced with a salt substitute. Many spices are included in the recipes, so that the replacement is relatively easy.

Specific Recommendations

1. Diets are ordered as salt (sodium chloride) or as sodium, which is about 40% of the weight of salt. Ordering *dietary prescriptions* by sodium content is more sensible because the "salt" content cannot actually be measured. The usual restrictions ordered are listed in Table 12-29.
2. Decrease the use of table salt and seasonings high in sodium (e.g., soy sauce, garlic salt, onion salt), and substitute herbs and other spices. If salt substitutes are used, make certain that the patient is not on medication that causes hyperkalemia (e.g., triamterene).
3. Limit intake of foods known to be high in sodium.

TABLE 12-29 Salt-Restricted Diets

Daily Intake (g)		Restrictions					
Sodium	Salt	Added Salt	Visibly Salted Items[a]	Processed Foods[b]	Milk, Bread[c]	Meat, Eggs	Practicality
5–6	12.5–15	Yes	Yes	Yes	Yes	Yes	Average US diet
4	10	No	Yes	Yes	Yes	Yes	Home use
3	7.5	No	No	Many	Yes	Yes	Home use
2	5.0	No	No	Few	Yes	Yes	Home use; needs cooperation
1	2.5	No	No	No	Salt-free bread	Yes	Needs great cooperation for home use
0.5	1.25	No	No	No	1 pt milk	4 oz meat, 1 egg	Hospital use

[a]Includes potato chips, pretzels, crackers or snacks, pickles, olives, and bacon.
[b]Includes most canned foods, dry cereals, prepared meats, ham, cheese, and prepared desserts.
[c]One hundred twenty milligrams of sodium per 8 oz of milk or 1 slice of bread.

4. Avoid less obvious sources of sodium, including foods that contain MSG, sodium saccharine, sodium nitrate (curing agent), and sodium benzoate (preservative). Some over-the-counter medications, such as antacids, laxatives, and sleeping pills, contain large quantities of sodium. For example, Alka-Seltzer effervescent antacid tablets contain 276 mg of sodium per tablet. Labels of over-the-counter products should be read carefully.
5. Modify recipes to include low-sodium ingredients—either prepared products labeled as such or fresh fruits, vegetables, meats, and fish. Particularly avoid canned products. Low-sodium cheese and peanut butter are available, as are unsalted crackers, low-sodium canned soups, and unsalted chips and popcorn.
6. When dining out, choose foods without sauces or gravies, use oil/vinegar dressing for salads, choose fresh fruit for dessert, and ask that no salt be added to individually prepared dishes (e.g., steak or fish). Avoid fast foods.

Side Effects

The low-sodium diet is not easy for some patients to follow because the intake of sodium in most Western diets is large. Care must be taken to maintain good protein intake. Because large amounts of fruits and vegetables are allowed, the intake of most vitamins and minerals is adequate. When a patient on a low-sodium diet also takes a diuretic, *hypokalemia* often develops. Potassium can be replaced by table foods or by medication (see Chapter 7).

Sodium depletion can develop in a patient on a low-sodium diet when urinary sodium losses are continuously high, as in chronic renal disease. Patients with obligatory sodium losses from ileostomies are also at risk for the development of sodium depletion if dietary sodium is restricted.

Supplements Required

Potassium may be needed if diuretics are used, but no other supplements are required.

Restriction of Serotonin-rich Foods

When a urinary collection for 5-hydroxyindoleacetic acid (5-HIAA) is ordered, the patient should not consume foods rich in serotonin or medications that react with the reagents used in the test. Foods to be avoided include avocado, bananas, butternut squash, eggplant, kiwi fruit, pecans, plantains, pineapple, plums, tomatoes, walnuts, and alcohol (281). Alcohol presumably stimulates the production of serotonin. Medications to be avoided are glyceryl guaiacolate, acetaminophen, and phenacetin; they interfere with the urinary and serum determinations.

Diet for Occult Blood Screening (Low-peroxidase Diet)

Screening for occult blood in stool is of proven efficacy. When standard low-sensitivity, peroxidase-based tests (e.g., Hemoccult) are used, the ingestion of red meat and uncooked peroxidase-rich plants (radish, turnip, broccoli) can produce false-positive results, although the effect is small. The low-meat diet and six mail-in stool sample cards are generally used, especially if the level of meat intake is high. The specificity of the available tests for routine fecal blood testing is affected by peroxidase-containing foods. The use of rehydrated Hemoccult or similar guaiac-impregnated cards increases the false-positive rate, and a low-peroxidase diet has been shown to reduce the false-positive rate from above 6% to 0.6% (161). Many clinicians have abandoned rehydrated guaiac techniques and ignore diet in their screening programs (282). However, a small increase in specificity can have a major impact on clinical decisions, so when outpatient screening for occult blood is performed, it seems prudent at the present time to recommend a meat-free, low-peroxidase diet when screening for CRC using guaiac-based tests (283).

A low-peroxidase diet is indicated when guaiac-containing cards are used to screen for colorectal neoplasms.

Practical Aspects
General Instructions

The low-peroxidase diet avoids red meat, raw or cooked. Although the peroxidase activity of most fruits and vegetables is destroyed completely by cooking at 100°C for 20 minutes, well-cooked red meat retains some activity. Because of the high level of peroxidase activity in red meat and uncertainty regarding how thoroughly cooked meat may be, all red meat is proscribed. Peroxidase-rich fruits and vegetables (categories 1 through 5, Table 12-30) are also eliminated.

Specific Recommendations

Foods in categories 1 to 5 (Table 12-29) are eliminated for 1 to 2 days before stool sampling begins and for 3 days consecutively, during which time one sample is collected per day. Aspirin-containing medications are not permitted, but it is not clear whether aspirin in modest doses increases fecal blood loss.

TABLE 12-30 Peroxidase Levels in Foods

Category	Peroxidase Activity[a] (mL of Blood Equivalent)	Food Items
1	>20	Broccoli, turnip[b]
2	10–20	Rare red meat, cantaloupe, cauliflower, red radish, parsnips
3	5–10	Bean sprouts, cucumber, green beans, mushrooms, parsley, zucchini, lemon rind
4	2–5	Grapefruit, carrot, cabbage, potato, pumpkin, fig
5	1–2	Peach, celery, lettuce, spinach, pickles
6	0.2–1.0	Blackberries, pineapple, watermelon, walnuts, sweet peppers
7	0.1–0.2	Banana, black grapes, pear, plum
8	<0.1	Well-cooked meat, apples, apricot, olives, raspberries
9	Peroxidase undetectable	Roast chicken, turkey, cooked fish, organ meats, pork, ham and bacon, white grapes, lemon, nectarine, orange, strawberries, tomato, raisins

[a]The peroxidase activity in 100 g of food is reported as the equivalent of "x" milliliters of blood.
[b]The data refer to uncooked vegetables. Adequate cooking destroys peroxidase activity.
Data from Caligore P, Macrae FA, St John DJ, et al. Peroxidase levels in food: relevance to colorectal cancer screening. *Am J Clin Nutr.* 1982;35:1487.

Vitamin K–Enriched Diet

Principle

Foods with a high content of vitamin K may interfere with the smooth control of anticoagulation. The dietary intake of vitamin K is only one of many factors influencing blood clotting in patients on long-term warfarin therapy. It is not clear whether the dietary intake of vitamin K is a significant factor because fecal flora produces the vitamin, and it can be absorbed in the colon.

Indication

This diet is used for patients receiving anticoagulant therapy when the regulation of anticoagulation is difficult or the patient is more resistant to warfarin therapy than expected.

Practical Aspects

All foods are allowed except those containing more than 100 mg of vitamin K per 100 g. These include broccoli, brussels sprouts, green or white cabbage, cauliflower, kale, lettuce, soybeans, spinach, turnip greens, beef liver or kidney, and pork liver. A more complete list of vitamin K content of foods can be found online, for example, htpp://www.inrtracker.com/resources/vitamin-k-foods.php.

Copper-Restricted Diet

Principle

Wilson disease is characterized by an increase in total body and hepatic copper. Treatment consists of a low copper intake plus chelating therapy. Other cholestatic liver diseases (e.g., primary biliary cirrhosis) are characterized by elevated levels of hepatic copper, but it is not clear that removal of copper alters the clinical course.

Indication

For patients with Wilson disease.

Practical Aspects

Milk, coffee, lemonade, carbonated beverages, and vanilla ice cream may be consumed freely. Regular table salt should be avoided. Analytic reagent-grade salt, available through the pharmacist, may be used as desired. Almost no foods are copper-free, so the more caloric and protein needs that can be met by low-copper foods, the better. A list of foods low in copper has been published (284). More recent lists of the copper content of foods in available online, for example, http://nutritiondata.self.com/foods. As Wilson disease is diagnosed earlier and effective drug therapy is used to create a negative copper balance, the strict use of low-copper diets becomes unnecessary. Obviously, the less copper ingested, the less drug theoretically needed to produce a negative copper balance, although this effect has not been quantified.

Fruit Juice and Drug Interactions

Grapefruit juice (but not other citrus juices), a good source of vitamin C, contains furanocoumarins (psoralens) that are competitive and mechanism-based inhibitors of the cytochrome P-450 isoform, CYP3A, and enhances the effect of some medications by down-regulating the intestinal cytochrome P-450 system, thereby increasing their bioavailability (285). Other citrus fruits also contain furanocoumarins, including pummelos and Seville oranges. Other juices have been investigated for drug–drug interactions, including cranberry, sweet orange, grape, pineapple, and pomegranate juice, but none have shown clear clinical inhibition (286). Pomegranate juice, like grapefruit juice, inhibits CYP3A4 and CYP2C9, but clinically significant interactions in humans have not yet been documented (286). Grapefruit, pummelo, and Seville orange juices are unique in that, when consumed in usual amounts, only enteric CYP3A is affected. However, the furanocoumarins cause an irreversible loss of enteric CYP3A protein, and the half-life of recovery is approximately 23 hours (3). Having said this, the vast majority of CYP3A substrate drugs have an AUC ratio after grapefruit juice ingestion that are below the cutoff value of 5.0 for "strong inhibition." In addition, when this ratio has been exceeded, it is usually with ingestion of greater than normal amounts of grapefruit juice, for example, three times a day of double-strength juice (285).

Other foods suspected to inhibit or induce intestinal CYP3A4 include red wine, broccoli, brussels sprouts, watercress, and cabbage (287). In general, ingestion of 200 to 250 mL of juice taken over a few days is needed to decrease enterocyte CYP3A4 activity, and this effect is greater in African Americans than in Caucasians (288). A partial list of medications that interacts with grapefruit juice include

- Calcium channel blockers: felodipine, nimodipine, nisoldipine, pranidipine
- Amiodarone
- Protease inhibitors: saquinavir
- Antihistamines: ebastine, loratadine, terfenadine
- Calcineurin antagonists: cyclosporine, tacrolimus
- HMG-CoA reductase inhibitors: atorvastatin, lovastatin, simvastatin
- Neuropsychiatric: buspirone, carbamazepine, clomipramine, diazepam, methadone, sertraline, trazolam, zaleplon
- Other: sildenafil, losartan
- See reference 288 for a more complete list.

Grapefruit juice also inhibits the drug transporters organic anion-transporting polypeptides (OATP) and P-glycoprotein, but by a different mechanism (289). The active ingredients are flavonoids, mostly naringin and hesperidin. Unlike the effect on CYP3A enzymes, the effect on transporters of the various juices in reversible and of short duration, with no effect noted after 4 hours of juice ingestion. In addition, this inhibition of transporters is seen with many other juices, including orange and apple juice (289). The effect on the OATP transporters might also have an effect in the liver as well, although data on this point are very limited in humans. The number of drugs reported to have reduced AUC values in the presence of grapefruit and other juices in limited, but includes atenolol, fexofenadine, and aliskiren (289). Many drugs are known substrates for OATP, but no data on low AUC have been reported for many of them, for example, statins (286).

Low-Purine Diet for Gout

Hyperuricemia is common, but most people with this finding do not have gout. Moreover, medical management of gout provides good prevention of acute attacks and their complications. Nonetheless, dietary components are risk factors for attacks, and diet is a component of gout prevention (290). Higher intake of meat, seafood, sugar-sweetened beverages, alcohol, and foods high in fructose increase the risk of a gout flare. Hypertension, diabetes, obesity, early menopause, and hyperuricemia also are risk factors. Diet may play an important role in gout prevention, but this section deals only with that dietary component that limits purine intake. It is not total purine content, but foods rich in the purine bases adenine and hypoxanthine that are uricogenic (291). Food lists that measure individual purine bases are few and limited, but confirm that most meat and fish contain higher levels of all purine bases (292). Hyoxanthine levels are dependent upon the freshness of meat and fish, and can double in amount after 10 to 20 days in storage (293,294).

Diets low in purines avoid foods with the highest purine content (>1,000 mg per 100 g portion) including organ meats, oily fish (e.g., anchovies, sardines, mackerel), meat extracts and gravies, and yeast extract (295,296). Food of moderate purine content (9 to 100 mg per 100 g portion) are allowed as one serving (203 oz per day), and include other meats (beef, lamb, portk) and other fish and shellfish, as well as legumes, mushrooms, asparagus, and cauliflower. Dairy products, most vegetables, cereals and breads, and juices are all allowed. More complete lists of purine content of foods are available online (297).

Diets for Selected Gastrointestinal Disorders

Inflammatory Bowel Disease

Enteral diets are useful in producing and maintaining remission in children with Crohn disease (298). The evidence is less compelling for adults or for patients of any age with UC. The rationale for the efficacy of elemental diets is not clear, but is presumed to improve the permeability of the bowel, providing decreased access of luminal antigens to the mucosa. Relapses of UC have been associated with intake of red meat, alcohol, and high sulfur/sulfate (299). However, the use of enteral nutrition (EN) in Crohn disease has not been shown superior to corticosteroids, not supporting the concept that "bowel rest" plus nutrition is a viable approach in adults (300). Thus, its use has been used mostly in children, in whom the diet is tolerated and the effects of corticosteroids on growth are avoided. Probiotics may have benefit, but the data are not yet sufficiently strong for recommendations (see Chapter 8, Probiotics). Use of diets in adults with IBD who do not have SBS is still empiric, and no standardized recommendations can be made at this time.

Acute Pancreatitis

The standard therapy for acute pancreatitis in the past was cessation of eating, to avoid the pain that was produced by food. However, because such patients are catabolic, starvation could worsen the course of the disease, and nutritional supplementation has been used extensively, at first by the parenteral route, but in recent years, by the enteral route. Meta-analyses of randomized trials show that EN leads to shorter hospital stays and lower infection rates than parenteral nutrition (301,302). Although these results seem clear, there are not enough data to determine whether EN improves overall outcome over standard therapy without artificial supplementation (203). There has been some suggestion of benefit from individual studies in which immune modulators (e.g., glutamine, arginine, and omega (ω)-3 PUFAs, were added to EN alone, but there are insufficient data to make specific recommendations. The mode (continuous or bolus) or site of delivery (gastric or jejunal) of the EN probably makes no difference in the clinical outcome. One randomized trial shows that mortality was nearly twice as high in the nasojejunal group, but the difference was not statistically significant (303).

Irritable Bowel Syndrome

The response of IBS patients to food is due to many factors. These include food intolerances (e.g., lactose) (304), food allergies (e.g., nuts), and possibly an alteration in bacterial flora with consequent changes in intestinal function (305). Diets containing yeast, milk, egg, wheat, and complex carbohydrates are often restricted in observational studies of diet in IBS, and these are foods that contain lactose or complex carbohydrates (FODMAPS) (see Low-Available-Carbohydrate Diet section, Chapter 12). The difficulty in determining the response to changes in diet or to food supplements resides in the overreporting of many IBS patients, related to somatization responses or multiple chemical sensitivity (306). None of these factors likely occurs in all patients with IBS, so it is difficult to predict whether dietary manipulation will improve symptoms in a consistent fashion. It is best to document as carefully as possible any food intolerance or allergy, but to expect only partial improvement to a dietary program that eliminates the offending agents. The traditional use of fiber to alleviate symptoms of IBS is not supported by most studies (307).

There is no diet that can be endorsed for IBS, but the patients are often convinced that diet is a key to their symptoms, probably because food ingestion increases gastrointestinal symptoms in any disease of the GI tract. It is probably best to follow the dietary and lifestyle advice provided by the British Dietetic Association, based on a comprehensive literature search (308). First-line treatment includes (a) establishment of a regular eating pattern and healthy-eating lifestyle, (b) maintenance of a high intake of noncaffeinated, noncarbonated, alcohol-free fluids, and (c) assessment of the dietary impact of milk and lactose, dietary fiber and complex carbohydrates, and fatty foods. If these measures fail, the guidelines recommend moving to symptom-specific dietary interventions, including a low–FODMAP diet and addition of probiotics. If all else fails, elimination diets can be tried. The evidence for restricting fermentable carbohydrates and for probiotics are based on moderate evidence (B-grade recommendation), but the other recommendations have rather little evidence to support them (D grade). Thus, improvement should not be expected in all patients.

Gastroparesis

The symptoms that can be attributed to delayed gastric emptying are not specific, but include bloating, nausea, and vomiting. When patients have chronic nausea and vomiting, initial therapy should ensure correction of fluid and micronutrient deficiencies. Dietary modifications have been developed to mitigate symptoms, and they benefit patients with mild or moderate symptoms who still have some degree of intact gastric emptying. These modifications include minimizing food components that delay gastric emptying (e.g., hyperosmotic foods, high protein, high fat), and employing tactics that may provide a mechanical basis for more rapid gastric emptying (e.g., eating small frequent meals, eating in the upright position, walking for 1 to 2 hours after meals, chewing food well, avoiding high-fiber–containing foods). Patients with delayed gastric emptying are at risk for developing phytobezoars, and should follow a diet that avoids high-risk foods (see Indications for Modified-Fiber Diets earlier in this chapter). These recommendations have been summarized for the American Motility Society and the International Foundation for Functional Gastrointesinal Disorders by Drs. Parrish, Soffer, and Parkman (http://www.motilitysociety.org/patient/pdf/Gastroparesis%20AMS%20 Dietary%20Recommendations%201%209%202006.pdf). For more information on a diet for gastroparesis (and other GI diets), go to the University of Virginia Health System Digestive Health Center website at www.healthsystem.virginia.edu/internet/digestive-health/nutrition/patientdu.cfm.

Liver Disease

Malnutrition is difficult to identify in patients with chronic liver disease, as both are characterized by loss of muscle mass and lean body weight. Thus, malnutrition is often overlooked. Causes of malnutrition can include a hypermetabolic state (~10% increase over expected), decreased glycogen stores that produce a starvation (catabolic) mode after only a few hours of fasting, anorexia, and ingestion of unpalatable diets too low in sodium and protein. Such patients require 35 to 40 kcal/kg/day, and sufficient protein for increased need (1.0 to 1.5 g/kg/day). This degree of protein intake does not help to prevent HE (309). The diet should be offered in small frequent meals, to avoid creating a starvation setting, including a supplement at bedtime. Patients benefit from a 2-g sodium diet to avoid requiring excessive diuretics, and may need multivitamin and mineral supplements for micronutrient deficiencies.

The treatment of NAFLD is primarily directed at weight loss (310). Although ingestion of caffeine and alcohol in limited amounts (2 drinks per day for men and 1 for women) have been suggested to decrease progression of NAFLD to NASH with fibrosis, the number of studies are not yet sufficient to make these dietary modifications as firm suggestions. In addition, the same caution should be made for the recommendation that vitamin E (800 IU per day) be given to nondiabetic patients with NASH, although the AASLD guidelines currently recommend this.

REFERENCES

1. American Dietetic Association, Dietitians of Canada. *Manual of Clinical Dietetics* [looseleaf]. 6th ed. Chicago, IL: American Dietetic Association; 2000.
2. Nelson JK, Moxness KE, Gastineau CF, et al. *Mayo Clinic Diet Manual: A Handbook of Nutritional Practice*. Rochester, MN: Mayo Medical Center, 1994.
3. USDA ChooseMyPlate. www.chooseMyPlate.gov
4. A Brief History of USDA Food Guides. http://www.choosemyplate.gov/food-groups/download/ MyPlate/A BriefHistoryOfUSDAFoodGuides.pdf.
5. Development of 2010 Dietary Guidelines for Americans. http://www.health.gov/dietaryguidelines/dga2010/dietaryguidelines2010.pdf.
6. American Dietetic Association; Dietitians of Canada. Position of the American Dietetic Association and Dietitians of Canada: vegetarian diets. *J Am Diet Assoc.* 2003;103:748.
7. Sabate J. The contribution of vegetarian diets to health and disease: a paradigm shift? *Am J Clin Nutr.* 2003;78(suppl):502S.
8. Lichtenstein AH, Appel LJ, Brands M, et al. Diet and lifestyle recommendations revision 2006: a scientific statement from the American Heart Association Nutrition Committee. *Circulation.* 2006;114:82. http://www.heart.org/idc/groups/heart-public/@wcm/@adv/documents/downloadable/ucm_312853.pdf
9. Singer AJ, Werther K, Nestle M. The nutritional value of university-hospital diets. *N Engl J Med.* 1996;335:1466.

10. Yarmolinsky DA, Zuker CS, Ryba NJP. Common sense about taste: from mammals to insects. *Cell.* 2009;139:234.
11. Tepper BJ. Nutritional implications of genetic taste variation: the role of PROP sensitivity and other taste phenotypes. *Annu Rev Nutr.* 2008;28:367.
12. Murphy C, Schubert CR, Cruickshanks KJ, et al. Prevalence of olfactory impairment in older adults. *JAMA.* 2002;288:2307.
13. Doty RL. Smell and the degenerating brain. *The Scientist.* 2013;10:33.
14. Bellisle F, Drewnowski A, Anderson GH, et al. Sweetness, satiation, and satiety. *J Nutr.* 2012;142:1149S.
15. Tolhurst G, Relmann F, Gribble FM. Intestinal sensing of nutrients. In: Joost HG, ed. *Appetite Control: Handbook of Experimental Pharmacology.* New York, NY: Springer, 2012;209:309.
16. Leitzmann C. Vegetarian nutrition, past, present, and future. *Am J Clin Nutr.* 2014;100(suppl 1):496S.
17. Lee JE, McLerran DF, Rolland B, et al. Meat intake and cause-specific mortality: a pooled analysis of Asian prospective cohort studies. *Am J Clin Nutr.* 2013;98:1032.
18. Mangels AR. Bone nutrients for vegetarians. *Am J Clin Nutr.* 2014;100(suppl 1):469S.
19. Hord NG, Tang Y, Bryan SN. Food sources of nitrates and nitrites: the physiologic context for potential health benefits. *Am J Clin Nutr.* 2009;90:1.
20. Authority EFS. Nitrate in vegetables: scientific opinion of the panel on contaminants in the food chain. *EFSA J. l* 2008;689:1.
21. Machha A, Schechter AN. Inorganic nitrate: a major player in cardiovascular health benefits of vegetables? *Nutr Rev.* 2012;70:367.
22. Hord NG. Dietary nitrates, nitrites, and cardiovascular disease. *Curr Atheroscler Rep.* 2011;13:484.
23. Nitrate (and potential endogenous formation of N-nitroso compounds). 2003. Joint Food and Agricultural Organization of the United States/World Health Organization committee on Food additives. WHO Food Additive series No:50.
24. Bach-Faig A, Berry EM, Lairon D, et al. Mediterranean diet pyramid today. Science and cultural updates. *Public Health Nutr.* 2011;14:2274.
25. Sofi F, Abbate R, Gensini GF, et al. Accruing evidence on benefits of adherence to the Mediterranean diet on health: an updated systematic review and meta-analysis. *Am J Clin Nutr.* 2010;92:1189.
26. Bere E, Brug J. Towards health-promoting and environmentally friendly regional diets—a Nordic example. *Public Health Nutr.* 2009;12:91.
27. Uusitupa M, Hermansen K, Savolainen MJ, et al. Effects of an isocaloric health Nordic diet on insulin sensitivity, lipid profile and inflammation markers in metabolic syndrome—a randomized study (SYSDIET). *J Intern Med.* 2013;274:52.
28. Larsen TM, Dalskov S, van Baak M, et al. The diet, obesity and genes (Diogenes) dietary study in eight European countries—a comprehensive design for long-term intervention. *Obesity Rev.* 2009;11:76.
29. Hancock G, Cresci G, Martindale R. The clear liquid diet: when is it appropriate? *Curr Gastroenterol Rep.* 2002;4:324.
30. Lewis SJ, Egger M, Sylvester PA, et al. Early enteral feeding versus "nil by mouth" after gastrointestinal surgery: systematic review and meta-analysis of controlled trials. *BMJ.* 2001;323:1.
31. Brown L, Heuberger R. Nothing by mouth at midnight: saving or starving? A literature review. *Gastroenterol Nurs.* 2014;17:14.
32. Albala K. Food for healing: convalescent cookery in the early modern era. *Stud Hist Philos Biol Biomed Sci.* 2012;43:323.
33. Charoenkwan K, Phillipson G, Vutyavanich T. Early versus delayed (traditional) oral fluids and food for reducing complications after major abdominal gynaecologic surgery. *Cochrane Database Syst Rev* 2007 Oct 17;(4):CD004508.
34. Warren J, Bhalla V, Cresci G. Postoperative diet advancement: surgical dogma vs evidence-based medicine. *Nutr Clin Pract.* 2011;26:115.
35. Lassen K, Soop M, Nygren J, et al. Consensus review of optimal perioperative care in colorectal surgery: Enhanced Recovery After Surgery (ERAS) Group recommendations. *Arch Surg.* 2009;144:961.
36. Meng WB, Li X, Li YM, et al. Three initial diets for management of mild acute pancreatitis: a meta-analysis. *World J Gastroenterol.* 2011;17:4235.
37. Popkin MB, Armstrong LE, Bray GM, et al. A new proposed guidance system for beverage consumption in the United States. *Am J Clin Nutr.* 2006;83:529.
38. Bray GA. Energy and fructose from beverages sweetened with sugar or high-fructose corn syrup pose a health risk for some people. *Adv Nutr.* 2013;4:220.

39. Renouf M, Guy PA, Marmet C, et al. Measurement of caffeic and ferulic acid equivalents in plasma after coffee consumption: small intestine and colon are key sites for coffee metabolism. *Mol Nutr Food Res.* 2010;54:760.
40. Higdon JV, Frei B. Coffee and health: a review of recent human research. *Crit Rev Food Sci Nutr.* 2006;46:101.
41. Emerson JL, Chappel CI. Health effects of coffee, tea, mate, cocoa, and their major methylxanthine components. In: Van der Heijden K, Younes M, Fishbein L, et al., eds. *International Food Safety Handbook.* New York: Marcel Dekker, 1999:141.
42. Paulson GW. Restless legs syndrome. How to provide symptom relief with drug and nondrug therapies. *Geriatrics.* 2000;55:35.
43. Cnattingius S, Signorello LB, Anneren G, et al. Caffeine intake and the risk of first-trimester spontaneous abortion. *N Engl J Med.* 2000;343:1839.
44. Greenwood DC, Alwan N, Boylan S, et al. Caffeine intake during pregnancy, late miscarriage and stillbirth. *Eur J Epidemiol.* 2010;25:275.
45. Floegel A, Lischon T, Bergmann MM, et al. Coffee consumption and risk of chronic disease in the European Prospective Investigation into Cancer and Nutrition (EPIC)-Germany study. *Am J Clin Nutr.* 2012;95:901.
46. Liu J, Sui X, Lavie CJ, et al. Association of coffee consumption with all-cause and cardiovascular disease mortality. *Mayo Clin Proc.* 2013;88:1066.
47. Aberegg SK. Coffee drinking and mortality [Correspondence]. *N Engl J Med.* 2012;367:575.
48. van Dam RM, Hu FB. Coffee consumption and risk of type 2 diabetes: a systematic review. *JAMA.* 2005;294:97.
49. Bhupathiraju SN, Pan A, Malik V, et al. Caffeinated and caffeine-free beverages and risk of type 2 diabetes. *Am J Clin Nutr.* 2013;97:155.
50. Michaels KB, Willett WC, Fuchs CS, et al. Coffee, tea, and caffeine consumption and incidence of colon and rectal cancer. *J Natl Cancer Inst.* 2005;97:282.
51. Peters U, Poole C, Arab L. Does tea affect cardiovascular disease? A meta-analysis. *Am J Epidemiol.* 2001;154:495.
52. Bravi F, Bosetti C, Tavani A, et al. Coffee reduces risk for hepatocellular carcinoma: an updated meta-analysis. *Clin Gastroenterol Hepatol.* 2013;11:1413.
53. Verster JC, Aufricht C, Alford C. Energy drinks mixed with alcohol: misconceptions, myths, and facts. *Int J Gen Med.* 2012;5:187.
54. Howland J, Rohsenow DJ. Risks of energy drinks mixed with alcohol. *JAMA.* 2013;309:245.
55. Sepkowitz KA. Energy drinks and caffeine-related adverse effects. *JAMA.* 2013;309:243.
56. Arria AM, O'Brien MC. The "high" risk of energy drinks. *JAMA.* 2011;305:600.
57. McLellan TM, Lieberman HR. Do energy drinks contain active components other than caffeine? *Nutr Rev.* 2012;70:730.
58. Saluja SS, Kaur N, Shrivastava UK. Enteral nutrition in surgical patients. *Surg Today.* 2002;32:672.
59. Pehl C, Waizenhoefer A, Wendl B, et al. Effect of low and high fat meals on lower esophageal sphincter motility and gastroesophageal reflux in healthy subjects. *Am J Gastroenterol.* 1999;94:1192.
60. Stephen AM, Cummings JH. The microbial contribution to human faecal mass. *J Med Microbiol.* 1980;13:45.
61. Kurasawa S, Haack VS, Marlett JA. Plant residue and bacteria as bases for increased stool weight accompanying consumption of higher dietary fiber diets. *J Am Coll Nutr.* 2000;19:426.
62. Achour L, Nancey S, Moussata D, et al. Faecal bacterial mass and energetic losses in healthy humans and patients with a short bowel syndrome. *Eur J Clin Nutr.* 2007;61:233.
63. The Definition of Dietary Fiber: report of the Dietary Fiber Definition Committee to the Board of Directors of the American Association of Cereal Chemists, January 10, 2001. *Cereal Foods World.* 2001;46:112.
64. Food and Nutrition Board, Institute of Medicine. *Dietary Reference Intakes for Energy, Carbohydrate, Fiber, Fat, Fatty Acids, Cholesterol, Protein, and Amino Acids (Macronutrients).* Washington DC: National Academies Press; 2005.
65. Howett JF, Betteridge VA, Champ M, et al. The definition of dietary fiber—discussions of the Ninth Vahouny Fiber Symposium: building scientific agreement. *Food Nutr Res.* 2010; 54:5750.
66. Jones JR, Lineback DM, Levine MJ. Dietary Reference Intakes: implications for fiber labeling and consumption: a summary of the International Life Sciences Institute North America Fiber Workshop, June 1–2, 2004, Washington, DC. *Nutr Rev.* 2006;64:31.

67. Canadian Food Inspection Agency. Dietary Fibre and Novel Fibre. *Canadian Food Directorate Guideline No. 9: Guidelines Concerning the Safety and Physiological Effects of Novel Fibre Sources and Food Products Containing Them*. Ottawa, ON: Canadian Food Inspection Agency, 2000.
68. Dhingra D, Michael M, Rajput H, Patil RT. Dietary fibre in foods: a review. *J Food Sci Technol.* 2012;49:255.
69. Englyst KN, Englyst HN. Carbohydrate availability. *Br J Nutr.* 2005;94:1.
70. Elleuch M, Bedigian D, Roiseux O, et al. Dietary fibre and fibre-rich by-products of food processing: characterization, technological functionality and commercial applications: a review. *Food Chem.* 2011;124:411.
71. Jenkins DJA, Kendall CWC. Resistant starches. *Curr Opin Gastroenterol.* 2000;16:178.
72. Fisher JJ. *Food Scientist's Guide to Dietary Fiber* [master's thesis]. Kansas State University, 2009. http://krex.k-state.edu/dspace/handle/2097/1454.
73. Misurcova L, Skrovankova S, Samek D, et al. Health benefits of algal polysaccharides in human nutrition. *Adv Food Nutr Res.* 2012;66:75.
74. Van Soest PJ, McQueen RW. The chemistry and estimation of fibre. *Proc Nutr Soc.* 1973;32:123.
75. Englyst HN, Quigley ME, Hudson GJ. Determination of dietary fibre as non-starch polysaccharides with gas-liquid chromatographic, high-performance liquid chromatographic or spectrophotometric measurement of constituent sugars. *Analyst.* 1994;119:1497.
76. Anderson JW, Bridges SR. Dietary fiber content of selected foods. *Am J Clin Nutr.* 1988;47:440.
77. Southgate DAT, Waldron K, Johnson LT, et al. *Dietary Fiber: Chemical and Biological Aspects*. Boca Raton, FL: CRC Press, 1991.
78. Cummings JH. Cellulose and the human gut. *Gut.* 1984:25:805.
79. Cummings JH, Englyst HN. Fermentation in the human large intestine and the available substrates. *Am J Clin Nutr.* 1987;45:1243.
80. National Health and Nutrition Examination Survey III, 1988–94. *NCHS CD-ROM series 11, No. 2A. ASCII version*. Hyattsville, MD: National Center for Health Statistics, April 1998.
81. Kritchevsky D, Bonfield C, Anderson JW eds. *Dietary Fiber*. New York: Plenum Publishing, 1990.
82. Slavin JL. Dietary fiber and body weight. *Nutrition.* 2005;21:411.
83. Howarth NC, Saltzman E, Roberts SB. Dietary fiber and weight regulation. *Nutr Rev.* 2001;59:129.
84. Saper RB, Eisenberg DM, Phillips RS. Common dietary supplements for weight loss. *Am Fam Phys.* 2004;70:1731.
85. Fogelholm M, Anderssen S, Gunnarsdottir I, et al. Dietary macronutrients and food consumption as determinants of long-term weight change in adult populations: a systematic literature review. *Food Nutr Res.* 2012;56.19103.
86. Satija A, Hu FB. Cardiovascular benefits of dietary fiber. *Curr Atheroscler Rep.* 2012;14:505.
87. Chuang SC, Norat T, Murphy N, et al. Fiber intake and total and cause-specific mortality in the European Prospective Investigation into Cancer and Nutrition cohort. *Am J Clin Nutr.* 2012;96:164.
88. Chandalia M, Garg A, Jutjohann D, et al. Beneficial effects of high dietary fiber intake in patients with type 2 diabetes mellitus. *N Engl J Med.* 2000;342:1392.
89. Brennan CS. Dietary fibre, glycaemic response, and diabetes. *Mol Nutr Food Res.* 2005;49:560.
90. Roberfroid MB. Fructo-oligosaccharide malabsorption: benefit for gastrointestinal functions. *Curr Opin Gastroenterol.* 2000;16:173.
91. Aldoori WH, Giovannucci EL, Rimm EB, et al. A prospective study of diet and the risk of symptomatic diverticular disease in men. *Am J Clin Nutr.* 1994;60:757.
92. AGA Clinical Practice and Practice Economics Committee. AGA technical review: impact of dietary fiber on colon cancer occurrence. *Gastroenterology.* 2000;118:1235.
93. Hill MJ. Cereals, cereal fibre and colorectal cancer risk: a review of the epidemiological literature. *Eur J Cancer Prev.* 1998;7(Suppl 2):S5.
94. Romaneiro S, Parekh N. Dietary fiber intake and colorectal cancer risk: weighing the evidence from epidemiologic studies. *Top Clin Nutr.* 2012;27:41.
95. Peters U, Sinha R, Chatterjee N, et al. Dietary fibre and colorectal adenoma in a colorectal cancer early detection programme. *Lancet.* 2003;361:1491.
96. Jacobs ET, Lanz E, Alberts DS, et al. Fiber, sex, and colorectal adenoma: results of a pooled analysis. *Am J Clin Nutr.* 2006;83:343.
97. Michels KB, Giovannucci E, Chan AT, et al. Fruit and vegetable consumption and colorectal adenomas in the Nurses' Health Study. *Cancer Res.* 2006;66:3942.
98. Park Y, Hunter DJ, Spiegelman D, et al. Dietary fiber intake and risk of colorectal cancer: a pooled analysis of prospective cohort studies. *JAMA.* 2005;294:2849.

99. Zuckerman MJ. The role of fiber in the treatment of irritable bowel syndrome: therapeutic recommendations. *J Clin Gastroenterol.* 2006;40:104.
100. Erkilla AT, Lichtenstein AH. Fiber and cardiovascular disease risk: how strong is the evidence? *J Cardiovasc Nurs.* 2006;21:3.
101. Brown L, Rosner B, Willett WW, et al. Cholesterol-lowering effects of dietary fiber: a meta-analysis. *Am J Clin Nutr.* 1999;69:30.
102. Levin EG, Miller VT, Muesing RA, et al. Comparison of psyllium hydrophilic mucilloid and cellulose as adjuncts to a prudent diet in the treatment of mild to moderate hypercholesterolemia. *Arch Intern Med.* 1990;150:1822.
103. Jenkins DJA, Kendall CWC, Vuksan V. Viscous fibers, health claims, and strategies to reduce cardiovascular risk. *Am J Clin Nutr.* 2000;71:401.
104. Kim YI. Short-chain fatty acids in ulcerative colitis. *Nutr Rev.* 1998;56:27.
105. Kaczmarczyk MM, Miller MJ, Freund GG. The health benefits of dietary fiber: beyond the usual suspects of type 2 diabetes mellitus, cardiovascular disease and colon cancer. *Metab Clin Exp.* 2012;61:1058.
106. Alaimo K, McDowell MA, Briefel RR, et al. Dietary intake of vitamins, minerals, and fiber of persons ages 2 months and over in the United States: Third National Health and Nutrition Examination Survey, phase 1, 1988–91. *Adv Data.* 1994;14:1.
107. Ladas SD, Kamberoglou D, Karamanalis G, et al. Systematic review: Coca-Cola can effectively dissolve gastric phytobezoars as a first-line treatment. *Aliment Pharmacol Ther.* 2013;37:169.
108. Lin HC, Zhao XT, Chu AW, et al. Fiber-supplemented enteral formula slows intestinal transit by intensifying inhibitory feedback from the distal gut. *Am J Clin Nutr.* 1997;65:1840.
109. Elia M, Engfer MB, Green CJ, et al. Systematic review and meta-analysis: the clinical and physiological effects of fibre-containing enteral formulae. *Aliment Pharmacol Ther.* 2008;27:120.
110. Brouns F, Senden J, Beckers EJ, et al. Osmolarity does not affect the gastric emptying rate of oral rehydration solutions. *JPEN J Parenter Enteral Nutr.* 1995;19:403.
111. Foster-Powell K, Holt SHA, Brand-Miller JC. International table of glycemic index and glycemic load values: 2002. *Am J Clin Nutr.* 2002;76:5.
112. Neuhouser ML, Tinker LF, Thomson C, et al. Development of a glycemic index database for food frequency questionnaires used in epidemiologic studies. *J Nutr.* 2006;136:1604.
113. Thomas D, Elliott EJ. Low glycaemic index, or low glycaemic load, diets for diabetes mellitus. *Cochrane Database Syst Rev.* 2009;21(1):CD006296.
114. Goff LM, Cowland DE, Hooper L, et al. Low glycaemic index diets and blood lipids: a systematic review and meta-analysis of randomized controlled trials. *Nutr Metab Cardiovasc Dis.* 2013;23:1.
115. Kelly S, Frost G, Whittaker V, et al. Low glycaemic index diets for coronary heart disease. *Cochrane Database Syst Rev.* 2004;18:CD004467.
116. Fung TT, van Dam RM, Hankinson SE, et al. Low-carbohydrate diets and all-cause and cause-specific mortality: two cohort studies. *Ann Intern Med.* 2010;153:289.
117. Foster GD, Wyatt HR, Hill JO, et al. Weight and metabolic outcomes after 2 years on a low-carbohydrate versus low-fat diet. *Ann Intern Med.* 2010;153:147.
118. Ukleja A. Dumping syndrome: pathophysiology and treatment. *Nutr Clin Pract.* 2005;20:517.
119. Lin HC, Zhao T, Wang L. Intestinal transit is more potently inhibited by fat in the distal (ileal brake) than in the proximal (jejunal brake) gut. *Dig Dis Sci.* 1997;42:19.
120. Matarese LE, O'Keefe SJ, Kandil HM, et al. Short bowel syndrome: clinical guidelines for nutrition management. *Nutr Clin Pract.* 2005;20:493.
121. Parrish CR. The clinician's guide to short bowel syndrome. *Pract Gastroenterol.* 2005;Sept:67, accessed at http://www.medicine.virginia.edu/clinical/departments/medicine/divisions/digestive-health/nutrition-support-team/nutrition-articles/September2005.pdf
122. Treem WR. Congenital sucrose-isomaltase deficiency. *J Pediatr Gastroenterol Nutr.* 1993;21:1.
123. Foster GD, Wyatt HR, Hill JO, et al. A randomized trial of a low-carbohydrate diet for obesity. *N Engl J Med.* 2003;248:2082.
124. Astrup A, Larsen MT, Harper A. Atkins and other low-carbohydrate diets: hoax or an effective tool for weight loss? *Lancet.* 2004;364:897.
125. O'Donnell K. Bariatric surgery: nutritional concerns on the weigh down. *Pract Gastroenterol.* 2004;18:33.
126. Thomas JR, Nanda R, Shu LH. A FODMAP diet update: craze or credible? *Pract Gastroenterol.* 2012;36:37.

127. Shepherd SJ, Parker FC, Muir JG, et al. Dietary triggers of abdominal symptoms in patients with irritable bowel syndrome: randomized placebo controlled evidence. *Clin Gastroenterol Hepatol.* 2008;6:765.
128. Staudacher HM, Whelan K, Irving PM, et al. Comparison of symptom response following advice for a diet low in fermentable carbohydrates (FODMAPs) versus standard dietary advice in patients with irritable bowel syndrome. *J Hum Nutr Diet.* 2011;24:487.
129. Heizer WD, Southern S, McGovern S. The role of diet in symptoms of irritable bowel syndrome in adults: a narrative review. *J Am Diet Assoc.* 2009;109:1204.
130. El-Salhy M, Ostgaard H, Gunderson D, et al. The role of diet in the pathogenesis and management of irritable bowel syndrome (review). *Int J Mol Med.* 2012;29:723.
131. Staudacher HM, Lomer MC, Anderson JL, et al. Fermentable carbohydrate restriction reduces luminal bifidobacteria and gastrointestinal symptoms in patients with irritable bowel syndrome. *J Nutr.* 2012;142:1510.
132. Morcos A, Quigley EM. Irritable bowel syndrome: role of food in pathogenesis and management. *J Dig Dis.* 2009;10:237.
133. LaTulippe MK, Skoog SM. Fructose malabsorption and intolerance: effects of fructose with and without simultaneous glucose ingestion. *Crit Rev Food Sci Nutr.* 2011;51:583.
134. Jones HF, Butler RN, Brooks DA. Intestinal fructose transport and malabsorption in humans. *Am J Physiol Gastrointest Liver Physiol.* 2011;300:6202.
135. Cheeseman C. GLUT7: a new intestinal facilitated hexose transporter. *Am J Physiol Endocrinol Metab.* 2008;295:E238.
136. Tappy L, Le KA, Tran C, et al. Fructose and metabolic diseases: new findings, new questions. *Nutrition.* 2010;26:1044.
137. Ha V, Jayalath VH, Cosma AI, et al. Fructose-containing sugars, blood pressure, and cardiometabolic risk: a critical review. *Curr Hypertens Rep.* 2013;15:281.
138. Ludwig DS. Examining the health effects of fructose. *JAMA.* 2013;310:33.
139. Riby JE, Fujisawa T, Kretchmer N. Fructose absorption. *Am J Clin Nutr.* 1993;58(suppl 5):748S.
140. Nobigrot T, Chasalow FI, Lifshitz F. Carbohydrate absorption from one serving of fruit juice in young children: age and carbohydrate composition effects. *J Am Coll Nutr.* 1997;16:152.
141. Elliott SS, Keim NL, Stern JS, et al. Fructose, weight gain, and the insulin resistance syndrome. *Am J Clin Nutr.* 2002;76:911.
142. American Dietetic Association. Position of the American Dietetic Association: use of nutritive and nonnutritive sweeteners. *J Am Diet Assoc.* 2004;104:255.
143. Kulczycki A. Aspartame-induced urticaria. *Ann Intern Med.* 1986;104:207.
144. Weihrauch MR, Diehl V. Artificial sweeteners-do they bear a carcinogenic risk? *Ann Oncol.* 2004;15:1460.
145. Brown RJ, Rother KI. Non-nutritive sweeteners and their role in the gastrointestinal tract. *J Clin Endocrinol Metab.* 2012;97:2597.
146. Pepino MY, Tiemann CD, Patterson BW, et al. Sucralose affects glycemic and hormonal responses to an oral glucose load. *Diabetes Care.* 2013;36(9):2530.
147. Pawar RS, Krynitsky AJ, Rader JI. Sweeteners from plants—with emphasis on *Stevia rebaudiana* (Bertoni) and *Siraitia grosvenarii* (Swingle). *Anal Bioanal Chem.* 2013;405:4397.
148. Ludwig DS. The glycemic index: physiological mechanism relating to obesity, diabetes, and cardiovascular disease. *JAMA.* 2002;287:2414.
149. Savaiano DA, Bouchey CJ, McCabe GP. Lactose intolerance symptoms assessed by meta-analysis: a grain of truth that leads to exaggeration. *J Nutr.* 2006;136:1107.
150. Byers KG, Savaiano DA. The myth of increased lactose intolerance in African-Americans. *J Am Coll Nutr.* 2005;24:569S.
151. Shaw AD, Davies GJ. Lactose intolerance: problems in diagnosis and treatment. *J Clin Gastroenterol.* 1999;28:208.
152. Di Stefano M, Missanelli A, Miceli E, et al. Hydrogen breath test in the diagnosis of lactose malabsorption: accuracy of new versus conventional criteria. *J Lab Clin Med.* 2004;144:313.
153. Heyman MB; Committee on Nutrition, American Academy of Pediatrics. Lactose intolerance in infants, children, and adolescents. *Pediatrics.* 2006;118:1279.
154. Kolars JC, Levitt MD, Aouji M, et al. Yogurt—an autodigesting source of lactose. *N Engl J Med.* 1984;310:1.
155. Martini MC, Savaiano DA. Reduced intolerance symptoms from lactose consumed during a meal. *Am J Clin Nutr.* 1988;47:57.

156. Eadala P, Waud P, Matthews SB, et al. Quantifying the 'hidden' lactose in drugs used for the treatment of gastrointestinal conditions. *Aliment Pharmacol Ther.* 2009;29:677.
157. Riserus U, Berglund L, Vessby B. Conjugated linoleic acid (CLA) reduced abdominal adipose tissue in obese middle-aged men with signs of the metabolic syndrome: a randomized controlled trial. *Int J Obes Relat Metab Disord.* 2001;25:1129.
158. German JB, Dillard CJ. Saturated fats: what dietary intake? *Am J Clin Nutr.* 2004;80:550.
159. Vesper H, Schmelz EM, Nikolova-Karakashian MN, et al. Sphingolipids in food and the emerging importance of sphingolipids to nutrition. *J Nutr.* 1999;129:1239.
160. American Dietetic Association. *Nutrition Trends Survey 1997.* Chicago: The American Dietetic Association, 1997.
161. Powell D. Approach to the patient with diarrhea, In: Yamada T, Alpers DH, Kaplowitz N, et al., eds. *Textbook of Gastroenterology,* 4th ed. Philadelphia: Lippincott–Raven Publishers, 2003:844.
162. Peretti N, Sassolas A, Roy CC, et al. Guidelines for the diagnosis and management of chylomicron retention disease based on a review of the literature and the experience of two centers. *Orpanet J Rare Dis.* 2010;5:24.
163. Bray GA. Is dietary fat important? *Am J Clin Nutr.* 2011;93:481.
164. Astrup A, Dyerberg J, Elwood P, et al. The role of reducing intakes of saturated fat in the prevention of cardiovascular disease: where does the evidence stand in 2010? *Am J Clin Nutr.* 2011;93:684.
165. Lawrence GD. Dietary fats and health: recommendations in the context of scientific evidence. *Adv Nutr.* 2013;4:294.
166. Rizos EC. Ntzani EE, Bika E, et al. Association between omega-3 fatty acid supplementation and risk of major cardiovascular diseases events: a systematic review and meta-analysis. *JAMA.* 2012;308:1024.
167. Anderson EJ, Taylor DA. Omega-3s: fishing for a mechanism. *The Scientist.* November 1, 2012:37.
168. Yaqoob P, Shaikh SR. The nutritional and clinical significance of lipid rafts. *Curr Opin Clin Nutr Metab Care.* 2010;13:156.
169. Gerberding JL. Safer fats for healthier hearts: the case for eliminating dietary artificial trans fat intake. *Ann Intern Med.* 209;151:137.
170. Angell SY, Silver LD, Goldstein GP, et al. Cholesterol control beyond the clinic: New York city's trans fat restriction. *Ann Intern Med.* 2009;151:129.
171. Mozaffarian D, Cao H, King IB, et al. Trans-palmitoleic acid, metabolic risk factors, and new-onset diabetes in U.S. adults. *Ann Intern Med.* 2010;153:790.
172. Jenkins DJA, Jones PJ, Lamarche R, et al. Effect of a dietary portfolio of cholesterol-lowering foods given at 2 levels of intensity of dietary advice on serum lipids in hyperlipidemia. *JAMA.* 2011;306:831.
173. Hendrich S. (n-3) fatty acids: clinical trials in people with type 2 diabetes. *Adv Nutr.* 2010;1:3.
174. Feskens EJM. The prevention of type 2 diabetes: should we recommend vegetable oils instead of fatty fish? *Am J Clin Nutr.* 2011;94:369.
175. Lucas M, Mirzaei F, O'Reilly EJ, et al. PUFA and depression. Oleagineux, Corps Gras, *Lipides* 2011;18:181.
176. Cusack L, De Buck E, Compernolle V, Vandekerckhove P. Blood type diets lack supporting evidence: a systematic review. *Am J Clin Nutr.* 2013;98:99.
177. Yilmaz Y. Review article: is non-alcoholic fatty liver disease a spectrum, or are steatosis and non-alcoholic steatohepatitis distinct conditions? *Aliment Pharmacol Ther.* 2012;36:815.
178. Musso G, Gambino R, Cassader M. Recent insights into hepatic lipid metabolism in non-alcoholic fatty liver disease (NAFLD). *Prog Lipid Res.* 2009;48:1.
179. Vuppalanchi R, Chalasani N. Nonalcoholic fatty liver disease and nonalcoholic steatohepatitis: selected practical issues in their evaluation and management. *Hepatology.* 2009;49:306.
180. Viljoen A, Wierzbicki AS. Diagnosis and treatment of severe hypertriglyceridemia. *Expert Rev Cardiovasc Ther.* 2012;10:505.
181. Lederle FA, Bloomfield HE. Drug treatment of asymptomatic hypertriglyceridemia to prevent pancreatitis: where is the evidence? *Ann Intern Med.* 2012;157:662.
182. Third report of the National Cholesterol Education Program (NCEP) Expert Panel on Detection, Evaluation, and Treatment of high blood cholesterol in adults (Adult Treatment Panel III) final report. *Circulation.* 2002;106:3143.
183. Akoh CC. Fat Replacers. *Food Technol.* 1998;52:47.
184. Bach A, Babayan VK. Medium-chain triglycerides—an update. *Am J Clin Nutr.* 1982;36:950.
185. Bach AC, Ingenbleek Y, Frey A. The usefulness of dietary medium-chain triglycerides in body weight control: fact or fancy? *J Lipid Res.* 1996;37:708.

186. Papamandjaris AA, MacDougall DE, Jones PJH. Medium chain fatty acid metabolism and energy expenditure: obesity treatment implications. *Life Sci.* 1998;62:1203.
187. Rego Costa AC, Rosado EL, Soares-Mota M. Influence of the dietary intake of medium chain triglycerides on body composition, energy expenditure and satiety; a systematic review. *Nutr Hosp.* 2012;27:103.
188. Sandler RS, Zorich NL, Filloon TG, et al. Gastrointestinal symptoms in 3181 volunteers ingesting snack food containing olestra or triglycerides. *Ann Intern Med.* 1999;130:253.
189. Balasekaran R, Porter JL, Santa Ana CA, et al. Positive results on tests for steatorrhea in persons consuming olestra potato chips. *Ann Intern Med.* 2000;132:279.
190. Neuhouser ML, Rock CL, Kristal AB, et al. Olestra is associated with slight reductions in serum carotenoids but does not markedly influence serum fat-soluble vitamin concentrations. *Am J Clin Nutr.* 2006;83:624.
191. Stead LM, Brosnan JT, Brosnan ME, et al. Is it time to reevaluate methyl balance in humans? *Am J Clin Nutr.* 2006;83:5.
192. Food and Nutrition Board, Institute of Medicine. *Dietary Reference Intakes for Thiamin, Riboflavin, Niacin, Vitamin B6, Folate, Vitamin B12, Pantothenic Acid, Biotin, and Choline*. Washington, DC: National Academies Press, 2000.
193. Zeisel SH, Caudill MA. Choline. *Adv Nutr.* 2010;1:46.
194. Fischer LM, da Costa KA, Kwock L, et al. Dietary choline requirements of women: effects of estrogen and genetic variation. *Am J Clin Nutr.* 2010;92:1113.
195. Guerrerio AL, Colvin RM, Schwartz AK, et al. Choline intake in a large cohort of patients with nonalcoholic fatty liver disease. *Am J Clin Nutr.* 2012;95:892.
196. Buchman AL, Ament ME, Sobel M, et al. Choline deficiency causes reversible hepatic abnormalities in patients receiving parenteral nutrition: proof of a human choline requirement: a placebo-controlled trial. *JPEN J Parenter Enteral Nutr.* 2001;25:260.
197. Shaw GM, Carmichael SL, Laurent C, Rasmussen SA. Maternal nutrient intakes and risk of orofacial clefts. *Epidemiology.* 2006;17:285.
198. Cummings JH, Pomare EW, Branch WJ, et al. Short chain fatty acids in human large intestine, portal, hepatic and venous blood. *Gut.* 1987;28:1221.
199. Thibault R, Blachier F, Darcy-Vrillon B, et al. Butyrate utilization by the colonic mucosa in inflammatory bowel diseases: a transport deficiency. *Inflamm Bowel Dis.* 2010;16:684.
200. Hamer HM, Jonkers D, Venema K, et al. Review article: the role of butyrate on colonic function. *Aliment Pharmacol Ther.* 2008;27:104.
201. Lawrance IC. Topical agents for idiopathic distal colitis and proctitis. *J Gastroenterol Hepatol.* 2011;26:36.
202. Hille A, Herrmann MK, Kertesz T, et al. Sodium butyrate enemas in the treatment of acute radiation-induced proctitis in patients with prostate cancer and the impact on late proctitis. *Strahlenther Onkol.* 2008;184:686.
203. Raqib R, Sarker P, Mily A, et al. Efficacy of sodium butyrate adjunct therapy in shigellosis: a randomized, double-blind, placebo-controlled clinical trial. *BMC Infect Dis.* 2012;12:111.
204. Zupec-Kania BA, Spellman E. An overview of the ketogenic diet for pediatric epilepsy. *Nutr Clin Pract.* 2008;23:589.
205. Pfeiffer H, Thiele EA. Low-glycemic-index treatment: a liberalized ketogenic diet for treatment of intractable epilepsy. *Neurology.* 2005;65:1810.
206. Kossoff EH, McGrogan JR, Blund RM, et al. A modified Atkins diet is effective for the treatment of intractable pediatric epilepsy. *Epilipsia.* 2006;47:421.
207. Paoli A, Rubini A, Volek JS, Grimaldi KA. Beyond weight loss: a review of the therapeutic uses of very-low-carbohydrate (ketogenic) diets. *Eur J Clin Nutr.* 2013;67:789.
208. Brosnan JT, Brosnan ME. Branched-chain amino acids: enzyme and substrate regulation. *J Nutr.* 2006;136:207S.
209. Klein S, Kinney J, Jeejeebhoy K, et al. Nutrition support in clinical practice: review of published data and recommendations for future research directions. *JPEN J Parenter Enteral Nutr.* 1997;21:133.
210. Stickel F, Hoehn B, Schuppan D, Seitz HK. Review article: nutritional therapy in alcoholic liver disease. *Aliment Pharmacol Ther.* 2003;18:357.
211. Als-Nielsen B, Koretz RL, Kjaergard LL, et al. Branched-chain amino acids for hepatic encephalopathy. *Cochrane Database Syst Rev.* 2004(2):CD001939
212. Charlton M. Branched-chain amino acid enriched supplements as therapy for liver disease. *J Nutr.* 2006;136:295S.

213. Marchesini G, Bianchi G, Merli M, et al. Nutritional supplementation with branched-chain amino acids in advanced cirrhosis: a double-blind, randomized trial. *Gastroenterology.* 2003;124:1792.
214. Pedrini MT, Levey AS, Lau J, et al. The effect of dietary protein restriction on the progression of diabetic and nondiabetic renal diseases: a meta-analysis. *Ann Intern Med.* 1996;124:627.
215. Sullivan DH, Sun S, Walls RC. Protein-energy undernutrition among elderly hospitalized patients: a prospective study. *JAMA.* 1999;281:2013.
216. Schurch MA, Rizzoli R, Slosman D, et al. Protein supplements increase serum insulin-like growth factor-I levels and attenuate proximal femur bone loss in patients with recent hip fracture. A randomized, double-blind, placebo-controlled trial. *Ann Intern Med.* 1998;128:801.
217. Ziegler TR, Mulligan K, eds. ASPEN research workshop: anabolic hormones in nutrition support. *JPEN J Parenter Enteral Nutr.* 1999;23(Suppl 6):S173.
218. Chadalavada R, Biyyani BS, Maxwell J, Mullen K. Nutrition in hepatic encephalopathy. *Nutr Clin Pract.* 2010;25:257.
219. Kachaamy T, Bajaj JS. Diet and cognition in chronic liver disease. *Curr Opin Gastroenterol.* 2011;27:174.
220. St Jeor ST, Howard BV, Prewitt E, et al. Dietary protein and weight reduction: a statement for healthcare professionals from the Nutrition Committee of the Council on Nutrition, Physical Activity, and Metabolism of the American Heart Association. *Circulation.* 2001;104:1869.
221. Katan MB. Alternatives to low-fat diets. *Am J Clin Nutr.* 2006;83:989.
222. Schugar RC, Crawford PA. Low-carbohydrate ketogenic diets, glucose homeostasis, and nonalcoholic fatty liver disease. *Curr Opin Clin Nutr Metab Care.* 2012;15:374.
223. Morenga LT, Mann J. The role of high-protein diets in body weight management and health. *Br J Nutr.* 2012;108(Suppl 2):S130.
224. American Heart Association, High-protein diets. http://www.heart.org/HEARTORG/Getting-Healthy/NutritionCenter/High-Protein-Diets_UCM_305989_Article.jsp.
225. Husby S, Koletzko S, Korpaonay-Szabo IR, et al. European Society for Pediatric Gastroenterology, Hepatology, and Nutrition Guidelines for the diagnosis of coeliac disease. *J Pediatr Gastroenterol Nutr.* 2012;54:136.
226. Lidvigsson JF, Leffler DA, Bai JC, et al. The Oslo definitions for coeliac disease and related terms. *Gut.* 2013;62:43.
227. Sapone A, Bai JC, Ciacci C, et al. Spectrum of gluten-related disorders: consensus on new nomenclature and classification. *BMC Med.* 2012;10:13.
228. Rubio-Tapia A, Hill ID, Kelly CP, et al. ACG Clinical Guidelines: diagnosis and management of celiac disease. *Am J Gastroenterol.* 2013;108:656.
229. Maki M. Lack of consensus regarding definitions of coeliac disease. *Nat Rev Gastroenterol Hepatol.* 2012;9:305.
230. Di Sabatino A, Corazza GR. Nonceliac gluten sensitivity: sense or sensibility? *Ann Intern Med.* 2012;156:309.
231. Biesiekierski JR, Newnham ED, Irving PM, et al. Gluten causes gastrointestinal symptoms in subjects without celiac disease: a double-blind randomized placebo-controlled trial. *Am J Gastroenterol.* 2011;106:508.
232. Iiesiekierski JR, Peters SL, Newnham ED, et al. No effects of gluten in patients with self-reported non-celiac gluten sensitivity after dietary reduction of low-fermentable, poorly absorbed, short-chain carbohydrates. *Gastroenterology.* 2013;145:320.
233. See J, Murray JA. Gluten-free diet: the medical and nutrition management of celiac disease. *Nutr Clin Pract.* 2006;21:1.
234. Hardman CM, Garioch JJ, Leonard JN, et al. Absence of toxicity of oats in patients with dermatitis herpetiformis. *N Engl J Med.* 1997;337:1884.
235. Janatuinen EK, Kemppainen TA, Julkunen RJ, et al. No harm from 5 year ingestion of oats in celiac disease. *Gut.* 2002;50:332.
236. Stoven S, Murray JA, Marietta E. Celiac disease: advances in treatment via gluten modification. *Clin Gastroenterol Hepatol.* 2012;10:859.
237. National Institutes of Health Consensus Development Conference Statement on Celiac Disease, June 28–30, 2004. *Gastroenterology.* 2005;128:S1.
238. Thompson T, Lee AR, Grace T. Gluten contamination of grains, seeds, and flours in the United States: a pilot study. *J Am Diet Assoc.* 2010;110:937.
239. Gilbert A, Kruizinga AG, Neuhold S, et al. Might gluten traces in wheat substitutes pose a risk in patients with celiac disease? A population-based probabilistic approach to risk estimation. *Am J Clin Nutr.* 2013;97:109.

240. Thompson T. Celiac disease: what gluten-free means today. *Pract Gastroenterol.* 2012;36:19.
241. Hlywiak KH. Hidden sources of gluten. *Pract Gastroenterol.* 2008;32:27.
242. Case S. The gluten free diet: how to provide effective education and resources. *Gastroenterology.* 2005;128:S128.
243. Marcason W. Where can I find information on the oxalate content of foods? *J Am Diet Assoc.* 2006; 106:627.
244. Siener R, Honow R, Voss S, et al. Oxalate content of cereals and cereal products. *J Agric Food Chem.* 2006;54:3008.
245. Bloch AS, Shils ME. Appendix. In: Shils ME, Olson JA, Shike M, et al., eds. *Modern Nutrition in Health and Disease,* 9th ed. Baltimore: Williams & Wilkins, 1999:A198.
246. Madsen C, Wuthrich B. Food sensitivities, allergic reactions, and food intolerances. In: van der Heijden K, Younes M, Fishbein L, et al., eds. *International Food Safety Handbook.* New York, NY: Marcel Dekker, 1999:447.
247. Frieri M, Kettelhut BV. *Food Hypersensitivity and Adverse Reactions: a Practical Guide for Diagnosis and Management.* New York, NY: Marcel Dekker, 1999.
248. Boyce JA, Assa'ad A, Burks AW, et al. Guidelines for the diagnosis and management of food allergy in the United States: summary of the NIAID-Sponsored Expert Panel Report. *J Allergy Clin Immunol.* 2010;126:1105.
249. Sampson HA. Food allergy. *JAMA.* 1997;278:1888.
250. Beyer K, Teuber SS. Food allergy diagnostics: scientific and unproven procedures. *Curr Opin Allergy Clin Immunol.* 2005;5:261.
251. Sicherer SH. Allergic disorders, In: Berdanier CD, ed. *Handbook of Nutrition and Food.* Boca Raton, FL: CRC Press, 2002:833.
252. FDA Food Allergen Labeling and Consumer Protection Act of 2004. http://www.fda.gov/Food/GuidanceRegulation/GuidanceDocumentsRegulatoryInformation/Allergens/ucm106187.htm.
253. Sampson HA, Sicherer SH, Birnbaum AH. AGA technical review on the evaluation of food allergy in gastrointestinal disorders. *Gastroenterology.* 2001;120:1026.
254. Hill DJ, Heine RG, Hosking CS. The diagnostic value of skin prick testing in children with food allergy. *Pediatr Allergy Immunol.* 2004;15:435.
255. Monsbakken KW, Vandvik PO, Farup PG. Perceived food intolerance in subjects with irritable bowel syndrome—etiology, prevalence, and consequences. *Eur J Clin Nutr.* 2006;60:667.
256. Hamilton RG, Franlin Adkinson N Jr. In vitro assays for the diagnosis of IgE-mediated disorders. *J Allergy Clin Immunol.* 2004;114:213.
257. Niggemann B, Rolinck-Werningaus C, Mehl A, et al. Controlled oral food challenges in children—when indicated, when superfluous? *Allergy.* 2005;60:865.
258. Kerschenlohr K, Darsow U, Burgdorf WH, et al. Lessons from atopy patch testing in atopic dermatitis. *Curr Allergy Asthma Rep.* 2004;4:285.
259. Dellon ES, Gibbs WB, Fritchie KJ, et al. Clinical, endoscopic, and histologic findings distinguish eosinophilic esophagitis from gastroesophageal reflux disease. *Clin Gastroenterol Hepatol.* 2009;7:1305.
260. Molina-Infante J, Ferrando-Lamana L, Ripoll C, et al. Esophageal eosinophilic infiltration responds to proton pump inhibition in most adults. *Clin Gastroenterol Hepatol.* 2011;9:110–117.
261. Spergel JM, Andrews T, Brown-Whitehorn TF, et al. Treatment of eosinophilic esophagitis with specific food elimination diet directed by a combination of skin prick and patch tests. *Ann Allergy Asthma Immunol.* 2005;95:336.
262. Penfield JD, Lang DM, Goldblum JR, et al. The role of allergy evaluation in adults with eosinophilic esophagitis. *J Clin Gastroenterol.* 2010;44:22.
263. Kagalwalla AF, Sentongo TA, Ritz S, et al. Effect of sea-food elimination diet on clinical and histologic outcomes i eosinophilic esophagitis. *Clin Gastroenterol Hepatol.* 2006;4:1097.
264. Atkinson W, Sheldon TA, Shaath N,Whorwell PJ. Food elimination based on IgG antibodies in irritable bowel syndrome. *Gut.* 2004;53:1459.
265. Aydinlar EI, Dikmen PY, Tiftikci A, et al. IgG-based elimination diet in migraine plus irritable bowel syndrome. *Headache.* 2012;53:514.
266. Ligaarden SC, Lyderson S, Farup PG. IgG and IgG4 antibodies in subjects with irritable bowel syndrome: a case control study in the general population. *BMC Gastroenterol.* 2012;12:186.
267. Mitchell N, Hewitt CE, Jayakody S, et al. Randomised controlled trial of food elimination diet based on IgG antibodies for the prevention of migraine like headaches. *Nutr J.* 2011;10:85.
268. Green TD, Burks AW. Oral food desensitization. *Curr Allergy Asthma Rep.* 2010;10:391.

269. Levitt MD, Bond JH. Flatulence. *Annu Rev Med.* 1980;31:127.
270. Alpha-galactosidase to prevent gas. *Med Lett Drugs Ther.* 1993;35:29.
271. Swain AR, Dutton P, Truswell AS. Salicylates in foods. *J Am Diet Assoc.* 1985;85:950.
272. Tiller JW, Dowling JT, Tung LH, et al. Tyramine-induced cardiac arrhythmias. *N Engl J Med.* 1985;313:266.
273. Rumore MM, Roth M, Orfanos A. Dietary tyramine restriction for hospitalized patients on linezolid: an update. *Nutr Clin Pract.* 2010;25:265.
274. Campbell HE, Escudier MP, Patel P, et al. Review article: cinnamon- and benzoate-free diet as a primary treatment for orofacial granulomatosis. *Aliment Pharmacol Ther.* 2011;34:687.
275. Campbell HE, Escudier P, Milligan P, et al. Development of a low phenolic diet for the management of orofacial granulomatosis. *J Hum Nutr Diet.* 2013;26:527.
276. Whelton PK, Appel LJ, Sacco RL, et al. Sodium, blood pressure, and cardiovascular disease: further evidence supporting the American Heart Association Sodium Reduction Recommendations. *Circulation.* 2012;126:2880.
277. Aburto NJ, Ziolkovska A, Hooper L, et al. Effect of lower sodium intake on health: systematic review and meta-analyses. *BMJ.* 2013;346:f136.
278. Appel LJ, Brands MW, Daniels SR, et al. Dietary approaches to prevent and treat hypertension: a scientific statement from the American Heart Association. *Hypertension.* 2006;47:296.
279. Reusser ME, McCarron DA. Reducing hypertensive cardiovascular disease risk of African Americans with diet: focus on the facts. *J Nutr.* 2006;136:1099.
280. Kuznetsova T, Staessen JA, Brand E, et al. Sodium excretion as a modulator of genetic associations with cardiovascular phenotypes in the European Project on Genes in Hypertension. *J Hypertens.* 2006;24:235.
281. Feldman JM, Lee EM, Castleberry CA. Catecholamine and serotonin content of foods: effect on urinary excretion of homovanillic and 5-hydroxyindoleactetic acid. *J Am Diet Assoc.* 1987;87:1031.
282. Simon JB. Occult blood screening for colorectal carcinoma: a critical review. *Gastroenterology.* 1985;88:820.
283. Fecal occult blood test for CRC screening-Ontario Health Technology Assessment Series 2009;9(10).
284. Pennington TH, Calloway DH. Copper content of foods. Factors affecting reported values. *J Am Diet Assoc.* 1993;63:143.
285. Hanley MJ, Cancalon P, Widmer WW, Greenblatt DJ. The effect of grapefruit juice on drug disposition. *Expert Opin Drug Metab Toxicol.* 2011;7:267.
286. Srinivas NR. Is pomegranate juice a potential perpetrator of clinical drug-drug interactions? Review of the in vitro, preclinical and clinical evidence. *Eur J Drug Metab Pharmacokinet.* 2013;38:223. doi:10.1007/s13318-013-0137-x.
287. Wilson T, Temple NJ, eds. *Beverages in Nutrition and Health.* Totowa, NJ: Humana Press, 2004.
288. Kiani J, Imam SZ. Medicinal importance of grapefruit juice and its interactions with various drugs. *Nutr J.* 2007;6:33.
289. Dolton MJ, Roiufogalis BD, McLachlan AJ. Fruit juices as perpetrators of drug interactions: the role of organic anion-transporting polypeptides. *Clin Pharm Ther.* 2012;92:622.
290. Singh JA, Reddy SB, Kundukulam J. Risk factors for gout and prevention: a systematic review of the literature. *Curr Opin Rheumatol.* 2011;23:192.
291. Brule D, Sarwar G, Savoie L. Changes in serum and urinary uric acid levels in normal human subjects fed purine-rich foods containing different amounts of adenine and hypoxanthine. *J Am Coll Nutr.* 1992;11:353.
292. Brule D, Sarwar G, Savoie L. Purine content of selected Canadian food products. *J Food Comp Anal.* 1988;1:130.
293. Yano Y, Katabo N, Watanabe M, et al. Evaluation of beef aging by determination of hypoxanthine and xanthine contents: application of a xanthine sensor. *Food Chem.* 1995;52:439.
294. Spinelli J, Eklund M, Miyauchi D. Measurement of hypoxanthine in fish as a method of assessing freshness. *J Food Sci.* 1964;29:710.
295. Boston University Medical Campus. Online Gout Study. https://dcc2.bumc.bu.edu/goutstudy/PurineContent.aspx.
296. Reliant Medical Group. Purine content of foods. www.reliantmedicalgroup/medical-services/nutrition/-/media/File/Nutrition/purine_content.ashx.
297. Acumedico. Various food types and their purine content. http://www.acumedico.com/purine.htm.

298. Griffiths AM. Enteral feeding in inflammatory bowel disease. *Curr Opin Nutr Metab Care.* 2006;9:314.
299. Jowett SL, Seal CJ, Pearce MS, et al. Influence of dietary factors on the clinical course of ulcerative colitis: a prospective cohort study. *Gut.* 2005;53:1479.
300. Yamamoto T. Dietary interventions in patients with inflammatory bowel disease. *Pract Gastroenterol.* 2011;36:10.
301. Marik PE, Zaloga GP. Meta-analysis of parenteral nutrition versus enteral nutrition in patients with acute pancreatitis. *BMJ.* 2004;238:1407.
302. McClave SA, Chang WK, Dhaliwal R, Heyland DK. Nutrition support in acute pancreatitis: a systematic review of the literature. *JPEN J Parenter Enteral Nutr.* 2006;30:143.
303. Eatock FC, Chong P, Menezes N, et al. A randomized study of early nasogastric versus nasojejunal feeding in severe acute pancreatitis. *Am J Gastroenterol.* 2005;100:432.
304. Lea R, Whorwell PJ. The role of food intolerance in irritable bowel syndrome. *Gastroenterol Clin North Am.* 2005;34:247.
305. O'Mahoney L, McCarthy J, Kelly P, et al. Lactobacillus and bifidobacterium in irritable bowel syndrome: symptom responses and relationship to cytokine profiles. *Gastroenterology.* 2005;128:541.
306. Alpers DH. Diet and irritable bowel syndrome. *Curr Opin Gastroenterol.* 2006;22:136.
307. Quartero AO, Meineche-Schmidt V, Muris J, et al. Bulking agents, antispasmodics and antidepressant medication for the treatment of irritable bowel syndrome (review). *Cochrane Database Syst Rev.* 2005;18:CD003460.
308. McKenzie YA, Alder A, Anderson W, et al. British Dietetic Association evidence-based guidelines for the dietary management of irritable bowel syndrome in adults. *J Hum Nutr Diet.* 2012;25:260.
309. Plauth M, Cabre E, Riggio O, et al. ESPEN guidelines on enteral nutrition: liver disease. *Clin Nutr.* 2006;25:285.
310. Mahady SE, George J. Management of nonalcoholic steatohepatitis: an evidence-based approach. *Clin Liver Dis.* 2012;16:631.

SECTION IV
Nutritional Management of Specific Diseases

13. Dietary Management of Diabetes, Renal Disease, and Hyperlipidemia

DIABETES
Introduction

In 2012, nearly 20.1 million Americans had diabetes, representing 9.3% of the adult population (1). Of these, 8.1 million cases (27%) were undiagnosed. Historical data have shown a disturbing temporal trend in diabetes prevalence. In 1980, there were about 5.6 million Americans with diagnosed diabetes. In 2005, this number had increased to nearly 21 million, and now the number of Americans with diabetes has further increased by more than one-third. Of Americans who are 20 years of age or older, nearly 16% of American Indians/Alaska Natives have diabetes, approximately 13% of Hispanics and non-Hispanic Blacks are diabetic, 9% of Asian Americans have diabetes, and 7.6% of non-Hispanic White adults are diabetic (1). Currently, based on fasting blood glucose or hemoglobin A1C levels, an additional 37% of Americans are estimated to have "prediabetes," distributed approximately equally among Hispanics, Hispanic Whites, and non-Hispanic Blacks (1). About 208,000 diabetics are less than 20 years old, representing 0.25% of the childhood and adolescent population (1). The vast majority has type 1 diabetes. Despite the high prevalence of obesity in children and adolescents, the overall prevalence of type 2 diabetes in children remains less than 1%, but the incidence of newly diagnosed type 2 diabetes is disturbing. In 2008 to 2009, the CDC estimated that somewhat more than 18,000 Americans younger than 20 years of age were newly diagnosed with type 1 diabetes on an annual basis and approximately 5,000 were diagnosed with type 2 diabetes annually. Of Children below the age of 10 years, few had type 2 diabetes, but type 2 diabetes represented a very significant fraction of newly diagnosed diabetes between the ages of 10 and 19 years of age, particularly among American Indians/Alaska Natives, Asians/Pacific Islanders, Hispanics and non-Hispanic Blacks (1).

Diabetes is the seventh leading cause of death in the United States. It is the leading cause of blindness in people between the ages of 20 and 74. Of diabetics who are aged 40 or older, about 4 million (approximately 28%) have diabetic retinopathy and more than 600,000 have advanced retinopathy of the degree that threatens vision (1). Diabetes is the leading cause of end-stage renal disease. In 2011, diabetes was responsible for 44% of new cases of renal failure and more than 225,000 people with renal failure due to diabetes were on dialysis or required a renal transplant (1). Diabetes is a principal cause of neuropathy and peripheral vascular disease. The relative risk for death from heart disease or stroke is increased nearly twofold in subjects with diabetes, and the overall all-cause mortality rate in diabetic adults is about 1.5 times greater in diabetic adults than in nondiabetic adults (1). In 2010, more than 70,000 nontraumatic lower-limb amputations in the United States, about 60% of all nontraumatic lower-limb amputations, were performed in diabetic adults. The overall total costs of diabetes in the United States were estimated to be $245 billion in 2012, with $176 billion representing direct medical costs of diabetes treatment and $69 billion representing the associated indirect costs due to disability, loss of work and productivity, and premature death.

Worldwide, the number of adults with diabetes increased from about 150 million people in 1980 to nearly 350 million in 2008, equivalent to a prevalence increase from 7.5% in 1980 to 9.2% in women and 9.8% in men in 2008 (2). In 2012, the International Diabetes Federation estimated that 371 million people worldwide had diabetes (3). Worldwide, the total number of excess deaths due to diabetes was almost 4 million in 2010, with approximately 6% of these occurring in Africa, nearly 10% occurring in South and Central America and the Western Pacific region, and from 11% to 15.7% occurring in Europe, the Eastern Mediterranean and the Middle East, Southeast Asia, and North America (4). The chronicity of the disease and its myriad complications make diabetes one of the most common problems encountered by physicians everywhere.

The National Institutes of Health Diabetes Control and Complications Trial (DCCT) that was conducted between 1983 and 1993 was the most important clinical trial conducted on type 1 diabetes (5–20). It was stopped 1 year early because the primary questions had been answered unequivocally: tight glycemic control prevented or delayed the appearance of background retinopathy and slowed the progression of early retinopathy to more advanced retinopathy (5,6,9). The trial also showed that prolonged near-normalization of blood glucose in persons with type 1 diabetes significantly reduced the development and progression of clinical neuropathy and nephropathy, although the number of cardiovascular events in the young subjects studied was too small to draw conclusions about preventing cardiovascular disease (5–20). When the active intervention ended, the study was continued as an observational study known as the Epidemiology of Diabetes Interventions and Complications (EDIC). This remarkable follow-up has now extended for 30 years, with data on 89% of the original cohort and 95% of the surviving cohort. The compelling result of this follow-up has been the realization that the beneficial effects of the early intensive active treatment period have carried over for two decades. In other words, microvascular complications of the eye, kidney, and nervous system were still better in the treatment group long than in the control group 20 years after the initial intensive treatment stopped (5–7,9,14–17). This phenomenon is referred to as "metabolic memory" by EDIC investigators, and there is now evidence that epigenetic mechanisms may play a role (20). Moreover, the additional lengthy follow-up permitted demonstration that early, intensive insulin treatment also reduced fatal and nonfatal cardiovascular consequences, including myocardial infarction and stroke, by approximately 40% (5,6,10,11). Furthermore, the available data also suggest that high levels of oxidized LDL and advanced glycation end products are contributing agents (12).

Unfortunately, however, even though the immunologic events that lead to destruction of pancreatic β-cells in type 1 diabetes begin, and can be identified, years before development of overt hyperglycemia, attempts to prevent a susceptible individual's progression to frank diabetes have largely proven unsuccessful (21,22).

On the other hand, a large number of trials have demonstrated convincingly that type 2 diabetes can be prevented in approximately 50% of nondiabetic obese individuals by intensive lifestyle changes that reduce caloric intake and increase physical activity, either alone or assisted by modest pharmacologic interventions (23–38). And, as with the DCCT trial, the United Kingdom Prospective Diabetes Study (UKPDS) in individuals with newly diagnosed type 2 diabetes showed that intensive glucose control not only reduced microvascular complications but also reaffirmed the "metabolic memory" effect uncovered in the DCCT by demonstrating a persistent beneficial effect of early normalization of blood glucose on reducing myocardial infarctions and deaths from any cause 10 years after the trial ended (39). On the other hand, in more adults with more established type 2 diabetes, the Look AHEAD study of intensive lifestyle intervention was able to achieve significantly greater weight loss in the intervention group, but was unable to show a beneficial effect on cardiovascular events, although a secondary analysis suggested that the incidence of chronic kidney disease was lowered (40–43).

The ability of lifestyle interventions to delay, prevent, or improve type 2 diabetes is largely due to effects of diet and physical activity on preventing weight gain. Like type 1 diabetes, type 2 diabetes has its pathophysiologic origins long before the frank development of overt diabetes. Thus, following the development of insulin resistance due to obesity, fasting blood glucose remains little changed as long as pancreatic β-cell insulin secretion can compensate. Eventually, β-cell function begins to fail. Even then, a 75% reduction in β-cell sensitivity to glucose is still associated with only a minor increase in blood glucose (44). Only after loss of the bulk of remaining β-cell function does frank diabetes become manifest (44). Therefore, lifestyle interventions that prevent weight gain or lead to successful weight loss during the lengthy course of pancreatic β-cell deterioration can prevent the development of diabetes by prolonging the adequacy of pancreatic β-cell insulin secretion. This principle has been repeatedly demonstrated by the various primary prevention studies cited above.

Role of Dietary Management

Control of dietary intake is a mainstay of prevention of type 2 diabetes and is one of the key elements of any diabetic treatment regimen aimed at normalizing blood glucose. It is also crucial in the management of obesity, hyperlipidemia, hypertension, and impaired renal function, all, unfortunately, common comorbidities. Diet plays a major role in regulating carbohydrate, fat, and protein homeostasis in patients with diabetes. Furthermore, proper dietary management is required for the safe and effective use of insulin.

As far as prevention is concerned, available evidence supports a conclusion that a variety of diets based on consumption of healthful foods and maintenance of healthy body weight are equally effective in preventing or delaying the onset of type 2 diabetes (45,46). Dietary patterns constructed with a predominance of plant foods are particularly recommended because of their overall health benefits. Various Mediterranean diets, vegetarian diet patterns, the dietary approaches to stop hypertension (DASH) diet plan, and dietary patterns constructed to conform to the Dietary Guidelines for Americans such as the Healthy Eating Index and the Alternative Healthy Eating Index are widely recommended (46). Recommendations based on inclusion or exclusion of specific foods or nutrients are largely based on the results of observational studies that demonstrate associations that often uncover compelling hypotheses (46). Nonetheless, such associations cannot themselves constitute proof of causal mechanisms because of the inability to account for all confounders, including the inability to completely separate other tightly associated, health-promoting lifestyle patterns from dietary intake patterns. There is absolutely no body of systematic evidence that any vitamin, mineral, dietary supplement, or herbal product can prevent either type 1 or type 2 diabetes.

While dietary advice was clearly effective in the intensive trials that delayed or prevented type 2 diabetes (as discussed above), there is only limited evidence from other prevention or treatment trials showing that dietary advice is effective in the treatment of diabetes, although dietary counseling can produce modest weight loss, an essential component in the treatment of individuals with type 2 diabetes (47–53). In fact, weight loss may be the most important therapeutic modality, since weight loss improves glycemic control (even to the extent of remission of diabetes in some case) and slows the progression of complications.

Like the results commonly observed in nondiabetic, obese subjects, it is usually very difficult to achieve significant weight loss in obese diabetic individuals. However, several decades of trials in obese individuals both with and without diabetes have consistently shown that a weight loss of only 5% to 10% body weight can lead to significant improvements in blood glucose, blood pressure, and plasma lipids (54). The likelihood of compliance is increased by adequate patient education and by intense efforts to tailor diets to the needs of individual patients in an effort to achieve prolonged compliance and a fundamental change in lifestyle (55). If a patient is offered no personal dietary instruction other than a preprinted guide to the diabetic diet, the chances of successful compliance are nil.

Most physicians have neither the time nor the knowledge to develop an individualized diet plan for each patient, educate each patient adequately, and follow the patient's dietary progress. Registered dietitians, certified diabetes educators, physician assistants, and other properly trained medical nutritionists and educators, who are either hospital-based, located in a physician's office or in private practice in the community, can formulate plans in cooperation with the physician and instruct patients. Local chapters of the American Diabetes Association (ADA) and the Juvenile Diabetes Research Foundation International can provide additional educational resources and support.

Diet Therapy

For practical purposes, the major divisions of type 1 (lean, insulin-requiring) and type 2 (overweight or obese, non–insulin-requiring) diabetes provide a means of classifying issues for dietary management. The goals of medical nutrition therapy for the prevention and treatment of diabetes are similar in most respects other than a greater emphasis on weight management in diets for type 2 diabetes and a particular focus on tailoring insulin treatment to match lifestyle and diet intake at meals in type 1 diabetes (56–60).

For individuals with risk of developing diabetes, the overriding principle of medical nutrition management is to decrease the risk of developing diabetes and its detrimental consequences by implementing the healthy lifestyle, food choice, and physical activity patterns that lead to moderate weight loss that is maintained over time (31–38, 45,46,53,56–58).

For persons who already have diabetes, the ADA has published recently an extensive guideline for the standards of medical care (58) and its detailed recommendations of the management of adults with diabetes (59). Although recommendations and guidelines published by various international groups may vary to some degree with respect to specifics, essentially all global diabetes recommendations are consistent with those of the ADA. Medical nutrition therapy is directed at lowering hemoglobin A1C levels to "below or around 7%" (58) because this goal "has been shown to reduce the microvascular complications of diabetes and, if implemented soon enough, is associated with a reduction in macrovascular disease." (58). Under this guiding principle, lifestyle, nutritional, and physical activity guidelines are essential adjuvants to pharmacologic therapy. Overall, the goals of nutrition therapy in adults with diabetes can be summarized as follows (59):

1. "To promote and support healthful eating patterns, emphasizing a variety of nutrient dense foods in appropriate portion sizes, in order to improve overall health and specifically to
   a. Attain individualized glycemic, blood pressure and lipid goals as follows:
      i. A1C < 7%
      ii. Blood Pressure < 140/80 mm Hg
      iii. LDL Cholesterol < 100 mg/dL; trygliceride < 150 mg/dL; HDL cholesterol > 40 mg/dL for men; HDL cholesterol > 50 mg/dL for women
      iv. Achieve and maintain body weight goals
      v. Delay or prevent complications of diabetes
2. "To address individual nutrition needs based on personal and cultural preferences, health literacy and numeracy, access to healthful food choices, willingness and ability to make behavioral changes, as well as barriers to change.
3. "To maintain the pleasure of eating by providing positive messages about food choices while limiting food choices only when indicated by scientific evidence.
4. "To provide the individual with diabetes with practice tools for day-to-day meal planning rather than focusing on individual macronutrients, micronutrients, or single foods."

Table 13-1 includes the full details of the ADA "Nutrition Therapy Recommendations for the Management of Adults with Diabetes" (59), a table that also provides a level of evidence rank for the individual recommendations according to an extensive evidence-based analysis and classification by the ADA (58). In the evidence-based hierarchy, *Level A* evidence is the highest level of evidence available and is equivalent to that which comes from well-conducted randomized controlled trials, well-conducted multicenter trials, meta-analyses that incorporate quality ratings in the analysis, and compelling nonexperimental evidence. *Level B* evidence is supportive evidence from well-conducted prospective cohort studies or meta-analyses of cohort studies, as well as well-conducted case–control studies. Levels of evidence below Level B are less-carefully controlled studies, studies with potential flaws that might bias or invalidate the results and, as well, recommendations based on expert consensus or clinical experience (58). Recommendations based on lower levels of evidence may, in fact, be correct. However, we are far less certain that this is the case and it is important to realize that not all of the ADA-specific

TABLE 13-1 Nutrition Recommendations for Diabetic Adults

Topic	Recommendation	Evidence Rating
Effectiveness of nutrition therapy	Nutrition therapy is recommended for all people with type 1 and type 2 diabetes as an effective component of the overall treatment plan.	A
	Individuals who have diabetes should receive individualized MNT as needed to achieve treatment goals, preferably provided by an RD familiar with the components of diabetes MNT.	A
	• For individuals with type 1 disbetes, participation in an intensive flexible insulin therapy education program using the carbohydrate counting meal planning approach can result in improved glycemic control.	A
	• For individuals using fixed daily insulin doses, consistent carbohydrate intake with respect to time and amount can result in improved glycemic control and reduce risk for hypoglycemia.	B
	• A simple diabetes meal planning approach such as portion control or healthful food choices may be better suited to individuals with type 2 diabetes identified with health and numeracy concerns. This may also be an effective meal planning strategy for older adults.	C
	People with diabetes should receive DSME according to national standards and diabetes self-management support when their diabetes is diagnosed and as needed thereafter.	B
	Because diabetes nutrition therapy can result in cost savings B and improved outcomes such as reduction in A1C A, nutrition therapy should be adequately reimbursed by insurance and other payers. E	B, A, E
Energy balance	For overweight or obese adults with type 2 diabetes, reducing energy intake while maintaining a healthful eating pattern is recommended to promote weight loss.	A
	Modest weight loss may provide clinical benefits (improved glycemia, blood pressure, and/or lipids) in some individuals with diabetes, especially those early in the disease process. To achieve modest weight loss, intensive lifestyle interventions (counseling about nutrition therapy, physical activity, and behavior change) with ongoing support are recommended.	A
Optimal mix of macronutrients	Evidence suggests that there is not an ideal percentage of calories from carbohydrate, protein, and fat for all people with diabetes B; therefore, macronutrient distribution should be based on individualized assessment of current eating patterns, preferences, and metabolic goals. E	B, E
Eating patterns	A variety of eating patterns (combinations of different foods or food groups) are acceptable for the management of diabetes. Personal preferences (e.g., tradition, culture, religion, heath beliefs and goals, economics) and metabolic goals should be considered with recommending one eating pattern over another.	E

(continued)

TABLE 13-1 Nutrition Recommendations for Diabetic Adults *(continued)*

Topic	Recommendation	Evidence Rating
Carbohydrates	Evidence is inconclusive for an ideal amount of carbohydrate intake for people with diabetes. Therefore, collaborative goals should be developed with the individual with diabetes.	C
	The amount of carbohydrates and available insulin may be the most important factor influencing glycemic response after eating and should be considered with developing the eating plan.	A
	Monitoring carbohydrate intake, whether by carbohydrate counting or experience-based estimation remains a key strategy in achieving glycemic control.	B
	For good health, carbohydrate intake from vegetables, fruits, whole grains, legumes, and dairy products should be advised over intake from other carbohydrate sources, especially those that contain added fats, sugars, or sodium.	B
Glycemic index and glycemic load	Substituting low-glycemic load foods for higher-glycemic load foods may modestly improve glycemic control.	C
Dietary fiber and whole grains	People with diabetes should consume at least the amount of fiber and whole grains recommended for the general public.	C
Substitution of sucrose for starch	While substitution sucrose-containing foods for isocaloric amounts of other carbohydrates may have similar blood glucose effects, consumption should be minimized to avoid displacing nutrient-dense food choices.	A
Fructose	Fructose consumed as "free fructose" (i.e., naturally occurring in foods such as fruit) may result in better glycemic control compared with isocaloric intake to sucrose or starch B, and free fructose is not likely to have detrimental effects on triglycerides as long as intake is not excessive (>12% energy). C	B, C
	People with diabetes should limit or avoid intake of SSBS (from any caloric sweetener including high fructose corn syrup and sucrose) to reduce risk for weight gain and worsening of cardiometabolic risk profile.	B
NNSs and hypocaloric sweeteners	Use of NNSs has the potential to reduce overall calorie and carbohydrate intake if substituted for caloric sweeteners without compensation by intake of additional calories from other food sources.	B
Protein	For people with diabetes and no evidence of diabetic kidney disease, evidence is inconclusive to recommend an ideal amount of protein intake for optimizing glycemic control or improving one or more CVD risk measures; therefore, goals should be individualized.	C

TABLE 13-1 Nutrition Recommendations for Diabetic Adults (continued)

Topic	Recommendation	Evidence Rating
	For people with diabetes and diabetic kidney disease (either micro- or macroabluminuria), reducing the amount of dietary protein below usual intake is not recommended because it does not alter glycemic measures, cardiovascular risk measures, or the course of GFR decline.	A
	In individuals with type 2 diabetes, ingested protein appears to increase insulin response without increasing plasma glucose concentrations. Therefore, carbohydrate sources high in protein should not be used to treat or prevent hypoglycemia.	B
Total fat	Evidence is inconclusive for an ideal amount of total fat intake for people with diabetes; therefore, goals should be individualized. C Fat quality appears to be far more important than quantity. B.	C, B
MUFAs/PUFAs	In people with type 2 diabetes, a Mediterranean-style, MUFA-rich eating pattern may benefit glycemic control and CVD risk factors and can therefore be recommended as an effective alternative to a lower-fat, higher-carbohydrate eating pattern.	B
Omega-3 fatty acids	Evidence does not support recommending omega-3 (EPS and DHA) supplements for people with diabetes for the prevention or treatment of cardiovascular events.	A
	As recommended for the general public, an increase in foods containing long-chain omega-3 fatty acids (EPS and DHA) (form fatty fish) and omega-3 linolenic acid (ALA) is recommended for individuals with diabetes because of their beneficial effects on lipoproteins, prevention of heart disease, and associations with positive health outcomes in observational studies.	B
	The recommendation for the general public to eat fish (particularly fatty fish) at least two times (two servings) per week is also appropriate for people with diabetes.	B
Saturated fat, dietary cholesterol, and *trans* fat	The amount of dietary saturated fat, cholesterol, and *trans* fat recommended for people with diabetes is the same as that recommended for the general population.	C
Plant stanols and sterols	Individuals with diabetes and dyslipidemia may be able to modestly reduce total and LDL cholesterol by consuming 1.6–3 g/d of plant stanols or sterols typically found in enriched foods.	C
Micronutrients and herbal supplements	There is no clear evidence of benefit from vitamin or mineral supplementation in people with diabetes who do not have underlying deficiencies.	C

(continued)

TABLE 13-1 Nutrition Recommendations for Diabetic Adults (continued)

Topic	Recommendation	Evidence Rating
	• Routine supplementation with antioxidants, such an vitamins E and C and carotene, is not advised because of lack of evidence of efficacy and concern related to long-term safety.	A
	• There is insufficient evidence to support the routine use of micronutrients such as chromium, magnesium, and vitamin D to improve glycemic control in people with diabetes.	C
	• There is insufficient evidence to support the use of cinnamon or other herbs/supplements for the treatment of diabetes.	C
	It is recommended that individualized meal planning included optimization of food choice to meet recommended dietary allowance/dietary reference intake for all micronutrients.	E
Alcohol	If adults with diabetes choose to drink alcohol, they should be advised to do so in moderation (one drink per day or less for adult women and two drinks per day or less for adult men).	E
	Alcohol consumption may place people with diabetes at increased risk for delayed hypoglycemia, especially if taking insulin or insulin secretagogues. Education and awareness regarding the recognition and management of delayed hypoglycemia is warranted.	C
Sodium	The recommendation for the general population to reduce sodium to less than 2,300 mg/day is also appropriate for people with diabetes.	B
	For individuals with both diabetes and hypertension, further reduction is sodium intake should be individualized.	B

(From Evert AB, Boucher JL, Cypress M, et al. Nutrition therapy recommendations for the management of adults with diabetes. *Diabetes Care.* 2014;37 (suppl 1):S120–S143.)

recommendations for medical nutrition therapy of diabetes are supported by Level A or Level B evidence (59). Along with the ADA nutritional recommendations and the basis for the evidence grading system, a full list of the citations supporting the level of evidence grade for each of the ADA nutrition therapy recommendations can be found at http://professional.diabetes.org/nutrition. An additional extensive set of evidence-documented guidelines for the care of people with diabetes mellitus was also published recently by the American Association of Clinical Endocrinologists (61), and detailed reviews of the principles and practice of dietary management of diabetics have been published recently (56,62).

From Table 13-1, selected recommendations for which are supported by the highest levels of evidence are discussed below, along with discussion of other closely related nutritional considerations.

Strategy of Diet Therapy for Obese, Type 2 Diabetics

Although the major goals of dietary therapy for the two types of diabetes are similar, the strategies for reaching these goals differ in some important ways (Table 13-2).

TABLE 13-2	Dietary Strategies for Patients with Type 1 and Type 2 Diabetes	
Strategy	Obese Diabetics Who do Not Require Insulin (Type 2)	Nonobese, Insulin-Dependent Diabetics (Type 1)
Decrease caloric intake	Yes	No
Protect or improve pancreatic β-cell function	Priority	Seldom important because β-cells are usually extinct
Increase frequency and number of feedings	Helpful	Yes
Maintain day-to-day consistency of intake of kilocalories, carbohydrate, protein, and fat	Not as crucial as dietary total energy and fat content	Very important
Maintain day-to-day consistency of ratios of carbohydrate, protein, and fat for each of the feedings	Helpful	Desirable
Time meals consistently	Not generally crucial	Very important
Allow extra food for unusual exercise	Not usually appropriate	Usually appropriate
Use food to treat, abort, or prevent hypoglycemia	Not generally necessary	Important
During complicating illness, provide small frequent feedings, or give carbohydrate IV to prevent starvation ketosis	Often not necessary because of resistance to ketosis	Important

(Adapted from West KM. Diet and diabetes. *Postgrad Med.* 1976;60(9):209–216.)

The primary therapeutic goal for patients with non–insulin-dependent diabetes is to maintain normal glucose, lipid, and blood pressure levels. Achieving this goal is facilitated by weight loss, which is a major focus of diet therapy in obese patients with type 2 diabetes. Although even relatively small amounts of weight loss, on the order of 5% to 10% are often sufficient to achieve major improvements in glycemic control and diabetes management, current strategies for achieving significant and sustained weight loss are often ineffective. For this reason, practical therapeutic approaches emphasize pharmacologic and other supportive approaches to control serum glucose, serum lipids, and blood pressure and use moderate caloric restriction paradigms to achieve and sustain at least a modest reduction of weight, in the range of 5% to 10% of initial body weight in individuals who are overweight or whose BMI are less than 35. Obviously, if additional weight loss is achievable, it is desirable. In diabetics who have BMI greater than 35 kg per m^2, a more aggressive weight management programs are often necessary, including consideration of bariatric surgery, an option that has been shown to be effective in improving control of diabetes (63,64). However, bariatric surgery is not without its own adverse consequences and surgical treatment of obesity is discussed in more detail in Chapter 14.

Regular clinical and biochemical monitoring is essential to evaluate the effects of various treatment regimens aimed at accomplishing the stated goals. For obese diabetics who are not taking insulin or oral hypoglycemic agents, the timing of meals, precise distribution of macronutrients, and day-to-day consistency in dietary patterns are, in general, somewhat less critical than they are in insulin-dependent subjects. However, consistency of meal content and timing is a clear adjunct to successful therapy in patients with type 2 diabetes, as it is in patients with type 1 diabetes.

Management should follow certain principles:

a. Food choices and dietary fat intake should be guided by the standards of a healthy diet as outlined in the *Dietary Guidelines for Americans* and the dietary intake recommendations of similar expert groups as discussed in Chapter 1 and detailed further for individuals with diabetes (59). On the whole, these expert recommendations aim for a modest total intake of dietary fat that is individualized for each patient according to their food habits and preferences because we do not know the ideal amount of fat that should be consumed either as a percent of energy consumed or as total daily amount. Likewise, we now realize that saturated fats, per se, can be relatively neutral in the average diet as far as cardiovascular complications are concerned and there are no longer specific recommendations aimed at significant reductions in dietary cholesterol intake because the relationship of dietary cholesterol intake, per se, to circulating plasma LDL-C levels is uncertain. However, dietary *trans* fats should be avoided and intake limited to the lowest amount practical because of known detrimental consequences of *trans* fats on cardiovascular disease risk. Furthermore, there is general agreement that replacing saturated fats in the diet by increasing polyunsaturated fat intake through the consumption of foods containing omega-3 fatty acids (DHA and EPA) is beneficial to health, but data do not support an effect of PUFA consumption on glycemic control (65). Additionally, adhering to the additional principles of DASH diet plan (Chapter 1) with increased consumption of fruits and vegetables will contribute additional benefits to weight and blood pressure control. On the other hand, increasing evidence suggests that replacing dietary saturated fats with carbohydrate may, in fact, increase cardiovascular risk. This issue is a very important one that requires extensive, additional evidence-based intervention data in diabetes. At the moment, there are no conclusive data on the ideal quantity of carbohydrate that should be recommended in a diabetic diet. Likewise, while there is body of evidence supporting the position that low glycemic index (GI) foods may improve glycemic control and clinical outcomes, the level of evidence for this position remains less than conclusive.

b. Long-term compliance with a weight loss diet is more likely if additional support for the behavioral and lifestyle changes necessary for long-term success are provided along with recommendations for caloric restriction and if the caloric restriction is not too stringent. Moderate caloric reductions to 250 to 500 kcal less than the subject's usual intake are appropriate. An overall calorie allowance of about 25 kcal per kg of ideal body weight allows gradual weight loss (on the order of 1–1.5 lb per week) without being so restrictive that compliance is unlikely. A detailed discussion of the principles of dietary management of weight reduction is presented in Chapter 14. These principles are not influenced to any significant degree by the presence of diabetes.

c. Adjuncts to dietary therapy often can improve both compliance and efficacy. Some patients are able to maintain a reduced dietary intake of energy if their caloric intake is spread throughout the day in the form of meals and snacks rather than three meals alone. Similarly, in addition to improving glycemic control, maintaining lean body mass, and enhancing a general feeling of well-being, regular physical activity augments energy expenditure and facilitates weight management. A diabetic patient who exercises can accelerate weight loss on a fixed intake of energy; conversely, the patient can maintain the same rate of weight loss on a smaller reduction in dietary energy intake.

d. The routine use of dietary supplements is not only unnecessary in most cases, but their use has been linked to detrimental consequences, especially in the case of the antioxidant vitamins A and E (59). Similarly, systematic reviews of the evidence have regularly failed to find any benefit from assorted vitamin, mineral, and herbal supplements of any kind, either in diabetics or in healthy individuals in the general public, as discussed in Chapter 1, Chapter 8, and elsewhere in this volume associated with the specific nutrient in question. The primary exceptions are those that apply to special populations of nondiabetic as well as diabetic persons. Thus, folic acid supplementation or the consumption of foods fortified with folic acid may be necessary for all diabetic women of childbearing age to achieve the CDCP recommendations for a daily folic acid intake of 400 µg. Secondly, elderly persons with diabetes are often advised to take supplemental vitamin B_{12} or foods fortified with vitamin B_{12} to achieve an adequate daily intake of that vitamin. Although no consensus recommendation has been made, diabetic women should consider taking a calcium supplement if their dietary calcium intake does not meet current recommended levels.

Dietary deficits of chromium and zinc have been reported in diabetic persons, but little systematic evidence is available to indicate that dietary zinc or chromium supplementation has any long-term benefit to diabetic patients or any role in the care of individuals with diabetes. Magnesium deficiency may follow sustained polyuria secondary to hyperglycemia or the use of diuretics, but this also is not a common problem or one that requires routine supplementation. Similarly, iron replacement should be reserved for patients with demonstrable iron deficiency.

e. Blood glucose control in diabetes requires matching dietary intake to the action of insulin or alternative pharmacologic agents. The general principles are discussed elsewhere (66–69). Achieving this match requires some knowledge of the carbohydrate content of the diet. There are two principal aids for accomplishing this in everyday practice. One is the long-used food exchange list system and the second what is commonly called "carbohydrate counting." Although the latter approach has become popular more recently, it was used in practice soon after insulin was discovered (68) and, in fact, both systems are merely variants of the same general approach and readily interchangeable.

The ADA food exchange system is one in which common measures of various foods are ordered into groups whose individual members have approximately equal contents of carbohydrate, protein, and fat (Table 13-3). The intent is to allow flexibility of food choices within groups while keeping the overall diet contents of macronutrients, especially carbohydrates, reasonably constant. However, although the exchange system is the one used most extensively for decades, it is merely one guide to understanding intelligent food choices within the context of a balanced diabetic diet. Currently, carbohydrate counting now appears to

TABLE 13-3 Nutritional Values of the Exchange Lists

	CHO	Protein	Fat	Calories
Carbohydrate group				
Starch	15	3	≤1	80
Fruit	15	—	—	60
Vegetables	5	2	—	25
Milk				
Skim	12	8	≤1	90
Low-fat	12	8	5	120
Whole	15	Varies	Varies	Varies
Meat and meat substitutes group				
Very lean	—	7	≤1	35
Lean	—	7	3	55
Medium-fat	—	7	5	75
High-fat	—	7	8	100
Fat group	—	—	5	45
Free foods group	<5	—	—	<20
Combination foods group	Varies	Varies	Varies	Varies
Fast foods group	Varies	Varies	Varies	Varies

CHO, carbohydrate.
(From the American Dietetic Association and the American Diabetes Association. *Exchange Lists for Meal Planning.* New York: American Diabetes Association; 1995.)

TABLE 13-4 Carbohydrate Counting

Equivalent 15 g carbohydrate servings
Starches: 1 slice of bread, 1/3 cup cooked pasta, ¾ cup dry cereal, or 4–6 crackers
Fruit: 1 small piece of fruit or ½ cup of fruit juice
Milk: 1 cup of nonfat (skim) milk or ¾ cup yoghurt
Desserts: 2 small cookies or ½ cup ice cream

Counting the Carbohydrates:

Amount of Carbohydrate	Carbohydrate Serving Count
0–5 g	0
5–10 g	½ serving
11–20 g	1 serving
21–25 g	1.5 servings
26–35 g	2 servings

(Data from Kulkarni KD. Carbohydrate counting: a practical meal-planning option for people with diabetes. *Clinical Diabetes.* 2005;23(3):120–122.)

be the most routinely used alternative approach (68–71) as shown in Table 13-4. It is based on the principle that only dietary carbohydrate affects blood glucose level and, thus, blood glucose control is primarily based on the amount of dietary carbohydrate consumed. These amounts are readily estimated from the known carbohydrate contents of various foods and from carbohydrate contents found on the nutrition facts label for commercially available foods (70). It should come as no surprise that the carbohydrate contents of the foods with carbohydrate counting approach are identical to the carbohydrate contents of foods in the exchange list system. That is, one can readily convert the exchange system to the carbohydrate counting system by just counting the amount of carbohydrate in each exchange. For example, a milk exchange is 12 g of carbohydrate, a fruit exchange is 15 g, a meat or fat exchange is 0 g. Either of these approaches allows great flexibility in diets consumed and, thus, more likely compliance with dietary diet plans developed for individual patients. Both permit reasonably consistent energy and macronutrient intake from day to day and facility matching insulin or oral agents to the glycemia anticipated after a meal. A step-by-step description of managing blood glucose using the calorie counting approach can be found at http://dbcms.s3.amazonaws.com/media/files/484c49b1-4af9-48dc-92f3-09d5fe0f878d/Ready,%20Set,%20Start%20Counting.pdf.

f. Choose dietary carbohydrates wisely. The management of dietary carbohydrate intake in diabetes had long focused on restricting the intake of simple sugars, primarily the disaccharides such as sucrose, but we now realize that this focus was misplaced. Foods containing simple sugars can generally be accommodated in a diabetic meal plan if adequately covered with appropriate glucose-lowering medications (38). At the same time, in some diabetics, restriction of the intake of simple sugars can be a helpful adjunct to dietary treatment and modest intakes must be maintained in order to avoid displacement of nutrient-dense foods in the diet. Thus, many experts recommend that sucrose and fructose be consumed only in moderation and the ADA recommends limitation of fructose intake (now largely consumed as high-fructose corn syrup in drinks) to less than 12% energy intake to avoid hypertriglyceridemia. The ADA also recommends limitation of sugar-sweetened beverages for this reason and to reduce the risk of weight gain because of the risk of excessive calorie intake. This principle, however, applies to excessive intake of the other macronutrients, protein, or fat as well.

Lately, all expert bodies have appreciated that the correct focus of dietary carbohydrate intake should be on the types of carbohydrates consumed. As discussed in the *Dietary Guidelines for Americans* (Chapter 1), the most healthful dietary carbohydrates are found in fruits, vegetables, whole grains, and legumes, and these should be the basis of carbohydrate intake in the diabetic diet. Additionally, although the evidence remains inconclusive as far as glycemic control and long-term outcomes are concerned, the consensus recommendation is that diabetics consume at least the dietary reference intake for fiber of 14 g per 1,000 kcal of dietary energy consumption, the same value recommended for the nondiabetic general population.

Despite a very large number of studies and despite some literature support (72–74) for the use of the GI and glycemic load in the management of diabetes, debate remains about whether there is a therapeutic advantage to using the GI of foods as an adjunct to improving postprandial hyperglycemia in diabetics. Thus, the ADA has concluded that there is only Level B evidence for "substituting low-glycemic load foods for high-glycemic load foods" in the management of diabetes (59, Table 13-1). In this context, it is important to remember that the mixed diet consumed by most Americans has a "medium" GI, so that studies comparing low GI foods with high GI foods may overestimate the actual effects that will be found in practice (see also the discussion of GI in Chapter 12, in "Low-Available Carbohydrate Diet").

g. In addition to diet and lifestyle interventions, employ appropriate drug therapy to ensure optimal control of hyperglycemia. The ADA, the American Association of Clinical Endocrinologists, and the International Diabetes Federation Guideline Development Group each has recently issued consensus guidelines for the successful pharmacologic management of glycemic control in persons with type 2 diabetes (58,60,61).

Strategy of Diet Therapy for Type 1 Diabetics

In persons who do not have diabetes, pancreatic insulin secretion changes abruptly and appropriately in response to a change in blood glucose. After a meal, insulin secretion increases as blood glucose starts to rise. Nondiabetics can vary their caloric intakes severalfold from day to day without becoming hyperglycemic or hypoglycemic because their insulin secretion is exquisitely responsive to changes in blood glucose and the blood glucose level is, thus, tightly regulated. On the other hand, individuals with type 1 diabetes are essentially completely insulin-deficient within, at most, several years, after their initial diagnosis. Thus, type 1 diabetics are unable to secrete insulin in response to a rise in blood glucose. In an attempt to anticipate and regulate glycemia after meals and during the course of normal daily activity, most type 1 diabetics inject, more than once daily, a combination of insulins with different time courses of action. The amount and proportions of the insulin dose are determined by preceding glycemia and anticipated glycemic response. Serum insulin levels are determined largely by the types of insulin injected and by the size and timing of the injected insulin dose. Herbst and Hirsch (75) have published a succinct, informative summary of insulin strategies used in caring for people with diabetes.

None of the currently available insulins, not even those called rapid-acting insulin, can provide a serum insulin profile to precisely match the immediate release of insulin that occurs in nondiabetic subjects following the ingestion of food and the minute-by-minute responsiveness of pancreatic insulin secretion that takes place in nondiabetic subjects. Additionally, no single insulin can match both the initial "first phase," virtually instantaneous pancreatic insulin release and the more-prolonged, and "second phase," sustained insulin release that follows carbohydrate ingestion. Thus, the timing of a meal following an injection of insulin is critical. Depending on the type of insulin used, meal ingestion may follow immediately, or almost so (as with the use of rapid-acting insulin), or delayed for 30 to 60 minutes (as with the use of short-acting insulin) in order to try to match the appearance of insulin into the systemic circulation with the absorption of glucose from the meal. Furthermore, it is imperative that the composition and distribution of meals be consistent with the composition and expected actions of the insulin injected. Because most patients with type 1 diabetes inject insulin on a relatively consistent schedule, they also consume meals on a relatively consistent schedule. Insulin doses should be adapted to the patient's lifestyle, schedule, eating preferences, and level of activity. Tailored regimens of this type are the rule for patients who monitor their blood glucose adequately. However, adjustment of the insulin dose is effective only if the caloric content is regular and the temporal distribution of food is consistent with the insulin regimen employed.

One should aim to achieve consistency in the composition of meals. Some regularity in the proportion of carbohydrates, proteins, and fats is necessary in each meal. The amount of insulin needed to "cover" a meal can be determined empirically, whatever the composition of the meal, and will remain fairly constant if the total number of ingested calories, the carbohydrate content, and the relative mix of the other macronutrients remain reasonably constant. The purpose of the exchange list and/or carbohydrate counting systems is to provide a practical degree of consistency yet allow flexible food choices and, based on the amount of dietary carbohydrate in a meal or snack, the amount and type(s) of injected insulin necessary to "cover" the postprandial glycemic response is estimated. This "insulin to carbohydrate ratio" is largely determined empirically and can vary widely based on the subject's sensitivity to insulin (and variables like body weight, physical activity, pregnancy, etc., known to alter insulin sensitivity), as well as on the presence (type 2 diabetes) or absence (type 1 diabetes) of the patient's own pancreatic insulin secretion. Scheiner (76) has written a very brief, entry-level primer describing the practical aspects of implementing insulin-to-carbohydrate ratios in diabetes care. However, there is no single algorithm that will accurately predict, a priori, the insulin to carbohydrate ratio for any specific subject. "First guess" estimates are in the range of about 1 unit of insulin to cover about 10 to 15 g of carbohydrate for adults. Children, particularly very young children, are likely to require much less insulin per gram of carbohydrate than adults. For children less than about 7 years of age, 1 unit of insulin may cover 30 g of carbohydrate and preadolescent children older than about seven may cover 20 g of carbohydrate with 1 unit of insulin.

a. The degree of flexibility in the diet that is consistent with good metabolic control varies from patient to patient. Some patients can vary their caloric intake and dietary composition from day to day and still tightly regulate their blood glucose level by paying careful attention to blood glucose monitoring and insulin dose adjustment. Others require a fixed regimen to control hyperglycemia. Whatever the case, the evidence basis for concluding that there is an unequivocal reduction in diabetic complications following prolonged "normalization" of blood glucose is now extensive. Good control should not be sacrificed for a more liberal diet.

b. The adverse consequences of rigid glycemic control include the risk for obesity because of diminished urinary loss of glucose calories and the antilipolytic effects of insulin. More importantly, however, tight control of blood glucose is associated with a large increased risk of significant, symptomatic hypoglycemia, an unwanted side effect that has now been reported consistently in studies that have achieved near normal blood glucose control. As a rule, the tighter the blood glucose control, the more one will experience clinically significant hypoglycemic episodes. Because we are unable to match plasma insulin and glucose profiles accurately, consistently, and precisely, diabetics who aim for normoglycemia are prone to episodes of serious hypoglycemia requiring the assistance of another person for resolution. Such episodes can lead to permanent detrimental consequences, both to the diabetic patient and others (e.g., auto accidents). Careful and regular monitoring for adverse effects is required, and the insulin dose and calorie intake must be adjusted as necessary. The clinical risk of hypoglycemia is increased when insulin doses are too large or not timed appropriately, when meals or snacks are missed, when physical activity is increased, and when insulin clearance is decreased as renal function declines. Cryer has recently summarized in great detail the evidence for balancing "glycemic goals in diabetes" as a "trade-off between glycemic control and iatrogenic hypoglycemia" (77). This assessment, which includes an exposition of the pathophysiology of hypoglycemia in diabetes, a summary of the evidence base for hypoglycemic risks, and a discussion of therapeutic goals that help minimize risk while preserving the benefit of diabetes control, is essential reading for all those responsible for managing individuals with diabetes (77).

The Dietary Prescription

It is important to individualize the diet prescription to accommodate the diabetic patient's lifestyle, eating habits, age, and concurrent disease. It is counterproductive to expect the opposite, that is that a patient will change their fundamental habits just to accommodate the diet prescription. The following list can be used to establish such a prescription (78):

1. In order of priority, what are the main general purposes (not strategies or methods) of this patient's prescription?
2. How much does the patient weigh? How much do the doctor, dietitian, and patient think the patient should weigh? How much would the patient like to weigh?
3. What is the appropriate level of caloric consumption for the patient?
4. Does the patient require insulin? If so, is the blood glucose level relatively stable, moderately labile, or severely labile? What kind of insulin is to be given? At what time? In what amount?
5. What, when, and how much would the patient like to eat if he or she did not have diabetes? Are there any special considerations relating to economic factors or to family or cultural dietary propensities?
6. Is the level of carbohydrate to be limited? To what level or range? To what extent and under what conditions, if any, are concentrated carbohydrates to be used?
7. Are there any special requirements concerning levels of protein?
8. Are there any specific or general requirements with respect to levels of dietary fat, either saturated or unsaturated?
9. How much alcohol is to be permitted? Under what conditions? Should alcohol be exchanged for food? If so, what kind and in what amount?
10. If the temporal distribution of food is of any importance, are there specific requirements concerning the following?
    a. The relative size and timing of each of the three main meals
    b. The timing, size, and characteristics of any extra feedings
11. To what degree is day-to-day consistency required in
    a. Total kilocalories?
    b. Size and characteristics of specific feedings, such as lunch?
12. Are dietary adjustments to be made for exercise or marked glycosuria? Of what nature?
13. Are there any special conditions unrelated to diabetes that require a special diet (e.g., gout, hyperlipidemia, renal or cardiac failure)?
14. Can all elements of the prescription be reconciled, and how should this be done? (For example, it is usually not feasible to construct a palatable diet for a lean diabetic if the prescription restricts both carbohydrate and fat.)
15. What kind and degree of changes are to be made subsequently by the dietitian without consulting the physician?
16. What should the patient do if it becomes necessary to postpone or modify a meal (e.g., when attending a dinner meeting or social affair)?
17. Tactical questions:
    a. How much precision is required in the various elements of this prescription?
    b. What foods can be freely allowed?
    c. What foods, if any, are to be weighed or measured?
    d. Are any modifications of the standard exchange system appropriate, such as simplification?
    e. In general, is food to be unmeasured, estimated, measured, or weighed?
    f. Is it necessary or desirable to instruct the patient about the carbohydrate, protein, and fat contents of the common foods?
    g. Under what circumstances are artificial sweeteners and diet drinks to be used?
18. Has the patient's understanding of dietary principles and methods been systematically evaluated?

Setting Up the Diabetic Diet

The first step in formulating the diabetic diet is to calculate the number of calories the patient requires to achieve or maintain a healthy body weight. This is no easy task because no simple approach to the accurate and precise estimation of a specific patient's energy requirements in a clinical setting is available. Caloric requirements are related to the patient's age, level of activity, and body weight. Basal metabolic rates (BMRs) are in the range of 21 to 29 kcal per kg daily for adults below the age of 60, with women, on average, having BMRs slightly lower than those for men. Above the age of 60, the daily BMR is in the range of 19 to 23 kcal per kg. It is most appropriate to start at the low end of these ranges to estimate energy expenditure (see also Chapter 5 for a more detailed discussion of energy expenditure).

A lean individual's estimated energy requirement (EER) in kilocalories per day can be estimated from his or her age, body weight in kilograms, and height in meters according to the following equations (79,80):

Men:
$$EER = 662 - (9.53 \times age) + PA \times [(15.91 \times wt) + (539.6 \times ht)]$$

Women:
$$EER = 354 - (6.91 \times age) + PA \times [9.36 \times wt) + (726 \times ht)]$$

PA is the subject's physical activity quotient. The value of PA assigned to the activities of usual daily living is 1.0. PA increases to 1.11 to 1.12 (for women and men, respectively) for the activities of daily life *plus* an additional 30 to 60 minutes of moderate activity daily, to 1.25 to 1.27 for at least an *additional* 60 minutes of moderate daily activity, and to 1.45 to 48 for the activities of daily life plus an *additional* 180 minutes of moderate activity or at least an *additional* 60 minutes of moderate daily activity plus an *additional* 60 minutes of vigorous activity (15,16).

For overweight and obese men and women, such as most type 2 diabetics, total daily energy expenditure for weight maintenance is better estimated using the following modifications of the above equations (79).

Men:
$$EER = 1086 - (10.1 \times age) + PA \times [(13.7 \times wt) + (416 \times ht)]$$

Women:
$$EER = 448 - (7.95 \times age) + PA \times [11.4 \times wt) + (619 \times ht)]$$

Sedentary men and women are assigned a PA of 1.0. Low active men and women are assigned the PA values of 1.12 for men and 1.16 for women. Active men and women are given PA values of 1.29 and 1.27, respectively; and very active men and women have PA values of 1.59 and 1.44, respectively. For most obese, type 2 diabetics, it is best to estimate activity level at the sedentary or low levels.

The next step in defining a diabetic diet is to determine the relative macronutrient contents. Various consensus guidelines today (56,59–61) are considerably less prescriptive than those in the past because of the realization that the evidence basis for former limits is not supported by more recent research. Thus, recommendations for the macronutrient contents of diets have evolved to lie within the bounds of healthful diets recommended for otherwise healthy adults as described in the *Dietary Guidelines for Americans* and its variants published by other expert bodies and discussed in detail in Chapters 1 to 3 as well as other individual sections of this book, including earlier in this chapter. Recommendations for the amounts and types of dietary carbohydrates, proteins, and fats consumed by diabetics are essentially no different from those for the general population. Likewise, as discussed earlier, carbohydrate choices made on the basis of GI or glycemic load have not been shown consistently and convincingly to improve the glycemic control and/or clinical outcomes of diabetics. Moreover, there is no simple algorithm that can predict the GI of individual foods consumed in a mixed diet. In general, the GIs of complex carbohydrates, especially in fiber-rich foods, are low. Soybeans and peanuts have very low GIs, but the GIs of lentils, chick peas, green peas, kidney beans, and pinto beans are two- to fourfold higher. The GI of fructose is equivalent to that of soybeans, the GI of honey is nearly equivalent to that of glucose, and the GI of table sugar (sucrose) is less than that of a baked potato. The blood glucose response after ingestion of a baked potato is essentially the same as that after oral glucose, but rice and pasta evoke a much lower blood glucose response. The reason for the differences in the glycemic response is not completely understood. The GI is influenced by the rate at which foods are digested and absorbed and the degree to which they raise the blood glucose level.

The rate of gastric emptying and the presence of fat and protein affect the glycemic response. The glycemic response in patients with type 2 diabetes is similar to that seen in normal persons, but the glycemic response in patients with type 1 diabetes is more variable. These individual variations limit the usefulness of the GI as a teaching tool for patients with diabetes. Also, in the context of mixed meals, the GI tends to lose its practical usefulness because the distinctions between individual foods are blurred. For these reasons, many experts do not consider the GI to be a valuable adjunct to diabetes management but prefer to simply regulate total carbohydrate intake using the carbohydrate counting method discussed earlier. Finally, and perhaps most importantly, the extra "work" of incorporating the GI into the overall diabetic diet prescription may neither necessary nor dramatically effective because all healthful diets such as the DASH diet, the Mediterranean diet, and the diet recommended in the *Dietary Guidelines for Americans* are fundamentally low GI diets, if implemented to their full extent.

One must next divide the daily diet prescription into meals. The distribution of calories during the day must be adjusted to the patient's lifestyle and insulin program. A typical diet provides 20% to 30% of calories at breakfast, 20% to 35% at lunch, 25% to 40% at supper, and none to 15% as snacks. Snacks are usually taken at mid-morning, at mid-afternoon, and near bedtime. Tight control of blood glucose is easier if snacks are part of the diet regimen. Mid-morning and mid-afternoon snacks may prevent hypoglycemia by providing calories at times when levels of regular and intermediate-acting insulin reach their peak. Similarly, a bedtime snack may prevent nighttime hypoglycemia. Snacks also reduce the number of calories that are taken at meals and thus help prevent episodes of postprandial hyperglycemia.

After estimating the patient's energy requirement and determining the meal distribution, a specific meal plan is formulated using the exchange list or carbohydrate counting algorithms. As detailed earlier, the purpose of both systems is to allow a patient to vary the foods eaten from day to day and still consume a reasonably constant number of calories with a relatively fixed distribution of calories among macronutrients and meals as shown in Tables 13-3 and 13-4.

A widespread misconception among diabetics is that by spending more money for special "diabetic foods" they can eat what they like and still control their disease. Although sugar alcohols such as sorbitol have, on average, about half the calories of nutritive sweeteners such as sucrose, most dietetic foods contain a significant number of calories. In fact, some products contain as many calories as the comparable regular foods. More importantly, however, is the fact that there is no evidence to indicate that such foods have any therapeutic advantage over regular foods in the care of, control of, or complications of diabetes. Nonnutritive sweeteners are commonly used as adjuncts in the management of both weight and glycemia. While these agents are generally recognized as safe by various expert scientific panels that have studied the issue, there remain somewhat mixed data of variable quality on whether their use, per se, is particularly helpful in achieving weight loss (81–84).

Alcohol is a component of the diet of many Americans. Most diabetics can consume limited amounts of alcohol, but several considerations peculiar to diabetes must be kept in mind. First, as with healthy people, daily alcohol intake should be limited to modest consumption, generally interpreted to mean no more than two drinks daily in men and one in women. Because alcohol contains a significant number of calories (7 kcal per g), it is difficult to fit much alcohol into a weight loss diet and still obtain adequate protein, vitamins, and minerals. In the obese diabetic, alcohol consumption should be minimized or eliminated until the excess weight is lost. Further some alcoholic beverages, especially beer and sweet wines, contain a substantial number of calories in the form of carbohydrate in addition to those in alcohol. These may contribute to hyperglycemia and must be considered in the diet. When using the exchange list system, alcohol is substituted for fat exchanges: 1 oz of whiskey is the equivalent of two to three fat exchanges; 12 oz of low-calorie beer is the equivalent of two fat exchanges.

It is also important to recognize the effect of alcohol consumption on blood glucose. This effect depends on such factors as time, consumption of other foods, and type of beverage. In fasting, insulin-dependent diabetics, the ingestion of a large amount of alcohol can induce profound hypoglycemia by inhibiting the release of glucose from the liver. Alcohol can also impair hepatic glucose production and, consequently, counter-regulation in insulin-induced hypoglycemia (79). This effect may be most pronounced in tightly controlled patients with an increased incidence of hypoglycemia. Because the symptoms of hypoglycemia closely resemble those of alcohol intoxication, the hypoglycemia may go unrecognized, leading to significant detrimental consequences. To minimize the risk of nocturnal hypoglycemia when taking insulin or oral hypoglycemic agents, diabetics should only consume alcohol with food. Alcoholism and insulin-dependent diabetes are an unfortunate combination of diseases.

Alcohol intake can also cause an increase in circulating triglyceride concentration and diabetes is frequently accompanied by hyperlipidemia. Fortunately, control of the blood glucose and achievement of ideal body weight may return the triglycerides levels to normal, so that moderate alcohol consumption can be allowed. Finally, some patients taking sulfonylureas experience flushing, nausea, dyspnea, and palpitations when they drink alcohol. This reaction, which resembles the effect of disulfiram (Antabuse), can be prevented by taking antihistamines before alcohol, although the preferred solution is abstinence.

Modifying the Diet for Illness

In both type 1 and type 2 diabetics who are acutely ill, two general principles always apply. First, insulin or oral hypoglycemic agents should be continued. Second, enhanced testing of plasma glucose and ketone values are necessary, as are drinking adequate amounts of fluids and ingesting sufficient amounts of carbohydrates. Cohen and Edelstein (85) have provided practical guidelines for sick-day management of individuals with diabetes, and Nyenwe and Abbas (86) have published extensive, evidence-based guidelines for the management of hyperglycemic crises in diabetics.

Acute illnesses are frequently accompanied by nausea, vomiting, and anorexia. In patients with type 2 diabetes, acute illness usually does not have a markedly adverse effect on diabetic control. For these patients, the major concern is avoiding dehydration by ensuring adequate fluid intake, usually by frequently ingesting small volumes of liquids and soft foods. Ingestion of at least 150 g of carbohydrate are recommended to reduce starvation ketosis. Occasionally, during an intercurrent illness such as influenza, insulin dependence develops in a patient with non–insulin-dependent diabetes; all diabetic patients should carefully monitor their blood glucose and their urine for the appearance of ketonuria during acute illness (85).

In individuals with type 1 diabetes, acute illness may result in profound hypoglycemia or in profound hyperglycemia and ketosis. Usually, the acute illness tends to increase insulin requirements. The only way to assess the insulin need is by frequent monitoring of blood glucose and urine ketones. The diabetic patient must take in enough carbohydrate (>150 g per day) to prevent starvation ketosis. To prevent hypoglycemia during bouts of illness when appetite is depressed, adequate carbohydrate can be obtained by the frequent ingestion of sweetened fluids and soft, easily digested foods such as ice cream, juices, sweetened Jell-O, and soups. The ingestion of small amounts of fluid on a 15- to 30-minute basis helps to prevent dehydration (see Tables 7-10 and 10-17 for selected oral rehydration solutions and Reference 86 for a detailed discussion of fluid management in hyperglycemic patients).

Modifying the Diet for Activity

Patients with non–insulin-dependent diabetes do not have to alter their diet to accommodate changes in exercise patterns. Exercise is a useful adjunct to caloric restriction in the attempt to lose weight. The overweight diabetic who begins an exercise program should gradually lose weight if the caloric intake is constant. However, it should be emphasized that daily regular physical activity of all kinds is beneficial to persons with type 2 diabetes. The diabetic patient should not be led to interpret "physical activity" as traditional "exercise" (e.g., running, tennis) but made to understand that all forms of nonsedentary behavior are valuable. Brisk walking is one of the most beneficial activities for obese diabetics and has been shown to be an effective adjunct in reducing the risk for coronary heart disease.

Changes in exercise patterns in patients with insulin-dependent diabetes, however, must be accompanied by adjustments in the diet and insulin doses. Obviously, regular exercise every day at a set time, at a set level of activity, for a set length of time is easily accommodated to the person's diabetic dietary regimen. Irregular exercise is a more difficult problem. An hour of moderate to vigorous exercise (e.g., cycling, basketball) will likely require extra dietary carbohydrate intake. If the exercise is to last for less than 2 hours, the consumption of extra food can be delayed until the exercise is complete and the patient determines whether any food is necessary by measuring the blood glucose. Often, however, depending on the subject's prior history of hypoglycemia with moderate exercise for this length of time, a snack of 10 to 15 g of carbohydrate may be consumed before exercise. Among the foods that may be eaten before exercise are low-fat cottage cheese, fruit, yogurt, bread, and crackers. These should be eaten about 30 minutes before exercise. If exercise is vigorous or of long duration, the athlete may need to consume a carbohydrate-rich snack every 30 minutes. The amount of food required to cover exercise depends on body size and the duration and intensity of activity.

Diabetes in Special Groups

Diabetes in Pregnant Women

Insulin-requiring diabetes is frequently more difficult to control during pregnancy, and pregnancy may cause glucose intolerance in a woman with previously normal glucose control. Special modifications of the diabetic diet are not needed to accommodate the additional requirements of pregnancy other than those recommended for pregnant women in general, as described in detail in Chapter 3. However, the normal consequences of pregnancy, such a morning sickness, may disrupt the patient's previously established eating patterns and established insulin regimens.

Weight gain during pregnancy is frequently excessive in diabetic patients and the consequences of obesity in pregnancy are substantial as discussed in Chapter 3. It is preferable to control body weight before pregnancy or, if not possible, to prevent excessive weight gain during pregnancy (Chapter 3). Excessive weight gain during pregnancy also magnifies the physiologic increase in insulin resistance that is a normal consequence of pregnancy. During the second and third trimesters, insulin requirements increase substantially, often as much as 50% to 100%, and additional dietary manipulations may be necessary to accommodate this increase. At the same time, the practitioner must be alert to the fact that the insulin requirement will drop immediately after delivery and the insulin dose lowered to prevent hypoglycemia.

Diabetes in Children

Diabetes is one of the most common serious chronic diseases of childhood. Whereas most adults with diabetes do not require insulin and are obese, 98% of children below the age of 10 with diabetes require insulin, and few are obese. More recently, however, as discussed earlier, the incidence and prevalence of obese, type 2 diabetics has increased substantially in adolescents.

The goals of dietary therapy in children with diabetes are the same as in adults with diabetes, but in addition, dietary therapy must promote normal growth and development. The calorie requirements for children are based on sex, age, size, growth rate, and physical activity and age and gender-specific energy intake recommendations are available elsewhere (79,80). Nevertheless, diets whose calculated energy intakes are constructed from these algorithms are only general guidelines and each child's actual caloric requirement must be determined individually by trial and error. During adolescence, caloric requirements increase with the rate of growth. The energy cost of growth is about 120 kcal per day at peak growth during adolescence, although this still represents only a small percent of the total energy requirement. The energy requirements of individual adolescents vary markedly. The total daily expenditure of energy in adolescent boys ranges from about 50 to 75 kcal per kg and in adolescent girls is between about 50 and 65 kcal per kg, respectively, depending on their resting metabolic rate and their habitual level of physical activity. The calorie allotments for children should be modified according to their longitudinal progress on their own, individual weight, and height charts. Many juvenile diabetics are underweight at the time of diagnosis. A common error is to place underweight children on a diet calculated to meet the needs of children of normal weight of the same age. Underweight children may require an additional several hundred calories per day to regain lost weight and maintain growth.

Diabetes in Patients with Hypertension, Hyperlipidemia, or Renal Disease

Diabetes is frequently associated with other chronic illnesses for which the management includes diet therapy. Chronic renal failure is a common complication of diabetes. Elevated plasma cholesterol and triglyceride levels are common among diabetics. Finally, hypertension, although not directly related to diabetes, is common among the obese, middle-aged patients who comprise the majority of the diabetic population. Because each of these illnesses is treated in part by dietary measures, the formulation of a diet for patients with more than one of these illnesses requires additional planning. Fortunately, the diets used in the management of these several illnesses do not conflict with, but frequently complement, each other.

Patients with Diabetes and Chronic Kidney Disease

Recently, the National Kidney Foundation reported clinical practice guidelines for individuals with diabetes and kidney disease (87) and the subject was also recently reviewed by others (88). For diabetics with kidney disease, other than end-stage renal disease, a target daily protein intake of 0.7 to 0.8 g per kg body weight is recommended, with additional protein intake, as necessary, to replace urinary protein losses in patients with significant albuminuria and minimize the risk of protein–energy wasting (89). Nonetheless, the results of the Modification of Diet in Renal Disease Study, the largest of its kind ever conducted, were inconclusive when attempting to show whether a reduction in dietary protein intake from 1.3 g/kg/d to 0.58 g/k/d would slow the progression of nondiabetic renal kidney disease (90). When consuming dietary protein intakes at the level of 0.8 g/kg/d, individuals must take care to consume dietary proteins of high biologic value, as described later in this chapter. In addition, patients must restrict their intakes of phosphorus, potassium, and sodium. None of these requirements should interfere with the recommended diabetic diet. The principal medical and pharmacologic therapeutic guidelines for the care of diabetics with kidney disease are directed toward control of hyperglycemia, hypertension, and hyperlipidemia. The dietary recommendations for nutritional control of these entities are fundamentally encompass the healthful diet patterns that are proposed for normal healthy adults (Chapters 1 to 3). In this context, one must be aware that the DASH and DASH-sodium diets that are fruit, vegetable, and grain-based diets that have been shown to be effective in reducing blood pressure are relatively high-protein diets with a daily protein intake on the order of 1.4 g/kg/d. Thus, applying the DASH diets to chronic kidney disease requires modification of the protein intake to comply with consensus recommendations (89), although modifications may not necessarily be especially restrictive based on the results of the Modification of Diet in Renal Disease Study (90).

Patients with Diabetes and Hyperlipidemia

Hypertriglyceridemia occurs in about 20% of patients with type 2 diabetes. Management regimens, including appropriate blood glucose control with insulin or oral agents, reduction of alcohol intake, and caloric restriction to attain ideal body weight, should result in reduced blood levels of both lipids and sugar. The dietary approach to hyperlipidemia is discussed in more detail later in this chapter.

Patients with Diabetes and Hypertension

The major dietary manipulations in the treatment of hypertension are caloric restriction, to help obese patients lose weight, sodium restriction (see Chapter 12) and the implementation of a healthful dietary pattern such as the DASH diet plan based on increased fruit and vegetable intake with elimination of foods that are both high in calories and in sodium, such as processed dinners and snacks, cold cuts, sausage, French fries, salted nuts, and snack chips. In this context, to be successful it is critical to read the nutrition facts label of every purchased product. Eliminating these items helps control both diabetes and hypertension (see Chapter 12 for a discussion of the low-sodium diet). Regular exercise and a reduced alcohol intake are also useful proven adjuncts in the treatment of hypertensive diabetics. The recommended pharmacologic approaches can be found in References 87 and 88.

RENAL DISEASE
General Principles

Diet therapy is an essential component of the management of renal disease. As mentioned above, although overall clinical practice evidence points to the fact that low-protein diets will retard the progression of chronic renal disease, unequivocal demonstration of this thesis remains elusive following the inconclusive (but largely negative) outcome of the largest systematic, randomized trial conducted to test this hypothesis (90,91). Mitch and Ikizler (92) and Kopple et al. (93)

have published the most recent, detailed analyses of nutritional management of individuals with impaired kidney function.

The goals of diet therapy are to (a) provide adequate nutrition, (b) minimize uremia and other metabolic derangements, (c) reduce the risk factors for cardiovascular disease and other comorbid conditions, and (d) delay the progression of renal failure. Improvement in the patient's metabolic status reduces the symptoms associated with uremia, including fatigue, nausea, pruritus, and anorexia.

A wasting syndrome in uremic patients is secondary to inadequate dietary intake of protein and energy, altered protein metabolism, and the endocrine abnormalities associated with renal failure (hyperparathyroidism, insulin resistance) (89,92,93). In addition, patients on dialysis lose nutrients into the dialysate, which further contributes to wasting. A major factor contributing to malnutrition in chronic renal failure is the *anorexia* caused by uremia. Uremia also diminishes taste acuity, so that food seems bland and unappealing. Proper nutrition may help reverse the wasting syndrome. For example, the correct manipulation of dietary protein can reduce the degree of uremia; if the patient's appetite improves, the caloric intake increases and wasting is reversed. Total parenteral nutrition (TPN) can be used in patients with chronic renal failure, whether they are managed conservatively or on dialysis, although this represents a management aid in complex rather than routine situations. The use of TPN in the renal patient is covered in Chapter 11 (Table 11-11). However, what has also become apparent in the last several years is that protein loss is associated with increased inflammatory cytokines that augment protein wasting by as yet incompletely understood mechanisms (94–96). As a consequence, trying to correct protein loss by simply feeding more protein is unsuccessful. Additionally, there is now substantial evidence that metabolic acidosis is a major contributor to both protein and bone loss in chronic kidney disease (97,98). The latter realization has led to therapeutic regimens aimed at treating the acidosis and raising serum bicarbonate levels into the normal range. Such treatment regimens have been shown to slow the loss of residual renal function (97). Perhaps as surprising is recognition that increasing dietary fruit and vegetable intakes as a means of decreasing metabolic acidosis are also effective and may provide a mechanism for the beneficial effects of the DASH diet plan (98).

The dietary management of chronic renal disease depends on the degree of renal failure and the need for dialysis. The National Kidney Foundation has published its clinical practice guidelines for chronic kidney disease that divides chronic renal disease into five stages (99):

Stage 1: Kidney damage with normal or increased glomerular filtration rate (GFR) ≥greater than or equal to 90 mL/min/1.73 m^2

Stage 2: Kidney damage with mildly decreased GFR between 60 and 89 mL/min/1.73 m^2

Stage 3: Moderately decreased GFR (30 to 59 mL/min/1.73 m^2)

Stage 4: Severely decreased GFR (15 to 29 mL/min/1.73 m^2)

Stage 5: Renal failure (GFR less than 15 mL/min/1.73 m^2) (or receiving dialysis)

While nutritional modifications are important in every stage of declining renal function, clearly the most stringent attention to nutrient intake must take place in Stage 5 renal disease when every aspect of nutrient ingestion and excretion are under conscious control of both the patient and the physician.

Phases of Management

Chronic Kidney Disease in Nondiaylzed Patients
Protein Quantity

In the predialysis phases of chronic kidney disease, renal function has not progressed to the point at which dialysis is indicated, but dietary therapy is a critically important component of medical care. Dietary protein intake is generally not restricted in people with Stage 1 or Stage 2 renal disease (GFR greater than 60 mL/min/1.73 m^2). For individuals with Stage 3 renal disease, recommendations for dietary protein restriction are somewhat variable since the data to support these recommendations are less clear. However, recommended dietary protein intakes in the range of 0.6 to 0.75 g protein/kg/d is generally the rule (92,93) with the initial goal toward the lower end of this range. It is important that the dietary proteins consumed are those of high biologic value such as found in meat, fish, and eggs. When renal disease progresses to Stage 4, dietary protein intake should be reduced to 0.60 g protein/kg/d (92,93). Available evidence supports the fact that this dietary approach can maintain good nutritional status, good metabolic status, limit symptoms of renal disease, and its secondary effects (e.g., renal osteodystrophy), while possibly slowing the progression of renal failure. Individuals with chronic renal disease who have nephrotic syndrome represent a special therapeutic category because of body protein loss via proteinuria. In these cases, dietary protein intake is liberalized somewhat to replace the irreversible loss of protein in the urine. Recommendations for protein intake average about 0.8 g protein/kg/d, but values range from about 0.7 g to 1.0 g (92,93). There is another very important modification of the dietary prescription, specifically recommended consumption of an additional 1.0 g of high biologic value protein per day for each gram of urinary protein lost above 5 g per day (93). In all instances above, compliance with dietary protein intake recommendations is followed by measuring urinary nitrogen excretion (92,93).

Protein Quality

As renal disease progresses, the ability of the kidneys to excrete urea diminishes. The load of urea presented to the kidneys is usually proportional to the amount of protein in the diet; however, even patients on a zero-protein diet produce some urea as a result of the breakdown of tissue proteins. If too much protein is included in the diet, the level of blood urea nitrogen (BUN) rises and symptoms of uremia develop. However, when dietary protein intake is restricted too much as a therapeutic or preventive strategy, the supply of essential amino acids required for the synthesis of necessary proteins becomes inadequate and protein malnutrition is the consequence. Further, it is not only important for a patient to consume an adequate *amount* of protein; it is also important that the protein be of the right *type* or *quality*. Dietary amino acids are classified as either nonessential or essential. Because the body cannot synthesize essential amino acids, they must come from the diet. Nonessential amino acids can be ingested or synthesized. In chronic renal failure, endogenous synthesis of the nonessential amino acids is preferable to ingestion for two reasons: The synthesis of an amino acid uses up an amino nitrogen that would otherwise go into urea, and the synthesis of an amino acid reduces the amount that amino acid that must be consumed in dietary protein. The net effect of both processes is diminished substrate for urea production. An alternative to this approach is the use of dietary α-keto acid analogues of essential amino acids. Via transamination, these keto acids are converted into the respective essential amino acids, so that an amino acid group is salvaged, while simultaneously an essential amino acid is provided. However, the evidence basis for whether this option can retard the progression of renal failure is largely negative and diets containing keto acid supplements are not recommended (93).

Essential amino acids, on the other hand, must be present in the diet (as protein) in quantities adequate to allow the required level of body protein synthesis. Moreover, in uremia, the conversion of phenylalanine to tyrosine is impaired and uremics also appear unable to synthesize enough histidine to meet their needs. Thus, these two amino acids (not normally essential in healthy individuals) become conditionally essential amino acids in patients with chronic kidney disease. The need to supply a sufficient amount of essential amino acids in the diet can become problematic in patients with chronic kidney disease since, to reduce generation of urea, they must restrict dietary protein intake. To accomplish both goals (sufficient essential amino acids and limited urea production) while maintaining adequate synthesis of body proteins, it is essential that the proteins these individuals consume have the maximum amounts of essential amino acids per gram of protein. Proteins of *high biologic value* meet this requirement, since most of the nitrogen is in the form of essential amino acids, all essential amino acids are present in the protein, and the essential amino acids are present in concentrations proportional to the minimum daily requirements. Eggs are the food with proteins of the highest biologic value. Other foods with proteins of high biologic value include fish, poultry, lean meat, and dairy products, while proteins of low biologic value are found in various grains, nuts, seeds, and legumes.

Other Diet and Lifestyle Recommendations

With few exceptions, such as dietary protein intake discussed above and the others discussed below, overall nutrition and lifestyle guidelines for individuals whose GFR are greater than about 30 mL/min/1.73 m^2 are largely consistent with those recommended in the *Dietary Guidelines for Americans* and the American Heart Association dietary guidelines (as discussed in Chapter 1), those discussed for people with diabetes earlier in this chapter, and the report of the Joint National Committee on Prevention, Detection, Evaluation and Treatment of High Blood Pressure (JNC 7) (100). Blood pressure control in patients with chronic renal disease is particularly important because lower systolic blood pressure is predictive of a more positive clinical outcome (101–105) and antihypertensive drug therapy is part of routine clinical care (106–107). Nonetheless, more recent data have questioned overly aggressive attempts to control blood pressure because very strict control of both systolic and diastolic blood pressures is associated with increased all-cause mortality in individuals with chronic kidney disease (108,109). Thus, some have recently recommended an optimal blood pressure range of 130 to 159 systolic and 70 to 89 diastolic in patients with chronic renal disease (108,109). In the context of blood pressure and extracellular fluid volume control, dietary sodium restriction has long served as a mainstay of the clinical management of patients with chronic renal disease (92,93). Like the data above suggesting moderation in blood pressure goals, recent dietary sodium intake data and their relationship with mortality, both in the general population and in patients with chronic renal disease, have suggested that more modest sodium restriction is the most prudent course of action in chronic renal disease subjects whose GFR are not extremely low, requiring dialysis (110–116).

In addition to the restricted protein and sodium intakes discussed above, individuals with chronic kidney disease require attention to their dietary intakes of potassium and phosphorus. Since the kidney is the predominant route for potassium excretion, one might expect that limitation of potassium intake is necessary once GFR begins to fall. However, as GFR falls, serum potassium levels tend to remain normal as long as urine volume is more than about 1 L daily (93) because both renal tubular and fecal excretion of potassium increase (92,93). Thus, it is generally not necessary to restrict dietary potassium intake until it is necessary to limit sodium intake in persons with chronic renal disease as the GFR declines. In fact, if hyperkalemia develops, one should be alert to the possibility of constipations, increased catabolism, academia, hyperaldosteronism, and unwanted side effects of antihypertensive drugs (92,93). As GFR declines to the lower levels found in Stage 3, potassium restriction to under about 4 g daily is sometimes necessary. In Stage 4, potassium intake is restricted to approximately 2 to 2.5 g daily (92,93).

Physicians are now increasingly recognizing the role of excess phosphate intake and hyperphosphatemia in elevating the risk of detrimental cardiovascular events in patients with chronic kidney disease (117,118). Furthermore, serum phosphorus control is a significant clinical issue because hyperphosphatemia can lead to the development of hyperparathyroidism as well as calcium phosphate deposits in soft tissues and arteries (92,93). Since phosphorus is widely present in foods, especially in animal products, as phytates in plants and as additives in a broad array of food products, reducing dietary phosphorus intake is no trivial undertaking. It is especially important to recognize what is now called "hidden phosphorus" present in many processed foods and popular beverages (119–131). Although there is some lack of consensus and because it is very difficult to keep a very-low-phosphorus diet, there is some lack of consensus on the optimal intake of phosphorous in clinical practice, but recommended intakes are largely in the range of 0.8 to 1.0 g phosphorus per day (92,93,99).

Table 13-5 shows a summary of the major nutritional recommendations for individuals with chronic kidney disease who do not require dialysis (93) and recommendations that are similar overall in principle, but not necessarily identical in practice, may be found in other expert assessments (Reference 92, for example). Thus, it is important to recognize that the values in Table 13-5 are only initial estimates. In clinical practice, it is essential to tailor dietary nutrient intakes on an individualized basis. This is particularly true because required essential nutrient intakes are not well defined in patients with chronic renal disease and because they are known to vary because of the progressive decline in GFR.

Chronic Kidney Disease Requiring Dialysis
Protein Intake

When the GFR falls to approximately 5 mL/1.73 m^2/min (advanced Stage 5 chronic kidney disease), dietary manipulation alone can no longer control the metabolic abnormalities associated with renal failure, and transplantation or dialysis is required. Even if the subject's GFR is in

TABLE 13-5 Nutritional Requirements for Patients with Chronic Renal Failure (93)

Dietary Nutrients	Chronic Kidney Disease Prior to Dialysis	Chronic Renal Failure Requiring Maintenance Dialysis
Protein	0.6–0.75 g/kg/d (of which ≥0.35 g/kg/d is protein of high biologic value)	Hemodialysis: 1.1–1.2 g/kg/d (≥50% high biologic value)
Peritoneal dialysis: 1.2–1.3 g/kg/d		
Energy	>35 kcal/kg/d[a]	>35 kcal/kg/d[a]
Fat	30%–40% energy	30%–40% energy
P:S fat ratio	1:1	1:1
Carbohydrate	Rest of nonprotein calories	Rest of nonprotein calories
Fiber	20–25 g/d	20–25 g/d
Fluids	Up to 3 L/d[b]	Usually 750–1,500 mL/d[b]
Sodium	1–3 g/d[b]	0.75–1.0 g/d[b]
Potassium	40–70 mEq/d	40–70 mEq/d
Phosphorus	5–10 mg/kg/d	8–17 mg/kg/d
Calcium	800 mg/d	800 mg/d
Magnesium	200–300 mg/d	200–300 mg/d
Iron	≥10–18 mg/d[c]	≥10–18 mg/d[c]
Zinc	15 mg/d	15 mg/d
Vitamin Supplements		
Thiamine	1.5 mg/d	1.5 mg/d
Riboflavin	1.8 mg/d	1.8 mg/d
Pantothenic acid	5 mg/d	5 mg/d
Niacin	20 mg/d	20 mg/d
Pyridoxine HCl	5 mg/d	5–10 mg/d
Vitamin A	0	0
Folic acid	1 mg/d	1 mg/d
Vitamin B_{12}	3 µg/d	3 µg/d
Vitamin C	70 mg/d	730 mg/d
Vitamin D	800 mg/d[d]	See text[d]
Vitamin E	15 mg/d[e]	15 mg/d[e]
Vitamin K	0	0

[a]Unless patient is overweight, obese, or is gaining unwanted weight. See Reference 93.
[b]Can be higher in patients with greater urinary or dialysis losses. See Reference 93.
[c]Ten milligrams for men and nonmenstruating women; 18 mg for menstruating women.
[d]Initial estimates only. Adjustments to intake recommendations are best made on the basis of circulating 25OHD levels. See Reference 93 for discussion.
[e]As α-tocopherol (includes *RRR*-α-tocopherol and the 2*R*-stereoisomeric forms).
(Data from Kopple JD, Ross AC, Caballerio B, et al. Nutrition, diet and the kidney. In: *Modern Nutrition in Health and Disease*. 11th ed. Philadelphia: Wolters Kluwer; 2014; see text.)

the upper ranges of Stage 5 chronic kidney disease, dialysis should be considered if nutritional status and body weight are difficult to maintain. The goals of diet therapy for patients on dialysis are to minimize metabolic abnormalities, correct for nutrients lost during dialysis, and provide sufficient nutritional support to prevent the protein–energy malnutrition that is commonly seen in patients undergoing maintenance dialysis (92,93,99).

In the absence of dialysis, the argument for limiting dietary protein intake is far more compelling in Stage 5 chronic renal disease. In this circumstance, a reduction in dietary protein intake not only reduces the generation of deleterious nitrogenous metabolic products but also leads to a concomitant reduction in the intake of both phosphorus and potassium, which generate additional deleterious metabolites. However, since these patients are at high risk of malnutrition and the long-term consequences of uremia, and since there is no evidence that withholding dialysis and limiting protein intake leads to a better outcome than instituting dialysis and providing a more liberal diet, most nephrologists recommend that maintenance dialysis (or renal transplantation) commence at this stage of deterioration of renal function.

When dialysis is successfully established, protein intake can be liberalized somewhat because of the nitrogen removed during dialysis. For patients undergoing maintenance hemodialysis, the recommended daily dietary protein intake is 1.2 g protein per kg body weight and for those undergoing peritoneal dialysis, it is 1.2 to 1.3 g protein per kg body weight (74,75) (Table 13-5). At least half of the dietary proteins consumed should be high-biologic-value proteins. This level of protein intake avoids the protein–energy malnutrition that can occur at lower intake levels due to the reduced capacity of these patients to conserve body proteins, amino acids, and other biologically important nitrogenous compounds are lost in the dialysate. In hemodialysis, losses are estimated to be as high as 1 g of free amino acids per hour and 3 g of total (free plus protein-bound) amino acids per hour. Thus, a standard 4-hour session of hemodialysis results in losses equivalent to 5 to 10 g of protein. Because a large proportion (30% to 40%) of the amino acids lost in the dialysate are essential amino acids, it is critical that at least half of the dietary protein be of high biologic value, as noted above. For similar reasons, patients undergoing long-term peritoneal dialysis may require even a greater intake of protein than patients on hemodialysis. The "pores" of the peritoneum are larger than those of dialysis tubing and so allow even larger proteins to be lost into the dialysate. On average, these patients lose 10 to 14 g of protein, peptides, and amino acids daily into the dialysate fluid.

Energy Intake

Daily maintenance energy intake in dialyzed patients is set at 35 kcal per kg body weight for those who are less than 60 years of age and 30 to 35 kcal per kg body weight for those older than 60. These are target values. If an individual is obese, overweight, or gaining weight at an accelerated rate, energy intake should be reduced. Likewise, individuals who are losing weight may require a higher energy intake.

An adequate intake of calories in the form of carbohydrates and fats is required to prevent the use of dietary or tissue protein as a source of energy. The catabolism of proteins results in increased urea production. The ideal calorie intake is whatever is required to achieve and maintain an ideal body weight. Patients who are below their ideal body weight need more calories. Unfortunately, the average calorie intake of dialysis patients is frequently lower than 30 kcal/kg/d and patients with chronic renal failure are often energy-deficient as manifested by weight loss, diminished adipose tissue, and loss of muscle mass. Because these patients also tend to be volume-expanded, their muscle mass and fat stores may be even lower than their weight might suggest.

Dietary instructions for renal patients must be complete, given by professionals, and reinforced regularly. Achieving an adequate caloric intake is a major problem in the management of patients with chronic renal failure. In some cases, compliance with other dietary restrictions must be sacrificed to attain an adequate caloric intake. The vigorous pursuit of perfect metabolic balance may result in a diet that is totally unpalatable and a patient with an inadequate calorie intake.

Because they are frequently anorectic and have difficulty in maintaining an adequate calorie intake, patients with chronic renal failure may require nutritional supplements that supply energy. Many commercial nutritional supplements are now available that are especially appropriate for patients with renal failure. In some supplements, the calories are all carbohydrate (e.g., G2 Gatorade) (Table 10-17). Other supplements are more specific to renal failure; they contain a mixture of fat and carbohydrate and are designed to be low in protein, phosphorus, sodium, and potassium for readily apparent reasons (e.g., Nepro). Table 10-4 lists the supplements specifically intended for patients with renal disease, and Table 10-5 provides the detailed nutritional content of some of them.

Water Intake

Water requirements are not usually a major problem for patients with chronic renal failure who are not receiving dialysis. Fluid intake should equal insensible loss (water lost from skin and lungs, which is usually 400 to 600 mL per day) plus urine volume. Most conservatively managed patients do well on 1.5 to 3.0 L per day. The goal of fluid (and salt) management in the patient who are receiving dialysis is to limit the rate of weight gain between dialysis treatments to 1 lb per day. This can be achieved with a diet containing 750 to 1,000 mg of sodium plus a water intake in the range of 750 to 1,000 mL daily (Table 13-5). A daily fluid allotment of 1,000 mL includes 500 mL for insensible losses and 500 mL for a 1-lb weight gain. Fluid in food must be subtracted from the fluid allotment. Any food that is liquid at room temperature (e.g., gelatin, ice cream) is counted as a fluid. Fruits and vegetables are 85% to 90% water, cooked cereals are 70% to 85% water, and meat is 45% to 60% water. It should be readily apparent that 1,000 mL per day is a severe fluid restriction; compliance is difficult for many patients.

In patients undergoing long-term peritoneal dialysis and in those on hemodialysis who have greater urinary losses, water and sodium intakes may be increased. Thus, in the absence of anuria, urinary salt and water losses can be added to the restrictive allowances above. Stringent salt restrictions may improve metabolic control but make the diet unpalatable. Nonetheless, patients with hypertension and congestive heart failure may have to reduce their salt intake.

Sodium Intake

Recommendations for dietary sodium intake are outlined in Table 13-5, and sodium-restricted diets are readily available. One must consider modest sodium restriction when possible because of the growing concern about the potentially detrimental consequences of severe sodium restriction as discussed earlier in this chapter. Little sodium is excreted in the feces, and as chronic renal disease progresses, the ability of the kidneys to respond to variations in sodium intake diminishes. The normal kidney responds to a low-sodium diet by reabsorbing virtually all the filtered sodium and responds to a high-sodium diet by reabsorbing less. The failing kidney progressively filters and reabsorbs less sodium and cannot adapt to changes in sodium intake. When this happens, edema, hypertension, and congestive heart failure may ensue. On the other hand, too little dietary sodium intake can result in dehydration, a reduced GFR, and acceleration of the deterioration in renal function. The goal is to have the daily sodium intake equal the fixed daily loss. Recently, Smyth et al. (132) systematically reviewed the data on sodium intake and renal outcomes in individuals with and without kidney disease. They concluded that high sodium intakes (more than 4.6 g per day) are likely detrimental, a conclusion supported by all of the data collected by others about adverse CVD outcomes in people without renal disease (110–114). Even so, the data in patients with renal disease are limited. On the other hand, Smyth et al. (132) found that the association of detrimental renal outcomes with low sodium intakes is uncertain due to inconsistent findings in available published reports. Again, this finding is consistent with other recent data on low dietary sodium intakes and adverse clinical outcomes (110–114).

Most patients with renal disease with GFR greater than 5 mL per minute will tolerate dietary sodium intakes in the range of 1 to 3 g per day (40 to 130 millimol per day), although the actual intake must be individualized to the patient. Further deterioration of renal function requires restriction and control over sodium intake to a level approximately half that immediately above. Following initiation of dialysis, the restriction may be liberalized somewhat because sodium output into the dialysate can be increased and managed to some degree. Patients with renal disease are often placed on diets in which the sodium restrictions are excessively stringent. A rising BUN may reflect dehydration instead of excessive protein intake. Further, not all forms of chronic renal failure affect sodium homeostasis in the same way. Pyelonephritis and polycystic kidney disease tend to be salt-wasting conditions requiring increased dietary sodium, and glomerulonephritis is associated with hypertension that might require a lower salt intake.

In any case, dietary sodium requirements change with nonurinary salt losses, primarily those in sweat. Sodium restrictions must be liberalized in warm climates for patients whose homes are not air-conditioned. Some patients require sodium bicarbonate for the treatment of acidosis, a management option that is now becoming more frequent because of demonstrated benefits

(97,98). In such cases, dietary sodium must be reduced to compensate for the sodium in the sodium bicarbonate if that is the alkalinizing agent used. Two grams of sodium bicarbonate contain the same amount of sodium as 1.5 g of salt.

Potassium Intake

For the reasons discussed above, individuals with chronic kidney disease do not require significant dietary potassium restriction until GFR and urine volume fall to very low levels, generally below about 15 to 20 mL per minute. Foods high in protein are usually also high in potassium, and, if patients with very low GFR, hyperkalemia may develop. The standard American diet contains 50 to 100 mEq of potassium per day. Patients with a GFR of less than 15 mL per minute usually require potassium restriction to 40 to 70 mEq per day. Hyperkalemia is less likely in those with a urine output of 1,000 mL or more per day. A 40-g protein diet (0.6 gm protein/kg/d for a 70-kg person) provides 50 to 60 mEq of potassium per day. Excessive dietary potassium can lead to hyperkalemia and the danger of cardiac arrhythmias. Patients with renal failure should not use salt substitutes that contain large amounts of potassium (Table 7-16). Similarly, they should not be given potassium supplements when treated with thiazides or furosemide. Hyperkalemia is exacerbated by acidosis and catabolic stress with muscle protein breakdown. These conditions should be prevented by proper medical management and corrected expeditiously when they occur. In some patients, potassium restriction may not be necessary, since, despite nearly normal serum potassium levels, the total body potassium is frequently low in chronic renal failure, since most potassium is located intracellularly. Thus, dietary potassium should not be appreciably restricted unless hyperkalemia is a problem and the urine output is below about 1,000 mL per day. Table 13-5 provides some general guidelines. The National Kidney Foundation provides guidelines on choosing foods to help regulate dietary potassium intake at http://www.kidney.org/atoz/content/potassium.

Phosphorus, Calcium, and Vitamin D Intakes

Renal osteodystrophy, a major problem in chronic renal disease, results from the abnormalities in calcium, phosphorus, parathyroid hormone (PTH), and vitamin D homeostasis brought on by renal failure (133–137). As the kidney fails, its ability to clear phosphate diminishes, and the serum phosphate level rises. Hyperphosphatemia is accompanied by hypocalcemia, which causes the release of PTH. Elevated levels of PTH result in increased renal phosphate clearance and bone resorption. The goals of therapy in renal osteodystrophy are to suppress secondary hyperparathyroidism and normalize osteoid mineralization by reducing phosphate absorption by decreasing dietary phosphate intake and using phosphate-binding gels, and by supplementing the diet with calcium and vitamin D. Table 13-5 shows the recommended phosphorus intakes for individuals with chronic kidney disease requiring dialysis.

PTH levels rise with the loss of as little as 25% of renal function. Thus, one of the earliest interventions required in renal failure is the reduction of phosphate absorption. Phosphate absorption is reduced by lowering the dietary intake of phosphate using specialized diets for that purpose and by administering phosphate-binding agents. The usual American diet contains 1.0 to 1.8 g of phosphorus per day. Intakes on the order of 1.0 to 1.2 g per day appear appropriate for individuals with GFR greater than 30 mL per minute, and these can be attained with modest dietary modifications and paying attention to the hidden sources of dietary phosphate discussed above (119–131). The elimination of milk, milk products, cheese, colas, and instant powdered beverages combined with protein restriction (40 g per day) can help reduce intake further, perhaps to the range of about 600 mg per day. Nonetheless, when the GFR falls below about 20 to 25 mL/min/d, this level of dietary phosphorus restriction is still not adequate to prevent hyperphosphatemia. The diet of patients on dialysis is higher in protein than that of conservatively managed patients, so that their dietary intake of phosphorus is also usually higher. The need for phosphate binders is just as great for dialysis patients as for nondialysis patients, and several commercial phosphate binders are available. The goal in using phosphate binders is to keep the serum phosphorus level in the range of 4 to 5 mg per dL. Most clinicians use phosphate-binding agents early in the course of renal disease before imposing any dietary restrictions. As mentioned earlier, data support the beneficial effects of such agents (138) and additional evidence-based meta-analyses support the efficacy of other therapeutic agents such as bisphosphonates on reduction of bone loss and fracture risk in patients with renal bone disease (139,140).

Calcium Intake

Although chronic renal failure causes a positive phosphorus balance, it results in a negative calcium balance. Several factors contribute to the negative calcium balance—hyperparathyroidism, calcium malabsorption secondary to vitamin D deficiency, and a diet low in calcium because phosphorus-rich dairy products are restricted. Patients with GFR greater than 30 mL per minute require calcium intakes of about 800 mg per day, although this value will vary depending on whether they are also taking vitamin D supplements. Patients with GFR less than about 15 mL per minute may require calcium intakes in the 1,000 to 1,600 mg per day range, and this will likely require use of calcium supplements. Because a diet with 40 g of protein provides about 300 to 400 mg of calcium daily, these subjects require approximately 0.8 to 1.3 g of calcium supplements daily.

Before calcium supplementation is started, it is important that the serum phosphorus be under control using phosphate binders such as sevelamer carbonate and lanthanum carbonate (93), but the data are insufficient to establish superiority of any one kind of binder on long-term outcomes like mortality (141). If calcium supplements are given in the face of hyperphosphatemia, one runs the risk of depositing calcium phosphate in soft tissues. The goal is to maintain serum calcium within the normal range (corrected for serum albumin level) (93).

Vitamin D Intake

The reduction in functioning renal mass in chronic renal failure is accompanied by a decreased conversion of 25-hydroxycholecalciferol (25OHD) to 1,25-dihydroxycholecalciferol (1,25OHD), the active metabolite of vitamin D. The decreased levels of 1,25-dihydoxycholecalciferol result in a decreased absorption of dietary calcium. Depending on one's definition of the level of circulating 25OHD that defines vitamin D deficiency, 50% to 100% of dialysis patients are vitamin D–deficient (142). While the metabolic consequences are clear, the long-term clinical benefits of vitamin D supplementation in chronic kidney disease are somewhat less clear. Several systematic reviews appear to confirm that vitamin D therapy can diminish proteinuria, delay the decline of renal function, and improve mortality, although some of the data analyzed come from observational trials (143–146), while other systematic assessment that focus only on the results of randomized controlled trials (147–149) can find no benefit of vitamin D supplementation.

In practice, vitamin D status can be monitored by measuring the plasma levels of 25OHD and intact PTH. Current guidelines for individuals with Stage 3 to Stage 5 chronic kidney disease recommend vitamin D supplementation of 800 IU per day, and if this dose does not increase serum 25OHD levels to less than 30 ng per mL, the vitamin D dose may be increased to 1,200 to 2,000 IU per day (93). Because it can be difficult to increase 25OHD levels, some have recommended even considerably higher doses of vitamin D (142). At the same time, because it is possible to induce hypercalcemia and hyperphosphatemia by giving calcium and vitamin D supplements, it is critical to confirm that circulating intact PTH, corrected calcium, and phosphorus values are in the target ranges for the stage of chronic kidney disease. Patients with Stage 5 chronic kidney disease who are receiving dialysis and who have serum levels of intact PTH greater than 300 pg per mL should receive a vitamin D supplement at a level that reduces serum PTH to within a target range of 150 to 300 pg per mL. In this case, intermittent, intravenous administration of calcitriol (1,25OHD) is more effective than oral administration.

Iron Intake

Twenty-five percent of nontransfused patients on long-term hemodialysis are deficient in iron. Iron intake (especially heme iron intake) is frequently low. A major cause of iron deficiency in these patients is the loss of 5 to 20 mL of blood left in the dialyzer after each treatment, which can amount to a loss of several hundred milligrams to a gram of iron per year. In addition, the heparin used as an anticoagulant may increase gastrointestinal and uterine blood loss and erythropoietin treatment will increase iron need due to increased erythropoiesis. For these reasons, many dialysis patients receive supplementation with 300 mg $FeSO_4$ up to three times daily (93).

Requirements for Other Vitamins

Patients with chronic renal failure are frequently vitamin-deficient because of their poor dietary intakes, either because of anorexia or because of iatrogenic dietary restrictions, and due to detrimental nutrient-drug interactions. However, the alterations in vitamin requirements caused by chronic renal failure are poorly defined, and the systematic data are insufficient to set new dietary reference intakes (DRIs) for vitamins. Supplementation with vitamin A should be avoided because chronic renal disease is associated with elevated levels of vitamin A. Vitamin K supplementation is not routinely required but may be necessary in patients who are receiving TPN and antibiotics. The loss of water-soluble vitamins into the dialysate in hemodialysis creates an additional demand. Nonetheless, although no consensus recommendations regarding the increased needs are available, many experts advise prudent supplementation of water-soluble vitamins (Table 13-5). One standard multivitamin plus 1 mg of folic acid per day should meet most requirements. The recommended vitamin supplementation is the same for both conservatively managed patients and those on dialysis.

Dietary Management of Concomitant Hyperlipoproteinemia and Hypertension

In chronic kidney disease, the catabolism of triglyceride-rich lipoproteins is diminished, leading to an increase in the circulating levels of the atherogenic apolipoprotein-B containing very-low-density lipoproteins (VLDL) and intermediate-density lipoproteins (IDLs), as well as a decrease in circulating high-density lipoproteins (HDL) (see later in this chapter). Clinical practice recommendations have been published for the management of hyperlipidemias in renal disease (150,151). The expert committee issuing these recommendations largely adopted the recommendations made by the National Cholesterol Education Task Force, Adult Treatment Panel III (ATP III) (152) as will be discussed later in this chapter. Saikumar and Kovesday (153) have recently discussed some of the ways that end-stage renal disease alters interpretation of traditional serum lipoprotein values. Hypertension is a common comorbidity in chronic kidney disease. The Eight Joint National Committee recently issued the current, evidence-based guidelines for the management of hypertension in patients with chronic kidney disease (154,155). Various additional recommendations and supporting data can be found throughout the medical literature (100–109). The goal of treatment is to maintain systolic blood pressure less than 140 mm Hg and diastolic blood pressure less than 90 mm Hg with the pharmaceutical mainstays of treatment being angiotensin-converting enzyme (ACE) inhibitors or angiotensin-receptor blockers (ARB) (154). Additionally, from the onset of treatment and maintained throughout, lifestyle change that includes maintaining a healthy body weight and increasing physical activity, a reduction of alcohol intake, a reduction in dietary sodium intake, and a focus on the DASH dietary intake pattern with an increased intake of fruits, vegetables, low-fat dairy products, whole grains, poultry, fish, and nuts (with modification of the high protein, potassium, and phosphorus intakes of the DASH diet pattern to accommodate the needs of patients with chronic kidney disease) form the foundation of the nonpharmaceutical management plan.

Practical Management Issues

1. In chronic renal failure, caloric intake is more likely to be inadequate than excessive; thus, caloric restriction is usually not appropriate. On the other hand, the proper dietary management of chronic renal failure is quite compatible with a diet low in sugars and alcohol and high in polyunsaturated fats.
2. A brief physical examination in addition to standard blood chemistry studies should make it possible to determine patient compliance and any needed changes in the diet. Various laboratory tests and other criteria assist in monitoring the adequacy of specific nutrients.
3. In patients who undergo dialysis three times a week, a reasonable goal is a BUN of 60 to 80 mg per dL after the longest interval between dialysis sessions (3 days). A higher BUN suggests excessive protein intake if weight is maintained or gained. It suggests protein catabolism if associated with recent weight loss.
4. Inability to achieve or maintain ideal body weight is a sign of poor caloric intake. A rising BUN may reflect protein catabolism in a patient with inadequate caloric intake.

5. Excessive weight gain between dialysis sessions with a normal serum sodium level reflects excess salt and water ingestion. Excessive weight gain with a low serum sodium level suggests excessive ingestion of fluids but not salt. Edema, congestive heart failure, and increasing blood pressure may be signs of excess sodium intake. Weight loss, diminished urine output, and a rising BUN all point to inadequate salt ingestion.
6. An elevated potassium level reflects increased potassium ingestion or acidosis.
7. An elevated phosphorus level may reflect either failure to take phosphate binders or excessive dietary phosphorus intake, usually in the form of dairy products.

Acute Renal Failure

There is no uniformly-agreed-upon practice plan for nutrition therapy of patients with acute renal failure (93). The goals of diet in acute renal failure are to provide adequate calories to maintain body weight and minimize catabolism of tissue proteins. The major difficulty in managing patients without dialysis is providing adequate calories without fluid overload. Whenever possible, the patient should receive nutrition via the enteral route, but if parenteral nutrition is required, the rationale and extensive discussion of recommendations for parenteral nutrition in patients with acute renal failure are available elsewhere (92,93).

The following are suggested guidelines for approaching the nutritional needs of patients with acute renal failure (93):

1. Fluids should be given in an amount totaling the sum of all measured sources of losses plus an additional amount (~400 mL per day) to account for contributions from insensible water loss and the water as a consequence of metabolic processes. The goal is a normal serum sodium level and no weight gain.
2. Desirable energy intake is initially estimated at about 30 kcal/kg/d with the goal of maintaining body weight and adjusting intake according to weight status. Obese subjects will require less caloric intake. However, since comorbidities such as inflammation and sepsis induce a hypercatabolic state, energy intake must often be increased. Unfortunately, there are no simple ways to estimate the total energy requirements of such patients at the bedside, so the changes in energy intake are largely estimated empirically with body weight change serving as a guide. About 10% to 20% of energy is supplied by lipid emulsions and sufficient glucose, at least 150 to 200 g per day should be supplied to minimize protein breakdown. The glucose is often given as a hypertonic solution because of the limited water tolerance of subjects with acute renal failure.
3. The protein/amino acid requirement in acute renal failure is a highly debated topic (93). If patients are otherwise adequately nourished and expected to regain renal function within a few weeks, 0.3 to 0.5 g of high-biologic-value protein or essential amino acids per kilogram per day is used. For patients who are highly catabolic, who have high levels of urinary nitrogen, or who are not expected to recover for more than 2 weeks, additional protein intake is advisable, up to 1.2 g/kg/d.
4. Salt intake should equal salt losses (urine, stool, gastric aspirate).
5. Because acute renal failure may be accompanied by substantial tissue destruction and acidosis, the possibility of rapidly developing hyperkalemia is greater than in chronic renal failure. Serum potassium should be monitored carefully and dietary potassium minimized.
6. In acute renal failure, dialysis makes it possible to control hyperkalemia, fluid overload, acidosis, and uremia. After the initiation of dialysis, less stringent restriction of protein, fluids, and potassium may be possible.

HYPERLIPOPROTEINEMIA
Introduction

Heart disease is the leading cause of death in both men and women in the United States. According to recent estimates (156), more than 83 million Americans have one or more forms of cardiovascular disease. Seventy-eight million are hypertensive and more than 15 million have coronary heart disease, including almost 8 million with myocardial infarction, nearly 8 million with angina pectoris, and about 6.8 million with stroke (156). Even though deaths from cardiovascular diseases have declined substantially, they still claimed nearly 800,000 lives in 2010, accounting for 35.3% of deaths (156). Coronary heart disease is the single leading cause of death in the United States today, accounting for about 380,000 deaths in 2010 (156).

More than 200 risk factors for cardiovascular disease have been identified, but the major factors are far fewer in number. Some, like male sex, increasing age, and genotype, cannot be modified. Others, such as increased plasma LDL-C, increased circulating triglycerides, low plasma HDL cholesterol (HDL-C), cigarette smoking, hypertension, obesity, and reduced physical activity, are theoretically reversible or at least modifiable to some extent. Reductions in LDL-C, hypertension, cigarette smoking, maintenance of a healthy body weight, and adequate physical activity have been shown repeatedly to lower risk. An increased HDL-C level is associated with lower CVD risk, but attempts to lower risk by interventions that increase HDL-C have not been successful in clinical trials. Because many of these risks are related to diet and lifestyle, a highly significant reduction in the risks for cardiovascular disease can be achieved through the nutritional practices outlined in various chapters throughout this volume, in the Dietary Guidelines for Americans (see Chapter 1), in recommendations issued by various expert groups (50,52,157–160) and from supporting data from a wide variety of both observational and interventional studies throughout the medical literature. Even though some of the individual recommendations differ in certain specifics, the overall recommendations and their guiding principles are largely the same across all expert groups and medical disciplines.

Definitions

Lipoproteins

By definition, lipids are insoluble in water. In order to be transported in the aqueous solution, plasma, triglycerides, and cholesterol are complexed with apoproteins (apo) and phospholipids to form solubilized particles, now called *lipoproteins*. The major lipoprotein classes are outlined in Table 13-6, and the metabolism of the lipoprotein classes is extensively reviewed elsewhere (161).

Chylomicrons

The major function of chylomicrons (161–165) is to carry exogenous dietary fat from the intestine to peripheral tissues. Chylomicrons are formed in the endoplasmic reticulum of enterocytes. During transit through the Golgi apparatus, they acquire apo A-I, A-II, A-IV, and B-48. After passing through the lacteals of the intestinal villi, the chylomicrons are transported through the thoracic duct into the bloodstream, where they acquire the additional apo C-II and apo E via

TABLE 13-6 Classes of Human Lipoproteins and Their Chemical Composition

	Surface Components		Core Lipids	
	Cholesterol	Phospholipids	Apolipoprotein	Triglycerides	Cholesteryl Esters
Chylomicrons	2	7	2	86	3
VLDL	7	18	8	55	12
IDL	9	19	19	23	29
LDL	8	22	22	6	42
HDL$_2$	5	33	40	5	17
HDL$_3$	4	25	55	3	13
Preβ$_1$-HDL	5	5	90	0	0

Surface components and core lipids are given as percentage of dry mass.
(Data from Havel RJ, Kane JP. Introduction: structure and metabolism of plasma lipoproteins. In: Valle D, Beaudet AL, Vogelstein B, et al., eds. *OMMBID: The Online Metabolic and Molecular Bases of Inherited Diseases*. New York, NY: McGraw-Hill; 2014.)

transfer from HDLs. Thereafter, the chylomicrons interact with the enzyme lipoprotein lipase (161,166,167), located on the endothelial surface of blood capillaries in many organs. Apo C-II is a required cofactor in the activation of lipoprotein lipase. Lipoprotein lipase hydrolyzes the chylomicron triglycerides into unesterified fatty acids and glycerol. At the same time, the apo A peptides are transferred to HDLs. The remaining, much smaller chylomicron particle, still containing apo B-48 and now called a *chylomicron remnant,* is taken up by a specific hepatic receptor that recognizes the apo E peptide on its surface.

Very-Low-Density Lipoproteins

Very-low-density lipoproteins (161,162), or VLDL, are synthesized by the liver. Their principal role is the transport endogenously synthesized triglycerides of hepatic origin to peripheral tissues. VLDL resemble chylomicrons in that they are rich in triglycerides (albeit somewhat smaller in size), receive small amounts of apo E and apo C-II from HDL, and lose their triglycerides via lipoprotein lipase-catalyzed hydrolysis. VLDL are unique in that they acquire apo B-100 during intrahepatic assembly. Although they are primarily triglyceride containing particles, VLDL also contain a modest amount of circulating cholesterol (VLDL cholesterol), and when VLDL concentrations are abnormally high, they may contribute significantly to the total circulating cholesterol level. VLDL triglyceride hydrolysis proceeds more slowly than that of chylomicrons and results in two lesser VLDL particles, the larger of which is called a *VLDL remnant* (removed by the hepatic LDL receptor) and the smaller of which is called an *intermediate-density lipoprotein* (IDL). Since VLDL remnants are VLDL particles that have had much of their triglyceride removed, they are relatively enriched in cholesterol and are atherogenic. About half of IDL are also taken up by hepatic receptors, but the remaining half are further converted to LDL, with apo B-100 as the predominant remaining peptide. In practice, IDL are included in the LDL fraction because they are small particles that are depleted in triglyceride, contain apo B-100, and are highly enriched in cholesterol, in other words much more like LDL than VLDL. Extensive review of the roles of triglyceride-rich lipoproteins in atherosclerotic cardiovascular disease can be found elsewhere (168–172).

Low-Density Lipoproteins

Low-density lipoproteins (161,162), or LDL, are the principal carrier of plasma cholesterol, accounting for approximately 60% to 70% of the total serum cholesterol level in normal persons (LDL-C). Half of the LDL particle is cholesterol; only 5% to 10% is triglyceride, and most of its protein is apo B-100 (Table 13-6). In normal individuals, more than 90% of apo B is found in LDL and the rest is associated with VLDL. LDL are the vehicles whereby cholesterol synthesized in the liver is delivered to peripheral tissues and to hepatocytes via the hepatic LDL receptor that clears about 60% to 80% of circulating LDL. The remaining LDL are cleared by other specific receptors, and oxidized LDL can be taken up by scavenger receptors on macrophages and vascular smooth muscle cells. When these macrophages become lipid-laden, they are called foam cells, which are a major component in the development of atherosclerosis. LDL are metabolized slowly over several days and are the major atherogenic lipoprotein. Additionally, when the little lipid in LDL is removed, they become a lipoprotein particle known as small dense LDL. This dense cholesterol–containing particle has a lower affinity for the LDL receptor and is more readily oxidized and removed by macrophages. Thus, small dense LDL are even more atherogenic than native LDL (173).

High-Density Lipoproteins

High-density lipoproteins (161,174–176), or HDL, are secreted in an immature, disc-like, nascent form largely by the liver but also by the intestine, containing as apo A-I as its principal apo. These disc-like particles can absorb free cholesterol from cells through the action of ATP-binding cassette transporter 1 and the apopeptides A-I and A-IV. Thereafter, through the action of a circulating cholesteryl ester transfer complex containing lecithin-cholesterol acyltransferase (LCAT) (98), an enzyme activated by apo A-I, HDL-C is esterified and carried back to the liver where it is removed by the LDL receptor or the hepatic scavenger receptor. Additionally, through the action of cholesteryl ester transfer protein (CETP), some cholesterol ester is transferred from HDL to apo B-100 containing triglyceride rich lipoproteins. The net effect is that cholesterol in peripheral tissues is transported back to the liver (so-called reverse cholesterol transport) and eventually removed by the liver. The liver, in turn, ultimately disposes of the cholesterol by excreting it in bile. The cholesterol content of HDL (HDL-C) is normally about 20% to 30% of the total serum cholesterol level.

Non–HDL Cholesterol

This term applies to a calculated value that is the difference between total plasma cholesterol and HDL-C. In other words, it represents the cholesterol content of LDL plus VLDL and includes all the lipoproteins that contain apo B, the atherogenic lipoproteins. Since it is easy to compute, this value has become a practical indicator of total atherogenic lipoproteins and is used as a surrogate for measuring apo B directly, a practical benefit because apo B measurements are not routinely available in many clinical laboratories. Another advantage of calculating non–HDL-C is that the subject does not have to be fasting for the measurement, since neither total plasma cholesterol nor HDL-C change appreciably after a meal.

Lipoprotein-Associated Cardiovascular Risks

Total and LDL Cholesterol

The US population distributions of serum total cholesterol, LDL-C, HDL-C, and triglyceride are given in Table 13-7 (177). An elevated serum LDL-C is the most significant lipoprotein

TABLE 13-7 Serum Total Cholesterol Levels (mg/dL) for Persons 20 Years of Age or Older in the United States

	Percentile				
	5th	25th	50th	75th	95th
Men					
≥20	139	173	200	228	273
20–34	131	161	183	209	253
35–44	143	180	205	232	267
45–54	154	191	214	242	283
55–64	154	189	214	243	282
65–74	149	186	209	237	284
75+	145	176	203	230	273
Women					
≥20	143	175	201	233	284
20–34	132	158	181	205	248
35–44	144	171	192	215	257
45–54	157	187	212	243	298
55–64	167	204	229	261	307
65–74	170	204	232	258	308
75+	161	198	228	258	305
Hispanic					
Men	137	171	197	224	272
Women	139	167	193	223	274
Non-Hispanic Black					
Men	136	169	195	222	275
Women	136	170	196	226	284
Non-Hispanic White					
Men	141	174	201	229	272
Women	144	177	203	235	284
Serum LDL Cholesterol Levels (mg/dL) for Persons 20 Years of Age or Older in the United States					
Men					
≥20	76	105	128	153	194
20–34	72	97	119	139	170

(continued)

TABLE 13-7 Serum Total Cholesterol Levels (mg/dL) for Persons 20 Years of Age or Older in the United States *(continued)*

	Percentile				
	5th	25th	50th	75th	95th
35–44	82	111	132	156	205
45–54	76	117	140	164	195
55–64	82	115	135	162	200
65–74	83	113	133	158	196
75+	86	109	128	151	194
Women					
≥20	69	98	121	147	190
20–34	63	90	109	130	170
35–44	70	96	115	137	171
45–54	70	106	129	153	190
55–64	80	121	143	167	209
65–74	76	119	144	166	203
75+	83	119	144	167	209
Hispanic					
Men	71	98	121	144	188
Women	67	93	115	137	178
Non-Hispanic Black					
Men	71	100	124	149	200
Women	63	97	119	145	193
Non-Hispanic White					
Men	79	106	129	154	194
Women	70	98	122	149	189

Serum HDL Cholesterol Levels (mg/dL) for Persons 20 Years of Age or Older in the United States

	5th	25th	50th	75th	95th
Men					
≥20	28	37	44	53	72
20–34	28	38	45	53	69
35–44	28	36	43	52	73
45–54	26	35	42	52	75
55–64	28	36	42	51	71
65–74	28	36	43	54	73
75+	28	37	44	54	75
Women					
≥20	34	44	53	64	83
20–34	34	45	53	64	83
35–44	34	44	53	64	79
45–54	36	45	55	65	84
55–64	33	44	53	65	89
65–74	33	45	54	65	84
75+	32	44	55	65	86
Hispanic					
Men	28	37	44	52	67
Women	33	42	51	60	77
Non-Hispanic Black					
Men	32	41	50	60	85
Women	35	46	55	66	86

TABLE 13-7 Serum Total Cholesterol Levels (mg/dL) for Persons 20 Years of Age or Older in the United States *(continued)*

	Percentile				
	5th	25th	50th	75th	95th
Non-Hispanic White					
Men	27	36	43	52	71
Women	34	45	54	64	84
Serum Triglyceride Levels (mg/dL) for Persons 20 Years of Age or Older in the United States					
Men					
≥20	53	83	118	173	318
20–34	46	70	94	139	256
35–44	53	82	126	180	307
45–54	62	100	135	201	366
55–64	64	101	144	228	396
65–74	64	99	137	190	319
75+	64	96	125	175	304
Women					
≥20	48	72	102	152	273
20–34	43	61	84	117	226
35–44	46	67	93	132	288
45–54	49	76	114	163	277
55–64	62	96	135	203	396
65–74	70	99	134	182	283
75+	64	94	130	178	274
Hispanic					
Men	53	83	120	184	361
Women	55	85	118	170	293
Non-Hispanic Black					
Men	45	64	89	135	245
Women	41	58	79	113	207
Non-Hispanic White					
Men	55	85	123	181	319
Women	49	75	104	156	274

(Data from National Cholesterol Education Program (NCEP) Expert Panel. Third Report of the National Cholesterol Education Program (NCEP) Expert Panel on Detection, Evaluation, and Treatment of High Blood Cholesterol in Adults (Adult Treatment Panel III) Final Report. National Cholesterol Education Program, National Heart, Lung, and Blood Institute, National Institutes of Health. NIH Publication No. 02-5215, September 2002.)

risk factor associated with the development of cardiovascular disease. The relationship between LDL-C and cardiovascular risk, a relationship verified in numerous population studies and clinical trials, is a log-linear one, even at the lowest serum LDL-C levels tested, with the relative risk = 1.0 level set at 40 mg per dL (178). From observational studies, people with LDL-C levels less than 100 mg per dL have very low risks of cardiovascular disease (179). Thus, these lower levels have been traditionally labeled as "optimal," a position supported initially by various early clinical trials that lowered LDL-C using lifestyle modification and drug therapy. However, the most recent aggressive drug trials have convincingly demonstrated the additional direct beneficial effect of reducing serum cholesterol to levels even lower than 100 mg per dL (Figures 13-1 and 13-2) (179–187). Two issues have arisen from these studies. First, as can be seen in Figures 13-1 and 13-2, the lowest LDL-C levels are achieved with the therapeutic use of statin drugs. Since these drugs appear to have a variety of beneficial effects themselves,

Statin
Placebo
Event (%)
LDL Cholesterol (mg/dL)
30
25
20
15
10
5
0
0
70
90
110
130
150
170
190
210
4S
4S
LIPID
LIPID
CARE
CARE
HPS
HPS
TNT (10 mg of atorvastatin)
TNT (80 mg of atorvastatin)

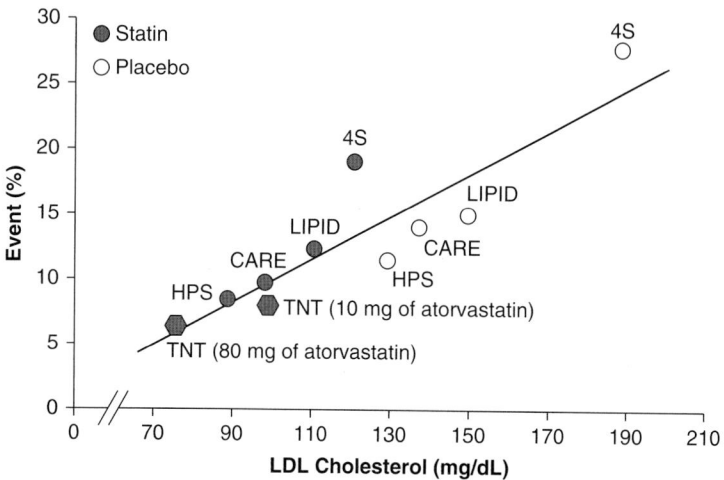

Figure 13-1. Event rates plotted against LDL cholesterol levels during statin therapy in secondary-prevention studies. (From LaRosa JC, Grundy SM, Waters DD, et al. Intensive lipid lowering with atorvastatin in patients with stable coronary disease. *N Engl J Med.* 2005;352:1425–1435.)

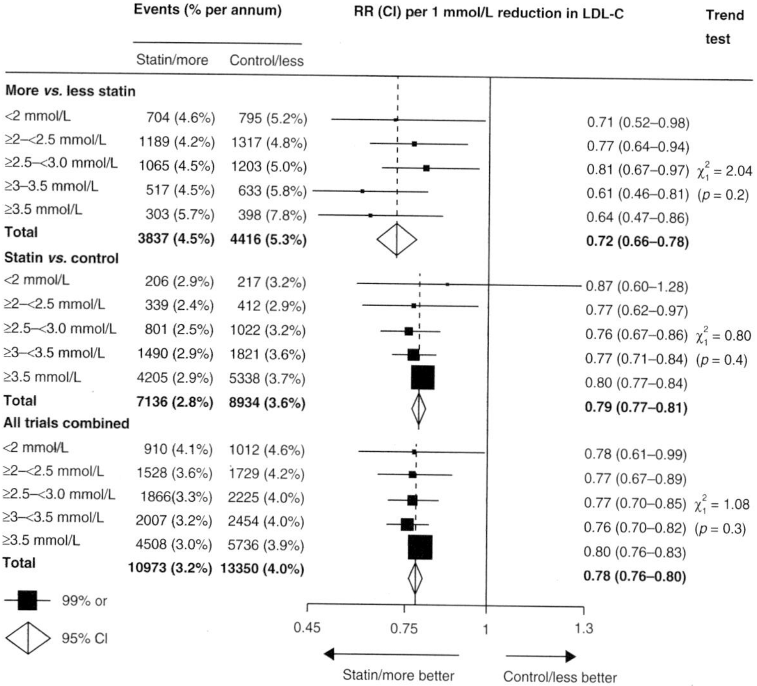

Events (% per annum)
Statin/more Control/less
RR (CI) per 1 mmol/L reduction in LDL-C
Trend test
More vs. less statin
<2 mmol/L 704 (4.6%) 795 (5.2%) 0.71 (0.52–0.98)
≥2–<2.5 mmol/L 1189 (4.2%) 1317 (4.8%) 0.77 (0.64–0.94)
≥2.5–<3.0 mmol/L 1065 (4.5%) 1203 (5.0%) 0.81 (0.67–0.97) χ^2_1 = 2.04
≥3–3.5 mmol/L 517 (4.5%) 633 (5.8%) 0.61 (0.46–0.81) (p = 0.2)
≥3.5 mmol/L 303 (5.7%) 398 (7.8%) 0.64 (0.47–0.86)
Total 3837 (4.5%) 4416 (5.3%) 0.72 (0.66–0.78)
Statin vs. control
<2 mmol/L 206 (2.9%) 217 (3.2%) 0.87 (0.60–1.28)
≥2–<2.5 mmol/L 339 (2.4%) 412 (2.9%) 0.77 (0.62–0.97)
≥2.5–<3.0 mmol/L 801 (2.5%) 1022 (3.2%) 0.76 (0.67–0.86) χ^2_1 = 0.80
≥3–<3.5 mmol/L 1490 (2.9%) 1821 (3.6%) 0.77 (0.71–0.84) (p = 0.4)
≥3.5 mmol/L 4205 (2.9%) 5338 (3.7%) 0.80 (0.77–0.84)
Total 7136 (2.8%) 8934 (3.6%) 0.79 (0.77–0.81)
All trials combined
<2 mmol/L 910 (4.1%) 1012 (4.6%) 0.78 (0.61–0.99)
≥2–<2.5 mmol/L 1528 (3.6%) 1729 (4.2%) 0.77 (0.67–0.89)
≥2.5–<3.0 mmol/L 1866(3.3%) 2225 (4.0%) 0.77 (0.70–0.85) χ^2_1 = 1.08
≥3–<3.5 mmol/L 2007 (3.2%) 2454 (4.0%) 0.76 (0.70–0.82) (p = 0.3)
≥3.5 mmol/L 4508 (3.0%) 5736 (3.9%) 0.80 (0.76–0.83)
Total 10973 (3.2%) 13350 (4.0%) 0.78 (0.76–0.80)
99% or
95% CI
0.45
0.75
1
1.3
Statin/more better
Control/less better

Figure 13-2. Relative risks of major cardiovascular events relative to baseline LDL-cholesterol. (From Cholesterol Treatment Trialists' (CTT) Collaboration. Efficacy and safety of more intensive lowering of LDL cholesterol: a meta-analysis of data from 170,000 participants in 26 randomised trials. *Lancet.* 2010;376:1670–1681.)

independent of their cholesterol lowering effects, the results of the statin trials do not convincingly prove that the cholesterol lowering, per se, is the sole or principal agent responsible for reducing CVD relative risk. Second, because statins also have side effects and because no RCT has tested the risk/benefit ratio of treating patients according to low LDL-C targets (187,188), the data have generated an ongoing and as yet unsettled debate about balancing the level of cholesterol lowering with the dose of statin that must be used to do so. While there is an increasing trend for moderation in this respect, many argue that the data are compelling enough and the side effect risks are low enough that therapeutic goals should be the lowest level of LDL-C that is achievable (179–186). Nonetheless, the most recent American College of Cardiology/American Heart Association guidelines on treating cholesterol to reduce CVD risk (158) did not find evidence "to support titrating cholesterol-lowering drug therapy to achieve optimal LDL-C or non–HDL-C levels because the clinical trials were essentially fixed-dose trials" and, thus, no recommendation on LDL-C targets were made (158). Rather, the expert committee addressed its recommendations to those that can be shown to reduce risk, a decision supported by others in the field (188–192).

Table 13-8 shows a traditional classification of serum total and LDL-C levels based on the ATP III recommendations (177). The equivalent non–HDL-C recommendations are 30 mg per dL higher than the values shown for LDL-C, since this is the approximate contribution of the cholesterol content of VLDL when triglyceride levels are normal. Because the risk for coronary artery disease decreases with serum cholesterol over the entire range of cholesterol levels found in the American population, it is difficult to define a "normal" cholesterol level and the lowest cholesterol levels are optimal ones. Based on the data from the 2009 to 2012 NHANES surveys, 13% to 14% of Americans have high circulating cholesterol levels (193).

Triglycerides

Over the last several decades (168), it has become increasingly clear that circulating triglyceride levels are also an independent risk factor for coronary heart disease (170–172) and that elevated nonfasting triglyceride levels are independently associated with an increased risk of cardiovascular events (194–196). Table 13-9 shows the ATP III classification of triglycerides for risk assessment and management, and various expert groups have outlined treatment guidelines for those with hypertriglyceridemia, generally defined as at serum triglyceride levels less than 150 mg per dL (197–199). In all cases, the initial approach to management deals with diet and lifestyle changes that are basically the same as those discussed for healthy adults in the *Dietary Guidelines for Americans*, recommendations that promote a healthy body weight, regular physical activity, and diets rich in plant foods as presented in various other chapters throughout this book. As discussed above, when triglyceride levels rise, VLDL remnants containing a significant amount of cholesterol contribute to the atherogenicity of plasma lipoproteins as estimated using the calculated non–HDL-C. This most prevailing view is that this cholesterol is the mechanism by

TABLE 13-8 ATP III Classification Total and LDL Cholesterol

Classification	Total Cholesterol (mg/dL)	LDL Cholesterol (mg/dL)
Optimal		<100
Near optimal/above optimal		100–129
Desirable	<200	
Borderline high	200–239	130–159
		<100 (optional)
High	≥240	160–189
Very High		≥190

(Adapted from National Cholesterol Education Program (NCEP) Expert Panel. Third Report of the National Cholesterol Education Program (NCEP) Expert Panel on Detection, Evaluation, and Treatment of High Blood Cholesterol in Adults (Adult Treatment Panel III) Final Report. National Cholesterol Education Program, National Heart, Lung, and Blood Institute, National Institutes of Health. NIH Publication No. 02-5215, September 2002.)

TABLE 13-9 Clinical Classification of Serum Triglyceride Levels

Triglyceride Category	ATP III Levels (mg/dL)
Normal	<150
Borderline-high	150–199
High	200–499
Very high	≥500

(From National Cholesterol Education Program (NCEP) Expert Panel. Third Report of the National Cholesterol Education Program (NCEP) Expert Panel on Detection, Evaluation, and Treatment of High Blood Cholesterol in Adults (Adult Treatment Panel III) Final Report. National Cholesterol Education Program, National Heart, Lung, and Blood Institute, National Institutes of Health. NIH Publication No. 02-5215, September 2002.)

which triglyceride-rich particles contribute to coronary heart disease risk. Thus, in the circumstances of hypertriglyceridemia, non–HDL-C is a better indicator of circulating atherogenic lipoproteins than is LDL-C.

HDL Cholesterol

There is extensive epidemiologic evidence linking low HDL levels to coronary heart disease and population studies show that coronary heart disease risk rises as HDL-C levels fall (174–176,200–203). Based on NHANES survey data (193), about 26% of American men and about 9% of American women have low HDL levels. However, as with LDL-C, there is a continuous inverse relationship between HDL-C and cardiovascular risk. Therefore, it is somewhat arbitrary to refer to a "low" or "normal" HDL, when one might more appropriately classify an HDL level as "better for risk" or "worse for risk." An average of 45 to 55 mg of cholesterol per deciliter of plasma is carried by HDL and, since cardiovascular risk declines as HDL-C increases, HDL-C is commonly called "good cholesterol." Nevertheless, although it is now abundantly clear from many well-controlled, randomized studies that lowering LDL-C decreases cardiovascular disease risk, it has not been possible to demonstrate in clinical trials that increasing circulating HDL-C diminishes the risk of coronary heart disease (201–203). For this reason, there is no specific target set for raising HDL-C in clinical management. LDL-C reduction remains the principal initial goal (157–159).

The Hyperlipoproteinemias

The term *hyperlipoproteinemia* describes a group of disorders in which serum lipoproteins are elevated on the basis of genetic abnormalities in lipoprotein metabolism (161,162,167,175,204–213). Because the concentrations of plasma lipids are continuous variables, any definition of hyperlipoproteinemia is somewhat arbitrary. Traditionally, these disorders were classified into six clinically useful phenotypes according to physical and biochemical presentation and the distribution of lipoprotein classes that were elevated (Table 13-10). Following identification of specific genetic defects that lead to the clinical phenotypes, this classification has fallen somewhat out of favor. However, because of its clinical practicality, the traditional method of classification remains in general use because the specific molecular bases for a large fraction of the clinically encountered hyperlipoproteinemias remain unknown and the identified Mendelian disorders account for only a small fraction of the variance in atherosclerosis disease susceptibility. As the availability of genotyping increases, the cost of genotyping decreases, and newer "next-gen" deep-sequencing methods that can detect an ever-growing number of gene abnormalities responsible for clinical disease phenotypes become more commonplace, the gap between known genetic defects and clinical lipoproteinemias will surely narrow significantly.

Each type of hyperlipoproteinemia is not a single disease, but rather a group of "genotypic" disorders marked by similar "phenotypic" abnormalities in circulating lipoproteins. Each type includes identified primary genetic defects and various secondary disorders. When

TABLE 13-10 Patterns of Lipid Abnormalities in the Traditional Approach to Classifying the Genetic Hyperlipoproteinemias

Type	Cholesterol	Triglycerides	Atherogenicity
I Chylomicronemia	Normal or slightly elevated	Very high	Uncertain
IIa Hypercholesterolemia	Elevated LDL cholesterol	Normal	+++
IIb Familial combined hyperlipemia	Elevated LDL cholesterol	Elevated	+++
III[a] Dsybetalipoprotinemia	Elevated	Elevated	+++
IV Hypertriglyceridemia	Normal or slightly elevated	Elevated	++
V Mixed hypertriglyceridemia	Moderately elevated	Markedly elevated	+

[a]Increased VLDL remnants or intermediate-density lipoproteins. A definitive diagnosis of type III requires lipoprotein ultracentrifugation and characterization of apo E isoforms.

the latter occur because of a specific underlying disease state, such as uncontrolled diabetes, treatment of the underlying disorder frequently corrects the lipid abnormality. Similarly, when the primary disorder is aggravated by obesity, alcohol consumption, or estrogen or glucocorticoid treatment, elimination of the aggravating factor facilitates diet therapy. Because obesity and excessive consumption of cholesterol, total fat, and saturated fat increase plasma lipoprotein concentrations in many people, diet is an important component of the management of hyperlipidemia.

Type I Hyperlipoproteinemia

Type I hyperlipoproteinemia (167) is characterized by fasting chylomicronemia. Plasma cholesterol is usually normal, and plasma triglycerides are markedly elevated, generally to values well above 1,000 mg per dL. Because chylomicrons do contain a small amount of cholesterol, when the chylomicron concentration is extremely high, a slight secondary elevation of plasma cholesterol may be found as well. The classic form of this disease is a rare autosomal recessive disorder with a prevalence of only about one per million people. The phenotype is caused by more than 220 identified mutations in the gene for the enzyme lipoprotein lipase (http://ghr.nlm.nih.gov/gene/LPL). It is usually identified in childhood by symptoms of eruptive xanthomata and pancreatitis. Chylomicronemia is less frequently caused by autosomal recessive defects in the gene for the apo C-II peptide activator of lipoprotein lipase (167). This defect is even rarer than lipoprotein lipase deficiency although at least 14 kindreds have been identified (167). Familial hepatic lipase deficiency, is an even more rare autosomal recessive disorder where chylomicrons may accumulate in plasma, although these subjects have additional dyslipidemia with accumulation of additional apo B containing lipoproteins representing incompletely metabolized VLDL (167). Deeb has discussed in detail the genetic variants in lipase genes and their relationships with plasma lipids and coronary artery disease (204).

Type IIa Hyperlipoproteinemia

Type IIa hyperlipoproteinemia (205,210–213), or familial hypercholesterolemia, is an autosomal dominant condition marked by high LDL levels and normal VLDL levels. Thus, plasma cholesterol is elevated but triglycerides are normal. Familial hypercholesterolemia results from a variety of genetic defects in the LDL cell surface receptor that controls the plasma removal of LDL (205). More than 1,600 different LDL receptor gene allelic variants have been found, and these account for more than 80% of patients with the phenotype of familial hypercholesterolemia (214). A small number of additional patients have this phenotype on the basis of a defective apolipoprotein B or other very rare abnormalities (211,214,215). The carrier frequency for this group of LDL receptor gene defects taken as a whole is approximately 1/500. Nevertheless, in about 10% of patients with a clinical diagnosis compatable with these monogenic hypercholesterolemias, no gene defect has been found.

Type IIb Hyperlipoproteinemia

Type IIb hyperlipoproteinemia (216,217) is the most common pattern found in families with premature coronary heart disease, is an autosomal dominant condition with variable penetrance, with a population prevalence of 1% to 5%. It is characterized by increases in both circulating VLDL and LDL; thus, plasma cholesterol and triglycerides are both elevated. Additionally, HDL levels tend to be reduced. No single gene defect has been found that results in this phenotype, called *familial combined hyperlipidemia*, and it is clearly a complex, polygenic disorder with coinheritance of various mutations that contribute to increasing triglyceride levels (216–219). The type IIb phenotype is aggravated by obesity or glucocorticoid treatment and also can be seen as a secondary consequence of the nephrotic syndrome.

What has now become clear through various GWAS studies is the polygenic nature not only of the phenotypic class of type IIb hyperlipoproteinemia discussed immediately above but also of the hypertriglyceridemia phenotypes III, IV, and V discussed immediately below (218,219). The following three lipidemic phenotypes will be discussed briefly for historical completeness sake and because they can be helpful in diagnostic assessment. However, we now appreciate that the same genetic variants are associated with phenotypes IIb, III, IV, and V. As comprehensive genetic diagnosis becomes more readily available, the classical clinical phenotypes defined by Donald Frederickson more than a half century ago will fade from view.

Type III Hyperlipoproteinemia

Type III hyperlipoproteinemia (206,318,220) is characterized by an accumulation of IDL due to impaired removal of triglyceride-rich lipoproteins. The result is combined cholesterolemia and triglyceridemia, usually to about the same degree. This condition is also called *remnant hyperlipoproteinemia*, *dysbetalipoproteinemia*, or *broad-β disease* because the accumulated IDLs are remnants of incompletely metabolized triglyceride-containing lipoproteins with a relatively high cholesterol content that migrate beyond the usual "β" or LDL-C band during electrophoresis.

Type III hyperlipoproteinemia is relatively uncommon, with a prevalence of about 0.2% in women and 0.4% to 0.5% in men. (220). Clinically, it is characterized by unusual xanthomata, called *planar xanthomata*, in the creases of the palms of the hand and by tuberous xanthomata over the elbows and knees. Diagnosis of this disorder requires identification of IDL by ultracentrifugation and confirmation of the homozygosity for the mutant apolipoprotein E_2 genotype, because more than 90% of people with type III hyperlipoproteinemia are homozygous for this apo E isoform that cannot bind effectively with the hepatic receptor responsible for removing apo E-containing lipoprotein remnant particles from plasma (206). The pathogenesis of dyslipidemia in type III hyperlipoproteinemia, however, is not completely understood since most people who are homozygous for apo E_2 are not hyperlipidemic, although, presumably, the elevated triglycerides are due to the genetic variants that increase the risk of hypertriglyceridemia in other hypertriglyceridemic conditions. Additionally, the development of clinical hyperlipidemia must be the result of interaction with these genes with environmental factors or comorbid conditions such as obesity, diabetes, and hypothyroidism.

Type IV Hyperlipoproteinemia

Type IV hyperlipoproteinemia is more commonly called *familial hypertriglyceridemia*. It is a relatively common problem, with a prevalence of about 5% to 10% and is characterized principally by an isolated increase in plasma triglycerides secondary to elevated VLDL, but HDL levels may be low. Although the principal genetic defect(s) have not been fully elucidated, GWAS studies show the contributing presence of common allelic variants responsible for all the common forms of hypertriglyceridemia (218,219). Hepatic VLDL overproduction appears to be the primary pathophysiologic mechanism, although some evidence for diminished removal has also been found. Elevated VLDL levels are seen commonly secondary to diabetes, uremia, nephrotic syndrome, alcohol ingestion, and glucocorticoid or estrogen treatment. Familial hypertriglyceridemia is associated with obesity, and obesity may aggravate VLDL elevations in subjects with primary hyperlipidemia. Nonetheless, obesity usually does not cause significant hypertriglyceridemia in persons with normal lipoprotein metabolism.

Chapter 13 • Dietary Management of Diabetes, Renal Disease, and Hyperlipidemia | 611

Type V Hyperlipoproteinemia

Type V hyperlipoproteinemia is a rare pattern marked by elevations in both chylomicrons and VLDL. Thus, triglycerides are significantly elevated, and the phenotype is often called *mixed hypertriglyceridemia* because the triglycerides are contained in both VLDL and chylomicrons. Mild elevations in cholesterol may be secondary to the cholesterol content of VLDLs and chylomicrons. Again, the underlying genetic causes appear to be coinheritance of allelic variants of genes known to influence triglyceride metabolism (218,219). The common feature in this disorder appears to be an inherent or acquired defect in the capacity to metabolize triglyceride-rich lipoproteins that have been produced in excess quantity by the liver in response to excessive fatty acid release by adipose tissue. Most patients have diabetes, renal failure, or other disorders, abuse alcohol, or are on various medication regimens.

Atherogenic Dyslipidemia

Atherogenic dyslipidemia is a particularly important constellation of lipoprotein abnormalities of great clinical significance appear to result from the coexistence of several defects, lipoprotein or otherwise, of lipid metabolism. The specific findings are (a) mild hypercholesterolemia, (b) mild to moderate hypertriglyceridemia, (c) the presence of circulating small, dense LDL particles, and (d) a low serum concentration of HDL-C. Although genotype and aging are strong contributors, three additional lifestyle factors are also apparently contributory or causative. These include obesity, physical inactivity, and diets high in fatty acids that increase serum cholesterol. Naturally, the latter three factors are clinically relevant because they are potentially modifiable. In this regard, the central pathophysiologic link is the presence of insulin resistance and the patient can improve insulin sensitivity by increasing physical activity and losing weight, two goals of almost every medical and public health recommendation for maintaining a healthy weight (see Chapter 1).

Diagnosis

Because of the association of hyperlipidemia with coronary heart disease, it is generally recommended that plasma cholesterol and triglycerides be measured periodically during adult life. If a family has a history of hyperlipidemia or, especially, premature deaths due to coronary heart disease, children should also be tested because familial hypercholesterolemia is an autosomal dominant disease.

Total serum cholesterol and serum HDL levels are relatively unaffected by eating. This is one of the reasons why the calculation of non–HDL-C is a particularly useful tool, as discussed above. However, a recent meal can cause a marked elevation of plasma triglycerides, due to the appropriate postprandial presence of chylomicrons in plasma. Triglycerides should be measured only after a 12- to 14-hour fast. Remember too that VLDL contain about 1 mg of cholesterol for every 4 mg of triglyceride, so that a person with significant hypertriglyceridemia may have a modestly increased total serum cholesterol value on the basis of the cholesterol content of his or her VLDL. A simple clinical approach to estimating VLDL cholesterol is to divide the triglyceride level by five, but the resulting quotient is only accurate when total serum triglycerides are less than 400 mg per dL. Thus, the calculation is not particularly helpful when it is most needed, that is in the case of severe hypertriglyceridemia. Plasma lipid values are best determined while patients are maintaining a steady weight and have been on their usual diet for several weeks. If abnormal values are found, before a firm diagnosis is made that may permanently affect the future course of a person's life, repeat fasting lipid levels should be measured on two or three occasions separated by 2- to 3-week intervals.

There are no routine clinical laboratory tests for the presence of chylomicrons in plasma, but a simple, practical approach to their detection is simply refrigerating the plasma overnight at 4°C. If chylomicrons are present, they will form a creamy layer on top of the plasma. The presence of chylomicrons in plasma drawn after a 12-hour fast is abnormal and indicative of familial chylomicronemia (type I lipoproteinemia), type V hyperlipoproteinemia, or a secondary abnormality caused by other diseases such as severe, insulin-deficient diabetes. Fasting chylomicronemia is usually seen only when plasma triglyceride levels are above 1,000 mg per dL.

The implications of elevated plasma cholesterol depend on the lipoprotein class with which the cholesterol is associated. As noted earlier, a risk for coronary heart disease is associated with an elevated level of apolipoprotein B containing particles carrying cholesterol. These are principally LDL and the various VLDL remnant particles. Both LDL and HDL-C can be measured specifically and directly in the clinical laboratory, and this is the preferred approach. Nonetheless, this is not done in every hospital and, often, LDL-C is estimated by taking the measured total cholesterol value and subtracting HDL-C and VLDL cholesterol (serum triglyceride concentration divided by five). As discussed above, this approach can be problematic when serum triglyceride values are significantly elevated (either as VLDL or as chylomicrons). Further, the calculation is incorrect if VLDL remnants are elevated as in type III hyperlipoproteinemia. All of the lipoprotein apo-peptides, such as apo B, can be measured directly and specifically as well, but these measurements are not readily available in most routine clinical laboratories. However, determining the apo E genotype is absolutely necessary for the diagnosis of type III hyperlipoproteinemia and for discriminating lipoprotein lipase deficiency from apo CII deficiency in the diagnosis of familial chylomicronemia (type I hyperlipoproteinemia). Sacks and his associates (221–224) have published extensively on the roles of the apo-peptides, particularly apo-CIII, and their relationship to coronary heart disease risk.

THERAPEUTIC APPROACHES
Nonlipid Risk Factors

In addition to the risk conferred through lipoproteins (high LDL and/or low HDL), the risk of coronary heart disease is changed by a number of other well-documented, nonlipid risk factors. Three of these, age (greater than 45 years in men and greater than 55 years in women), male gender, and a family history of premature coronary heart disease are not modifiable by the patient or physician. The remaining factors that increase cardiovascular risk, on the other hand, are theoretically modifiable at least to some extent. These include obesity, physical inactivity, a diet pattern that promotes atherogenesis, cigarette smoking, LDL-C and HDL-C, diabetes, hypertension, and emerging risk variables associated the prothrombotic and proinflammatory factors (158,177,225). As discussed earlier, the newest American College of Cardiology/American Heart Association treatment guidelines for blood cholesterol control are founded on reduction of cardiovascular disease risks (158) (Figure 13-3). For the purposes of calculating one's risk of stroke and coronary heart disease events, a downloadable risk calculator is provided at http://my.americanheart.org/cvriskcalculator. Additionally, in the iTunes App Store, the American College of Cardiology provides a free app called "ASCVD Risk Estimator" that performs the same calculation. The app also provides physicians with various lifestyle and treatment advice for their patients based on the risk score and the treatment guidelines found in Reference 158 (Figure 13-3). Likewise, the app provides advice to patients based on their estimated risk.

The presence of obesity is not included in the risk calculation because the prevailing opinion is that CVD risks due to obesity operate through the comorbidity risks associated with obesity (i.e., hypertension, hyperlipidemia, and diabetes). Physical activity level is also not included because its principal beneficial effect is not on lowering LDL-C, the primary lipoprotein goal. A person is considered at high risk if he or she has two of more of the remaining risk factors that are known to increase the likelihood of coronary heart disease and stroke.

A healthy lifestyle is the primary foundation on which lowering risk is based. The rationale, evidence base, and explicit guidelines are provided in detail elsewhere (157). The principal goal of a preventive or therapeutic approach is to attempt to reduce the modifiable, nonlipid risk factors by convincing the patient to cease smoking, by controlling blood pressure, and by improving nutrition and physical activity to maintain a healthy body weight or to accomplish weight reduction if the person is overweight or obese. The foundation for this approach is behavior change–mediated lifestyle intervention. Although a full discussion of behavioral change is beyond the scope of this book, Foreyt and his associates have provided the rationale and the specific essential components of behavioral modification elsewhere (226–228). Behavioral change is essential in order to ensure that lifestyle modifications are maintained throughout the person's lifetime, even if it becomes necessary to introduce pharmacologic treatment to ensure that cholesterol, blood pressure, and blood glucose goals are met. It should come as no surprise that the recommended nutrition and lifestyle recommendations are largely

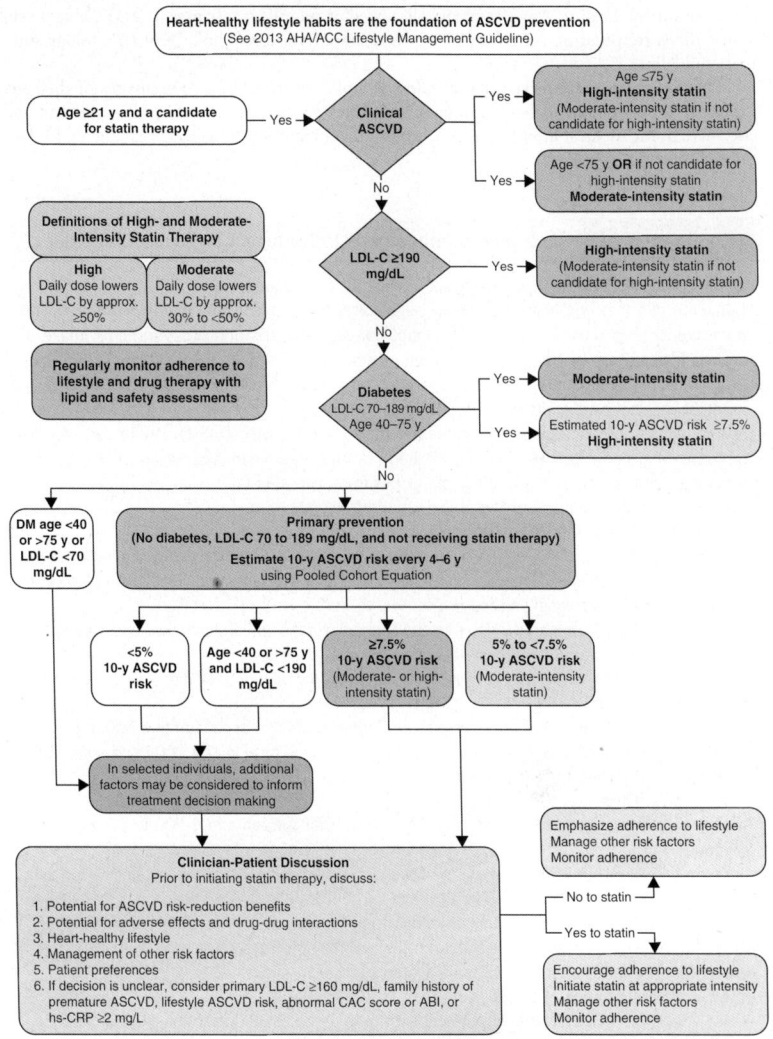

Figure 13-3. American College of Cardiology/American Heart Association algorithm for the treatment of blood cholesterol to reduce the risk of arteriosclerotic heart disease. (From Stone NJ, Robinson JG, Lichtenstein AH, et al. 2013 ACC/AHA guideline on the treatment of blood cholesterol to reduce atherosclerotic cardiovascular risk in adults—a report of the American College of Cardiology/American Heart Association Task Force on practice guidelines. *JACC*. 2014;63:2889–2934.)

those found for healthy Americans and discussed at length in Chapter 1, and Table 13-11 shows the corresponding American Heart Association/American College of Cardiology summary guidelines.

There is now an extensive array of effective lipid-lowering drugs. Discussion of their use is beyond the scope of this book and guidelines can be found in References 158 and 159 and elsewhere in the medical literature. Our discussion will focus on the aspects of reducing LDL-C through nutritional means.

TABLE 13-11 Lifestyle Management to Reduce Cardiovascular Risk

Diet recommendations for low-density lipoprotein cholesterol lowering
Consume diet that emphasizes intake of vegetables, fruits, and whole grains; include low-fat dairy products, poultry, fish, legumes, nontropical vegetable oils and nuts; and limit intake of sweets, sugar-sweetened beverages, and red meats.
Adapt diet to calorie requirements, personal and cultural food preferences, and nutrition therapy for other medical conditions (including diabetes mellitus).
Follow plans such as Dietary Approaches to Stop Hypertension (DASH) dietary pattern, US Department of Agriculture (USDA) Food Pattern, or American Heart Association (AHA) Diet.
Aim for a diet that achieves 5% to 6% of calories from saturated fat.
Reduce percent of calories from saturated fat and trans fat.
Diet recommendations for BP lowering
Consume diet that emphasizes intake of vegetables, fruits, and whole grains; include low-fat dairy products, poultry, fish, legumes, nontropical vegetable oils, and nuts; limit intake of sweets, sugar-sweetened beverages, and red meats.
Adapt diet to calorie requirements, personal and cultural food preferences, and nutritional therapy for other medical conditions (including diabetes mellitus).
Follow plans such as DASH dietary pattern, USDA Food Pattern, or AHA diet (COR: I, LOE: A).
Lower sodium intake
Consume no more than 2,400 mg/d of sodium. Further reduction of sodium to 1,500 mg/d can result in greater reduction in BP. Even reducing sodium intake by at least 1,000 mg/d lowers BP.
Combine DASH dietary pattern with lower sodium intake.
Diets for weight loss
Aim for a daily energy intake of 1,200 to 1,500 kcal/d for women and 1,500 to 1,800 kcal/d for men.
Aim for a 500 kcal/d or 750 kcal/d energy deficit in women and men, respectively.
Limit intakes of certain food types (such as high-carbohydrate foods, low-fiber foods, or high-fat foods) to create the energy deficit since evidence supports their efficacy in achieving weight goals.
Design the specific diet with the assistance of professional nutritional counseling, if possible, and based on the patient's personal food preferences and health status.
Physical activity recommendations
Advise adults to engage in aerobic physical activity to reduce LDL-C and non–HDL-C: three to four sessions a week, average 40 minutes per session, involving moderate-to-vigorous intensity physical activity.
Advise adults to engage in aerobic physical activity to lower blood pressure: three to four sessions a week, average 40 minutes per session, involving moderate-to-vigorous intensity physical activity.

(Adapted from Eckel RH, Jakicic JM, Ard JD, et al. 2013 AHA/ACC Guideline on Lifestyle Management to Reduce Cardiovascular Risk: A Report of the American College of Cardiology/American Heart Association Task Force on Practice Guidelines. *Circulation*. 2014;129(25, suppl 2):S76–S99; and Stone NJ, Robinson JG, Lichtenstein AH, et al. 2013 ACC/AHA Guideline on the Treatment of Blood Cholesterol to Reduce Atherosclerotic Cardiovascular Risk in Adults—A Report of the American College of Cardiology/American Heart Association Task Force on Practice Guidelines. *JACC*. 2014;63:2889–2934.)

Dietary Therapy
General Principles

Dietary therapy is the mainstay of lifestyle-altering treatment of all the hyperlipoproteinemias, and nutritional approaches to serum lipoprotein reduction have been an active area of nutrition research and practice for decades. Although the responses of serum lipids to dietary manipulations are well described, the relationships are often difficult to interpret in the context of human health benefits due to the complex nature of mixed diets and the biochemical/metabolic adaptations to dietary changes, since, at least for the macronutrients, it is not possible to change one component (e.g., fat) without making a change in one of the other macronutrients (e.g., CHO or protein) in order to keep the diet isocaloric. Despite the fact that most cholesterol circulating in the blood stream is of endogenous origin rather than of dietary origin, alterations in dietary cholesterol and saturated fat intakes can change serum cholesterol levels. However, the effect of dietary alterations on serum cholesterol varies greatly from person to person and the American Heart Association concluded recently that "There is insufficient evidence to determine whether lowering dietary cholesterol reduces LDL-C" (158). Dietary changes that cause a marked fall in cholesterol in one person may have little or no effect in another. The reduction in serum cholesterol is most marked when dietary cholesterol is reduced to a very low level (less than 100 mg per day). In severe dietary cholesterol restriction, the diet consists largely of cereals, legumes, fruits, and vegetables, with only small allowances of meat and dairy products. The intensive degree of dietary restriction required to significantly reduce circulating cholesterol by dietary means alone is unlikely to be adopted by the vast majority of the population. Additionally, the fall in serum cholesterol is not directly proportional to the degree of dietary restriction. A substantial reduction in dietary cholesterol (e.g., from 600 to less than 300 mg per day) usually results in only a modest reduction in serum cholesterol.

What has also been appreciated in recent years is the fact that the relationships of total and saturated fat intakes to cardiovascular risk are more complicated than initially thought. Reduction in total fat intake itself has not been shown to reduce cardiovascular risk or other speculated clinical risks and previous guidelines that recommended reduction in total dietary fat have largely been abandoned. In large part, this has been due to the realization that the macronutrient that replaces fat in the diet to maintain caloric balance has a profound influence on subsequent health risks as discussed below. Also recognized in recent years is the fact that relationships of saturated fats intake to cardiovascular outcomes is more complicated than previously assumed (229–246). Specifically, while all fats that replace carbohydrates in the diet increase HDL-C, the increase caused by saturated fats is greater than that caused by mono- or polyunsaturated fats. Additionally, although the saturated fatty acid, stearic acid has essentially no effect on LDL-C, the saturated fatty acids lauric, myristic, and palmitic acids increase LDL-C. But since they also increase HDL-C, they have little significant effect on the circulating ratio of the "good" and "bad" forms of cholesterol. Additionally, conclusions about clinical consequences are not easy to derive from the data, since the population of LDL circulating in plasma is not a uniform one. The distribution of different LDL subpopulations varies among people and is independent of the total LDL-C level. Small dense LDL particles are the most atherogenic, but the principal effect of saturated fat ingestion is to increase the larger, less dense, less-atherogenic LDL particles (234,247–249,173).

There is general agreement from controlled trials that replacing dietary saturated fats with mono- or polyunsaturated fats lowers LDL-C, although, unfortunately, HDL-C also declines albeit to a somewhat lesser extent (157). Polyunsaturated fats also lower circulating triglycerides, but monounsaturated fats tend to increase triglycerides slightly. While a variety of controlled clinical trials have shown that substitution of dietary saturated fats by polyunsaturated fats reduces coronary heart disease risks, recent analyses have questioned the comprehensive nature of this conclusion by finding no relationships among consumption of various mono- and polyunsaturated fats and CVD risks (231,232,240,242, 250–254). Additionally, one of the largest, double-blind randomized clinical trials ever conducted to directly test the hypothesis that increasing the ratio of polyunsaturated to saturated fats (P:S) in the diet was unable to find a reduction in "cardiovascular events, cardiovascular deaths, or total mortality" over the 4.5 year follow-up period (255). Nonetheless, essentially every expert committee report recommends the replacement of dietary saturated fats with mono- or polyunsaturated fats because of the large body of evidence accumulated over the last several decades showing that this strategy can reduce CVD risk. Moreover, there is also general agreement that *trans*-fatty acids increase LDL-C and represent a significant factor in increased risk for cardiovascular disease (158,256). For this reason, all current recommendations call for reduction in *trans* fat intakes to the lowest level possible.

Omega-3 polyunsaturated fatty acids appear to be a unique class of polyunsaturated fats. The omega-3 fatty acid, α-linolenic acid, is found in soybean and canola oil (and in walnuts), while fish oils contain the longer-chain omega-3 fatty acids, eicosapentaenoic acid (EPA) and docosahexaenoic acid (DHA). Historically, a wide variety of studies have shown that omega-3 fatty acids from fish consumption or fish oil supplementation reduce the risks of cardiovascular disease (also see discussion in Chapter 8). For this reason, essentially all expert bodies recommend substituting fish for meat products in the diet. Additionally, some have suggested that omega-3 fatty acid supplements will complement therapy with statins, particularly when the patient has elevations in both cholesterol and triglycerides, because increased consumption of polyunsaturated fats lowers hepatic VLDL secretion. Nonetheless, recommendations to increase consumption of omega-3 fatty acids have also come under close scrutiny recently because a large meta-analysis was unable to show that omega-3 consumption was associated with a decrease in all-cause mortality, cardiovascular events or deaths, or stroke (235). In addition, this study showed that as the subject sample size increased over the last two decades, the size of the omega-3 effect on mortality has steadily diminished (235), a phenomenon seen with a wide variety of medical therapeutic interventions.

Carbohydrates

Perhaps the most important modification to earlier dietary recommendations comes from the appreciation that replacement of dietary saturated fats by carbohydrates does not reduce heart disease risk but, in fact, contributes to increased CVD risk, since such replacement lowers HDL-C, increases small dense LDL particles, and increases circulating triglycerides (243–245). For this reason, current dietary recommendations focus on a moderate carbohydrate intake in which the majority of carbohydrates are consumed as the complex carbohydrates in whole grains, fruits, and vegetables. This will also ensure an adequate intake of dietary fiber that should be consumed at an intake level of about 14 g of fiber for each 1,000 calories of energy.

Plant Stanols/Sterols

Recent studies indicate that plant sterols and plant-derived stanols or stanol esters can reduce LDL-C when consumed in the amounts of about 2 g daily (range 1 to 3 g per day) (257–259). These are found naturally to some degree in all plant foods and particularly in fruits, vegetables, seeds, nuts, and many vegetable oils; that is, all components of a wide variety of healthy diet patterns. Current plant sterol/stanol intakes in the United States are only about 0.5 g per day and moving to healthier, plant-based dietary patterns would clearly increase their intake. However, these substances are now added to several margarines, salad dressings, yoghurts, snack bars, and at least one brand of orange juice. Not unexpectedly, plant sterols and stanols are now constituents of a wide variety of dietary supplement products.

Soy Protein

While there are some data that soy protein can cause small reductions in LDL-C (260), the average effect tends to be small, and even this small reduction requires intakes on the order of 30 g per day. The most recent systematic review of randomized controlled trials in hypercholesterolemic adults (261) was unable to demonstrate an effect on total or LDL-C. On the whole, there appears to be little compelling reason to recommend increasing soy protein intake or substituting soy protein for other dietary proteins on the basis of cardiovascular health benefits.

Wine

In populations, light to moderate alcohol intake is associated with a reduced cardiovascular risk, although it is not clear whether there is any particular benefit of wine compared to other forms of alcohol (262). On the other hand, there is also considerable epidemiologic evidence that more substantial alcohol intakes are associated with increased risks of hypertension and stroke. Because of the potential for excess consumption, there is agreement on a way to calculate the risk/benefit ratio for a public health recommendation. Overall, the American Heart Association advisory statement concludes that "...there is little current justification to recommend alcohol (or wine specifically) as a cardioprotective strategy. The American Heart Association maintains its recommendation that alcohol use should be an item of discussion between physician and patient" (262).

Vitamin and Mineral Supplements

Other than a routine daily multivitamin taken for "nutrition insurance," the use of vitamin B_{12} supplements in elderly individuals, the recommendation for calcium supplements in women unable to achieve an adequate intake of calcium, and the public health recommendation for folic acid supplements in women of childbearing age, there is no evidence that any dietary supplements have benefit in preventing cardiovascular disease (263). In fact, there is some evidence that β-carotene, vitamin A, and vitamin E supplements may actually increase, rather than decrease, mortality (263). Likewise, there is no evidence that herbal or other botanical supplements have any beneficial effect in reducing the risk for coronary heart disease.

Other comorbidities must be taken into account when a cholesterol-lowering diet is designed. For example, as described earlier in this chapter, if renal disease is present, it may be necessary to lower dietary protein, potassium and phosphorus intakes and, if the patient has hypertension, further limitation of the salt intake may be required. The DASH diet plan accomplishes both blood pressure reduction and lipid reduction and can improve body weight. However, as discussed earlier in this chapter, the DASH diet plan must be modified if applied to individuals with renal disease.

Obesity (with or without diabetes) and alcohol consumption both commonly precipitate hypertriglyceridemia. The major determinant of chylomicron production and VLDL production is the rate of synthesis of triglycerides in the enterocytes and hepatocytes, respectively. The rate of triglyceride synthesis in enterocytes is determined by the intake of fat. The rate of triglyceride synthesis in hepatocytes is determined by total caloric intake and fat intake. Thus, caloric restriction reduces both chylomicron and VLDL production by reducing the synthesis of triglycerides. Thus, caloric-restriction–induced weight loss (even only 5% to 10% of initial body weight) usually reduces the hypertriglyceridemia associated with obesity. In many patients with hypertriglyceridemia, a pronounced rise in triglyceride levels occurs after alcohol ingestion. Elimination or marked curtailment of alcohol results in decreased triglycerides. Thus, weight-reduction diets and elimination of alcohol are essential steps in managing hypertriglyceridemia.

When high plasma levels of triglycerides are secondary to other diseases, therapy should be directed first toward the underlying disorder. Non–insulin-dependent diabetes, when poorly controlled, is a common cause of hypertriglyceridemia; treatment with caloric restriction, exercise, or insulin often normalizes triglyceride concentrations. When hypothyroidism is associated with hypertriglyceridemia, patients usually are obese and may have a familial form of hyperlipidemia; with this combination of disorders, thyroid hormone therapy alone may not correct the hypertriglyceridemia completely. An additional approach in severe hypertriglyceridemia is to restrict fat intake to 10% to 15% of energy intake, but this is only a temporizing measure and can be problematic in the long term, both from the standpoint of compliance and because the necessarily increased carbohydrate content of the diet might lead to increased synthesis of VLDL triglycerides. Along with a restriction in dietary saturated fat and energy intakes, omega-3 fatty acid supplements may improve plasma triglyceride levels.

Practical Dietary Management

The most important message that has come from the last decade of studies addressing the relationships of diets and cardiovascular disease risks is that overall healthy diet patterns are more important than the focus on any individual food or nutrient component of the diet. Thus, in almost all expert recommendations today, the guidelines are couched in terms of whole foods and their use in constructing overall health diet patterns. This is precisely the principle discussed in Chapter 1 in reference to the Dietary Guidelines for Americans, and the latter expert recommendations apply to individuals who are attempting to limit their risk of cardiovascular disease. Likewise, the American Heart Association/American College of Cardiology guidelines on lifestyle management to reduce cardiovascular risk are similarly composed with recommendations to achieve a healthy eating pattern based on the DASH diet pattern, the USDA food pattern, or the AHA diet (157). Every pattern, while different in certain specifics, "emphasizes the intake of vegetables, fruits, and whole grains; includes low-fat dairy products, poultry, fish, legumes, nontropical vegetable oils and nuts; and limits the intake of sweets, sugar-sweetened beverages and red meats" (158).

Although reducing dietary cholesterol intake, per se, is no longer a mainstay of dietary recommendations to lower LDL-C levels, it may be an adjunct to lifestyle management particularly in individuals with borderline cholesterol values who are reluctant to take statin drugs. The most recent population data from NHANES show that the average American man consumes slightly more than 300 mg of cholesterol daily, while American women consume consumes about 225 mg day. These values are significantly lower than those in the second half of the 20th century and can be reduced further by eliminating high-fat meats (beef, lamb, pork, ham), organ meats, butter fat, lard, and margarines high in *trans* fats, and by substituting skim milk for whole milk (Table 13-12). The cholesterol contents of some common foods are as follows: a large egg, 215 mg; 1 tbsp of butter, 30 mg; a hamburger made with a quarter of a pound of beef, 85 mg; one strip of bacon, 16 mg; and 1 cup of whole milk, 34 mg. Although eggs contain cholesterol (less now than in the 20th century), they are relatively "poor" in saturated fatty acids and studies

TABLE 13-12 Lipid Content of Selected Foods

Specific Food (100 g)	Total Fat (g)	P:S Ratio[a]	Cholesterol (g)
Beef, lean, cooked	14.9	0.1	80
Beef, fatty, cooked	29.8	0.1	85
Chicken and turkey (light meat, no skin)	3.9	0.8	77
Frankfurter, all beef, cooked	28.5	0.1	61
Bologna, salami, cold cuts	30.0	0.1	85
Bacon, regular, cooked	49.0	0.3	85
Fish (cod)	1.5	1.7	68
Shrimp	1.1	1.54	195
Clams, mussels, cooked	1.9	2.9	67
Tuna, canned, water-packed	0.8	1.5	30
Eggs (equivalent to two whole)	10.5	0.4	425
Egg, yolk	30.9	0.4	1,281
Egg, white	0	—	0
Milk, whole	3.5	0.1	13.6
Milk, 1% fat	1.1	0.1	4
Milk, skim	0.2	0.1	2
Cheese, cheddar, American	33.1	0.1	105
Cheese, cottage, low-fat	1.9	0.1	8
Ice cream, regular (11% fat)	11	0.1	44
Butter	81.0	0.1	219
Oils			
Corn	100.0	4.6	0
Cottonseed	100.0	2.0	0
Safflower	100.0	8.2	0
Sesame	100.0	2.9	0
Soybean, partially hydrogenated	100.0	2.5	0
Olive	100.0	0.6	0
Peanut	100.0	1.9	0
Coconut	100.0	0.1	0
Peanut butter	50.6	1.6	0

[a]P:S ratio is the ratio of polyunsaturated fatty acids to saturated fatty acids; values less than 0.1 have been rounded to 0.1. For dairy products, the values average closer to 0.05, and for coconut oil, the P:S ratio is closer to 0.02.

show that, by themselves, eggs do not increase LDL-C when consumed in the modest quantities. Fish, shellfish, and poultry intakes are encouraged. Although the cholesterol content of shrimp is high, they contain many noncholesterol sterols (e.g., sitosterol) that compete for absorption and the amount of shrimp eaten is generally considerably less than the amount of beef consumed. Meat substitutes, made from a variety of vegetable sources are now widely available in virtually every supermarket and in almost every meat product configuration, including "bacon," "sausage," "ground beef," and "turkey." Surimi, a form of processed pollock that is low in fat and cholesterol, is sold as imitation crabmeat and is a reasonably priced substitute for meat protein.

Except for cottage cheese and farmer's cheese, most cheeses are high in cholesterol. Fat-modified cheeses are now commonly available in supermarkets. The calorie content of low-fat or nonfat cheeses is reduced in comparison to that of regular cheese, and cheeses made from vegetable fats rather than animal fats have no cholesterol and a high ratio of polyunsaturated fats to saturated fats, although their caloric content is about the same as that of natural cheese. Some whole milk substitutes, made for lactose-intolerant patients, are composed entirely of vegetable products and oils (e.g., soy "milk") are acceptable substitutes. However, in the context of weight maintenance, it is important to remember that these products may contain as many calories as whole milk.

Many homemade and commercially prepared baked goods contain significant amounts of saturated fat in the form of butter, lard, and whole milk in addition to the cholesterol of egg yolks. These products include waffles, pancakes, muffins, pastries, French toast, potato chips, cakes, and pies. Low-cholesterol baked goods can be made at home, with either egg whites or egg substitutes used instead of whole eggs, skim milk instead of whole milk, and soft margarine instead of butter and lard. A variety of low-fat, low-cholesterol bakery products is now available commercially.

A significant part of today's recommendations for cardiovascular health involve increased consumption of dietary polyunsaturated fats. The P:S ratio in the usual American diet is less than 1.0. Most polyunsaturated fats come from vegetable oils, whereas most saturated fat comes from meat and dairy products. Traditional margarines were all made by partially hydrogenating vegetable oils that increases fatty acid saturation and, therefore reduces, the P:S ratio. During the hydrogenation process, some fatty acids are converted to *trans*-fatty acids, products that are as atherogenic, or even more atherogenic, than saturated fats. All expert bodies recommend reducing the intake of *trans* fats to as low as possible. This goal is made easier every day, since most manufacturers are removing all (or nearly all) man-made *trans* fats from their products. When buying margarine, it is critical to read the label, since *trans* fats are listed. Many margarine products are now *trans* fat–free and others have added healthy fats and unsaturated oils to decrease the atherogenic properties. In particular, these use vegetable oils and are, thus, soft margarines, generally sold in tubs, rather than the stick margarines. Further, given the listing of grams of saturated and unsaturated fats on the label, one can calculate the P:S ratio, which is best when above 2.0. Also, when reading the label, pay attention to the type of vegetable fat, since this term may refer to coconut oil or other oils that are high in saturated fats. Of all the vegetable oils, safflower oil has the highest P:S ratio. Other vegetable oils with a high P:S ratio are corn, soybean, and sunflower oils. The P:S ratio for olive oil (0.6) is lower than that for most other vegetable oils because olive oil is predominantly a monounsaturated oil. The P:S ratios for palm oil (0.2) and coconut oil (0.2) are even lower, and these are not effective cholesterol-lowering oils.

Most regular commercially prepared baked goods, including crackers for snacks, cookies, cakes, and pies, have low P:S ratios because they are made with animal fats or hydrogenated vegetable fats. Commercial cake mixes have low P:S ratios for the same reason. At least in part, this is due to the fact that baked goods of this type require some fats that are solid at room temperature in order to rise properly when baked and to maintain their shape and final form after baking.

The P:S ratios for vegetable products are generally high and fish and poultry have higher P:S ratios than do other animal products. To raise the P:S ratio of the diet, one must reduce the consumption of meat, eggs, butter, and whole milk and increase the consumption of foods and oils with a high P:S ratio. The dietary changes that decrease cholesterol intake also generally lower the intake of saturated fat because, in the American diet, the foods that are high in cholesterol are tend to be high in saturated fat (e.g., meat, butter, and dairy products made from whole milk). Many recipes call for saturated fats; Table 13-13 provides a list of polyunsaturated substitutes for these saturated fats but, for the reasons stated above, such substitutions will change the character of baked goods.

TABLE 13-13 Polyunsaturated Substitutes for Saturated Fats Useful in Changing a Recipe That May Be High in Saturated Fat to One That Is High in Polyunsaturted Fat

Saturated Fat	Polyunsaturated Fat
1 oz chocolate	= 2 tbsp cocoa + 2 tsp margarine
1 egg	= 1 tbsp flour for thickening
1 egg	= 2 egg whites
1 cup butter	= 1 cup margarine
1 cup sour cream	= 1 cup yogurt
1 cup whole milk	= 1 cup skim milk + 2 tsp margarine
1 tbsp butter	= 3/4 tbsp oil
1 1/4 cup butter	= 1 cup oil

Data from the Washington University Lipid Research Center.

ADDITIONAL RESOURCES

The following government-sponsored website can serve as an additional resource for patient and professional information on diet, healthy weight, hypertension, cholesterol, and coronary heart disease: http://www.nhlbi.nih.gov/health/resources/.

REFERENCES

1. U.S. Centers for Disease Control and Prevention. National Diabetes Statistics Report, 2014. National Center for Chronic Disease Prevention and Health Promotion, Division of Diabetes Translation; 2014. http://www.cdc.gov/diabetes/pubs/statsreport14/national-diabetes-report-web.pdf
2. Danaei G, Finucane MM, Lu Y, et al; on behalf of the Global Burden of Metabolic Risk Factors of Chronic Diseases Collaborating Group (Blood Glucose). National, Regional, and Global Trends in Fasting Plasma Glucose and Diabetes Prevalence Since 1980: Systematic Analysis of Health Examination Surveys and Epidemiological Studies with 370 Country-years and 2.7 Million Participants. *Lancet*. 2011;378:31–40.
3. International Diabetes Federation. IDF Diabetes Atlas. 5th ed. 2012 Update. http://www.idf.org/sites/default/files/5E_IDFAtlasPoster_2012_EN.pdf
4. Roglic G, Unwin N. Mortality attributable to diabetes: estimates for the year 2010. *Diabetes Res Clin Pract*. 2010;87:15–19.
5. Nathan DM, Bayless M, Cleary P, et al.; for the DCCT/EDIC Research Group. Diabetes control and complications trial/epidemiology of diabetes interventions and complications study at 30 years: advances and contributions. *Diabetes*. 2013;62:3976–3986.
6. Kilpatrick ES, Rigby AS, Atkin SL. The Diabetes Control and Complications Trial: the gift that keeps giving. *Nat Rev Endocrinol*. 2009;5:537–545.
7. Nathan, DM; for the DCCT/EDIC Research Group. The diabetes control and complications trial/epidemiology of diabetes interventions and complications study at 30 years: overview. *Diabetes Care*. 2014;37:9–16.
8. Fullerton B, Jeitler K, Seitz M, et al. Intensive glucose control versus conventional glucose control for type 1 diabetes mellitus. *Cochrane Database Syst Rev*. 2014;2:CD009122.
9. Aiello LP; for the DCCT/EDIC Research Group. Diabetic retinopathy and other ocular findings in the diabetes control and complications trial/epidemiology of diabetes interventions and complications study. *Diabetes Care*. 2014;37:17–23.
10. Lachin JM, Orchard TJ, Nathan DM; for the DCCT/EDIC Research Group. Update on cardiovascular outcomes at 30 years of the diabetes control and complications trial/ epidemiology of diabetes interventions and complications study. *Diabetes Care*. 2014;37:39–43.
11. Brown A, Reynolds LR, Bruemmer D. Intensive glycemic control and cardiovascular disease: an update. *Nat Rev Cardiol*. 2010;7:369–375.
12. Hunt KJ, Baker N, Cleary P, et al.; DCCT/EDIC Research Group. Oxidized LDL and AGE-LDL in circulating immune complexes strongly predict progression of carotid artery IMT in type 1 diabetes. *Atherosclerosis*. 2013;231:315–322.

13. Gubitosi-Klug RA; for the DCCT/EDIC Research Group. The diabetes control and complications trial/epidemiology of diabetes interventions and complications study at 30 years: summary and future directions. *Diabetes Care.* 2014;37:44–49.
14. de Boer IH; for the DCCT/EDIC Research Group. Kidney disease and related findings in the diabetes control and complications trial/epidemiology of diabetes interventions and complications study. *Diabetes Care.* 2014;37:24–30.
15. deBoer IH, Sun W, Gao X, et al.; for the DCCT/EDIC Research Group. Effect of intensive diabetes treatment on albuminuria in type 1 diabetes: long-term follow-up of the diabetes control and complications trial and epidemiology of diabetes interventions and complications study. *Lancet Diabetes Endocrinol.* 2014 (in press).
16. Martin CL, Albers JW, Pop-Busui R; for the DCCT/EDIC Research Group. Neuropathy and related findings in the diabetes control and complications trial/epidemiology of diabetes interventions and complications study. *Diabetes Care.* 2014;37:31–38.
17. Pop-Busui R, Herman WH, Feldman EL, et al.; for the DCCT/EDIC Research Group. DCCT and EDIC studies in type 1 diabetes: lessons for diabetic neuropathy regarding metabolic memory and natural history. *Curr Diab Rep.* 2010;10:276–282.
18. Nathan DM, McGee P, Steffes MW, et al.; for the DCCT/EDIC Research Group. Relationship of glycated albumin to blood glucose and HbA1c values and to retinopathy, nephropathy, and cardiovascular outcomes in the DCCT/EDIC study. *Diabetes.* 2014;63:282–290.
19. Purnell JQ, Hokanson JE, Cleary PA, et al; for the DCCT/EDIC Research Group. The effect of excess weight gain with intensive diabetes treatment on cardiovascular disease risk factors and atherosclerosis in type 1 diabetes: results from the Diabetes Control and Complications Trial/Epidemiology of Diabetes Interventions and Complications Study (DCCT/EDIC) study. *Circulation.* 2013;127:180–187.
20. Pirola L. The DCCT/EDIC study: epigenetic clues after three decades. *Diabetes.* 2014;63:1460–1462.
21. Wherrett DK. Trials in the prevention of type 1 diabetes: current and future. *Can J Diabetes.* 2014;38:279–284.
22. Atkinson MA, Eisenbarth GS, Michels AW. Type 1 diabetes. *Lancet.* 2014;383:69–82.
23. Tuomilehto J, Lindström J, Eriksson JG, et al. Prevention of type 2 diabetes mellitus by changes in lifestyle among subjects with impaired glucose tolerance. *N Engl J Med.* 2001;344:1343–1350.
24. Knowler WC, Barrett-Connor E, Fowler SE, et al. Reduction in the incidence of type 2 diabetes with lifestyle intervention of metformin. *N Engl J Med.* 2002;346:393–403.
25. Chiasson J-L, Josse RG, Gomis R, et al. Acarbose for prevention of type 2 diabetes mellitus: the STOP-NIDDM randomised trial. *Lancet.* 2002;359:2072–2077.
26. Buchanan TA, Xiang AH, Peters RK, et al. Preservation of pancreatic β-cell function and prevention of type 2 diabetes by pharmacological treatment of insulin resistance in high-risk Hispanic women. *Diabetes.* 2002;51:2796–2803.
27. Penn L, White M, Lindström J, et al. Importance of weight loss maintenance and risk prediction in the prevention of type 2 diabetes: analysis of European diabetes prevention study RCT. *PLos One.* 2013;8:e57143.
28. Torgerson JS, Hauptman J, Boldrin MN, et al. Xenical in the prevention of diabetes in obese subjects (XENDOS) study: a randomized study of orlistat as an adjunct to lifestyle changes for the prevention of type 2 diabetes in obese patients. *Diabetes Care.* 2004;27:155–161.
29. Pan XR, Li GW, Hu YH, et al. Effects of diet and exercise in preventing NIDDM in people with impaired glucose tolerance: the Da Qing IGT and Diabetes Study. *Diabetes Care.* 1997;20:537–544.
30. Ramachandran A, Snehalatha C, Mukesh MS, et al.; Indian Diabetes Prevention Programme (IDPP). The Indian Diabetes Prevention Program shows that lifestyle modification and metformin prevent type 2 diabetes in Asian Indian subjects with impaired glucose tolerance (IDPP-1). *Diabetologia.* 2006;49:289–297.
31. Gong Q, Gregg EW, Wang J, et al. Long-term effects of a randomised trial of a 6-year lifestyle intervention in impaired glucose tolerance on diabetes-related microvascular complications: the China Da Qing Diabetes Prevention Outcome Study. *Diabetologia.* 2011;54:300–307.
32. Li G, Zhang P, Wang J, et al. Cardiovascular mortality, all-cause mortality, and diabetes incidence after lifestyle intervention with people with impaired glucose tolerance in the Da Qing Diabetes Prevention Study: a 23-year follow-up study. *Lancet Diabetes Endocrinol.* 2014;2:474–480.
33. Li G, Zhang P, Wang, J, et al. The long-term effect of lifestyle interventions to prevent diabetes in the China Da Qing Diabetes Prevention Study: a 20-year follow-up study. *Lancet.* 2008;371:1783–1789.
34. Saaristo T, Moilanen L, Korpi-Hyövälti E, et al. Lifestyle intervention for prevention of type 2 diabetes in primary health care. *Diabetes Care.* 2010;33:2146–2151.

35. Diabetes Prevention Program Research Group. 10-year follow-up of diabetes incidence and weight loss in the Diabetes Prevention Program Outcomes Study. *Lancet.* 2009;374:1677–1686.
36. Yoon U, Kwok LL, Magkidis A. Efficacy of lifestyle interventions in reducing diabetes incidence in patients with impaired glucose tolerance: a systematic review of randomized controlled trials. *Metabolism.* 2013;62:303–314.
37. Schellenberg ES, Dryden DM, Vandermeer B, et al. Lifestyle interventions for patients with and at risk for type 2 diabetes: a systematic review and meta-analysis. *Ann Intern Med.* 2013;159:543–551.
38. Merlotti C, Morabito A, Pontiroli AE. Prevention of type 2 diabetes; a systematic review and meta-analysis of different intervention strategies. *Diabetes Obes Metab.* 2014;16:719–727.
39. Holman RR, Paul SK, Bethel MA, et al. 10-year follow-up of intensive glucose control in type 2 diabetes. *N Engl J Med.* 2008;359:1577–1589.
40. The Look AHEAD Research Group. Cardiovascular effects of intensive lifestyle intervention in type 2 diabetes. *N Engl J Med.* 2013;369:145–154.
41. The Look AHEAD Research Group. Eight-year weight losses with an intensive lifestyle intervention: the look AHEAD study. *Obesity.* 2014;22:5–13.
42. Wing RR; for the Look AHEAD Research Group. Implications of look AHEAD for clinical trials and clinical practice: invited review article. *Diabetes Obes Metab.* 2014 (in press).
43. The Look AHEAD Research Group. Effect of a long-term behavioural weight loss intervention on nephropathy in overweight or obese adults with type 2 diabetes: a secondary analysis of the look AHEAD randomised clinical trial. *Lancet Diabetes Endocrinol.* 2014 (in press).
44. Buchanan TA. (How) can we prevent type 2 diabetes? *Diabetes.* 2007;56:1502–1507.
45. Esposito K, Chiodini P, Maiorino MI, et al. Which diet for prevention of type 2 diabetes? A meta-analysis of prospective studies. *Endocrine.* 2014;47:107–116.
46. Ley SH, Hamdy O, Mohan V, et al. Prevention and management of type 2 diabetes: dietary components and nutritional strategies. *Lancet.* 2014;383:1999–2007.
47. Moore H, Summerbell C, Hooper L, et al. Dietary advice for treatment of type 2 diabetes mellitus in adults. *Cochrane Database Syst Rev.* 2004;2:CD004097. Update in *Cochrane Database Syst Rev.* 2004;3:CD004097.
48. Nield L, Moore HJ, Cruickshank JK, et al. Dietary advice for treatment of type 2 diabetes mellitus in adults. *Cochrane Database Syst Rev.* 2007;3:CD004097.
49. Nield L, Summerbell CD, Hooper L, et al. Dietary advice for the prevention of type 2 diabetes mellitus in adults. *Cochrane Database Syst Rev.* 2008;3:CD005102.
50. Moyer VA; on behalf of the U.S. Preventive Services Task Force. Behavioral counseling interventions to promote a healthful diet and physical activity for cardiovascular disease prevention in adults: U.S. Preventive Services Task Force recommendation statement. *Ann Intern Med.* 2012;157:367–372.
51. Robertson C, Archibald D, Avenell A, et al. Systematic reviews of and integrated report on the quantitative, qualitative and economic evidence base for the management of obesity in men. *Health Technol Assess.* 2014;18:v–vi, xxiii–xxix.
52. Lin JS, O'Connor E, Evans CV, et al. Behavioral counseling to promote a healthy lifestyle in persons with cardiovascular risk factors: a systematic review for the U.S. Preventive Services Task Force. *Ann Intern Med.* 2014 (in press).
53. Dunkley AJ, Bodicoat DH, Greaves CJ, et al. Diabetes prevention in the real world: effectiveness of pragmatic lifestyle interventions for the prevention of type 2 diabetes and of the impact of adherence to guideline recommendations: a systematic review and meta-analysis. *Diabetes Care.* 2014;37:922–933.
54. Henry RR, Chilton R, Garvey WT. New options for the treatment of obesity and type 2 diabetes mellitus (narrative review). *J Diabetes Complications.* 2013;27:508–518.
55. Franz MJ, Boucher JL, Evert AB. Evidence-based diabetes nutrition therapy recommendations are effective: the key is individualization. *Diabetes Metab Syndr Obes.* 2014;7:65–72.
56. Jaacks LM, Wylie-Rosett J, Mayer-Davis EJ. Diabetes. In Erdman JW Jr, Macdonald IA, Zeisel SH, eds. *Present Knowledge in Nutrition.* 10th ed. Ames, IA: Wiley; 2012.
57. Bantle JP, Wylie-Rosett J, Albright AL, et al; for the American Diabetes Association. Nutrition recommendations and interventions for diabetes: a position statement of the American Diabetes Association. *Diabetes Care.* 2008;31(suppl 1):S61–S78.
58. American Diabetes Association. Standards of medical care in diabetes—2014. *Diabetes Care.* 2014;37(suppl 1).
59. Evert AB, Boucher JL, Cypress M, et al. Nutrition therapy recommendations for the management of adults with diabetes. *Diabetes Care.* 2014;37(suppl 1):S120–S143.
60. International Diabetes Federation Guideline Development Group. Global guideline for type 2 diabetes. *Diabetes Res Clin Pract.* 2014;104:1–52.

61. Handelsman Y, Mechanick JI, Blonde L, et al. American Association of Clinical Endocrinologists Medical Guidelines for Clinical Practice for developing a diabetes mellitus comprehensive care plan. *Endocr Pract.* 2011;17(suppl 2):1–53.
62. Oh S, Kalyani RR, Dobs A, et al. Nutritional management of diabetes. In: *Modern Nutrition in Health and Disease*, 11th ed. Philadelphia: Wolters Kluwer; 2014.
63. Schauer PR, Bhatt DL, Kirwan JP, et al. Bariatric surgery versus intensive medical therapy for diabetes—3-year outcomes. *N Engl J Med.* 2014;370(21):2002–2013.
64. Ricci C, Gaeta M, Rausa E, et al. Long-term effects of bariatric surgery on type II diabetes, hypertension and hyperlipidemia: a meta-analysis and meta-regression study with 5-year follow-up. *Obes Surg.* 2014 (in press).
65. Hartweg J, Perera R, Montori V, et al. Omega-3 polyunsaturated fatty acids (PUFA) for type 2 diabetes mellitus. *Cochrane Database Syst Rev.* 2008;(1):CD003205.
66. Sheard NF, Clark NG, Brand-Miller J, et al. Dietary carbohydrate (amount and type) in the prevention and management of diabetes: a statement by the American Diabetes Association. *Diabetes Care.* 2004;27(9):2266–2271.
67. Wheeler ML, Xavier P-S. Carbohydrate issues: type and amount. *J Am Diet Assoc.* 2008:108:S34–S39.
68. Gillespie SJ, Kulkarni KD, Daley AE. Using carbohydrate counting in diabetes clinical practice. *J Am Diet Assoc.* 1998;98:897–905.
69. Chiesa G, Piscopo MA, Rigamonti A, et al. Insulin therapy and carbohydrate counting. *Acta Biomed.* 2005;76(suppl 3):44–48.
70. Kulkarni KD. Carbohydrate counting: a practical meal-planning option for people with diabetes. *Clinical Diabetes.* 2005;23(3):120–122.
71. Bell KJ, Barclay AW, Petocz P, et al. Efficacy of carbohydrate counting in type 1 diabetes: a systematic review and meta-analysis. *Lancet Diabetes Endocrinol.* 2014;2(2):133–140.
72. Ajala O, English P, Pinkney J. Systematic review and meta-analysis of different dietary approaches to the management of type 2 diabetes. *Am J Clin Nutr.* 2013;97(3):505–516.
73. Thomas D, Elliott EJ. Low glycaemic index, or low glycaemic load, diets for diabetes mellitus. *Cochrane Database Syst Rev.* 2009;(1):CD006296.
74. Wheeler ML, Dunbar SA, Jaacks LM, et al. Macronutrients, food groups, and eating patterns in the management of diabetes: a systematic review of the literature, 2010. *Diabetes Care.* 2012;35:434–445.
75. Herbst KL, Hirsch IB. Insulin strategies for primary care providers. *Clinical Diabetes.* 2002;20(1):11–17.
76. Scheiner G. Insulin-to-carb ratios made easy. www.healthcentral.com, November 2007.
77. Cryer PE. Glycemic goals in diabetes: trade-off between glycemic control and latrogenic hypoglycemia. *Diabetes.* 2014;63:2188–2195.
78. West KM. Diet and diabetes. *Postgrad Med.* 1976;60(9):209–216.
79. Food and Nutrition Board, Institute of Medicine, National Academy of Sciences. *Dietary Reference Intakes for Energy, Carbohydrate, Fiber, Fat, Fatty Acids, Cholesterol, Protein, and Amino Acids.* Washington, DC: National Academy Press; 2005.
80. Institute of Medicine, National Academy of Sciences. *Dietary Reference Intakes: The Essential Guide to Nutrient Requirements.* Washington, DC: National Academy Press; 2006.
81. Shankar P, Ahuja S, Sriram K. Non-nutritive sweeteners: review and update. *Nutrition.* 2013;29(11-12):1293–1299.
82. Miller PE, Perez V. Low-calorie sweeteners and body weight and composition: a meta-analysis of randomized controlled trials and prospective cohort studies. *Am J Clin Nutr.* 2014;100(3):765–777.
83. Hill JO. What do you say when your patients ask whether low-calorie sweeteners help with weight management? *Am J Clin Nutr.* 2014;100(3):739–740.
84. Massougbodji J, Le Bodo Y, Fratu R, et al. Reviews examining sugar-sweetened beverages and body weight: correlates of their quality and conclusions. *Am J Clin Nutr.* 2014;99(5):1096–1104.
85. Cohen AS, Edelstein EL. Sick-day management for the home care client with diabetes. *Home Healthc Nurse.* 2005;23(11):717–724.
86. Nyenwe EA, Abbas EK. Evidence-based management of hyperglycemic emergencies in diabetes mellitus. *Diabetes Res Clin Pract.* 2011;94:340–351.
87. National Kidney Foundation KDOQI. KDOQI clinical practice guideline for diabetes and CKD: 2012 update. *Am J Kidney Dis.* 2012;60(5):850–886.
88. Gosmanov AR, Wall BM, Gosmanova EO. Diagnosis and treatment of diabetic kidney disease. *Am J Med Sci.* 2014;347(5):406–413.

89. Kovesdy CP, Kopple JD, Kalantar-Zadeh K. Management of protein-energy wasting in non-dialysis-dependent chronic kidney disease: reconciling low protein intake with nutritional therapy. *Am J Clin Nutr.* 2013;97:1163–1177.
90. Levey AS, Greene T, Sarnak MJ, et al. Effect of dietary protein restriction on the progression of kidney disease: long-term follow-up on the Modification of Diet in Renal Disease (MDRD) Study. *Am J Kidney Dis.* 2006;48(6):879–888.
91. Klahr S, Levey AS, Beck GJ, et al. The effects of dietary protein restriction and blood-pressure control on the progression of chronic renal disease. Modification of Diet in Renal Disease Study Group. *N Engl J Med.* 1994;330(13):877–884.
92. Mitch WE, Ikizler TA. In: *Handbook of Nutrition and the Kidney*, 6th ed. Philadelphia, PA: Wolters Kluwer/Lippincott, Williams & Wilkins; 2010.
93. Kopple JD, Ross AC, Caballerio B, et al. Nutrition, diet and the kidney. In: *Modern Nutrition in Health and Disease*, 11th ed. Philadelphia, PA: Wolters Kluwer; 2014.
94. Zhang L, Rajan V, Lin E, et al. Pharmacological inhibition of myostatin suppresses systemic inflammation and muscle atrophy in mice with chronic kidney disease. *FASEB J.* 2011;25:1653–1663.
95. Zhang L, Pan J, Dong Y, et al. Stat3 activation links a C/EBPdelta to myostatin pathway to stimulate loss of muscle mass. *Cell Metab.* 2013;18:368–379.
96. Zhang L, Du J, Hu Z, et al. IL-6 and serum amyloid a synergy mediates angiotensin II-induced muscle wasting. *J Am Soc Nephrol.* 2009;20:604–612.
97. de Brito-Ashurst I, Varagunam M, Raftery MJ, et al. Bicarbonate supplementation slows progression of CKD and improves nutritional status. *J Am Soc Nephrol.* 2009;20:2075–2084.
98. Goraya N, Simoni J, Jo C, et al. Dietary acid reduction with fruits and vegetables or bicarbonate attenuates kidney injury in patients with a moderately reduced glomerular filtration rate due to hypertensive nephropathy. *Kidney Int.* 2012;81:86–93.
99. National Kidney Foundation. K/DOQI clinical practice guidelines for bone metabolism and disease in chronic kidney disease. *Am J Kidney Dis.* 2003;42(4, suppl 3):S1–S201.
100. Chobanian AV, Bakris GL, Black HR, et al. Seventh report of the joint national committee on prevention, detection, evaluation, and treatment of high blood pressure. *Hypertension.* 2003;42(6):1206–1252.
101. Jafar TH, Schmid CH, Landa M, et al. Angiotensin-converting enzyme inhibitors and progression of nondiabetic renal disease. A meta-analysis of patient-level data. *Ann Intern Med.* 2001;135:73–87.
102. Jafar TH, Start PC, Schmid CH, et al. Progression of chronic kidney disease: the role of blood pressure control, proteinuria, and angiotensin-converting enzyme inhibition: a patient-level meta-analysis. *Ann Intern Med.* 2003;139:244–252.
103. Wright JT Jr, Bakris G, Greene T, et al. Effect of blood pressure lowering and antihypertensive drug class on progression of hypertensive kidney disease: results from the AASK trial. *JAMA.* 2002;288:2421–2431.
104. Fink HA, Ishani A, Taylor BC, et al. Screening for, monitoring, and treatment of chronic kidney disease stages 1 to 3: a systematic review for the U.S. Preventive Services Task Force and for an American College of Physicians Clinical Practice Guideline. *Ann Intern Med.* 2012;156:570–581.
105. Lv J, Ehteshami P, Sarnak MJ, et al. Effects of intensive blood pressure lowering on the progression of chronic kidney disease: a systematic review and meta-analysis. *CMAJ.* 2013;185:949–957.
106. Ptinopoulou AG, Pikilidou MI, Lasaridis AN. The effect of antihypertensive drugs on chronic kidney disease: a comprehensive review. *Hypertens Res.* 2013;36:91–101.
107. Van Buren PN, Toto RD. The pathogenesis and management of hypertension in diabetic kidney disease. *Med Clin North Am.* 2013;97:31–51.
108. Kovesdy CP, Bleyer AJ, Molnar MZ, et al. Blood pressure and mortality in U.S. veterans with chronic kidney disease: a cohort study. *Ann Intern Med.* 2013;159:233–242.
109. Kovesdy CP, Lu JL, Molnar MZ, et al. Observational modeling of strict vs conventional blood pressure control in patients with chronic kidney disease. *JAMA Intern Med.* 2014;174:1442–1449.
110. Graudal N, Jürgens G, Baslund B, et al. Compared with usual sodium intake, low- and excessive-sodium diets are associated with increased mortality: a meta-analysis. *Am J Hypertens.* 2014;9:1129–1137.
111. Mente A, O'Donnell MJ, Rangarajan S, et al. Association of urinary sodium and potassium excretion with blood pressure. *N Engl J Med.* 2014;371:601–611.
112. O'Donnell M, Mente A, Rangarajan S, et al. Urinary sodium and potassium excretion, mortality, and cardiovascular events. *N Engl J Med.* 2014;371:612–623.

113. Mozaffarian D, Fahimi S, Singh GM, et al. Global sodium consumption and death from cardiovascular causes. *N Engl J Med.* 2014;371:624–634.
114. Oparil S. Low sodium intake—cardiovascular health benefit or risk? *N Engl J Med.* 2014;371:677–679.
115. Humalda JK, Navis G. Dietary sodium restriction: a neglected therapeutic opportunity in chronic kidney disease. *Curr Opin Nephrol Hypertens.* 2014 (in press).
116. Sanghavi S, Vassalotti JA. Dietary sodium: a therapeutic target in the treatment of hypertension and CKD. *J Ren Nutr.* 2013;23:223–227.
117. Gonzalez-Parra E, Tuñón J, Egido J, et al. Phosphate: a stealthier killer than previously thought? *Cardiovasc Pathol.* 2012;21:372–381.
118. Ellam TJ, Chico TJA. Phosphate: the new cholesterol? The role of the phosphate axis in non-uremic vascular disease. *Atherosclerosis.* 2012;220:310–318.
119. Benini O, D'Alessandro C, Gianfaldoni D, et al. Extra-phosphate load from food additives in commonly eaten foods: a real and insidious danger for renal patients. *J Ren Nutr.* 2011;21:303–308.
120. Kalantar-Zadeh K, Gutekunst L, Mehrotra R, et al. Understanding sources of dietary phosphorus in the treatment of patients with chronic kidney disease. *Clin J Am Soc Nephrol.* 2010;5:519–530.
121. Uribarri J. Phosphorus additives in food and their effect in dialysis patients. *Clin J Am Soc Nephrol.* 2009;4:1290–1292.
122. Murphy-Gutekunst L. Hidden phosphorus: where do we go from here? *J Ren Nutr.* 2007;17:e31–e36.
123. Wickham E. Phosphorus content in commonly consumed beverages. *J Ren Nutr.* 2014:24:e1–e4.
124. Murphy-Gutekunst L. Hidden phosphorus in popular beverages: Part 1. *J Ren Nutr.* 2005;15:e1–e6.
125. Murphy-Gutekunst L. Hidden phosphorus in popular beverages. *Nephrol Nurs J.* 2005;32:443–445.
126. Murphy-Gutekunst L, Barnes K. Hidden phosphorus at breakfast: Part 2. *J Ren Nutr.* 2005;15:e1–e6.
127. Sherman RA, Mehta O. Phosphorus and potassium content of enhanced meat and poultry products: implications for patients who receive dialysis. *Clin J Am Soc Nephrol.* 2009;4:1370–1373.
128. Murphy-Gutekunst L, Uribarri J. Hidden phosphorus-enhanced meats: Part 3. *J Ren Nutr.* 2005;15:e1–e4.
129. Karalis M, Murphy-Gutekunst L. Enhanced foods: hidden phosphorus and sodium in foods commonly eaten. *J Ren Nutr.* 2006;16:79–81.
130. Sarathy S, Sullivan C, Leon JB, et al. Fast food, phosphorus-containing additives, and the renal diet. *J Ren Nutr.* 2008;18:466–470.
131. Butt S, Leon JB, David CL, et al. The prevalence and nutritional implications of fast food consumption among patients receiving hemodialysis. *J Ren Nutr.* 2007;17:264–268.
132. Smyth A, O'Donnell MJ, Yusuf S, et al. Sodium intake and renal outcomes: a systematic review. *Am J Hypertens.* 2014;27:1277–1284.
133. Salam SN, Eastell R, Khwaja A. Fragility fractures and osteoporosis in CKD: pathophysiology and diagnostic methods. *Am J Kidney Dis.* 2014;63:1049–1059.
134. Sprague SM. Renal bone disease. *Curr Opin Endocrinol Diabetes Obes.* 2010;17:535–539.
135. Lewis R. Mineral and bone disorders in chronic kidney disease: new insights into mechanism and management. *Ann Clin Biochem.* 2012;49(Pt 5):432–440.
136. Zhang R, Chouhan KK. Metabolic bone diseases in kidney transplant recipients. *World J Nephrol.* 2012;1:127–133.
137. Miller PD. Chronic kidney disease and osteoporosis: evaluation and management. *BoneKEy Reports.* 2014;3. Article Number 542.
138. Zhang J, Wen J, Li Z, et al. Efficacy and safety of lanthanum carbonate on chronic kidney disease-mineral and bone disorder in dialysis patients: a systematic review. *BMC Nephrol.* 2013;14:226.
139. Palmer SC, Strippoli GF, McGregor DO. Interventions for preventing bone disease in kidney transplant recipients: a systematic review of randomized controlled trials. *Am J Kidney Dis.* 2005;45:638–649.
140. Mitterbauer C, Schwarz C, Haas M, et al. Effects of biophosphonates on bone loss in the first year after renal transplantation—a meta-analysis of randomized controlled trials. *Nephrol Dial Transplant.* 2006;21:2275–2281.
141. Navaneethan SD, Palmer SC, Craig JC, et al. Benefits and harms of phosphate binders in CKD: a systematic review of randomized controlled trials. *Am J Kidney Dis.* 2009;54:619–637.
142. Singer RF. Vitamin D in dialysis: defining deficiency and rationale for supplementation. *Semin Dial.* 2013;26:40–46.

143. de Borst MH, Hajhosseiny R, Tamez H, et al. Active vitamin D treatment for reduction of residual proteinuria: a systematic review. *J Am Soc Nephrol.* 2013;24:1863–1871.
144. Pilz S, Iodice S, Zittermann A, et al. Vitamin D status and mortality risk in CKD: a meta-analysis of prospective studies. *Am J Kidney Dis.* 2011;58:374–382.
145. Duranton F, Rodriguez-Ortiz ME, Duny Y, et al. Vitamin D treatment and mortality in chronic kidney disease: a systematic review and meta-analysis. *Am J Nephrol.* 2013;37:239–248.
146. Zheng Z, Shi H, Junya J, et al. Vitamin D supplementation and mortality risk in chronic kidney disease: a meta-analysis of 20 observational studies. *BMC Nephrol.* 2013;14:199.
147. Palmer SC, McGregor DO, Craig JC, et al. Vitamin D compounds for people with chronic kidney disease not requiring dialysis. *Cochrane Database Syst Rev.* 2009;4:CD008175.
148. Palmer SC, McGregor DO, Craig JC, et al. Vitamin D compounds for people with chronic kidney disease requiring dialysis. *Cochrane Database Syst Rev.* 2009;4:CD005633.
149. Theodoratou E, Tzoulaki I, Zgaga L, et al. Vitamin D and multiple health outcomes: umbrella review of systematic reviews and meta-analyses of observational studies and randomised trials. *BMJ.* 2014;348:g2035.
150. Kidney Disease Outcomes Quality Initiative (K/DOQI) Group. K/DOQI Clinical Practice Guidelines for Management of Dyslipidemias in Patients with Kidney Disease. *Am J Kidney Dis.* 2003;41(4, suppl 3):I–IV, S1–S91.
151. Kasiske B, Cosio FG, Beto J, et al. Clinical practice guidelines for managing dyslipidemias in kidney transplant patients: a report from the Managing Dyslipidemias in Chronic Kidney Disease Work Group of the National Kidney Foundation Kidney Disease Outcomes Quality Initiative. *Am J Transplant.* 2004;4(suppl 7):13–53.
152. National Cholesterol Education Program. Third report of the National Cholesterol Education Program (NCEP) Expert Panel on Detection, Evaluation, and Treatment of High Blood Cholesterol in Adults (Adult Treatment Panel III). Final report. *Circulation.* 2002;106:3143–3421.
153. Saikumar JH, Kovesdy CP. What is the role of lipid measurements in end-stage renal disease? *Semin Dial.* 2014 (in press).
154. James PA, Oparil S, Carter BL, et al. 2014 Evidence-based guideline for the management of high blood pressure in adults: report from the Panel Members Appointed to the Eighth Joint National Committee (JNC 8). *JAMA.* 2014;311:507–520.
155. Feldman H, Zuber K, Davis JS. Staying up to date with the JNC 8 hypertension guideline. *JAAPA.* 2014;27:44–49.
156. Go AS, Mozaffarian D, Roger VL, et al. Executive summary: heart disease and stroke statistics—2014 update: a report from the American Heart Association. *Circulation.* 2014;129:399–410.
157. Eckel RH, Jakicic JM, Ard JD, et al. 2013 AHA/ACC Guideline on lifestyle management to reduce cardiovascular risk: a report of the American College of Cardiology/American Heart Association Task Force on practice guidelines. *Circulation.* 2014;129(25, suppl 2):S76–S99.
158. Stone NJ, Robinson JG, Lichtenstein AH, et al. 2013 ACC/AHA Guideline on the treatment of blood cholesterol to reduce atherosclerotic cardiovascular risk in adults—a report of the American College of Cardiology/American Heart Association Task Force on practice guidelines. *JACC.* 2014;63:2889–2934.
159. Jellinger PS, Smith DA, Mehta AE, et al. American Association of Clinical Endocrinologists' guidelines for management of dyslipidemia and prevention of atherosclerosis. *Endocr Pract.* 2012;18(suppl 1):1–78.
160. Morris PB, Ballantyne CM, Birtcher KK, et al. Review of clinical practice guidelines for the management of LDL-related risk. *JACC.* 2014;64:196–206.
161. Havel RJ, Kane JP. *Introduction: structure and metabolism of plasma lipoproteins.* In: Valle D, Beaudet AL, Vogelstein B, et al, eds. OMMBID—The Online Metabolic and Molecular Bases of Inherited Diseases. New York, NY: McGraw-Hill; 2014.
162. Kane JP, Havel RJ. *Disorders of the biogenesis and secretion of lipoproteins containing the B apolipoproteins.* In: Valle, D, Beaudet AL, Vogelstein B, et al, eds. OMMBID—The Online Metabolic and Molecular Bases of Inherited Diseases. New York, NY: McGraw-Hill; 2014.
163. Lambert JE, Parks EJ. Postprandial metabolism of meal triglyceride in humans. *Biochim Biophys Acta.* 2012;1821:721–726.
164. Changting X, Lewis GF. Regulation of chylomicron production in humans. *Biochim Biophys Acta.* 2012;1821:736–746.
165. Kindel T, Lee DM, Tso P. The mechanism of the formation and secretion of chylomicrons. *Atheroscler Suppl.* 2010;11:11–16.

166. Kersten S. Physiological regulation of lipoprotein lipase. *Biochim Biophys Acta.* 2014;1841:919–933.
167. Brunzell JD, Deeb SS. *Familial lipoprotein lipase deficiency, apo C-II deficiency, and hepatic lipase deficiency.* In: Valle D, Beaudet AL, Vogelstein B, et al, eds. OMMBID—The Online Metabolic and Molecular Bases of Inherited Diseases. New York, NY: McGraw-Hill; 2014.
168. Havel RJ. Triglyceride-rich lipoproteins and plasma lipid transport. *Arterioscler Thromb Vasc Biol.* 2010;30:9–19.
169. Varbo A, Nordestgaard BG. Remnant cholesterol and ischemic heart disease. *Curr Opin Lipidol.* 2014;25:266–273.
170. Talayero BG, Sacks FM. The role of triglycerides in atherosclerosis. *Curr Cardiol Rep.* 2011;13:544–552.
171. Nordestgaard BG, Varbo A. Lipids and cardiovascular disease 3—triglycerides and cardiovascular disease. *Lancet.* 2014;384:626–635.
172. Stauffer ME, Weisenfluh L, Morrison A. Association between triglycerides and cardiovascular events in primary populations: a meta-regression analysis and synthesis of evidence. *Vasc Health Risk Manag.* 2013;9:671–680.
173. Krauss RM. All low-density lipoprotein particles are not created equal. *Arterioscler Thromb Vasc Biol.* 2014;959–961.
174. Rye K-A, Barter PJ. Regulation of high-density lipoprotein metabolism. *Circ Res.* 2014;114:143–156.
175. Tall AR, Breslow JL, Rubin EM. *Genetic disorders affecting plasma high-density lipoproteins.* In: Valle D, Beaudet AL, Vogelstein B, et al, eds. *OMMBID—The Online Metabolic and Molecular Bases of Inherited Diseases.* New York, NY: McGraw-Hill; 2014.
176. Oldoni F, Sinke RJ, Kuivenhoven JA. Mendelian disorders of high-density lipoprotein metabolism. *Circ Res.* 2014;114:124–142.
177. National Cholesterol Education Program (NCEP) Expert Panel. Third Report of the National Cholesterol Education Program (NCEP) Expert Panel on Detection, Evaluation, and Treatment of High Blood Cholesterol in Adults (Adult Treatment Panel III). Final Report. National Cholesterol Education Program, National Heart, Lung, and Blood Institute, National Institutes of Health. NIH Publication No. 02-5215, September 2002.
178. Grundy SM, Cleeman JI, Merz CN, et al. Implications of recent clinical trials for the National Cholesterol Education Program Adult Treatment Panel III Guidelines. *Circulation.* 2004;110:227–239.
179. Kostis WJ. How low an LDL-C should we go with statin therapy? *Curr Atheroscler Rep.* 2014;16:388.
180. LaRosa JC, Grundy SM, Waters DD, et al. Intensive lipid lowering with atorvastatin in patients with stable coronary disease. *N Engl J Med.* 2005;352:1425–1435.
181. Sherbet DP, Garg P, Brilakis ES, et al. Low-density lipoprotein cholesterol: how low can we go? *Am J Cardiovasc Drugs.* 2013;13:225–232.
182. Bulbulia R, Armitage J. LDL cholesterol targets—how low to go? *Curr Opin Lipidol.* 2012;23:265–270.
183. Karalis DG. Intensive lowering of low-density lipoprotein cholesterol levels for primary prevention of coronary artery disease. *Mayo Clin Proc.* 2009;84:345–352.
184. La Rosa JC, Pedersen TR, Somaratne R, et al. Safety and effect of very low levels of low-density lipoprotein cholesterol on cardiovascular events. *Am J Cardiol.* 2013;111:1221–1229.
185. Cholesterol Treatment Trialists' (CTT) Collaboration. Efficacy and safety of more intensive lowering of LDL cholesterol: a meta-analysis of data from 170,000 participants in 26 randomised trials. *Lancet.* 2010;376:1670–1681.
186. Study of the Effectiveness of Additional Reductions in Cholesterol and Homocysteine (SEARCH) Collaborative Group. Intensive lowering of LDL cholesterol with 80 mg versus 20 mg simvastatin daily in 12,064 survivors of myocardial infarction: a double-blind randomised trial. *Lancet.* 2010;376:1658–1669.
187. Kearney PM, Baigent C. Statins: are any questions unanswered. *Curr Opin Lipidol.* 2006;17:418–425.
188. Hayward RA, Krumholz HM. Three reasons to abandon low-density lipoprotein targets: an open letter to the Adult Treatment Panel IV of the National Institutes of Health. *Circ Cardiovasc Qual Outcomes.* 2012;5:2–5.
189. Krumholz HM. The new cholesterol and blood pressure guidelines: perspective on the path forward. *JAMA.* 2014;311:1403–1405.

190. Krumholz HM. Target cardiovascular risk rather than cholesterol concentration. *BMJ.* 2013;347:f7110.
191. Kohli P, Whelton SP, Yancy CW, et al. Clinician's guide to the updated ABCs of cardiovascular disease. *J Am Heart Assoc.* 2014;3.
192. Ledford H. Cholesterol limits lose their lustre. *Nature.* 2013;494:410–411.
193. Carroll MD, Kit BK, Lacher DA, et al. Total and high-density lipoprotein cholesterol in adults: National Health and Nutrition Examination Survey, 2011-2012. US Department of Health and Human Services, Centers for Disease Control and Prevention, National Center for Health Statistics. *NCHS Data Brief.* 2013; No. 132.
194. McBride PE. Triglycerides and risk for coronary heart disease. *JAMA.* 2007;298:336–338.
195. Nordestgaard BG, Benn M, Schnor P, et al. Nonfasting triglycerides and risk of myocardial infarction, ischemic heart disease, and death in men and women. *JAMA.* 2007;298:299–308.
196. Bansal S, Buring JE, Rifai N, et al. Fasting compared with nonfasting triglycerides and risk of cardiovascular events in women. *JAMA.* 2007;298:309–316.
197. Berglund L, Brunzell JD, Goldberg AC, et al. Evaluation and treatment of hypertriglyceridemia: An Endocrine Society clinical practice guideline. *J Clin Endocrinol Metab.* 2012;97:2969–2989.
198. Hegele RA, Ginsberg HN, Chapman MJ, et al. The polygenic nature of hypertriglyceridaemia: implications for definition, diagnosis, and management. *Lancet Diabetes Endocrinol.* 2014;2:655–666.
199. Chapman MJ, Ginsberg HN, Amarenco P, et al. Triglyceride-rich lipoproteins and high-density lipoprotein cholesterol in patients at high risk of cardiovascular disease: evidence and guidance for management. *Eur Heart J.* 2011;32:1345–1361.
200. Rader DJ, Hovingh GK. Lipids and cardiovascular disease 2—HDL and cardiovascular disease. *Lancet.* 2014;384:618–625.
201. Tuteja S, Rader DJ. High-density lipoproteins in the prevention of cardiovascular disease: changing the paradigm. *Clin Pharmacol Ther.* 2014;96:48–56.
202. Kingwell BA, Chapman MJ, Kontush A, et al. HDL-targeted therapies: progress, failures and future. *Nat Rev Drug Discov.* 2014;13:445–464.
203. Subedi BH, Joshi PH, Jones SR, et al. Current guidelines for high-density lipoprotein cholesterol in therapy and future directions. *Vasc Health Risk Manag.* 2014;10:205–216.
204. Deeb SS. Association of variants in the lipase genes with lipid levels and coronary artery disease. In: Valle D, Beaudet AL, Vogelstein B, et al, eds. *OMMBID—The Online Metabolic and Molecular Bases of Inherited Diseases.* New York, NY: McGraw-Hill; 2014.
205. Goldstein JL, Hobbs HH, Brown MS. Familial hypercholesterolemia. In: Valle D, Beaudet AL, Vogelstein B, et al, eds. *OMMBID—The Online Metabolic and Molecular Bases of Inherited Diseases.* New York, NY: McGraw-Hill; 2014.
206. Mahey RW, Rall SC. Type III hyperlipoproteinemia (dysbetalipoproteinemia): the role of apolipoprotein E in normal and abnormal lipoprotein metabolism. In: Valle D, Beaudet AL, Vogelstein B, et al, eds. *OMMBID—The Online Metabolic and Molecular Bases of Inherited Diseases.* New York, NY: McGraw-Hill; 2014.
207. Assmann G, von Eckardstein A, Bryan Brewer HH. Familial analphalipoproteinemia: tangier disease. In: Valle D, Beaudet AL, Vogelstein B, et al, eds. *OMMBID—The Online Metabolic and Molecular Bases of Inherited Diseases.* New York, NY: McGraw-Hill; 2014.
208. Santamarina-Fojo S, Hoeg JM, Assmann G, et al. Lecithin cholesterol acyltransferase deficiency and fish eye disease. In: Valle D, Beaudet AL, Vogelstein B, et al, eds. *OMMBID—The Online Metabolic and Molecular Bases of Inherited Diseases.* New York, NY: McGraw-Hill; 2014.
209. Utermann G. Lipoprotein(a). In: Valle D, Beaudet AL, Vogelstein B, et al, eds. *OMMBID—The Online Metabolic and Molecular Bases of Inherited Diseases.* New York, NY: McGraw-Hill; 2014.
210. Nair DR, Sharifi M, Al-Rasadi K. Familial hypercholesterolaemia. *Curr Opin Cardiol.* 2014;29:381–388.
211. Raal FJ, Santos RD. Homozygous familial hypercholesterolemia: current perspectives on diagnosis and treatment. *Atherosclerosis.* 2012;223:262–268.
212. Sniderman AD, Tsimikas S, Fazio S. The severe hypercholesterolemia phenotype: clinical diagnosis, management, and emerging therapies. *JACC.* 2014;63:1935–1947.
213. Kwiterovich PO Jr. Diagnosis and management of familial dyslipoproteinemias. *Curr Cardiol Rep.* 2013;15:371.
214. Hopkins PN, Toth PP, Ballantyne CM, et al. Familial hypercholesterolemias: prevalence, genetics, diagnosis and screening recommendations from the National Lipid Association Expert Panel on familial hypercholesterolemia. *J Clin Lipidol.* 2011;5(3, suppl):S9–S17.

215. Marais AD. Review article: familial hypercholesterolaemia. *Clin Biochem Rev.* 2004;25:49–68.
216. Brouwers MCGJ, van Greevenbroek MMJ, Stehouwer CDA, et al. The genetics of familial combined hyperlipidaemia. *Nat Rev Endocrinol.* 2012;8352–8362.
217. Talmud PJ, Futema M, Humphries SE. The genetic architecture of the familial hyperlipidaemia syndromes: rare mutations and common variants in multiple genes. *Curr Opin Lipidol.* 2014;25:274–281.
218. Johansen CT, Hegele RA. Genetic bases of hypertriglyceridemic phenotypes. *Curr Opin Lipidol.* 2011;22:247–253.
219. Hegele RA, Ban MR, Hsueh N, et al. A polygenic basis for four classical frederickson hyperlipoproteinemia phenotypes that are characterized by hypertriglyceridemia. *Hum Mol Genet.* 2009 18:4189–4194.
220. Hopkins PN, Brinton EA, Nanjee MN. Hyperlipoproteinemia type 3: the forgotten phenotype. *Curr Atheroscler Rep.* 2014;16:440.
221. Sacks FM. The apolipoprotein story. *Atheroscler Suppl.* 2006;7:23–27.
222. Zheng C, Khoo C, Furtado J, et al. Apolipoprotein C-III and the metabolic basis for hypertriglyceridemia and the dense low-density lipoprotein phenotype. *Circulation.* 2010;121: 1722–1734.
223. Mendivil CO, Rimm EB, Chiuve SE, et al. Low-density lipoproteins containing apolipoprotein C-III and the risk of coronary heart disease. *Circulation.* 2011;124:2065–2072.
224. Jensen MK, Rimm EB, Furtado JD, et al. Apolipoprotein C-III as a potential modulator of the association between HDL-cholesterol and incident coronary heart disease. *J Am Heart Assoc.* 2012;1(2):1–10.
225. Eckel RH, Cornier M-A. Update on the NCEP ATP-III emerging cardiometabolic risk factors. *BMC Med.* 2014;12:115.
226. Foreyt JP. Need for lifestyle intervention: how to begin. *Am J Cardiol.* 2005;96(4A):11E–14E.
227. Foreyt JP. The role of lifestyle modification in dysmetabolic syndrome management. In: Bantle JP, Slama G, eds. *Nutritional Management of Diabetes Mellitus and Dysmetabolic Syndrome. Nestlé Nutr Workshop Ser Clin Perform Programme.* 2006;11:197–206.
228. Johnston CA, Tyler C, Foreyt JP. Behavioral management of obesity. *Curr Atheroscler Rep.* 2007;9:448–453.
229. Astrup A, Dyerberg J, Elwood P, et al. The role of reducing intakes of saturated fat in the prevention of cardiovascular disease: where does the evidence stand in 2010? *Am J Clin Nutr.* 2011;93:684–688.
230. Baum, SJ, Kris-Etherton PM, Willett WC, et al. Fatty acids in cardiovascular health and disease: a comprehensive update. *J Clin Lipidol.* 2012;6:212–234.
231. Chowdhury R, Warnakula S, Kunutsor S, et al. Association of dietary, circulating, and supplement fatty acids with coronary risk: a systematic review and meta-analysis. *Ann Intern Med.* 2014;160:398–406.
232. De Goede J, Verschuren WM, Boer JM, et al. N-6 and N-3 fatty acid cholesteryl esters in relation to fatal CHD in a Dutch adult population: a nested case-control study and meta-analysis. *PLoS One.* 2013;8:e59408.
233. DiNicolantonio JJ. The cardiometabolic consequences of replacing saturated fats with carbohydrates or Ω-6 polyunsaturated fats: do the dietary guidelines have it wrong? *Open Heart.* 2014;1:e000032. doi:10.1136/openhrt-2013-000032.
234. Dreon DM, Fernstrom HA, Campos H, et al. Change in dietary saturated fat intake is correlated with change in mass of large low-density-lipoprotein particles in men. *Am J Clin Nutr.* 1998;67:828–836.
235. Jakobsen MU, O'Reilly EJ, Heitmann BL, et al. Major types of dietary fat and risk of coronary heart disease: a pooled analysis of 11 cohort studies. *Am J Clin Nutr.* 2009;89:1425–1432.
236. Lawrence GD. Dietary fats and health: dietary recommendations in the context of scientific evidence. *Adv Nutr.* 2013;4:294–302.
237. Mensink RP, Zock PL, Kester AD, et al. Effects of dietary fatty acids and carbohydrates on the ratio of serum total to HDL cholesterol and on serum lipids and apolipoproteins: a meta-analysis of 60 controlled trials. *Am J Clin Nutr.* 2003;77:1146–1155.
238. Micha R, Mozaffarian D. Saturated fat and cardiometabolic risk factors, coronary heart disease, stroke, and diabetes: a fresh look at the evidence. *Lipids.* 2010;45:893–905.
239. Mozaffarian D, Micha R, Wallace S. Effects on coronary heart disease of increasing polyunsaturated fat in place of saturated fat: a systematic review and meta-analysis of randomized controlled trials. *PLoS Med.* 2010;7(3) e1000252.

240. Ravnskov U, DiNicolantonio JJ, Harcombe Z, et al. The questionable benefits of exchanging saturated fat with polyunsaturated fat. *Mayo Clin Proc.* 2014;89:451–453.
241. Sanders TAB. Conference on dietary strategies for the management of cardiovascular risk: reappraisal of SFA and cardiovascular risk. *Proc Nutr Soc.* 2013;72:390–398.
242. Schwingshackl L, Hoffman G. Dietary fatty acids in the secondary prevention of coronary heart disease: a systematic review, meta-analysis and meta-regression. *BMJ Open.* 2014;4:e004487. doi:10.1136/bmjopen-2013-004487.
243. Siri-Tarino PW, Sun Q, Hu FB, et al. Saturated fat, carbohydrate, and cardiovascular disease. *Am J Clin Nutr.* 2010;91:502–509.
244. Siri-Tarino, PW, Sun Q, Hu FB, et al. Meta-analysis of prospective cohort studies evaluating the association of saturated fat with cardiovascular disease. *Am J Clin Nutr.* 2010;91:535–546.
245. Siri-Tarino PW, Sun Q, Hu FB, et al. Saturated fatty acids and risk of coronary heart disease: modulation by replacement nutrients. *Curr Atheroscler Rep.* 2010;12:384–390.
246. Dalen JE, Devries S. Diets to prevent coronary heart disease 1957-2013: what have we learned? *Am J Med.* 2014;127:364–369.
247. Berneis KK, Krauss RM. Metabolic origins and clinical significance of LDL heterogeneity. *J Lipid Res.* 2002;43:1363–1379.
248. Griffin BA, Freeman DJ, Tait GW, et al. Role of plasma triglyceride in the regulation of plasma low density lipoprotein (LDL) subfractions: relative contribution of small, dense LDL to coronary heart disease risk. *Atherosclerosis.* 1994;106:241–253.
249. Hoogeveen RC, Gaubatz JW, Sun W, et al. Small dense low-density lipoprotein-cholesterol concentrations predict risk for coronary heart disease. The Atherosclerosis Risk in Communities (ARIC) study. *Arterioscler Thromb Vasc Biol.* 2014;34:1069–1077.
250. Kotwal S, Jun M, Sullivan D, et al. Omega 3 fatty acids and cardiovascular outcomes: systematic review and meta-analysis. *Circ Cardiovasc Qual Outcomes.* 2012;5:808–818.
251. Ramsden CE, Zamora D, Leelarthaepin B, et al. Use of dietary linoleic acid for secondary prevention of coronary heart disease and death: evaluation of recovered data from the Sydney Diet Heart Study and updated meta-analysis. *BMJ.* 2013;346:e8707.
252. Rizos EC, Ntzani EE, Bika E, et al. Association between omega-3 fatty acid supplementation and risk of major cardiovascular disease events: a systematic review and meta-analysis. *JAMA.* 2012;308:1024–1033.
253. Ramsden CE, Hibbeln JR, Majchrzak SF, et al. n-6 Fatty acid-specific and mixed polyunsaturate dietary interventions have different effects on CHD risk: a meta-analysis of randomised controlled trials. *Br J Nutr.* 2010;104:1586–1600.
254. Michas G, Micha R, Zampelas A. Dietary fats and cardiovascular disease: putting together the pieces of a complicated puzzle. *Atherosclerosis.* 2014;234:320–328.
255. Frantz ID Jr, Dawson EA, Ashman PL, et al. Test of effect of lipid lowering by diet on cardiovascular risk. The Minnesota Coronary Survey. *Arterioscler Thromb Vasc Biol.* 1989;9:129–135.
256. Nestel P. Trans fatty acids: are its cardiovascular risks fully appreciated? *Clin Ther.* 2014;36:315–321.
257. Gylling H, Plat J, Turley S, et al. Plant sterols and plant stanols in the management of dyslipidaemia and prevention of cardiovascular disease. *Atherosclerosis* 2014;232:346–360.
258. Ras RT, Hiemstra H, Lin Y, et al. Consumption of plant sterol-enriched foods and effects on plasma plant sterol concentrations—a meta-analysis of randomized controlled studies. *Atherosclerosis.* 2013;230:336–346.
259. Ras RT, Geleijnse JM, Trautwein EA. LDL-cholesterol-lowering effect of plant sterols and stanols across different dose ranges: a meta-analysis of randomised controlled studies. *Br J Nutr.* 2014;112:214–219.
260. Anderson JW, Bush HM. Soy protein effects on serum lipoproteins: a quality assessment and meta-analysis of randomized, controlled studies. *J Am Coll Nutr.* 2011;30:79–91.
261. Qin Y, Niu K, Zeng Y, et al. Isoflavones for hypercholesterolaemia in adults. *Cochrane Database Syst Rev.* 2013;6:CD009518.
262. Goldberg IJ, Mosca L, Piano MR, et al. Wine and your heart: a science advisory for healthcare professionals from the nutrition committee, council on epidemiology and prevention, and council on cardiovascular nursing of the American Heart Association. *Circulation.* 2001;103:472–475.
263. Lichtenstein AH. Nutrient supplements and cardiovascular disease: a heartbreaking story. *J Lipid Res.* 2009;50 suppl:S429–S433.

14 Obesity

DEFINITION

Adipose tissue. Adipose tissue triglycerides are the body's major fuel reserve. A lean adult has about 35 billion adipocytes and each adipocyte contains about 0.5 µg of triglyceride, whereas an extremely obese adult can have four times as many adipocytes (125 billion), each containing twice as much lipid (~1.0 µg of triglyceride) (1). The high energy density and hydrophobic nature of triglycerides make it a much more energy-dense and compact fuel than glycogen. Triglycerides liberate 9.3 kcal per gram when oxidized and are stored as an oil inside the fat cell, accounting for 85% of adipocyte weight. Glycogen produces only 4.1 kcal per gram when oxidized and is stored intracellularly as a gel containing approximately 2 g of water for every gram of glycogen. Therefore, adipose tissue provides an effective fuel-storage mechanism that permits mobility and survival during periods of food deprivation. When adequate fluids are provided, the duration of survival during starvation depends on the amount of endogenous body fat. In lean men, death occurs after approximately two months of starvation when more than 35% (~25 kg) of body weight is lost (2). In contrast, obese persons have undergone therapeutic fasts for prolonged periods without adverse consequences; the longest reported fast is that of a 207-kg man who lost 61% (126 kg) of his initial body weight after fasting for 382 days, consuming only acaloric fluids, vitamins, and minerals (3).

Body mass index. Obesity represents an unhealthy excess in body fat mass. However, the threshold value that defines how much body fat is "unhealthy" is not clear, and is influenced by sex, age, ethnicity, race, fitness, fat distribution, lifestyle factors, and unknown genetic factors. Moreover, the ability to reliably measure body fat mass requires specialized equipment that is not readily available in a typical clinical setting. Therefore, a classification system has been developed to categorize weight status based on body mass index (BMI), which represents the relationship between weight and height (weight in kilograms divided by height in meters squared [kg per m^2], or weight in pounds multiplied by 704 and divided by height in inches squared). Table 14-1 provides an estimate of BMI values based on height in inches and weight in pounds; an automated BMI calculator can be found at http://www.nhlbi.nih.gov/guidelines/obesity/BMI/bmicalc.htm. Although BMI correlates with percent body fat mass in a curvilinear fashion (4), there is considerable variability at any given BMI value. In fact, some people can have a normal amount of body fat but an "obese" BMI value because of increased muscle mass, whereas others can have excessive body fat but a "lean" BMI value because of decreased muscle mass.

BMI and mortality. Data from epidemiological studies that evaluated the relationship between BMI and mortality rates (Figure 14-1), primarily in Caucasians living in the United States, have been used to categorize people as "normal weight" or "pre-obese" (BMI = 18.5–24.9 kg per m^2), "overweight" (BMI = 25.0–29.9 kg per m^2), and "obese" (BMI >30 kg per m^2) (Table 14-2) (5). The severity of obesity itself is further characterized by subclassifications: class I obesity (BMI 30.0–34.9 kg per m^2), class II obesity (BMI 35.0–39.9 kg per m^2), and class III obesity (BMI ≥40 kg per m^2). In addition, a BMI greater than 40 kg per m^2 is also known as "extreme obesity," and "morbid obesity" is a term used to define patients who meet criteria for bariatric surgery (BMI ≥40 kg/m^2, or BMI 35.0–39.9 kg/m^2 and one or more severe obesity-related medical complications, such as hypertension, type 2 diabetes mellitus, heart failure, or sleep apnea) (6).

The current perception of mortality risk associated with the current BMI classifications has recently been challenged by a careful evaluation of data from the National Health and Nutrition Examination Surveys (NHANES) collected between 1971 and 2000, and a systematic review and meta-analysis of reported all-cause mortality hazard ratios for overweight and obesity relative to normal weight in 97 population studies (7,8). These data demonstrated that persons who were overweight had a lower all-cause mortality and those with class 1 obesity did not have a

TABLE 14-1 Body Mass Index Calculator

	Normal							Overweight							Obese												Extreme Obesity									
BMI	19	20	21	22	23	24	25	26	27	28	29	30	31	32	33	34	35	36	37	38	39	40	41	42	43	44	45	46	47	48	49	50	51	52	53	54
Height (inches)																	Body Weight (pounds)																			
58	91	96	100	105	110	115	119	124	129	134	138	143	148	153	158	162	167	172	177	181	186	191	196	201	205	210	215	220	224	229	234	239	244	248	253	258
59	94	99	104	109	114	119	124	128	133	138	143	148	153	158	163	168	173	178	183	188	193	198	203	208	212	217	222	227	232	237	242	247	252	257	262	267
60	97	102	107	112	118	123	128	133	138	143	148	153	158	163	168	174	179	184	189	194	199	204	209	215	220	225	230	235	240	245	250	255	261	266	271	276
61	100	106	111	116	122	127	132	137	143	148	153	158	164	169	174	180	185	190	195	201	206	211	217	222	227	232	238	243	248	254	259	264	269	275	280	285
62	104	109	115	120	126	131	136	142	147	153	158	164	169	175	180	186	191	196	202	207	213	218	224	229	235	240	246	251	256	262	267	273	278	284	289	295
63	107	113	118	124	130	135	141	146	152	158	163	169	175	180	186	191	197	203	208	214	220	225	231	237	242	248	254	259	265	270	278	282	287	293	299	304
64	110	116	122	128	134	140	145	151	157	163	169	174	180	186	192	197	204	209	215	221	227	232	238	244	250	256	262	267	273	279	285	291	296	302	308	314
65	114	120	126	132	138	144	150	156	162	168	174	180	186	192	198	204	210	216	222	228	234	240	246	252	258	264	270	276	282	288	294	300	306	312	318	324
66	118	124	130	136	142	148	155	161	167	173	179	186	192	198	204	210	216	223	229	235	241	247	253	260	266	272	278	284	291	297	303	309	315	322	328	334
67	121	127	134	140	146	153	159	166	172	178	185	191	198	204	211	217	223	230	236	242	249	255	261	268	274	280	287	293	299	306	312	319	325	331	338	344
68	125	131	138	144	151	158	164	171	177	184	190	197	203	210	216	223	230	236	243	249	256	262	269	276	282	289	295	302	308	315	322	328	335	341	348	354
69	128	135	142	149	155	162	169	176	182	189	196	203	209	216	223	230	236	243	250	257	263	270	277	284	291	297	304	311	318	324	331	338	345	351	358	365
70	132	139	146	153	160	167	174	181	188	195	202	209	216	222	229	236	243	250	257	264	271	278	285	292	299	306	313	320	327	334	341	348	355	362	369	376
71	136	143	150	157	165	172	179	186	193	200	208	215	222	229	236	243	250	257	265	272	279	286	293	301	308	315	322	329	338	343	351	358	365	372	379	386
72	140	147	154	162	169	177	184	191	199	206	213	221	228	235	242	250	258	265	272	279	287	294	302	309	316	324	331	338	346	353	361	368	375	383	390	397
73	144	151	159	166	174	182	189	197	204	212	219	227	235	242	250	257	265	272	280	288	295	302	310	318	325	333	340	348	355	363	371	378	386	393	401	408
74	148	155	163	171	179	186	194	202	210	218	225	233	241	249	256	264	272	280	288	295	303	311	319	326	334	342	350	358	365	373	381	389	396	404	412	420
75	152	160	168	176	184	192	200	208	216	224	232	240	248	256	264	272	279	287	295	303	311	319	327	335	343	351	359	367	375	383	391	399	407	415	423	431
76	156	164	172	180	189	197	205	213	221	230	238	246	254	263	271	279	287	295	304	312	320	328	336	344	353	361	369	377	385	394	402	410	418	426	435	443

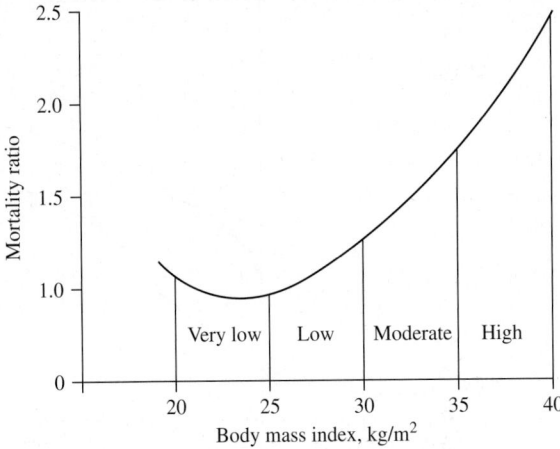

Figure 14-1. Relationship between body mass index and mortality risk in adult men and women in the United States. (Bray GA. Obesity: basic considerations and clinical approaches. Dis Mon 1989;35:454.)

higher mortality than normal-weight people. In older adults (age ≥70 years), even class II and III obesity were not associated with higher mortality.

Obesity paradox. The relationship between BMI and mortality risk is also complicated by the presence of certain concomitant diseases. Being overweight or obese in patients with cardiovascular disease (CVD; myocardial infarction, congestive heart failure, hypertension and coronary heart disease, coronary artery bypass graft surgery, heart transplant), end-stage renal disease, hip fracture, rheumatoid arthritis, and tuberculosis is associated with lower mortality rates than patients with normal BMI values (9–17). The reason for this phenomenon, known as the "obesity paradox", is not known.

BMI and disease. The relationship between BMI and disease risk differs from the relationship between BMI and mortality risk. Therefore, overweight can be a risk factor for certain medical conditions without being a risk factor for mortality. In fact, the risk of developing an obesity-related disease, such as diabetes, begins to increase at BMI values that are within the normal-weight range (23 kg per m² in women and 24 kg per m² in men) (Figure 14-2) (18,19). Other factors, such as body fat distribution (intrahepatic triglyceride content, intra-abdominal fat volume, and waist circumference) (20–22), level of cardiopulmonary fitness (23,24), and ethnic/racial background (25,26), also modify BMI-related risk. For example, at the same BMI values as Caucasians, Asian-Pacific populations are at increased risk for the development of

TABLE 14-2	Body Mass Index (BMI)–Associated Mortality Risk	
	Obesity Class	**BMI (kg/m²)**
Underweight		<18.5
Normal		18.5–24.9
Overweight		25.0–29.9
Obesity	I	30.0–34.9
	II	35.0–39.9
Extreme obesity	III	≥40.0

Adapted from National Institutes of Health, National Heart, Lung, and Blood Institute. Clinical Guidelines on the Identification, Evaluation, and Treatment of Overweight and Obesity in Adults—The Evidence Report. Bethesda (MD): National Heart, Lung, and Blood Institute; 1998 Sep. Report No.: 98-4083.

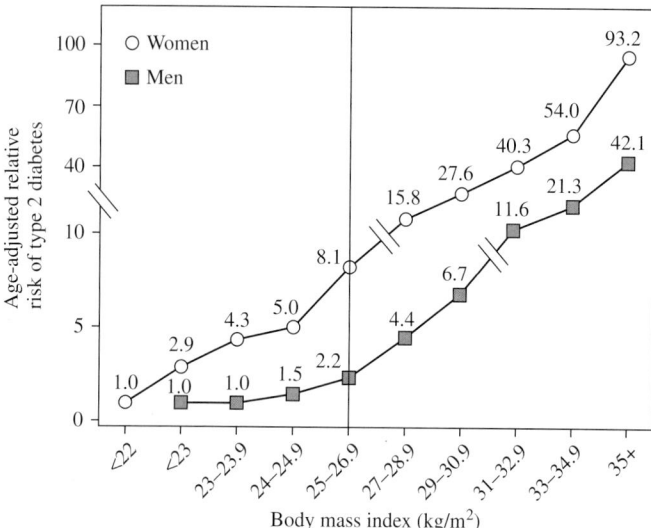

Figure 14-2. Relationship between body mass index and type 2 diabetes in men and women. The vertical line separates lean from overweight and obese persons. Data from: Colditz GA, Willett WC, Rotnitzky A, et al. Weight gain as a risk factor for clinical diabetes mellitus in women. *Ann Intern Med.* 1995;122:481–486; Chan JM, Rimm EB, Colditz GA, et al. Obesity, fat distribution, and weight gain as risk factors for clinical diabetes in men. *Diabetes Care.* 1994;17:961–969.

diabetes and CVD. Accordingly, the World Health Organization has proposed maintaining the current BMI cutoff points as international classifications in Southeast Asian populations, but reducing the BMI cutoffs for potential public health action to 17.5 to 22.9 kg per m² as "normal weight", 23.0 to 27.4 kg per m² as "overweight," and greater than or equal to 27.5 kg per m² as "obese" (27).

Childhood obesity. In children, the BMI normal range changes with age and is different in boys and girls. In infants (birth to 36 months), "obesity" is defined as weight more than 95th percentile for length and sex (Figure 14-3A and B). In children and adolescents (age 2–20 years), "obesity" is defined as BMI greater than 95th percentile for age and sex (Figures 14-3C and D) (www.cdc.gov/growthcharts). Obesity-related diseases that typically are seen in adults, such as type 2 diabetes mellitus, hyperlipidemia, hypertension, orthopedic complications, sleep apnea, gallbladder disease, and nonalcoholic steatohepatitis, are now being seen with increasing frequency in children. In addition, early-onset obesity is associated with an increased chance of being an obese adult and an increased risk of obesity-related diseases (28,29).

PREVALENCE

The global prevalence of obesity in children and adults has continued to increase from 1980 to 2013 in both developed and developing countries, although the rates have markedly slowed in some developed countries such as the United States. Island nations in the Pacific and the Caribbean and countries in the Middle East and Central America have the highest prevalence rates of obesity (30). Data from the 2011–2012 NHANES found that 16.9% of youth (age 2–19 years) and 34.9% of adults (age ≥20 years) in the United States were obese (31). Although the overall prevalence of obesity did not differ between men and women, it was much higher in non-Hispanic Black women (57%) than men (37%). In addition, the prevalence of obesity was higher among non-Hispanic Black (48%), Hispanic (43%), and non-Hispanic White (33%) adults than among non-Hispanic Asian adults (11%).

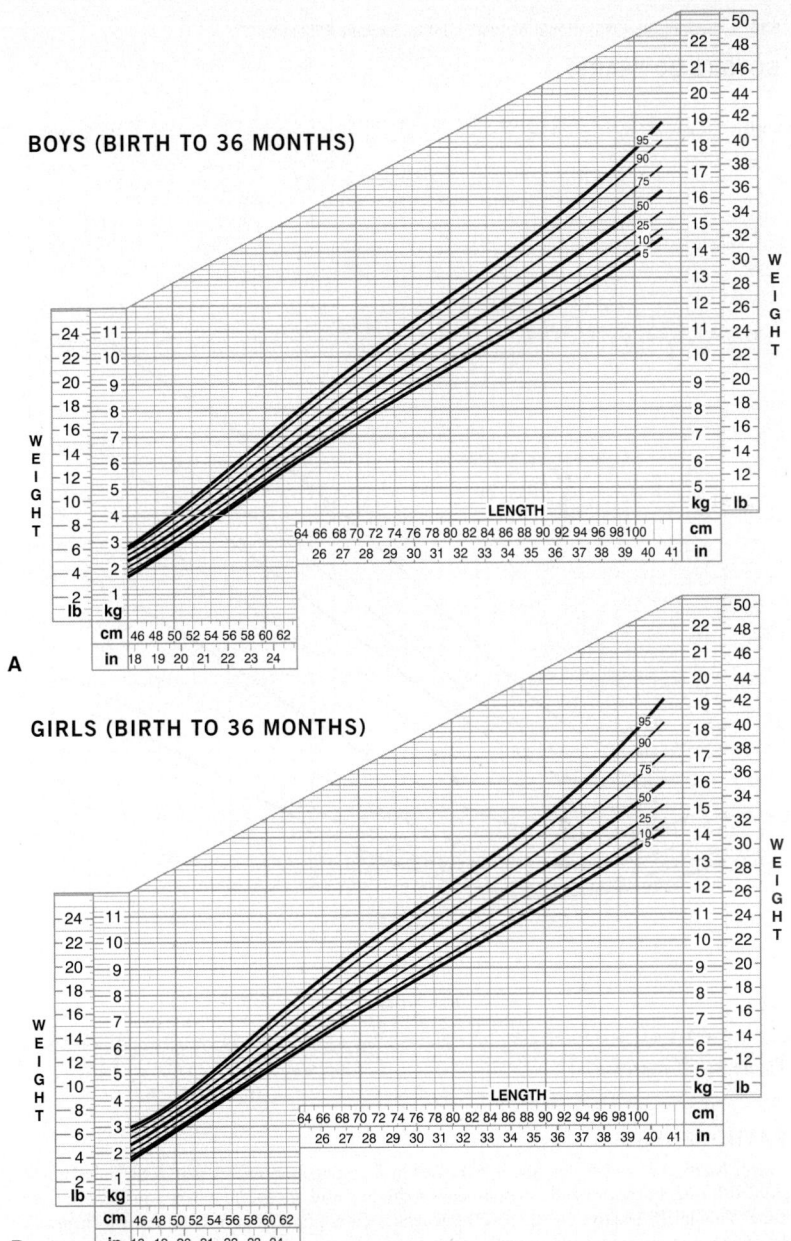

Figure 14-3. Growth charts for children. Obesity is defined as weight greater than or equal to 95th percentile for length and sex in infants (birth to 36 months): boys (A) and girls (B). Obesity is defined as BMI greater than or equal to 95th percentile for age and sex for children and adolescents (age 2–20 years): boys (C) and girls (D) (www.cdc.gov/growthcharts).

(continued)

BOYS (2-20 YEARS)

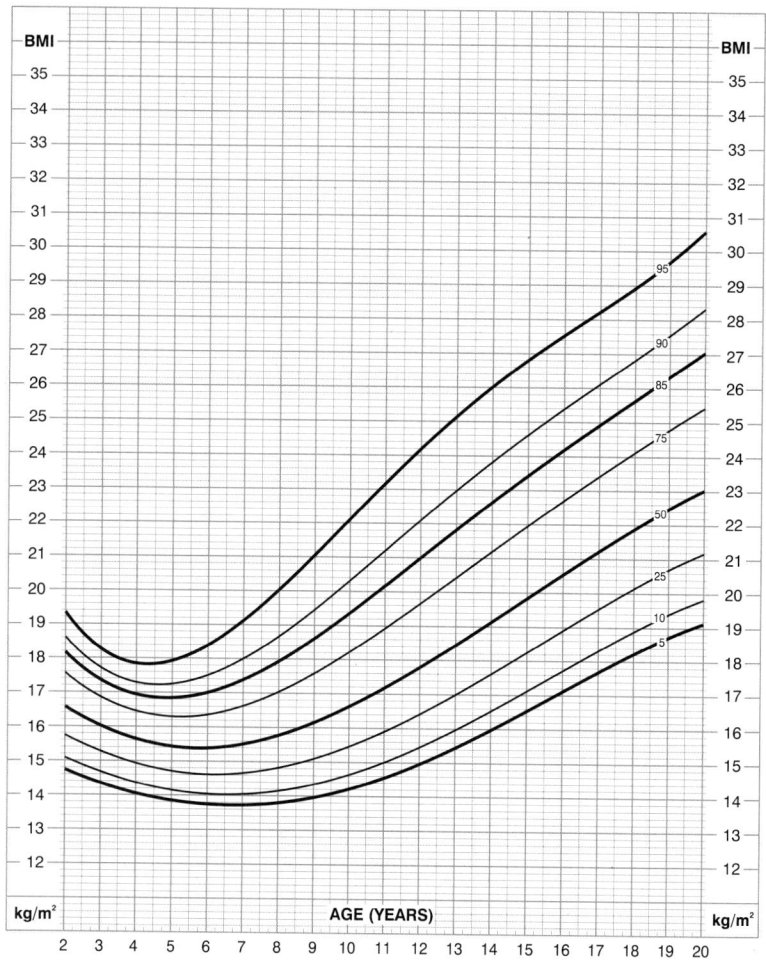

Figure 14-3. *(continued)*

PATHOGENESIS

Energy balance. In all persons, obesity is caused by ingesting more energy than is expended (and needed for organ growth and development in children and adolescents) over a long period of time. This initial positive energy balance generates an accumulation of body fat, which must be maintained by continued adequate energy intake. However, the mechanisms responsible for ultimate body weight involve a complex interaction among genetic, endocrine, neurologic, psychologic, behavioral, developmental, and environmental factors, and differ among individuals.

Dietary energy components are comprised of carbohydrate, protein, and fat, and a smaller component from alcohol. However, not all ingested calories are absorbed; approximately 5% of energy intake is lost in feces, but the exact amount of energy absorbed from the diet depends on

GIRLS (2-20 YEARS)

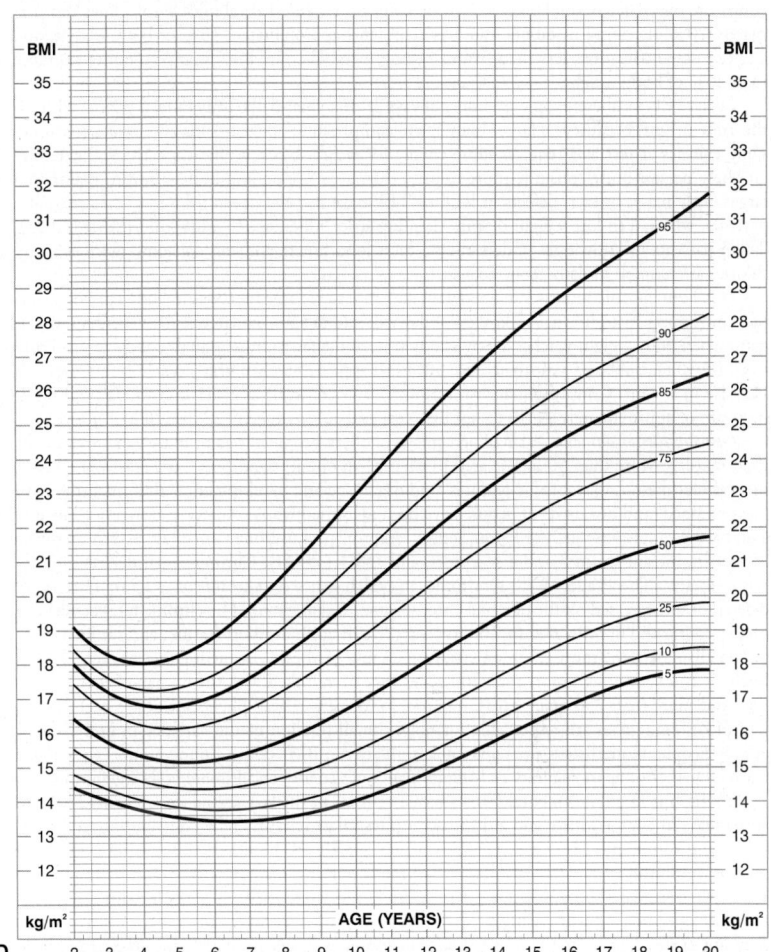

Figure 14-3. *(continued)*

the specific foods eaten, food preparation, mastication, and intestinal factors. Daily total energy expenditure (TEE) is comprised of (1) resting energy expenditure (REE, i.e., energy expended for normal cellular and organ function during postabsorptive resting conditions; approximately 70% of TEE), (2) thermic effect of food (i.e., the increase in energy expenditure associated with digestion, absorption, and increased sympathetic nervous system activity after eating a meal; approximately 10% of TEE), and (3) energy expended in physical activity (i.e., energy cost of volitional mechanical work, such as exercise and daily activities, and nonvolitional activity, such as fidgeting, spontaneous muscle contractions, and maintaining posture; approximately 20% of TEE). Energy requirements differ among body tissues. Highly active organs, such as the liver, gut, brain, kidney, and heart, have the highest energy requirements per gram of tissue. In a lean adult, these organs account for approximately 75% of the resting metabolic rate, although they constitute only 10% of total body weight. In contrast, resting skeletal muscle consumes approximately 20% of resting metabolic rate but represents approximately 40% of body weight, and adipose tissue consumes less than 5% of resting metabolic rate but usually accounts for more than 20% of body weight.

Daily TEE in obese people is almost always greater than daily TEE in lean people who are the same height, because the larger body mass, comprised of active organs and tissue, consumes more calories at rest and requires more energy for weight-bearing physical activity. Therefore, an obese person must consume more calories than a corresponding lean person to maintain a larger body mass. In fact, defects in REE or TEE have not even been found in "diet-resistant" patients, who fail to lose weight despite claiming strict adherence to a low-calorie diet (32,33). These patients unknowingly underestimate their food intake and can consume twice as many calories as recorded in daily food records.

Small but chronic increases in energy intake can lead to large increases in body fat. For example, consuming an additional 10 kcal every day will lead to approximately 1 lb of eventual weight gain, when body weight reaches a new steady state and energy intake equals energy expenditure (34). It will take about 1 year to achieve 50% and approximately 3 years to achieve 95% of this increase in weight. Consuming an extra candy bar (~220 kcal) as a snack every day will result in a gain of approximately 11 lbs (5 kg) in 1 year and approximately 22 lbs (10 kg) in 3 years.

Genes and environment. A small percentage of obese people have a primary genetic cause for their obesity. More than 50 loci related to Mendelian obesity syndromes, often associated with mental retardation, dysmorphic features, and organ-specific developmental abnormalities, have been mapped, and hundreds of people have been identified whose obesity is the consequence of single-gene mutations, such as leptin, leptin receptor, prohormone convertase 1, pro-opiomelanocortin, melanocortin 3 and 4 receptors, and SIM1 (35–41). Chromosomal defects can also cause obesity. The Prader–Willi syndrome, in which genes on chromosome 15 (q 11–13) are deleted or unexpressed on the paternal chromosome, is characterized by chronic hunger with excessive eating and life-threatening obesity, cognitive disabilities, short stature, and secondary hypogonadism; it is the most common syndromic cause of obesity, occurring in 1 of every 25,000 births (42). Even though more than 200 genes have been linked with the human obesity phenotype and more than 250 quantitative trait loci for obesity-related phenotypes have been identified (43), these genes are responsible for only a small fraction of the variance in body weight among people. Nonetheless, the remarkable similarity in BMI values among monozygotic twins reared together or apart suggests a strong influence of genetics on ultimate body weight (44,45).

Alterations in environmental factors have occurred in the last several decades that facilitate an increase in energy intake and a decrease in physical activity, thereby contributing to the development of obesity. More meals are now eaten outside the home, there is greater availability and consumption of convenience and snack foods, serving sizes are larger, and daily physical activity has decreased because of sedentary lifestyle and work activities. Persons with certain genetic backgrounds are particularly predisposed to weight gain and obesity-related diseases when they are exposed to a "modern" lifestyle. For example, Pima Indians living in Arizona have experienced a dramatic change in their lifestyle, which has led to an epidemic of obesity and diabetes in the last 60 years (46). These Pimas now eat a high-fat, high-calorie diet rather than their traditional low-fat diet and are much more sedentary than when they lived as farmers. In contrast, Pima Indians who live in the Sierra Madre Mountains of Northern Mexico have been isolated from Western influences, eat a traditional Pima diet, and are physically active as farmers and sawmill workers. The Pimas of Mexico have a much lower incidence of obesity and diabetes than those who live in Arizona.

Early life factors. The in utero environment can affect the future risk of obesity and obesity-related metabolic diseases in adulthood. Adults who were small for gestational age at birth, defined by a low birth weight, low ponderal index (birth weight/length^3), or small head circumference, are more likely to have a higher BMI, the metabolic syndrome, and coronary artery disease than men and women who were normal-sized at birth (47,48).

Both childhood and parental obesity affect the risk of obesity in adulthood (49). The probability of a child becoming an obese adult increases based on the age and severity of obesity in childhood and whether one or both parents are obese. For example, an obese child at 1 or 2 years of age who has lean parents does not have an increased risk of obesity in adulthood, whereas being obese after 6 years of age is associated with more than a 50% chance of being an obese adult. In addition, the presence of obesity in one or both parents increases the risk of obesity in their offspring. If neither parent is obese, the offspring have a 10% chance of becoming obese, whereas having one obese parent increases the risk for obesity to 40%, and the risk increases to 80% if both parents are obese.

Circadian rhythm and sleep: Many physiological processes are influenced by internal recurrent daily rhythms, which likely represent an adaptation to the Earth's rotation around the sun and the recurrent 24-hour light–dark cycles in the external environment. These circadian rhythms are important for maintaining health; disruption of circadian rhythm can have adverse effects on body weight and metabolic function. Inadequate sleep is associated with an increased risk of developing obesity. Experimentally-induced sleep restriction increases hunger and appetite, and data from both prospective and cross-sectional epidemiological studies show an association between short-duration and/or poor-quality sleep and the prevalence of obesity and the cardiometabolic complications associated with obesity (diabetes, metabolic syndrome, hypertriglyceridemia, and hypertension) (50,51).

MEDICAL COMPLICATIONS OF OBESITY

Obesity is an important risk factor for many serious medical complications (Table 14-3), which lead to impaired quality of life, considerable morbidity, premature death, and economic burden (52). The most common complications of obesity involve alterations in metabolic function that are risk factors for CVD, namely insulin resistance, diabetes, dyslipidemia (increased serum TG and decreased serum HDL-cholesterol), and increased blood pressure (53). However, not all obese persons develop metabolic complications, and approximately 25% of obese adults are "metabolically normal" based on insulin sensitivity measured by using the hyperinsulinemic euglycemic clamp technique (54). In addition, data from the 1994 to 2004 NHANES found that about one-third of obese adults were metabolically normal, defined as having less than one cardiometabolic abnormality (based on blood pressure, homeostasis model assessment of insulin resistance [HOMA-IR] value, and plasma glucose, triglyceride, HDL-cholesterol, and C-reactive protein [CRP] concentrations) (55). Metabolically-normal obesity, also known as "metabolically healthy but obese," "uncomplicated obesity," and "metabolically benign obesity," is further

TABLE 14-3 Medical Complications Associated with Obesity

Endocrine/metabolic	Insulin resistance, prediabetes, type 2 diabetes, dyslipidemia, metabolic syndrome, polycystic ovary syndrome
Cardiovascular	Hypertension, coronary heart disease, congestive heart failure, dysrhythmias, pulmonary hypertension, ischemic stroke, venous stasis, deep vein thrombosis, pulmonary embolus
Respiratory	Abnormal pulmonary function, obstructive sleep apnea, obesity hypoventilation syndrome
Gastrointestinal	Gallstones, pancreatitis, abdominal hernia, nonalcoholic fatty liver disease, gastroesophageal reflux disease
Musculoskeletal	Osteoarthritis, gout, low back pain
Gynecologic	Abnormal menses, infertility
Genitourinary	Urinary stress incontinence
Ophthalmologic	Cataracts
Neurologic	Idiopathic intracranial hypertension
Cancer	Liver, pancreas, stomach, esophagus, colon, gallbladder, kidney, prostate, multiple myeloma, postmenopausal breast, uterus, cervix, ovary, non-Hodgkins lymphoma
Postoperative events	Atelectasis, pneumonia, deep vein thrombosis, pulmonary embolus

characterized by less visceral and liver fat compared with metabolically-abnormal obese persons (56,57). Moreover, metabolically-normal obese persons are at lower risk of developing future diabetes and CVD than metabolically-abnormal obese or metabolically-abnormal lean persons, but are usually at higher risk than metabolically-normal lean people (58,59).

WEIGHT MANAGEMENT APPROACH TO THE OBESE PATIENT

Clinical Evaluation

The medical evaluation (history, physical examination, and blood tests) should include (1) a history of body weight, previous attempts at weight loss and lifestyle (dietary activity and sleep) habits to assess effectiveness of previous weight loss efforts and help identify potential lifestyle factors that contribute to the person's obesity; (2) a review of family history of obesity and obesity-related diseases; (3) an assessment of medications (Table 14-4) and medical conditions (e.g., Cushing syndrome) that can increase body weight; and (4) an evaluation to determine the presence and severity of obesity-related disease risk factors for disease, active medical diseases, and functional quality of life (Table 14-5). This approach provides important information that can help guide therapeutic options and align the intensity and type of weight loss therapy with the medical need to lose weight and the treatment options that are likely to have the most success. In addition, an understanding of the patient's obesity-related health risks and complications helps define clinical targets that indicate successful weight loss outcomes rather than simply the amount of weight loss itself.

Therapy

General Principles

The key to obesity therapy is to eat fewer calories than are expended in order to consume endogenous fat stores as fuel. Decreasing daily energy intake by 10 kcal will result in about a 1 lb weight loss; it will take approximately 1 year to achieve 50% and approximately 3 years to achieve 95% of this weight loss (34). The decrease in body mass induced by a negative energy balance results in a decrease in daily TEE. At some point, the reduced-energy diet consumed will equal energy expended, so weight loss will stop and body weight will plateau at a new lower level. Successful weight management strategies should appreciate the following 10 principles: (1) the major goals of weight loss therapy are to improve or eliminate obesity-related health risk factors, comorbidities, and/or improve physical function and quality of life; (2) obesity is a chronic illness that requires long-term treatment for long-term success; (3) even compliant patients will stop losing weight and reach a weight plateau (usually after ~6 months of therapy), so further weight loss will require a greater reduction in energy intake or increase in energy expenditure, or both; (4) a patient must be willing and ready to make lifestyle changes to achieve successful weight loss; (5) a slow rate of weight loss (<2% body weight loss per week) achieved by consuming a low-calorie diet is associated with less risk of developing weight loss–induced gallstones than rapid rate of weight

TABLE 14-4 Prescription Drugs Associated with Weight Gain

Psychotropic medications
    Second-generation antipsychotics (atypical antipsychotics):
    High risk: clozapine, olanzapine
    Medium risk: iloperidone, paliperidone, quetiapine, risperidone
    Low risk: aripiprazole, asenapine, lurasidone, ziprasidone
    Antidepressants: paroxetine, mirtazapine, tricyclics, monoamine oxidase inhibitors
    Mood stabilizer: lithium
Antiseizure medications: valproic acid, divalproex, carbamazepine, gabapentin
Diabetes medications: meglitinides, thiazolidinediones, sulfonylureas, insulin
Antihypertensives: clonidine, amlodipine,
β-Adrenergic blockers: propranolol, atenolol, metoprolol
Steroid and sex hormones: prednisone, methyl prednisolone, tamoxifen, estrogen, progestins
Antihistamines: diphenhydramine, cetirizine, fexofenadine
Protease inhibitors

TABLE 14-5 Indications for Intensive Obesity Therapy

Obesity-Related Risk Factors for Cardiometabolic Disease:
Poor glycemic control: impaired fasting glucose, impaired glucose tolerance, HbA1c 6%–6.5%
Abnormal lipid profile: increased triglyceride, decreased HDL-cholesterol, increased small dense LDL
Increased blood pressure
Metabolic syndrome
Family history of diabetes and cardiovascular disease
Common Obesity-Related Diseases:
Diabetes
Hypertension
Hypertriglyceridemia
Nonalcoholic fatty liver disease
Pulmonary dysfunction: obstructive sleep apnea, obesity hypoventilation syndrome
Cardiovascular disease
Osteoarthritis
Infertility
Obesity-Related Effects on Quality of Life and Function:
Joint pain
Impaired mobility
Poor endurance
Impaired quality of life

loss achieved by consuming a very-low-calorie diet (VLCD; <800 kcal per day); (6) behavioral therapy, particularly encouraging self-monitoring, is necessary for long-term lifestyle changes; (7) exercise has important metabolic, cardiovascular, functional, and psychological benefits, but does not produce effective weight loss in most people; (8) attempts to change a patient's medications from those that cause weight gain to those that are weight neutral or induce weight loss should be made, if medically acceptable; (9) minimal weight loss (as little as 2%) can have therapeutic cardiometabolic benefits, and greater weight loss results in progressive dose–response improvement in health outcomes; and (10) more aggressive therapy (greater dietary restrictions and meal replacements, more intensive behavioral therapy, pharmacotherapy, and bariatric surgery) should be initiated in patients who are unable to achieve weight loss targets with current therapy.

Consideration of Specific Treatment Options

The current therapeutic options available for weight management include lifestyle intervention (diet, physical activity, behavior modification), pharmacotherapy, and surgery. In general, the weight loss efficacy of pharmacotherapy is greater than lifestyle intervention (dietary intervention, physical activity, behavior modification), and the weight loss efficacy of bariatric surgery is greater than pharmacotherapy, and these modalities can be used alone or in combination with each other. However, the increase in treatment efficacy is associated with increased costs and risks of complications. The indications for using specific weight loss therapies, based on the clinical guidelines developed by an expert panel convened by the National Heart, Lung and Blood Institute, was published as a monograph in October 2000 (Table 14-6) (60). This approach was focused on the prevention and treatment of CVD. The composite of body weight classification (based on BMI), current cardiovascular illnesses, and risk factors for future coronary heart disease (identified by the medical examination) is used to determine the need for and aggressiveness of obesity therapy. An effective treatment plan must also consider patients' willingness to undergo therapy, their ability to comply with specific treatment approaches, access to skilled caregivers, and financial considerations. Weight loss therapy is not recommended for patients with a BMI less than 25 kg per m^2; however, providing recommendations for a healthy lifestyle, including dietary and physical activity modification, is reasonable for lean persons who have, or are at increased risk for, metabolic and CVDs. An algorithm for the evaluation and treatment of the obese patient was recently developed by The Obesity Society, the American College of Cardiology, and the American Heart Association (Figure 14-4) (61). This algorithm incorporates

TABLE 14-6 Criteria for Specific Weight Loss Therapy Based on Body Mass Index and Risk Factors

Treatment	BMI Category (kg/m^2)				
	25.0–26.9	27.0–29.9	30.0–34.9	35.0–39.9	≥ 40.0
Diet and physical activity	With risk factor	With risk factor	Yes	Yes	Yes
Pharmacotherapy[a]		With obesity-related disease	Yes	Yes	Yes
Surgery[b]			With obesity-related disease (LAGB only)	With obesity-related disease	Yes

[a]Pharmacotherapy should be considered in patients who are not able to achieve adequate weight loss by available conventional therapy (diet, physical activity, and behavior therapy).
[b]Bariatric surgery should only be considered in patients who are unable to lose weight by available conventional therapy.
Examples of obesity-related risk factors and diseases are listed in Table 14-5.
LAGB, laparoscopic adjustable gastric banding.
Adapted from National Institutes of Health, National Heart, Lung, and Blood Institute. Clinical Guidelines on the Identification, Evaluation, and Treatment of Overweight and Obesity in Adults—The Evidence Report. Bethesda (MD): National Heart, Lung, and Blood Institute; 1998 Sep. Report No.: 98-4083

a chronic disease model into the treatment of obesity and uses a stepwise series of questions to guide evaluation and therapy. The algorithm is disease-focused, rather than simply weight-focused, in that it highlights the need to identify and treat obesity-related medical complications, incorporates an assessment of health risk in the need to lose weight, and includes both health targets and weight loss targets as treatment goals.

Lifestyle Intervention

Although many obese persons can achieve short-term weight loss by making lifestyle changes in dietary intake and physical activity, successful long-term weight maintenance is much more difficult to achieve and most people who lose weight regain their lost weight over time. Collaboration with other health-care professionals (e.g., an experienced weight management dietitian or behaviorist) for additional counseling should be considered to provide more effective therapy. The initial goal of therapy should not simply be to reach a targeted body weight, but also provide goals related to specific health outcomes and quality of life. The effectiveness of even intensive lifestyle therapy and a low-calorie diet is moderate, and usually results in 5% to 10% weight loss in one year. Nonetheless, this amount of weight loss can have considerable medical benefits. However, these results are derived from studies conducted in obese subjects who are ready to lose weight and have enrolled in weight loss trials.

Diet Therapy

Decreasing energy intake is the cornerstone of weight loss therapy, and is most effective when diet education is provided in conjunction with behavioral therapy. Most diets proposed for losing weight vary in energy content and macronutrient composition. However, the energy content, not the relative macronutrient composition of the diet, is the primary determinant of weight loss. The calorie content of selected common foods is provided in Table 5-9, Chapter 5. A balanced–deficit diet of conventional foods usually contains less than 1,500 kcal per day and an appropriate balance of macronutrients. Low-calorie diets contain 800 to 1,500 kcal per day and are consumed as liquid formula, nutritional bars, conventional food, or a combination of these items. VLCDs contain less than 800 kcal per day and are usually high in protein (70 to 100 g per day) and low in fat (<15 g per day). These diets can be consumed as a liquid formula, nutritional bars, and/or conventional foods of mostly lean meat, fish, or fowl. The use of a VLCD causes rapid weight loss; patients lose 15% to 20% of initial weight by 12 to 16 weeks of treatment

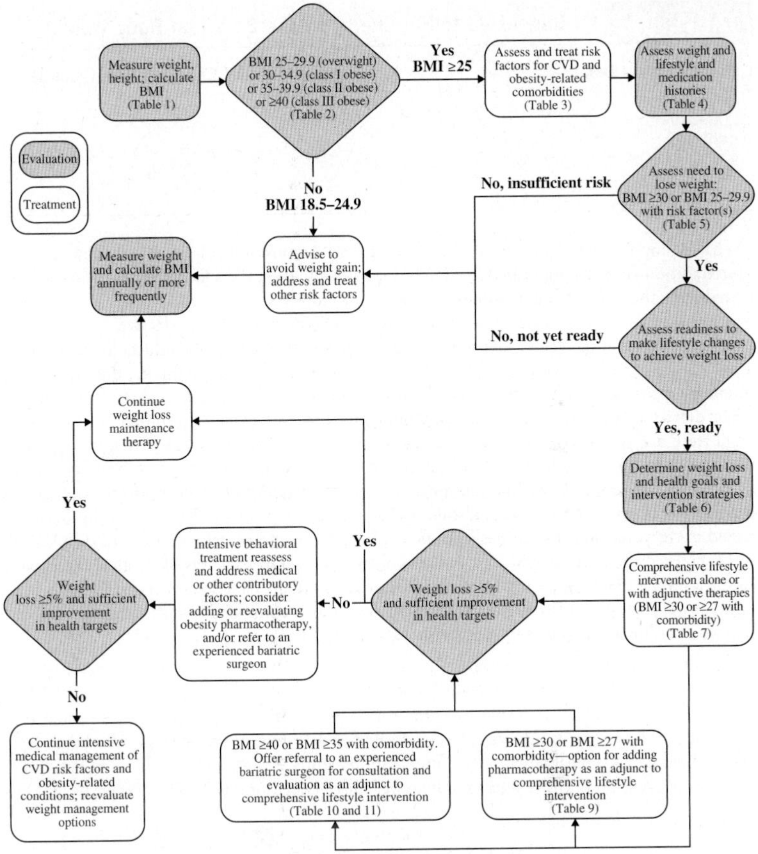

Figure 14-4. Weight management evaluation and treatment algorithm proposed by The Obesity Society, the American College of Cardiology, and the American Heart Association (Adapted from Jensen MD, Ryan DH, Donato KA, et al. 2013 AHA/ACC/TOS Guideline for the Management of Overweight and Obesity in Adults: A Report of the American College of Cardiology/American Heart Association Task Force on Practice Guidelines and The Obesity Society. *J Am Coll Cardiol.* 2014;63(25_PA):2960-2984).

(62). However, therapy with a VLCD requires more intense medical monitoring than treatment with a low-calorie diet, and is associated with high costs, high attrition rates, and a high probability of regaining 50% or more of lost weight so weight loss at 1 to 2 years is not different from those randomized to a low-calorie diet.

A diet that produces an energy deficit of 500 to 1,000 kcal per day has been recommended for treating obesity by many expert panels (60,61). However, this approach is difficult to execute in practice, because measuring TEE is not possible in clinical practice, estimates of total daily energy requirements made by using standard equations (63,64) (see Chapter 5 for detailed review) are imprecise, estimates of daily energy intake obtained from diet history and food records are often unreliable, and the ability to formulate a diet that has a precise energy content is poor. A suggested initial energy intake shown in Table 14-7 provides a simple approach for starting diet therapy, with the understanding that the weight loss response will dictate further dietary adjustments.

TABLE 14-7 Suggested Initial Energy Intake Based on Body Weight

Body Weight (lbs)	Suggested Initial Energy Intake (kcal/d)
150–199	1,200
200–249	1,500
250–299	1,800
300–349	2,200
>350	2,500

Many popular diets differ in their macronutrient composition (Figure 14-5). Low-fat diets have traditionally been prescribed for weight loss, because these diets facilitate energy restriction by reducing the intake of energy-dense triglycerides. However, data from a series of randomized controlled trials (RCTs) have shown that a low-carbohydrate diet is as effective, or even more effective, in generating weight loss as a low-fat diet (65–68). Weight loss induced by consuming a low-carbohydrate diet can be explained by a decrease in total energy intake, not an increase in energy expenditure (69), but the mechanism responsible for decreased energy consumption when dietary carbohydrates are restricted while fats and proteins are unlimited is not known. Data from a 2-year RCT found that a calorie-restricted Mediterranean diet (rich in vegetables and low in red meat, and up to 35% of calories from fat, primarily from olive oil and nuts) is just as effective as a low-carbohydrate, unrestricted-calorie diet and resulted in greater weight loss than conventional low-fat, restricted-calorie diet therapy (70). In another RCT, four diets that varied in the percentage of calories from fat, carbohydrate, and protein were evaluated (71). All diets achieved the same weight loss, but compliance was poor, so it was likely all subjects were eating a similar diet by the end of the study. In summary, these data demonstrate that there is no optimal weight loss diet for obese people. Therefore, diet recommendations should consider the patient's preferences and previous experiences with diet therapy.

Commercial Weight Loss Programs

Commercial programs facilitate weight loss (72,73). However, few long-term (≥1 year) RCTs have evaluated the weight loss efficacy of these programs. Only four programs were evaluated in RCTs of at least 1 year in duration: face-to-face lifestyle intervention (Weight Watchers), face-to-face lifestyle with meal replacement intervention (Jenny Craig), online structured behavioral lifestyle intervention (Vtrim), and a self-help website (e.Diets.com) (72). The average weight loss

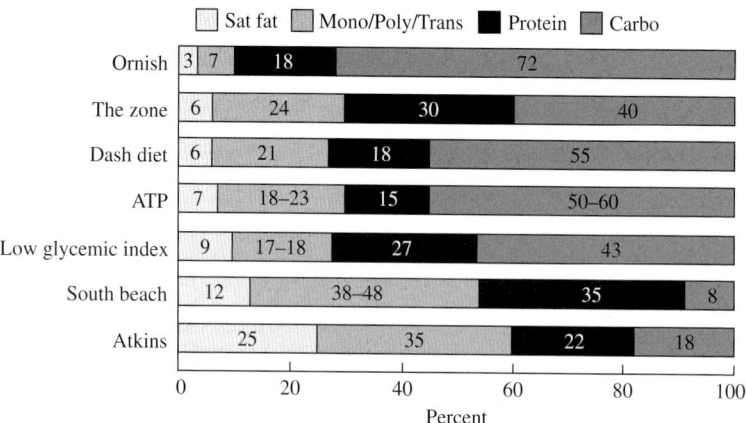

Figure 14-5. Macronutrient composition of selected popular weight-reduction diets. (From Wadden TA, Butryn ML, Wilson C. Lifestyle modification for the management of obesity. *Gastroenterology.* 2007;132:2226, with permission.)

(greater than the control group) is generally greater in a program that provides meal replacement at 1 year (-7 kg) than those that do not (2–3 kg).

Advice on choosing a commercial weight loss program can be found online from The National Institutes of Health, http://win.niddk.nih.gov/publications/choosing.htm.

Physical Activity

Increasing physical activity alone is not an effective initial weight loss therapy. The energy expended during physical activity or programmed exercise is small (Table 14-8) (Chapter 5, Table 5-6) compared with the energy deficit that can be achieved by dieting. Moreover, the energy consumed during exercise will have little impact on daily energy balance if it causes subsequent fatigue and sedentary behavior, or if it stimulates food intake. However, physical activity might facilitate successful long-term weight management. Obese subjects who are successful in maintaining long-term (≥ 1 year) weight loss engage in regular exercise. However, the amount of exercise that is associated with weight-loss maintenance is considerable and requires expending approximately 2,500 kcal per week (74). This level of energy expenditure requires vigorous activity (aerobics, cycling, or jogging) for approximately 30 minutes per day or more moderate activity (brisk walking) for 60 to 75 minutes per day.

Physical activity has additional health benefits that are independent of weight loss itself. Endurance and resistance exercise increases insulin sensitivity, and endurance exercise improves aerobic fitness. Physical activity and aerobic fitness are associated with a decrease risk of developing diabetes (24) and dying from CVD (23). In addition, exercise attenuates the loss of fat-free mass that occurs with weight loss (75), and improves physical function, which is particularly important in obese older adults (76).

TABLE 14-8 Energy Expenditure from Exercise Activities in a Lean Man and Woman

Activity	Energy Expended (kcal/kg/min)	Energy Expended (kcal/30 min) Reference Woman (5 ft 5 in/128 lbs)	Reference Man (5 ft 9 in/154 lbs)
Badminton	0.097	170	205
Basketball	0.138	240	290
Canoeing	0.044	75	90
Cycling			
5.5 mph	0.064	110	135
9.4 mph	0.100	175	210
Dancing, ballroom	0.051	90	90
Field hockey	0.134	235	280
Golf	0.085	150	180
Gymnastics	0.066	115	140
Horseback riding	0.110	190	230
Jogging (9 min/mile)	0.193	335	405
Judo, karate	0.195	340	410
Running (6 min/mile)	0.252	460	535
Skiing			
Cross-country	0.143	250	300
Downhill	0.098	190	230
Squash	0.212	370	445
Swimming, slow crawl	0.128	225	270
Tennis	0.109	190	230
Volleyball	0.050	90	105
Walking (15 min/mile)	0.080	140	165

Adapted from Katch F, McArdle W. *Nutrition, Weight Control and Exercise.* Boston: Houghton-Mifflin, 1983.

Behavior Modification

The purpose of behavior modification therapy is to help patients identify and then modify their lifestyle habits that contribute to their obesity. The main principles of behavioral therapy include (1) identifying specific and realistic goals that can be easily measured, (2) developing a reasonable plan for achieving goals so that planning, not willpower, is the focus, and (3) setting small and achievable goals and continue to build on successful experiences. The components of behavior modification strategies include stimulus control (avoiding the cues that prompt eating), self-monitoring (keeping daily records of food intake and physical activity), problem-solving skills (developing a systematic manner of analyzing a problem and identifying possible solutions), cognitive restructuring (correcting irrational thoughts that undermine weight control efforts, such as catastrophizing ["I've blown it"] and having unrealistic goals ["I won't be happy until I can wear a size 2 dress"]), social support (cooperation from family members and friends in altering lifestyle behavior), and relapse prevention (methods to promote recovery from bouts of overeating or weight regain).

Providing effective behavior therapy for obesity within a typical clinical practice setting is not realistic, because physicians usually do not have the time or expertise to provide this care. Therefore, involving professionals who are trained in behavior counseling for obesity is useful, if available. Behavior therapy can be provided in either group or individual sessions. In addition, lifestyle counseling can be provided by regular telephone contact or by using Internet-based programs, where patients get personal feedback from experienced professionals.

Pharmacotherapy

General Principles

The difficulty in achieving long-term weight management with lifestyle modification has led to the need for effective pharmacotherapy for obesity. The use of pharmacotherapy should be considered as part of a chronic disease–care approach. Accordingly, pharmacotherapy should not be considered a short-term treatment to "get patients going," because patients who lose weight with drug therapy usually regain weight when the therapy is stopped. Therefore, effective pharmacotherapy for obesity is likely to require long-term, if not life-long, treatment. Even with drug therapy, weight loss usually plateaus at 6 to 9 months of treatment, and weight begins to increase after approximately 1 year despite continued drug treatment. Pharmacotherapy alone is not as effective as pharmacotherapy given in conjunction with a comprehensive weight management program. Therefore, patients given drug treatment without the other standard approaches to weight management, including behavior modification and diet education, are exposed to the full risks of drug treatment without the full medical benefits. Some obese patients are refractory to drug therapy. If a patient does not respond to drug treatment for obesity in the first 12 weeks by losing at least 5% body weight, long-term success is unlikely and discontinuation of treatment or increased dosing should be considered.

Medications Approved by the United States Food and Drug Administration

The Food and Drug Administration (FDA) has proposed that a drug can be considered effective for weight loss if the results of a 1-year prospective randomized, double-blind, controlled trial, conducted in a total of approximately 3,000 subjects randomized to active doses of the drug and no fewer than 1,500 subjects randomized to placebo, demonstrate that (1) weight loss with drug treatment is more than 5% greater than, and statistically significantly different from, weight loss with placebo, and (2) the proportion of subjects who lose more than 5% of baseline body weight in the drug-treated group is at least 35%, is approximately double the proportion in the placebo-treated group, and the difference between groups is statistically significant (http://www.fda.gov/downloads/Drugs/…/Guidances/ucm071612.pd.).

Weight loss pharmacotherapy is approved for patients who have no contraindications to therapy and who have a BMI greater than 30.0 kg per m^2, or a BMI between 27.0 and 29.9 kg per m^2 and an obesity-related medical condition, such as type 2 diabetes, hypertension, dyslipidemia, sleep apnea, or CVD. All currently approved weight-loss drugs act as anorexiants with the exception of orlistat, which inhibits the absorption of dietary fat. Orlistat, phentermine–topiramate extended release (ER), lorcaserin, and naltrexone-bupropion are the only medications currently approved by the FDA for long-term use (>12 weeks) in the management of

TABLE 14-9	History of Medications Approved by the US Food and Drug Administration to Treat Obesity	
Year Approved	Generic Name (Trade name)	Year Withdrawn
1947	Desoxyephedrine/methamphetamine	
1956	Phenmetrazine (Preludin)	
1959	Phentermine (Adipex, Ionamin)	
1959	Diethylpropion (Tenuate)	
1959	Phendimetrazine (Bontril, Prelu-2)	
1960	Benzphetamine (Didrex)	
1972	Fenfluramine (Pondimin)	1997
1973	Mazindol (Sanorex)	
1996	Dexfenfluramine (Redux)	1997
1997	Sibutramine (Meridia)	2010
1999	Orlistat (Xenical)[a]	
2012	Phentermine-topiramate extended release (Qsymia)	
2012	Lorcaserin (Belviq)	
2014	Naltrexone-bupropion (Contrave)	

[a]Approved as an over-the-counter medication at half the prescription dose in 2007

obesity. However, phentermine–topiramate ER and lorcaserin are not marketed in Europe because of safety concerns of the European Medicines Agency. The history of drugs approved by the US FDA for the treatment of obesity is shown in Table 14-9. Three drugs have been withdrawn from the market because of the increased incidence of valvular heart disease (fenfluramine and dexfenfluramine) or cardiovascular events (sibutramine) associated with their use. The most commonly prescribed medications for obesity is phentermine.

Phentermine
Phentermine stimulates the release of norepinephrine, and to a lesser extent stimulates the release of serotonin and dopamine, from nerve terminals. Only one RCT, which was published in 1968, evaluated the effect of at least 8 months of phentermine therapy on body weight (77). In that study, 108 obese women were randomized to receive a low-calorie diet and treatment with either daily phentermine (30 mg per day), daily phentermine every other month alternating with daily placebo every other month, or daily placebo for 36 weeks. Of the 64 subjects who completed the study, those randomized to either continuous or every-other-month phentermine therapy achieved the same 13% weight loss, which was greater than the 5% weight loss observed in the placebo group. In a more recent RCT, subjects who completed 28 weeks of therapy with one-half (15 mg per day) or one-fourth (7.5 mg per day) the usual dose of phentermine had a 7.4% and 6.7% weight loss, respectively, compared with 2.3% weight loss in the placebo group (78).

Phentermine Side Effects
The most common side effects of phentermine are dry mouth, insomnia, and constipation. Although all sympathomimetic agents can increase blood pressure and heart rate, these abnormalities usually do not occur with phentermine therapy in the presence of weight loss.

Orlistat
Orlistat is a synthetic derivative of lipstatin, a product made by the Streptomyces toxytricini mold, which inhibits most mammalian lipases. Orlistat binds to lipases in the gastrointestinal tract and blocks the digestion of dietary triglycerides. The degree of fat malabsorption is directly related to the dose of orlistat administered. The recommended prescribed dose of 120 mg three times daily with meals causes malabsorption of approximately 30% of ingested triglycerides, which is near the maximum effect; ingesting more than 120 mg of orlistat with a meal is unlikely to increase the malabsorption of ingested fat. Orlistat has no effect on systemic lipases because less than 1% of the administered dose is absorbed.

Several long-term (1 to 4 years) RCTs evaluated orlistat therapy for obesity. Data from meta-analyses of orlistat RCTs found that subjects treated with orlistat for 1 to 2 years lost about 3%

(3 kg) more weight than those randomized to placebo (79,80). In a categorical analysis, about twice as many subjects randomized to orlistat lost at least 5% and 10% of their initial body weight, compared with those randomized to placebo. In the longest orlistat RCT, weight loss was 5% greater (11% versus 6%) at 1 year and 3% greater (7% versus 4%) at 4 years for subjects treated with orlistat compared with those treated with placebo (81).

Orlistat Side Effects

The most common side effects experienced with orlistat therapy are gastrointestinal events related to orlistat's mechanism of action (e.g., oily stool, oily spotting, increased defecation, fecal urgency, flatulence, and abdominal discomfort), which occur in most patients. These events usually occur early (within the first 4 weeks), are of mild or moderate intensity, are usually limited to one or two episodes, and resolve despite continued orlistat treatment. Another concern with orlistat therapy is the potential malabsorption of fat soluble vitamins and the malabsorption of lipophilic drugs if they are taken with orlistat. It is recommended that all patients who are treated with orlistat be given a daily multivitamin supplement that is taken at a time when orlistat is not being ingested. In addition, orlistat should not be taken for at least 2 hours before or after the ingestion of lipophilic drugs, and plasma drug concentrations should be followed to ensure appropriate dosing if possible.

Phentermine–Topiramate ER

Phentermine–topiramate ER is a combination drug containing phentermine and topiramate, an anticonvulsant that has an unknown mechanism for reducing food intake. These two agents were combined in an effort to get successful weight loss by using lower doses than usually required for each drug alone, and thereby reduce the adverse side effects of each medication when given at their normal full dose. Four different doses of phentermine and ER topiramate are available: (1) starting dose (3.75 mg per 23 mg), (2) recommended dose (7.5 mg per 46 mg), (3) transition dose (11.25 mg per 69 mg), and (4) top dose (15 mg per 92 mg). The suggested treatment approach is (1) begin with the starting dose for 2 weeks, (2) advance to the recommended dose, (3) if less than 3% weight loss after 12 weeks, either discontinue or advance to top dose by providing the transition dose for 2 weeks, and (4) if less than 5% weight loss after 12 weeks on full dose, plan to stop treatment by taking the medication every other day for one week and then discontinue completely.

Phentermine–topiramate ER has been evaluated in two large RCTs (82,83). Weight loss at 1 year demonstrated a dose–response relationship, and was similar in both studies. An intention-to-treat analysis of the 1-year placebo-subtracted weight loss was approximately 9% for the top dose, and approximately 6.5% for the recommended dose. A third study evaluated the potential weight loss efficacy at 2 years of therapy; 78% of participants from one of the 1-year RCTs continued to receive their blinded treatment for an additional year, and demonstrated the weight loss achieved at the end of year 1 was maintained through year 2.

Phentermine–Topiramate ER Side Effects

The most common adverse effects were dry mouth, dizziness, dysgeusia, constipation, insomnia, and paresthesias. In addition, cognitive impairment (attention or memory deficits) can occur, and there is a potential risk of fetal toxicity in pregnant women treated with topiramate (topiramate monotherapy exposure during pregnancy is associated with two- to fivefold increased prevalence of oral clefts), acute myopia, and secondary-angle closure glaucoma.

Lorcaserin

Lorcaserin is a selective 5-HT2C receptor agonist that is thought to decrease food intake through the pro-opiomelanocortin system in the brain. The recommended dose is 10 mg b.i.d.; if a patient has not lost at least 5% of baseline body weight by 12 weeks, it is recommended to discontinue drug treatment. The results from two RCTs in subjects without diabetes (84,85) and one RCT in subjects with type 2 diabetes (86) demonstrated that the 1-year placebo-subtracted weight loss was only 2% to 4%, which did not meet the FDA-proposed guidelines, but did meet the FDA criteria for adequate categorical ($\geq$5%) weight loss.

Lorcaserin Side Effects

The most frequent adverse effects of lorcaserin in these studies were headache, dry mouth, dizziness, and nausea. There was no difference in the development of FDA-defined valvulopathy between drug-treated and placebo-treated subjects at 1 or 2 years, which supports the selectivity of lorcaserin for the 5-HT2C receptor, because the activation of the 5-HT2B receptors expressed on cardiac valvular interstitial cells was likely responsible for the valvulopathy induced by two previous weight loss drugs, fenfluramine and dexfenfluramine.

Naltrexone-bupropion

Naltrexone-bupropion is a combination drug containing extended-release forms of naltrexone HCl and bupropion HCl. Naltrexone is an opioid receptor antagonist and bupropion inhibits neuronal reuptake of dopamine and norepinephrine. The rationale for using this combination is based on the synergistic effect of bupropion and naltrexone on pro-opiomelanocortin (POMC) neurons to inhibit food intake. Post-translational processing of POMC in the arcuate nucleus of the hypothalamus generates two primary peptides: 1) α-melanocyte–stimulating hormone (α-MSH), which is a potent anorexiant, and 2) β-endorphin, which causes opioid receptor-induced inhibition of POMC neurons and stimulates food intake. Bupropion stimulates POMC neurons and naltrexone blocks feedback inhibition from β-endorphin, resulting in an increase in α-MSH action. The doses of naltrexone HCl (8 mg) and bupropion HCL (90 mg) in each tablet are lower than that available for either agent alone. The recommended dosing involves an escalated approach to reduce side effects: one tablet in the morning during week 1, one tablet in the morning and one in the evening during week 2, two tablets in the morning and one in the evening during week 3, and two tablets in the morning and two in the evening (total daily dose naltrexone/bupropion 32 mg/360 mg) during week 4 and thereafter.

Naltrexone-bupropion should not be used in patients treated with opiates or monoamine oxidase inhibitors, and use of alcohol should be minimized when taking this medication. In addition, bupropion inhibits CYP2D6, so it can increase the concentrations of drugs metabolized by CYP2D6, such as certain antidepressants (e.g. selective serotonin reuptake inhibitors and tricyclics), antipsychotics, (e.g. haloperidol risperidone, thioridazine) beta-blockers (e.g. metoprolol), and type 1C antiarrhythmics (e.g. propafenone, flecainide)

Naltrexone-bupropion has been evaluated in four large RCTs (87-90). An intention-to-treat analysis of the 1-year placebo-subtracted weight loss was ~2% in the study that only included for patients with type 2 diabetes (87) and ~3-4% in other obese cohorts (88-90).

Naltrexone-bupropion Side Effects

The most common adverse effects were nausea, constipation, headache, vomiting, dizziness, insomnia, and dry mouth. In addition, Naltrexone-bupropion treatment attenuates the beneficial effects of weight loss on lowering blood pressure and heart rate.

Bariatric Surgery

Types of Procedures

There are currently five different standard bariatric surgery procedures: (1) Roux-en-Y gastric bypass, (2) laparoscopic adjustable gastric banding, (3) sleeve gastrectomy, (4) biliopancreatic diversion, and (5) biliopancreatic diversion with duodenal switch (Figure 14-6) (91). Roux-en-Y gastric bypass involves the creation of a small gastric pouch (<30 mL) that is connected to a segment of jejunum, which has been transected at 30 to 75 cm from the ligament of Treitz, to form a Roux-en-Y limb. Bowel continuity is restored via an anastomosis between the "Roux" limb and the excluded biliopancreatic limb approximately 75 to 150 cm distal to the gastrojejunostomy. Laparoscopic adjustable gastric banding involves placing a silicone ring with an inflatable inner tube around the upper stomach, just distal to the gastroesophageal junction. The inner tube is connected to a subcutaneous port, which is used to inject or withdraw saline to adjust the band diameter. Typically, six adjustments are made in the first year after band placement, as needed to enhance weight loss. Sleeve gastrectomy involves dividing the stomach along its vertical length, removing approximately 75% of the stomach, and creating a banana-shaped sleeve. This procedure was originally intended as a first-stage procedure of biliopancreatic diversion with duodenal switch in high-risk patients, but has now become a stand-alone operation. Biliopancreatic diversion involves a horizontal gastrectomy, leaving behind 200 to 500 mL of stomach, which is anastomosed to the small intestine, 250 cm from the ileocecal valve. The excluded biliopancreatic limb is anastomosed to the ileum, 50 cm from the ileocecal valve. The distal 50-cm common channel is where digestive secretions from the biliopancreatic limb mix with the ingested food delivered by

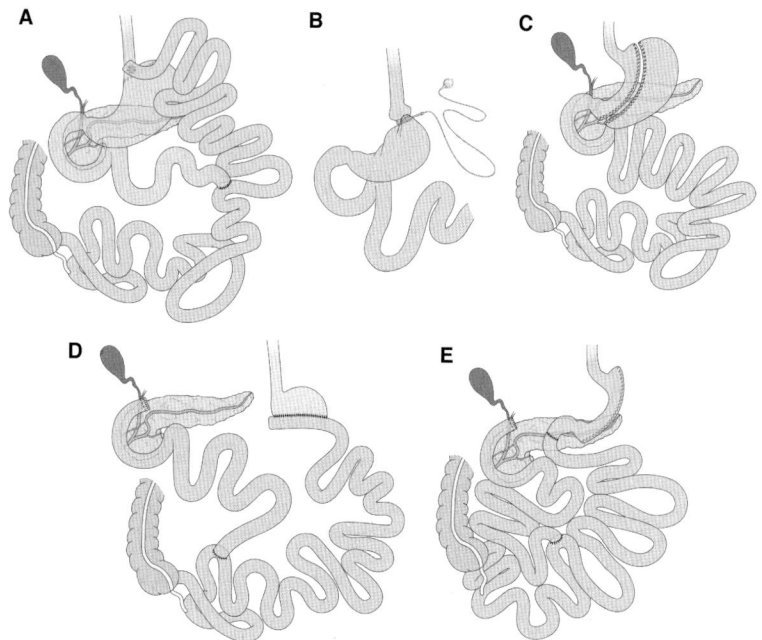

Figure 14-6. Standard bariatric surgery procedures: (A) Roux-en-Y gastric bypass, (B) laparoscopic adjustable gastric banding, (C) sleeve gastrectomy, (D) biliopancreatic diversion, (E) biliopancreatic diversion with duodenal switch (Bradley D, Magkos F, Klein S. Effects of bariatric surgery on glucose homeostasis and type 2 diabetes. *Gastroenterology.* 2012;143:897–912).

the alimentary limb. Biliopancreatic diversion with duodenal switch involves constructing a 150 to 200 mL volume vertical sleeve gastrectomy with preservation of the pylorus and formation of a duodenal-ileal anastomosis. The excluded biliopancreatic limb is anastomosed to the ileum, 100 cm from the ileocecal valve, where digestive secretions and nutrients mix. Both biliopancreatic diversion and biliopancreatic diversion with duodenal switch cause considerable malabsorption.

Criteria for Surgery

The indications for bariatric surgery were established in 1991 by a consensus conference sponsored by the National Institutes of Health 6), and approval to lower the BMI requirement for laparoscopic adjustable gastric banding was established by the FDA in 2011 (Table 14-10). The NIH guidelines were established before (1) improved technical expertise reduced perioperative risks, (2) minimally invasive laparoscopic adjustable gastric banding, Roux-en-Y gastric, bypass, and sleeve gastrectomy procedures were used, and (3) data from long-term observational studies and randomized clinical trials were available to carefully assess the risk: benefit of bariatric surgery. Therefore, the indications for bariatric surgery should be updated to focus more on the potential clinical benefits in patients who are unable to achieve targeted weight loss–induced clinical benefits by lifestyle therapy (diet and behavioral treatment) with or without pharmacotherapy.

Weight Loss Efficacy

Bariatric surgery is the most effective available weight loss therapy and results in long-term (20 years) successful weight loss in most patients (92,93). However, weight loss is not the same among procedures (Table 14-11) (94,95). Weight loss after Roux-en-Y gastric bypass, laparoscopic adjustable gastric banding, and sleeve gastrectomy is primarily due to a decrease in energy intake because there is little or no malabsorption after these procedures, and weight loss

TABLE 14-10   Clinical Criteria for Selecting Patients for Bariatric Surgery

1. Body mass index:
   BMI ≥40 kg/m^2
   BMI ≥35 kg/m^2 and significant obesity comorbidity (e.g., hypertension, diabetes, sleep apnea, incapacitating osteoarthritis)
   BMI 30–34 kg/m^2 and significant obesity comorbidity (laparoscopic adjustable gastric band only)
2. Additional patient criteria:
   Unable to achieve targeted weight loss with nonsurgical therapy
   Ability to comprehend the expected changes in dietary intake necessary after surgery to achieve sustained weight loss
   Willingness to maintain continued medical management after surgery, including visits to registered dietitians, internists
   Absence of drug addiction or serious psychiatric illness that would affect clinical outcome
   Acceptable operative risk

TABLE 14-11   Effect of Different Bariatric Surgical Procedures on Body Weight

	Approximate Weight Loss (%)	Approximate Excess Weight Loss (%)
Laparoscopic adjustable gastric banding	20	40
Sleeve gastrectomy	30	55
Roux-en-Y gastric bypass	30	65
Biliopancreatic diversion	35	70
Biliopancreatic diversion + duodenal switch	35	70

after biliopancreatic diversion with or without duodenal switch is likely due to a combination of decreased energy intake and malabsorption. Moreover, not all patients lose a lot of weight, and some patients who lose weight initially regain most or all of their lost weight over time (96).

Therapeutic Efficacy

Bariatric surgery–induced weight loss has potent therapeutic effects in both preventing and treating the medical complications associated with obesity. In particular, bariatric surgery is much more effective than any other approach for preventing (97) and treating (98–100) type 2 diabetes. Procedures that involve anatomical diversion of the upper gastrointestinal tract (e.g., Roux-en-Y gastric bypass and biliopancreatic diversion) have greater therapeutic effects in patients with diabetes than those that maintain intestinal continuity (e.g., laparoscopic adjustable gastric banding and sleeve gastrectomy). For example, most patients with diabetes who are treated with Roux-en-Y gastric bypass surgery achieve remission of their diabetes, defined as maintaining normal or near-normal blood glucose concentrations and HbA1c without the use of diabetes medications. Even those who do not achieve diabetes remission usually experience a marked improvement in glycemic control. Accordingly, bariatric surgery should be considered a part of standard therapy for type 2 diabetes.

Complications

Bariatric surgery is associated with both early (within 30 days of surgery) and late postoperative complications. The overall early and late mortality rate is about 0% to 2%; the risk of complications and mortality is influenced by the type of procedure, experience of the surgeon, presence of a competent bariatric surgery team and hospital, and medical status of the patient. Most complications that occur with any gastrointestinal surgical procedure also occur after bariatric

TABLE 14-12. Risk of Selected Micronutrient Deficiencies after Bariatric Surgery

Nutrient	LAGB	SG	RYGB	BPD/BPD + DS
Thiamine	+	+	+	+
Vitamin B_{12}		+++	+++	+
Vitamin A			+	+++
Vitamin D	+	++	+++	+++
Iron	+	+	++	++

LAGB, laparoscopic adjustable gastric banding; SG, sleeve gastrectomy; RYGB, Roux-en-Y gastric bypass; BPD, biliopancreatic diversion; BPD + DS, biliopancreatic diversion with duodenal switch. Adapted from Mechanick JI, Youdim A, Jones DB, et al; American Association of Clinical Endocrinologists; Obesity Society; American Society for Metabolic & Bariatric Surgery. Clinical practice guidelines for the perioperative nutritional, metabolic, and nonsurgical support of the bariatric surgery patient—2013 update: cosponsored by American Association of Clinical Endocrinologists, The Obesity Society, and American Society for Metabolic & Bariatric Surgery. *Obesity.* 2013;21 (Suppl 1):S1–27.

TABLE 14-13. Suggested Nutritional Evaluations after Bariatric Surgery

Test	Timing After Surgery	LAGB	LSG	RYGB	BPD/BPD + DS
Bone density (DXA)	2 years	X	X	X	X
24-h urinary calcium excretion	6 months and then every 1 year	X	X	X	X
Iron				X	X
Folic acid				X	X
Vitamin B_{12}	Every 1 year	X	X	X	X
25-vitamin D iPTH				X	X
Vitamin A	Every 1 year				X

LAGB, laparoscopic adjustable gastric banding; SG, sleeve gastrectomy; RYGB, Roux-en-Y gastric bypass; BPD, biliopancreatic diversion; BPD + DS, biliopancreatic diversion with duodenal switch.
Adapted from Mechanick JI, Youdim A, Jones DB, et al; American Association of Clinical Endocrinologists; Obesity Society; American Society for Metabolic & Bariatric Surgery. Clinical practice guidelines for the perioperative nutritional, metabolic, and nonsurgical support of the bariatric surgery patient—2013 update: cosponsored by American Association of Clinical Endocrinologists, The Obesity Society, and American Society for Metabolic & Bariatric Surgery. *Obesity.* 2013;21 (Suppl 1):S1–27.

surgery, including atelectasis, pneumonia, deep vein thrombosis, pulmonary embolism, anastomotic leak with peritonitis, wound infection, gastrointestinal bleeding, and internal hernias. Dumping syndrome and hypoglycemia specifically occur in a subset of patients after Roux-en-Y gastric bypass surgery, and can usually be controlled with dietary management. Specific nutritional deficiencies can also occur (Table 14-12), so guidelines for routine monitoring have been suggested (Table 14-13) (101).

REFERENCES

1. Hirsch J, Knittle JL. Cellularity of obese and non-obese human adipose tissue. *Fed Proc.* 1970;29:1516–1521.
2. Leiter LA, Marliss EB. Survival during fasting may depend on fat as well as protein stores. *JAMA.* 1982;248:2306–2307.
3. Stewart WK, Fleming LW. Features of a successful therapeutic fast of 382 days duration. *Postgrad Med J.* 1973;49:203–209.

4. Gallagher D, Heymsfield SB, Heo M, et al. Health percentage body fat ranges: an approach for developing guidelines based on body mass index. *Am J Clin Nutr.* 2000;72:694–701.
5. National Institutes of Health, National Heart, Lung, and Blood Institute. Clinical guidelines on the identification, evaluation, and treatment of overweight and obesity in adults—the evidence report. *Obes Res.* 1998;6 (Suppl 2):51S–209S.
6. NIH Conference. Gastrointestinal surgery for severe obesity: Consensus Development Conference Panel. *Ann Intern Med.* 1991;115:956–961.
7. Flegal KM, Graubard BI, Williamson DF, et al. Excess deaths associated with underweight, overweight, and obesity. *JAMA.* 2005;293:1861.
8. Flegal KM, Kit BK, Orpana H, et al. Association of all-cause mortality with overweight and obesity using standard body mass index categories: a systematic review and meta-analysis. *JAMA.* 2013;309:71–82.
9. Kragelund C, Hassager C, Hildebrandt P, et al. TRACE study group: impact of obesity on long-term prognosis following acute myocardial infarction. *Int J Cardiol.* 2005;98:123–131.
10. McAuley P, Myers J, Abella J, et al. Body mass, fitness and survival in veteran patients: another obesity paradox? *Am J Med.* 2007;120:518–524.
11. Uretsky S, Messerli FH, Bangalore S, et al. Obesity paradox in patients with hypertension and coronary artery disease. *Am J Med.* 2007;120:863–870.
12. Oreopoulos A, Padwal R, Norris CM, et al. Effect of obesity on short- and long-term mortality postcoronary revascularization: a meta-analysis. *Obesity (Silver Spring).* 2008;16:442–450.
13. Mano A, Fujita K, Uenomachi K, et al. Body mass index is a useful predictor of prognosis after left ventricular assist system implantation. *J Heart Lung Transplant.* 2009;28:428–433.
14. Lea JP, Crenshaw DO, Onufrak SJ, et al. Obesity, end-stage renal disease, and survival in an elderly cohort with cardiovascular disease. *Obesity (Silver Spring).* 2009;17:2216–2222.
15. Beck TJ, Petit MA, Wu G, et al. Does obesity really make the femur stronger? BMD, geometry, and fracture incidence in the Women's Health Initiative—Observational Study. *J Bone Miner Res.* 2009;24:1369–1379.
16. Van der Helm-van Mil AH, van der Kooij SM, Allaart CF, et al. A high body mass index has a protective effect on the amount of joint destruction in small joints in early rheumatoid arthritis. *Ann Rheum Dis.* 2008;67:769–774.
17. Leung CC, Lam TH, Chan WM, et al. Lower risk of tuberculosis in obesity. *Arch Intern Med.* 2007;167:1297–1304.
18. Colditz GA, Willet WC, Rotnitzky A, et al. Weight gain as a risk factor for clinical diabetes mellitus in women. *Ann Intern Med.* 1995;122:481–486.
19. Chan JM, Rimm EB, Colditz GA, et al. Obesity, fat distribution, and weight gain as risk factors for clinical diabetes in men. *Diabetes Care.* 1994;17:961–969.
20. Fabbrini E, Mohammed BS, Magkos F, et al. Intrahepatic triglyceride, not visceral fat, is associated with metabolic complications of obesity in human subjects. *Proc Natl Acad Sci.* 2009;106:15430–15435.
21. Pouliot MC, Despres JP, Lemieux S, et al. Waist circumference and abdominal saggital diameter: best simple anthropometric indices of abdominal visceral adipose tissue accumulation and related cardiovascular risk in men and women. *Am J Cardiol.* 1994;73:460–468.
22. Rimm EB, Stampfer MJ, Giovannucci E, et al. Body size and fat distribution as predictors of coronary heart disease among middle-aged and older US men. *Am J Epidemiol.* 1995;141:1117–1127.
23. Lee CD, Blair SN, Jackson AS. Cardiorespiratory fitness, body composition, and all-cause and cardiovascular disease mortality in men. *Am J Clin Nutr.* 1999;69:373–380.
24. Wei M, Gibbons L, Mitchell T, et al. The association between cardiorespiratory fitness and impaired fasting glucose and type 2 diabetes mellitus in men. *Ann Intern Med.* 1999;130:89–96.
25. International Diabetes Institute, World Health Organization. *The Asia-Pacific Perspective: Redefining Obesity and Its Treatment.* Geneva: World Health Organization, 2000:1. http://www.wpro.who.int/nutrition/documents/docs/Redefiningobesity.pdf?ua=1
26. Yoon K-H, Lee J-H, Kim J-W, et al. Epidemic obesity and type 2 diabetes in Asia. *Lancet.* 2006;368:1681–1688.
27. WHO Expert Consultation. Appropriate body-mass index for Asian populations and its implications for policy and intervention strategies. *Lancet.* 2004;363:157–163.
28. Serdula MK, Ivery D, Coates R, et al. Do obese children become obese adults? *Prev Med.* 1993;22:167–177.
29. Guo SS, Huang C, Maynard LM, et al. Body mass index during childhood, adolescent and young adulthood in relation to adult overweight and adiposity: the Fels Longitudinal Study. *Int J Obes Relat Metab Disord.* 2000;24:1628–1635.

30. Ng M, Fleming T, Robinson M, et al. Global, regional, and national prevalence of overweight and obesity in children and adults during 1980–2013: a systematic analysis for the Global Burden of Disease Study 2013. *Lancet.* 2014;384(9945):766–781.
31. Ogden CL, Carroll MD, Kit BK, et al. Prevalence of childhood and adult obesity in the United States, 2011–2012. *JAMA.* 2014;311:806–814.
32. Skov AR, Toubro S, Buemann B, et al. Normal levels of energy expenditure in patients with reported "low metabolism." *Clin Physiol.* 1997;17:279–285.
33. Lichtman SW, Pisarka K, Berman ER, et al. Discrepancy between self-reported and actual caloric intake and exercise in obese subjects. *N Engl J Med.* 1992;327:1893–1898.
34. Hall KD, Sacks G, Chandramohan D, et al. Quantification of the effect of energy imbalance on body weight. *Lancet.* 2011;378:826–837.
35. Rankinen T, Zuberi A, Chagnon YC, et al. The human obesity gene map: the 2005 update. *Obesity.* 2006;14:529.
36. Farooqi IS, Wangensteen T, Collins S, et al. Clinical and molecular genetic spectrum of congenital deficiency of the leptin receptor. *New Engl J Med.* 2007;356:237.
37. Lee YS, Poh LK, Loke KY. A novel melanocortin 3 receptor gene (MC3R) mutation associated with severe obesity. *J Clin Endocrinol Metab.* 2002;87:1423.
38. Farooqi IS, Keogh JM, Yeo GSH, et al. Clinical spectrum of obesity and mutations in the melanocortin 4 receptor gene. *N Engl J Med.* 2003;348:1085.
39. Challis BG, Pritchard LE, Creemers JW, et al. A missense mutation disrupting a dibasic prohormone processing site in pro-opiomelanocortin (POMC) increases susceptibility to early-onset obesity through a novel molecular mechanism. *Hum Mol Genet.* 2002;11:1997.
40. Jackson RS, Creemers JW, Ohagi S, et al. Obesity and impaired prohormone processing associated with mutations in the human prohormone convertase 1 gene. *Nat Genet.* 1997;16:303.
41. Holder JL Jr, Butte NF, Zinn AR. Profound obesity associated with a balanced translocation that disrupts the SIM1 gene. *Hum Mol Gene.* 2000;9:101.
42. Goldstone AP. Prader-Willi syndrome: advances in genetics, pathophysiology and treatment. *Trends Endocrinol Metab.* 2004;15:12–20.
43. Waalen J. The genetics of human obesity. *Transl Res.* 2014;pii: S1931–5244(14)00197–2.
44. Allison DB, Heshka S, Neale MC, et al. A genetic analysis of relative weight among 4,020 twin pairs, with an emphasis on sex effects. *Health Psychol.* 1994;4:362.
45. Allison DB, Kaprio J, Korkeila M, et al. The heritability of body mass index among an international sample of monozygotic twins reared apart. *Int J Obes Res Relat Metab Disord.* 1996;6:501.
46. Pratley RE. Gene-environment interactions in the pathogenesis of type 2 diabetes mellitus: lessons learned from the Pima Indians. *Proc Nutr Soc.* 1998;57:175–181.
47. Barker DJP. The fetal origins of diseases of old age. *Eur J Clin Nutr.* 1992;46:S3–S9.
48. Martorelli R, Stein AD, Schroeder DG. Early nutrition and later adiposity. *J Nutr.* 2001;131:874S–880S.
49. Whitaker RC, Wright JA, Pepe MS, et al. Predicting obesity in young adulthood from childhood and parental obesity. *N Engl J Med.* 1997;337:869–873.
50. Gangwisch JE. Epidemiological evidence for the links between sleep, circadian rhythms and metabolism. *Obes Rev.* 2009;10 (Suppl 2):37–45.
51. Spiegel K, Tasali E, Leproult R, et al. Effects of poor and short sleep on glucose metabolism and obesity risk. *Nat Rev Endocrinol.* 2009;5:253–261.
52. Klein S, Wadden T, Sugerman HJ. AGA technical review on obesity. *Gastroenterology* 2002;123:882–932.
53. Brochu M, Tchernof A, Dionne IJ, et al. What are the physical characteristics associated with a normal metabolic profile despite a high level of obesity in postmenopausal women? *J Clin Endocrinol Metab.* 2001;86:1020–1025.
54. Ferrannini E, Natali A, Bell P, et al. Insulin resistance and hypersecretion in obesity. European Group for the Study of Insulin Resistance (EGIR). *J Clin Invest.* 1997;100:1166–1173.
55. Wildman RP, Muntner P, Reynolds K, et al. The obese without cardiometabolic risk factor clustering and the normal weight with cardiometabolic risk factor clustering: prevalence and correlates of 2 phenotypes among the US population (NHANES 1999–2004). *Arch Intern Med.* 2008;168:1617–1624.
56. Karelis AD. Metabolically healthy but obese individuals. *Lancet.* 2008;372:1281–1283.
57. Stefan N, Kantartzis K, Machann J, et al. Identification and characterization of metabolically benign obesity in humans. *Arch Intern Med.* 2008;168:1609–1616.
58. Kramer CK, Zinman B, Retnakaran R. Are metabolically healthy overweight and obesity benign conditions?: a systematic review and meta-analysis. *Ann Intern Med.* 2013;159:758–769.

59. Bell JA, Kivimaki M, Hamer M. Metabolically healthy obesity and risk of incident type 2 diabetes: a meta-analysis of prospective cohort studies. *Obes Rev.* 2014;15:504–515.
60. National Institutes of Health, National Heart, Lung and Blood Institute and North American Association for the Study of Obesity. *Practical Guide to the Identification, Evaluation, and Treatment of Overweight and Obesity in Adults.* 2000. NIH publication number 00-4084.
61. Jensen MD, Ryan DH, Donato KA, et al. Executive summary: guidelines (2013) for the management of overweight and obesity in adults: A Report of the American College of Cardiology/American Heart Association Task Force on Practice Guidelines and The Obesity Society Published by The Obesity Society and American College of Cardiology/American Heart Association Task Force on Practice Guidelines. Based on a systematic review from the The Obesity Expert Panel, 2013. *Obesity.* 2014;22 (Suppl 2):S5–S39.
62. Tsai AG, Wadden TA. The evolution of very-low-calorie diets: an update and meta-analysis. *Obesity.* 14:1283–1293.
63. Harris JA, Benedict FG. Standard basal metabolism constants for physiologists and clinicians. In: *A Biometric Study of Basal Metabolism in Man.* [The Carnegie Institute of Washington. Publication 279]. Philadelphia: JB Lippincott; 1919.
64. World Health Organization. WHO/FAO/UNO report: energy and protein requirements. WHO Technical Report Series No. 724; 1985
65. Foster GD, Wyatt HR, Hill JO, et al. A randomized trial of a low-carbohydrate diet for obesity. *N Engl J Med.* 2003;348:2082–2090.
66. Samaha FF, Iqbal N, Seshadri P, et al. A low-carbohydrate as compared with a low-fat diet in severe obesity. *N Engl J Med.* 2003;348:2074–2081.
67. Brehm BJ, Seeley RJ, Daniels SR, et al. A randomized trial comparing a very low carbohydrate diet and a calorie-restricted low fat diet on body weight and cardiovascular risk factors in healthy women. *J Clin Endocrinol Metab.* 2003;88:1617–1623.
68. Foster GD, Wyatt HR, Hill JO, et al. Effects of low-carbohydrate and low-fat diets on body weight and coronary heart disease risk factors: a two-year, multi-center randomized trial. *Ann Intern Med.* 2010;153:147–157.
69. Boden G, Sargrad K, Homko C, et al. Effect of a low-carbohydrate diet on appetite, blood glucose levels, and insulin resistance in obese patients with type 2 diabetes. *Ann Intern Med.* 2005;142:403–411.
70. Shai I, Schwarzfuchs D, Henkin Y, et al. Dietary Intervention Randomized Controlled Trial (DIRECT) Group. Weight loss with a low-carbohydrate, Mediterranean, or low-fat diet. *N Engl J Med.* 2008;359:229–241.
71. Sacks FM, Bray GA, Carey VJ, et al. Comparison of weight-loss diets with different compositions of fat, protein, and carbohydrates. *N Engl J Med.* 2009;360:859–873.
72. Finkelstein EA, Kruger E. Meta- and cost-effectiveness analysis of commercial weight loss strategies [Epub ahead of print]. *Obesity* 2014;22:1942-1951.
73. Tsai AD, Wadden TA. Systematic review: an evaluation of major commercial weight loss programs in the United States. *Ann Intern Med.* 2005;142:156.
74. Schoeller DA, Shay K, Kushner RF. How much physical activity is needed to minimize weight gain in previously obese women? *Am J Clin Nutr.* 1997;66:551–556.
75. Garrow JS, Summerbell CD. Meta-analysis: effect of exercise, with or without dieting, on the body composition of overweight subjects. *Eur J Clin Nutr.* 1995;49:1–10.
76. Villareal DT, Chode S, Parimi N, et al. Weight loss, exercise, or both and physical function in obese older adults. *N Engl J Med.* 2011;364:1218–1229.
77. Munro JF, MacCuish AC, Wilson EM, et al. Comparison of continuous and intermittent anorectic therapy in obesity. *Br Med J.* 1968;1:352–356.
78. Aronne LJ, Wadden TA, Peterson C, et al. Evaluation of phentermine and topiramate versus phentermine/topiramate extended-release in obese adults. *Obesity.* 2013;21:2163–2171.
79. Padwal R, Li SK, Lau DC. Long-term pharmacotherapy for overweight and obesity: a systematic review and meta-analysis of randomized controlled trials. *Int J Obes Relat Metab Disord.* 2003;27:1437–1446.
80. Li Z, Maglione M, Tu W, et al. Meta-analysis: pharmacologic treatment of obesity. Ann Intern Med. 2005;142:532–546.
81. Torgerson JS, Hauptman J, Boldrin MN, et al. XENical in the Prevention of Diabetes in Obese Subjects (XENDOS) study: a randomized study of orlistat as an adjunct to lifestyle changes for the prevention of type 2 diabetes in obese patients. *Diabetes Care.* 2004;27:155–161.

82. Allison DB, Gadde KM, Garvey WT, et al. Controlled-release phentermine/topiramate in severely obese adults: a randomized controlled trial (EQUIP). *Obesity*. 2012;20:330–342.
83. Gadde KM, Allison DB, Ryan DH, et al. Effects of low-dose, controlled-release, phentermine plus topiramate combination on weight and associated comorbidities in overweight and obese adults (CONQUER): a randomized, placebo-controlled, phase 3 trial. *Lancet*. 2011;377:1341–1352.
84. Smith SR, Weissman NJ, Anderson CM, et al. Multicenter, placebo-controlled trial of lorcaserin for weight management. *N Engl J Med*. 2010;363:245–256.
85. Fidler MC, Sanchez M, Raether B, et al. A one-year randomized trial of lorcaserin for weight loss in obese and overweight adults: the BLOSSOM trial. J Clin Endocrinol Metab. 2011;96:3067–3077.
86. O'Neil PM, Smith SR, Weissman NJ, et al. Shanahan WR. Randomized placebo-controlled clinical trial of lorcaserin for weight loss in type 2 diabetes mellitus: the BLOOM-DM study. *Obesity*. 2012;20:1426–1436.
87. Hollander P, Gupta AK, Greenway F, et al., COR-Diabetes Study Group. Effects of naltrexone sustained-release/bupropion sustained-release combination therapy on body weight and glycemic parameters in overweight and obese patients with type 2 diabetes. *Diabetes Care*. 2013;36:4022–9.
88. Greenway FL, Fujioka K, Plodkowski RA, et al., for the COR-I Study Group. Effect of naltrexone plus bupropion on weight loss in overweight and obese adults (COR-I): a multicenter, randomised, double-blind, placebocontrolled, phase 3 trial. *Lancet*. 2010; 376:595–605.
89. Apovian CM, Aronne L, Rubino D, et al. COR-II Study Group. *Obesity*. 2013;21:935–43.
90. Wadden TA, Foreyt J, Foster GD, et al. Weight loss with Naltrexone SR/Bupropion SR combination therapy as an adjunct to behavior modification: The COR-BMOD Trial. *Obesity*. 2011;19:110–120.
91. Bradley D, Magkos F, Klein S. Effects of bariatric surgery on glucose homeostasis and type 2 diabetes. *Gastroenterology*. 2012;143:897–912.
92. Sjöström L, Peltonen M, Jacobson P, et al. Bariatric surgery and long-term cardiovascular events. *JAMA*. 2012;307:56–65.
93. Buchwald H, Avidor Y, Braunwald E, et al. Bariatric surgery: a systematic review and meta-analysis. *JAMA*. 2004;292:1724–1737.
94. Boza C, Gamboa C, Salinas J, et al. Laparoscopic Roux-en-Y gastric bypass versus laparoscopic sleeve gastrectomy: a case-control study and 3 years of follow-up. *Surg Obes Relat Dis*. 2012;8:243–249.
95. Courcoulas AP, Christian NJ, Belle SH, et al. Longitudinal Assessment of Bariatric Surgery (LABS) Consortium. Weight change and health outcomes at 3 years after bariatric surgery among individuals with severe obesity. *JAMA*. 2013;310:2416–2425.
96. Carlsson LM, Peltonen M, Ahlin S, et al. Bariatric surgery and prevention of type 2 diabetes in Swedish obese subjects. *N Engl J Med*. 2012;367:695–704.
97. Dixon JB, O'Brien PE, Playfair J, et al. Adjustable gastric banding and conventional therapy for type 2 diabetes: a randomized controlled trial. *JAMA*. 2008;299:316–323.
98. Schauer PR, Kashyap SR, Wolski K, et al. Bariatric surgery versus intensive medical therapy in obese patients with diabetes. N Engl J Med. 2012;366:1567–1576.
99. Mingrone G, Panunzi S, De Gaetano A, et al. Bariatric surgery versus conventional medical therapy for type 2 diabetes. *N Engl J Med*. 2012;366:1577–1585.
100. Ikramuddin S, Korner J, Lee WJ, et al. Roux-en-Y gastric bypass vs intensive medical management for the control of type 2 diabetes, hypertension, and hyperlipidemia: the Diabetes Surgery Study randomized clinical trial. *JAMA*. 2013;309:2240–2249.
101. Mechanick JI, Youdim A, Jones DB, et al. American Association of Clinical Endocrinologists; Obesity Society; American Society for Metabolic & Bariatric Surgery. Clinical practice guidelines for the perioperative nutritional, metabolic, and nonsurgical support of the bariatric surgery patient—2013 update: cosponsored by American Association of Clinical Endocrinologists, The Obesity Society, and American Society for Metabolic & Bariatric Surgery. *Obesity*. 2013;21 (Suppl 1): S1–27.

15 Nutritional Considerations in Chronic Diseases

GENERAL CONSIDERATIONS
Cachexia

Many chronic diseases are associated with weight loss and decreased muscle mass, although the relationships of these changes to alterations in nutrition vs. the underlying disease process are difficult if not impossible to separate. Cachexia has been variably defined, but it is a syndrome of multifactorial cause, characterized by decreased body weight, loss of muscle and fat, and increased protein catabolism (1). Because cachexia is the result of the underlying disease and disease-related metabolic changes, its phenotype differs from that of starvation, although losses in body weight and muscle mass may be similar (Table 15-1). Cachexia is characterized by increased protein degradation, even in the presence of adequate nutrient intake.

Anorexia frequently accompanies the cachexia of cancer. Proposed mediators of cachexia have included hypothalamic serotonin, leptin, proinflammatory cytokines (tumor necrosis factor-α [TNF-α], interleukin-1 [IL-1], IL-6, interferon-γ [IFN-γ]), prostaglandins, and tumor-specific products (2). Many of these circulating catabolic factors can be produced by either the host or tumor itself. However, none of these has been documented to be causative in the anorexia of cancer (3). Starvation is characterized by an excessive loss of nutrients, but cachexia is associated with the acute-phase responses that are part of underlying inflammatory or malignant conditions. Thus, feeding does not reverse the macronutrient deficiency. Body compartment analysis in cachexia, in contrast to starvation, shows increases in resting energy expenditure, protein degradation, and serum insulin and cortisol levels (4). These changes lead to increases in urinary nitrogen loss, skeletal protein breakdown, and lipolysis and to glucose intolerance. Despite aggressive caloric replacement, lean body mass decreases in critically ill patients with underlying infection or tumor (3).

Sarcopenia

Sarcopenia is defined as an "age-associated loss of skeletal muscle mass and function" (5). Muscle mass can be lost alone or in conjunction with increased fat mass (Table 15-1). The causes of sarcopenia include chronic disease, disuse, altered endocrine function, and/or nutritional

TABLE 15-1 Nutritional Alterations in Starvation, Cachexia, and Sarcopenia

Variable	Starvation	Cachexia	Sarcopenia
Body weight	↓	0/↓	↓
Caloric intake	↓↓↓	↓↓	↓
Total energy expenditure	↓↓	↓	↓
Resting energy expenditure	↓↓	↑↑	↓
Muscle mass & function	↓↓	↓	↓
Protein synthesis	↓↓↓	↓↑	↓
Muscle protein synthesis	↓	↑	↑
Protein degradation	↓↓↓	↑↑↑	↑↓
Body fat	↓↓↓	↓↓	↑
Insulin resistance	↑↓	↑	↑
Serum cortisol	↑↓	↑↑	↑↓

Adapted from Kotler DP. Cachexia. *Ann Intern Med*. 2000;133:622; Evans WJ. Skeletal muscle loss: cachexia, sarcopenia, and inactivity. *Am J Clin Nutr*. 2010;91(Suppl):1123S.

deficiency. While cachexia always has loss of muscle mass, not all elderly subjects with sarcopenia have cachexia or even chronic disease. Loss of muscle strength is a consistent feature of subjects with sarcopenia, with loss of strength occurring at a rate of 3% to 4%/year for men and 2.5% to 3%/year for women (6). However, the definitions of sarcopenia and cachexia are working definitions of syndromes, as the etiology is usually multifactorial and variable from patient to patient. Furthermore, most patients will progress from muscle wasting to altered muscle function to a more severe clinical status with loss of weight, but there are no clear cutoff values to define each step in this progression (7). Muscle function can also be defined by strength (e.g., hand grip), power (e.g., leg extension), or overall physical performance (e.g., usual gait speed). It is thought that 5% to 13% of elderly subjects age 60 to 70 would qualify for sarcopenia. Because the clinical syndrome definitions are not precise and the etiologies are many, the treatment of decreased muscle mass and function has been difficult to validate, and the role of nutrition in this treatment program is even more open to question. The only certain role for nutritional supplementation is for malnutrition due to decreased intake and/or absorption of nutrients.

Role of Nutrition in Management of Chronic Diseases with Cachexia and/or Sarcopenia

There are two roles for nutrition in the management of chronic diseases: first, to prevent the disease, and second, to manage it once it is established. The first approach tries to take advantage of epidemiologic dietary associations, especially when the etiology is complex or unknown. These studies lead to prospective intervention studies, but these may not be equivalent to the diet itself or studied in patients who manifest nutritional deficiencies that may have influenced the original epidemiologic association. The second approach is usually focused on stimulating food intake of a balanced diet and reversing any micronutrient deficiencies that develop on the basis of an inadequate intake of food.

There are multiple problems in trying to develop a reasonable evidence base for studies of diet. It is unusual for randomized studies of diet to be accomplished, and when they are, it is not usual for only a single component to be altered. Meta-analyses are often used to "settle" the issue, but in many cases, they are not suitable to do so, either because the entry criteria do not allow inclusion of all the "relevant" papers or because meta-analyses were designed in part to demonstrate areas of uncertainty, not to finalize clinical decisions. In addition, nutrition studies, unlike those using drug interventions, can rarely control or document the nutrient under investigation, making the conduct of meta-analysis of randomized trials even more challenging. These problems are highlighted by two examples. In the first, two Cochrane systematic reviews on nutrition in cardiovascular disease reached largely negative conclusions that have not been endorsed or adopted by expert committees (8). This result may have been complicated by bias on the part of the expert committees, but nonetheless, the results of the meta-analyses have not yet been accepted. In the second example, a large prospective study as part of the Women's Health Initiative have led to disappointment about nutritional intervention for all patients with osteoporosis (9). Although calcium and vitamin D supplementation did achieve a modest improvement in bone-mineral density but without a change in fracture rates, this result was obtained in patients allowed to take at least the dietary reference intake (DRI) for those nutrients. It seems quite possible that patients who were deficient in either nutrient in their diet and/or body stores might have shown a change in fracture rates. Nonetheless, this is an example of a well-designed and large study that demonstrated how difficult it is to document a benefit of "standard" dietary programs across an unselected population.

The above discussion might suggest that providing a defined diet or dietary supplements may not be useful. The value of providing only dietary advice as opposed to advice plus oral nutritional supplements has been reviewed (10). Sixteen trials in patients with illness-related malnutrition were examined, showing that provision of oral supplements led to more energy intake and more weight gain. Once again, however, this systematic review was not designed to provide definitive answers, but forms the background to future large interventional trials.

CANCER
Dietary Guidelines to Minimize Cancer Risk
Much epidemiologic evidence is available to suggest that environmental and dietary factors play a role in the development of carcinomas in a variety of organs (11–13). Individual dietary

components have been examined as part of an effort to compile recommendations for reducing the risk for cancer (Table 15-2). All reports suggest increasing one's intake of fruits, vegetables, and grains and cereals; decreasing one's intake of fatty meats, fats and oils, saturated fats, and refined sugars; and avoiding excessive salt. All reports also suggest maintaining a healthful body weight, engaging in physical activity, and limiting one's intake of alcohol to less than two drinks a day for men, or one for women. Excess body weight and obesity continue to be independent risk factors for cancer in many organs, including those of the gastrointestinal (GI) tract (14). Excessive weight may also be a risk factor for premalignant conditions, such as colorectal adenomas.

The National Research Council of the National Academy of Sciences concluded that the human diet contains anticarcinogens and protective factors, most of which have not been identified. It also contains carcinogens. The precise role of diet in reducing cancer risk is poorly defined, but 30% of cancers may be affected. The recommendations for a prudent diet are included in the reports of the Council (11,13). The recommendations are not novel, and their effectiveness has never been prospectively demonstrated (15,16). There were trends suggesting protection in the study with the low-fat diet for breast cancer if the patients had been followed up for longer than 6 years (15). However, the existing recommendations are sensible guidelines for sound nutrition, and their use can certainly be encouraged (see below and the sections on folate and vitamins C, A, and E in Chapter 6).

Although altering many aspects of the diet at the same time would make the most sense for cancer prevention, such an intervention is not as practical as changing a single component or adding a specific supplement. Many specific foods have been implicated in cancer risk, but although many single studies report quite large effects, the effect size shrinks with meta-analysis (17). There are some suggestions that a global approach may be useful. In the Lyon Diet Heart Study, prospective use of a Mediterranean-type diet (more bread and cereals, more fresh fruit and vegetables, more legumes and fish, less beef and pork, no butter and cream, and replacement with an experimental canola oil margarine) was associated with a reduced cancer death rate in comparison with the step 1 American Heart Association prudent diet (18). Nearly 600 patients with colonic adenomas (part of the European Cancer Prevention [ECP] Intervention Study of calcium and fiber supplementation) completed a dietary questionnaire that identified three patterns: Mediterranean, sweets and snacks, and high fat and proteins (19). In women, the Mediterranean-pattern diet had high consumption of olive oil, vegetables, fruits, fish, and lean meat, and had a reduced adenoma incidence. A review of over 12,000 cases of cancer in Northern Italy between 1983 and 1998 showed a lower relative risk of developing cancers in the digestive tract, breast, urinary tract, and female genital tract (20). However, there is still not enough epidemiologic evidence that change of the entire diet will be protective for cancers (21). Thus, large prospective trials are needed, especially in Mediterranean countries where delivering such a diet would be practical. The issue of the length of such trials is important, as data on the regular use of multivitamins were protective in the Cancer Prevention Study II Nutrition Cohort of 145,260 men and women, but the use had to have occurred more than 10 years before the study began (22). If the lag time to see an effect on cancer prevention is greater than a decade, the existing studies may not be providing us with a complete data set on which to alter the general recommendations in Table 15-2.

American Cancer Society 2012 Guidelines on Nutrition and Physical Activity for Cancer Prevention

The American Cancer Society (ACS) Nutrition and Physical Activity Guidelines Advisory Committee updated the ACS guidelines in 2012 (23) (Table 15-3). These recommendations are more focused on cancer than the general recommendations for healthy populations, especially regarding food preparation and preservation, but the general restrictions regarding the composition of the diet are very similar. In general, the guidelines have been more strategic and less prescriptive than earlier versions.

Additional information for patients regarding diets and cancer can be obtained from the American Cancer Society, 90 Park Avenue, New York, New York 10016 (www.cancer.org), and from the American Institute for Cancer Research, Washington, DC 20069.

Increase Intake of Fruits and Vegetables (The Antioxidant Hypothesis)

The best epidemiologic evidence at present involves foods containing β-carotenes, vitamin A, and vitamin C (24–26) (Table 15-4).

TABLE 15-2 Recommendations to Modify Dietary Components Associated with Reducing the Risk of Cancer (1989–2005)[a]

Report	Veg/Fruit (servings/day)	Starch/Grains (servings/day)	Meat (servings/day)	Fiber (g/day)	CHO (% energy)	Fats/oils (% energy)	Sat/unsat (% energy)	Refined Sugar	Salt (g/day)
US NAS 1989	≥5	≥6	Lean	Yes	>55	<30	<10	Ind	<6
WHO 1990	>400 g	Ind	NS	16–24	50–75	15–30	0–10	0–10	<6
US DHHS 1991	≥5	≥6	NC	Ind	Ind	<30	<10	NC	Mod
CCS 1992	Yes	Yes	NC	Ind	NS	<30	NS	NC	Mod
SO 1993	3+	Ind	↓	>16	<40	<35	<11	<10	4
ESO 1994	5	6	NC	Ind	Ind	<30	<10	NS	6
US ACS 1996	5	3+	Lean	NS	NC	↓	↓	NC	NS
US HR 1996	>5	Ind	<1/week	NS	↑ Complex	No	↓ Animal	↓	Mod
WCRF 1997	5	7	<3 oz/day	38/25 g for M/F	45–65	15–30	Limit animal fat	Limit intake	<6 g
US ACS 2001	5	Whole grains	Lean	NS	NC	30	Limit animal fat	NC	NS
WHO/FAO 2003	>400g	Whole grain esp	NS	>25 g	55–75	15–30	<10 S, <1 trans, 6–10 PUFA	<10	5–6 iodized
USDA/DHHS 2005	>5, all five groups	3 whole grain	Lean meat	Fiber-rich foods	Ind	25–30	<10 SFA, limit trans fat	Limit sugar and sweeteners	<2.3 (1 tsp)

ACS, American Cancer Society; CCS, Canadian Cancer Survey; DHHS, Department of Health and Human Services; ESO, European States Organization; HR, Harvard Report on Cancer Prevention; and, restriction/increase indicated but not quantified; NAS, National Academy of Science; NC, not counted; NS, not stated; SO, Scotland; USDA/DHHS, US Department of Agriculture/Department of Health and Human Services: *Dietary Guidelines for Americans 2005*, Government Printing Office, Washington DC; WCRF, World Cancer Research Fund/American Institute for Cancer Research: *Food, Nutrition and the Prevention of Cancer*, Washington DC; WHO/FAO, World Health Organization: *Diet, Nutrition and the Prevention of Chronic Diseases*, Report of a Joint FAO/WHO Expert Consultation, WHO Technical report Series 916.

[a]The US reports offer recommendations for individuals. The European reports offer percentages of population limits. Adapted from National Research Council, Commission on Life Sciences, Food and Nutrition Board, Committee on Diet and Health. *Diet and Health Implications for Reducing Chronic Disease Risk*. Washington, DC: National Academies Press, 1989, and from Kolonel L, Global Health & Environment Monitor, CECHE (Center for Communications, Health & the Environment) 2006;14:1 (www.ceche.org).

TABLE 15-3   2012 American Cancer Society (ACS) Guidelines on Nutrition and Physical Activity for Cancer Prevention: Recommendations for Individual Choice

Achieve and Maintain a Healthy Weight Throughout Life

Be as lean as possible throughout life without being underweight.

Avoid excess weight gain at all ages. For those who are currently overweight or obese, losing even a small amount of weight has health benefits and is a good place to start.

Engage in regular physical activity and limit consumption of high-calorie foods and beverages as key strategies for maintaining a healthy weight.

Adopt a Physically Active Lifestyle

Adults should engage in at least 150 minutes of moderate-intensity or 75 minutes of vigorous-intensity activity each week, or an equivalent combination preferably spread throughout the week.

Children and adolescents should engage in at least 1 hour of moderate- or vigorous-intensity activity each day, with vigorous activity occurring at least 3 days each week.

Limit sedentary behavior such as sitting, lying down, watching television, or other forms of screen-based entertainment.

Doing some physical activity above usual activities, no matter what one's level of activity, can have many health benefits.

Consume a Healthy Diet, with an Emphasis on Plant Food

Choose foods and beverages in amounts that help achieve and maintain a healthy weight.

Limit consumption of processed meat and red meat.

Eat at least 2.5 cups of vegetables and fruits each day.

Choose whole grains instead of refined grain products.

If You Drink Alcoholic Beverages, Limit Consumption

Drink no more than 1 drink per day for women or 2 drinks per day for men.

Adapted from Kushi LH, Doyle C, McCullough M, et al. American Cancer Society Guidelines on Nutrition and Physical Activity for cancer prevention. *CA Cancer J Clin.* 2012;62:30.

Most of the evidence to support a relationship between diet and cancer (or other chronic disease) prevention comes from consumption of foods, not dietary supplements. There is a substantial body of evidence that a diet rich in fruits and vegetables is important in disease prevention, yet a causal link between these factors has never been established (26). Among the antioxidants, the epidemiologic evidence for β-carotene has been the most complete. A review of carotenoid intake and lung cancer risk in North America and Europe showed that β-carotene intake was not associated with lung cancer, and only β-cryptoxanthin intake was inversely related to lung cancer (27). However, in the Polyp Prevention Trial, baseline dietary intake of α-carotene and vitamin A was inversely related to colorectal polyp recurrence in nonsmokers and nondrinkers (28). This result might be related to healthy lifestyle factors other than the diet. It is also possible that cruciferous vegetables contain other, undefined inhibitors of carcinogens. Most of the data in humans are from case–control and cohort studies showing an inverse correlation between cancer rates and dietary intake or serum vitamin levels, nearly all of them within the normal range.

Intervention trials with these vitamins have not demonstrated a protective effect to date, and in fact β-carotene may increase risk of lung cancer in intervention studies (29). Some of the data suggest prevention, but in general the data are negative, especially when specific interventions are attempted (see Chapter 6 for information on vitamins and Chapter 12 for a discussion of fiber). Some cohort studies continue to suggest a role for vitamin intake, but most do not (30–32). Even when premalignant endpoints are examined, such as colorectal polyps, the data for the role of increased fiber, prospectively provided, are negative (31). The relative risk of pooled data shows a value near unity for all interventions, but the 95% confidence intervals (CIs) are very large. For esophageal cancer, where the pooled risk with β-carotene supplementation is 0.15 and

TABLE 15-4 Epidemiologic Evidence for Associations between Diet, Lifestyle, and Cancer Prevention

Level of Evidence	Decreases Risk	Increases Risk
Convincing	Physical activity (colorectal, breast)	Overweight/obesity (esophagus, colorectal, breast (postmenopausal), endometrium, kidney)
		Alcohol (oral cavity, pharynx, larynx, esophagus, liver, breast)
		Aflatoxin (liver)
		Salted fish, Chinese or Japanese style (nasopharynx)
		Tobacco (lung, oropharynx, esophagus)
		Sedentary life style (colorectal, breast, endometrium)
Possible	Fruits and vegetables (oral cavity, lung, esophagus, stomach, colorectum)	Preserved meat and red meat (colorectum)
		Salt preserved foods and salt itself (stomach)
	Selenium (prostate, colorectum)	Very thermally hot foods and drinks (oral cavity, pharynx, esophagus)
	Folate-containing multivitamins (colorectum)	High-dose antioxidants in susceptible high-risk patients (lung, digestive system)
Insufficient	Soy components, ω-3 fatty acids, carotenoids, vitamins B_2, B_6, folate, C, D, E, calcium, zinc, nonnutrient plant components (e.g., flavonoids, isoflavones, allium compounds)	Animal fats, heterocyclic amines, polycyclic aromatic hydrocarbons, nitrosamines
		Sugar (stomach, colorectal)

Data from Williams MT, Hord NG. The role of dietary factors in cancer prevention: beyond fruits and vegetables. *Nutr Clin Pract.* 2005;20:451.

apparently protective, the 95% CIs were 0.01 to 3.72 (29). The addition of the antioxidants vitamin E, β-carotene, and vitamin C has been extensively studied in prevention of prostate cancer as part of the Prostate, Lung, Colorectal, and Ovarian (PLCO) Cancer Screening Trial (33). There is not strong evidence for an effect of high-dose supplementation in 1,338 cases of prostate cancer among 29,361 men, although vitamin E supplements in smokers and β-carotene supplements in those with low dietary intake were associated with reduced risk of disease. The effect of supplementation with selenium (200 μg per day) has been studied over a decade in the Nutritional Prevention of Cancer Trial. No effect was found on the incidence of cancers of the lung, colon and rectum, and skin, but there was a protective effect on prostate cancer in males with a lower baseline plasma selenium concentration (34).

In vitro and in vivo animal studies continue to support the antioxidant theory of cancer prevention, although the human data are much less supportive (35). The current debate is whether a "whole foods" concept or single agents/foods are better for cancer prevention, although the evidence supports the former concept somewhat better (36). Another issue that is being addressed is whether any strategy is appropriate for the general population or for a specific subset of subjects, although such subsets have not been consistently defined. These concepts have been supported by work on antioxidants and prevention of GI cancers (37). The sum of studies does not support the role for antioxidants in prevention of GI cancers in the general population, but some evidence suggests that they may play a role in populations at high risk for gastric and esophageal cancers.

Drink Alcoholic Beverages Only in Moderation

The carcinogenic effect of alcohol is associated with a large intake, especially when combined with cigarette smoking. Intake should be limited to no more than two drinks per day for men and one for women. One drink is equal to 12 oz of beer, 5 oz of wine, or 1.5 oz of 80-proof distilled liquor.

Unresolved Issues in Cancer Prevention

Calcium and Vitamin D

The epidemiologic data suggesting an association are reasonable. These two components are intimately associated, and separating them may prove difficult. Addition of calcium and vitamin D supplements did not alter the risk for colorectal cancer (CRC) (38). In the Poly Prevention Trial, no association was found between adenoma recurrence and dietary calcium or vitamin D intake (39). Studies suggest that intake of vitamin D above the usual recommended dietary intake of 200 to 400 IU may be necessary to decrease the risk of colorectal (and other) cancer (40). Also, vitamin D status at baseline may influence the course of the disease. This is a recurrent theme in cancer chemoprevention, that is, identification of a group most likely to respond to nutrient intervention.

A meta-analysis of 12 population-based studies found an inverse relationship of 25(OH) D levels with all-cause mortality, with a pooled HR of 0.92 (CI 0.89 to 0.05) for a 20 nmol/L increase in 25(OH)D levels (41). The potential mechanism for such an association is the finding that low vitamin D status has been linked to a variety of chronic diseases, including hypertension, cardiovascular disease, type 2 diabetes (42), and several types of cancer. However, a meta-analysis of 3 randomized controlled trials (RCTs) and 28 observational studies for cancer outcomes only suggested a reduction in CRC risk, but no effect for prostate or breast cancer (43). Every 10 nmol/L increase in blood 25(OH)D levels accounted for a 6% decrease in CRC risk, but higher blood levels might be associated with an increase in cancer risk. Most participants were elderly women, so even these tepid results cannot be extrapolated to the general population. A separate analysis of the breast cancer data showed no dose response, but suggested that the lowest risk was associated with a vitamin D intake of 400 IU/day and serum vitamin D levels of approximately 30 ng/mL (44). In contrast to earlier reports, no association was found between vitamin D levels and bladder cancer (45). The data overall are not sufficiently robust to make recommendations on the role of benefit or harm of supplemental D in prevention of cancer.

Meat Consumption

There is a positive relationship between meat consumption and the risk of CRC (46). An even larger study in 478,040 adults in the European EPIC study showed similar findings, but when controlled for covariates, showed significance only for processed meats and not red meat (47). Yet another study showed no relationship after following 45,496 women for a decade (48). It seems safe to conclude that there is some relationship between meat intake and CRC, but the data are not strong enough to recommend a change in diet, or if so, what change. Some experts recommend a conservative compromise, a modest meat intake as part of an overall dietary strategy, replacing meat protein (especially processed and well-done meats) with that from fish, nuts, poultry, and legumes (49). In fact, the relationship between meat intake and lung cancer appears from observational studies to depend on the type of meat consumed, with red meat increasing the risk by approximately 30%, and poultry decreasing it by approximately 10% (50). The roles for cooking technique, meat mutagens, and heme iron are still obscure. It is still unclear, however, what the relationship is between high consumption of fish and marine fatty acids and the risk of cancer (51). Although higher concentrations of chemical carcinogens have been recorded during preparation of poultry and fish meat, the CRC risk is not increased (52). Countries with low beef intake have low risks of CRC (e.g., Japan and Korea), but post-WWII undercooked beef consumption was associated with an increase in the incidence of CRC. This risk has been considered possibly to be related to contaminating bovine viruses, although this remains just a hypothesis (52). However, along with changes in consumption of beef are changes in other dietary components, such as resistant starch, a component that has been suggested to have a role in prevention of CRC (53).

Deficiencies in insulin-like growth factor 1 (IGF-1) in mice and humans produce major decreases in age-related diseases, including cancer. Protein restriction reduces IGF-1 levels and its corresponding growth-promoting activities. One population of 8,381 adults age above 50 years from NHANES III was studied to identify those with a high protein intake (20% or more of calories from protein), a moderate intake (10% to 19%), or a low intake (<10%). Subjects with a high protein intake had a fourfold increase in cancer death risk during 18 years of follow-up, but this increased risk was nearly abolished if the proteins were plant-derived, or the subjects were aged 65 or older (54). IGF-1 levels were correlated with the degree of protein intake. These are the first data suggesting that a low protein intake during middle age might be important for preventing cancer, possibly by regulation of circulating IGF-1. This would translate into following the minimum requirement recommended by the Food and Nutrition Board (0.7 to 0.8 g of protein/kg body weight/day), in contrast with the observed intake of adults on a Western diet (1.0 to 1.3g/kg/day). This study confirms the concept that not all calories are the same in regard to cancer risk, but the lack of the effect of low protein in older subjects is unexplained. While it appears sensible to limit protein intake to no more than is necessary, this result will need to be replicated before firm recommendations can be made.

Diets low in fat may also protect against premalignant conditions, such as colorectal adenomas (55). Processed meat consumption in the large European Prospective Investigation into Cancer & Nutrition (EPIC) was associated with increased all-cause mortality, most of which was due to cardiovascular disease and cancer (56). One problem with meat epidemiologic studies is the imprecision with which the databases can identify red or processed meat, so the exact degree of association, if real, is often not clear. Another confounder of such studies is the degree to which trans-fatty acids (TFAs) have replaced animal fat in the diets. Biodegraded TFAs from ruminant-derived foods (beef, lamb, dairy) are associated with increased cardiovascular diseases and cancer (57). Consumption of high amounts of TFAs from all sources (hydrogenated vegetable oils and ruminant fat) is also associated with premalignant colorectal adenomas (58). These findings are reinforced by a lower all-cause mortality rate in patients with cardiovascular disease on a Mediterranean-style diet (59). While none of these associations have yet been shown by prospective studies to be causal, more associations continue to appear between Mediterranean-style (low meat) diets and other clinical outcomes, such as minimal cognitive impairment (60). Randomized clinical trials will be needed to resolve the causal relationship of these associations, before recommendations can be supported and implemented with confidence.

Polyphenols

Polyphenols contain more than one phenol ring and include flavonoids. In tea, catechins comprise the majority of the polyphenols. Green tea is steamed or pan-fried, preserving the catechins, whereas black tea is dried first and then fermented, converting the catechins to other polyphenols with different properties. A cup of black tea contains 24 to 40 mg of catechins (166 to 193 mg of polyphenols), but a cup of green tea has up to 200 mg of catechins. Mean polyphenol intake in the United States is 1.1 g per day (100 to 2000 mg range) (61). The literature is full of publication bias with no large trials (62,63); larger and better studies are needed. The amount of green tea needed for benefit, if any, is not known. Ingestion of 6 to 10 cups has been suggested (64), but other dietary differences between Western and Japanese or Chinese diets are so great that no conclusions can be made.

There are a large number of phytochemicals, mostly polyphenols, for which cell and animal data suggest a role as inhibitors of cell proliferation. These include genistein (soy), resveratrol (red grapes, peanuts, berries, red wine), epigallocatechin gallate (green tea), lycopene (tomato), capsaicin (chili pepper), bromelain (pineapple), curcumin (turmeric), indole-3-carbinol (cruciform vegetables), D-limonene (citrus fruits), and diallyl sulfide (garlic) (65). Nearly all of the work suggesting a role in control of cell proliferation and/or cancer comes from cell or animal studies. Moreover, nonhuman primates do not demonstrate carcinogenicity for many of the compounds that produce tumors in rodents (66), so the value of anticancer activity of compounds in rodents is difficult to translate to humans. On the other hand, metabolites of ellagitannins produced by intestinal flora yield urolithins, which persist for a long time in the pig and humans, due largely to an enterohepatic circulation (67). Thus, it is possible that this group of phytochemicals could have a prolonged biological role. The most common phytochemicals associated with cancer risk in epidemiological studies are phytoestrogens and carotenoids, although phytosterols, isothiocyanates, and chlorophyll have also been studied. Most reviews report no association between individual phytochemicals and cancer risk (68). Berries contain a complex mixture of flavonoids and other antioxidants. Studies, mostly in animals, suggest a protective role for berries against cancer and cardiovascular disease (69). Many polyphenolic compounds have been found in wine and beer, including resveratrol, but the data suggesting a possible role in cancer prevention of these beverages is compounded by factors such as diet, smoking, hormone-replacement therapy, and family history (70). Thus, the available data do not support any recommendations regarding the role of any phytochemicals in prevention of human cancers (see further discussion on polyphenol supplementation in Chapter 8).

Folate

Mandatory folate fortification to prevent neural tube defects has produced increased serum folate levels, but the data are still mixed on whether folate supplements help or worsen cancers (71). The rationale for a protective role of folate in cancer is based on the effects of low cellular folate, including DNA strand breaks, genomic instability, and impaired DNA repair, effects that might lead to mutations. The World Cancer Research Fund (WCRF) report of 2007 showed a significant protection of dietary folate for pancreatic cancer, with a suggestion for esophageal cancer (72). The data for CRC are more mixed. Studies using supplemental folate are examined by meta-analysis, there is a borderline significant increase in frequency of cancer in the folic acid–supplemented group, but only prostate cancer showed an increased risk (73). Suggestive evidence seems to be present, therefore, for a U-shaped curve, with increased cancer risk at low and very high intake. Thus, the data support the use of dietary folate to prevent the increased cancers associated with folate deficiency, and there is reason to avoid folate supplementation of more than 1 mg/day. Similar hypotheses have been suggested for vitamin B_{12} ingestion, because of the presence of transcobalamin receptors on tumor cells, but only limited and not yet reproducible human data are available to support any association with cancer at high intake levels of vitamin B_{12} (74).

Diagnosis of Nutritional Abnormalities in Cancer Patients

Nonspecific Findings

A number of findings in patients with advanced cancer are related to nutrition but are often difficult to treat with specific nutritional intervention. The most prevalent of these are weight loss and a decreased intake of food (75). Abnormal carbohydrate metabolism is characterized by glucose intolerance and insulin resistance. Body fat tends to become more depleted relative to protein loss, and lipolysis is increased. Protein turnover in the entire body increases as the disease progresses, with a reduced fractional synthetic rate in muscle. The protein kinetics in cancer patients with weight loss resembles those in persons with trauma and infection; patients with these clinical conditions cannot easily be brought into positive nitrogen balance, even with total parenteral nutrition (TPN). When sepsis develops, serum levels of TNF increase, but high levels, such as are seen in childhood leukemias, have not been reproducibly found in patients with solid tumors (2). Up to 80% of patients with advanced malignancies develop the cancer cachexia syndrome (CCS), characterized by depletion of energy and muscle (76). However, unlike the case in starvation, the weight loss with CSS cannot be reversed by provision of nutrients alone.

There are multiple factors that produce unintentional weight loss in cancer patients. These include obstruction of the GI tract, malabsorption due to hormones (e.g., VIP) or nutritional deficiency (e.g., vitamin D), and anorexia. Anorexia can be related to altered taste, depression, or altered metabolism of substances that affect appetite, especially hormones (e.g., ghrelin, leptin) or neuropeptides (e.g., neuropeptide Y) (75). The hormones synthesized by some tumors cause clinical syndromes that appear to be nutritionally based (e.g., weight loss, bone disease) but are not. These include carcinoid syndrome, Zollinger–Ellison syndrome, hypercalcemia, and oncogenic osteomalacia secondary to renal phosphate wasting and decreased levels of plasma dihydroxyvitamin D, parathyroid hormone, and calcium. These syndromes must be identified and the manifestations of increased hormone production treated with available (nonnutritional) methods.

Nutritional Management of Patients with Malignancy

The first thing that must be done is to identify weight loss early enough so that intervention might have a chance to be effective (77). Nutrition screening involves gathering data about height, weight, weight change, and stage of disease and comorbid conditions (76) (see also Chapter 5). Evidence of increased inflammation at the time of admission to hospital may predict an increase in mortality, and provide an explanation for nonnutrient-related causes of weight loss. The modified Glasgow Prognostic Score has been used for this purpose, with a cutoff value of 10 mg/L for C-reactive protein, and an albumin level of 35 g/L (3).

Providing dietary advice alone is not sufficient, and the data suggest that dietary supplements are needed as part of the program to maintain good nutrition (10). Many studies have shown that a loss of body weight or lean body mass is associated with an increase in mortality. However, no data indicate that wasting is the cause of death or that nutritional support reverses wasting. It is just as likely that wasting is a measure of disease severity. The use of nutritional support does not improve the condition of patients with cancer (78,79) or AIDS (80). A conference examining the current evidence concluded that the routine use of short-term enteral or parenteral feeding does not decrease complications or mortality in patients with cancer, and that it does not reverse wasting syndrome in patients with HIV infection if decreased food intake alone is not the cause of wasting (80). Despite the hope that formal nutrition assessment would identify patients at risk for nutrient-related complications, this approach has not been validated. Moreover, the link between identification of such patients and improvement with nutrient provision is also lacking (76). Thus, the only guideline approved by ASPEN is to screen to identify patients with cancer who might benefit from more formal assessment.

Oral nutritional intervention in malnourished cancer patients does not lead to significant improvements in weight and energy intake (81). However, a few studies show that when nutritional intervention is individualized, a significant improvement in long-term prognosis can be demonstrated, as in the case of CRC (82). Recommendations for nutrition support perioperatively are reserved only for patients who are moderately or severely malnourished, and who cannot take nutrients orally (83). Similar recommendations are included in the guidelines for nutrition support therapy during anticancer treatment in adults (84). The use of immune-enhancing enteral formulas is also recommended (containing glutamine, arginine, nucleic acids, and essential fatty acids), but studies using these formulas have shown mostly improved immune parameters and "soft" clinical outcomes such as length of hospital stay, but some have shown decreased infection rate (see discussion later in this chapter).

Many attempts have been made to alter anorexia and cachexia pharmacologically with steroids, antiserotoninergics (cyproheptadine), and hydrazine sulfate, but these have not been successful. The ideal agent should have sustained effects on the appetite, lead to repletion of body cell mass, and have few adverse effects on the host or on tumor therapy. None of the available agents comes close to this ideal profile. The progestational agents megestrol acetate and dihydroxyprogesterone acetate inconstantly improve appetite (3) (see later discussion in this chapter) and increase weight, but the weight gain represents increases in fat, not fat-free tissue. Both these agents produce side effects, including venous thrombosis and peripheral edema, the latter finding supporting the observation that the weight gain does not represent an increase in lean tissue mass. Growth hormone has not yet been shown to be useful in managing cachexia. However, anabolic steroids (e.g., 20 mg of oxandrolone per day in conjunction with a high intake of protein and physical therapy) do increase fat-free mass (4,85). Although inhibition of proinflammatory cytokines has not been shown to increase weight, such treatment may decrease protein breakdown and be clinically useful. For example, the use of thalidomide in HIV-infected patients being treated for tuberculosis can promote weight gain (4), and 200 mg per day produced weight gain in patients with advanced pancreatic cancer, but no change in survival (86). Thus, nutrition may not be a critical variable in advanced cancer, but improved nutrition may contribute to quality of life. Preliminary studies of a combination of a progestational agent and nonsteroidal anti-inflammatory drugs have reported some success, but no recommendation can be made from such early data. The administration of 6 g of eicosapentaenoic acid per day or 2 g of fish oil (FO) per day appeared to stabilize the weight of patients with cancer cachexia when added to a protein- and energy-dense diet (87).

Nutritional intervention is sometimes appropriate when a specific cancer causes a clinical syndrome or problem that can be reversed. Most often, calories or fluid is provided when oral intake becomes limited, either by the cancer itself or by the side effects of medication. In such situations, nutritional intervention may resolve the immediate problem, but in most instances, the effect on the eventual outcome is small. The metabolic alterations caused by the tumor

TABLE 15-5 Nutritional Consequences of Cancer and Its Treatment

Problem	Pathophysiology	Nutritional intervention
Weight loss	Decreased intake	Table foods, calorie supplements
Nausea	Multifactorial	Encourage oral intake, antiemetics limited except at chemotherapy
Enterocutaneous fistula	Fluid/electrolyte loss	Replacement, orally if possible
Protein-losing enteropathy	Lymphatic blockage	Low-fat diet
Anemia	Blood loss (iron), ↓ intake (folate)	Iron, folate supplements, orally if possible
Abdominal radiation	Diarrhea, malabsorption	Opiates as needed
Oral/mediastinal radiation	Ulcers, dysphagia, stricture	Full liquid diets, avoid TPN or gastrostomy, if possible
Vagotomy	Steatorrhea	Limit fat intake
Gastrectomy	Loss of reservoir, intrinsic factor, dumping syndrome	Small meals, antidumping diet, vitamin B_{12} supplement
Ileal resection	↓ Bile salt pool, bile salt/fatty acid diarrhea	Low fat intake, Ca/Mg supplements, cholestyramine
Ileostomy/colostomy	↓ Salt, fluid absorption	Replace orally, if possible
Pancreatectomy	↓ Pancreatic enzymes	Limit fat intake
Corticosteroids	Salt retention	Limit salt intake
Chemotherapy	Nausea, diarrhea, anorexia	None, use serotonin-receptor antagonists
Surgery	↓ Catabolism in severely malnourished patients	Limited benefit (up to 10% ↓ survival) of TPN given perioperatively

TPN, total parenteral nutrition.

usually blunt or prevent the effects of nutritional intervention. Thus, nutritional intervention must be undertaken with a full understanding on the part of both patient and physician of the limited goals of such therapy. Table 15-5 outlines some of the more common nutritionally related problems that develop in cancer patients.

A frustrating situation is created when decreased food intake, vomiting, weight loss, and chronic fluid loss develop in a patient undergoing chemotherapy. With a malnourished patient, there is often little choice but to intervene, provided the intervention does not create a distasteful situation (e.g., gastrostomy) that will continue after the course of chemotherapy is over. A meta-analysis of 12 randomized studies of normally nourished patients receiving chemotherapy showed no benefit of TPN (88). Even though enteral feeding causes fewer complications than TPN does, it is unlikely that enteral nutrition (EN) would produce a different long-term result. In severely malnourished patients who are undergoing major surgery, analysis of the available data suggests a very modest improvement in survival (~10%) when TPN is given perioperatively (80).

Nutritional Management of Treatment-induced GI Mucositis

The mucosa of the mouth and GI tract turns over relatively rapidly, and is at risk for being damaged by radiation or chemotherapy used to treat cancers, when no specific tumor target can be identified. Mucositis is a troublesome complication, because the symptoms are those of pain and inability to eat. Many treatments have been tried with the view to replace nutrients that will help to preserve mucosal cell mass, or help it to regenerate. Glutamine has been used in large doses (1 to 2 g per m^2 intravenously, or 8 to 30 g per day orally) as it has been suggested that glutamine supply may be limited in acute stress. A review of the literature from 1980 to 2003 revealed some instances where glutamine improved either mouth pain or diarrhea, but not in all studies (89). Some double-blind randomized studies showed a protective effect after radiation on the symptoms of mucositis by α-tocopherol 400 mg (90) and of zinc sulfate 50 mg as elemental zinc t.i.d. (91). However, most studies are small (<50 patients). A subsequent review could not support the evidence in favor of glutamine, but does provide data supporting the use of *Lactobacillus* spp.

for prevention of chemoradiation treatment–induced diarrhea (92). Placebo-controlled larger studies are needed to know if any of these nutritional supplements will be of value in managing treatment-related mucositis.

HIV INFECTION
Weight Loss: Scope of the Problem

At the start of the AIDS epidemic, weight loss and malnutrition were commonly seen, and careful nutritional assessment and therapy were considered essential to aid recovery. AIDS and its complications remain a national concern and a major priority in health-care management. Patients infected with HIV are still malnourished, and the causes of protein–energy malnutrition in patients with AIDS are multiple. Wasting is usually defined according to weight loss as mild (<5%), moderate (6% to 10%), or severe (>10%). Weight loss and wasting still occur in patients who are treated successfully with Highly Active Antiretroviral Therapy (HAART), including those who respond or fail on HAART. About 18% of patients report a body weight of less than 10%, and 21% a loss of less than 5% (93). About 8% of patients had a BMI less than 18, the cutoff for malnutrition. The loss in weight appears to be a combination of lean body and fat mass. Generalized malnutrition may explain some of the immune dysfunction, as more protein is lost during acute periods of weight loss than could be predicted from starvation alone (94).

Etiology of Nutritional Deficiency in Patients with HIV Infection

A person's nutritional status represents a balance of caloric and nutrient intake, absorption or malabsorption, and energy expenditure, which are altered by hormonal and metabolic factors. Weight loss is the most frequent finding associated with HIV infection. Weight loss may be caused by inadequate oral intake, intestinal malabsorption, altered metabolism, or a combination of these factors (93). Major factors that predict wasting in HIV-positive patients are heavy alcohol use, cocaine or crack use, and protease inhibitor treatment (95).

A loss of appetite may be caused by myriad reasons, including systemic infection and fever, depression, and side effects of medication. Alterations in taste sensation resulting from medications or oral infections may decrease salivation and appetite. Ulcerative gastritis or duodenitis also may cause anorexia. Nausea, vomiting, anorexia, abdominal discomfort, or diarrhea may compound the loss of appetite. These symptoms may be secondary to drugs or to the underlying medical process. The intake of food may be decreased by a complete loss of appetite, early satiety, or fear of pain or diarrhea. Women are more vulnerable to inadequate intake than men, explained in part by lower socioeconomic status, particularly in former or current intravenous drug users (92). Because lower intake occurs in about one-third of women, and can be explained by socioeconomic, not clinical, factor, early recognition of these concerns is important in preventing malnourishment.

Causes of weight loss other than decreased intake still occur in the HAART era, but are less common than formerly. Oral pain and discomfort can be secondary to oral candidiasis, oral herpes, cytomegalovirus (CMV) infection, aphthous ulcers, oral hairy leukoplakia, or oropharyngeal bulky tumors of Kaposi's sarcoma or non-Hodgkin lymphoma. HIV–associated gingivitis and HIV–associated periodontitis can be rapidly destructive and may resist therapy. Esophageal odynophagia and dysphagia may be caused by ulceration from CMV, herpes simplex virus (HSV), or candidal infection. Pharyngeal or esophageal lesions of Kaposi's sarcoma may cause dysphagia through obstruction. Nausea and vomiting may be secondary to GI or central nervous system (CNS) malignancies or infections. Symptoms also may be exacerbated by any of the commonly used therapeutic agents. HIV–associated dementia, CNS pathogens, weakness, debilitation, and depression also may contribute to a decreased oral intake. CNS disease processes include CMV infection, HIV encephalitis, cryptococcal meningitis, primary lymphomas, and progressive multifocal leukoencephalopathy. Cytokines such as TNF may cause anorexia by decreasing GI motility. IL-1 and α- and γ-IFNs have been shown to contribute to anorexia. TNF and α- and γ-IFNs have been reported to induce nausea and vomiting during therapeutic trials, although their precise role in causing anorexia in clinical disease is not known.

In the HAART era, diarrhea is no longer such a significant factor in the etiology of weight loss as it was previously. However, in intravenous drug users opportunistic infections and hepatitis C still occur with regularity (96). In the Nutrition for Healthy Living (NFHL) cohort studied longitudinally from 1995 to 2005 to assess the impact of nutrition on patients with HIV, 88% of subjects had at least one abnormality in GI function, and 40% had at least one episode of diarrhea (93). However, increased energy requirements related to infections or malignancies contributed only in a small way to weight loss.

Altered Metabolism

Hypermetabolism was considered a significant contributor to the wasting syndrome in the past. However, when caloric intake and resting energy expenditure were examined in HIV–infected patients with weight loss at various stages of disease, only the patients with secondary infections lost weight (97). In patients without infection, only those with a decreased intake lost weight, and only in those patients was total energy expenditure decreased (98). Thus, it now appears that weight loss in HIV–infected patients is caused by decreased food intake, not hypermetabolism. A similar observation has been made in cancer patients (2). Although the metabolic rate can be extremely high (e.g., because of fever), food intake is invariably diminished in such patients.

These observations translate into practical considerations. When the provision of calories was increased (by TPN) in patients with AIDS wasting, the increased caloric intake led to weight gain (99). When weight loss was secondary to malabsorption or GI disease, the administration of TPN increased body cell mass. However, patients with AIDS wasting who had infection but not malabsorption continued to lose weight on TPN therapy (100).

Protease Inhibitors

Antiretroviral therapy stabilizes weight and lessens the severity of malnutrition (95,13). However, body cell mass is decreased even in patients on protease inhibitors; some patients do not respond optimally, and some gain weight on treatment, even though their lean body mass does not increase (101). Residual nutrition-related abnormalities in HIV–infected patients treated with protease inhibitors include subcutaneous and visceral accumulation of fat, hypertriglyceridemia and hypercholesterolemia, and peripheral insulin resistance (102). These effects were initially considered to be caused by protease inhibitors, but clearly they can occur in patients not taking protease inhibitors (103). In the HAART era, lean tissue wasting (lipodystrophy) that may not be reflected in weight change per se can still occur. Fat accumulates in the abdomen, dorsocervical, and breast areas, with loss of fat in limbs and the face. The optimal management of these patients requires the same working knowledge and skillful management of nutrition that is required in the management of others, plus a knowledge of the numerous symptoms, complications, and infections associated with progressive HIV infection.

Effects of Malnutrition

Protein–calorie Malnutrition

In AIDS patients, body cell mass depletion is increased out of proportion to total weight loss. Body cell mass, measured by total body potassium, is more depleted than body fat mass in immunodeficient patients (104). A linear relationship can be found between the degree of body mass depletion and time to death. The loss of body cell mass correlates with time to death when the body cell mass is depleted by about 50% and the body weight is decreased by about 33%. The time to death does not correlate with body fat depletion. Thus, it has been surmised that the time to death in AIDS patients with wasting may be more closely related to the degree of body cell mass depletion than to its underlying cause (105).

Both malnourishment and overnourishment affect immune status. Nutritional deficiencies, seen most commonly in some Third World countries, are linked with decreased immune function and increased rates of infection. However, no solid scientific data are available to prove that malnutrition per se predisposes HIV–infected patients to AIDS. Body cell mass correlates better than immune function (assessed by CD4+ lymphocyte count) with physical performance (106).

Micronutrient Deficiencies

Any patient with weight loss and wasting is at risk for deficiency of an individual micronutrient but some have been reported with some frequency in AIDs patients. Pyridoxine deficiency may result from decreased food intake or from treatment with pyridoxine antagonists such as isoniazid or hydralazine. Symptoms of peripheral neuropathy, seborrheic dermatitis, and oral lesions, including glossitis, angularis stomatitis, and cheilosis, may be present. Deficiency of vitamin B_{12}

is present in 16% to 33% of patients with AIDS (107). Vitamin B_{12} deficiency may be secondary to malabsorption resulting from ileal dysfunction, bacterial overgrowth with bacterial binding of vitamin B_{12}, or intrinsic factor deficiency (103). Symptoms include anorexia, loss of taste, glossitis, diarrhea, hair loss, impotence, and anemia, which may result in weakness, fatigue, and dyspnea. Neurologic symptoms include paresthesias, loss of sensory and motor function, irritability, and memory disturbances. Many of these patients do not have megaloblastic changes; however, when deficiency is suspected, it should be documented with elevated serum methylmalonic acid and homocysteine levels (see Chapter 7). If the diagnosis remains in doubt, treatment should not be withheld. Folate levels are low in one-third of patients. Absorption may be decreased by inhibition of the dihydrofolate reductase enzyme by drugs, including methotrexate, trimethoprim, pyrimethamine, and triamterene. Supplements should be administered when a deficient state is suspected or when these drugs are used. It is essential to include vitamin B_{12} replacement when deficiencies of both vitamins are expected.

Low 25(OH)D levels are common in over half of AIDS patients, as they are in the general population (<30 ng/mL). Associated with these low levels are many factors, including obesity, advanced AIDS, substance abuse, HAART, and skeletal and cardiovascular function (108). Low vitamin D has also been associated with high viral loads and low CD4 counts, but these have not been studied prospectively or reversal demonstrated yet by vitamin D supplementation. Excess amounts of vitamin D have been shown to decrease T-cell function. It is important to monitor for additional regimens that patients may be taking, including megadoses of certain vitamins and minerals.

Iron deficiency favors *Candida* and *Salmonella* infections. The prevalence of iron deficiency is higher in adults with recurrent HSV infections than in matched controls. However, current data do not indicate that correction of this deficiency protects against infection. Deficiency results in depletion of storage iron, a decrease in circulating iron, and a hypochromic, microcytic anemia. Iron-containing substrates such as muscle myoglobin and mitochondrial cytochromes are also affected, which may account for symptoms of weakness. Zinc deficiency is secondary to decreased absorption and increased losses in chronic diarrhea. Zinc deficiency itself may cause diarrhea in addition to poor wound healing, dysgeusia, skin rashes, and apathy. Selenium deficiency is common in HIV–infected patients and may play a role in the pathogenesis of cardiomyopathy. It also is an independent factor associated with decreased survival (109). However, data to support an effect of selenium supplementation are lacking (110).

Treatment for Specific Complications of HIV Infection Contributing to Malnutrition

The management of HIV depends upon two agreed tenets: first, that HAART prolongs life and controls the infection, and second, that food and proper nutrition are essential to full health (111). A WHO workshop in 2010 agreed on nutrient-specific recommendations for patients with HIV. Table 15-6 outlines the nutrition-related treatment recommendations for HIV–infected adults; multiple micronutrient supplements appear to decrease mortality and morbidity, especially when uncomplicated by pulmonary tuberculosis (112). However, the trials with micronutrient supplementation are sufficiently heterogeneous in design and results that no change is recommended from the 2003 values for RDAs for each micronutrient (113) (see Chapters 6 and 7 for details).

No standard of nutritional management in AIDS is universally accepted. The American Dietetic Association and the Dietitians of Canada have endorsed a position statement that supports the following: maintaining optimal weight and preventing rapid weight loss, reducing or discontinuing smoking and alcohol consumption, reducing or balancing intake of foods and beverages rich in calcium and vitamin D and protein, supplementing with calcium when needed, minimizing side effects of HAART, and use of regular weight-bearing or resistance exercises (94). In general, patients who are not malnourished do not require nutritional supplements. However, they do need an adequate intake of macronutrients and micronutrients from a balanced diet of table foods. The use of nutritional supplements in HIV–infected patients has produced small and variable effects, although the studies were small and were done around the time HAART was introduced (114). Most are safe to give, but no claims can be made for efficacy. Many websites are available to obtain information on nutrition in AIDS (Table 15-7).

TABLE 15-6 Nutrition-Specific Recommendations for Adult AIDS Patients

Nutrient	Conclusion & Comments
Energy	Prior recommendations to provide an extra 10% of daily caloric intake are warranted in asymptomatic patients. There is little evidence to support increasing this energy provision in patients with symptoms or active opportunistic infections.
Macronutrients (protein, fat, carbohydrate)	Ensure that macronutrients are provided at recommended amounts for uninfected adults (see Chapter 5). While insufficient evidence is available to recommend increased protein intake, there is no evidence against that recommendation. No recommendations are made regarding the type or amount of fat.
Weight loss, decreased food intake	Give appetite-stimulating drugs.
Micronutrients (vitamins, minerals)	Due to heterogeneity of study design and results, it is not possible to recommend anything except the current RDA/DRI for a given nutrient, or a standard multivitamin/mineral preparation. High intake should not be encouraged to avoid toxicity (e.g., vitamin A that may increase viral replication).

DRI, dietary reference intake; RDA, recommended dietary allowance.
From Pitney CL, Royal M, Klebert M. Selenium supplementation in HIV-infected patients: is there any potential clinical benefit? *J Assoc Nurses in AIDS Care.* 2009;20:326.

TABLE 15-7 Websites with Nutrition Information for AIDS Patients

Organization	Material offered	URL
American Dietetic Association	A Guide to Nutrition (2003)	www.eatright.org
Assoc. of Nutrition Services Providers (ANSA)	Materials for AIDS meal providers	www.aidsnutrition.org
Canadian AIDS Treatment Information Exchange (CATIE)	Fact sheets, treatment information	www.catie.ca
Gay Men's Health Crisis (GMHC)	Client education	www.gmhc.org
Health Resources and Services Administrations, HIV/AIDS bureau	Client education and nutrition manual	www.aids-etc.org
HIV/AIDS Dietetic Practice Group	Dietetics professionals' resources	www.idndpg.org

Dietary Recommendations

1. Optimal oral and dental hygiene is essential to prevent infections, oral discomfort, and changes in taste.
2. Patients who are at risk for aspiration because of oropharyngeal dysfunction should be evaluated by a speech pathologist or ear, nose, and throat specialist.
3. Meals and the administration of medication should be timed to avoid anticipatory vomiting. Drugs that induce nausea or vomiting should be administered long before meals.
4. Foods should be thoroughly cooked and stored with adequate refrigeration. Leftover foods should be completely reheated. Bacterial food contamination can be fatal in the immunocompromised patient. Raw or undercooked shellfish and seafood, meat, poultry, and unpasteurized milk products (e.g., steak tartare and sushi) should be avoided because they may lead to enteric infections with *Salmonella, Campylobacter, Listeria,* and *Escherichia coli.* Separate cutting boards should be used for uncooked meats, fruits, and vegetables. Neutropenic diets, in which uncooked fruits and vegetables are avoided, are advisable for patients whose white blood cell counts are low.

5. Avoidance of significant alcohol consumption is advisable. Ethanol abuse decreases function in multiple components of the immune system and further compromises nutrient absorption, utilization, storage, and secretion (115).
6. Patients with diarrhea or fat malabsorption should limit intake of fatty foods.
7. For anorectic patients, meals should be served in an appetizing fashion in a well-lit environment free from distractions. Frequent small meals served on small plates are often best tolerated. Providing nutrient-dense foods may help in these situations. Variety in the temperatures of food is welcomed by some. Offering favorite foods in a pleasant atmosphere in the presence of family members or companions may help.
8. Foods served at cool temperatures may be more soothing. Foods with strong aromas and spices should be avoided.
9. Fluid intake during meals, which causes early satiety, should be avoided. The remainder of the fluid requirement should be ingested between meals.
10. For patients with dysgeusia, serving liquids at meal time and altering the texture and temperatures of foods may stimulate sensory feedback. Serving foods with small amounts of liquids may aid chewing and swallowing. Sour candy may stimulate salivation in patients with dry mouth.
11. Enteral nutritional supplementation is best given at times other than meal times, such as just before bedtime, to allow for optimal appetite during meals. Iso–osmolar formulas with an increased fat content may be better tolerated by patients with sepsis who are glucose intolerant. Patients with malabsorption may benefit from low-fat diets or diets containing medium-chain triglycerides. The use of these supplemental diets may be limited because of their potentially adverse effects of hyperosmolarity and diarrhea. The intake of carbohydrate and fat in both table foods and enteral supplements should be adjusted to reduce symptoms of diarrhea.

Appetite Stimulants and Anabolic Agents

These should be reserved for patients with weight loss and decreased food intake (Table 15-8).

Megestrol Acetate

The progestational agent megestrol acetate may increase appetite and promote weight gain in AIDS patients without any clear underlying cause of weight loss. Similar benefits have been seen in some cancer patients. In two trials in which 800 mg of megestrol acetate was given daily for 12 weeks to AIDS patients with anorexia and cachexia, a weight gain of 3 to 4 kg was reported (116,117). The optimal dosing of megestrol acetate remains to be determined. No significant

TABLE 15-8 Anabolic Treatments for Patients with AIDS Wasting

Treatment	Usual Dose	Demonstrated Result
Appetite-stimulating drugs	400–800 mg/day	Improved appetite, weight gain (mostly fat) in 30% of patients, may take 4–6 week
Megestrol acetate		
Dronabinol	5 mg/day	
		Improve appetite, increase weight
Testosterone and analogs	300 mg q 3 week	↑ lean body mass
Testosterone, IM Testosterone, transdermal Oxandrolone, oral	5 mg/day	
	20 mg/day	No significant effect
Nandrolone, IM	150 mg q 2 week	Weight gain, ↑ lean body mass
Recombinant human growth hormone	6 mg/day	Weight gain, ↑ lean body mass (short term)
Exercise training	Individualized	↑ Lean body mass
Cytokine modulators		
Thalidomide	200–400 mg/day	Weight gain

Data from Corcoran C, Grinspoon S. Treatments for wasting in patients with the acquired immunodeficiency syndrome. *N Engl J Med*. 1999;340:1740; Gibson RJ. Keefe DMK, Lalla RV, et al. Systematic review of agents for the management of gastrointestinal mucositis in cancer patients. *Support Care Cancer*. 2013;21:313.

side effects were observed during the course of therapy. Long-term effects on weight gain, repletion of body cell mass, and quality of life are not yet known. Consistent with its glucocorticoid action, the drug can exacerbate diabetes (118) and cause adrenal insufficiency on withdrawal. Fat deposition may be the major component of weight gain.

Dronabinol (Δ-9-tetrahydrocannabinol)
The active agent in marijuana has been shown to enhance appetite, but weight gain is very slight (119). The body composition of this weight gain has yet to be evaluated. It may function as an antiemetic to improve appetite. Side effects include drowsiness, anxiety, poor coordination, and confusion.

Anabolic Steroids
These have been useful only in men, producing a modest increase in lean body mass and a weight gain of about 1 kg over control during 12 to 14 weeks (101). Both oxandrolone (20 to 80 mg per day) and oxymetholone (10 to 150 mg per day) are active orally and are 5 to 10 times more active than testosterone, with fewer side effects (120). However, not all trials with oxandrolone have shown efficacy (93).

Growth Hormone
Patients with weight loss may have some resistance to endogenous growth hormone, perhaps related to malnutrition or underlying HIV infection. In an uncontrolled 3-month study, an increase in weight of 3 kg was achieved by giving 5 mg subcutaneously every other day. Other studies showed an improved exercise capacity and a confirmed modest weight gain in comparison with controls (121). However, the recombinant drug is very expensive, and side effects include edema, arthralgias/myalgias, and decreased glucose tolerance.

Thalidomide
The use of thalidomide in treating cancers and inflammatory conditions is well documented (122). The drug acts via an active metabolite by interfering with TNF-α or IL-1 β-induced activation of IκK, with subsequent suppression of NFκB. In randomized, placebo-controlled trials of patients with painful oral ulcers, over half responded to doses of 100 to 200 mg per day. Several trials in HIV+/AIDS patients showed improved weight gain over short periods (122). Usual doses range from 100 to 1,200 mg per day. Adverse effects include sedation, peripheral neuropathy, and teratogenicity, but rash, dizziness, constipation, tremor, mood changes, and headache are also common. The effects may be related to its effect on inflammation produced by chemotherapy, as a randomized trial of thalidomide showed no difference from placebo in patients with weight loss not on active chemotherapy (123). The study was very small, however. Thalidomide has been used largely in combination with other drugs for malignant disease, but is effective as monotherapy in inflammatory disorders, particularly of the skin and gut.

L-carnitine
Carnitine is a quaternary ammonium metabolite that transports fatty acids into the mitochondrial matrix and improves energy in the skeletal muscle. Patients with cancer have decreased activity of mitochondrial carnitine O-palmitoyltransferases that are responsible for β-oxidation of long-chain fatty acids. Low levels of serum and muscle carnitine have been documented in patients with cancer cachexia (124). One RCT of L-carnitine (4 g) vs. placebo in patients with advanced pancreatic cancer showed an increase in BMI by 3.4%, along with increased body cell mass (125). In a trial of patients with cancer cachexia carnitine at 4 g/day was compared with megestrol (320 mg/day), eicosapentaenoic acid, and thalidomide (200 mg/d), but lean body mass and fatigue improved only in the treatment arm containing all agents (126). Another trial testing carnitine (2 g/day) for its effect on fatigue in patients with invasive malignancies showed no effect (127). Thus, it is unclear whether carnitine has any role in the patient with symptoms from cancer wasting (for further discussion on L-carnitine supplementation, see chapter 8).

NUTRITIONAL SUPPORT IN PATIENTS IN CRITICALLY ILL PATIENTS

The role of nutrition support in critically ill patients is still controversial, with little agreement about how many calories to give, when to give them, and whether to include agents to improve immune function (see next section). A major part of the problem is that all patients from well-nourished to malnourished are analyzed together. A meta-analysis of well-designed trials with intention-to-treat end points showed a significant reduction in mortality in patients receiving parenteral nutrition (PN), although there were more infectious complications in the group with parenteral feeding (11). Subsequent reviews of PN and EN of all randomized trials found that efficacy was not often found, and when it was, it was in less well-designed studies in which bias could have been important (128,129). However, the issue of benefit for a select population (critically ill, malnourished patients) was raised again by an observational report from 167 ICUs in 37 countries, that reported that an increase of 1,000 kcal/day was associated with reduced 60-day mortality rate (RR 0.76) for patients with BMI less than 25 or greater than 35 (130).

The same issues seen in critically ill patients have been reproduced in studies of surgical patients. Although weight loss may not have occurred following acute surgical procedures, the net catabolic state is similar to those that produce weight loss. When the patient at baseline has lost weight and is malnourished, as is often the case with surgical patients and chronic medically ill patients, the need for nutritional support seems quite logical. Perioperative nutritional support is most often provided for patients with cancer and appears to be of benefit if the patient is malnourished at baseline (80,131). The definition of malnutrition versus catabolic state in the face of chronic illness can be difficult, however (see Chapter 5), as malnutrition implies a response to exogenous nutrients. Perhaps the reason why more studies have not been positive is that it takes approximately 7 days or more of preoperative positive nitrogen balance to reduce infectious complications when patients are malnourished, and most patients do not receive such a prolonged preoperative treatment (132). Studies do not show a benefit when supplements are provided postoperatively. For patients with distal bowel surgery, it is now clear that oral feeding is possible and desirable because the gut recovers within a few days in most patients (133). When oral nutrition was compared with enteral or parenteral supplements in cancer patients (with weight loss) during postoperative recovery, no difference was seen in outcome, except that the supplemented groups had more complications (134). Thus, oral nutrition is probably preferred postoperatively. In patients who have short-bowel syndrome the requirement for PN, especially at night, may be ameliorated by the use of a GLP-2 analog (teduglutide), designed to increase remaining small intestinal mucosal mass (135).

Because many clinical aspects of clinical nutrition are linked to gastroenterology, the presence of GI symptoms in ICU patients with or without diseases of the GI tract has attracted attention. The presence of GI signs or symptoms (including abnormal bowel sounds, vomiting, high gastric residual volume, diarrhea) is associated with increased mortality in ICU patients (136). Infection with *C. difficile* produces colitis in many ICU patients, but nutrition support with EN is not contraindicated in these patients (137). The role of nutrition in acute pancreatitis has been confusing, because bowel rest was the standard of care for many years. In addition, most patients with mild or even moderate pancreatitis will resolve spontaneously and do not need nutrition support during their stay in the ICU. However, if resumption of feeding in severe pancreatitis is delayed, EN is usually recommended, although it is not clear if earlier intervention will improve outcomes (138). Patients with inflammatory bowel disease (IBD) who are hospitalized will need correction of any nutrient deficiencies, especially when intake is low (folate), the small bowel is involved (calcium, vitamin D, magnesium, vitamin B_{12}), bleeding is present (iron), or diarrhea is significant (zinc) (139). The addition of probiotics does not yet appear to have support from existing studies (140). EN may have a role in preventing relapses, especially in children, but chronic use of EN is usually not well tolerated in adults (141).

The use of omega-3 fatty acids along with antioxidants have been proposed to modulate the systemic inflammatory response. Although a few small trials suggest some efficacy in IBD patients (139), no effect was found in a prospective trial in patients with acute lung injury (142). Moreover, parenteral supplementation with omega-3 fatty acids does not improve mortality and morbidity in critically ill patients (143). In advanced cancer, there are limited data suggesting a role in preservation of muscle mass and function during radiation/chemotherapy, but there is no evidence that clinical response is altered (144).

IMMUNONUTRITION

Immune modulation has been proposed to benefit patients under intense stress. In addition, the innate immune system ages, with reduced neutrophil and NK cell activity predicting increased mortality in older adults (145). The rationale is that key nutrients, normally not essential, are made conditionally essential when the rate of consumption or need is increased. The nutrients suggested for such a role include glutamine (a nutrient for immune cells and gut barrier protector), arginine (an NO precursor), nucleotides (improve T lymphocyte function), sulfur-containing amino acids (enhance antioxidation via glutathione production), and n-3 fatty acids (anti-inflammatory, suppress cytokine production) (146). However, there are no definitive data in humans to confirm the conditionally essential role for these nutrients, most especially for glutamine (147) or arginine (148) where the most data have been gathered. Nonetheless, commercial products have been developed and used, particularly in patients who are critically ill. The data using these products have shown mixed results, but also suggest that harm can be produced by their use.

A meta-analysis of the use of "immune-modulating" products (available before 2001) in 22 studies revealed that they were associated with fewer infections but no change in mortality (149). Results were markedly heterogeneous, and surgical patients had lower infection rates than critically ill patients, contrary to the hypothesis that more stress produces conditional deficiencies. Most of the studies were small, few were blinded, few had any follow-up data, and all were compared with "standard" nutrition support that varied between studies. But standard nutrition support may be harmful in itself, as n-6 fatty acids are proinflammatory (150). Standard lipid emulsions contain only 4% to 11% of the lipid as n-3 linolenic acid. To deliver enough nutrients to improve immune function (at least theoretically), a large volume (>800 mL) is needed, and the studies often do not provide such volume (151). In addition, sepsis in the patients was often severe, and nutrition was not delivered early. Most of the oral/enteral products currently available in the USA and advertised to be immune-modulating contain arginine, glutamine, and n-3 fatty acids (many providing 30% to 50% of the lipid in this form), in addition to the more standard n-6 fatty acids (Table 15-9). The data suggesting that arginine-rich products might decrease infection rates in critically ill patients led to cautious recommendations for their use (152,153). They have been found useful in surgical patients during the preoperative period (154). Not all experts agree that these products should be used (149,151,155). Parenteral FO emulsions enriched in n-3 fatty acids have been used for a variety of purposes (Table 15-9) (156). When compared with soybean oil–based emulsions (n-6 fatty acids) the FO emulsions

TABLE 15-9 Oral/Enteral Immune-Modulating Products

Product	Source	kcal/mL	arg (g/L)	gln (g/L)	Nucleotide (g/L)	n-3 FA (g/L)	n-6 FA (g/L)
AlitraQ	Abbott	1.0	3.0	14.2	0	0.02	6.6
Crucial	Nestle	1.5	12	0	0	3.6	7.7
Impact Glutamine	Novartis	1.3	16.3	15	1.6	2.7	3.9
Impact 1.5	Novartis	1.5	18.7	0	1.8	2.6	3.8
Impact Recover	Novartis	1.0	16.9	11.2	1.6	4.1	4.6
Oxepa	Abbott	1.5	0	0	0	10.2	18.8
Perative	Abbott	1.3	6.5	0	0	1.2	6.8
Pivot 1.5	Abbott	1.5	0	0	0^a	0	48^c
Peptamen AF	Nestle	1.1	0	0	0^b	0	54^c

^{a}Contains L-carnitine 144 g/L
^{b}Contains L-carnitine 120 g/L
^{c} Total lipid
Arg, arginine; gln, glutamine; FA, fatty acid.

TABLE 15-10 Characteristics of Four Lipid Emulsions Containing 10 g fat/100 ml Emulsion

Characteristic	Intralipid	ClinOleic	SMOF Lipid	Omegaven
Manufacturer	Baxter	Baxter Healthcare	Fresenius Kabi	Fresenius Kabi
	Fresenius Kabi			
Oil source (g)				
Soybean	10	2	3	0
MCT	0	0	3	0
Olive oil	0	8	2.5	0
Fish oil	0	0	1.5	10
α-Tocopherol (mg/L)	38	32	200	150–296

Data from Koretz RL. Immunonutrition: fact, fantasy, and future. *Curr Gastroenterol Reports.* 2002;4:322.

appear to shorten hospital and intensive care unit stays (157). Enteral diets containing arginine and FO (Table 15-10) also seemed to confer a similar benefit on high-risk surgical patients (158). Another systematic review examined 24 studies of critically ill patients and found that only the three using an enteral FO preparation showed an effect on lower mortality, rate of infection, and length of stay (159). However, each study had significant methodological problems, and study design and outcome end points were very different. Thus, it is not possible to make a recommendation for treatment based on the available data (160). A separate systematic review of the use of enteral and parenteral n-3 fatty acids in 14 RCTs in cancer, surgery, and critical care also concluded that the data were too inconsistent for any conclusions (161). Enteral supplements maintained body weight in cancer and critical care patients but not in surgical patients, whereas results with PN were inconsistent. When specific types of diseases were examined, inconsistency of results was found in patients with GI cancer (162) and head and neck cancers (163). However, the one use for which FO emulsions have proven their worth is in the treatment of intestinal failure associated liver disease, where replacement of soy oil–based emulsions with FO-based emulsions produces dramatic improvement in bilirubin and transaminase values, in children especially (156).

There are no data available regarding the use of these products in any situation but that of acute medical or surgical stress. However, some patients are immunosuppressed chronically and might benefit from measures to prevent stress to their immune systems. It is standard procedure following hematopoietic stem cell transplantation to use a diet low in microbial content (164). The most commonly restricted foods are fresh fruits and fruit juices, fresh vegetables, and raw eggs. Also restricted are raw and undercooked meat, unpasteurized milk or cheeses, aged or blue cheeses, unroasted nuts or nuts in the shell, uncooked raw grains, raw honey, all miso products, sun tea, and herbal preparations and nutrient supplements. Guidelines for safe food handling practices can be found at www.foodsafety.gov, www.fda.gov, www.fsis.usda.gov, and www.cdc.gov.

REFERENCES

1. Muscaritoli M, Anker SD, Argiles J, et al. Consensus definition of sarcopenia, cachexia and pre-cachexia: joint document elaborated by Special Interest Groups (SIG) "cachexia-anorexia in chronic wasting diseases" and "nutrition in geriatrics." *Clin Nutr.* 2010;29:154.
2. Esper DH, Harb WA. The cancer cachexia syndrome: a review of metabolic and clinical manifestations. *Nutr Clin Pract.* 2005;20:369.
3. Suzuki H, Asakawa A, Amitani H, et al. Cancer cachexia–pathophysiology and management. *J Gastroenterol.* 2013;48:574.
4. Barber MD. The pathophysiology and treatment of cancer cachexia. *Nutr Clin Pract.* 2002;17:203.
5. International Working Group on Sarcopenia. Sarcopenia: an undiagnosed condition in older adults. Current consensus definition: prevalence, etiololgy, and consequences. *J Am Med Dir Assoc.* 2011;12:249.

6. Mitchell WK, Williams J, Atherton P, et al. Sarcopenia, dynapenia, and the impact of advancing age on human skeletal muscle size and strength; a quantitative review. *Front Physiol.* 2012;3:260.
7. von Hachling S, Morley JE, Anker SD. From muscle wasting to sarcopenia and myopenia: update 2012. *J Cachexia Sarcopenia Muscle.* 2012;3:213.
8. Truswell AS. Some problems with Cochrane reviews of diet and chronic disease. *Eur J Clin Nutr.* 2005;(Suppl 1):S150.
9. Jackson RD, LaCroix AZ, Gass M, et al. Calcium plus vitamin D supplementation and the risk of fractures. *N Eng J Med.* 2006;354:669.
10. Baldwin C, Parsons T, Logan S. Dietary advice for illness-related malnutrition in adults. *Cochrane Database Syst Rev.* 2001;(2):CD002008.
11. Chief Medical Officers' Committee on Medical Aspects of Food. *Nutritional Aspects of the Development of Cancer.* London: Stationery Office, 1998. Department of Heath report on health and social subjects No. 48.
12. Forman MR, Hursting SD, Umar A, et al. Nutrition and cancer prevention: a multidisciplinary perspective on human trials. *Annu Rev Nutr.* 2004;24:223.
13. National Research Council, Commission on Life Sciences, Food and Nutrition Board, Committee on Diet and Health. *Diet and Health: Implications for Reducing Chronic Disease Risk.* Washington DC: National Academies Press, 1989.
14. Kant P, Hull MA. Excess body weight and obesity—the link with gastrointestinal and hepatobiliary cancer. *Nat Rev Gastroenterol Hepatol.* 2011;8:224.
15. Prentice RL, Caan B, Chlebowski RT, et al. Low-fat dietary pattern and risk of invasive breast cancer: the Women's Health Initiative randomized controlled dietary modification trial. *JAMA.* 2006;295:629.
16. Beresford SAA, Johnson KC, Ritenbaugh C, et al. Low-fat dietary pattern and risk of colorectal cancer: the Women's Health Initiative randomized controlled dietary modification trial. *JAMA.* 2006;295:643.
17. Schoenfield JD, Ioannidis JPA. Is everything we eat associated with cancer? A systematic cookbook review. *Am J Clin Nutr.* 2013;97:127.
18. de Logeril M, Salen P, Martin JL, et al. Mediterranean dietary pattern in a randomized trial. *Arch Intern Med.* 1998;158:1181.
19. Cottet V, Bonithon-Kopp C, Kronborg O, et al. Dietary patterns and the risk of colorectal adenoma recurrence in a European intervention trial. *Eur J Cancer Prev.* 2005;14:21.
20. La Vecchia C. Mediterranean diet and cancer. *Public Health Nutr.* 2004;7:965.
21. Martinez-Gonzalez MA, Estruch R. Mediterranean diet, antioxidants and cancer: the need for randomized trials. *Eur J Cancer Prev.* 2004;13:327.
22. Jacobs EJ, Connell CJ, Chao A, et al. Multivitamin use and colorectal cancer incidence in a US cohort: does timing matter? *Am J Epidemiol.* 2003;158:621.
23. Kushi LH, Doyle C, McCullough M, et al. American Cancer Society Guidelines on nutrition and physical activity for cancer prevention. *CA Cancer J Clin.* 2012;62:30.
24. Williams MT, Hord NG. The role of dietary factors in cancer prevention: beyond fruits and vegetables. *Nutr Clin Pract.* 2005;20:451.
25. Lee KW, Lee HJ, Surh YJ, et al. Vitamin C and cancer chemoprevention: reappraisal. *Am J Clin Nutr.* 2003;78:1074.
26. Stanner SA, Hughes J, Kelly CNM, et al. A review of the epidemiological evidence for the 'antioxidant hypothesis.' *Public Health Nutr.* 2003;7:407.
27. Mannisto S, Smith-Warner SA, Spiegelman D, et al. Dietary carotenoids and risk of lung cancer in a pooled analysis of seven cohort studies. *Cancer Epidemiol Biomarkers Prev.* 2004;13:40.
28. Steck-Scott S, Forman MR, Sowell A, et al. Carotenoids, vitamin A and risk of adenomatous polyp recurrence in the polyp prevention trial. *Int J Cancer.* 2004;112:295.
29. Bjelakovic G, Nikolava D, Simonetti RG, et al. Antioxidant supplements for prevention of gastrointestinal cancers: a systematic review and meta-analysis. *Lancet.* 2004;364:1219.
30. Cummings JH, Bingham SA. Diet and the prevention of cancer. *BMJ.* 1998;317:1636.
31. Janne PA, Mayer RJ. Chemoprevention of colorectal cancer. *N Engl J Med.* 2000;342:1960.
32. Biasco G, Paganelli GM. European trials on dietary supplementation for cancer prevention. *Ann N Y Acad Sci.* 1999;889:152.
33. Kirsh VA, Hayes RB, Mayne ST, et al. Supplemental and dietary vitamin E, β-carotene, and vitamin C intakes and prostate cancer risk. *J Natl Cancer Inst.* 2006;98:245.

34. Duffield-Lillico AJ, Reid ME, Turnbull BW, et al. Baseline characteristics and the effect of selenium supplementation on cancer incidence in a randomized clinical trial: a summary report of the Nutritional Prevention of Cancer Trial. *Cancer Epidemiol Biomarkers Prev*. 2002;11:630.
35. van Gils CH, Peeters PHM, Bueno-de-Mesquita HB, et al. Consumption of vegetables and fruits and risk of breast cancer. *JAMA*. 2005;203:183.
36. Ahmad N, Mukhtar H. Antioxidants meet molecular targets for cancer prevention and therapeutics. *Antioxid Redox Signal*. 2013;19:85.
37. Williams CD. Antioxidants and prevention of gastrointestinal cancers. *Curr Opin Gastroenterol*. 2013;29:195.
38. Wactawski-Wende J, Kotchen JM, Anderson GL, et al. Calcium plus vitamin D supplementation and the risk of colorectal cancer. *N Engl J Med*. 2006;354:684.
39. Hartman TJ, Albert PS, Snyder K, et al. The association of calcium and vitamin D with risk of colorectal adenomas. *J Nutr*. 2005;135:252.
40. Giovannucci E. The epidemiology of vitamin D and colorectal cancer: recent findings. *Curr Opin Gastroenterol*. 2006;22:24.
41. Schottker B, Ball D, Geleert C, et al. Serum 25-hydroxyvitamin D levels and overall mortality. A systematic review and meta-analysis of prospective cohort studies. *Ageing Res Rev*. 2013;12:708.
42. Gorouhi NG, Ye Z, Rickard AP, et al. Circulating 25-hydroxyvitamin D concentration and the risk of type 2 diabetes: results from the European Prospective Investigation into Cancer (EPIC)-Norfolk cohort and updated meta-analysis of prospective studies. *Diabetologia*. 2012;55:2173.
43. Chung M, Lee J, Terasaw T, et al. Vitamin D with or without calcium supplementation for prevention of cancer and fractures: an updated meta-analysis for the U.S. Preventive Services Task Force. *Ann Intern Med*. 2011;155:827.
44. Hong Z, Tian C, Zhang X. Dietary calcium intake, vitamin D levels, and breast cancer risk: a dose-response analysis of observational studies. *Breast Cancer Res Treat*. 2012;136:309.
45. Mondul AM, Weinstein SJ, Horst RL, et al. Serum vitamin D and risk of bladder cancer in the Prostate, Lung, Colorectal, and Ovarian (PLCO) cancer screening trial. *Cancer Epidemiol Biomarkers Prev*. 2012;21:1222.
46. Chao A, Thun MJ, Connell CJ, et al. Meat consumption and risk of colorectal cancer. *JAMA*. 2005;293:172.
47. Norat T, Bingham S, Ferrari P, et al. Meat, fish, and colorectal cancer risk: the European Prospective Investigation into cancer and nutrition. *J Natl Cancer Inst*. 2005;97:906.
48. Flood A, Velie EM, Sinha R, et al. Meat, fat, and their subtypes as risk factors for colorectal cancer in a prospective cohort of women. *Am J Epidemiol*. 2003;158:59.
49. Willett WC. Diet and cancer: an evolving picture. *JAMA*. 2005;293:233.
50. Yang WS, Wong MY, Voghmann E, et al. Meat consumption and risk of lung cancer: evidence from observational studies. *Ann Oncol*. 2012;23:3163.
51. Terry PD, Rohan TE, Wolk A. Intakes of fish and marine fatty acids and the risks of cancers of the breast and prostate and of other hormone-related cancers: a review of the epidemiologic evidence. *Am J Clin Nutr*. 2003;77:532.
52. zur Hausen H. Red meat consumption and cancer: reasons to suspect involvement of bovine infectious factors in colorectal cancer. *Int J Cancer*. 2012;130:2475.
53. Higgins JA, Brown IL. Resistant starch: a promising dietary agent for the prevention/treatment of inflammatory bowel disease and bowel cancer. *Curr Opin Gastroenterol*. 2013;29:190.
54. Levine ME, Suarez JA, Brandhorst S, et al. Low protein intake is associated with a major reduction in IGF-1, cancer, and overall mortality in the 65 and younger but not older population. *Cell Metab*. 2014;19:407.
55. Austin GL, Adair LS, Galanko JA, et al. A diet high in fruits and low in meats reduces the risk of colorectal adenomas. *J Nutr*. 2007;137:999.
56. Richmann S, Overvad K, Bueno-de-Mesquita HB, et al. Meat consumption and mortality—results from the European Prospective Investigation into Cancer and Nutrition. *BMC Med*. 2013;11:63.
57. Gebauer SK, Chardigny JM, Jakobsen MU, et al. Effects of ruminant trans fatty acids on cardiovascular disease and cancer: a comprehensive review of epidemiological, clinical, and mechanistic studies. *Adv Nutr*. 2011;2:332.
58. Vinikoor LC, Schroeder JC, Millikan RC, et al. Consumption of trans-fatty acid and its association with colorectal adenomas. *Am J Epidemiol*. 2008;168:289.
59. Lopez-Garcia E, Rodriguez-Aralejo F, Li TY, et al. The Mediterranean-style diet pattern and mortality among men and women with cardiovascular disease. *Am J Clin Nutr*. 2014;99:172.

60. Scarmeas N, Stern Y, Mayeux R, et al. Mediterranean diet and mild cognitive impairment. *Arch Neurol*. 2009;66:216.
61. Hakim IA, Hartz V, Harris RB, et al. Reproducibility and relative validity of a questionnaire to assess intake of black tea polyphenols in epidemiological studies. *Cancer Epidemiol Biomarkers Prev*. 1002;10:667.
62. Arab L, Il'yasova D. The epidemiology of tea consumption and colorectal cancer incidence. *J Nutr*. 2003;133:3310S.
63. Rietveld A, Wiseman S. Antioxidant effects of tea: evidence from human clinical trials. *J Nutr*. 2003;133:3285S.
64. Weisburger JH, Chung FL. Mechanisms of chronic disease causation by nutritional factors and tobacco products and their prevention by tea polyphenols. *Food Chem Toxicol*. 2002;40:1145–1154.
65. Singh M, Singh P, Shukla Y. New strategies in cancer chemoprevention by phytochemicals. *Front Biosci*. 2012;E4:426.
66. Schoeffner DJ, Thorgeirsson UP. Susceptibility of nonhuman primates to carcinogens of human relevance. *In Vivo*. 2000;14:149.
67. Espin JC, Gonzalez-Barrio R, Cerda B, et al. Iberian pig as a model to clarify obscure points in the bioavailability and metabolism of ellagitannins in humans. *J Agric Food Chem*. 2007;55:10476.
68. Miller PE, Snyder DC. Phyochemicals and cancer risk: a review of the epidemiological features. *Nutr Clin Pract*. 2012;27:599.
69. Anonymous. Berries of many colours. *Arbor Clin Nutr*. 2009;311:1.
70. Arranz S, Chiva-Vlanch G, Valderas-Martinez P, et al. Wine, Beer, Alcohol and polyphenols on cardiovascular disease and cancer. *Nutrients*. 2012;4:759.
71. Kim YI. Will mandatory folic acid fortification prevent or promote cancer? *Am J Clin Nutr*. 2004;80:1123.
72. WCRF/AICR. *Food, Nutrition, Physical Activity and the Prevention of Cancer: A Global Perspective*. Washington, DC: AICR, 2007. http://www.dietandcancerreport.org/.
73. Wien TN, Pike E, Wisloff T, et al. Cancer risk with folic acid supplements: a systematic review and meta-analysis. *BMJ Open*. 2012:2:e000653.
74. Sharp L, Carsin AE, Cantwell MM, et al. Intake of dietary folate and other B vitamins are associated with rates of esophageal adenocarcinoma, Barrett's esophagus, and reflex esophagitis. *J Nutr*. 2013;143:1966.
75. Mattox TW. Treatment of unintentional weight loss in patients with cancer. *Nutr Clin Pract*. 2005;20:400.
76. Huhmann MB, August DA. Review of American Society for Parenteral and Enteral Nutrition (A.S.P.E.N.) clinical guidelines for nutrition support in cancer patients: nutrition screening and assessment. *Nutr Clin Pract*. 2008;23:182.
77. Capra S, Bauer J, Davidson W, et al. Nutritional therapy for cancer-induced weight loss. *Nutr Clin Pract*. 2002;17:210.
78. Klein S, Koretz RL. Nutrition support in patients with cancer: what do the data really show? *Nutr Clin Pract*. 1994;9:91.
79. McGeer AJ, Detsky AS, O'Rourke KO. Parenteral nutrition in cancer patients undergoing chemotherapy: a meta-analysis. *Nutrition*. 1990;6:233.
80. Klein S, Kinney J, Jeejeebhoy K, et al. Nutrition support in clinical practice: review of published data and recommendations for future research directions. *JPEN J Parenter Enteral Nutr*. 1997;21:133.
81. Baldwin C, Spiro A, Ahern R, et al. Oral nutritional interventions in malnourished patients with cancer: a systematic review and meta-analysis. *J Natl Cancer Inst*. 2012;104:371.
82. Ravasco P, Monteiro-Grillo I, Camilo M. Individualized nutrition intervention is of major benefit to colorectal cancer patients: long-term follow-up of a randomized controlled trial of nutritional therapy. *Am J Clin Nutr*. 2012;96:1346.
83. Huhmann MB, August DA. Perioperative nutrition support in cancer patients. *Nutr Clin Pract*. 2012;27:586.
84. August DA, Huhmann MB. A.S.P.E.N. clinical guidelines: nutrition support therapy during adult anticancer treatment and in hematopoietic cell transplantation. *JPEN J Parenter Enteral Nutr*. 2009;33:472.
85. Orr R, Singh MF. The anabolic androgenic steroid oxandrolone in the treatment of wasting and catabolic disorders. *Drugs*. 2004;64:72.
86. Gordon JN, Trebble TM, Ellis RD, et al. Thalidomide in the treatment of cancer cachexia: a randomized placebo controlled trial. *Gut*. 2005;54:540.

87. Fearon KC, von Meyenfeldt MF, Moses AG, et al. Effect of a protein and energy dense N-3 fatty acid enriched oral supplement on loss of weight and lean tissue in cancer cachexia: a randomized double blind trial. *Gut.* 2003;52:1479.
88. American College of Physicians. Parenteral nutrition in patients receiving cancer chemotherapy. *Ann Intern Med.* 1989;110:734.
89. Savarese DMF, Savy G, Vahdat L, et al. Prevention of chemotherapy and radiation toxicity with glutamine. *Cancer Treat Rev.* 2003;29:501.
90. Ferreira PR, Fleck JF, Diehl A, et al. Protective effect of alpha-tocopherol in head and neck cancer radiation-induced mucositis: a double-blind randomized trial. *Head Neck.* 2004;26:313.
91. Ertekin MV, Koc M, Karslioglu I, et al. Zinc sulfate in the prevention of radiation-induced oropharyngeal mucositis: a prospective, placebo-controlled, randomized study. *Int J Radiat Oncol Biol Phys.* 2004;58:167.
92. Gibson RJ, Keefe DMK, Lalla RV, et al. Systematic review of agents for the management of gastrointestinal mucositis in cancer patients. *Support Care Cancer.* 2013;21:313.
93. Mangili A, Murman DH, Zampini AM, et al. Nutrition and HIV infection: review of weight loss and wasting in the era of highly active antiretroviral therapy from the nutrition for healthy living cohort. *Clin Infect Dis.* 2006;42:836.
94. Fields-Gardner C, Fergusson P; American Dietetic Association; Dietitians of Canada. Position of the American Dietetic Association and the Dietitians of Canada: nutrition intervention in the care of persons with human immunodeficiency infection. *J Am Diet Assoc.* 2004;104:1425.
95. Campa A, Yang Z, Lai S, et al. HIV-related wasting in HIV-infected drug users in the era of highly active antiretroviral therapy. *Clin Infect Dis.* 2005;41:1179.
96. Hendricks KM, Erzen HD, Wanke CA, et al. Nutrition issues in the HIV-infected injection drug user: findings from the nutrition for healthy living cohort. *J Am Coll Nutr.* 2010;29:136.
97. Grunfeld C, Pang M, Shimizu L, et al. Resting energy expenditure, caloric intake, and short-term weight change in human immunodeficiency virus infection and AIDS. *Am J Clin Nutr.* 1992;55:455.
98. Macallan DC, Noble C, Baldwin C, et al. Energy expenditure and wasting in human immunodeficiency virus infection. *N Engl J Med.* 1995;333:83.
99. Melchior J, Chastang C, Gelas P, et al. Efficacy of 2-month total parenteral nutrition in AIDS patients: a controlled randomized prospective trial. *AIDS.* 1996;10:379.
100. Suttmann U, Ockenga O, Selberg O, et al. Incidence and prognostic value of malnutrition and wasting in human immunodeficiency virus-infected outpatients. *J Acquir Immune Defic Syndr Hum Retrovirol.* 1995;8:239.
101. Flexner C. HIV-protease inhibitors. *N Engl J Med.* 1998;338:1281.
102. Corcoran C, Grinspoon S. Treatments for wasting in patients with the acquired immunodeficiency syndrome. *N Engl J Med.* 1999;340:1740.
103. Lo JC, Mulligan K, Tai VW, et al. Buffalo hump in men with HIV-1 infection. *Lancet.* 1998;351:867.
104. Kotler DP, Wang J, Pierson RN. Body composition studies in patients with the acquired immunodeficiency syndrome. *Am J Clin Nutr.* 1985;42:1255.
105. Kotler DP, Tierney AR, Wang J, et al. Magnitude of body-cell-mass depletion and the timing of death from wasting in AIDS. *Am J Clin Nutr.* 1989;50:444.
106. Ott M, Fischer H, Polat H, et al. Bioelectrical impedance analysis as a predictor of survival in patients with human immunodeficiency virus infection. *J Acquir Immune Defic Syndr Hum Retrovirol.* 1995;9:20.
107. Harriman GR, Smith PD, Horne MK. Vitamin B_{12} malabsorption in patients with acquired immunodeficiency syndrome. *Arch Intern Med.* 1989;149:2039.
108. Griffin AT, Arnold FW. Review of metabolic, immunologic, and virologic consequences of suboptimal vitamin D levels in HIV infection. *AIDS Patient Care STDS.* 2012;28:516.
109. Baum MK, Shor-Posner G, Lai S, et al. High risk of HIV-related mortality is associated with selenium deficiency. *J Acquir Immune Defic Syndr Hum Retrovirol.* 1997;15:370.
110. Pitney CL, Royal M, Klebert M. Selenium supplementation in HIV-infected patients: is there any potential clinical benefit? *J Assoc Nurses in AIDS Care.* 2009;20:326.
111. Raiten DJ, Mulligan K, Papathakis P, et al. Executive summary-nutritional care of HIV-infected adolescents and adults, including pregnant and lactating women: what do we know, what can we do, and where do we go from here? *Am J Clin Nutr.* 2011;94(Suppl):1667S.

112. Jiang S, He J, Zhao X, et al. The effect of multiple micronutrient supplementation on mortality and morbidity of HIV-infected adults: a meta-analysis of randomized controlled trials. *J Nutr Sci Vitaminol*. 2012;58:105.
113. Forrester JE, Sztam KA. Micronutrients in HIV/AIDS: is there evidence to change the WHO 2003 recommendations? *Am J Clin Nutr*. 2011;94(Suppl):1683S.
114. Keithley JK, Swanson B. Oral nutritional supplements in human immunodeficiency virus disease: a review of the evidence. *Nutr Clin Pract*. 2001;16:98.
115. Watzl B, Watson RR. Role of alcohol abuse in nutritional immunosuppression. *J Nutr*. 1992;122:733.
116. Von Roenn JH, Armstrong D, Kotler DP, et al. Megestrol acetate in patients with AIDS-related cachexia. *Ann Intern Med*. 1994;121:393.
117. Oster MH, Enders SR, Samuels SJ, et al. Megestrol acetate in patients with AIDS and cachexia. *Ann Intern Med*. 1994;121:400.
118. Henry K, Rathgaber S, Sullivan C, et al. Diabetes mellitus induced by megestrol acetate in a patient with AIDS and cachexia. *Ann Intern Med*. 1992;116:53.
119. Beal JE, Olson R, Laubenstein L, et al. Dronabinol as a treatment for anorexia associated with weight loss in patients with AIDS. *J Pain Symptom Manage*. 1995;10:89.
120. Gervasio J. Anabolic agents: adjuncts to nutrition support. *Nutr Clin Pract*. 2004;19:263.
121. Gullett NP, Hebbar G, Ziegler TR. Update on clinical trials of growth factors and anabolic steroids in cachexia and wasting. *Am J Clin Nutr*. 2010;91(Suppl):1143S.
122. Franks ME, Macpherson GR, Figg WD. Thalidomide. *Lancet*. 2004;363:1802.
123. Yennurajalingam S, Willey JS, Palmer JL, et al. The role of thalidomide and placebo for the treatment of cancer-related anorexia-cachexia symptoms: results of a double-blind placebo-controlled randomized study. *J Palliative Med*. 2012;15:1059.
124. Szefel J, Kruszewski WJ, Ciesielski M, et al. L-carnitine and cancer cachexia, I: L-carnitine distribution and metabolic disorders in cancer cachexia. *Oncol Rep*. 2012;28:319.
125. Kraft M, Kraft K, Gartner S, et al. L-carnitine supplementation in advanced pancreatic cancer (CARPAN)—a randomized multicenter trial. *Nutr J*. 2012;11:52.
126. Mantovani G. Randomised phase III clinical trial of 5 different arms of treatment on 332 patients with cancer cachexia. *Eur Rev Med Pharmacol Sci*. 2010;14:292.
127. Cruciani RA, Zhang JJ, Manola J, et al. L-carnitine supplementation for the management of fatigue in patients with cancer: an eastern cooperative oncology group phase III, randomized, double-blind, placebo-controlled trial. *J Clin Oncol*. 2012;30:3864.
128. Simpson F, Doig GS. Parenteral vs enteral nutrition in the critically ill patient: a meta-analysis of trials using the intention to treat principle. *Intensive Care Med*. 2005;31:12.
129. Koretz RL. Do data support nutrition support? Part I: intravenous nutrition. *J Am Diet Assoc*. 2007;107:988.
130. Koretz RL. Do data support nutrition support? Part II: enteral artificial nutrition. *J Am Diet Assoc*. 2007;107:1374.
131. Van Way CW III. Perioperative nutritional support as an adjunct to surgical therapy for cancer. *Nutr Clin Pract*. 2002;17:214.
132. Howard L, Ashley C. Nutrition in the perioperative patient. *Annu Rev Nutr*. 2003;23:263.
133. Naslund E, Hellstrum PM, Kral JG. The gut and food intake: an update for surgeons. *J Gastrointest Surg*. 2001;5:556.
134. Hyltander A, Bosaeus I, Svedlund J, et al. Supportive nutrition on recovery of metabolism, nutritional state, health-related quality of life, and exercise capacity after major surgery: a randomized study. *Clin Gastroenterol Hepatol*. 2005;3:466.
135. Buchman AL. Teduglutide and short bowel syndrome: every night without parenteral fluids is a good night. *Gastroenterol*. 2012;43:1416.
136. Reintam A, Parm P, Cern H, et al. Gastrointestinal symptoms in intensive care patients. *Acta Anaesthesiol Scand*. 2009;53:318.
137. DeLegge MH, Berry A. Enteral feeding: should it be continued in the patient with *Clostridium difficile* enterocolitis? *Pract Gastroenterol*. 2009;33:40.
138. Spanier BWM, Bruno MJ, Mathus-Vliegen MH. Enteral nutrition and acute pancreatitis: a review. *Gastroenterol Res Pract*. 2011; doi:10.1155/2011/857949.
139. Naik AS, Venu N. Nutritional care in adult inflammatory bowel disease. *Pract Gastroenterol*. 2012;36:18.

140. Zigra PI, Maipa VE, Alamanos YP. Probiotics and remission of ulcerative colitis: a systematic review. *Neth J Med*. 2007;41:411.
141. Yamamoto T. Nutrition and diet in inflammatory bowel disease. *Curr Opin Gastroenterol*. 2013;29:216.
142. Rice TW, Wheeler AP, Thompson BT, et al. Enteral omega-e fatty acid, γ-linolenic acid, and antioxidant supplementation in acute lung injury. *JAMA*. 2011;306:1574.
143. Palmer AJ, Clement KM, Ajibola O, et al. The role of ω-3 faty acid supplemented parenteral nutrition in critical illness in adults: a systematic review and meta-analysis. *Crit Care Med*. 2013;41:307.
144. Laviano A, Rianda S, Molfino A, et al. Omega-3 fatty acids in cancer. *Curr Opin Clin Nutr Metab Care*. 2013;16:156.
145. Panda A, Arjona A, Sapey E, et al. Human innate immunosenescence: causes and consequences for immunity in old age. *Trends Immunol*. 2009;30:325.
146. Grimble RF. Immunonutrition. *Curr Opin Gastroenterol*. 2005;21:216.
147. Alpers DH. Glutamine: do the data support the cause for glutamine supplementation in humans? *Gastroenterology*. 2006;130:S106.
148. Zaloga GP, Siddiqui R, Terry C et al. Arginine: mediator or modulator of sepsis? *Nutr Clin Pract*. 2004;19:201.
149. Heyland DK, Novak F, Drover JW, et al. Should immunonutrition become routine in critically ill patients? *JAMA*. 2001;286:944.
150. Griffiths RD. Specialized nutrition support in critically ill patients. *Curr Opin Crit Care*. 2003;9:249.
151. McCowen KC, Bistrian BR. Immunonutrition: problematic or problem solving? *Am J Clin Nutr*. 2003;77:764.
152. Montejo JC, Zarazaga A, Lopez-Martinez J, et al. Immunonutrition in the intensive care unit. A systematic review and consensus statement. *Clin Nutr*. 2003;22:221.
153. Martindale MD, Miles J. Is immunonutrition ready for prime time? Two points of view. *Nutr Clin Pract*. 2003;18:489.
154. Sacks GS, Genton L, Kudsk KA. Controversy of immunonutrition for surgical critical-illness patients. *Curr Opin Crit Care*. 2003;9:300.
155. Koretz RL. Immunonutrition: fact, fantasy, and future. *Curr Gastroenterol Rep*. 2002;4:322.
156. Chang MI, Puder M, Gura KM. The use of fish oil emulsion in the treatment of intestinal failure associated liver disease (IFALD). *Nutrients*. 2012;4:1828.
157. Waitzberg DL, Torrinhas RS. Fish oil lipid emulsions and immune response: what clinicians need to know. *Nutr Clin Pract*. 2009;24:487.
158. Marik PE, Zaloga GP. Immunonutrition in high-risk surgical patients: a systematic review and analysis of the literature. *JPEN J Parenter Enteral Nutr*. 2010;34:378.
159. Marik PE, Zaloga GP. Immunonutrition in critically ill patients: a systematic review and analysis of the literature. *Intensive Care Med*. 2008;34:1980.
160. Peterik A, Milbrandt EB, Darby JM. Immunonutrition in critical illness: still fishing for the truth. *Crit Care*. 2009;13:305.
161. van der Meij BS, van Bokhorst-de van der Schueren MA, Langius JA, et al. n-3 PUFAs in cancer, surgery, and critical care: a systematic review on clinical effects, incorporation, and washout of oral or enteral compared with parenteral supplementation. *Am J Clin Nutr*. 2011;94:1248.
162. Zhang Y, Gu Y, Guo T, et al. Perioperative immunonutrition for gastrointestinal cancer: a systematic review of randomized controlled trials. *Surg Oncol*. 2012;21:e87.
163. Rodera PC, de Luis DA, Candela CG, et al. Immunoenhanced enteral nutrition formulas in head and neck cancer surgery: a systematic review. *Nutr Hosp*. 2012;27:681.
164. Lipkin AC, Lenssen P, Dickson BJ. Nutrition issues in hematopoietic stem cell transplantation: state of the art. *Nutr Clin Pract*. 2005;20:423.
165. Kotler DP. Nutritional alterations associated with HIV infection. *J Immune Defic Syndr*. 2000;25 Suppl 1:S81.
166. Alberda C, Gramlich L, Jones N, et al. The relationship between nutritional intake and clinical outcomes in critically ill patients: results of an international multicenter observational study. *Intensive Care Med*. 2009;35:1728.

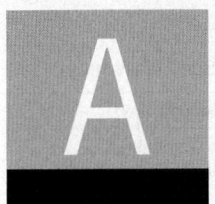

Facts and Formulas Commonly Used in Nutritional Therapeutics

Caloric Value of Macronutrients

1 g dietary fat = 9 kcal
1 g carbohydrate = 4 kcal
1 g protein = 4 kcal
1 g ethanol = 7 kcal
1 g medium-chain triglycerides = ~8 kcal
1 g IV dextrose monohydrate = 3.4 kcal
1 mL 10% fat emulsion = 1.1 kcal

Caloric Value of Alcohol-Containing Beverage

$$0.8 \times \frac{\text{Proof of beverage}}{2} \times \text{Volume of beverage (dl)} = \text{Weight of alcohol (g)} \times 7 = \text{kcal}$$

Estimation of Nitrogen Content in Dietary Protein

$$\text{Nitrogen (g)} = \frac{\text{Protein (g)}}{6.25}$$

Estimation of Basal (Resting) Energy Needs (kcal/day)
Harris–Benedict Method for Calculating Basal Metabolic Rate

$$BMR \text{ (women)} = 665 + (9.6 \times W) + (1.8 \times H) - (4.7 \times A)$$
$$BMR \text{ (men)} = 66 + (13.7 \times W) + (5 \times H) - (6.8 \times A)$$

where W = weight (kg)
H = height (cm)
A = age (y)

World Health Organization/Food and Agriculture Organization of the United Nations Equations for Estimating Resting Energy Expenditure

Age (y)	Male	Female
0–3	$(60.9 \times W^a) - 54$	$(61.0 \times W) - 51$
3–10	$(22.7 \times W) - 495$	$(22.5 \times W) + 499$
10–18	$(17.5 \times W) + 651$	$(12.2 \times W) + 746$
18–30	$(15.3 \times W) + 679$	$(14.7 \times W) + 996$
30–60	$(11.6 \times W) + 879$	$(8.7 \times W) + 829$
>60	$(13.5 \times W) + 987$	$(10.5 \times W) + 596$

^{a}Weight in kilograms.

Estimate of Energy Requirements for Patients Based on Body Mass Index[a]

BMI (kg/m^2)	Energy requirements (kcal/kg/day)	
	Critically ill patients (RMR)	Other patients (RMR + TEF + TEA)
<15	35–40	35–40 + 20%
15–19	30–35	30–35 + 20%
20–29	20–25	20–25 + 20%
≥30	15–20[b]	15–20

[a]Use the Harris–Benedict or World Health Organization equation to estimate the requirement for patients whose estimate by this method is less than 1,200 kcal/day.
[b]Do not exceed 2,000 kcal/day.
RMR, resting metabolic rate; TEF, thermal energy of food; TEA, thermal energy of activity.

Estimation of Recommended Daily Protein Intake

Clinical condition	Protein requirements (g/kg IBW/day)
Normal	0.75
Metabolic "stress/illness/injury"	
Mild/moderate	1.0–1.25
Moderate/severe	1.25–1.5
Severe with extra losses (e.g., skin, urine)	1.5–[a]
Renal failure, acute (undialyzed)	0.8–1.0
Hemodialysis	1.2–1.4
Peritoneal dialysis	1.3–1.5
Hepatic encephalopathy	0.4–0.6

[a]Upper limit determined from measured losses.
IBW, ideal body weight.

Estimation of Ideal Body Weight for Adults
Woman with medium frame: 120 lb for first 5 ft of height + 3 lb/in
Man with medium frame: 130 lb for first 5 ft of height + 3 lb/in
Small frame: Subtract 10 lb from above
Large frame: Add 10 lb to above

Conversion factors for calories
1 kcal = 4.184 kjoules
1 kjoule = 0.239 kcal
1 lb of weight lost = ~3,400 kcal

Body Mass Index
BMI = W (kg)/H^2 (m), or = W (lb)/H^2 (in) × 703

Conversion Factors for Major Minerals

1 mEq Na = 1 mmol Na = 23 mg Na
1 g Na = 43 mEq Na = 43 mmol Na
1 mEq K = 1 mmol K = 39 mg K
1 g K = 26 mEq K = 26 mmol K
1 mEq Ca = 0.5 mmol Ca = 20 mg Ca
1 g Ca = 50 mEq Ca = 25 mmol Ca
1 mEq Mg = 0.5 mmol Mg = 12 mg Mg
1 g Mg = 82 mEq Mg = 41 mmol Mg
1 mmol P = 2 mEq HPO_3 = 31 mg P
1 mEq Cl = 1 mmol Cl = 35 mg Cl
1 g Cl = 29 mEq Cl = 29 mmol Cl

Major Mineral Content in Various Compounds and Solutions

1 g NaCl = 393 mg Na = 17 mEq Na
1 g $NaHCO_3$ = 273 mg Na = 12 mEq Na
1,000 mL saline solution = 9 g NaCl = 3.5 g Na = 154 mEq Na
1,000 mL lactated Ringer's solution = 3 g Na = 130 mEq Na
1 ampule (50 mL) 7.5% $NaHCO_3$ = 1 g Na = 44 mEq Na
1 g KCl = 524 mg K = 13 mEq K
1 g $CaCl_2$-$2H_2O^a$ = 273 mg Ca = 13.6 mEq Ca
1 g calcium gluconate[b] = 93 mg Ca = 4.6 mEq Ca
1g $MgSO_4$-$7H_2O^a$ = 99 mg Mg = 8.1 mEq Mg
1 g Mg gluconate-$2H_2O^a$ = 54 mg Mg = 4.4 mEq Mg
1 g $CaCO_3$ = 400 mg Ca = 20 mEq Ca
1 g $FeSO_4$−$7H_2O^a$ = 201 mg Fe
1 g Fe gluconate-$2H_2O^a$ = 116 mg Fe
1 mL Fe dextran = 50 mg Fe

Liquid Measure Equivalents: Volume

Apothecary	Metric (mL)	Household
1 fluid gram	4	1 teaspoon (tsp)
1/2 fluid ounce (oz)	15	1 tablespoon (tbsp) (3 tsp)
1 oz	30	2 tbsp (1/8 cup)
4 oz	118	8 tbsp (1/2 cup)
8 oz	237	16 tbsp (1 cup)
16 oz	473	1 pint (pt)
32 oz	947	1 quart (qt) (2 pt)
128 oz	3,785	1 gallon (gal) (4 qt)

[a]When weighed in hydrated forms, as indicated.
[b]Small amounts of calcium D-saccharate may be added for stabilization and contribute to the total calcium content.

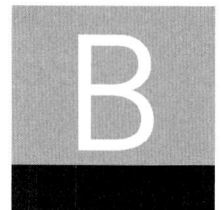

Food Labeling

REGULATIONS

Both the Food and Drug Administration (FDA) and the US Department of Agriculture Food Safety and Inspection Service (FSIS) have established regulations for food labeling (*Code of Federal Regulations*; Title 21, Vol. 2, Parts 100 to 169, 4/1/99). The FDA rules comply with the provisions of the Nutrition Labeling and Education Act of 1990, and the FSIS rules are coordinated with the FDA rules. The FDA rules became effective May 8, 1994, and apply to most processed foods. Nutritional information is also available for fresh fruits and vegetables and raw fish at the point of purchase. The FSIS rules became effective July 6, 1994, and apply to meat and poultry products. Labeling for trans fat content was added in January 2006; advice for reducing allergen risk was published on January 23, 2009. Gluten-free label guidelines were suggested in August 2013.

NUTRITION PANEL

The FDA food label has a nutrition panel that is headed "Nutrition Facts." The dietary components appear on the nutrition panel (Table B-1). These mandatory and voluntary components

TABLE B-1   Mandatory and Voluntary Dietary Components of the Nutrition Panel

Total calories
Calories from fat
Calories from saturated fat
Total fat
Saturated fat
Polyunsaturated fat
Monounsaturated fat
Trans fat
Cholesterol
Sodium
Potassium
Total carbohydrate
Dietary fiber
Soluble fiber
Insoluble fiber
Sugars
Sugar alcohol (e.g., the sugar substitutes xylitol, mannitol, and sorbitol)
Other carbohydrates (difference between total carbohydrate and the sum of dietary fiber, sugars, and sugar alcohol if declared)
Protein
Vitamin A
Vitamin C
Calcium
Iron
Other essential vitamins and minerals

are the only ones allowed on the nutrition label and must be presented in the order given. "Voluntary" nutrients can be included if the manufacturer chooses; however, if a claim is made about them, or if a food is fortified or enriched with them, then they must be listed. Trans fats have been added, as this class of nutrients leads to elevated LDL cholesterol. Foods introduced after 2006 must disclose trans fat content, but for older products, this disclosure is voluntary. Even so, if the food contains more than 0.5g/serving, the content may not be declared on the label. "Gluten-free" has now been defined as containing less than 20 ppm of gluten. This term is also synonymous with "no gluten," "free of gluten," and "without gluten." Food allergens that may be included on labels include milk or egg products, peanuts, tree nuts, soybeans, wheat, fish, and shellfish, as these include more than 90% of the offending foods that produce allergy (see also Chapter 12).

This list of nutrients has been chosen because it reflects health concerns in the population. Nutrients are listed in the order of priority of current dietary recommendations. Thiamine, riboflavin, and niacin, which were required elements on the old nutrition label, are not required now, because they are no longer considered to be of public health significance; however, they can be listed voluntarily.

Data for each of the nutrients must be presented as grams (or milligrams) per serving and as percentage of daily value (Figure B-1, left side). Daily values are a new way of presenting

Nutrition Facts
Serving Size 2/3 cup (55g)
Servings Per Container About 8

Amount Per Serving	
Calories 230	Calories from Fat 40

	% Daily Value*
Total Fat 8g	**12%**
Saturated Fat 1g	**5%**
Trans Fat 0g	
Cholesterol 0mg	**0%**
Sodium 160mg	**7%**
Total Carbohydrate 37g	**12%**
Dietary Fiber 4g	**16%**
Sugars 1g	
Protein 3g	
Vitamin A	10%
Vitamin C	8%
Calcium	20%
Iron	45%

* Percent Daily Values are based on a 2,000 calorie diet. Your daily value may be higher or lower depending on your calorie needs.

	Calories:	2,000	2,500
Total Fat	Less than	65g	80g
Sat Fat	Less than	20g	25g
Cholesterol	Less than	300mg	300mg
Sodium	Less than	2,400mg	2,400mg
Total Carbohydrate		300g	375g
Dietary Fiber		25g	30g

Nutrition Facts
8 servings per container
Serving Size 2/3 cup (55g)

Amount per 2/3 cup
Calories 230

% DV*	
12%	**Total Fat** 8g
5%	Saturated Fat 1g
	Trans Fat 0g
0%	**Cholesterol** 0mg
7%	**Sodium** 160mg
12%	**Total Carbs** 37g
14%	Dietary Fiber 4g
	Sugars 1g
	Added Sugars 0g
	Protein 3g
10%	Vitamin D 2mcg
20%	Calcium 260mg
45%	Iron 8mg
5%	Potassium 235mg

* Footnote on Daily Values (DV) and calories reference to be inserted here.

Figure B-1 Representative nutrition panel—left side, current nutrition label; right side, label showing proposed changes. The major differences in the new label on the right are that the number of calories is much more prominent, and the category of 'added sugars' is included.

nutritional information. Percentage of daily value expresses the amount of a nutrient in a serving of a particular food as a percentage of the amount of the nutrient that would be consumed in a 2,000-calorie balanced diet. Daily values are based on two sets of new dietary standards, daily reference values (DRVs) and reference daily intakes (RDIs); however, only the term *daily value* appears on the label. DRVs have been established for fat, carbohydrate, protein, cholesterol, sodium, and potassium. DRVs for the energy-producing nutrients (fat, carbohydrates, and protein) are based on the number of calories consumed per day. The daily values that appear at the top of the nutrition label are based on a 2,000-calorie diet. Adjustments for other caloric intakes are included at the bottom of the label. The proposed changes to the label (Figure B-1, right side), emphasize the calorie content more, and require notation of added sugar content. These changes are open to public comment until June 2, 2014. Once passed, companies will have 2 years to comply.

The DRVs for Macronutrients Are Calculated as Follows:

1. Fat is based on 30% of calories.
2. Saturated fat is based on 10% of calories.
3. Carbohydrates are based on 60% of calories.
4. Protein is based on 10% of calories.
5. Fiber is based on 11.5 g per 1,000 calories.

The DRVs for Some Nutrients Represent the Upper Limits of the Desirable Range Based on Public Health Recommendations:

1. Total fat should be less than 65 g.
2. Saturated fat should be less than 20 g.
3. Cholesterol should be less than 300 mg.
4. Sodium should be less than 2,400 mg.
5. Trans fat should be less than 0.5 g per serving.

Reference Daily Intakes

The RDIs are reference values for vitamins and minerals; *RDI* replaces the term *US–recommended dietary allowance (RDA)*. The values for the RDIs are the same as those for the old US RDAs. The required data for vitamin A, vitamin C, calcium, and iron are presented as a percentage of the RDI. Voluntary data for other vitamins and minerals are presented in the same way.

Daily values may be confusing for consumers because some of the data, such as those for vitamin A, vitamin C, iron, and calcium, are presented as a percentage of the smallest desirable daily intake, whereas other data, such as those for fat, cholesterol, and sodium, are presented as a percentage of the maximum recommended daily allowance. Thus, consumers may misinterpret the labels as indicating that at least 300 mg of cholesterol and at least 2,400 mg of sodium should be consumed, rather than no more than 300 mg of cholesterol and no more than 2,400 mg of sodium.

All the data in the nutrition label are presented in relation to a defined serving size (which is presented in both household and metric measures); the same serving sizes must be used by all manufacturers. Under the old regulations, serving sizes were defined by the food manufacturer; under the new regulations, the serving sizes are defined by the FDA and represent amounts that people actually consume.

NUTRIENT CONTENT DESCRIPTORS

The regulations define terms that may be used to describe the level of a nutrient in a food.

Free

The term *free* means that a product does not contain the nutrient, or contains only a trivial or "physiologically inconsequential" amount. *Calorie-free* means less than 5 calories per serving. *Sugar-free* and *fat-free* both mean less than 0.5 g per serving.

Low

The general definition for *low* is that it is possible to consume a food low in a nutrient frequently during the course of a day without exceeding the dietary guidelines.

1. *Low in fat* means 3 g or less per serving.
2. *Low in saturated fat* means 1 g or less per serving.
3. *Low in sodium* means less than 140 mg per serving.
4. *Very low in sodium* means less than 35 mg per serving.
5. *Low in cholesterol* means less than 20 mg per serving.
6. *Low in calories* means 40 calories or less per serving.

Lean and Extralean

These terms are used to describe meats, poultry, and seafood. *Lean* means less than 10 g of fat, less than 4 g of saturated fat, and less than 95 mg of cholesterol per serving and per 100 g. *Extralean* means less than 5 g of fat, less than 2 g of saturated fat, and less than 95 mg of cholesterol per serving and per 100 g.

High

High means that a single serving of a food contains 20% or more of the daily value for a particular nutrient.

Good Source

The term *good source* means that one serving of a food contains 10% to 19% of the daily value for a particular nutrient.

Reduced

The term *reduced* means that a nutritionally altered product contains 25% less of a nutrient or 25% fewer calories than the regular (unaltered) product. A claim that a product is *reduced* cannot be made if the reference food already meets the requirements for a *low* claim.

Less

The term *less* means that a food contains 25% less of a nutrient or 25% fewer calories than the reference food. Pretzels with 25% less fat than potato chips can carry the *less* claim.

Light

The term *light* can mean that an altered product contains one-third fewer calories or half the fat of the reference item. If more than 50% of the calories in a food are derived from fat, then the fat must be reduced by 50% if the food is to qualify for a *light* claim. *Light* can also mean that the sodium content of a low-calorie, low-fat food has been reduced by 50%. A claim of *light in sodium* may be used on foods in which the sodium content has been reduced by 50%. The term *light* also can be applied to color and texture, in such terms as *light brown sugar*, as long as the meaning is clear.

More

The term *more* means that the quantity of a nutrient in a serving of food is at least 10% greater than the daily value of the reference food. The terms *enriched*, *fortified*, and *added* also can be used if the quantity of a nutrient is at least 10% greater than the daily value of the reference food, and in this case, the food must be altered.

Percentage Fat-free

To qualify for this claim, a product must meet the definition for *low in fat* or *fat-free*. In addition, the value for *percentage fat-free* must reflect the amount of fat in 100 g of the food. Thus, if a claim is to be made that a food is *95% fat-free*, 100 g of the food must contain no more than 5 g of fat.

Implied

Claims cannot be made when they wrongfully imply that a food contains or does not contain a meaningful level of a nutrient. Thus, one cannot claim that a food is "made with oat bran," implying that the food is a good source of fiber, unless the product contains enough oat bran to meet the definition for a *good source* of fiber.

Meals and Main Dishes

Claims for the amount of sodium or cholesterol in a meal or main dish must meet the same requirements as those for individual foods. Some other definitions are more relaxed; *low-calorie*, when applied to a meal or main dish, means that the meal or main dish contains no more than 120 calories per 100 g.

Healthy

The term *healthy* can be used to describe a food that is low in fat and saturated fat and that contains no more than 480 mg of sodium and no more than 60 mg of cholesterol per serving.

Fresh

When the term *fresh* is used to suggest that a food is raw or unprocessed, it can be used only to refer to a food that has never been frozen or heated and that contains no preservatives (irradiation at low levels is allowed). The term *fresh-frozen* can be used for foods that are quickly frozen while still fresh. Brief scalding before freezing (blanching) is allowed.

HEALTH CLAIMS

The FDA allows health claims for relationships between several nutrients and risk for a particular disease (see also Chapter 8). The claims for the food product must meet the requirements for authorized health claims. They cannot state the degree of risk reduction and must use the word *may* or *might* in discussing the relationship between the nutrient and the disease. The claims also must phrase the relationship between the nutrient and the disease in a way that the consumer can understand. An example of an appropriate claim is the following: "While many factors affect heart disease, diets low in saturated fat and cholesterol may reduce the risk for heart disease." Claims for the following nutrient–disease relationships are allowed on food labels:

Calcium and Osteoporosis

A food must contain 20% or more of the daily value for calcium (200 mg) per serving, as much or more calcium than phosphorus, and a form of calcium that is readily absorbed. The claim must name the target groups most in need of an adequate calcium intake (teenagers and young, adult White and Asian women) and state the requirement for exercise and a healthy diet to prevent osteoporosis. A product that contains 40% or more of the daily value for calcium must state on the label that a total dietary intake of more than 200% of the daily value for calcium ($\geq 2,000$ mg) is not known to be of additional benefit.

Fat and Cancer

To carry this claim, a food must meet the requirements for *low in fat* or, if the food is fish or a game meat, for *extralean*.

Saturated Fat and Cholesterol in Coronary Heart Disease

This claim may be used if the food meets the requirements for the descriptors *low in saturated fat*, *low in cholesterol*, and *low in fat*, or, if the food is fish or a game meat, for *extralean*. It may mention the link between a reduced risk for coronary heart disease and lower intakes of saturated fat and cholesterol to lower blood cholesterol levels.

Fiber-containing Grain Products, Fruits, and Vegetables and Cancer

To carry this claim, a food must be or contain a grain product, fruit, or vegetable, meet the requirements for the descriptor *low in fat*, and be a *good source* of dietary fiber without fortification.

Fruits, Vegetables, and Grain Products That Contain Fiber and Risk for Coronary Heart Disease

To carry this claim, a food must be or contain fruits, vegetables, or grain products. It also must meet the requirements for the descriptors *low in saturated fat*, *low in cholesterol*, and *low in fat* and contain, without fortification, at least 0.6 g of soluble fiber per serving.

Sodium and Hypertension

To carry this claim, a food must meet the requirements for the descriptor *low in sodium*.

Fruits and Vegetables in Cancer

This claim may be made for fruits and vegetables that meet the requirement for the descriptor *low in fat* and that, without fortification, are a *good source* of at least one of the following: dietary fiber, vitamin A, or vitamin C. This claim relates diets low in fat and rich in fruits and vegetables (and thus vitamins A and C and dietary fiber) to a reduced risk for cancer.

Folate and Neural Tube Defects

When pregnant women consume a diet containing a minimum of 400 µg of folate per day, the risk for neural tube defects in the fetus is reduced. Foods containing 400 µg of folate can make this claim.

Sugar Alcohols and Dental Caries

Between-meal consumption of foods high in sugars promotes tooth decay. Foods containing sugar alcohols, such as sorbitol, can claim an association with a reduced risk for tooth decay.

Soluble Fiber from Oats or Psyllium and Coronary Artery Disease

Foods that provide 3 g or more of B-glucan soluble fiber from whole oats per day or 7 g of soluble fiber from psyllium seed husk per day can claim an association with a reduced risk for coronary artery disease.

Soy Protein and Coronary Artery Disease

Foods containing at least 6.25 g of soy protein per serving can claim an association with a reduced risk for coronary artery disease.

Index

Page numbers followed by a *t* refer to tables; those followed by an *f* refer to figures.

A

Acacia gum 501
Acceptable daily intake (ADI) 65
Acesulfame potassium, low-available carbohydrate diet and 517
Acetyl-l-carnitine (Alcar) 382
Acid-base balance, diet and effect on 245
Acquired immunodeficiency syndrome (AIDS)
 breast feeding and 48
 malnutrition and 669–670
ACS. *See* American Cancer Society cancer recommendations
*Actinobacteri*a 387
Acute disease-related malnutrition 399
ADA. *See* American Diabetic Association
Additives, food 60–63, 62*t*
 regulations 64–66
Adequate intakes (AIs) 55–57, 55*t*
Adipocyte 141, 631
Adipose tissue 84, 104, 127, 192, 199, 631
Adolescence
 calcium intake and 9–10
 pregnancy during 43
 protein requirements 98–100
Adults
 BMI for 55*t*
 daily values for 54*t*
 osteomalacia in 200
Age
 chronologic 13
 obesity and 634
 population distribution 14, 16*f*
 vitamin deficiency and 190
Aging 13
 pathobiology 16–18
 pathophysiologic consequences of 18–19
 theories 16–18, 17*t*
AHA. *See* American Heart Association
AIDS. *See* Acquired immunodeficiency syndrome
β-Alanine 383
AIs. *See* Adequate intakes
Albumin 108–109. *See also* Thyroxine-binding prealbumin
Alcohol. *See also* Sugar alcohols
 caloric content of 95, 683
 consumption 9
 dietary guidelines for 489, 490*t*
 folate deficiency and 158
 pregnancy and 9, 44–45
Alcoholic liver disease, protein intake for 534–535, 534*t*

Aldehydes 370
Alkaline phosphatase 275
Alkalosis 274
All-*trans*-retinoic acid (ATRA) 189
Allergy
 diagnostic tests for 545
 elimination diets for 544–548, 545*t*
  diagnosis for 546
  practical aspects of 547–548
 food 547
  diets for 544–548, 545*t*
  gluten-restricted diet and 538
  milk 547
  restricted diets for 548–551
  supplementation in 549
Alzheimer disease, vitamin E deficiency and 216
American Cancer Society (ACS)
 cancer recommendations 10, 659–663, 661*t*
 guidelines on nutrition and physical activity 4*t*
American Diabetic Association (ADA) 573–574
American Heart Association (AHA) 3*t* 10, 159, 489
American Society for Parenteral and Enteral Nutrition (ASPEN) 116, 453
 mineral requirements 462–463, 463*t*
Amino acids 379
 arginine 380–381
 creatine 382–383
 glutamine 379–380
 L-Carnitine 381–382
 PN therapy and solutions for 464–466, 465*t*, 466*t*, 467*t*
 requirements 98
 taurine 281
 vegetarian sources of 483, 483*t*
Aminopterin, folate and 38
Amitriptyline 76, 138, 379, 521
Anabolic agents, HIV malnutrition and 672–673
Anemia
 copper deficiency and 333
 iron deficiency and 310
 megaloblastic, folate and 38, 45
 pregnancy and 38, 45
Anergy 112
Anorexia
 HIV and 668
 nutritional therapy for chronically ill patients with associated 412

694 | Index

Anthropomorphic measurements 65. *See also* Height; Weight
Antioxidants
 for cancer 368–369, 659–663
 for chronic diseases 368–369
 circulating levels of, enteral nutritional therapy and 424
 elderly and 20–21
 system, vitamin E and compensation in 217
 theory, vitamin E 211–212
AOAC method. *See* Association of Official Analytical Chemists method
Arachidonic acid 386
Arginine
 enteral nutritional therapy and 424
 parenteral nutritional therapy and 380–381
Ascorbic acid. *See* Vitamin C
Aspartame, low-available carbohydrate diet and 517
ASPEN. *See* American Society for Parenteral and Enteral Nutrition
Association of Official Analytical Chemists (AOAC) method 502
Atherogenesis 371
Atherogenic dyslipidemia 611
Atopy patch tests (APTs) 546
Atorvastatin, grapefruit juice and 557
ATRA. *See* All-*trans*-retinoic acid
Avocados 484–485
Axona 531
Azathioprine, cobalamin deficiency and 169

B

Bacterial overgrowth, HIV and 670
Bacteroidetes 386
Balanced diet 489
Bariatric surgery procedures
 complications 651–652, 652*t*
 criteria for surgery 650, 651*t*
 micronutrient deficiencies after 652*t*
 nutritional evaluations after 652*t*
 postoperative low-available carbohydrate diet for 511
 therapeutic efficacy 651
 types of 649–650, 650*f*
 weight loss efficacy 650–651, 651*t*
Basal energy expenditure (BEE) 81
 BMI estimates for 88–89, 88*t*
 hospitalized patient estimate for 88–89
Basal energy needs, estimation of 683
Basal energy requirement (BER) 81
Basal metabolic rate (BMR) 81
 assessment of 83–89
 body size/age method for estimating 85*t* 90
 body surface area estimation of 84, 85*t*
 calculating methods for 84–89
 FAO equation 86–88
 Harris-Benedict equation for estimating 85–86
 malnutrition and 85
 obesity and estimating 87*t*
 WHO equation 86–88
 Wilmore's equation for estimating 88
Basic Four Food Guide 485
BCAAs. *See* Branched-chain amino acids
BEE. *See* Basal energy expenditure
Behavior modification therapy, for obesity 646
Benfotiamine 134
Benign prostatic hypertrophy (BPH)
 saw palmetto used to treat 378–379
Benzoate-cinnamon-free diet 551
BER. *See* Basal energy requirement
Beverage Guidance Panel 492
Beverages. *See also specific beverages*
 caffeine content of 493–496
 caloric-containing 492–493
 as source of polyphenols 369–370
BIA. *See* Bioelectrical impedance analysis
Bile acid malabsorption 544
Biliopancreatic diversion 649–650, 650*f*
Bioavailability 126
Bioelectrical impedance analysis (BIA) 106
Biotin 178–179
Biotinidase deficiency 179
Black currant oil 386
Bland diet 498
BMD. *See* Bone density measurement
BMR. *See* Basal metabolic rate
Body composition
 aging and 18
 assessment of 102–110
 bioelectrical impedance analysis of 106
 functional, to supplement BMI 108
Body mass index (BMI) 55, 55*t*, 112–113, 634*f*, 684
 anthropomorphic assessment by 102–104
 BEE 88–89, 88*t*
 calculating 103, 105*t*, 632*t*
 childhood 631
 dietary plan and 5
 energy requirements for patients based on 684
 functional body composition to supplement 108
 mortality and 631–633, 633*f*, 633*t*
 for overweight patients 104*t*
Body weight 103, 313
 initial energy intake based on 643, 644*t*
Bone
 biopsy 277
 densitometry, vitamin D assessment and 198

density, postmenopausal women 275–276
disease
   metabolic, HPN and 479
   PN therapy and 473
health
   calcium and 19–20, 271–273
   elderly and 19–20
   phosphorus and 19–20
   vitamin D and 19–20, 202
   vitamin K and 19–20, 222
Bone density measurement (BMD) 275–276
   guidelines for 276
   method 276–277
Borage oil 386
Bottle-fed infants, folate deficiency and 157
Branched-chain amino acids (BCAAs) 534–535
Breast feeding recommendations 46–48. *See also* Lactating women
Buspirone, grapefruit juice and 557
Butyrate 533

C

C-section. *See* Cesarean section
Cachexia 65
   cancer and 665
   definition 657
   nutritional alterations in 657*t*
   role of nutrition in management of 658
Caffeine 371, 383, 493–496
   beverage content of 493–496
   cocoa content of 495
   food and drug contents of 493–496, 494*t*
   health consequences of 495
   pregnancy and 495
Calcifediol. *See* 25-Hydroxyvitamin D_3
Calcium 271–281
   absorption 274, 277–278
      interference with 281
      vitamin D and 198
   adolescence and 9–10
   alkaline phosphatase and 275
   assessment 274–276
   BMD and 275–276
      guidelines for 276
      method for 276–277
   bone biopsy 277
   bone health and 19–20, 271–273
   cancer and 663
   colon cancer and 281
   deficiency 278–279
   determination 274–275
   dietary sources 9–10, 273–274
   DRI 272–273, 272*t*
   enteroenteric circulation 278
   food sources 273–274
   fortification 41, 273
   hypercalcemia and 278, 281
   hypertension and 280–281
   hypocalcemia and treatment with 279
   intake 9–10, 11, 14, 274
   lactating women and 41–43
   malabsorption 279
   metabolism, vitamin D and 42
   nutritional deficiency and 280
   oral preparations 281, 282*t*
   osteoporosis and 9, 201, 280, 690
   phosphorus ratio to 289, 289*t*
   physiology 277–278
   pregnancy and 41–43
   premenstrual syndrome and 281
   renal disease, chronic and 597–598
   requirements 271–272
   serum 274, 274*t*
   supplementation 41, 274
   toxicity 281
   treatment 279–281
   twenty-four-hour urinary excretion of, vitamin D assessment and 197
   urinary excretion of 197, 271, 274
   vitamin D 42, 197–198, 279
Calcium carbonate 274
Calcium gluconate, potassium toxicity 270
Calderol. *See* 25-Hydroxyvitamin D_3
Calories
   activity level and 89–92, 91*t*
   alcohol 95, 683
   assessment 81–120
   beverages containing 492–493
   conversion factors for 684
   cooking oil content of 95
   diets low in 125
   empty 489
   enteral nutritional therapy formulas and 421
   food content of 92–93, 93*t*–94*t*
   intake 81–120
      estimation of 92–96
      food distribution among 485
      pregnancy and 43
      restricting 17
      vitamin deficiency and low 125
   macronutrient 683
   needs, patient 404, 406
   obtained 96
   PA and burning 5, 6*t*
   PN therapy 460
   requirements 81–120
      estimating normal daily 81–83
      protein and 101–102, 101*t*
   support plan 407–409
Calorimetry, indirect 83–84, 89

Cancer. *See also specific cancers*
  ACS recommendations for 659–663, 661*t*
  antioxidants for 368–369, 659–663
  calcium and 663
  diets for preventing 488, 658–659, 660*t*
  fat and 690
  fiber and 690
  folate and 665
    deficiency of 159–160
  malignancy, nutritional management of 665–667
  meat consumption and 663–664
  nutritional abnormalities in 665–668
  nutritional considerations 658–668
  nutritionally-related problems in 667, 667*t*
  polyphenols and 664–665
  prevention
    diets for 488, 658–659, 660*t*
    issues in 663–665
    physical activity for 659–663
    vitamins 659, 662*t*
  risk, dietary guidelines to minimize 658–659, 660*t*
  selenium and 662
    treatment with 344–345
  vitamin D therapy and 203, 663
  vitamin E and
    deficiency in 213, 214*t*–215*t*
    prevention with 211–212, 214*t*–215*t*
Carbamazepine 179
  folate and 38
  grapefruit juice and 557
Carbohydrates 483. *See also* Low-available carbohydrate diet; Resistant short-chain carbohydrates
  counting 582*t*
  dietary therapy 616
  diets low in 509–519, 518
  modulars 416
  proteins modified by 220
  thiamine intake and 132
Carboxylase deficiency 179
Carcinoid syndrome, niacin deficiency and 142
Cardiovascular disease
  copper deficiency and 333
  diets and 489
  lipoproteins associated with 603–608
  low-available carbohydrate diet for 511
  vitamin D deficiency and 203–204
  vitamin E deficiency and 213, 214*t*–215*t*
Carnitine 523, 673
Carnitor. *See* Levocarnitine
Carotenoids
  food sources 184, 185*t*
  function 188
  HPLC 184
Cassia senna 379

Catabolic conditions, nutritional support for 118*t*, 119, 674
Cataracts, vitamin E deficiency and 216
Catechins 371
Catheters. *See also* Central venous catheter
  aseptic 459–460
  maintenance 459–460
  occlusive dressing 459
  peripheral, PN 459
  PN 459–460
  related function, management of 458*t*
  tubing 459
Causal inference 78*t*
Causation, inference for 77, 78*t*
Cellulose 499–500
Central parenteral nutrition (CPN) 455
Central venous catheter (CVC)
  catheter complications 457–458, 458*t*
  complications 457–458, 458*t*
  infections 458–459, 458*t*
  parenteral 459
  PN therapy, ordering/initiation of 473–477, 474*t*, 475*f*, 476*t*
Ceruloplasmin, copper assessment and 330
Cesarean section (C-section) 37
Chemotherapy
  clear liquid diet and 492
  nutrition and 667, 668
CHI. *See* Creatinine-height index
Childhood obesity 634, 635*f*–636*f*
Children. *See also* Adolescence; Infancy
  BMI for 55*t*, 631
  daily values for 54*t*
  diabetes in 589
  iron intoxication in 38
  nutrient in 487*t*
  rickets in 200
Chitin 501
Chitosan 501
Chloride salts 76, 248–262. *See also* Sodium
  serum 253–254
Chocolate, modified-fiber diet and 372
Cholecalciferol (Vitamin D_3) 204–205
Cholesterol 7–8
  coronary heart disease and 690
  dietary 615
  disease management and 618–620
  fiber and lowering levels of 505
  HDL 608
  LDL 603–607, 603*t*–605*t*
  non-HDL 603
  total 603–607, 607*t*
Choline 533
Chondroitin sulfate 374–375
Chromium 340–342
  assessment 340–341
  deficiency 341

DRI 340, 341*t*
food sources 340
physiology 341
toxicity 342
treatment 342
Chronic diseases
  anorexia and, nutritional therapy for associated 412
  antioxidants for 368–369
  dietary guidelines for preventing 55*t*–57*t*, 69, 488
    vegetarian 488
  magnesium treatment for 288
  nutritional considerations in 657–676
  nutritional supplements for prevention of 372–375
    chondroitin sulphate and glucosamine 374–375
    immune-modulating polysaccharides 374
    minerals 373–374
    vitamins 373–374
  people at risk for, vitamin requirements 124–125
  related malnutrition 399
  systemic, pregnancy and 45
  vitamin A and preventing 189–190
  vitamin C and preventing 177
Chronologic age 13
Chylomicrons 601
Circadian rhythm and sleep 639
Clear liquid diet 492–496, 493*t*
Clinical practice, diets and dietary components in 483–559
Clomipramine, grapefruit juice and 557
Clonidine, SBS 446
Clostridium difficile diarrhea 387
Cobalamin (vitamin B_{12}) 161–172
  absorption 22–23, 168
  assessment 162–163
    absorption 162–163
    intake 162–163
  body stores 163–172, 164*t*
    in elderly 165
    holo-TCII and 166–167
    homocysteine levels and 165–166
    methylmalonic acid, serum and 165–166
    screening 167
    vegetarians and 164
  coenzyme conversion of 168
  deficiency 167–169, 169*t*
    cognitive decline and 159
    dementia and 170
    hyperhomocysteinemia and 171
    infancy 125
    multiple sclerosis and 170
    neuropsychiatric presentation of 170, 170*t*
    persons at risk for 167
    vegetarians and 161, 164, 167
  DRI 161, 162*t*
  elderly and 22–23
  food sources 161–162, 163*t*
  fortification 39
  HIV and 669–670
  intake 16
    assessment 162–163
  physiology 168
  RDA 22
  treatment 171–172
  vegetarians and 161, 164, 167
Cocoa, caffeine content of 494*t*, 495
Codex Committee on Nutrition and Foods for Special Dietary Uses 499
Coenzyme Q_{10} (CoQ_{10}) supplements 181–182, 373–374
Coffee ingestion 495–496
Cognitive decline
  cobalamin deficiency and 159
  folate deficiency and 159
  homocysteine levels and 159
Cognitive function, use of antioxidant in 369
Cold, zinc treatment of 327
Colitis, inflammatory 505
Colon cancer, calcium and 281
Colonic disorders, high-fiber diet and 504–505, 505*t*
Colorectal cancer 148–149, 663
Commercial weight loss programs 644–645
Complete bowel rest, PN therapy for 453–455
Constipation
  pregnancy and 46
  TF and 438
Cooking preparations
  folate food sources and 150
  vegetable nutrients and 7
Copper 328–334
  absorption 331, 332
  assessment 329–330
  deficiency 332–333
    in disease 332
  DRI 328, 329*t*
  excretion 332
    urinary 330
  food sources 329, 330*t*
  functions 332
  intake 16
  metabolism, intracellular 331
  metallothionein and 332
  organ distribution 331
  physiology 331
  plasma 329–330
  requirement 328
  restricted diet 556

Copper (*continued*)
    therapy 333
    toxicity 333–334
    urinary excretion 330
Corn bran 501
Coronary artery disease 691
Coronary heart disease 4, 594, 612
    cholesterol and 690
    high-fiber diet and 504, 691
    saturated fat and 690
CPN. *See* Central parenteral nutrition
Creatine 382–383
    excretion 107, 107*t*
Creatinine-height index (CHI) 106–107
Crohn's disease
    PN therapy for 454, 455*t*
    small bowel, TF for 414
Crude fiber 499, 502
Curcumin 375
CVC. *See* Central venous catheter
Cyanobacteria 379
Cyclosporine, grapefruit juice and 557
Cyclosporine A, zinc toxicity 328
Cysteine dioxygenase (CDO) 381
Cysteine sulfinate decarboxylase (CSD) 381
Cytokines, HIV and 668

D

Daily food plan 488*t*
Daily reference values (DRVs) 54–55
    macronutrient 688
    nutrient 688
Daily values, for adults and children 54*t*
Dairy products. *See specific dairy products*
DASH. *See* Dietary Approaches to Stop Hypertension
DCCT. *See* Diabetes Control and Complications Trial
DCH. *See* Delayed cutaneous hypersensitivity
Dehydration
    clear liquid diet and 492
    nutrient deficiency and 69
Delayed cutaneous hypersensitivity (DCH) reactions 110, 111–112
Dementia, cobalamin deficiency and 170
Dental caries, sugar consumption and 8, 691
Depression
    of circulating lymphocyte 111
    folate deficiency and 159
DEQAS. *See* Vitamin D Quality Assessment Scheme
DETERMINE checklist 115
DEXA. *See* Dual-energy X-ray absorptiometry
Dexamethasone, retinoic acid syndrome 191
Dextrose, PN therapy solution and 466

DFEs. *See* Dietary folate equivalents
DGAC. *See* Dietary Guidelines Advisory Committee
DHT. *See* Dihydrotachysterol
Diabetes. *See also* American Diabetic Association; Epidemiology of Diabetes Interventions and Complications
    adults, nutrition recommendations for 575*t*–578*t*
    childhood 589
    diet
        activity modification for 588–589
        illness modification for 588
        management 571–590
        setting up 585–588
        therapy 574–585
    enteral nutritional therapy formulas for 423
    high-fiber diet and 504
    hyperlipidemia and 589–590
    hypertension and 589–590
    incidence 571
    niacin and 142
    nutrition therapy 574
    obesity and 571
    pregnancy and 44, 589
    prevalence 571–572
    renal disease and 589–590
    in specific groups 589–590
    trials 572–573
    type1, diet therapy for 574, 583–584
    type2
        diet therapy 574, 578–583, 581*t*
        prevention of 572
    vitamin C and 177
    vitamin D deficiency and 204
    weight loss and 573
Diabetes Control and Complications Trial (DCCT) 572
Dialysis, chronic renal disease 593–599
Diarrhea
    clear liquid diet and 492
    HIV and 668
    sodium reabsorption and 255–257
    TF and 438
    zinc treatment for 326
Diazepam, grapefruit juice and 557
Diet(s). *See also specific diets*
    acid-base balance and 245
    alcohol consumption and 489, 489*t*
    altered consistency and 492–509
    bland 498
    BMI and 5
    cancer-preventing 488, 658–659, 660*t*
    cardiovascular disease 489
    chronic disease prevention and 69
    clear liquid 492–496
    in clinical practice 483–559

DASH 5
diabetes 571–591
  activity modification for 588–589
  illness modification for 588
  setting up 585–588
  type1, 583–584
  type2, 578–583, 581*t*
  disease management with 618–620
  enteral nutritional therapy, pancreatic
    disease 440, 442
  gastrointestinal disorder-specific 557–559
  heart disease-preventing 488
  high-fiber 503–505
  HIV malnutrition 670–672
  hyperlipoproteinemia managed
    with 600–612
  hypertension managed with 599
  individual components restricted/
    supplemented by 509–559
  liquid 412
  low-calorie nutritionally balanced 125
  mechanical soft 497–498
  medical illnesses managed by 69, 72
  mediterranean 491
  modified-fiber 498–509
    content of 499
    fermentation and 502–503
    measurement of 501
  nordic 491–492
  normal 483–485
  nutritional therapy
    disease 615–617
    enteral, and modifying 411, 412
  occult blood screening 555, 555*t*
  placebo effect 72
  practical aspects of 489
  pregnancy and 44
  renal acid excretion and 245
  renal disease managed with 590–600
    phases of 591–599
  restricted 483
  SBS therapy with 444–445
  smell and 489–490
  soft 412
  taste and 489–490
  therapy 69–72, 615–617
  vegetarian 483, 483*t*, 490–491
  vitamin K-enriched 556
  weighing 96
  weight loss on controlled 97
  zinc content of 320
Diet pyramids 10–11. *See also* MyPyramid
    food guidance system
  alternative 11
Dietary Approaches to Stop Hypertension
  (DASH) 552
  diet plan 5
  sodium and 249

Dietary fiber, ingredients high in 501
Dietary folate equivalents (DFEs) 39, 152
Dietary guidelines 57–65
  for Americans 1, 2*t*–3*t*, 5, 57, 486–489,
    488*t*
  chronic disease prevention 55*t*–58*t*, 488
  implementation 10–11
  pyramids 10–11
Dietary Guidelines Advisory Committee
  (DGAC) 57
Dietary intakes 14–16
  24-hour recall of 96
  assessing, methods for 96
Dietary reference intakes (DRIs) 52–54,
  53*t*, 123, 124
  biotin 178
  calcium 272–273, 272*t*
  chromium 340, 341*t*
  cobalamin 161, 162*t*
  copper 328, 329*t*
  energy 97
  folate 150*t*, 152
  manganese 340
  phosphorus 289
  protein 99
  selenium 342–343, 342*t*
  vitamin A 182, 183*t*
  vitamin C 173, 173*t*
  vitamin D 193–194, 193*t*
  vitamin E 207, 208*t*
  vitamin K 217–218, 218*t*
  zinc 319, 319*t*
Dietary Supplement Health and Education
  Act (DSHEA) 63, 361
Dietary supplements 361–388, 557–559
  commercial 413
  definition 363
  fat 527–532
  functional foods and
    supplements 362–388
  gluten-restricted diet 543
  individual components and 509–559
  lactose-free 413
  low-protein diet 537
  oral 413
  protein 537–543
  regulation of 361–362
  selected nutritional 363, 364*t*–375*t*
Dihomo-γ-linolenic acid (DGLA) 386
Dihydrofolate reductase, inhibition 158
Dihydrotachysterol (DHT) 205
1,25-Dihydroxyvitamin D_3, 197, 205–206
Disease. *See also specific diseases*
  copper, hepatic content in 332
  nutritional management of
    specific 571–620
    dietary therapy for 615–617
    nonlipid risk factors of 612–614

Disease (*continued*)
practical dietary management 617–620
therapeutic approaches to 612–620
obesity and risks of 633–634
prevention
nutrition and 658–659
Divalent cations 245
Docosahexaenoic acid (DHA) 383–384
Donepezil 376
Double-blind oral control challenge 546
Double-blind, randomized controlled trials (DBRCT) 368, 378
Doxorubicin, vitamin E therapy and 217
DRIs. *See* Dietary reference intakes
Dronabinol 673
Drugs. *See also specific drugs*
action 75–76, 77*t*
addiction, pregnancy and 44–45
associated with weight gain 640*t*
caffeine content of 493–496, 494*t*
elderly and 24–25
food intake alterations and 76, 78*t*
gluten in 543
micronutrient metabolism and effects of 75
mineral status affected by 345–346, 345*t*
nutrients and 24–25, 26*t*, 27*t*, 74–76
oral manifestations induced by 67*t*–68*t*
DRVs. *See* Daily reference values
DSHEA. *See* Dietary Supplement Health and Education Act
Dual-energy X-ray absorptiometry (DEXA) 106–107
Dumping syndrome, low-available carbohydrate diet for 510
Dysgeusia, drug-causing 76
Dyslipidemia, atherogenic 611
Dysphagia, HIV and 668

E

E. sinica 377
EAR. *See* Estimated average requirement
Ebastine, grapefruit juice and 557
Echinacea 376, 379
Eclampsia, maternal weight gain and 36
Edema, pregnancy and 46
EDIC. *See* Epidemiology of Diabetes Interventions and Complications
EEA. *See* Energy expenditure of activity
EER. *See* Estimated energy requirements
EFA. *See* Essential fatty acids
Eicosanoids 385
Eicosapentaenoic acid (EPA) 383, 384, 666
Eldepryl. *See* Selegiline HCl
Elderly
antioxidants and 20–21
bone health in 19–20
cobalamin and 22–23
body stores of 165
treatment for 172
dietary intakes 14–16
drugs and 24–25
energy expenditure and 25, 27
fiber and 21–22
folate and 22–23
food access/selection in 19
iodine and 23–24
iron and 23–24
magnesium and 23–24
minerals and 23–24
MNA 69
niacin and 23
nutrition 13–29, 28*t*
advice for 25–29, 28*t*
deficiency 65
intake 25, 25*t*
issues in 19–25
pyridoxine and 22–23
recommendations for healthy 13–29
riboflavin and 23
thiamine and 23
vegetarians, cobalamin and 22
vitamin A and 23
vitamin C levels in 177
vitamin D deficiency in 201–202
vitamin requirements 124
zinc and 23–24
Electrolytes. *See also* Monitor Serum Electrolytes; Serum electrolyte concentration
nutrition monitoring and 407
PN therapy and
additives of 470–471
administered via PN solution 462*t*
preparations for 470–471
TF and disturbances in 437–438
Empty calories 489
Emsam. *See* Transdermal selegiline
Endocrine organs 18, 440, 684
Energy. *See also* Basal energy expenditure; Basal energy requirement; Resting energy expenditure
balance 96–97
DRI 97
evaluation, assessment for 116*t*, 119
requirements
illness 92
lactating women and 100
pregnancy and 92
special 92
weight loss and needs of 92
Energy dense foods 6
Energy equation 81–83

Energy expenditure 97
  elderly and 25, 27
  obesity and 637–638
  PAL 89–92, 90*t*
Energy expenditure of activity (EEA) 89–92
Energy intake
  recommended daily 97
  renal disease, chronic and 595
  thiamine requirements and 129
Energy medicine 365
Enhanced Recovery After Surgery (ERAS) Group 492
Enrichment
  niacin 139
  riboflavin 135
Enteral nutritional therapy 411–446, 411*f*
  administration sets for 428
  diet modifications for 411, 412
  feeding access devices 425–427, 427*t*
  feeding containers for 428
  feeding equipment for 428
  feeding methods 427
  feeding pumps for 428
  forced TF and 412
    caloric density of formulas for 417, 421
    definitions 417–420
    diabetes formulas of 423
    disease specific formulas for 422–423
    elemental formulas for 421–422
    fiber-containing formulas for 420–421
    formulas for 416–425, 417*t*, 418*t*–420*t*
    hepatic disease formulas for 422
    immune modulating formulas for 423–425
    low-residue formulas for 412
    nonprotein calorie ratio to nitrogen and 417–420
    osmolality and formulas for 417
    pulmonary disease formulas for 422
    renal disease formulas for 423
    semi-elemental formulas for 421–422
    standard formulas for 420–421
  indications 412–415
  initiation of 435–436, 435*f*
    maintaining 45-degree elevation and 435–436
  modular products, supplementation with commercially available 416
  oral, methods of providing 415–416
  oral supplements for 412, 413
  pancreatic disease 440–443
  pancreatitis, acute 443
  pancreatitis, chronic 440–443
    diet and 440, 442
    enzyme replacement for 442, 442*t*
    vitamin supplementation for 442–443
  short-bowel syndrome 444–446
    adaptation after massive resection, following 444–446
    adjunctive medications for 446
    antimotility agents for 446
    control gastric hypersecretion and 446
    intestinal adaptation after massive resection and 444
    oral rehydration solutions and 446, 446*t*
  TF
    aspirate 436
    bolus 436
    choosing product for 425–437, 426*f*
    constant-infusion technique for 436
    feeding formulas for 436
    insertion site care for 433–434, 434*t*
    intermittent 436
    long-term access for 433
    monitoring patients for 436–437, 437*t*
    percutaneous endoscopic gastrostomy technique for 433
    short silicone post low-profile tube for 433
    short-term access for 429, 432*f*
    tip location for 428–429, 428*t*
    tube insertion for 429–435, 430*t*–431*t*
    tube patency maintenance and 434–435, 435*t*
  whole food supplementation in 415–416, 415*t*
Enterocutaneous fistulas
  PN therapy for 454–455
  TF for 414
Enzymes
  low-lactose diet and replacing 521, 522*t*
  pancreatic disease enteral nutrition therapy replacement of 442, 442*t*
Eosinophilic esophagitis (EoE) 546
Ephedra 379
Ephedra sinica. See Ma huang
Ephedrine 377
EPIC. *See* European Prospective Investigation of Cancer and Nutrition
Epidemiology of Diabetes Interventions and Complications (EDIC) 572
Epinephrine 317
Ergocalciferol. *See* Vitamin D_2
Ergosterol. *See* Vitamin D_2
Erythrocyte hemolysis, vitamin E 208–209
Esophageal ulcer, TF and 438
Esophagitis, TF and 438
ESPEN. *See* European Society for Parenteral and Enteral Nutrition
Essential fatty acids (EFA) 523–524
  manifestations of 464
  omega-3, 525
  PN therapy 463–464

Estimated average requirement
(EAR) 52
  iron, pregnancy and 37–38
  nitrogen 99
  protein 9
  thiamine 23
  vitamin A 23
  vitamin E 23
Estimated energy requirements
(EER) 5, 82–83
  dietary intakes and 14
  lactating women 34–35
  method, choice of 83
  pregnancy and 34–35
Ethane, breath 210
Ethnicity/race
  diabetes and 571
  lactose intolerance and 519
  life expectancy 14
  obesity and 638
European Prospective Investigation of Cancer and Nutrition (EPIC) 160, 370
European Society for Parenteral and Enteral Nutrition (ESPEN) 115
Evening primrose oil 386
Evodia ruaecarpa 379
Exercise 8–9. *See also* Physical activity

F

Falls, vitamin D therapy and 202–203
FAO. *See* Food and Agriculture Organization
Fast food 489
Fat(s) 483. *See also* Fatty acids; Low-fat diet; *specific fats*
  cancer and 690
  content 523, 528*t*–530*t*
  distribution 631
  grams of 11
  healthy 619
  intake 523–525
  malabsorption 524
  modular 416
  percentage of calories from 11
  replacers 532*t*
  saturated 7–8
  stores 104–106
  substitutes 527
  supplements 527–532
  types 523–524
Fat mass (FM) 97
Fat-free mass (FFM) 97
Fat-free, nutrient content descriptor 689
Fatty acids. *See also specific fatty acids*
  dietary therapy 615, 616
  fiber fermentation and volatile 503
FDA. *See* Food and Drug Administration
Felodipine, grapefruit juice and 557
Ferritin 304–305, 304*t*
Ferrlecit. *See* Sodium ferric gluconate
Ferumoxytol (Feraheme) 317
FFM. *See* Fat-free mass
Fiber 7. *See also* High-fiber diet; Lowfiber diet; Modified-fiber diet
  cancer and 690
  cholesterol levels lowered by 505
  classes of 499, 500*t*
  colitis, inflammatory treated with 505
  content 499, 507*t*–508*t*
  coronary artery disease and 691
  coronary heart disease and 691
  crude 499, 502
  dietary 498
    functions of 503–505
    modified 498–509
  elderly and 21–22
  enteral nutritional therapy formulas and 420–421
  fermentation 502–503
  intake 503, 505*t*
  sources 508
  stool weight and 503, 504*t*
  total 498–499
Fick equation 83
Firmicutes 386
Fish oil 384, 385
Five food groups 485
  balanced diet and 485
Flavocoxid 379
Flavonoids 370
  dietary 134, 135
Fluid retention, pregnancy and 45–46
Fluorine
  assessment 337
  deficiency 338
  food sources 337
  physiology 338
  requirement 337
  toxicity 338
  treatment 338
  urinary excretion 337–338
Fluorosis, systemic 338
FM. *See* Fat mass
FODMAP elimination diet 516–517
Folacin. *See* Folate
Folate (folic acid, folacin, pteroylglutamic acid) 149–161. *See also* Dietary folate equivalents
  absorption 154–155
  anemia, megaloblastic and 38, 45
  assessment 152–154
    absorption 152–154
    assays 154
    intake 152–154
    serum homocysteine 154, 156*t*
    status, interpretation of 152, 153*t*
    tissue stores 153*t*, 154

body stores 40
cancer and 159–160, 665
deficiency 156–160
  cancer and 159–160
  cognitive decline and 159
  depression and 159
  hyperhomocysteinemia and 158–159
  neural tube defects and 157
diet content of, average 152
dietary sources 39–40
DRI 150t, 152
drug interfering with metabolism of 38
elderly and 22–23
food processing and 40
food sources 41, 150, 151t
  availability 151–152
  cooking preparations and 150
fortification 22, 39, 152, 160–161
HIV and 670
intake 16
  assessment 152–154
medication 161
metabolism, intracellular 156
monoglutamate forms 151
neural tube defects and 157, 691
physiology 154–156
polyglutamate forms 151
pregnancy deficiency of 125
protein binding of 156
reabsorption 156
requirements 149–150
  estimation, difficulty 149–150
  pregnancy 38–41
supplementation 40–41, 159, 160
synthetic 152
toxicity 161
treatment 160–161
Folic acid. *See* Folate
Food. *See also* Serotonin-rich foods, restriction of
additives
  adverse reactions to 548
  restricted diets for 548–551
allergies 547
  diets for 544–548, 545t
caffeine content of 493–496, 494t
caloric content of 92–93, 93t–94t
elderly and 19
groups 5–6, 485
high-fiber diet and decreased 503
induced reactions, classification of 545t
intake, drug-induced alterations of 76, 78t
intolerance to 544–545
low-available carbohydrate diet 512–513, 514t–515t
osmolarity, low-available carbohydrate diet and 513, 513t
variety 5–7

Food Additives Amendment 64
Food Allergen and Consumer Protection Act 543
Food Allergen Labeling and Consumer Protection Act of 2004 (FALCPA) 546
Food and Agriculture Organization (FAO) 86–88
Food and Drug Act of 1906, 64
Food and Drug Administration (FDA)
  dietary supplement regulation by 361
  drug regulation by 361
  health claims approved by 551, 690–691
  herbal product regulation by 361–362
Food composition 57–65, 58t, 59t
Food, Drug, and Cosmetic Act of 1938, 64, 362
Food groups, caloric content of 95t, 97
Food guide pyramid 10–11, 485
Food preparation 552
  iron and 300
  supplements and 300
Food processing 58–60, 60t
  folate and 40
  nutrient loss and 59, 61t
  potassium and 263, 264t
  sodium and effect of 250–252, 251t
  zinc and 320
Food Pyramid guide 485
Food Wheel 485
Fortification
  advantage 62
  calcium 41, 273
  cobalamin 39
  folate 22, 39, 160–161
  food 62–63
  iron 300
  nutrient 63–64, 63t
  vitamin D 42, 192
Fractures, bone health and 202
Free erythrocyte protoporphyrin, iron assessment and 303–304
Free radicals, antioxidants and 20
Free, nutrient content descriptor 688
Fresh, nutrient content descriptor 690
Fructose
  intolerance 512
  low-available carbohydrate diet and 516
Fructus Psoraleae 379
Fruit
  juice, drug interactions and 556–557
  nutrients 6–7, 7t
  as source of polyphenols 369–370
  variety 6–7
Functional foods
  definition 362
  physiologically active compounds in 367t

Furanocoumarins 556
Furazolidone (Furoxone) 549
Furoxone. *See* Furazolidone

G

G. biloba 376
Galactosemia, low-lactose diet and 520
α-galactosidase (Beano) 548
Gastric bypass, low-available carbohydrate diet, postoperative for 511
Gastric hypersecretion, control 446
Gastrointestinal (GI) tract
　HIV and infections of 659
　PN therapy and 453
　protein loss through 102
Gastrointestinal disorders
　diets for, specific 557–559
　nutritional support for 117*t*, 119
　pregnancy and 46–47
　selenium treatment of 344
　vitamin deficiency treatment in 125
Gastroparesis, diet 558–559
Genetics, obesity and 638
German Federal Institute for Drugs and Medicinal Devices 362
GI. *See* Glycemic index
GI tract. *See* Gastrointestinal tract
Ginkgolides 376
Ginseng 376–377
b-Glucan 501
Glucosamine 374–375
Glucose, potassium toxicity 270
Glutamine (Gln) 379–380, 424, 667
Gluten
　drug product 543
　when eating out 543
　grain product content of 538, 539*t*
　grains classification based on 539*t*
Gluten-free diet (GFD) 537–538
Gluten-restricted diet
　allergy relationship to 538
　commercial products for 543
　cookbooks for 542–543
　definitions 537–538
　duration 539
　general instructions 539–542
　indications 539
　patient support groups for 542
　practical aspects 536*t*, 539–542, 540*t*–541*t*
　safe commercial products 543
　side effects 543
　specific recommendations 542–543
　supplements 543
Glutena, sources of 540*t*–541*t*
Glycemic index (GI)
　definition 510
　low-available carbohydrate diet and 518–519

Good source, nutrient content descriptor 689
Gout, low-purine diet for 557
Grain products
　gluten content 538, 539*t*
　phosphorus in 290–291
　toxic 538
　variety 6–7
　whole 6
Grapefruit juice 556–557
Green tea 370–371
Growth hormone 673

H

Hair. *See also* Menkes kinky hair syndrome
　copper assessment and 330
　zinc in 322
Hallervorden-Spatz syndrome 180
Harris-Benedict equation 85–86, 683
Hartnup disease, niacin deficiency and 142
Harvard School of Public Health 11
HDLs. *See* High density lipoproteins
Health claims 690–691
Healthy, nutrient content descriptor 690
Heart disease. *See also* Coronary heart disease
　diets for preventing 488
　fish oil for 384
　L-carnitine and 382
Heartburn, pregnancy and 46
Height 55. *See also* Creatinine-height index
Hemicelluloses 500
Hemodialysis 598
Hemoglobin, iron assessment and 301, 302*t*, 303
Hemorrhagic disease, newborn 222
Heparin
　hemodialysis and 598
　PN therapy and 471
Hepatic disease 422
Hepatic encephalopathy 414
Hepcidin 305–306
Herbae pulvis standardisatus 379
Herbal medicines 365
　adverse effects of 379
Herbal products 375–379
　adverse effects of 378–379
　Curcumin 375
　Echinacea 376
　G. biloba 376
　ginseng 376–377
　Hoodia 377
　labeling of 361–362
　Ma Huang 377
　Phytosterols 377–378
　saw palmetto berry 378–379
　soy protein 378
　St. John's wort 379

High density lipoproteins (HDLs) 602–603. *See also* Non-HDL cholesterol
cholesterol 608
High fat (ketogenic) diet 533–534
High-fiber diet 505*t*, 508–509
  clinical effects of 503–505
  food intake, decrease and 503
High, nutrient content descriptor 689
High-pressure liquid chromatography (HPLC)
  carotenoid 184
  niacin 130
  thiamine 130
  vitamin C 175, 175*t*
High-protein diet 537
Highly Active Antiretroviral Therapy (HAART) 668
HIV. *See* Human immunodeficiency virus
Holo-TCII, cobalamin and 166–167
Home parenteral nutrition (HPN) 478
  bone disease, metabolic and 478–479
  liver dysfunction and 476*t*, 479
  long-term, complications of 478–479
  sepsis, line and 478
Homeopathic products 366
Homocysteine
  cobalamin and levels of 165–166
  cognitive decline and 159
  pyridoxine body stores and 146, 146*t*
  serum, folate 154, 156*t*
Homocysteine Lowering Trialists' Collaboration 158
*Hoodia Gordoni*i 377
Hospital house diet 489
Hospitalized patients
  BEE estimates for 88–89
  low-protein diet for 535
  REE estimates for 89, 89*t*
  surgical procedure preparations for 412–414
  test preparations for 412–414
  TF, indications for 414–415
HPLC. *See* High-pressure liquid chromatography
HPN. *See* Home parenteral nutrition
Human immunodeficiency virus (HIV)
  breast feeding and 48
  malnutrition and
    anabolic agents for 672–673
    appetite stimulants for 672–673
    dietary recommendations for 671–672
    disorders accompanying 673
    effects of 669–670
    treating 670–672, 671*t*
  metabolism, altered in 668
  micronutrients, individual and 669–670
  nutritional deficiency in 668–669
  nutritional management of 668–673

protease inhibitors 669
  vitamin deficiency treatment in 125
  weight loss 668
Huperzia serrata 379
Hutchinson–Gilford progeria syndrome 17
25-Hydroxycholecalciferol (25-OHD) 42
5-Hydroxytryptophan (5-HTP) 383
25-Hydroxyvitamin D (25OHD) 195–197
25-Hydroxyvitamin D_3 (calcifediol, Calderol) 206
Hypercalcemia 278
  calcium toxicity and 281
  PN therapy and 473
Hyperhomocysteinemia
  AHA screening recommendations for 159
  cobalamin deficiency and 171
  folate deficiency and 158–159
Hyperhomocysteinuria, pyridoxine deficiency and 147
Hypericum perforatum 379
Hyperkalemia 268
Hyperlipidemia
  diabetes and 589–590
  diagnosis 611–612
Hyperlipoproteinemia 599, 608–612, 609*t*
  definitions 601–603
  dietary management 600–612
  familial 610
  type 608–609
  type I 609
  type IIa 609–610
  type IIb 610
  type III 610
  type IV 610
  type V 611
Hypermagnesemia 288
Hypernatremia, sodium toxicity and 261
Hyperosmolarity syndrome
  PN therapy and 473
  TF and 438
Hyperoxaluria 543–544
Hyperproteinemia 274
Hypertension
  calcium and 280–281
  diabetes and 589–590
  dietary management 599
  sodium and 691
Hypertriglyceridemia 590
  mixed 611
  to prevent pancreatitis 526
Hyperuricemia 557
Hypervitaminosis A 190
Hypoalbuminemia 115
Hypocalcemia 279
Hypoglycemia, low-available carbohydrate diet for 510–511

Hyponatremia, sodium depletion and 258, 258*t*
Hypophosphatemia
 mild 295
 moderate 295
 phosphorus treatment of 295–296
 severe 295–296

I

IBS. *See* Irritable bowel syndrome
Ice cream substitutes 521–522
IgE–mediated reactions 546–547
Ileostomy, SBS 445
Ill patients, nutrition monitoring in 406–407
Illness
 energy requirements during 92
 medical, diets for managing 69, 72
 protein estimation during 101–102
 protein requirements and 102, 102*t*
Immune system
 abnormalities 110
 enteral nutritional therapy formulas for modulating 423–425
 function, zinc and 325
 nutrition and 669
 tests 110–112, 111*t*
Immune-modulating polysaccharides 374
Immune-modulating products 675*t*
Immunocompetence, nutritional assessment and 110–112
Immunonutrition 675–676, 675*t*, 676*t*
Implementation guidelines 10–11
 suggestions for 11
Implied, nutrient content descriptor 690
Infancy
 premature
  copper deficiency and 333
  vitamin E and 217
 protein requirements 99–100
 vitamin C requirement and 173
 vitamin deficiency treatment in 125
Infant Formula Act 363
Infant formulas, folate deficiency and 157
InFeD. *See* Iron dextran
Inflammatory bowel disease
 diets for 557–558
 fish oil for 385
Institute of Medicine (IOM)
 on folate supplementation 41
 on maternal weight 36
Insulin
 diabetes 572
 PN therapy and 471
 potassium toxicity 270
Intensive obesity therapy, indications for 641*t*

Intestinal symptoms, nonspecific 524–525
Intestines, sodium reabsorption in 255–257, 257*t*
Intravenous fat emulsions (IVFE) 466–469, 468*t*
Involutional osteoporosis, vitamin D deficiency and 201
Iodine
 assessment 334–335
 deficiency 336
 elderly and 23–24
 food sources 334
 medication content of 336, 336*t*
 physiology 335
 PN therapy and 471
 requirement 334
 toxicity 336
 treatment 336
 urinary excretion 334, 335, 335*t*
Ion excretion, sodium 255
Iron 294–319. *See also* Neurodegeneration with brain iron accumulation
 absorption 308
  estimated 301
  factors affecting 308–309
  rate of 297
 assessment 301–306, 302*t*
  ferritin and 304–305, 304*t*
  free erythrocyte protoporphyrin and 303–304
  hepcidin 305–306
  sTfR and 305
  summary 306–307
  transferrin and 303
 body stores 308
 deficiency 310–312
  blood loss and 311
  gastrointestinal loss 311
  increased utilization and 310–311
  iron-refractory iron-deficiency anemia 312
  other medical conditions 311–312
  restless leg syndrome 312
  screening for 307, 308*t*
 EAR, pregnancy and 37
 elderly and 23–24
 food preparation and 300
 food sources 298–301, 299*t*
 fortification 300
 hemoglobin and 301, 302*t*, 303
 HIV and 670
 intake 15, 300–301
  inadequate 311
 losses 307–308
  daily 297
 malabsorption 311
 oral 312–313, 314*t*
 overload 318
  screening for 307

oxidation of absorbed 309
parenteral 313–316, 315t
  dose calculation for 316
  indications for 313, 315t
  intramuscular route for 316
  intravenous route for 316
phlebotomy and 319
physiology 307–310
PN therapy and 470–471
pregnancy and 37–38, 45
RDA 297–298
  pregnancy 37
renal disease, chronic and 598
requirements 297–298, 298t
  pregnancy and 37–38
serum 303
stores, direct methods for assessing 306
  therapy response and 306
supplementation, gastrointestinal side effects of 38
toxicity 318
  children and 38
  diagnosis 319
transcellular, transport 309–310
transport of absorbed 309
treatment 312–318
  hypersensitivity reactions 318
  response to 317–318
vitamin C and absorption of 177–178
Iron carboxymaltose (Ferinject, Injectafer) 317
Iron dextran (InFeD) 316–317
Iron isomaltoside (Monofer) 317
Iron sucrose (Venofer) 317
Iron-refractory iron-deficiency anemia (IRIDA) 312
Irritable bowel syndrome (IBS) 366, 558
Isocarboxazid (Marplan) 549
Isoflavones 378
IVFE. *See* Intravenous fat emulsions

J
Jejunostomy, SBS 445
Junk food 489

K
Kaposi's sarcoma, HIV and 668
Kayexalate. *See* Polystyrene sulfonate
Kidney 265–266. *See also* Renal acid excretion; Renal disease; Renal failure

L
L-Carnitine 381–382, 673. *See also* Acetyl-l-carnitine; Propionyl-l-carnitine
Labeling
  of dietary supplements 361–362
  food 686–691
    nutrition panel and 686–688, 686t, 687f
    regulations for 686

nutrient content descriptors and 688–691
reading labels and 11
sodium 553
Lactating women 34–48
  calcium and 41–43
  EER for 34–35
  energy requirements 34–36, 100
  folate requirements 39–40
  nutrition 46–47
    requirements for 37–43, 40t, 47
    special considerations for 47–48
  phosphorus and 41–43
  protein requirements 34–36
  thiamine requirements in 129
  vitamin D and 41–43
  zinc and 41–43
Lacto-ovo-vegetarians 490
Lacto-vegetarians 490
Lactose. *See also* Low-lactose diet
  dietary sources of 516t, 521
  free supplements 522
  intolerance 41
    ethnicity/race and 519
    low-lactose diet and 519–520
  SBS enteral nutritional therapy and 445
  substitutes 521–522
Laparoscopic adjustable gastric banding 649, 650f
Larrea tridentata 379
LCT. *See* Long-chain triglycerides
LDLs. *See* Low density lipoproteins
Lean body mass 106
Lean/extralean, nutrient content descriptor 689
Legumes 7
Less, nutrient content descriptor 689
Levocarnitine (Carnitor) 382
Life expectancy 14
Light, nutrient content descriptor 689
Lignin 369–370, 498–502
Limbrel 379
Linezolid (Zyvox) 549
α-Linolenic acid 385
γ-Linolenic acid (GLA) 386
Lipid(s)
  conditionally essential 533–534
  food content of 618, 618t
  profile, supplements and foods to improve 383–386
Lipid emulsions
  PN therapy 468–469, 468t
  soybean-based 468–469, 468t
Lipoproteins 601, 601t. *See also* High density lipoproteins; Low density lipoproteins; Very low density lipoprotein
  cardiovascular risk associated with 603–608
Liquid diet, full 496–497. *See also* Clear liquid diet

Liquid measure equivalents 685
Liver biopsy, iron store assessment and 306
Liver disease 414. *See also* Alcoholic liver disease, protein intake for; Nonalcoholic fatty liver disease
  malnutrition 559
  vitamin D deficiency and 204
Liver dysfunction
  HPN and 476*t*, 479
  PN therapy and 479
Long-chain triglycerides (LCT) 416
Loperamide, SBS 446
Loratadine, grapefruit juice and 557
Lorcaserin, for obesity
  management 648–649
Losartan, grapefruit juice and 557
Lovastatin, grapefruit juice and 557
Lovaza 385
Low birth weight
  food restriction during pregnancy and 44
  maternal weight gain and 36
Low density lipoproteins (LDLs) 602
  cholesterol 603–607, 603*t*–605*t*
Low, nutrient content descriptor 689
Low-available carbohydrate diet 509–519
  indications 510–512
  practical aspects of 512–519
  principles 509–510
  side effects 519
  supplements 519
Low-fat diet 523–527
  general instructions 526–527
  indications 524–526
  practical aspects 526–527
  principles 523–524
  recommendations for, specific 527, 528*t*–530*t*
  side effects 527
Low-fiber diet 506, 509
  partial 505*t*, 506
  side effects 509
  supplements for 509
Low-lactose diet 519–522
  enzyme replacement and 521, 522*t*
  indications 519–520
  practical aspects 520–522
  principles 519
  side effects 522
  supplements 522
  websites 522
Low-oxalate diet
  indications 544
  principles 543–544
Low-protein diet 534–537
  indications 535
  instructions 535–537, 536*t*
  pathophysiology 534–535, 534*t*
  practical aspects 535–537
  principles 534–535
  side effects 537
  supplements required for 537
Low-sodium diet 551–553
  cookbooks 553
  general instructions 552–553
  indications 552
  practical aspects 552–553
  principles 551–552
  recommendations, specific 553–554, 554*t*
  side effects 554
Lung disease, vitamin D deficiency and 204

M

Ma Huang 377
Macronutrients 483, 484*t*
  caloric value 683
  DRV 688
  food contents of, obesity and 642
  food sources 483, 484*t*
Macrosomia, fetal 37
Macular degeneration, zinc treatment 327
Magnesium 282–289
  absorption 283–284, 285
  assessment 283–285, 284*t*
  body stores 284, 284*t*
  deficiency 286–287
    causes of 286–287, 287*t*
    clinical manifestations of 286, 286*t*
  EAR for 43
  elderly and 23–24
  food sources 282–283
  function 285
  intake 283–284
  oral 287, 288*t*
  parathyroid hormone response 286
  parenteral 287
  physiology 285–286
  requirements 282, 283*t*
  toxicity 288–289
  treatment 287–288
  urinary excretion 285
Main dishes, nutrient content descriptor 690
Malabsorption
  bile acid 544
  energy requirements 92
  fat, predominantly 524
  "global", 524
  HIV and 668, 669
  low-fat diet for 524
  vitamin D deficiency and 200–201
Malnourished patients
  HIV and 668
  nutritional therapy, intensive for 112–116

Malnutrition 399, 400f
  AIDS patients and 670
  BMR 85
  classification 399
  concept of 65
  copper deficiency and 333
  HIV and
    anabolic agents for 672–673
    appetite stimulants for 672–673
    dietary recommendations for 671–672
    disorders accompanying 673
    effects of 669–670
    treating 670–672, 671t
  in hospitalized patients 400f
  obesity and 1
  protein-calorie 669
  screening tests for 113–116
Malnutrition Screening Tool (MST) 399
Malnutrition Universal Screening Tool (MUST) 115
Manganese 338–340
  absorption 339
  assessment 339
  deficiency 339
  DRI 338
  food sources 339
  function 339
  physiology 339
  PN therapy and 471
  requirement 338–339
  toxicity 340
  treatment 340
Marplan. See Isocarboxazid
Marrow staining, iron store assessment and 306
Maternal weight gain 36–37
Matrix-Gla protein (MGP) 220
Matulane. See Procarbazine
MCT. See Medium-chain triglycerides
Meals, nutrient content descriptor 690
Meat consumption, cancer and 663–664
Mechanical soft diet 497–498
Medical disorders, osteoporosis in 280
Medical food 362, 531
Medications. See also specific medications
  iodine content in 336, 336t
  PN therapy and 471, 472t
  sodium in 252
Mediterranean-pattern diet 249, 491, 659
Medium-chain triglycerides (MCT) 416, 416t, 527, 530–531
Megestrol acetate 672–673
Menkes kinky hair syndrome 333
Mephyton. See Phytonadione
6-Mercaptopurine, cobalamin deficiency and 169
3-Methylhistidine excretion 108

Metabolic disorders, polyphenols for 369–372
  chocolate 372
  green tea 370–371
  olive oil 371–372
Metabolism
  complications
    PN therapy-associated 471–473
    TF 437–438
  HIV and altered 668
  micronutrient, drug effects on 75
Metallothionein, copper and 332
Metals 247–248. See also specific metals
Methadone, grapefruit juice and 557
Method of Southgate 502
Methotrexate therapy, folate and 38, 160
Methylmalonic acid, serum 165–166
MGP. See Matrix-Gla protein
Micronutrients 483–484
  food sources 483–485, 485t, 486t
  HIV and individual 669–670
  metabolism, drug effects on 75
Mid-upper arm circumference (MUAC) 106
Mifflin-St Jeor equation 406
Milk
  allergy 547
  low-available carbohydrate diet and 512, 513, 516t
  phosphorus in 290
  products, enteral nutrition therapy and 415
  substitutes 521
Mind-body medicine 366
Mineral(s) 245–346. See also specific minerals
  body stores 245
  content 685
  conversion factors of major 685
  deficiency
    clinical manifestations of 245, 246t
    evaluation of 245–247
    factors involved in 245–248
    treatment of 248
  drug action and effect on 75–76, 77t
  drugs that affect status of 345–346, 345t
  elderly and 23–24
  food sources 483–485, 486t
  high-fiber diet and availability of 504
  intestinal absorption/secretion of 245
  major 248–297
  overload 247–248
    factors involved in 245–255
  for prevention of chronic disease 373–374
  requirements
    ASPEN 461, 463t
    PN therapy 461, 462t, 463t
  supplements
    dietary therapy 617
    elderly and 29

Mineral(s) (*continued*)
  toxicity 55, 56*t*–57*t*, 247–248
  trace 297–345
    PN therapy and 470–471
    TF and deficiencies in 438
Mini Nutritional Assessment (MNA) 69, 113*t*–114*t*, 116
MNA. *See* Mini Nutritional Assessment
Modified-fiber diet 498–509
  consumption levels, current and 505–506
  definition 498–499
  fiber in
    content of 499
    fermentation and 502–503
    indications 505–506
    intake, recommended and 505*t*, 506
    measurement of 501
    practical aspects of 506–509
Modular products, enteral nutritional therapy supplemented with commercially available 416
Molybdenum, PN therapy and 471
Monitor serum electrolytes, SBS 444
Mono-fatty acids, dietary therapy 615–616
Monoamine oxidase, drugs inhibiting 549
Monosodium glutamate (MSG) 551
Monovalent cations 245
More, nutrient content descriptor 689
Mortality
  body mass index and 631–633, 633*f*, 633*t*
  rate, vitamin D deficiency and 203
Mottled teeth, fluorine and 338
MSG. *See* Monosodium glutamate
Mucositis 667–668
Multiple sclerosis, cobalamin deficiency and 170
Multivitamin supplements, elderly and 29
Muscle
  function, vitamin D therapy and 202–203
  maintenance, creatine for 382–383
  mass, estimates 107
MUST. *See* Malnutrition Universal Screening Tool
MVI-Adult 461*t*, 470, 476*f*
Myeloneuropathy, copper deficiency and 333
MyPlate tool 10, 66, 485–486
MyPyramid food guidance system 485–486, 488*t*

N

NAFLD. *See* Nonalcoholic fatty liver disease
Nails, zinc in 322
Nardil. *See* Phenelzine sulfate
National Cholesterol Education Program (NCEP) 378
National Cholesterol Education Program Adult Treatment Panel III (ATPIII) 526
National Health and Nutrition Examination Surveys (NHANES) 1, 14, 96
National Institute of Allergy and Infectious Diseases (NIAID) 545
National Labeling Education Act 362
Nausea
  HIV and 668
  pregnancy and 46
NBIA. *See* Neurodegeneration with brain iron accumulation
Neotame, low-available carbohydrate diet and 517
Neural tube defects, folate deficiency and 39, 157, 691
Neurodegeneration with brain iron accumulation (NBIA) 180
Neutral detergent residues 502
Neutrophos treatment 346
NHANES. *See* National Health and Nutrition Examination Surveys
Niacin (vitamin B_3) 138–143
  assessment 139–140
    absorption 139–140
    body stores 140, 141*t*
    intake 139–140
  deficiency 141–142
    carcinoid syndrome and 142
    Hartnup disease and 142
    pellagra and 141–142
    pyridoxine deficiency and 143
  elderly and 23
  enrichment 139
  food sources 139, 140*t*
  intake 16, 23
  pharmacologic effects 142–143
  physiology 140–141
  requirements 23, 138–139, 139*t*
  toxicity 143
  treatment 142
  urinary excretion 139–140, 141*t*
Nicotinamide 141
Nicotinic acid 141
Nimodipine, grapefruit juice and 557
Nisoldipine, grapefruit juice and 557
Nitrates, vegetable source in 491
Nitrite, vegetable source in 491
Nitrogen 99
  protein content of 683
Non–alcoholic fatty liver disease (NAFLD) 213–216, 526, 559
Non–alcoholic steatohepatitis (NASH) 526
Non–celiac gluten sensitivity (NCGS) 538
Non-HDL cholesterol 603
Noncellulose polysaccharides 502–503

Nordic diet 491–492
Normal diet 483–485
NRS. *See* Nutritional Risk Screening
Nut-derived oils, lipid
 content of 523*t*
Nutrient(s). *See also* Macronutrients;
 Malnutrition; *specific nutrients*
 adequate 1
 clear liquid diet of 493, 493*t*
 content descriptors of 688–691
 deficiency
  anthropomorphic measurements and 65
  approach to 51–79
  dehydration and 69
  general assessment of 65–69
  laboratory tests 69, 75*t*, 76*t*
  physical examination and 66–69,
   70*t*–71*t*
  signs/symptoms of 70*t*–71*t*
  taste, decreased and 66, 67*t*–68*t*
 dense foods 6
 deposition, pregnancy and 35, 35*t*
 disease managed with
  dietary therapy for 612–617
  nonlipid risk factors of 612–614
  practical dietary management 617–620
  specific 571–620
  therapeutic approaches to 612–620
 distribution of, among food
  groups 485, 487*t*
 DRIs 52–54, 53*t*
 drugs and 24–25, 26*t*, 27*t*, 74–76
 DRV 54–55, 56*t*–57*t*, 688
 elderly and advice for 25–29, 25*t*
 FDA-approved health
  claims for 366*t*
 fortification 63–64, 63*t*
 fruits 6–7, 7*t*
 history 65–66, 66*t*
 HIV and intake of 668
 individual, component 81–122
 lactating women and
  requirements 37–43, 40*t*
 loss, food processing and 59, 61*t*
 pregnancy and
  requirements for 37–43, 40*t*
  risk factors of 43–46
 RDAs 51, 52
 related Internet sites 59*t*
 requirements
  PN therapy 460–464, 461*t*
  renal disease, chronic 591–593, 594*t*
 screening tools 69, 74*t*
 sufficiency, definitions of 51–57
 supplements 60–63
 toxicity 55, 56*t*–57*t*
 vegetables 6–7, 7*t*
Nutrient Content of the U.S. Food Supply 64

Nutrition
 American Cancer Society
  guidelines on 4*t*
 assessment 400–401, 400*f*, 401*t*, 402*t*
  immunocompetence in 110–112
  pregnancy 43
  serum protein used for 108*t*
  status, clinical applications of 112–120
 cancer and 658–668
  malignancy of 665–667
 cancer problems related to 667*t*, 668
 catabolic condition 118*t*, 119, 674
 chemotherapy and 668, 677
 chronic diseases and 657–676
 for diabetic adults 575*t*–578*t*
 disease and 658–659
 elderly 13–29, 28*t*
 for healthy elderly adults 13–29
 for healthy young adults 1–11
 HIV and
  deficiency in 668–669
  managing 668–673
 immune system and 669
 intervention 401–406, 403*f*
 lactating women 46–47
  requirements for 40*t*, 47
  special considerations for 47–48
 malnourished patients 402–403
 monitoring 406–407
  electrolytes and 407
  plan for 406–407
 pregnancy and 34–37
  assessing 43
  risk factors for 43–46
 screening
  questions for 399, 400*t*
  successful 399
 support for critically ill
  patients 401–406, 403*f*, 673–674
  avenues of 403*f*
  decision making 399–409
  definition of 399
  enteral 403–404, 404*f*
  intensive 404, 405*f*, 406
  malnourished patients 402–403
  parenteral 403–404, 404*f*
  specific indications for 116, 117*t*, 118*t*
  time length for 403, 404*t*
 therapeutic 399
Nutrition Care Process 399
Nutrition panel 686–688, 686*t*, 687*f*
Nutritional Effects Foundation
 (NEF) 526–527
Nutritional Risk Screening (NRS) 115
Nutritional supplements, for prevention of
 chronic disease 372–375
Nutritional therapeutics, facts/
 formulas 683–685

Nutritional therapy. *See also* Enteral nutritional therapy; Parenteral nutritional therapy
  diabetes 574
  malnourished patient 112–116
  oral supplementation and 411, 412, 413*t*

O

Oat bran 501
Obesity 1, 4, 631–652
  bariatric surgery for 649–652, 650*f*, 651*t*–652*t*
  BMR estimates for 87*t*
  childhood 634, 635–636
  definition 631–634
  diabetes and 571, 578–583, 581*t*
  dietary plan for 4–5, 489
  disease risks in, relative 631–633
  energy expenditure and 637–638
  energy intake and 638
  environmental factors and 638
  genetics 638
  health risks 4
  low-available carbohydrate diet for 511
  macronutrient content of foods and 642, 644*f*
  maternal 36
  medical complications of 639–640, 639*t*
  pathogenesis 636–639
  pharmacotherapy 646–649, 647*t*
  prevalence 4, 635
  weight loss and 97
  weight management approaches to 640–652, 640*t*, 641*t*, 642*t*, 643*f*, 644*f*, 644*t*
Occult blood screening, diet for 555, 555*t*
  general instructions 555, 555*t*
  specific recommendations 554*t*, 555
25OHD. *See* 25-Hydroxyvitamin D
Olestra 531
Olive oil 371–372
Omega-3 fatty acids (n-3 lipids) 468, 525, 674
  dietary therapy 616
  enteral nutritional therapy and 425
Opium, SBS 446
Oral contraceptives, vitamin C and 177
Oral immunotherapy 547
Oral manifestations
  drug-induced 67*t*–68*t*
  nutrient deficiency and 69, 73*t*
Oral mucosa, nutrient deficiency and 69, 73*t*
Organ system function, aging and 18–19
Organic anion-transporting polypeptides (OATP) 557
Orlistat, for obesity management 647–648
Orofacial granulomatosis (OFG) 551
γ-*Oryzanol*. *See* Phytosterols

Osteodystrophies, vitamin deficiency treatment in 125
Osteomalacia 41
  vitamin D deficiency and 200
Osteoporosis
  calcium and 201, 280, 690
  intake of 9–10
  medical disorder 280
  vitamin A toxicity and 191
  vitamin D deficiency and 201
Overfeeding syndromes 116–117, 119*t*
Ovo-vegetarians 490
Ox-LDL. *See* Oxidation of low-density lipoprotein particles
Oxalate, food 544. *See also* Low-oxalate diet
Oxidation of low-density lipoprotein particles (Ox-LDL) 371
Oxygen
  consumption 83–84
  uptake, measuring 83

P

P. ginseng 377
PA. *See* Physical activity
PAL. *See* Physical activity level
Pancreatic disease, enteral nutritional therapy 440–443
Pancreatitis, acute
  diets for 558
  enteral nutritional therapy 443
    diet for 443
  severe
    PN therapy for 455
    TF for 414–415
Pancreatitis, chronic, enteral nutritional therapy 440–443
  diet and 440, 442
  enzyme replacement for 442, 442*t*
  vitamin supplementation for 442–443
Pancreatitis, clear liquid diet and 492
Pantothenic acid (vitamin B_5) 179–180
Parathyroid hormone, magnesium and response of 286
Parenteral nutritional (PN) therapy 453–479. *See also* Central parenteral nutrition; Home parenteral nutrition
  background 453
  CVC, ordering/initiation of 473–477, 475*f*, 476*t*
  cycling 477
  discontinuing 475–477
  EFA 463–464
  electrolytes in
    additives of 470
    preparations for 470–471
  general principles 453–455
  home 478–479
  indications/contraindications 453–455, 454*t*

insulin and 471
lipid emulsions 468–469, 468*t*
medications in 471, 472*t*
metabolic complications associated
with 471–473
mineral requirements 461, 462*t*, 463*t*
monitoring patients on 475, 476*t*
nutrient requirements
during 460–464, 461*t*
calories 460
fluid requirements and 460
nonprotein calories 460
peripheral
ordering/initiating 477–478, 478*t*
osmolarity of 477–478, 478*t*
planning 477–478, 478*t*
venous catheters for 459
SBS 444–446
solution for, designing 464–472
additives, other 471
amino acids and 464–465, 465*t*, 466*t*, 467*t*
dextrose and 466
IVFE and 466–469, 468*t*
TNA 469–470
trace minerals and
preparations for 470–471
supplements of 470–471
types of 455
venous access 455–460, 456*t*–457*t*
central 455–459
peripheral venous catheters for 459
vitamins and 470
requirements for 460–462, 461*t*
Parenteral replacement, sodium 258–259
Parkinson disease, vitamin E deficiency
and 216
Parnate. *See* Tranylcypromine
Partial low-fiber diet 505*t*, 506
Peanut butter, enteral nutrition therapy
and 415
Pellagra 141–142
Penicillin, potassium 268
Pentane 210
Percutaneous endoscopic gastrostomy
technique 433
Peroxidase levels, in foods 555*t*
Pharmacotherapy, for obesity 646–649
general principles 646
Lorcaserin 648–649
medications approved by food and drug
administration 646–647, 647*t*
Orlistat 646, 647–648
phentermine 646–647
phentermine–topiramate ER 648
Phenelzine sulfate (Nardil) 549
Phenobarbital, folate and 38
Phenolic acids 370, 551

Phentermine, for obesity
management 646–647
Phentermine–topiramate ER, for obesity
management 648
Phenytoin, folate and 38
Phlebotomy 319
iron store assessment and 306
Phosphate
absorption, vitamin D and 198
homeostasis 293–294
plasma 291, 292*t*
PN therapy and 462–463
urinary 291
Phosphorus 289–297
absorption 291–292
assessment 291
phosphate and 291, 292*t*
bone health and 19–20
calcium ratio to 289, 289*t*
deficiency 294
causes of 294
clinical manifestations of 294–295
hypophosphatemia and 294
DRI 289
food sources 289–290, 290*t*
function 294
intake 16, 19–20
lactating women and 41–43
metabolism, vitamin D and 42
phosphate and 291, 292*t*
homeostasis of 293–294
physiology 291–294
pregnancy and 41–43
renal disease, chronic and 597–598
requirements 289
toxicity 296
treatment, hypophosphatemia and 295
urinary excretion 292–293, 293*t*
Physical activity (PA) 5
American Cancer Society guidelines on 4*t*
calories burned by 5, 6*t*
daily 5
weight loss therapy and 645, 645*t*
Physical activity level (PAL) 81–82, 82*t*
calculations based on 89–92, 91*t*
energy expenditure of 89–92, 90*t*
Physical examination, nutrient deficiency
and 66–69, 70*t*–71*t*
Physical medicine 366
Phytoestrogens. *See* Soy protein
Phytonadione (Mephyton) 222
Phytosterols 377–378
Piper methysticum 379
PIVKA. *See* Protein-induced by vitamin K
absence
Placebo effect, diet 72
Plant stanols/sterols, dietary therapy 616
Plasma phosphate 291, 292*t*

Plasma phylloquinone 219–220
PLCO Cancer Screening Trial. *See* Prostate, Lung, Colorectal, and Ovarian Cancer Screening Trial
PLP. *See* Pyridoxal-5′-phosphate
PMS. *See* Premenstrual syndrome
PN therapy. *See* Parenteral nutritional therapy
Polydextrose 501
Polyp Prevention Trial 661
Polyphenols
  cancer and 664–665
  sources 369–372
Polysaccharides, nonstructural 500
Polystyrene sulfonate (Kayexalate) 270
Polyunsaturated fatty acids 523, 523*t*, 620*t*
  dietary therapy 616
Pomegranate juice 556
Population trends 14
Postmenopausal women, bone density measurements and 274–275
Potassium 262–271
  absorption 265–266
  assessment 263–265
  bodily removal of 270–271
  body stores 263
  deficiency 266–267
  excretion 263–265
  food processing and 263, 264*t*
  food sources 263, 264*t*
  intake, increased 268
  ionic, measuring 263–265
  losses, bodily 263–265
    tests measuring 265, 266*t*
  penicillin 268
  physiology 265–266
  reabsorption 265–266
  renal disease, chronic and 597
  renal excretion 263–265
    impaired 268
  requirements 262
    PN therapy and 462
  serum 263
  supplementation 267–268, 269*t*
    sodium and 267–268
  toxicity 268
    causes of 268
    signs/symptoms of 268–270
    treatment of 270–271
  treatment 267
  urinary excretion 263–265
PPD. *See* Purified protein derivative
Prader–Willi syndrome 638
Pranidipine, grapefruit juice and 557
Prealbumin. *See* Transthyretin
Preeclampsia, maternal weight gain and 36

Pregnancy 34–48
  adolescent 43
  alcohol consumption and 9, 44–45
  anemia and 38, 45
  caffeine consumption and 495
  calcium and 41–43
  diabetes and 44, 589
  drug addiction and 44–45
  economic deprivation and 44
  EER for 34–35
  energy cost of 35*t*
  energy requirements 34–36, 92
  folate requirements during 38–41, 157
  food restriction and 44
  gastrointestinal problems in 46–47
  iron requirements during 37–38, 45
  multiple, within 2 years 43
  neural tube defects and 39
  nutrition during 34–37
    assessing 43
    deposition 35, 35*t*
    requirements 37–43, 40*t*
  nutritional risk factors and 43–46
  phosphorus and 41–43
  protein requirements 34–36, 100
  reproductive performance, poor and 43
  smoking during 44–45
  thiamine requirements in 129
  tissue deposition during 35, 35*t*
  vitamin A toxicity and 190
  vitamin C requirement and 173
  vitamin D and 41–43
  vitamin deficiency treatment in 125
  weight gain during 36–37, 36*t*
    excessive 45–46
    inadequate 45
  zinc and 41–43
Premature infants
  copper deficiency and 333
  vitamin E and 217
Premenstrual syndrome (PMS)
  calcium and 281
  γ-Linolenic acid treatment of 386
Primidone, folate and 38
Pro-oxidants, vitamin E therapy and 217
Probiotic(s) 386, 558
  in allergic disease 387
  definition 386
  digestive disease and 387
  food 367*t*–368*t*
  for metabolic condition 388
  in United States of America 367*t*–368*t*
Procarbazine (Matulane) 549
Produce, shopping for 11
Propionyl-l-carnitine 382
Prostate, Lung, Colorectal, and Ovarian (PLCO) Cancer Screening Trial 662

Protein. *See also* High-protein diet; Low-protein diet; Purified protein derivative; Retinol-binding protein; Soy protein
  alcoholic liver disease intake of 534–535, 534*t*
  animal sources 9
  assessment 81–120
  biochemical assessment of 108–110
  calorie requirement for 101–102, 101*t*
  circulating 108–110, 108*t*
  content of foods 536*t*
  DRI 99
  EAR 9
  enteral feeding, forced and 417–420
  evaluation, assessment for 116*t*, 119
  illness and estimation of 101–102
  intake 9, 14, 17, 81–120
    estimation of recommended daily 684
  loss
    bodily fluid 102
    conditions characterized by excessive 101–102
    gastrointestinal tract 102
    lungs 102
    skin 102
    urinary 101–102
  metabolism, aging and 18
  modulars 416
  needs, patient 404, 406
  nitrogen content in 683
  for nutritional assessment 108*t*
  RDA 9, 99
    lactating women and 35
    pregnancy and 35
  renal disease, chronic and 591–595
  requirements 81–120
    estimating normal daily 81–83
    estimation of 98–100
    illness and 102, 102*t*
    lactating women 34–36
    life stages and 99, 99*t*
    pregnancy and 34–36
  stores 106–108
  supplements 537–543
  support plan 407–409
Protein-induced by vitamin K absence (PIVKA) 220
Protein-losing enteropathies 102
Prothrombin time 220
P:S ratio 619
Pseudoephedrine 377
Psyllium powders, commercial 506, 508
Psyllium/ispaghula 501
Pteroylglutamic acid. *See* Folate
ω-3 PUFA 383–384
  prescription forms of 385
  source of 385
Pulmonary disease, enteral nutritional therapy formulas for 422
Purified protein derivative (PPD) 112
Pyridoxal-5′-phosphate (PLP) 145–146
Pyridoxine (vitamin B_6) 143–149
  antagonists 147–148
  assessment 144
  body stores
    homocysteine and 146, 146*t*
    PLP and 145–146
    transaminases and 145
    xanthurenic acid excretion and 146
  colorectal cancer and 148–149
  deficiency 147
  elderly and 22–23
  food sources 143–144, 145*t*
  HIV and 669–670
  intake 16, 22–23
  pharmacologic doses of 149
  physiology 147
  RDA 23
  requirements 143, 144*t*
  syndromes dependent on 148, 148*t*
  therapy 149
  toxicity 149
  urinary excretion 144, 146*t*

Q

Q-SYMBIO trial 374

R

Radiation therapy, clear liquid diet and 492
RBP. *See* Retinol-binding protein
RDAs. *See* Recommended dietary allowances
RDIs. *See* Reference daily intakes
Recommended dietary allowances (RDAs) 16, 51, 52
  cobalamin 22
  iron 297–298
    pregnancy and 37
  protein 9, 99–100
    lactating women 35
    pregnancy and 35
  pyridoxine 23
  thiamine 23
  vitamin 123, 124
Red blood cell production 308
Reduced, nutrient content descriptor 689
REE. *See* Resting energy expenditure
Refeeding syndromes 116–117
  clinical characteristics of 117, 119*t*
  PN therapy and 489–490
  TF and 438
Reference daily intakes (RDIs) 688
Reference weights 55
Rehydration solution, oral 446, 446*t*
Relative dose-response assay, vitamin A 187
Renal acid excretion, diet and effect on 245

Renal disease
  chronic
    calcium intake and 597–598
    diabetes and 589–590
    dialysis required by 593–599
    dietary management for 591
    energy intake and 595
    iron intake and 598
    managing, practical issues with 599–600
    nondiaylzed patient 591–593
    nutritional requirements 591–593, 594t
    phosphorus intake and 597–598
    potassium intake and 597
    protein and 591–595
    sodium intake and 596–597
    vitamin D intake and 597–598
    vitamin requirements for 599
    water intake and 596
  diabetes and 589–590
  dietary management 590–600
    phases of 591–599
  enteral nutritional therapy
    formulas for 423
Renal failure
  acute 600
  chronic, low-protein diet for 535
  patients with 413–414
Resistant short-chain carbohydrates (RSCCs) 500
Resting energy expenditure (REE) 81
  for critically ill 404
  estimating 683
  in hospitalized patients 89, 89t
Resting metabolic rate (RMR) 81
Restless leg syndrome (RLS) 312
Resveratrol 370
Retinoic acid. *See also* All-*trans*-retinoic acid
  enterohepatic circulation of 188
  syndrome 191
Retinol
  body stores 184–185
  physiology 188
  vitamin A and equivalents of 182–184
Retinol-binding protein (RBP) 110
  body stores 187
Riboflavin (vitamin B$_2$) 134–138
  assessment 136
    status, interpretation of 136, 137t
  coenzyme function 137
  colonic bacteria 135
  deficiency 137–138
  elderly and 23
  enrichment 135
  excretion 137
  food sources 135, 136t
  intake 16, 23
    assessment 136
  nondeficiency states 138
  physiology 137
  requirements 134–135, 135t
  toxicity 138
  treatment 138
  urinary excretion 136, 137
Rice bran 501
Rickets
  calcium and 280
  vitamin D deficiency and 200
RLS. *See* Restless leg syndrome
RMR. *See* Resting metabolic rate
Roux-en-Y gastric bypass 649, 650f
RSCCs. *See* Resistant short-chain carbohydrates

S

Saccharin, low-available carbohydrate diet and 517
Salicylates, restricted diets for 548
Salt consumption 8–9
Salt-restricted diets 554t
Saquinavir, grapefruit juice and 557
Sarcopenia
  definition 658
  role of nutrition in management of 658
Saturated fatty acids 7–8, 523, 618–619, 620t
  coronary heart disease and 690
  dietary therapy 615–616
  disease management and 617–620
Saw palmetto berry 378–379
SBS. *See* Short-bowel syndrome
Schilling test, cobalamin assessment and 162, 163
Scurvy, vitamin C and 172
  deficiency of 176
  therapy for 176–177
Selegiline HCl (Eldepryl) 549
Selenium 342–346
  antioxidant 21
  assessment 343
  cancer and 662
  deficiency 344
  DRI 342–343, 342t
  food sources 343
  HIV and 670
  intake 16, 21–22
  physiology 343–344
  requirement 342–343
  toxicity 21, 345
  treatment 344–345
    deficiency 344
    gastrointestinal disease 344
SELenium and vitamin E Cancer prevention Trial (SELECT) 213
Sepsis, HPN and line 478
Serenoa repens 378
Serotonin-rich foods, restriction of 554
Sertraline, grapefruit juice and 557

Serum alkaline phosphatase 197–198
Serum electrolyte concentration, PN therapy and 473
Sex
 life expectancy 14
 population distribution 14, 16f
SGA. *See* Subjective Global Assessment
Short-bowel syndrome (SBS)
 without a colon, low-available carbohydrate diet for 511
 adaptation after massive resection, following
  diet therapy for 444–445
  enteral nutritional therapy for 444–446
 enteral nutritional therapy 444–446
  adaptation after massive resection, following 444–446
  adjunctive medications for 446
  antimotility agents for 446
  control gastric hypersecretion and 446
  intestinal adaptation after massive resection and 444
  lactose and 445
  oral rehydration solutions and 446, 446t
 intestinal adaptation after massive resection and 444
 monitor 444
 TPN 444
Sildenafil, grapefruit juice and 557
Simplesse 531
Simvastatin 142, 143, 379
 grapefruit juice and 557
Sitosterol esters 378
Skinfold measurement 105
SKSD. *See* Streptokinase streptodornase
Sleeve gastrectomy 649, 650f
Small-bowel adaptation, TF for 414
Smell, diet and 489–490
Smokers
 folate deficiency and 159
 vitamin C levels in 177
Smoking 9
 pregnancy and 44–45
Snacks 489
Sodium 8, 248–262. *See also* Low-sodium diet
 absorption 254–255
 assessment 253–254
 content 553
 deficiency 257–258
 depletion 258
 food processing effect on 250–252, 251t
 food sources 250–252, 251t, 252t
 hypernatremia and 261
 hypertension and 691
 hyponatremia and 258, 258t
 intake
  adequate 248–249
  UL, tolerable 249–250
 intestinal reabsorption 255–257, 257t
 ion excretion and 255
 labeling 553
 laboratory evaluation 254
 medications 252
 oral replacement 259–261, 260t
  food-based solutions for 261
  vasopressin receptor antagonists 261
 parenteral replacement 258–259
 physiology 254–257
 potassium supplementation and 267–268
 prepared food 252
 renal disease, chronic and 596–597
 requirements 248–250
 retention, abnormal 262
 seasonings, alternative 262, 262t
 serum 253–254
 therapy 258–259
 toxicity 261
 transport 254–255
 water 252
Sodium bicarbonate, potassium toxicity 270
Sodium ferric gluconate (Ferrlecit) 317
Soluble gel-forming fiber 505
Soluble plasma transferrin receptor (sTfR) 305
Soy bran 501
Soy protein 378
 coronary artery disease and 691
 dietary therapy 616
St. John's wort 379
Starches
 digestibility 510
 resistant 500–501
Starvation 65
 related malnutrition 399
 weight loss during 97
Steatorrhea 440, 442, 442t
Sterols, dietary therapy 616
Stevia rebaudiana (Bertoni), low-available carbohydrate diet and 518
sTfR. *See* Soluble plasma transferrin receptor
Stool weight, fiber and factors related to 503, 504t
Streptokinase streptodornase (SKSD) 112
Subjective Global Assessment (SGA) 69, 113, 115f
Sucralose, low-available carbohydrate diet and 517–518
Sucrose–isomaltase deficiency 511
Sugar alcohols
 dental caries and 8–9, 691
 low-available carbohydrate diet and 518
Sugar consumption 8–9
Sulfasalazine, folate deficiency and 158

Sulfites, restricted diets for 549–551
Sunlight exposure, vitamin D and 42, 191
Supplement groups 365–367
Supplementation. *See also* Dietary supplements; Multivitamin supplements, elderly and
 allergy diet 548
 calcium 41, 274
 dietary therapy 617
 enteral nutritional therapy 411, 412
 excessive 10
 folate 40–41, 159, 160
 food 60–63
 food additive diet 549
  folate 159, 160
  thiamine 134
  vitamin 126–127
  vitamin E 213
 iron, gastrointestinal side effects of 38
 liquid diet, full 497
 low-available carbohydrate diet and 519
 low-lactose diet 522
 mineral, elderly 29
 modified-fiber diet 509
 nutrient 60–63
 nutritional therapy, enteral 413t
 potassium 267–268, 269t
 safety issues 63
 zinc 327–328
Survey in Europe on Nutrition and the Elderly, a Concerned Action (SENECA) Study 372
Swedish Mammography Cohort, folate deficiency and 160
Sweeteners, low-available carbohydrate diet and 517–518. *See also specific sweeteners*
Swingle (*S. prosverorii*), low-available carbohydrate diet and 518

T

Tacrolimus, grapefruit juice and 557
Tardive dyskinesia, vitamin E deficiency and 216
Tartrazine, restricted diets for 548–549
Taste
 decreased, nutrient deficiency and 67t–68t
 diet and 489–490
Taurine 381
Taurolidine 381
TBPA. *See* Thyroxine-binding prealbumin
TEA. *See* Thermal effect of activity
Teratogenicity, vitamin A 190
Terbutaline 551
Terfenadine, grapefruit juice and 557
Tetracycline, zinc and absorption of 328
TF. *See* Tube feeding
Thalidomide 673
"The Healthy Eating Plate", 11

Theaflavins 371
Thearubigins 371
Theobromine 495
Therapeutic Lifestyle Change (TLC) diet 378
Thermal effect of activity (TEA) 81–82
Thiamine (vitamin B_1) 129–134
 antithiamine factors 133
 assessment
  absorption 129
  intake 129
  status, interpretation of 132t
 carbohydrate intake and 132
 deficiency
  mechanisms of 133
  presentation, usual 133
 EAR 23
 elderly and 23
 food sources 129, 131t
 function 132
 inborn errors 134
 intake 16, 23
  assessment 129
 metabolism 133
 nondeficiency states 134
 physiology 131–132
 preventive therapy 134
 RDA 23
 requirements 129, 132t
 supplementation 134
 toxicity 134
 treatment 134
 urinary excretion 129
Thromboembolism, pyridoxine and venous 148
Thrombosis, catheter 457–458
Thyroxine-binding prealbumin (TBPA) 110
Ticrynafen, vitamin K and 222
Tissue. *See also* Adipose tissue
 damage, vitamin E deficiency and 210
 deposition 35, 35t
TLC. *See* Total lymphocyte count
TNA. *See* Total nutrient admixture
Total daily energy expenditure (TDEE) 97
Total iron-binding capacity (TIBC) 109
Total lymphocyte count (TLC) 111
Total nutrient admixture (TNA)
 advantages/disadvantages 469, 469t
 emulsion deterioration 469–470
 PN therapy 469–470
Total parenteral nutrition (TPN) 88, 311, 408, 444, 591
Toxemia, pregnancy and 45
TPN. *See* Total parenteral nutrition
Trace minerals 297–345
 PN therapy and
  preparations of 470–471
  supplements of 470–471
 TF and deficiencies in 438

Trans fatty acids 523, 616
Transaminases, pyridoxine body stores and 145
Transdermal selegiline (Emsam) 549
Transferrin 109–110, 303
Transthyretin (prealbumin) 187
Tranylcypromine (Parnate) 549
Trazolam grapefruit juice and 557
Triamterene, folate and 38
Triceps skin fold thickness (TSF) 105
Triglycerides 607–608, 608t
Trimethoprim, folate and 38
Tryptophan 138
Tube feeding (TF)
  aspirate 436
  bolus 436
  complications 437–438
    metabolic 437–438
    nonmetabolic 438
  constant-infusion technique 436
  constipation and 438
  diarrhea and 438
  electrolyte disturbances and 437–438
  enteral product for, choosing 425–437, 426f
  esophageal ulcer and 438
  feeding formulas for 436
  forced enteral 412
  hyperosmolarity syndrome and 438
  indications for 414–415
  insertion site care 433–434, 434t
  intermittent 436
  long-term access for 433
  maintaining 45-degree elevation and 435–436
  medication administration through
    administration of 439–440
    drug and 438–439
    drugs with specific requirements and 440, 441t
  monitoring patients and 436–437, 437t
  percutaneous endoscopic gastrostomy technique 433
  refeeding syndrome and 438
  short silicone post low-profile tube 433
  short-term access for 429, 432t
  stylets for 427
  tip location for 428–429, 428t
    gastric 428–429, 428t
    small bowel 428t, 429, 432t
  trace mineral deficiencies and 438
  tube for 439
  tube insertion for 429–435, 430t–431t
  tube length/diameter 425
  tube material 425
  tube patency maintenance and 434–435, 435t
  tungsten tips for 427
  warfarin resistance and 438
  Y-ports for 427
Tyramine
  drugs inhibit monoamine oxidase 549
  population at risk 549
  restricted diets for 549, 550t

U

UL intake. *See* Upper level intake
Ulcerative colitis, PN therapy for 454
Upper level (UL) intake, sodium 249–250
Urinary excretion
  calcium 197, 271, 274
  copper assessment and 330
  fluorine 337–338
  iodine 334, 335, 335t
  magnesium 285
  niacin 139–140, 141t
  nitrogen 99
  phosphorus 292–293, 293t
  potassium 263–265
  protein 101–102
  pyridoxine 144, 146t
  riboflavin 136, 137
  thiamine 129
  zinc 322, 325
Urinary nitrogen loss 98
U.S. Department of Agriculture (USDA) 57, 485–486
  food groups defined by 5
USDA. *See* U.S. Department of Agriculture

V

Vanillin 370
Vascular health, vitamin K deficiency and 222
Vasopressin receptor antagonists (VAPTANS) 261
Vegans
  diet 490
    risks of 490
  lactation and 47
  pregnancy and 44
Vegetables
  cooking preparations and 7
  nutrients 6–7, 7t
  variety 6–7
Vegetarians
  amino acid sources 483, 483t
  cobalamin and 22
    body stores of 164
    deficiency of 161, 169
  diet 483, 490–491
    chronic condition prevention and 488
    risks of 490
  elderly, cobalamin and 22
Venofer. *See* Iron sucrose
Very-low-calorie diets (VLCDs) 642–643

Very low density lipoprotein (VLDL) 602
Vescapa 385
Vitamin(s) 123–223. *See also specific vitamins*
  bioavailability 124
  cancer prevention and 659, 662*t*
  daily allowances 123
  deficiency 124–126, 126*t*
    clinical manifestations of 71*t*–72*t*, 127, 128*t*
    evaluation of 123–129
    onset of clinical 127
    therapeutic supplementation and 127, 129
    treatment of 126*t*
  drug action and effect on 75–76, 77*t*
  fat-soluble 182–223
  food sources 483–485, 485*t*
  intake, evaluation of 123–129
  pancreatic disease enteral nutrition therapy and 442–443
  PN therapy 470
    requirements for 460–462
  for prevention of chronic disease 373–374
  RDAs 123, 124
  requirements 124–125
    for chronic disease patient 124–125
    for elderly people 124
    for physically active people 124
    PN therapy 460–462
    renal disease, chronic 599
  status
    assessment of 129
    drug effects on 223, 223*t*
  supplements
    dietary therapy 617
    for gastrointestinal disorders 125
    for HIV patients 125
    for infancy 125
    for low-calorie intake/diets 125
    for osteodystrophies 125
    during pregnancy 125
  toxicity 55, 56*t*–57*t*
  water-soluble 129–182
Vitamin A 182–191
  assessment 184–187
    absorption 184
    body stores 184–187, 186*t*
    functional assays 187
    intake 184
    relative dose-response assay 187
  deficiency 189
  DRI 182, 183*t*
  EAR 23
  elderly and 23
  food sources 184, 185*t*
  infection prevention and 190
  intake 16, 23
  physiology 187–188
  requirements 182–184
  teratogenicity 190
  therapy 189
  toxicity 190–191
Vitamin B$_1$. *See* Thiamine
Vitamin B$_{12}$. *See* Cobalamin
Vitamin B$_2$. *See* Riboflavin
Vitamin B$_3$. *See* Niacin
Vitamin B$_5$. *See* Pantothenic acid
Vitamin B$_6$. *See* Pyridoxine (vitamin B6)
Vitamin C (ascorbic acid) 172–178
  absorption 175–176
  antioxidant 21
  assessment 174–175
    absorption 174–175
    body stores 175
    HPLC 175, 175*t*
    intake 174–175
    status, interpretation of 174, 175*t*
  chronic disease prevention and 177
  deficiency 176
  DRI 173, 173*t*
  food sources 173–174, 174*t*
  intake 20
    assessment 174–175
  iron absorption and 177–178
  metabolic function 176
  physiology 175–176
  requirements 172–173
  scurvy and 172, 176–177
  therapy 176–178
    scurvy and 176–177
  toxicity 178
Vitamin D 191–206. *See also* 1,25-Dihydroxyvitamin D$_3$; 25-Hydroxyvitamin D
  assessment 195–198, 196*t*
    bone densitometry and 198
    calcium urinary excretion, twenty-four-hour and 197
    serum alkaline phosphatase and 197–198
  bone health and 19–20
  calcium and 197–198
    deficiency of 279
    metabolism of 42
  cancer and 663
  deficiency 199–200, 199–204
    adult osteomalacia 200
    age and 193
    bone health and fractures 202
    cancer and 203
    cardiovascular disease and 203–204
    diabetes mellitus and 204
    in elderly and hospitalized patients 201–202
    involutional osteoporosis 201
    liver disease and 204

lung disease and 204
malabsorption 200–201
mortality rate 203
muscle function and falls 202–203
osteomalacia and 200
osteoporosis and 201
rickets and 200
DRI 193–194, 193t
food sources 194–195, 195t
fortification 42, 192
functions 198–199
HIV and 670
infancy deficiency of 125
intake 10, 16
lactating women and 41–43
metabolism 199
oral 192
phosphorus metabolism and 42
physiology 198–199
pregnancy and 41–43
preparations 204–206, 205t
renal disease, chronic
  and 597–598
requirements 191–192
sunlight exposure and 42
synthetic analogs 206
toxicity 206
types 191–192
Vitamin D Quality Assessment Scheme
  (DEQAS) 196
Vitamin D_2 (ergosterol, ergocalciferol) 205
Vitamin E 207–217
absorption 211
antioxidant 20–21, 211–212
assessment 208–210
  erythrocyte hemolysis 208–209
  status, interpretation of 210, 210t
cancer prevention and 211–212, 214t–215t
chemical forms 207
deficiency
  cancer and 213, 214t–215t
  cardiovascular disease and 213,
    214t–215t
  isolated 213
  medical conditions and 212
  nonalcoholic fatty liver disease 213–216
  persons at risk for 212
  therapy 216–217
  tissue damage in 210
DRI 207, 208t
EAR 23
food sources 207–208, 209t
function 210–211
infancy deficiency of 125
intake 16, 208
physiology 210–212
PUFAs and ratio to 208
requirements 207

serum 209–210
supplementation 213
therapy
  deficiency states and 216–217
  pro-oxidant effects and 217
toxicity 217
Vitamin K 217–223. *See also*
Protein-induced by vitamin K absence
absorption 220
assessment 219–220
  body stores 220
  intake 219–220
bone health and 19–20, 222
deficiency 221–222
  bone health and 222
  drug interference and 221–222
  hemorrhagic disease of newborn and 222
diet enriched with 556
DRI 217–218, 218t
food sources 218–219, 219t
function 221
infancy deficiency of 125
lipid emulsions and 470
metabolism 220
physiology 220–221
PN therapy 470
requirements 217–218
therapy 222
tissue stores 220–221
toxicity 222–223
vascular health and 222
VLCDs. *See* Very-low-calorie diets
VLDL. *See* Very low density lipoprotein
Vomiting
  HIV and 668
  pregnancy and 46

W

Warfarin
  resistance, TF and 438
  vitamin K and 219, 221, 222
Wasting syndrome 591. *See also* Chronic
  diseases, nutritional considerations in
Water
  balance 247
  fluorine in 337
  renal disease, chronic and 596
  requirements 247
  sodium in 252
WBC. *See* White blood count
Weighed diet 97
Weight. *See also* Obesity
  beverages containing calories and 492–493
  gain
    adulthood 638–639
    amitriptyline and 76
    drugs associated with 640t
    maternal 36–37, 36t, 45

Weight (*continued*)
 healthy 103
 ideal, estimation of 684
 loss 103
  diabetes and 573
  diet and controlled 97
  energy needs and 92
  HIV and 668
  obesity and 97
  starvation and 97
 management 1–5
 ranges, healthy 633*t*
 reference 55
Weight loss programs. *See also* Diet(s)
 commercial 644–645
Weight loss, supplements for 368
Weight loss therapy
 criteria for 642*t*
Weight management, approach to obese patient 640–652
 clinical evaluation 640, 640*t*
 lifestyle intervention 642–646
  behavior modification 646
  commercial weight loss programs 644–645
  diet therapy 642–644, 644*f*, 644*t*
  physical activity 645
 specific treatment options 641–642, 642*t*, 643*f*
 strategies for 640
 therapy 640–642
 treatment algorithm 643*f*
Wheat bran 501
White blood count (WBC) 111
WHO. *See* World Health Organization
Whole foods 1
 calorie supplementation with 415–416
 enteral nutrition therapy supplemented with 415–416, 415*t*
Wilmore's equation 88
Wilson disease 556
 zinc treatment 327

Wine 616–617
World Health Organization (WHO) 86–88

X
Xanthurenic acid excretion 146

Z
Zaleplon, grapefruit juice and 557
Zinc 319–328
 absorption 323–324
 assessment 320–323
 binding 324–325
 cellular update 324–325
 deficiency
  acute diarrhea in children 326
  candidate syndromes of 326–327
  clinical manifestations of 325–326, 325*t*
  syndromes of 325–327
 diet content of 320
 DRI 319, 319*t*
 elderly and 23–24
 excretion 325
 food processing and 320
 food sources 320, 321*t*
 hair 322
 HIV and 670
 immune function and 325
 intake, decreased dietary 327
 lactating women and 41–43
 nails 322
 physiology 323–325
 plasma 321–322, 322*t*
 PN therapy and 470
 pregnancy and 41–43
 requirements 319–320
 supplementation 327–328
 toxicity 328
 treatment 327–328
 urinary excretion 322, 325
Zyvox. *See* Linezolid